BRIEF CONTENTS

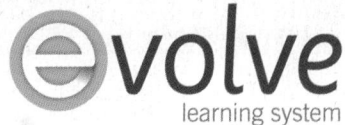
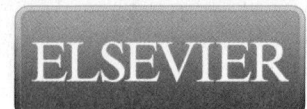
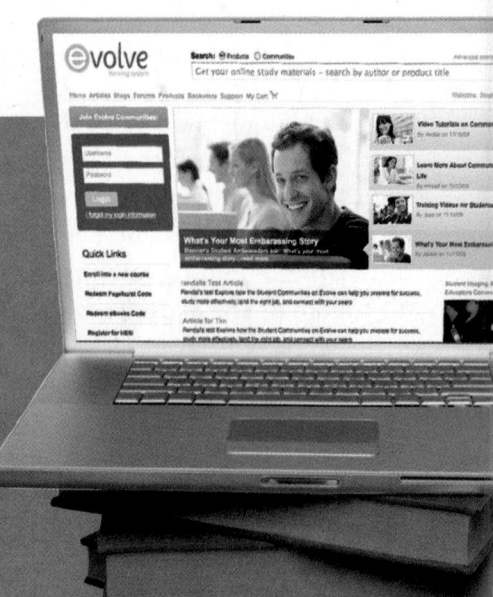

Mosby's TEXTBOOK FOR
Nursing Assistants

Eighth Edition

SHEILA A. SORRENTINO, PhD, RN
Curriculum and Health Care Consultant
Anthem, Arizona

LEIGHANN N. REMMERT, MS, RN
Health Occupations Instructor
Lincolnland Technical Education Center
Lincoln, Illinois

ELSEVIER

ELSEVIER
MOSBY

3251 Riverport Lane
St. Louis, Missouri 63043

MOSBY'S TEXTBOOK FOR NURSING ASSISTANTS

ISBN: 978-0-323-08068-2 (Hard Cover)
ISBN: 978-0-323-08067-5 (Soft Cover)

Notices

Previous editions copyrighted 2008, 2004, 2000, 1996, 1992, 1987, 1984

Library of Congress Cataloging-in-Publication Data

Sorrentino, Sheila A.
  Mosby's textbook for nursing assistants / Sheila A.
Sorrentino, Leighann N. Remmert. -- 8th ed.
       p. ; cm.
  Textbook for nursing assistants
  Includes index.
  ISBN 978-0-323-08068-2 (hardcover. : alk. paper) -- ISBN 978-0-323-08067-5
(pbk. : alk. paper)
  I. Remmert, Leighann N. II. Title. III. Title: Textbook for nursing assistants.
  [DNLM: 1. Nurses' Aides. 2. Nursing Care. WY 193]
  610.7306'98--dc23
                                                                        2011037263

Content Strategist: Nancy O'Brien
Senior Content Development Specialist: Maria Broeker
Publishing Services Manager: Jeff Patterson
Project Manager: Bill Drone
Designer: Jessica Williams

Printed in the United States of America

Last digit is the print number: 9 8 7 6 5 4 3 2 1

To the cycle of life, with its joys and sorrows . . .

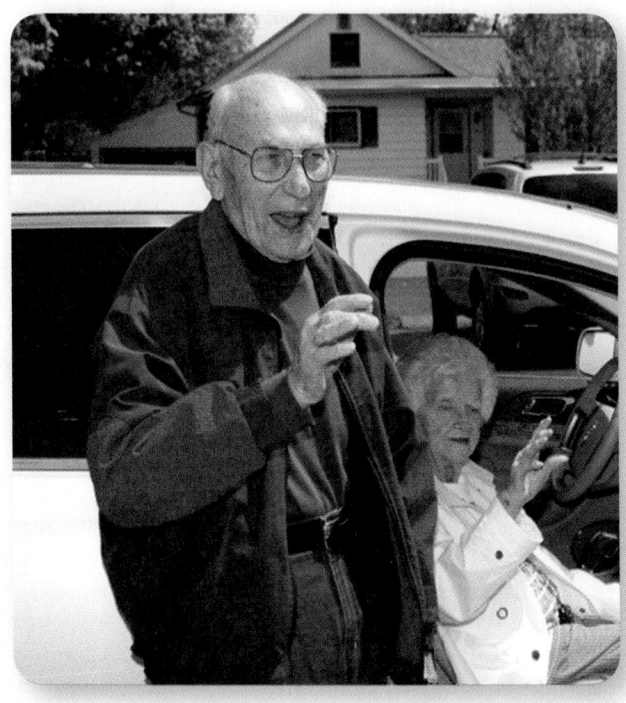

In memory of my dad
January 1, 1920-April 23, 2011
A remarkable man of simple pleasures
and admirable values
With love and sadness
Sheila

In celebration of new life
Olivia Louise Remmert
Born September 13, 2011
The blessing of this life has forever changed mine
Leighann (Mom)

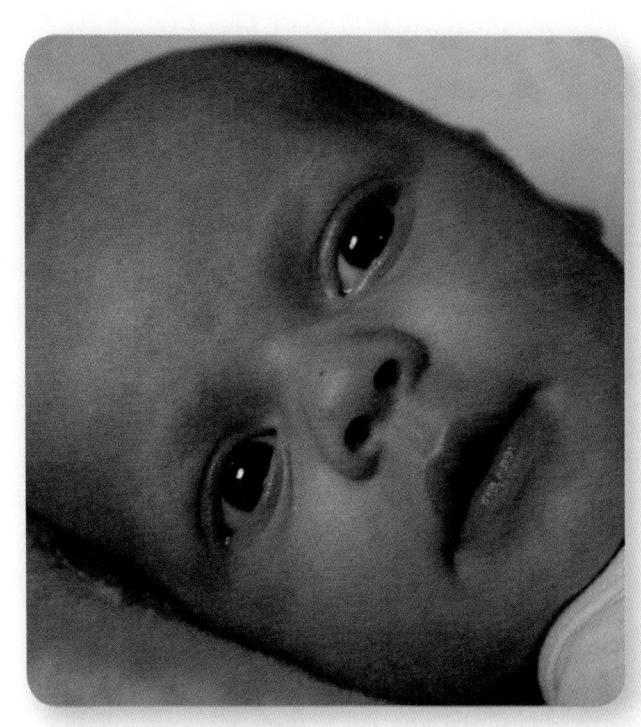

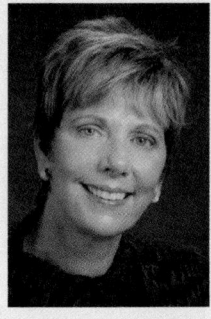

Sheila A. Sorrentino is currently a curriculum and health care consultant focusing on effective delegation and partnering with assistive personnel in hospitals, long-term care centers, and home care agencies.

Dr. Sorrentino was instrumental in the development and approval of CNA-PN-ADN programs in the Illinois community college system and has taught in nursing assistant, practical nursing, associate degree, and baccalaureate and higher degree programs. Her career includes experiences as a nursing assistant, staff nurse, charge nurse, head nurse, nursing educator, assistant dean, dean, and consultant.

A Mosby author since 1982, Dr. Sorrentino is the author of *Mosby's Textbook for Long-Term Care Nursing Assistants (6e)* and several other textbooks for nursing assistive personnel. She was also involved in the development of *Mosby's Nursing Assistant Skills Videos* and *Mosby's Nursing Skills Videos*, winner of the 2003 AJN Book of the Year Award (electronic media). An earlier version of nursing assistant skills videos won the 1992 International Medical Films Award on caregiving.

Dr. Sorrentino has a Bachelor of Science degree in nursing, a Master of Arts degree in education, a Master of Science degree in community nursing, and a PhD in higher education administration. She is a member of Sigma Theta Tau International, the Honor Society of Nursing and the Rotary Club of Anthem (Anthem, Arizona). She is a former member of the Provena Senior Services Board of Directors (Mokena, Illinois) and a former member and chair of the Central Illinois Higher Education Health Care Task Force. She also served on the Iowa-Illinois Safety Council Board of Directors and the Board of Directors of Our Lady of Victory Nursing Center in Bourbonnais, Illinois.

In 1998 she received an alumni achievement award from Lewis University for outstanding leadership and dedication in nursing education. In 2005 she was inducted into the Illinois State University College of Education Hall of Fame. Her presentations at national and state conferences focus on delegation and other issues relating to nursing assistive personnel.

Dr. Sorrentino sponsors two nursing scholarships. One is for a senior high school student from her high school alma mater intending to major in nursing. The other is for a nursing assistant intending to major in nursing and working at one of the three agencies in which she worked during and after college (Heritage Health-Therapy and Senior Care, Peru, Illinois; Illinois Valley Community Hospital, Peru, Illinois; and St. Margaret's Hospital, Spring Valley, Illinois).

Mike Spinelli Photography, Phoenix, Arizona

Leighann N. Remmert is a Health Occupations Instructor at Lincolnland Technical Education Center in Lincoln, Illinois. She teaches high school nursing assistant students in the clinical setting and instructs nursing assistant courses for adult learners.

Graduating with highest honors, Leighann received a Bachelor of Science degree in nursing from Bradley University in Peoria, Illinois. She was selected as the student representative to address the faculty, families, and classmates in attendance at the nursing department's pinning ceremony for her graduating class. Leighann earned a Master of Science degree in nursing education from Southern Illinois University Edwardsville and received a certificate of achievement for academic honors upon graduation. She is a member of Sigma Theta Tau International, the Honor Society of Nursing.

Leighann's clinical background includes the roles of nursing assistant/tech, nurse extern, staff nurse, charge nurse, nurse preceptor, and trauma nurse specialist. She acquired diverse clinical experience in the areas of general medical, intermediate care, pediatric, cardiac, oncology, emergency, and post-surgical nursing as a nursing assistant/tech and extern at St. John's Hospital in Springfield, Illinois. As a registered nurse, Leighann concentrated in the area of emergency nursing at Memorial Medical Center in Springfield, Illinois.

Leighann has supervised, instructed, and evaluated student learning in various long-term care and acute care settings as a clinical nursing instructor at the Capital Area School of Practical Nursing in Springfield, Illinois. In her current position at Lincolnland Technical Education Center, Leighann guides students in acquiring the skills and knowledge needed to succeed as nursing assistants. Through her teaching, she emphasizes the importance of professionalism and work ethics, safety, teamwork, communication, and accountability. Valuing the role of the nursing assistant and treating the person with dignity, care, and respect are integral to her instruction in the classroom and clinical settings.

Leighann is co-author of *Mosby's Textbook for Medication Assistants* and *Mosby's Essentials for Nursing Assistants (4e)*. She was a consultant on *Mosby's Textbook for Long-Term Care Nursing Assistants (6e)*.

Leighann and her husband, Shane, volunteer as senior high youth sponsors and are active in leadership at Elkhart Christian Church in Elkhart, Illinois. Leighann is certified as a basic life support instructor and teaches CPR and First Aid training courses for the church and community.

Terry Farmer Photography, Springfield, Illinois

ACKNOWLEDGMENTS

Many individuals and agencies have contributed to this new, eighth edition of *Mosby's Textbook for Nursing Assistants* by providing information, insights, and resources. We are especially grateful and appreciative of the efforts of:

- Rose Mary Carrico (Director of Medical/Surgical and ICU Services), Illinois Valley Community Hospital (Peru, Illinois), for her outstanding efforts in coordinating our photo shoot. We were in awe of her creativity and problem solving abilities.
- Illinois Valley Community Hospital (Peru, Illinois) for once again hosting a photo shoot.
- Lori Walsh (Administrator) and Deb Boyd (Director of Nursing) at Heritage Health–Therapy and Senior Care (La Salle, Illinois) for coordinating and hosting our photo shoot. Their efforts allowed us to move through the session with ease.
- Abraham Lincoln Memorial Hospital (Lincoln, Illinois) for providing electronic charting samples.
- All family, friends, and volunteers who participated in the photo shoot:
  - Anthony and Frances Sorrentino
  - Jodi Reeder
  - Ty Reeder
  - Jerry and Joanne Orlandini
  - Larry Huffman
  - Roger Tidaback
  - Pat Wlodarchak
  - John Apitado
  - Sue Fiesel
  - Michelle Lucas
  - Macee Lentz
  - Chuck Kellett
  - Kenneth Greening
  - Brianna Rebholz
  - Kayla Funtsinn
  - Tamara Cobb
  - Bekki Prokup
  - Miles McFadin
  - Maureen Rebholz
- Mary Beth Sorrentino Herron for providing clerical and technical support.
- The artists at Graphic World (St. Louis, Missouri) for their talented work.
- Photographer Mike DeFilippo (St. Louis, Missouri) for his great photos. He is very patient, cooperative, and flexible during photo shoots.
- Sandra L. Allen, Cynthia Bartlau, Charlotte Browe, Sally Christiansen, Colleen Cucchiara Flick, Michelle Dionne-Vahalik, Linda Greer, and Clare Kostelnick for reviewing the manuscript and for their candor and suggestions. They have contributed to the thoroughness and accuracy of this book.
- Kimberly Gibbs, Mary Beth Herron, Kimberly Little, and Teresa Novy for their tireless work on the various ancillaries associated with the textbook.
- Susan Broadhurst (Rochester, New York) for serving as copy editor. It was a pleasure talking to her.
- Jody McBride (Temple, TX) for her proofreading efforts and attention to detail throughout the production process.
- And finally, to the talented and dedicated Elsevier/Mosby staff, especially:
  - Sally Schrefer (Managing Director of Nursing and Health Professions) is an amazing, perceptive, and supportive woman. Sally is always willing to listen and problem solve.
  - Nancy O'Brien (Editor) gave guidance and kept the project on track. She is genuine, caring, and supportive.
  - Editors Suzi Epstein (retired) and Tamara Myers for their efforts early in the planning and development processes.
  - Maria Broeker (Senior Developmental Editor) handled numerous details, manuscript needs, tasks, and issues. She always has an empathetic ear and time to listen to author wants, needs, and frustrations. She is beyond terrific.
  - Jacqueline Kiley (Editorial Assistant) provided supportive assistance. Welcome to our team.
  - Jeff Patterson (Publishing Services Manager), Bill Drone (Project Manager), and Kathy Teal (Production Assistant) for their production efforts. With all of the design elements and layout considerations inherent in this book, they produced a user-friendly and attractive text.
  - Jessica Williams (Book Designer) took all of our ideas, some rather abstract, and created a unique and colorful book and cover design. As always, this book is distinctive from the rest.
  - Jason Gonulsen (Senior Producer) for coordinating all of the efforts involved in updating the Nursing Assistant Companion CD.

And to all those who contributed to this effort in any way, we are sincerely grateful.

Sheila A. Sorrentino
Leighann N. Remmert

The eighth edition of *Mosby's Textbook for Nursing Assistants* prepares students to function as nursing assistants in acute care, long-term care, and home settings. It serves the needs of students and instructors in all educational settings offering nursing assistant courses. This book is a valuable resource for the competency test review as well as a useful reference as the working nursing assistant seeks to review or learn information for safe care.

Foundational principles are presented in specific chapters and values, objectives, and organizational strategies are intertwined and integrated in content and key features throughout the book (see pages xiii–xv of the Student Preface). Key content and features include:

- Describing the work setting and the individuals in that setting. See *Chapter 1: Introduction to Health Care Agencies, Chapter 8: Understanding the Person,* and *Focus on Long-Term Care and Home Care* boxes.
- Respecting patients and residents, across the life-span, as *persons* with dignity and value who have a past, a present, and a future and who have basic needs and protected rights. This includes persons with bariatric needs. See *Chapter 2: The Person's Rights, Focus on Children and Older Persons* boxes, the *Quality of Life* section in procedure boxes, and *Focus on PRIDE: The Person, Family, and Yourself* at the end of each chapter.
- Describing the legal principles affecting the nursing assistant role. Federal and state laws define the role, range of functions, and limitations that vary among states and agencies. Therefore nursing assistant responsibilities, limitations, professional boundaries, and the legal and ethical aspects of the role are emphasized. This includes reporting abuse. See *Chapter 3: The Nursing Assistant, Chapter 4: Ethics and Laws,* and *Focus on PRIDE: The Person, Family, and Yourself.*
- Stressing effective delegation in relation to nursing assistant functions and role limits. Building on the delegation principles (Chapter 3), *Delegation Guidelines* boxes empower the student to seek information from the nurse and the care plan about critical aspects of a procedure and the observations to report and record. Step 1 of most procedures refers the student to the appropriate *Delegation Guidelines* boxes. Also see *Focus on PRIDE: The Person, Family, and Yourself* at the end of each chapter.
- Appreciating the role of cultural heritage and religion in health and illness practices. See *Caring About Culture* boxes.
- Understanding that knowledge about body structure and function is needed for safe care and to perform nursing skills safely. See *Chapter 9: Body Structure and Function* and the *Body Structure and Function Review* boxes presented in relation to various procedures and medical-surgical problems and disorders.
- Emphasizing the core values of safety and comfort. *Chapter 12: Safety, Chapter 13: Preventing Falls,* and *Chapter 14: Restraint Alternatives and Safe Restraint Use* focus on safety. *Promoting Safety and Comfort* boxes direct the student's attention on the need to be safe and cautious and to promote comfort when giving care. Step 1 of most procedures refers the student to the appropriate *Promoting Safety and Comfort* boxes.
- Encouraging work ethics, teamwork, time management, and communication skills to be a productive, efficient member of the nursing team and to communicate effectively with patients, residents, and families. See *Chapter 5: Work Ethics, Teamwork and Time Management* boxes, *Focus on Communication* boxes, and *Focus on PRIDE: The Person, Family, and Yourself.*
- Recognizing that besides safety, other concepts and functions are foundational to safe care. See *Chapter 15: Preventing Infection* and *Chapter 16: Body Mechanics.*
- Embracing the nursing process as the basis for planning and delivering nursing care and the role that nursing assistants play in assisting with the process. See *Chapter 7: Assisting With the Nursing Process.*

To enhance learning, the *Nursing Assistant Companion CD* in this book presents key procedures using video clips and animations along with interactive exercises. The CD also includes an audio glossary and a Spanish vocabulary and phrases audio glossary as well as Body Spectrum, an interactive review of anatomy and physiology terms.

Content Issues

Every edition requires revision and content decisions. Changes in laws or in guidelines and standards issued by government or accrediting agencies make the decisions easy. So do state curricula and competency tests. Every attempt is made to publish an up-to-date book. Sometimes changes are made right before publication.

Student learning needs and abilities, instructor desires, work-related issues, course/program and book length, and cost to the student are among the many factors considered. With such issues in mind, new and expanded content and figures include:

New Chapters
- Chapter 2: The Person's Rights
- Chapter 34: Pressure Ulcers

New Content
- Persons Needing Bariatric Care
- The Lymphatic System
- Bariatric-Safe Equipment
- Color-Coded Wristbands
- Bariatric Beds
- Persons With Bariatric Needs (*Chapter 20: Personal Hygiene*)
- Applying Incontinence Products
- Checking Pedal Pulses
- Dressings (*Chapter 34: Pressure Ulcers*)

- Complications (*Chapter 34: Pressure Ulcers*)
- Dysrhythmias
- Sleep Apnea
- Lymphedema
- Lymphoma
- Cirrhosis
- Binge-Eating Disorder
- Paranoia
- Communication Problems (*Chapter 46: Confusion and Dementia*)
- Screaming (*Chapter 46: Confusion and Dementia*)
- Rummaging and Hiding Things (*Chapter 46: Confusion and Dementia*)
- Fragile X Syndrome
- Rescue Breathing
- Types of Care (*Chapter 52: End-of-Life Care*)
- Breathing Problems
- Mental and Emotional Needs

New Boxes

- Box 15-2 Possible Healthcare-Associated Infections
- Box 22-3 Guidelines for Applying Incontinence Products
- Box 24-7 Common Causes of Dehydration
- Box 26-1 Factors Affecting Vital Signs
- Box 26-3 Glass Thermometers
- Box 39-4 Signs and Symptoms of Vision Problems
- Box 40-1 Some Signs and Symptoms of Cancer
- Box 40-2 Safety Measures During Chemotherapy
- Box 43-3 Persons At Risk for Hepatitis
- Box 43-4 Care of the Person With Cirrhosis
- Box 45-6 Symptoms of An Alcohol Use Disorder
- Box 46-4 Signs and Symptoms of Delirium
- Box 46-6 Alzheimer's Disease and Normal Age-Related Changes
- Box 46-8 Communication Measures for Persons With AD and Other Dementias
- Box 46-10 Family Caregivers—Taking Care of Yourself

New Focus on Communication Boxes

- Your Role ("Meeting Standards" in *Chapter 1: Introduction to Health Care Agencies*)
- Information
- Activities
- The Training Program
- Informed Consent
- Reporting Abuse
- Attendance
- Harassment
- Reporting and Recording
- Assignment Sheets
- Effective Communication
- Behavior Issues
- Applying Restraints
- Isolation Precautions
- Positioning the Person
- Noise
- Bariatric Beds
- Skin and Scalp Conditions

- Urinals
- Applying Incontinence Products
- Assisting With IV Therapy
- Using a Stethoscope
- Normal and Abnormal Blood Pressures
- Ambulation
- Pain
- Weight and Height
- Preparing the Person (*Chapter 30: Assisting With the Physical Examination*)
- The Midstream Specimen
- Tape
- Pressure Ulcers
- Deep Breathing and Coughing
- Communication (*Chapter 38: Rehabilitation and Restorative Care*)
- Psychological and Social Aspects (*Chapter 38: Rehabilitation and Restorative Care*)
- The Person's Needs (*Chapter 40: Cancer, Immune System, and Skin Disorders*)
- Schizophrenia
- Suicide
- Care and Treatment
- Communication Problems (*Chapter 46: Confusion and Dementia*)
- Chain of Survival for Adults
- Performing Adult CPR
- Culture and Spiritual Needs

New Focus on Long-Term Care and Home Care Boxes

- Effects of Illness and Disability
- Elder Abuse
- Preventing Poisoning (Home Care)
- Lead Poisoning
- Disasters (Home Care)
- Causes and Risk Factors for Falls (Home Care)
- Fecal Impaction
- Pressure Ulcers

New Focus on Children and Older Persons Boxes

- Preventing Burns
- Carbon Monoxide Poisoning
- The Person's Needs (*Chapter 52: End-of-Life Care*)

New Promoting Safety and Comfort Boxes

- Paying for Health Care
- Reporting and Recording Time
- Preventing Poisoning
- Applying Incontinence Products
- Safety and Comfort (*Chapter 23: Bowel Elimination*)
- Diarrhea
- Suppositories
- Radiation Therapy
- Lymphedema
- Urinary Diversions
- Behaviors and Problems

New Delegation Guidelines Boxes
- Applying Incontinence Products
- Suppositories

New Procedures
- Using an Alcohol-Based Hand Rub
- Applying Incontinence Products

New Teamwork and Time Management Boxes
- Persons With Bariatric Needs (*Chapter 20: Personal Hygiene*)

New Caring About Culture Boxes
- Communication Problems (*Chapter 46: Confusion and Dementia*)

New Body Structure and Function Review Boxes
- The Ear
- The Eye
- The Immune System
- The Integumentary System
- The Nervous System
- The Musculo-Skeletal System
- The Cardiovascular System
- The Respiratory System
- The Lymphatic System
- The Digestive System
- The Endocrine System
- The Reproductive System

New Figures
Chapter 9
- **9-9** Pyloric sphincter.
- **9-18** The lymphatic system.

Chapter 10
- **10-1** Changes from birth to maturity.

Chapter 12
- **12-1** Door knob cover.
- **12-3** Outlet cover.
- **12-29** The MSDS 800 hotline number.
- **12-36** Color-coded wristbands.

Chapter 13
- **13-12** Applying a transfer/gait belt.

Chapter 14
- **14-10** The restraint is secured to the moveable part of the bed frame.

Chapter 15
- **15-3** Sneezing into the upper arm.
- **15-6** The fingers are interlaced for a good lather.
- **15-10** Using an alcohol-based hand rub.

Chapter 17
- **17-25** Bariatric ceiling lift.
- **17-28** Lateral transfer device with slide board.

Chapter 18
- **18-13** Bariatric bed.
- **18-15** The bariatric chair.

Chapter 20
- **20-4** Baby bottle tooth decay.
- **20-12, C** Brushing denture chewing surfaces.

Chapter 21
- **21-2** Beauty shop in a nursing center.

Chapter 22
- **22-2** Color chart for urine.
- **22-5** Bariatric bedpan.
- **22-10, C** Bariatric commode.
- **22-11** Disposable garment protectors.
- **22-12** Applying a complete incontinence brief.
- **22-13** Applying a pad and undergarment.
- **22-14** Applying pull-on underwear.

Chapter 23
- **23-2** Bowel elimination record.

Chapter 25
- **25-13** IV sites in children.

Chapter 26
- **26-1, H** Pacifier thermometer.
- **26-20** The pedal pulse.
- **26-23, D** Wrist monitor.
- **26-24, B** The cuff arrow is aligned with the brachial artery.
- **26-25** Reading the manometer.
- **26-26** Charting sample.

Chapter 29
- **29-4, C** Wheelchair scale.
- **29-6** Balance scale.
- **29-8** Reading the height measurement.
- **29-10** This resident is being discharged.

Chapter 31
- **31-14** The bar code on the bottle of reagent strips is scanned.

Chapter 33
- **33-2** Excoriation.
- **33-27** Compression garment.

Chapter 34
- **34-4, A** Suspected deep tissue injury.
- **34-4, F** Unstageable pressure ulcer.
- **34-5** Turn clock.
- **34-13** Braden Scale.

Chapter 36
- **36-19** Cannula prongs are inserted.

Chapter 37
- **37-6** Tracheostomy tube is suctioned.

Chapter 42
- **42-7** Pacemaker.

Chapter 43
- **43-2** Hiatal hernia.
- **43-7** Liver damage from alcohol.
- **43-8** Ascites.

Chapter 44
- **44-2, A** Normal prostate size.
- **44-2, B** Enlarged prostate.

Chapter 46
- **46-2, A** Normal brain.
- **46-2, B** Dark patches show damage to brain tissue.
- **46-3, A** Very early AD.
- **46-3, B** Mild to moderate AD.
- **46-3, C** Severe AD.
- **46-7** Safety covers on stove knobs.

Sheila A. Sorrentino, BSN, MA, MSN, PhD, RN
Leighann N. Remmert, BSN, MS, RN

This book was designed for you. It was designed to help you learn. The book is a useful resource as you gain experience and expand your knowledge.

This preface gives study guidelines and helps you use the book. For a reading assignment, do you read from the first page to the last page without stopping? What do you remember? To learn more, use a study system with these steps:

- Survey or preview
- Question
- Read and record
- Recite and review

Preview

First, preview or survey the reading assignment for a few minutes. This gives an idea of what the assignment covers. It also helps in recalling what you know about the subject. Carefully look over the assignment. Preview the chapter title, objectives, key terms and abbreviations, headings, subheadings, and key ideas in italics. Also survey the boxes and review questions at the end of the chapter.

Question

Next, form questions to answer while reading. Questions should relate to how the information applies to giving care or what might be asked on a test. Use the headings and subheadings to form questions. Questions starting with what, how, or why are helpful. Avoid questions with one-word answers. If a question does not help you study, just change the question. Questioning sets a purpose for reading. Changing a question makes this step more useful.

Read and Record

Reading is the next step. You read to:
- Gain new information.
- Connect new information to what you know already.
- Find answers to your questions.

Break the assignment into small parts. Then answer your questions as you read each part. Also underline or highlight important information. This reminds you of what you need to learn. Review the marked parts later. Also make notes for more immediate learning. To make notes, write down important information in the margins or in a notebook. Use words and statements to jog your memory about the material.

To remember what you read, work with the information. Organize information into a study guide. Study guides have many forms. Diagrams or charts show relationships or steps in a process. Note taking in outline format is also very useful. The following is a sample outline.

1. Main heading
   a. Second level
   b. Second level
      i. Third level
      ii. Third level
2. Main heading

Recite and Review

Finally, recite and review. Use your notes and study guides. Answer your questions and others that came up when reading and answering the "Review Questions" at the end of a chapter. Answer all questions out loud (recite).

Reviewing is more about when to study rather than what to study. You decided what to study during the preview, question, and reading steps. It is best to review right after the first study session, one week later, and before a quiz or test.

This book was designed to help you study. Special features are described on the next pages.

We hope you enjoy learning and your work. You and your work are important. You and the care you give make a difference in the person's life!

Sheila A. Sorrentino
Leighann N. Remmert

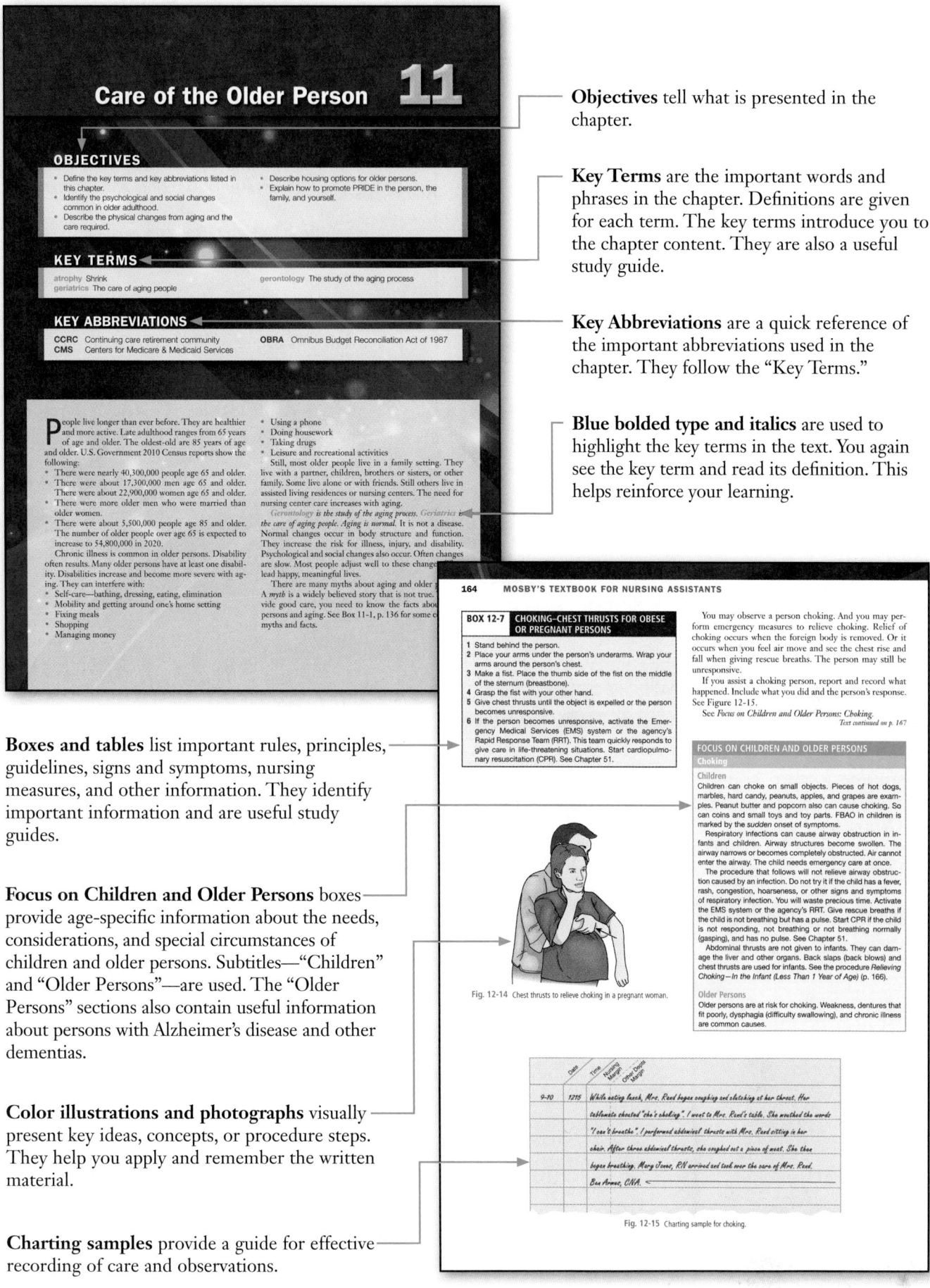

Objectives tell what is presented in the chapter.

Key Terms are the important words and phrases in the chapter. Definitions are given for each term. The key terms introduce you to the chapter content. They are also a useful study guide.

Key Abbreviations are a quick reference of the important abbreviations used in the chapter. They follow the "Key Terms."

Blue bolded type and italics are used to highlight the key terms in the text. You again see the key term and read its definition. This helps reinforce your learning.

Boxes and tables list important rules, principles, guidelines, signs and symptoms, nursing measures, and other information. They identify important information and are useful study guides.

Focus on Children and Older Persons boxes provide age-specific information about the needs, considerations, and special circumstances of children and older persons. Subtitles—"Children" and "Older Persons"—are used. The "Older Persons" sections also contain useful information about persons with Alzheimer's disease and other dementias.

Color illustrations and photographs visually present key ideas, concepts, or procedure steps. They help you apply and remember the written material.

Charting samples provide a guide for effective recording of care and observations.

Care of the Older Person 11

OBJECTIVES

- Define the key terms and key abbreviations listed in this chapter.
- Identify the psychological and social changes common in older adulthood.
- Describe the physical changes from aging and the care required.
- Describe housing options for older persons.
- Explain how to promote PRIDE in the person, the family, and yourself.

KEY TERMS

atrophy Shrink
geriatrics The care of aging people
gerontology The study of the aging process

KEY ABBREVIATIONS

CCRC Continuing care retirement community
CMS Centers for Medicare & Medicaid Services
OBRA Omnibus Budget Reconciliation Act of 1987

People live longer than ever before. They are healthier and more active. Late adulthood ranges from 65 years of age and older. The oldest-old are 85 years of age and older. U.S. Government 2010 Census reports show the following:

- There were nearly 40,300,000 people age 65 and older.
- There were about 17,300,000 men age 65 and older. There were about 22,900,000 women age 65 and older.
- There were more older men who were married than older women.
- There were about 5,500,000 people age 85 and older. The number of older people over age 65 is expected to increase to 54,800,000 in 2020.

Chronic illness is common in older persons. Disability often results. Many older persons have at least one disability. Disabilities increase and become more severe with aging. They can interfere with:

- Self-care—bathing, dressing, eating, elimination
- Mobility and getting around one's home setting
- Fixing meals
- Shopping
- Managing money

- Using a phone
- Doing housework
- Taking drugs
- Leisure and recreational activities

Still, most older people live in a family setting. They live with a partner, children, brothers or sisters, or other family. Some live alone or with friends. Still others live in assisted living residences or nursing centers. The need for nursing center care increases with aging.

Gerontology is the study of the aging process. Geriatrics is the care of aging people. Aging is normal. It is not a disease. Normal changes occur in body structure and function. They increase the risk for illness, injury, and disability. Psychological and social changes also occur. Often changes are slow. Most people adjust well to these changes and lead happy, meaningful lives.

There are many myths about aging and older persons. A *myth* is a widely believed story that is not true. To provide good care, you need to know the facts about older persons and aging. See Box 11-1, p. 136 for some common myths and facts.

---

164 MOSBY'S TEXTBOOK FOR NURSING ASSISTANTS

BOX 12-7 CHOKING—CHEST THRUSTS FOR OBESE OR PREGNANT PERSONS

1 Stand behind the person.
2 Place your arms under the person's underarms. Wrap your arms around the person's chest.
3 Make a fist. Place the thumb side of the fist on the middle of the sternum (breastbone).
4 Grasp the fist with your other hand.
5 Give chest thrusts until the object is expelled or the person becomes unresponsive.
6 If the person becomes unresponsive, activate the Emergency Medical Services (EMS) system or the agency's Rapid Response Team (RRT). This team quickly responds to give care in life-threatening situations. Start cardiopulmonary resuscitation (CPR). See Chapter 51.

You may observe a person choking. And you may perform emergency measures to relieve choking. Relief of choking occurs when the foreign body is removed. Or it occurs when you feel air move and see the chest rise and fall when giving rescue breaths. The person may still be unresponsive.

If you assist a choking person, report and record what happened. Include what you did and the person's response. See Figure 12-15.

See *Focus on Children and Older Persons: Choking.*

Text continued on p. 167

FOCUS ON CHILDREN AND OLDER PERSONS
Choking

Children
Children can choke on small objects. Pieces of hot dogs, marbles, hard candy, peanuts, apples, and grapes are examples. Peanut butter and popcorn also can cause choking. So can coins and small toys and toy parts. FBAO in children is marked by the *sudden* onset of symptoms.

Respiratory infections can cause airway obstruction in infants and children. Airway structures become swollen. The airway narrows or becomes completely obstructed. Air cannot enter the airway. The child needs emergency care at once.

The procedure that follows will not relieve airway obstruction caused by an infection. Do not try it if the child has a fever, rash, congestion, hoarseness, or other signs and symptoms of respiratory infection. You will waste precious time. Activate the EMS system or the agency's RRT. Give rescue breaths if the child is not breathing but has a pulse. Start CPR if the child is not responding, not breathing or not breathing normally (gasping), and has no pulse. See Chapter 51.

Abdominal thrusts are not given to infants. They can damage the liver and other organs. Back slaps (back blows) and chest thrusts are used for infants. See the procedure *Relieving Choking—In the Infant (Less Than 1 Year of Age)* (p. 166).

Older Persons
Older persons are at risk for choking. Weakness, dentures that fit poorly, dysphagia (difficulty swallowing), and chronic illness are common causes.

Fig. 12-14 Chest thrusts to relieve choking in a pregnant woman.

Date	Time	Nursing Margin	Other Data Margin	
9-10	1215	While eating lunch, Mrs. Reed began coughing and clutching at her throat. Her tablemate shouted "she's choking". I went to Mrs. Reed's table. She mouthed the words "I can't breathe". I performed abdominal thrusts with Mrs. Reed sitting in her chair. After three abdominal thrusts, she coughed out a piece of meat. She then began breathing. Mary Jones, RN arrived and took over the care of Mrs. Reed. Bea Armes, CNA.		

Fig. 12-15 Charting sample for choking.

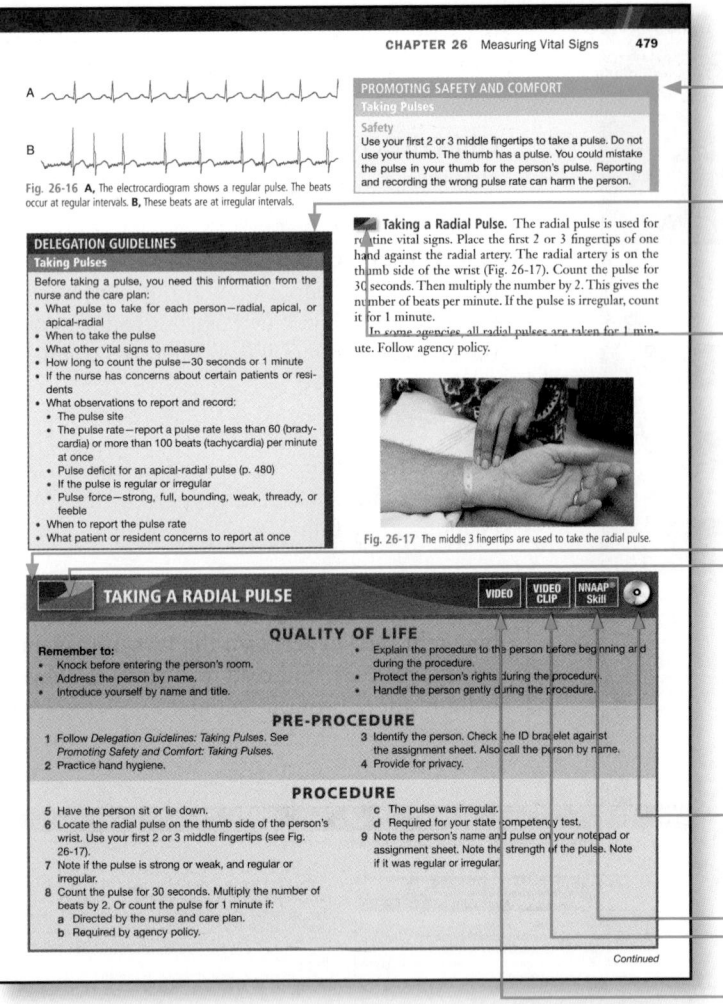

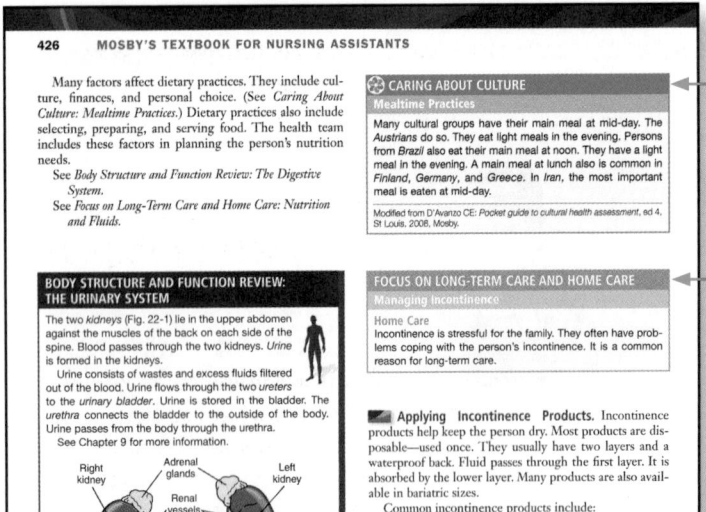

Promoting Safety and Comfort boxes focus your attention on the need to be safe and cautious and promote comfort when giving care. "Safety" and "Comfort" subtitles are used.

Delegation Guidelines describe the information you need from the nurse and care plan before performing a procedure. They also tell you the observations to report and record.

Heading icons alert you to associated procedures. Procedure boxes contain the same icon.

Procedures boxes are written in a step-by-step format. They are divided into *Quality of Life*, *Pre-Procedure*, *Procedure*, and *Post-Procedure* sections for easy studying. The *Quality of Life* section lists 6 simple courtesies that show respect for the patient or resident as a person.

Procedure icons in the title bar alert you to associated content areas. Heading icons and procedure icons are the same.

CD icons appear in the procedure box title bar for the skills included on the CD-ROM in the book.

NNAAP® in the procedure title bar alerts you to the skills that are part of the National Nurse Aide Assessment Program (NNAAP®). Note: Not all states participate in NNAAP®. Ask your instructor for a list of the skills tested in your state.

Video clip icons in the procedure title bar alert you to related video clips available on-line on *Evolve Student Learning Resources*.

Video icons in the procedure title bar alert you to procedures included in *Mosby's Nursing Assistant Video Skills 3.0*.

Caring About Culture boxes contain information about the various practices of other cultures.

Focus on Long-Term Care and Home Care boxes highlight information for safe functioning in long-term care and home care settings. "Long-Term Care" and "Home Care" subtitles are used.

Body Structure and Function Review boxes provide a review of body systems as they relate to various procedures and medical-surgical problems and conditions.

---

538 MOSBY'S TEXTBOOK FOR NURSING ASSISTANTS

FOCUS ON COMMUNICATION
Assisting With the Exam

Each examiner has a routine. He or she does things in a certain order. To better assist, ask the examiner to explain the routine to you. Also ask him or her to tell you what equipment and supplies are needed. For example:
- "Dr. Weaver, I want to help in the best way that I can. Please tell me how you will start the exam and how you will proceed."
- "Ms. Carrigan, please ask for equipment and supplies as you need them. That way I can hand you the correct item."

FOCUS ON CHILDREN AND OLDER PERSONS
Assisting With the Exam

Children
A parent is present when children are examined. If the child is uncooperative, the parent may need to hold him or her still during some parts of the exam. Being kept still may frighten an infant. The child may fear harm or separation from the parent. A calm, comforting manner helps the child and parent. The parent may have fears too.

The equipment used for children is like that for the adult exam. Toys are used to assess development. Vaginal speculums are not used.

Older Persons
Persons with dementia may resist the examiner's efforts. The person may be agitated and aggressive from confusion and fear. Do not restrain or force the person to have the exam. The exam is tried another time. Sometimes a family member can calm the person. The doctor may order drugs to help the person relax. The person's rights are always respected.

After the Exam
After the exam, the person dresses or returns to bed. Lubricant was used to examine the vagina or rectum. The area is wiped or cleaned before the person dresses or returns to the room. Assist as needed. You also need to:
- Discard disposable items.
- Replace supplies so the tray is ready for the next exam.
- Clean re-usable items. Follow agency policy. Return items to the tray or storage area. This includes the otoscope and ophthalmoscope tips and stethoscope.
- Send a re-usable speculum to the supply department. It needs to be sterilized.
- Cover the exam table with a clean drawsheet or paper.
- Label specimens. Take them to the designated area with a requisition slip. See Chapter 31.
- Clean and straighten the person's unit or exam room.
- Follow agency policy for soiled linens.
See *Teamwork and Time Management: After the Exam.*

TEAMWORK AND TIME MANAGEMENT
After the Exam

Make sure that the exam room is clean and that supplies and equipment are ready for the next exam. Otherwise you delay the patient or resident, examiner, and the staff member assisting.

You may find an exam room that is not clean. Or you may find that exam equipment and supplies are not ready. Call for the nurse before you start to prepare the room and ready supplies and equipment. The nurse needs to see the problem. The nurse can find out who last used the room or tray. The nurse can then talk to the staff members involved.

FOCUS ON PRIDE
The Person, Family, and Yourself

Personal and Professional Responsibility
Physical, mental, and social discomfort are common during the physical exam. Often only a gown is worn. Sometimes an uncomfortable position is required. Private body parts (breasts, vagina, penis, and rectum) may be examined. Anxiety and fear are common feelings.

The person needs to feel safe, secure, and protected from exposure. The person should feel comfortable with the examiner and the person assisting. Be professional and courteous at all times. Provide care in a way that promotes dignity, self-esteem, and well-being.

Rights and Respect
The person has the right to privacy. Protect the person from exposure. Only the examiner and the person assisting have the right to see the person's body. The person must consent for others to be present. This includes family. Proper draping and screening are needed. Keep the person covered. Expose only the body part being examined.

Independence and Social Interaction
Fears about the exam affect the person's well-being. These fears are common:
- Who will perform the exam? How will the exam be done?
- Why is the exam needed?
- Will an illness be found? Is it cancer?
- Will surgery be needed? Will more drugs be needed? Will I die?
  To ease the person's fears:
- Greet the person. Introduce yourself by name and title.
- Talk with the person. Be pleasant.
- Tell the person good things about the examiner or agency. For example: "Dr. Foster will examine you today. She is very kind and thorough."
  Your interactions affect the person's mental comfort. Caring, kindness, and a positive attitude ease worries.

CHAPTER 30 Assisting With the Physical Examination **539**

Delegation and Teamwork
When preparing for an exam, make sure needed supplies are in the room. Check that equipment works properly. If not, the examiner and person must wait while you get the supplies or new equipment. The person may be in an uncomfortable position. The delay causes more discomfort.

Know where to find supplies and equipment. If you need an item, you can get it quickly. If you do not know, ask a co-worker where to find the item. Thank your co-worker for helping you.

Ethics and Laws
Information discussed during the exam is confidential. Only staff involved in the person's care need to know the reason for the exam and its results. If the person consents, the doctor tells the family. The person can share the information with others if he or she wants to.

You must keep the person's information confidential. Talking about an exam with family, friends, or staff not involved in the person's care violates the Health Insurance Portability and Accountability Act of 1996 (HIPAA). HIPAA protects the privacy and security of the person's health information. Failure to follow HIPAA rules can result in fines, penalties, and criminal action.

REVIEW QUESTIONS
Circle the BEST answer.
1 The otoscope is used to examine
  a Internal eye structures
  b The external ear and the eardrum
  c Reflexes
  d The vagina
2 You are preparing a person for an exam. You should do the following except
  a Ask the person to void
  b Ask the person to undress
  c Drape the person
  d Go tell the nurse when the person is ready
3 Which part of an exam can you do?
  a Test reflexes
  b Inspect the mouth, teeth, and throat
  c Measure weight, height, and vital signs
  d Observe the perineum and rectum
4 A person is supine. The hips are flexed and externally rotated. The feet are supported in stirrups. The person is in the
  a Dorsal recumbent position
  b Lithotomy position
  c Knee-chest position
  d Sims' position
5 You will assist with Mrs. Janz's exam. Which is *false*?
  a Hand hygiene is practiced before and after the exam
  b Instruments are placed near the examiner
  c A male nursing team member stays in the room
  d Privacy is provided by screening, closing the door, and proper draping

Answers to these questions are on p. 833.

Focus on Communication boxes suggest what to say and questions to ask when interacting with patients, residents, visitors, and the nursing team.

Teamwork and Time Management boxes suggest ways to efficiently work with and help nursing team members.

Focus on PRIDE: The Person, Family, and Yourself boxes build on the concepts and principles presented in the chapter to help you promote pride in the person, family, and yourself. PRIDE is spelled out in the first letter of each section:

- **Personal and Professional Responsibility**—how you can have pride in yourself through personal and professional behaviors and development.

- **Rights and Respect**—how to promote the person's rights and respect him or her as a person with dignity.

- **Independence and Social Interaction**—ways to help the person remain or attain independence and interact socially with others.

- **Delegation and Teamwork**—how to work efficiently with and help other nursing team members.

- **Ethics and Laws**—laws affecting nursing care and doing the right thing when dealing with patients, residents, and co-workers.

Review Questions are useful study guides. They help in reviewing what you have learned. You can also use them to study for a test or for the competency evaluation. Answers are given at the back of the book. See p. 832.

CONTENTS

PROCEDURES

Procedures with this icon [●] are also on the CD-ROM in this book.

Procedures with this icon [VIDEO CLIP] are also on the Evolve Student Resources for this book.

Procedures with this icon [VIDEO] are available in *Mosby's Nursing Assistant Video Skills 3.0*.

Procedures with this icon [NNAAP® Skill] are NNAAP® (National Nurse Aide Assessment Program) skills.

Introduction to Health Care Agencies

1

OBJECTIVES

- Define the key terms and key abbreviations listed in this chapter.
- Describe the types, purposes, and organization of health care agencies.
- Describe members of the health team and nursing team.

- Describe the nursing service department.
- Describe four nursing care patterns.
- Describe the programs that pay for health care.
- Explain why standards are met.
- Explain how to promote PRIDE in the person, the family, and yourself.

KEY TERMS

acute illness A sudden illness from which a person is expected to recover

assisted living residence (ALR) Provides housing, personal care, support services, health care, and social activities in a home-like setting to persons needing help with daily activities

case management A nursing care pattern; a case manager (an RN) coordinates a person's care from admission through discharge and into the home or long-term care setting

chronic illness An ongoing illness, slow or gradual in onset; it has no known cure; it can be controlled and complications prevented with proper treatment

functional nursing A nursing care pattern focusing on tasks and jobs; each nursing team member has certain tasks and jobs to do

health team The many health care workers whose skills and knowledge focus on the person's total care; interdisciplinary health care team

hospice A health care agency or program for persons who are dying

licensed practical nurse (LPN) A nurse who has completed a 1-year nursing program and has passed a licensing test; called *licensed vocational nurse (LVN)* in some states

licensed vocational nurse (LVN) See "licensed practical nurse (LPN)"

nursing assistant A person who has passed a nursing assistant training and competency evaluation program; performs delegated nursing tasks under the supervision of a licensed nurse

nursing team Those who provide nursing care—RNs, LPNs/LVNs, and nursing assistants

patient-focused care A nursing care pattern; services are moved from departments to the bedside

primary nursing A nursing care pattern; an RN is responsible for the person's total care

registered nurse (RN) A nurse who has completed a 2-, 3-, or 4-year nursing program and has passed a licensing test

team nursing A nursing care pattern; a team of nursing staff is led by an RN who decides the amount and kind of care each person needs

terminal illness An illness or injury from which the person will not likely recover

KEY ABBREVIATIONS

ALR	Assisted living residence		**LVN**	Licensed vocational nurse
DON	Director of nursing		**PPO**	Preferred provider organization
HMO	Health maintenance organization		**RN**	Registered nurse
LPN	Licensed practical nurse		**SNF**	Skilled nursing facility

---

BOX 1-1 **TYPES OF HEALTH CARE AGENCIES**

- Hospitals
- Long-term care centers (nursing homes, nursing facilities, nursing centers)
- Memory care facilities
- Home care agencies; home health care agencies
- Out-patient surgery centers
- Adult day-care centers
- Assisted living residences
- Board and care homes
- Rehabilitation and subacute care facilities
- Hospices
- Doctors' offices
- Clinics
- Centers for persons with mental illnesses
- Centers for persons with developmental disabilities
- Drug and alcohol treatment centers
- Crisis centers for rape, abuse, suicide, and other emergencies

---

Health care agencies offer services to persons needing health care (Box 1-1). Agencies vary in size, services, hours open, and staff. The *person* is always the focus of care.

Staff members have special talents, knowledge, and skills. All work to meet the person's needs.

AGENCY PURPOSES

Services range from simple to complex. Some agencies have one purpose and offer one service. Out-patient surgery centers are an example. Surgeries and medical procedures are done in a non-hospital setting. The person returns home the same day or the next day. Other agencies have many purposes. They offer many services.

The purposes of health care are:

- *Health promotion.* The goal is to reduce the risk of physical or mental illnesses. People receive teaching and counseling about healthy living. This includes diet, exercise, and the warning signs and symptoms of illness. They learn how to manage and cope with health problems.
- *Disease prevention.* Risk factors and early warning signs of disease are identified. Measures are taken to reduce risk factors and prevent disease. Immunizations prevent some infectious diseases. Polio, measles, mumps, smallpox, and hepatitis B are examples. Simple life-style changes can prevent health problems. For example, high blood pressure can lead to heart attacks and strokes. Diet and exercise can help lower blood pressure.
- *Detection and treatment of disease.* This involves diagnostic tests, physical exams, surgery, emergency care, and drugs. Often respiratory, physical, and occupational therapies are needed. The nursing team observes signs and symptoms, gives care, and follows the doctor's orders.

- *Rehabilitation and restorative care.* The goal is to return persons to their highest possible level of physical and mental functioning and to independence. *Independence* means not relying on or needing care from others. The rehabilitation process starts when the person first seeks health care. The person learns or re-learns skills needed to live, work, and enjoy life. Maintaining function is important. Help is given with making needed changes at home.

These purposes are related. For example, Mr. Parker has chest pain and problems breathing. He goes to a hospital emergency department. After an exam and tests, the doctor diagnoses a heart attack. Mr. Parker is admitted to the hospital for treatment. He receives teaching and counseling about heart attack risk factors and healthy living. The goals are to promote health and prevent another heart attack. He begins a rehabilitation program. Activity starts slowly and may progress from walking to jogging and swimming. Teaching and counseling focus on diet, drugs, life-style, activity, and how to cope with fears and concerns. Successful rehabilitation promotes health and may prevent another heart attack.

Student Learning

Many agencies are learning sites for students. (See "The Health Team" on p. 4.) Students assist in the purposes of health care. They are involved with and provide care.

TYPES OF AGENCIES

Nursing assistants work in many settings. Some work in doctors' offices and clinics. Most work in the following agencies.

Hospitals

Hospital services include emergency care, surgery, nursing care, x-ray procedures and treatments, and laboratory testing (Fig. 1-1). Services also include respiratory, physical, occupational, speech, and other therapies.

People of all ages need hospital care. They go to have babies, for physical and mental health problems, for surgery, to heal broken bones, or to die. They have acute, chronic, or terminal illnesses:

- *Acute illness is a sudden illness from which the person is expected to recover.*
- *Chronic illness is an on-going illness that is slow or gradual in onset. There is no known cure. The illness can be controlled and complications prevented with proper treatment.*
- *Terminal illness is an illness or injury from which the person will not likely recover. The person will die (Chapter 52).*

Rehabilitation and Subacute Care Agencies

Hospital stays are often short. This is because of insurance coverage. Some people do not need hospital care but are too sick to go home. Medical and nursing care and rehabilitation are needed. Care needs fall between hospital care and long-term care. Complex equipment and care measures are needed. See Chapter 38 for common rehabilitation programs.

Some hospitals and long-term care centers have rehabilitation and subacute care units. Some are separate agencies. Many persons fully recover and return home. Others need long-term care.

Long-Term Care Centers

Some persons cannot care for themselves at home but do not need hospital care. Long-term care centers (nursing homes, nursing facilities, nursing centers) can help them. Care needs range from simple to complex. Medical, nursing, dietary, recreation, rehabilitation, and social services are provided. So are housekeeping and laundry services.

Persons in long-term care centers are called *residents*. They are not *patients*. This is because the center is their temporary or permanent home.

Most residents are older. They may have chronic diseases, poor nutrition, memory problems, or poor health. Long-term care centers are designed to meet their needs (Chapter 11).

Not all residents are old. Some are disabled from birth defects, accidents, or diseases. Hospital patients are often discharged while still sick or recovering from surgery. Some need home care. Others need long-term care until able to go home. Others need care until death.

Skilled Nursing Facilities. Skilled nursing facilities (SNFs) provide more complex care than do nursing centers. They are part of hospitals or nursing centers. SNF residents need rehabilitation or time to recover from illness or surgery. Often they return home after a short stay. Others remain nursing center residents.

Assisted Living Residences

An *assisted living residence (ALR) provides housing, personal care, support services, health care, and social activities in a home-like setting for persons needing help with daily activities* (Chapter 50). Some ALRs are part of nursing centers or retirement communities (Chapter 11).

The person has a room or an apartment. Three meals a day are provided. So are housekeeping, laundry, and transportation services. Help is given with personal care and drugs. Social and recreational activities are provided. There is access to health and medical care.

Mental Health Centers

Mental health centers are for persons with mental health problems. Some persons have problems with life events. Others present dangers to themselves or others because of how they think and behave. Out-patient care is common. Some need short-term or life-long in-patient care.

Home Care Agencies

Many services are provided to people where they live. Services are provided by nurses and nursing assistants and other health team members. Services range from health teaching and supervision to bedside nursing care. Physical therapy, rehabilitation, and food services are common. Hospitals, health care systems, public health departments, and private businesses offer home care services.

People of all ages need home health care. So do some persons who are dying.

Hospices

A *hospice is a health care agency or program for persons who are dying*. Such persons no longer respond to treatments aimed at cures. Usually they have less than 6 months to live.

The physical, emotional, social, and spiritual needs of the person and family are met. The focus is on comfort, not cure. Children and pets can visit. Family and friends can assist with care.

Hospice care is provided by hospitals, nursing centers, and home care agencies. Hospice services are often provided in the home setting.

Health Care Systems

Agencies join together as one provider of care. A system usually has hospitals, nursing centers, home care agencies, hospice settings, and doctors' offices (Fig. 1-2). An

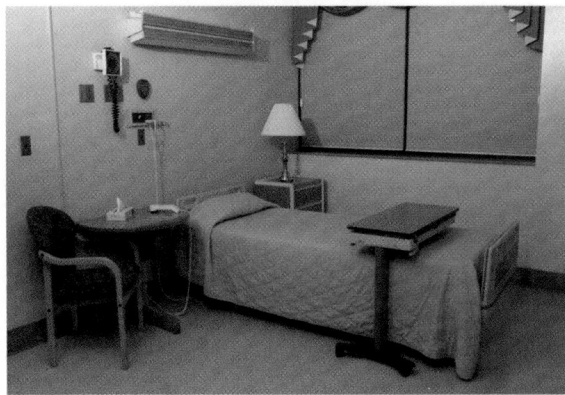

Fig. 1-1 Furniture and equipment in a hospital room.

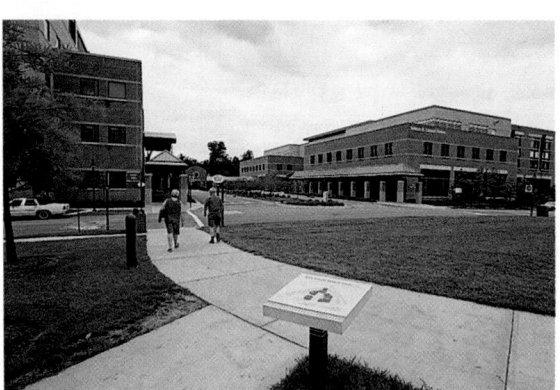

Fig. 1-2 The hospital and doctors' offices are part of a health care system.

A health care system owns Mercy Hospital. Dr. Moore and Dr. Gills work there. The hospital has:
- A rehabilitation unit
- A home care service
- An ambulance service
- A medical supply store
- A nursing center

June Adams is 78 years old. She sees Dr. Moore in his office. She complains of tightness in her chest, dizziness, and a "pounding heart." She is having a heart attack. Dr. Moore admits her to the hospital. Dr. Gills, a heart specialist, takes over her care. A few days later she has a stroke. She cannot move her left side. She is given needed medical care. When stable, she transfers to the rehabilitation unit.

Mrs. Adams spends 2 weeks on the rehabilitation unit. She needs home care if she returns home. Or she can go to a nursing center. She wants to go home. Her family wants to help care for her. They need a hospital bed, commode, bedpan, wheelchair, and other items. They rent some items and buy others at the medical supply store.

Mrs. Adams is transported home by the ambulance service. The hospital's home care agency provides home care services. A nursing assistant visits every day to help with hygiene and grooming needs. A nurse visits three times a week.

A month later Mrs. Adams has another stroke. She returns to the hospital by the ambulance service. After 8 days, she transfers to the rehabilitation unit. The second stroke has caused more disabilities. Dr. Gills suggests nursing center care. Mrs. Adams and her family agree with him.

The nurse arranges for Mrs. Adams to be admitted to the nursing center. She is transferred there by the ambulance service.

ambulance service and medical supply store for home care are common. The system may serve a community or a large region.

The goal is to serve all health care needs. A person uses system providers as needed (Box 1-2).

ORGANIZATION

An agency has a governing body called the *board of trustees* or *board of directors*. The board makes policies. It makes sure that safe care is given at the lowest possible cost. Local, state, and federal laws are followed.

An administrator manages the agency. He or she reports directly to the board. Directors or department heads manage certain areas (Fig. 1-3).

See *Focus on Long-Term Care and Home Care: Organization.*

The Health Team

The *health team* involves the many health care workers whose skills and knowledge focus on the person's total care (Table 1-1). (In nursing centers, it is called the *interdisciplinary health care team*.) The goal is to provide quality care. The person is the focus of care (Fig. 1-4, p. 7).

Many team members are involved in the care of each person. Coordinated care is needed. An RN leads this team.

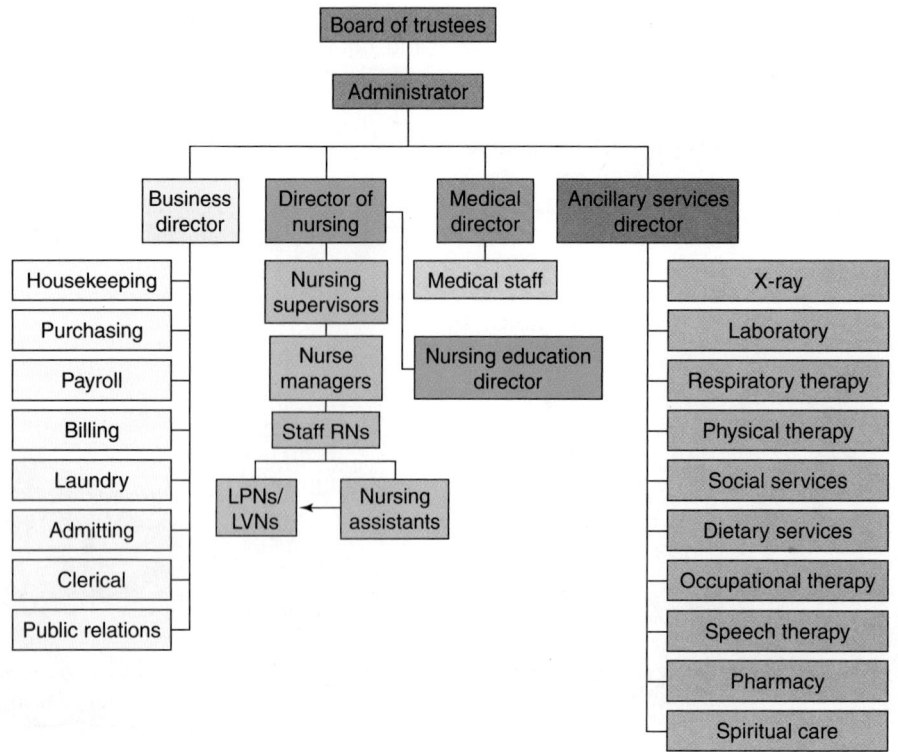

Fig. 1-3 Sample organizational chart of a health care agency. Titles and department names may vary among states and agencies.

FOCUS ON LONG-TERM CARE AND HOME CARE
Organization

Long-Term Care

Nursing centers are usually owned by an individual or a corporation. Some are owned by county health departments.

Each center has an administrator. Department directors report to the administrator. Nursing centers have nursing, therapy, and food service departments. They also have housekeeping, maintenance, and laundry departments. A human resources director handles personnel matters such as hiring staff. A finance director handles billing. A social services director meets the social needs of residents and families. An activities director plans resident activities.

By law, nursing centers must have a medical director. This person is a doctor. This doctor consults with the staff about medical problems not handled by a resident's doctor. Guidance is given about resident care policies and programs.

TABLE 1-1 HEALTH TEAM MEMBERS

Title	Description	Credentials
Activities director	Assesses, plans, and implements recreational needs	Varies with state and/or employer; ranges from no training to bachelor's degree
Audiologist	Tests hearing; prescribes hearing aids; works with persons who are hard-of-hearing	Master's degree or higher; state license
Cleric (clergyman; clergywoman)	Assists with spiritual needs	Priest, minister, rabbi, sister (nun), deacon, or other pastoral training
Clinical laboratory technologist	Performs complicated laboratory tests on blood, urine, and other body fluids, secretions, and excretions; organizes, supervises, and performs diagnostic analyses	Bachelor's degree; national certification test; license in some states
Clinical nurse specialist	Provides nursing care and consults in a nursing specialty—geriatrics, critical care, diabetes, rehabilitation, and wound care are examples	RN with master's degree or doctorate as a clinical nurse specialist
Dental hygienist	Focuses on preventing dental disorders; supervised by a licensed dentist	Completion of a dental hygiene program; state license
Dentist	Prevents and treats disorders and diseases of the teeth, gums, and oral structures	Doctor of dental science (DDS) or doctor of dental medicine (DMD); state license
Dietitian and nutritionist	Assesses and plans for nutritional needs; teaches good nutrition, food selection, and preparation	Bachelor's degree; registered dietitian (RD) must pass a national registration test; license or certification in some states
Home health aide	Assists persons in their own homes (see "Nursing assistant")	See "Nursing assistant"
Homemaker	Provides light housekeeping and homemaking tasks—laundry, bedmaking, shops for food, plans and prepares meals; assists with hygiene, dressing, and grooming	Varies from state to state; on-the-job training
Licensed practical/vocational nurse (LPN/LVN)	Provides direct nursing care, including giving drugs, under the direction of an RN	State-approved program (usually 1 year in length); licensing exam and state license
Medical or clinical laboratory technician	Collects samples and performs laboratory tests on blood, urine, and other body fluids, secretions, and excretions	Associate's degree; national certifying test; license in some states
Medical records and health information technician	Maintains medical records; transcribes medical reports; files records; completes required reports	Associate's degree; credentialing test
Medication assistant-certified (MA-C)	Gives drugs as allowed by state law under the supervision of an RN or LPN/LVN	Certified nursing assistant with additional education and training required by state law; state certification

Modified from Bureau of Labor Statistics, U.S. Department of Labor, *Occupational Outlook Handbook, 2010-11 Edition.*

Continued

TABLE 1-1	HEALTH TEAM MEMBERS—cont'd	
Title	**Description**	**Credentials**
Nurse practitioner	Plans and provides care with the health team; does physical exams, health assessments, and health education	RN with master's degree or higher and clinical experience in a nursing area; certification test may be required
Nursing assistant	Assists nurses and gives nursing care; supervised by an RN or LPN/LVN	Completion of a state-approved training and competency evaluation program to work in long-term care or in home care agencies receiving Medicare funds; state registry; state certification or license
Occupational therapist registered (OTR)	Assists persons to learn or retain skills needed to perform daily activities; designs adaptive equipment for daily living	Master's degree or higher; national certification exam; state license
Occupational therapy assistant	Performs tasks and services supervised by an OTR	Associate's degree; national certification; license in some states
Pharmacist	Fills drug orders written by doctors; monitors and evaluates drug interactions; consults with doctors and nurses about drug actions and interactions	Pharm.D. degree; state license
Physical therapist (PT)	Assists persons with musculo-skeletal problems to restore function and prevent disability	Master's degree or higher; state license
Physical therapy assistant	Performs tasks and services supervised by a PT	Associate's degree; national certification or license in some states
Physician (doctor)	Diagnoses and treats diseases and injuries	Medical school graduation (MD, DO), residency, and national board certification; state license
Physician's assistant (PA)	Assists in diagnosis and treatment; performs medical tasks supervised by a doctor	Master's degree; national certification exam; license in some states
Podiatrist	Prevents, diagnoses, and treats foot disorders	Doctor of podiatric medicine (DPM); state license
Radiographer/radiologic technologist	Takes x-rays; processes film for viewing	Associate's degree or higher; license in some states
Registered nurse (RN)	Assesses, makes nursing diagnoses, plans, implements, and evaluates nursing care; supervises LPNs/LVNs and nursing assistants	Associate's degree, diploma, or bachelor's degree; licensing exam and state license
Respiratory therapist (RT)	Assists in treating lung and heart disorders; gives respiratory treatments and therapies	Associate's degree or higher; national certification test; license in most states
Social worker	Deals with social, emotional, and environmental issues affecting illness and recovery; coordinates community agencies to assist patients, residents, and families	Bachelor's degree or higher; 2 years supervised work experience for clinical social workers; license, certification, or registration
Speech-language pathologist	Evaluates speech and language and treats persons with speech, voice, hearing, communication, and swallowing disorders	Master's degree; supervised work experience and national test for licensure in most states

Nursing Service

Nursing service is a large department. The director of nursing (DON) is an RN. (*Director of nursing services, chief nurse executive, vice president of nursing,* and *vice president of patient services* are some other titles used.) Usually a bachelor's or higher degree is required. The DON is responsible for the entire nursing staff. This includes giving safe care.

Nursing supervisors and nurse managers (usually RNs) assist the DON. They manage and carry out nursing department functions. Shift managers coordinate nursing

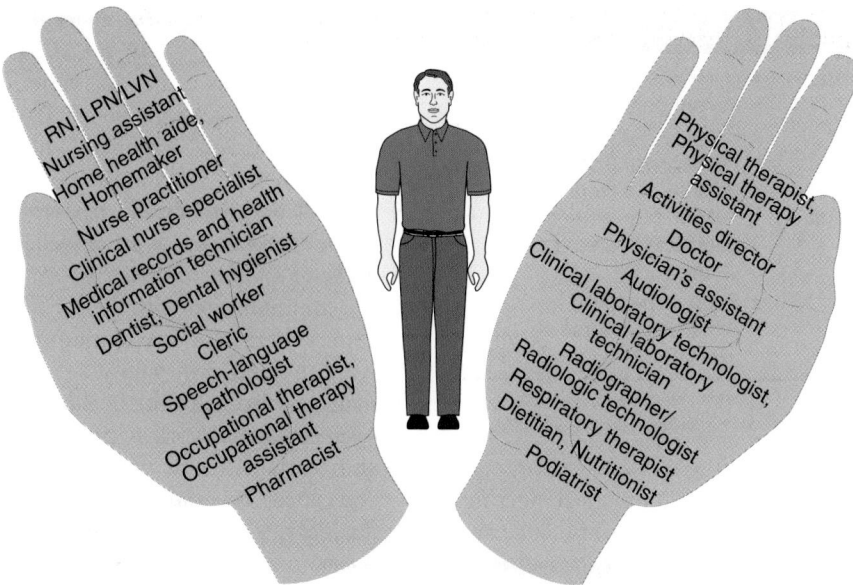

Fig. 1-4 Members of the health team. The person is the focus of care.

care for a certain shift. Hospital nursing areas include surgical, medical, intensive care, pediatric, and mental health units. They also include operating and recovery areas, an emergency department, and a maternity department.

Other nurse supervisors or managers focus on a nursing area or a certain function. Staff development, restorative nursing, infection control, and continuous quality care are examples. Nurse supervisors or managers are responsible for all nursing care and the actions of nursing staff in their areas.

Nursing areas usually have charge nurses for each shift. They are usually RNs. In some states, LPNs/LVNs are charge nurses. The charge nurse is responsible for all nursing care and for the actions of nursing staff during that shift. Staff RNs report to the charge nurse. LPNs/LVNs report to staff RNs or to the charge nurse. You report to the nurse supervising your work.

Nursing education (staff development) is part of nursing service. Nursing education staff:
- Plan and present educational programs (in-service programs).
- Share new and changing information with the nursing team.
- Show how to use new equipment and supplies.
- Review key policies and procedures on a regular basis.
- Educate and train nursing assistants.
- Conduct new employee orientation programs.
- Provide programs that meet federal and state educational requirements.

THE NURSING TEAM

The *nursing team involves those who provide nursing care—RNs, LPNs/LVNs, and nursing assistants.* Their roles and responsibilities differ. All focus on the physical, social, emotional, and spiritual needs of the person and family.

Registered Nurses

A *registered nurse (RN) has completed a 2-, 3-, or 4-year nursing program and has passed a licensing test:*
- Community college programs—2 years
- Hospital-based diploma programs—2 or 3 years
- College or university programs—4 years

Nursing and the biological, social, and physical sciences are studied. Graduate nurses take a licensing test offered by their state board of nursing. They receive a license and become *registered* when the test is passed. RNs must have a license recognized by the state in which they work.

RNs assess, make nursing diagnoses, plan, implement, and evaluate nursing care (Chapter 7). They develop care plans, provide care, and make sure care plans are followed. They also delegate (Chapter 3) nursing care and tasks to the nursing team. They evaluate how the care plans and nursing care affect each person. RNs teach the person and family how to improve health and independence.

RNs follow the doctor's orders. They may delegate the orders to LPNs/LVNs or nursing assistants. RNs do not prescribe treatments or drugs. However, RNs can become *clinical nurse specialists* or *nurse practitioners.* These RNs have limited diagnosing and prescribing functions.

RNs work as staff nurses, nurse supervisors or managers, DONs, agency administrators, and instructors. Other career options depend on education, abilities, and experiences.

Licensed Practical Nurses and Licensed Vocational Nurses

A *licensed practical nurse (LPN) has completed a 1-year nursing program and has passed a licensing test.* Hospitals, community colleges, vocational schools, and technical schools offer programs. Some programs are 10 months long; others take 18 months. Some high schools offer 2-year programs.

BOX 1-3	NURSING ASSISTANT TITLES
• Certified nursing assistant (CNA)	• Nursing support technician
	• Patient care assistant
• Clinical technician	• Patient care attendant
• Health care assistant	• Patient care monitor
• Health care technician	• Patient care technician
• Licensed nursing assistant (LNA)	• Patient care worker
	• Registered nurse aide (RNA)
• Nurse's aide	• Support partner
• Nurse extender	• State tested nurse aide (STNA)
• Nurse technician	
• Nursing care partner	

Graduates take a licensing test for practical nursing. After passing the test, they receive a license to practice and the title of *licensed practical nurse*. *Licensed vocational nurse (LVN) is used in some states*. LPNs/LVNs must have a license required by the state in which they work.

LPNs/LVNs are supervised by RNs, licensed doctors, and licensed dentists. They have fewer responsibilities and functions than RNs do. They need little supervision when the person's condition is stable and care is simple. They assist RNs in caring for acutely ill persons and with complex procedures.

Nursing Assistants

A *nursing assistant has passed a nursing assistant training and competency evaluation program (NATCEP)*. Nursing assistants *perform delegated nursing tasks under the supervision of a licensed nurse*. Box 1-3 lists some titles for nursing assistants. The title depends on the setting, roles, functions, and state laws.

Community colleges, technical schools, and high schools offer nursing assistant courses. So do hospitals and nursing centers. Nursing assistants are discussed in Chapter 3.

NURSING CARE PATTERNS

Nursing care is given in many ways. The pattern used depends on how many persons need care, the staff, and the cost.

- *Functional nursing focuses on tasks and jobs. Each nursing team member has certain tasks and jobs to do.* For example, one nurse gives all drugs. Another gives all treatments. Nursing assistants give baths, make beds, and serve meals.
- *Team nursing involves a team of nursing staff led by an RN.* Called the "team leader," *the RN decides the amount and kind of care each person needs.* The team leader delegates the care of certain persons to other nurses. Some tasks and procedures are delegated to nursing assistants. Delegation is based on the person's needs and team member abilities. Team members report observations and the care given to the team leader.
- *Primary nursing involves total care. The primary nurse (an RN) is responsible for the person's total care.* The nursing team assists as needed. The RN gives nursing care and makes discharge plans. If needed, home care or long-term care is arranged. The RN teaches and counsels the person and family.
- *Case management is like primary nursing. A case manager (an RN) coordinates a person's care from admission through discharge and into the home or long-term care setting.* He or she communicates with the person's doctor and the health team. There also is communication with the insurance company and community agencies as needed. The case manager also helps the health team work together. Some case managers work with certain doctors. Others deal with certain health problems. Heart diseases, diabetes, and cancer are examples.
- *Patient-focused care is when services are moved from departments to the bedside.* The nursing team performs basic skills usually done by other health team members. For example, an RN may draw a blood sample. The number of people caring for each person is reduced. This reduces care costs.

PAYING FOR HEALTH CARE

Health care is a major focus in society. The goals are to provide health care to everyone and to reduce the high cost of care. Health care is costly. So are drugs, medical supplies, and therapies. Most people cannot afford these costs. Some avoid health care because they cannot pay. Others pay doctor bills but go without food or drugs. Health care bills cause worry, fear, and emotional upset. If the person has insurance, some costs are covered. Rarely is the total cost of care covered.

These programs help pay for health care:

- *Private insurance* is bought by individuals and families. The insurance company pays for some or all health care costs.
- *Group insurance* is bought by groups or organizations for individuals. This is often an employee benefit.
- *Medicare* is a federal health insurance program for persons 65 years of age or older. Some younger people with certain disabilities are covered. Part A pays for some hospital, SNF, hospice, and home care costs. Part B helps pay for doctors' services, out-patient hospital care, physical and occupational therapists, some home care, and many other services. Part B is voluntary. The person pays a monthly premium.
- *Medicaid* is a health care payment program. Sponsored by the federal government, it is operated by the states. People with low incomes usually qualify. So do some children and some older, blind, and disabled persons. There is no insurance premium. The amount paid for covered services is limited.

See *Promoting Safety and Comfort: Paying for Health Care.*

PROMOTING SAFETY AND COMFORT
Paying for Health Care

Safety
Some conditions can be prevented with proper care. Medicare pays a lower rate for such conditions if they are acquired during a hospital stay. Pressure ulcers (Chapter 34) and certain types of falls, trauma, and infections are examples. You must assist the nursing and health teams in preventing such conditions.

BOX 1-4 TYPES OF MANAGED CARE

Health Maintenance Organization (HMO). For a pre-paid fee, the person receives needed services offered by the HMO. Some have a yearly physical exam. Others need hospital care. HMOs stress preventing disease and maintaining health. Keeping someone healthy costs far less than treating illness.

Preferred Provider Organization (PPO). A group of doctors and hospitals provides health care at reduced rates. Usually the agreement is between the PPO and an employer or an insurance company. Employees or those insured have reduced rates for the services used. The person can choose any doctor or hospital in the PPO.

Prospective Payment Systems

Prospective payment systems limit the amount paid by insurers, Medicare, and Medicaid. Prospective means *before* care. The amount paid for services is determined before giving care.

- Medicare severity-adjusted diagnosis-related groups (MS-DRGs) are for hospital costs.
- Resource utilization groups (RUGs) are for SNF payments.
- Case mix groups (CMGs) are used for rehabilitation centers.
- Home health resource groups (HHRGs) are used for home health care.

Length of stay and treatment costs are determined for each group. If costs are less than the amount paid, the agency keeps the extra money. If costs are greater, the agency takes the loss.

Managed Care

Managed care deals with health care delivery and payment (Box 1-4). Insurers contract with doctors and hospitals for reduced rates or discounts. The insured person uses doctors and agencies providing the lower rates. If others are used, care is covered in part or not at all. The person pays for costs not covered by insurance.

Managed care limits the choice of where to go for health care. It also limits the care that doctors provide. Many states require managed care for Medicaid and Medicare coverage.

Managed Care as Pre-Approval for Services. Many insurers must approve the need for health care services. If the need is approved, the insurer pays for the services. If not approved, the person pays for the costs. The pre-approval process depends on the insurer.

This pre-approval process is also called *managed care*. It includes monitoring care. The purpose is to reduce unneeded services and procedures. The insurer decides what to pay. With HMOs and PPOs, the insurer may decide where the person goes for services.

MEETING STANDARDS

Health care agencies must meet certain standards. Standards are set by the federal and state governments. They also are set by accrediting agencies. Standards relate to

policies and procedures, budget and finances, and quality of care. An agency must meet standards for:

- *Licensure.* A license is issued by the state. An agency must have a license to operate and provide care.
- *Certification.* This is required to receive Medicare and Medicaid funds.
- *Accreditation.* This is voluntary. It signals quality and excellence.

The Survey Process

Surveys are done to see if the agency meets set standards. A survey team will:

- Review policies and procedures.
- Review medical records.
- Interview staff, patients and residents, and families.
- Observe how care is given.
- Observe if dignity and privacy are promoted.
- Check for cleanliness and safety.
- Review budgets and finances.
- Make sure the staff meet state requirements. (Are doctors and nurses licensed? Are nursing assistants on the state registry?)

The survey team decides if the agency meets the standards. If standards are met, the agency receives a license, certification, or accreditation.

Sometimes problems are found. A problem is called a *deficiency*. The agency usually has 60 days to correct the problem. Sometimes less time is given. The agency can be fined for uncorrected or serious deficiencies. Or it can lose its license, certification, or accreditation.

Your Role

You have an important role in meeting standards and in the survey process. You must:

- Provide quality care.
- Protect the person's rights.
- Provide for the person's and your own safety.
- Help keep the agency clean and safe.
- Conduct yourself in a professional manner.
- Have good work ethics.
- Follow agency policies and procedures.
- Answer questions honestly and completely.
  See *Focus on Communication: Your Role*, p. 10.

FOCUS ON COMMUNICATION
Your Role

A surveyor may approach you to ask questions. If so, be polite. Avoid seeming annoyed or upset about being asked. Answer the questions honestly and as thoroughly as you can. If you do not understand a question, ask the surveyor to rephrase it. If you do not know an answer, do not guess. Tell the surveyor where you would go to find the answer. You can say: "I am unsure, but I would ask the nurse."

For example, you are approached by a surveyor:
Surveyor: "Do you have a moment? May I ask you a few questions?"
You: "Yes. I would be happy to answer your questions."
Surveyor: "Thank you. First, when should you practice hand hygiene?"

You: "I wash my hands before and after contact with a patient. I also wash my hands when they are dirty and after I take off my gloves."
Surveyor: "Thank you. Next, what are two appropriate patient identifiers?"
You: "I am not sure I understand the question. Can you rephrase it?"
Surveyor: "Yes. Name two things you can use to identify a patient."
You: "Okay. Thank you. I can use the patient's full name and date of birth. I cannot use the room number."
Surveyor: "Thank you. I have one last question. In case of a disaster, where would you find the Emergency Preparedness Plan?"
You: "Well, I'm not sure where the plan is located. I could ask my supervising nurse or the charge nurse where to find it."

FOCUS ON PRIDE
The Person, Family, and Yourself

Personal and Professional Responsibility

Health care is a rewarding profession. The health team works hard to provide quality care to patients and residents. You are an important part of that team. You will spend most of your shift giving care. Remember to show patience, compassion, dignity, and respect. You have a great impact on the quality of care each person receives.

Rights and Respect

Many health care agencies conduct employee satisfaction surveys. The surveys are used to gather information about how employees feel about their jobs. Yearly surveys are common.

All staff members are expected to complete and return the form. You may need to note the area you work in or your role in the agency. Other information, such as your name, is usually not given. This helps protect your identity. You have the right to voice your true feelings on a survey. When filling out a survey:
- Be honest. Positive and negative feedback are important.
- Take the survey seriously. Do not rush. Answer the questions completely.
- Finish and return the form in a timely manner.

Surveys are one way health care agencies show respect for employees. Feedback is used to make changes. Take pride in your ideas to improve your agency. Take part in employee satisfaction surveys. Your thoughts matter.

Independence and Social Interaction

People who must rely on others for care often feel frustrated, useless, sad, and a burden to others. A common goal is to return persons to their highest level of functioning. Physical, occupational, and speech therapists work together with doctors, nurses, nursing assistants, and others to promote independence (see Table 1-1). Independence promotes feelings of improvement and success. Help the person take pride in working to restore independence.

Delegation and Teamwork

The health team has many different members. Each has a certain role. Everyone must work together to provide quality care. Offer to help team members when you can. Helping others shows you are dependable and value teamwork.

Ethics and Laws

Nursing team members have different levels of training and responsibilities. RNs, LPNs/LVNs, and nursing assistants all have different roles. Federal and state laws determine the legal limits of these roles. See Chapter 3 for the role limits for nursing assistants. Functions may also vary among agencies. A job description (Chapter 3) describes the agency's expectations. To protect yourself and others, know the limits of your role in your state and agency.

REVIEW QUESTIONS

Circle the BEST answer.

1 Helping persons return to their highest physical and mental function is called
   a Maintaining independence
   b Promoting health
   c Preventing disease
   d Rehabilitation

2 Rehabilitation starts when the
   a Person is ready to leave the agency
   b Person first seeks health care
   c Doctor writes the order
   d Health team thinks the person is ready

3 A health care program for dying persons is a
   a Hospice
   b Assisted living residence
   c Skilled nursing facility
   d Home care agency

4 Who controls policy in a health care agency?
   a The survey team
   b The board of directors
   c The health team
   d Medicare and Medicaid

5 Who is responsible for the entire nursing staff and safe nursing care?
   a The case manager
   b The director of nursing
   c The charge nurse
   d The RN

6 You are a member of
   a The health team and the nursing team
   b The health team and the medical team
   c The nursing team and the medical team
   d An HMO and a PPO

7 The nursing team does *not* include
   a Doctors
   b LPNs/LVNs
   c Nursing assistants
   d RNs

8 Nursing assistants are supervised by
   a Licensed nurses
   b Other nursing assistants
   c The health team
   d The medical director

9 The nursing assistant's role is to
   a Meet Medicare and Medicaid standards
   b Perform delegated tasks
   c Follow the doctor's orders
   d Manage care

10 Nursing tasks are delegated according to a person's needs and staff member abilities. This nursing care pattern is called
   a Team nursing
   b Functional nursing
   c Case management
   d Primary nursing

11 Medicare is for persons who
   a Are 65 years of age or older
   b Need nursing center care
   c Have group insurance
   d Have low incomes

12 Which is required for an agency to operate and provide care?
   a A license
   b Certification
   c Accreditation
   d A survey

13 Which is voluntary for health care agencies?
   a Licensure
   b Certification
   c Accreditation
   d Surveys

14 A survey team member asks you some questions. You should
   a Refer all questions to the nurse
   b Answer as the DON tells you to
   c Give as little information as possible
   d Give honest and complete answers

Answers to these questions are on p. 832.

2 The Person's Rights

OBJECTIVES

- Define the key terms and key abbreviations listed in this chapter.
- Explain the purpose of *The Patient Care Partnership: Understanding Expectations, Rights, and Responsibilities.*
- Describe the purpose and requirements of the Omnibus Budget Reconciliation Act of 1987 (OBRA).

- Identify the person's rights under OBRA.
- Explain how to protect the person's rights.
- Explain the ombudsman role.
- Explain how to promote PRIDE in the person, the family, and yourself.

KEY TERMS

involuntary seclusion Separating a person from others against his or her will, keeping the person to a certain area, or keeping the person away from his or her room without consent

ombudsman Someone who supports or promotes the needs and interests of another person

representative Any person who has the legal right to act on the resident's behalf when he or she cannot do so for himself or herself

treatment The care provided to maintain or restore health, improve function, or relieve symptoms

KEY ABBREVIATIONS

AHA American Hospital Association

OBRA Omnibus Budget Reconciliation Act of 1987

People want information about their health problems and treatment. They also want better care at lower costs. They want to understand and be involved in treatment decisions. They do not accept the doctor's advice without question. As patients and residents, they have certain rights.

PATIENTS' RIGHTS

In April 2003 the American Hospital Association (AHA) adopted *The Patient Care Partnership: Understanding Expectations, Rights, and Responsibilities* (Box 2-1). The document explains the person's rights and expectations during hospital stays. The relationship between the doctor, the health team, and the patient is stressed.

RESIDENTS' RIGHTS

In 1987 the U.S. Congress passed the Omnibus Budget Reconciliation Act (OBRA). This federal law applies to all 50 states. OBRA requires that nursing centers provide care in a manner and in a setting that maintains or improves each person's quality of life, health, and safety. It also

When you need hospital care, your doctor and the nurses and other professionals at our hospital are committed to working with you and your family to meet your health care needs. Our dedicated doctors and staff serve the community in all its ethnic, religious, and economic diversity. Our goal is for you and your family to have the same care and attention we would want for our families and ourselves.

The sections below explain some of the basics about how you can expect to be treated during your hospital stay. They also cover what we will need from you to care for you better. If you have questions at any time, please ask them. Unasked or unanswered questions can add to the stress of being in the hospital. Your comfort and confidence in your care are very important to us.

What to Expect During Your Hospital Stay

- **High quality hospital care.** Our first priority is to provide you the care you need, when you need it, with skill, compassion, and respect. Tell your caregivers if you have concerns about your care or if you have pain. You have the right to know the identity of your doctors, nurses, and others involved in your care, and you have the right to know when they are students, residents, or other trainees.
- **A clean and safe environment.** Our hospital works hard to keep you safe. We use special policies and procedures to avoid mistakes in your care and keep you free from abuse or neglect. If anything unexpected and significant happens during your hospital stay, you will be told what happened, and any resulting changes in your care will be discussed with you.
- **Involvement in your care.** You and your doctor often make decisions about your care before you go to the hospital. Other times, especially in emergencies, those decisions are made during your hospital stay. When decision-making takes place, it should include:
  - *Discussing your medical condition and information about medically appropriate treatment choices.* To make informed decisions with your doctor, you need to understand:
    - The benefits and risks of each treatment.
    - Whether your treatment is experimental or part of a research study.
    - What you can reasonably expect from your treatment and any long-term effects it might have on your quality of life.
    - What you and your family will need to do after you leave the hospital.
    - The financial consequences of using uncovered services or out of network providers.

    Please tell your caregivers if you need more information about your treatment choices.
  - *Discussing your treatment plan.* When you enter the hospital, you sign a general consent to treatment. In some cases, such as surgery or experimental treatment, you may be asked to confirm in writing that you understand what is planned and agree to it. This process protects your right to consent to or refuse a treatment. Your doctor will explain the medical consequences of refusing recommended treatment. It also protects your right to decide if you want to participate in a research study.
  - *Getting information from you.* Your caregivers need complete and correct information about your health and coverage so

What to Expect During Your Hospital Stay—cont'd

that they can make good decisions about your care. That includes:
- Past illnesses, surgeries, or hospital stays.
- Past allergic reactions.
- Any medicines or dietary supplements (such as vitamins and herbs) that you are taking.
- Any network or admission requirements under your health plan.

- *Understanding your health care goals and values.* You may have health care goals and values or spiritual beliefs that are important to your well-being. They will be taken into account as much as possible throughout your hospital stay. Make sure your doctor, your family, and your care team know your wishes.
- *Understanding who makes decisions when you cannot.* If you have signed a health care power of attorney stating who should speak for you if you become unable to make health care decisions for yourself, or a "living will" or "advance directive" that states your wishes about end-of-life care, give copies to your doctor, your family, and your care team. If you or your family need help making difficult decisions, counselors, chaplains, and others are available to help.

- **Protection of your privacy.** We respect the confidentiality of your relationship with your doctor and other caregivers and the sensitive information about your health and health care that are part of that relationship. State and federal laws and hospital operating policies protect the privacy of your medical information. You will receive a Notice of Privacy Practices that describes the ways that we use, disclose, and safeguard patient information and that explains how you can obtain a copy of information from our records about your care.
- **Preparing you and your family for when you leave the hospital.** Your doctor works with the hospital staff and professionals in your community. You and your family also play an important role in your care. The success of your treatment often depends on your efforts to follow medication, diet, and therapy plans. Your family may need to help care for you at home. You can expect us to help you identify sources of follow-up care and let you know if our hospital has a financial interest in any referrals. As long as you agree we can share information about your care with them, we will coordinate our activities with your caregivers outside the hospital. You can also expect to receive information and, where possible, training about the self-care you will need when you go home.
- **Help with your bill and filing insurance claims.** Our staff will file claims for you with health care insurers or other programs such as Medicare and Medicaid. They also will help your doctor with needed documentation. Hospital bills and insurance coverage are often confusing. If you have questions about your bill, contact our business office. If you need help understanding your insurance coverage or health plan, start with your insurance company or health benefits manager. If you do not have health coverage, we will try to help you and your family find financial help or make other arrangements. We need your help with collecting needed information and other requirements to obtain coverage or assistance.

While you are here, you will receive more detailed notices about some of the rights you have as a hospital patient and how to exercise them. We are always interested in improving. If you have questions, comments, or concerns, please contact
_____.

requires nursing assistant training and competency evaluation (Chapter 3). Resident rights are a major part of OBRA.

Residents have rights as United States citizens. For example, they have the right to vote. They also have rights relating to their everyday lives and care in a nursing center. These rights are protected by federal and state laws. Nursing centers must protect and promote such rights. The center cannot interfere with a resident's rights.

Some residents are incompetent (not able). They cannot exercise their rights. A representative (partner, adult child, court-appointed guardian) does so for them. A *representative is any person who has the legal right to act on the resident's behalf when he or she cannot do so for himself or herself.*

Nursing centers must inform residents of their rights. Centers must also inform residents of all rules about their conduct and responsibilities in the center. This is done orally and in writing. Such information is given before or during admission to the center, as needed during the person's stay, and when laws (state or federal) or center rules change. It is given in the language the person uses and understands.

- Medical terms are avoided to the extent possible.
- An interpreter is used if the person speaks and understands a foreign language or communicates by sign language.
- Written translations are provided in the foreign languages common in the center's geographic area.
- Sign language and other communication aids are used as necessary.
- Large print texts are available for persons with impaired vision.

Resident rights (Box 2-2) are posted throughout the center. Those affecting your role are described in this chapter.

Information

The *right to information* means access to all records about the person. They include the medical record, contracts, incident reports, and financial records. The request can be oral or written.

The person has the right to be fully informed of his or her health condition. Information is given in a language and in words the person can understand. Interpreters are used as needed. Sign language or other aids are used for those with hearing losses.

The person must also have information about his or her doctor. This includes the doctor's name, specialty, and how to contact the doctor.

Report any request for information to the nurse. *You do not give the information described above to the person or family* (Chapter 3).

See *Focus on Communication: Information.*

Refusing Treatment

The person has the *right to refuse treatment. Treatment means the care provided to maintain or restore health, improve function, or relieve symptoms.* A person who does not give consent (Chapter 4) or refuses treatment cannot be treated against his or her wishes. The center must find out what the person is refusing and why. For example, a person learned to walk after a hip fracture. However, the person refuses to walk. The center must:

- Find out the reason for the refusal.
- Educate the person about the problems that can result from not walking.
- Offer other treatment options.
- Continue to provide all other services.

Advance directives are part of the right to refuse treatment (Chapter 52). They include living wills and instructions about life support. *Advance directives are written instructions about health care when the person is not able to make such decisions.*

Report any treatment refusal to the nurse. The nurse may change the person's care plan.

Privacy and Confidentiality

Residents have the *right to personal privacy.* Staff must provide care in a manner that maintains privacy of the person's body. Expose the person's body only as necessary. Only staff directly involved in care and treatment are present. The person must give consent for others to be present. For example, a student wants to observe a treatment. The person's consent is needed for the student to observe.

A person has the right to use the bathroom in private. Privacy is maintained for all personal care measures. Bathing, dressing, and elimination are examples. Protect privacy by:

- Closing privacy curtains, doors, and window coverings.
- Removing residents from public view.
- Providing clothes or draping the person to prevent unnecessary exposure of body parts.
- Practicing the measures listed in Chapter 4. See "Invasion of Privacy" in Chapter 4.

Leaving the person without a gown, clothing, or bed covers violates the person's right to privacy. So does leaving the room door open when the person uses the bathroom or a bedpan.

Residents have the right to visit with others in private—in areas where others cannot see or hear them.

BOX 2-2 RESIDENT RIGHTS

- To be treated with dignity and respect. And to receive quality care.
- To exercise his or her rights as a center resident and as a citizen of the United States.
- To be informed orally and in writing of his or her rights and center rules. This is done in a language the person understands.
- To access all records about himself or herself, including current clinical records.
- To obtain copies of his or her records. This is at the resident's expense.
- To refuse treatment.
- To refuse to take part in experimental research. This is the development and testing of new treatments and drugs.
- To make advance directives (Chapter 52).
- To be informed of Medicare benefits and services. This includes costs and charges covered and not covered.
- To file complaints with the appropriate state agency about abuse, neglect, and the mis-use of his or her property.
- To be informed of center services and of the charges for those services.
- To choose his or her doctor.
- To know the name, specialty, and how to contact the doctor responsible for his or her care.
- To be fully informed of his or her total health status, including his or her medical condition.
- To be informed of:
  - Any accident or injury that may need medical attention
  - A change in the person's physical, mental, or psycho-social status
  - The need to stop, change, or add a treatment
  - A decision to transfer or discharge the person
  - A change in the person's room or roommate
  - A change in the person's rights under federal or state law
- To manage his or her personal and financial affairs.
- To be fully informed in advance about his or her care and treatment. This includes changes in care and treatment.
- To privacy and confidentiality:
  - Of personal and medical records
  - Of treatment and personal care
  - Of written and phone communications
  - During visits with family and friends
  - When meeting with resident groups

- To voice grievances and have them solved promptly.
- To see the results of federal and state surveys. The person also has the right to see the plans to correct problems or areas of weakness.
- To perform services for the center or to refuse to perform services.
- To send and receive mail that is not open. To buy supplies to send mail.
- To receive information from his or her doctor and community and state agencies responsible for protecting developmentally disabled and mentally ill persons.
- To have and use personal items and clothing.
- To share a room with his or her spouse (husband, wife) when married residents live in the same center (Chapter 48).
- To take his or her drugs without help if able.
- To refuse to change to a different room.
- To be free from physical and chemical restraints (Chapter 14).
- To be free from abuse (verbal, sexual, physical), bodily punishment, and involuntary seclusion (Chapter 4).
- To be cared for in a manner and in a setting that maintains or enhances quality of life.
- To choose activities, schedules, and health care that meets his or her interests and needs.
- To interact with community members inside and outside of the center.
- To make choices about his or her life in the center.
- To organize and take part in resident groups.
- To take part in social, religious, and community activities.
- To a setting and services that consider his or her needs and choices.
- To be informed of his or her health and medical condition in a language that he or she understands. That language is used when he or she takes part in care planning.
- To a clean, comfortable, and home-like setting. This includes temperature, lighting, and sound levels.
- To attain or maintain his or her highest level of function.
- To closet space.
- To visit with his or her spouse, family, and friends at any reasonable hour.

If requested, the center must provide private space. Offices, chapels, dining rooms, and meeting rooms are used as needed.

Residents have the right to make phone calls in private (Fig. 2-1, p. 16). The calls must not be where they can be overheard. Therefore phones are not used in offices or at the nurses' station. Centers provide cordless phones or phone jacks in resident rooms. Phones are at the correct height for use by persons in wheelchairs. Phones for hearing impaired persons are also available. Some residents have their own wireless phones.

The right to privacy also involves mail. The person has the right to send and receive mail without others interfering.

No one can open mail the person sends or receives without his or her consent. Un-opened mail is given to the person within 24 hours of delivery to the center. Mail the person sends is delivered to the postal service within 24 hours on days of regular delivery or pick-up service.

Information about the person's care, treatment, and condition is kept confidential. So are medical and financial records. Consent is needed to release them to other agencies or persons.

You must provide privacy and protect confidentiality. Doing so shows respect for the person. It also protects the person's dignity. Privacy and confidentiality are discussed in Chapters 4 and 5.

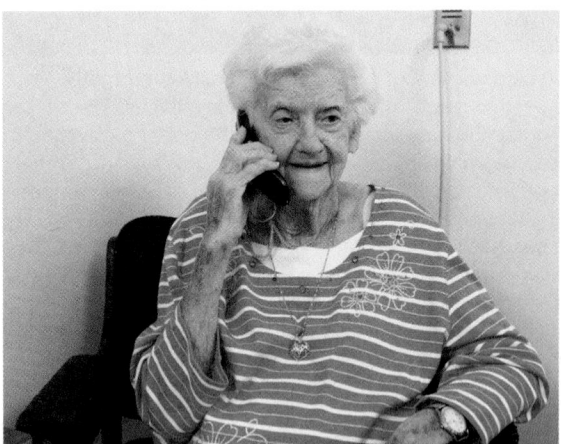

Fig. 2-1 A resident is talking privately on the phone.

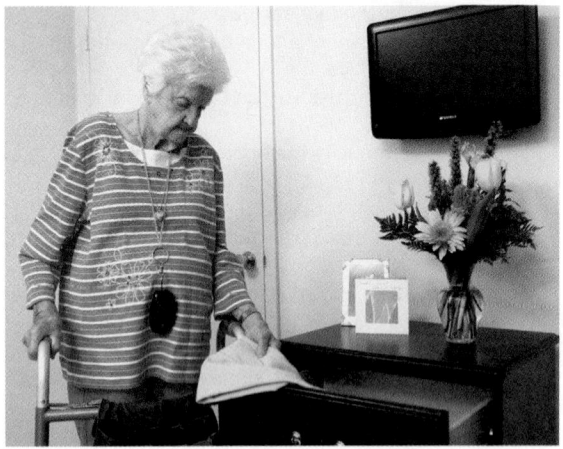

Fig. 2-2 A resident is choosing what clothing to wear.

Personal Choice

Residents have the *right to make their own choices*. They can choose their own doctors. They also have the right to take part in planning and deciding about their care and treatment. They can choose activities, schedules, and care based on their preferences. They can choose when to get up and go to bed, what to wear, how to spend time, and what to eat (Fig. 2-2). They can choose friends and visitors inside and outside the center.

Personal choice promotes quality of life, dignity, and self-respect. You must allow personal choice whenever safely possible.

Grievances

Residents have the *right to voice concerns, questions, and complaints about treatment or care*. The problem may involve another person. It may be about care that was given or not given. The center must promptly try to correct the matter. No one can punish the person in any way for voicing the grievance.

Work

The person does not work for care, care items, or other things or privileges. The person is not required to perform services for the center.

However, the person has the *right to work or perform services if he or she wants to*. Some people like to garden, repair or build things, clean, sew, mend, or cook. Other persons need work for rehabilitation or activity reasons. The desire or need for work is part of the person's care plan. Residents volunteer or are paid for their services.

Taking Part in Resident Groups

The person has the *right to form and take part in resident groups*. Families have the right to meet with other families. These groups can discuss concerns and suggest center improvements. They also can support each other, plan activities, and take part in educational activities.

Residents have the *right to take part in social, cultural, religious, and community events*. They have the *right to help in getting to and from events of their choice*.

Personal Items

Residents have the *right to keep and use personal items*. This includes clothing and some furnishings. The type and amount of personal items allowed depend on space needs and the health and safety of others.

Treat the person's property with care and respect. The items may not have value to you. However, they have meaning to the person. They also relate to personal choice, dignity, a home-like setting, and quality of life.

The person's property is protected. Items are labeled with the person's name. The center must investigate reports of lost, stolen, or damaged items. Police help is sometimes needed. The person and family are advised not to keep jewelry and other costly items in the center.

Protect yourself and the center from being accused of stealing a person's property. Do not go through a person's closet, drawers, purse, or other space without the person's knowledge and consent. A nurse may ask you to inspect closets and drawers. Center policy should require that a co-worker and the person or legal representative be present. The co-worker is a witness to your activities. Follow center policy for reporting and recording the inspection.

Freedom From Abuse, Mistreatment, and Neglect

Residents have the *right to be free from verbal, sexual, physical, and mental abuse* (Chapter 4). *Abuse* means:
- The willful infliction of injury, unreasonable confinement, intimidation (to threaten to hurt or punish), or punishment that results in physical harm, pain, or mental anguish.
- Depriving the person of the goods or services needed to attain or maintain well-being.

They also have the right to be free from *involuntary seclusion:*
- *Separating the person from others against his or her will*
- *Keeping the person to a certain area*
- *Keeping the person away from his or her room without consent*

No one can abuse, neglect, or mistreat a resident. This includes center staff, volunteers, and staff from other agencies or groups. It also includes other residents, family members, friends, visitors, and legal representatives. Nursing centers must investigate suspected or reported cases of abuse. They cannot employ persons who:
- Were found guilty of abusing, neglecting, or mistreating others by a court of law.
- Have a finding entered into the state's nursing assistant registry (Chapter 3) about abuse, neglect, mistreatment, or wrongful acts involving the person's money or property. A *finding* means that a state has determined that the employee abused, neglected, mistreated, or wrongfully used the person's money or property.

Freedom From Restraint

Residents have the *right not to have body movements restricted.* Restraints and certain drugs can restrict body movements. Some drugs can restrain the person because they affect mood, behavior, and mental function. Sometimes residents are restrained to protect them from harming themselves or others. A doctor's order is needed for restraint use. Restraints are not used for staff convenience or to discipline a person. They are used only if required to treat the person's medical symptoms. Restraints are discussed in Chapter 14.

Quality of Life

Residents have the *right to quality of life.* They must be cared for in a manner and in a setting that promotes dignity and respect for self. This means that staff must provide care in a manner that maintains or enhances the person's self-esteem and feelings of self-worth. Staff must promote physical, mental, and social well-being. Protecting resident rights promotes quality of life. It shows respect for the person.

You must be polite and courteous when speaking to the person. Good, honest, and thoughtful care enhances the person's quality of life. Box 2-3 lists OBRA-required actions that promote dignity and privacy.

See *Focus on Communication: Quality of Life,* p. 18.

BOX 2-3 **OBRA-REQUIRED ACTIONS TO PROMOTE DIGNITY AND PRIVACY**

Courteous and Dignified Interactions
- Use the right tone of voice.
- Use good eye contact.
- Stand or sit close enough as needed.
- Use the person's proper name and title. For example: "Mrs. Crane."
- Gain the person's attention before interacting with him or her.
- Use touch if the person approves.
- Respect the person's social status.
- Listen with interest to what the person is saying.
- Do not yell at, scold, or embarrass the person.

Courteous and Dignified Care
- Groom hair, beards, and nails as the person wishes.
- Assist with dressing in the right clothing for time of day and personal choice.
- Promote independence and dignity in dining.
- Respect private space and property. For example, change radio or TV stations only with the person's consent.
- Assist with walking and transfers. Do not interfere with independence.
- Assist with bathing and hygiene preferences. Do not interfere with independence.
  - Appearance is neat and clean.
  - The person is clean shaven or has a groomed beard and mustache.
  - Nails are trimmed and clean.
  - Dentures, hearing aids, eyeglasses, and other devices are used correctly.
  - Clothing is clean.
  - Clothing is properly fitted and fastened.
  - Shoes, hose, and socks are properly applied and fastened.
  - Extra clothing is worn for warmth as needed. Sweaters and lap blankets are examples.

Privacy and Self-Determination
- Drape properly during care and procedures to avoid exposure and embarrassment.
- Drape properly in chair.
- Use privacy curtains or screens during care and procedures.
- Close the room door during care and procedures as the person desires. Also close window coverings.
- Knock on the door before entering. Wait to be asked in.
- Close the bathroom door when the person uses the bathroom.

Personal Choice and Independence
- Person smokes in allowed areas.
- Person takes part in activities according to his or her interests.
- Person takes part in scheduling activities and care.
- Person gives input into the care plan about preferences and independence.
- Person is involved in room or roommate change.
- The person's items are moved or inspected only with the person's consent.

FOCUS ON COMMUNICATION

Quality of Life

Every person deserves to be addressed in a manner that conveys dignity and respect. When speaking with a patient or resident, address the person by his or her title and last name. For example: Mr. Baker, Mrs. Harty, or Dr. Collins. Do not address a person by his or her first name or another name unless the person requests it. Avoid the use of terms like *Sweetheart*, *Honey*, *Grandpa*, and *Dear*.

TEAMWORK AND TIME MANAGEMENT

Activities

Residents may need help getting to and from activity programs. Know when an activity begins and ends. Before assisting residents to activity areas:

- Assist with elimination needs and hand washing.
- Assist with grooming measures such as brushing and combing hair. A person may want to apply some perfume or make-up.
- Make sure the person wears the correct clothing and footwear for the activity.
- Make sure the person has needed assistive devices. Eyeglasses, hearing aids, canes, and walkers are examples.

Allow 15 to 20 minutes to assist residents to and from the activity area. Help your co-workers as needed.

You may have to help residents with activities (Fig. 2-3). If not, use the activity time wisely. Provide needed care and visit residents who cannot leave their rooms. You can also clean and straighten rooms, bathrooms, shower rooms, and utility rooms.

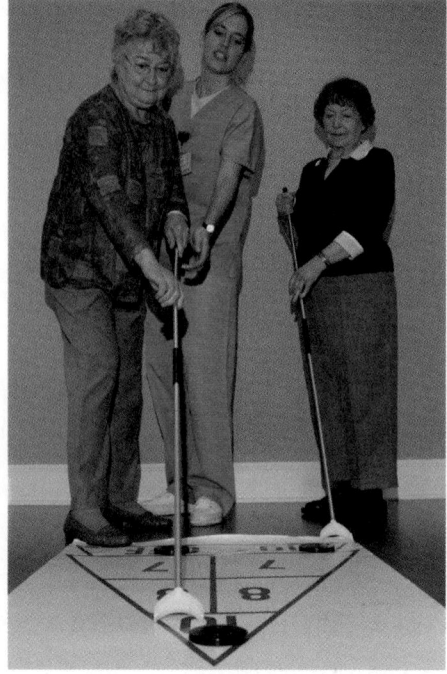

Fig. 2-3 A nursing assistant is helping residents in an activity program.

FOCUS ON COMMUNICATION

Activities

You may need help assisting residents to and from activity programs. Politely ask a co-worker to help you. Share the following with your co-worker:

- What time you need the help.
- How much of the co-worker's time you need.
- The residents you need help with.
- If the person walks or uses a wheelchair.
- What assistive devices are used. Eyeglasses, hearing aids, canes, and walkers are examples.

Always say "please" when asking for help. And thank the person for helping you. For example: "Jane, can you please help me assist two residents to the concert? It starts at 1:00, so I'll need your help at 12:45. Mr. Harris needs his glasses and hearing aid. He'll use a walker. Mrs. Janz uses a wheelchair. She needs her glasses and a blanket for her lap. The blanket is in her wheelchair. The concert is over at 2:00. Can you help me then, too? Thanks so much for helping me."

Activities

Residents have the *right to activities that enhance each person's physical, mental, and psycho-social well-being.* The intent is to promote self-esteem, pleasure, comfort, education, creativity, success, and independence. They must have a purpose and relate to the person's needs, interests, culture, and background. Centers also provide religious services for spiritual health. Activities must have meaning for the person. They are meaningful when they:

- Reflect the person's interests and lifestyle.
- Are enjoyed by the person.
- Help the person feel useful or produce something useful.
- Provide a sense of belonging.

Activities may involve large or small groups. A concert is a large group activity. A card game is a small group activity. Other activities involve two people. Or the person does something alone. Writing a letter and playing a computer game are examples.

You assist residents to and from activity programs. You may need to help them with activities.

See *Teamwork and Time Management: Activities.*
See *Focus on Communication: Activities.*

Environment

Residents have the *right to a safe, clean, comfortable, and home-like setting.* The person is allowed to have and use personal items to the extent possible.

The center must provide a setting and services that meet the person's needs and preferences. The setting and staff must promote the person's independence, dignity, and well-being. The center must try to change schedules, call systems, and room arrangements to meet the person's desires and needs.

For example, the center must make changes when a person:
- Refuses a bath because he or she prefers a shower.
- Prefers to have a shower at a different time or day.
- Refuses a shower because of the fear of falling.
- Is uneasy about the staff assigned to help him or her.
- Is worried about falling.
- Cannot reach or use the signal light.
- Cannot reach personal items.
- Does not like the food served.

OMBUDSMAN PROGRAM

The Older Americans Act is a federal law. It requires a long-term care ombudsman program in every state. An *ombudsman is someone who supports or promotes the needs and interests of another person.* Long-term care ombudsmen are employed by a state agency. Some are volunteers. They are not nursing center employees. They act on behalf of persons receiving health care at home and in hospitals, nursing centers, assisted living residences, adult day care, and other settings.

Ombudsmen protect a person's health, safety, welfare, and rights. They:
- Investigate and resolve complaints.
- Provide services to assist the person.
- Assist persons on Medicare with hospital access or discharge concerns.
- Provide information about long-term care services.
- Monitor nursing center care.
- Monitor nursing center conditions.
- Provide support to resident and family groups.
- Help the person and family resolve conflicts within the family.
- Help the center manage difficult problems.
- Educate persons, families, and the public about long-term care issues and concerns.
- Represent older persons' interests before local, state, and federal governments.

Residents have the right to voice grievances and disputes. They also have the right to communicate privately with anyone of their choice. They can share concerns with anyone outside the center.

OBRA requires that nursing centers post the names, addresses, and phone numbers of local and state ombudsmen. This information must be posted where residents can easily see it.

A resident or family may share a concern with you. You must know state and center policies and procedures for contacting an ombudsman. Ombudsman services are useful when:
- There is concern about a person's care or treatment.
- Someone interferes with a person's rights, health, safety, or welfare.

FOCUS ON PRIDE

The Person, Family, and Yourself

Personal and Professional Responsibility

OBRA is concerned with the quality of life, health, and safety of residents. All care must maintain or improve each person's quality of life. You are responsible for the care you give. To provide quality care:
- Protect the person's rights.
- Provide for safety (Chapter 12).
- Help keep the agency clean and safe.
- Act in a professional manner.
- Have good work ethics (Chapter 5).
- Follow agency policies and procedures.

Take pride in the work you do. The care you give helps improve each person's quality of life, health, and safety.

Rights and Respect

Every person has the right to refuse treatment. This does not mean that all treatment stops. The health team offers other treatment options. For example, the doctor suggests short-term placement in a nursing center. The person refuses. The family agrees to help the person at home. A social worker helps the person and family arrange for home health care and respite care (Chapter 8).

Independence and Social Interaction

Many patients and residents feel a loss of independence and social interaction. Help promote independence by allowing the person to choose food, clothing, visitors, activities, and schedules. Encourage social interaction by telling the person about center activities and offering help to and from activities. Also, respect the person's right to privacy when visiting with others and making phone calls. These actions help improve independence, self-worth, and quality of life.

Delegation and Teamwork

Health care agencies must meet the person's needs and preferences. Schedules, care assignments, and room arrangements may need to change to meet the person's needs. Flexibility, good teamwork, and communication are required to provide quality care.

For example, Mrs. Gordon needs help with bathing. She likes to bathe at night. She says bathing at night helps her to rest better. However, the day shift gives baths. You share her preference with the nurse. The daytime and evening staffs work together so Mrs. Gordon can bathe when she chooses.

Ethics and Laws

Every person has the right to keep his or her personal information private. This includes information about health care. The Health Insurance Portability and Accountability Act of 1996 (HIPAA) protects the privacy and security of a person's health information. HIPAA is discussed further in Chapter 4.

Follow agency policies and procedures for protecting health information. Only staff directly involved in the person's care can discuss the person's treatment. Direct any questions to the nurse.

REVIEW QUESTIONS

Circle the BEST answer.

1 *The Patient Care Partnership: Understanding Expectations, Rights, and Responsibilities* is concerned with
   a Hospital care
   b Home care
   c Long-term care
   d All health care agencies and settings

2 A hospital patient has the right to the following *except*
   a Respectful care
   b Treatment information
   c Refuse treatment
   d Free care

3 OBRA is a
   a State law
   b Federal law
   c State agency
   d Federal agency

4 A son has the legal right to act on his mother's behalf. The son is his mother's legal
   a Ombudsman
   b Representative
   c Caregiver
   d Health care provider

5 A daughter wants to read her father's medical record. What should you do?
   a Give her the medical record.
   b Ask the resident if you can give the daughter the record.
   c Tell the nurse.
   d Tell her that she cannot do so.

6 A resident refuses to have a shower. What should you do?
   a Tell her that she cannot refuse a shower.
   b Tell her daughter.
   c Comply, but tell her she must have a shower tomorrow.
   d Tell the nurse.

7 Which violates the person's right to privacy?
   a Closing the bathroom door when the person uses the bathroom
   b Opening the window blinds when assisting with bathing
   c Covering the person when giving personal care
   d Asking the person's permission to observe a treatment

8 A resident has a phone in his room. He wants to make a phone call. What should you do?
   a Leave the room.
   b Tell the nurse.
   c Ask him to use the phone at the nurses' station.
   d Close the privacy curtain so you can stay in the room to finish your tasks.

9 Who decides how to style a person's hair?
   a The person
   b The nurse
   c You
   d The ombudsman

10 Residents do *not* have the right to
   a A private room
   b Refuse treatment
   c Contact an ombudsman
   d Make personal choices

11 A person brought furniture and other items from home. They are
   a Sent home with the family
   b Labeled with the person's name
   c Arranged as you prefer
   d Shared with other residents

12 Residents have the right to be free from the following *except*
   a Disease
   b Abuse
   c Involuntary seclusion
   d Neglect

13 Who selects activities for a resident?
   a The nurse
   b You
   c The person's representative
   d The person

14 A nursing center must provide the following *except*
   a A safe and clean setting
   b A comfortable setting
   c A home-like setting
   d A noise-free setting

15 A long-term care ombudsman
   a Is employed by the nursing center
   b Investigates resident complaints
   c Grants a nursing center a license or certification
   d Can prevent a resident from leaving the center

16 Which action does *not* promote a person's dignity?
   a Restraining the person
   b Providing privacy during personal care
   c Making sure the person has needed assistive devices
   d Listening to the person

17 Which is the correct way to address a person?
   a "Hello, sweetie."
   b "Hello, Mrs. Smith."
   c "Hello, Jim."
   d "Hello, Grandpa."

18 Which does *not* promote dignity or privacy?
   a Knocking before entering the person's room
   b Closing the bathroom door when the person uses the bathroom
   c Assisting with bathing and hygiene preferences
   d Moving the person's items as you prefer

Circle T if the statement is TRUE or F if it is FALSE.

19 T F *The Patient Care Partnership: Understanding Expectations, Rights, and Responsibilities* is a federal law.

20 T F OBRA applies to all 50 states.

21 T F Nursing center residents have rights as U.S. citizens.

22 T F Residents are informed of their rights only in writing.

23 T F You should open the person's mail within 24 hours of it being delivered to the center.

24 T F A resident complains about the food. The center must try to provide desired foods.

25 T F Residents must provide some type of work for the center.

26 T F Resident groups can discuss ideas for activity programs.

27 T F An employee was found guilty of abusing a resident. The center can continue to employ the person.

28 T F You can restrain a resident to provide care.

Answers to these questions are on p. 832.

The Nursing Assistant

OBJECTIVES

- Define the key terms and key abbreviations listed in this chapter.
- Explain the history and current trends affecting nursing assistants.
- Explain the laws that affect nursing assistants.
- List the reasons for denying, suspending, or revoking a nursing assistant's certification, license, or registration.
- Describe the training and competency evaluation requirements for nursing assistants.
- Identify the information in the nursing assistant registry.
- Explain how to obtain certification, a license, or registration in another state.
- Describe what nursing assistants can do and their role limits.
- Describe the standards for nursing assistants developed by the National Council of State Boards of Nursing.
- Explain why a job description is important.
- Describe the delegation process.
- Explain your role in the delegation process.
- Explain how to accept or refuse a delegated task.
- Explain how to promote PRIDE in the person, the family, and yourself.

KEY TERMS

accountable Being responsible for one's actions and the actions of others who performed the delegated tasks; answering questions about and explaining one's actions and the actions of others

delegate To authorize another person to perform a nursing task in a certain situation

job description A document that describes what the agency expects you to do

nursing task Nursing care or a nursing function, procedure, activity, or work that can be delegated to nursing assistants when it does not require an RN's professional knowledge or judgment

responsibility The duty or obligation to perform some act or function

KEY ABBREVIATIONS

CNA	Certified nursing assistant; certified nurse aide		**NCSBN**	National Council of State Boards of Nursing
LNA	Licensed nursing assistant		**OBRA**	Omnibus Budget Reconciliation Act of 1987
LPN	Licensed practical nurse			
LVN	Licensed vocational nurse		**RN**	Registered nurse
NATCEP	Nursing assistant training and competency evaluation program		**RNA**	Registered nurse aide
			STNA	State tested nurse aide

Federal and state laws and agency policies combine to define the roles and functions of each health team member. Everyone must protect patients and residents from harm. To do so, you need to know:

- What you can and cannot do
- Your legal limits

Laws, job descriptions, and the person's condition shape your work. So does the amount of supervision you need.

HISTORY AND CURRENT TRENDS

For decades, nursing assistants have helped nurses with basic nursing care. Often called *nurse's aides*, they gave baths and made beds. They helped with grooming, elimination, and other needs. Their work was similar in hospitals and nursing centers. Until the 1980s, training was not required by law. Nurses gave on-the-job training. Some hospitals, nursing centers, and schools offered nursing assistant courses.

Before the 1980s, team nursing was common. A registered nurse (RN) was the team leader. The RN assigned care to nurses and nursing assistants. Care was assigned according to each person's needs and condition. It also depended on the staff member's education and experiences.

Primary nursing was common in the 1980s. RNs planned and gave care. Many hospitals hired only RNs. Meanwhile, nursing centers relied on nursing assistants for resident care.

Home care increased during the 1980s. Prospective payment systems limit health care payments (Chapter 1). To reduce care costs, hospital stays are shorter. Therefore patients are discharged earlier than in the past. Often they are still quite ill and need home care.

Efforts to reduce health care costs include:

- *Hospital closings.* Many do not make enough money to stay open.
- *Hospital mergers.* Hospitals merge to share resources and to avoid the same costly services. For example, one hospital offers heart surgery. The other serves women and children.
- *Health care systems.* Agencies join together as one provider of care. See Chapter 1.
- *Managed care.* Insurers have contracts with doctors, hospitals, and health care systems for reduced rates. See Chapter 1.
- *Staffing mix.* Hospitals hire RNs, licensed practical nurses/licensed vocational nurses (LPNs/LVNs), and nursing assistants. Most hospitals require a state-approved nursing assistant training and competency evaluation for employment. More training is given for tasks not in the training program.

- *Patient-focused care.* Services are moved from departments to the bedside. Staff members are cross-trained to perform the basic skills of other health team members. For example, the doctor orders a blood test for Ms. Tyler. The nurse tells the unit secretary, who calls the laboratory. The laboratory secretary tells a technician, who then goes to Ms. Tyler's room to draw the blood sample. Five people are involved so far. With patient-focused care, a nursing team member draws the blood when the order is given. Ms. Tyler does not wait for laboratory staff. She is served faster by fewer staff members, which lowers costs.

FEDERAL AND STATE LAWS

The U.S. Congress makes federal laws for all 50 states to follow. State legislatures make state laws. For example, the Maine legislature makes state laws for Maine. The Ohio legislature makes state laws for Ohio. You must know the federal and state laws that affect your work. They provide direction for what you can do.

See Chapter 4 for other laws affecting your work.

Nurse Practice Acts

Each state has a nurse practice act. It protects the public's welfare and safety by regulating nursing practice in that state. A nurse practice act:

- Defines RN and LPN/LVN.
- Describes the scope of practice for RNs and LPNs/LVNs.
- Describes education and licensing requirements for RNs and LPNs/LVNs.
- Protects the public from persons practicing nursing without a license. Persons who do not meet the state's requirements cannot perform nursing functions.

The law allows for denying, revoking, or suspending a nursing license. The intent is to protect the public from unsafe nurses. Reasons include:

- Being convicted of a crime in any state
- Selling or distributing drugs
- Using the person's drugs for oneself
- Placing a person in danger from the over-use of alcohol or drugs
- Demonstrating grossly negligent nursing practice
- Being convicted of abusing or neglecting children or older persons
- Violating a nurse practice act and its rules and regulations
- Demonstrating incompetent behaviors
- Aiding or assisting another person to violate a nurse practice act and its rules and regulations
- Making medical diagnoses
- Prescribing drugs and treatments

Nursing Assistants. A state's nurse practice act is used to decide what nursing assistants can do. Some nurse practice acts also regulate nursing assistant roles, functions, education, and certification requirements. Other states have separate laws for nursing assistants.

Legal and advisory opinions about nursing assistants are based on the state's nurse practice act. So are any state laws about their roles and functions. If you do something beyond the legal limits of your role, you could be practicing nursing without a license. This creates serious legal problems for you, your supervisor, and your employer.

Nursing assistants must be able to function with skill and safety. Like nurses, nursing assistants can have their certification denied, revoked, or suspended. (See "Certification" on p. 24.)

The Omnibus Budget Reconciliation Act of 1987

The Omnibus Budget Reconciliation Act of 1987 (OBRA) is a federal law. Its purpose is to improve the quality of life of nursing center residents.

OBRA sets minimum training and competency evaluation requirements for nursing assistants. Each state must have a nursing assistant training and competency evaluation program (NATCEP). A nursing assistant must successfully complete a NATCEP to work in a nursing center, hospital long-term care unit, or home care agency that receives Medicare funds.

The Training Program. OBRA requires at least 75 hours of instruction. Some states have more hours. Classroom and at least 16 hours of supervised practical training are required (Fig. 3-1). Such training occurs in a laboratory or clinical setting. Students perform nursing tasks on another person. A nurse supervises this practical training (clinical practicum or clinical experience).

The training program includes the knowledge and skills needed to give basic nursing care. Areas of study include:
- Communication
- Infection control
- Safety and emergency procedures
- Residents' rights
- Basic nursing skills
- Personal care skills
- Feeding methods
- Elimination procedures
- Skin care
- Transferring, positioning, and turning methods
- Dressing
- Helping the person walk
- Range-of-motion exercises
- Signs and symptoms of common diseases
- How to care for cognitively impaired persons (those who have problems with thinking and memory)

See *Focus on Communication: The Training Program.*

Competency Evaluation. The competency evaluation has a written test and a skills test (Appendix A, p. 836). The written test has multiple-choice questions. Each has 4 choices. Only 1 answer is correct. The number of questions varies from state to state.

FOCUS ON COMMUNICATION

The Training Program

In many training programs, clinical experiences take place in a real clinical setting. Care is practiced on real patients or residents. The patient or resident has the right to know who is providing care. When you meet the person, introduce yourself. Tell the person you are a student. For example: "Hello! My name is Jennifer Smith. I am a nursing assistant student. I will be working with your nurse, Mr. Kline, today."

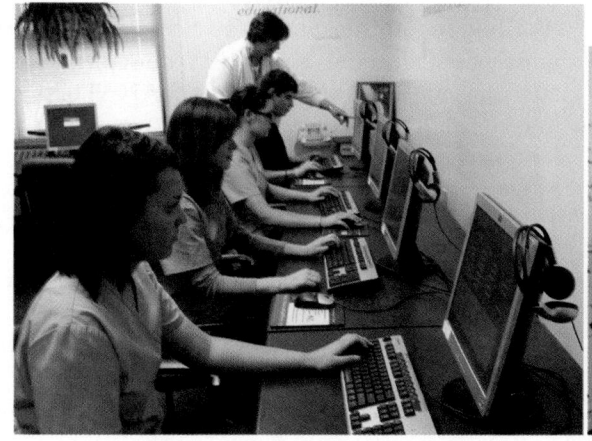
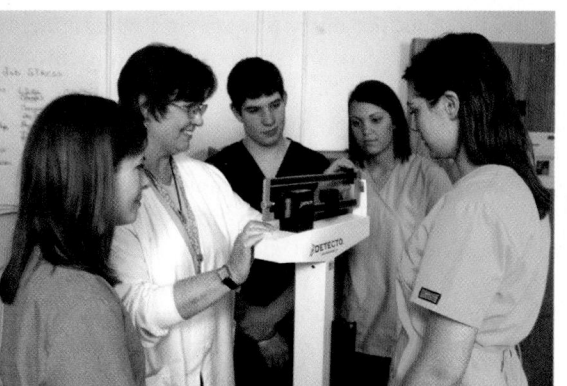

Fig. 3-1 Nursing assistant training program. **A,** Students study in a classroom setting. **B,** An instructor demonstrates a skill in a laboratory setting.

The skills test involves performing nursing skills. You will perform certain skills learned in your training program.

You take the competency evaluation after your training program. Your instructor tells you the testing service used in your state and when and where the tests are given. He or she helps you complete the application. Or you can go to the testing service website to complete the application on-line. The evaluation has a fee. If working in a nursing center, the employer pays the fee. You are told the place and time of the tests after your application is processed. Some states give a choice of test dates and sites.

Your training prepares you for the competency evaluation. If you listen, study hard, and practice safe care, you should do well. If the first attempt was not successful, you can retest. OBRA allows at least 3 attempts to successfully complete the evaluation.

Nursing Assistant Registry. OBRA requires a nursing assistant registry in each state. It is an official record or listing of persons who have successfully completed that state's approved NATCEP. The registry has information about each nursing assistant:

- Full name, including maiden name and any married names.
- Last known home address.
- Registry number and the date it expires.
- Date of birth.
- Last known employer, date hired, and date employment ended.
- Date the competency evaluation was passed.
- Information about findings of abuse, neglect, or dishonest use of property. It includes the nature of the offense and supporting evidence. If a hearing was held, the date and its outcome are included. The person has the right to include a statement disputing the finding. All information stays in the registry for at least 5 years.

Any health care agency can access registry information. You also receive a copy of your registry information. The copy is sent when the first entry is made and when information is changed or added. You can correct wrong information.

Other OBRA Requirements. Re-training and a new competency evaluation program are required for nursing assistants who have not worked for 24 months. It does not matter how long you worked as a nursing assistant before. What matters is how long you did *not* work. States can require:

- A new competency evaluation
- Both re-training and a new competency evaluation

Agencies covered under OBRA must provide 12 hours of educational programs to nursing assistants every year. Performance reviews also are required. That is, your work is evaluated. These requirements help ensure that you have the current knowledge and skills to give safe, effective care.

See *Teamwork and Time Management: Other OBRA Requirements.*

TEAMWORK AND TIME MANAGEMENT
Other OBRA Requirements

Educational programs are commonly called *in-service programs* or *in-service training*. Some are required; others are optional. Program announcements and schedules are posted on bulletin boards on nursing units, in staff locker rooms and lounges, by the time clock, and on websites. Some are included with your paycheck. Know where your agency posts in-service information. Check those areas often.

Such training is scheduled before your shift begins, during your shift, or after your shift. If scheduled before work, plan to arrive early. If scheduled after work, plan to stay late. Arrange for transportation and childcare as needed (Chapter 5).

If the program is during your shift, plan with your co-workers. Some staff stay on the unit while others attend the program. Staff on the unit tend to all patients and residents. A person may have special care needs while you are off the unit. Share this information with the staff that will provide such care. When you return to the unit, thank your co-workers for helping you. Help your co-workers when they leave the unit to attend in-service programs.

Certification

Each state's NATCEP must meet OBRA requirements. Some states require more training hours. And each state has its own competency evaluation program. After successfully completing your state's NATCEP, you have the title used in your state:

- Certified nursing assistant (CNA) or certified nurse aide (CNA). CNA is used in most states.
- Licensed nursing assistant (LNA).
- Registered nurse aide (RNA).
- State tested nurse aide (STNA).

Nursing assistants can have their certification (licenses, registration) denied, revoked, or suspended. See Box 3-1 for the reasons listed by the National Council of State Boards of Nursing (NCSBN).

Working in Another State. To work in another state, you must meet that state's NATCEP requirements. First, contact the state agency responsible for NATCEPs and the nursing assistant registry. To find that agency, do one of the following:

- Contact your current nursing assistant registry.
- Go to the NCSBN website. Find the link to the state agency.

Then apply to the state agency to be a CNA (LNA, RNA, STNA). The state uses one of these terms: *endorsement*, *reciprocity*, or *equivalency*. The terms mean that:

- Your application for CNA (LNA, RNA, STNA) is reviewed to see if you meet the state's requirements:
  - Your certification (license, registration) is current and in good standing.
  - You meet that state's education, work, and legal requirements.
- Certification (a license, registration) is granted if the requirements are met.

BOX 3-1	REASONS FOR LOSING CERTIFICATION, A LICENSE, OR REGISTRATION

The National Council of State Boards of Nursing (NCSBN) lists these reasons for doing so:

- Substance abuse or dependency.
- Abandoning, abusing, or neglecting a person.
- Fraud or deceit. Examples include:
  - Filing false personal information
  - Providing false information when applying for initial certification, re-instatement, or renewal
- Violating professional boundaries (Chapter 4).
- Giving unsafe care.
- Performing acts beyond the nursing assistant role.
- Misappropriation (stealing, theft) or mis-using property.
- Obtaining money or property from a patient or resident. This can be done through fraud, falsely representing oneself, or by force.
- Being convicted of a crime. Examples include murder, assault, kidnapping, rape or sexual assault, robbery, sexual crimes involving children, criminal mistreatment of children or a vulnerable adult (Chapter 4), drug trafficking, embezzlement (to take a person's property for one's own use), theft, and arson (starting fires).
- Failing to conform to the standards of nursing assistants (p. 26).
- Putting patients and residents at risk for harm.
- Violating a person's privacy.
- Failing to maintain the confidentiality of patient or resident information.

BOX 3-2	RULES FOR NURSING ASSISTANTS

- You are an assistant to the nurse.
- A nurse assigns and supervises your work.
- You report observations about the person's physical and mental status to the nurse (Chapter 7). Report changes in the person's condition or behavior at once.
- The nurse decides what is done for a person. The nurse decides what should not be done for a person. You do not make these decisions.
- Review directions and the care plan with the nurse before going to the person.
- Perform only those nursing tasks that you are trained to do.
- Ask a nurse to supervise you if you are not comfortable performing a nursing task.
- Perform only the nursing tasks that your state and job description allow.

Follow the application instructions. Expect to:

- Complete the required forms.
- Provide proof of successfully completing a NATCEP. You may need to send a copy of the certificate of completion from your NATCEP. Do not send the original.
- Request written registry verification from the state in which you are currently certified (licensed, registered). Pay the required fee.
- Provide fingerprints.
- Pay the required application fee.

A criminal background check is done. Registry information is checked. Expect an investigation if the check shows a criminal history. Or if the registry check shows findings of abuse, neglect, dishonest use of property, or other action against you.

You must be truthful. False or misleading information may result in:

- Denial of certification (a license, registration)
- Disciplinary action
- A fine

The application review results in one or more of the following:

- Being granted or denied certification (a license, registration).
- Having to take a competency test. This may be the written test, the skills test, or both.
- Having to take a NATCEP in that state.

ROLES AND RESPONSIBILITIES

Nurse practice acts, OBRA, state laws, and legal and advisory opinions direct what you can do. To protect persons from harm, you must understand what you can do, what you cannot do, and the legal limits of your role. In some states, this is called *scope of practice*. The NCSBN calls it *range of functions*.

Licensed nurses supervise your work. You assist them in giving care. You also perform nursing tasks related to the person's care. A *nursing task is the nursing care or a nursing function, procedure, activity, or work that can be delegated to nursing assistants when it does not require an RN's professional knowledge or judgment.* Often you function without a nurse in the room. At other times you help nurses give care. In some agencies, you assist doctors with procedures. The rules in Box 3-2 will help you understand your role.

The range of functions for nursing assistants varies among states and agencies. Before you perform a nursing task make sure that:

- Your state allows nursing assistants to do so.
- It is in your job description.
- You have the necessary education and training.
- A nurse is available to answer questions and to supervise you.

You perform nursing tasks to meet the person's hygiene, safety, comfort, nutrition, exercise, and elimination needs. You also move and transfer persons, make observations, and collect specimens. You help admit and discharge patients and residents. You also measure temperatures, pulses, respirations, and blood pressures. And you help promote the person's mental comfort.

Box 3-3 on p. 26 describes the limits of your role—the tasks that you should never do. State laws differ. Know what you can do in the state in which you are working. For example, you move from Vermont to Texas. You must learn the laws and rules in Texas. Or you might work in two

| BOX 3-3 | ROLE LIMITS FOR NURSING ASSISTANTS |

- **Never give drugs.** This includes drugs given orally, rectally, vaginally, and by injection. It also includes drugs given by application to the skin, eyes, ears, and nose. Nor do you give drugs directly into the bloodstream or through an intravenous (IV) line. Nurses give drugs. Many states allow nursing assistants to give drugs after completing a state-approved medication assistant training program. The function must be in your job description. And you must have the necessary supervision.
- **Never insert tubes or objects into body openings. Do not remove them from the body.** You must not insert tubes into a person's bladder, esophagus, trachea, nose, ears, bloodstream, or surgically created body openings. Exceptions to this rule are the procedures you will study during your training. Giving enemas is an example. To perform them, they must be in your job description. And you must have the necessary supervision.
- **Never take oral or phone orders from doctors.** Politely give your name and title, and ask the doctor to wait for a nurse. Promptly find a nurse to speak with the doctor.
- **Never perform procedures that require sterile technique.** With sterile technique, all objects in contact with the person are free of microorganisms (Chapter 15). Sterile technique and procedures require skills, knowledge, and judgment beyond your training. You can assist a nurse with a sterile procedure. However, do not perform the procedure yourself.
- **Never tell the person or family the person's diagnosis or medical or surgical treatment plans.** This is the doctor's responsibility. Nurses may clarify what the doctor has said.
- **Never diagnose or prescribe treatments or drugs for anyone.** Doctors diagnose and prescribe.
- **Never supervise others, including other nursing assistants.** This is a nurse's legal responsibility. You will not be trained to supervise others. Supervising others can have serious legal problems.
- **Never ignore an order or request to do something. This includes nursing tasks that you can do, those you cannot do, and those that are beyond your legal limits.** Promptly and politely explain to the nurse why you cannot follow the order or request. The nurse assumes you are doing what you were told to do unless you explain otherwise. You cannot neglect the person's care.

FOCUS ON LONG-TERM CARE AND HOME CARE
Roles and Responsibilities

Home Care

You provide personal care and home services. Home services depend on the needs of the person and family. They may include:

- Laundry. You wash, iron or fold, and mend clothing and linens. This may include family laundry.
- Shopping for groceries and household items.
- Preparing and serving meals. You plan menus, follow diets, and feed the person if necessary.
- Light housekeeping. You do not do heavy housekeeping. This includes moving heavy furniture, waxing floors, shampooing carpets, washing windows, and cleaning rugs or drapes. You do not carry firewood, coal, or ash containers.

| BOX 3-4 | NURSING ASSISTANT STANDARDS |

The nursing assistant:
- Performs nursing tasks within the range of functions allowed by the state's nurse practice act and its rules.
- Is honest and shows integrity in performing nursing tasks. (*Integrity* involves following a code of ethics. See Chapter 4.)
- Bases nursing tasks on his or her education and training. Also bases them on the nurse's directions.
- Is accountable for his or her behavior and actions while assisting the nurse and helping patients and residents.
- Performs delegated aspects of the person's nursing care.
- Assists the nurse in observing patients and residents. Also assists in identifying their needs.
- Communicates:
  - Progress toward completing delegated nursing tasks
  - Problems in completing delegated nursing tasks
  - Changes in the person's status
- Asks the nurse to clarify what is expected when unsure.
- Uses educational and training opportunities as available.
- Practices safety measures to protect the person, others, and self.
- Respects the person's rights, concerns, decisions, and dignity.
- Functions as a member of the health team. Helps implement the care plan (Chapter 7).
- Respects the person's property and the property of others.
- Protects confidential information unless required by law to share the information.

Modified from National Council of State Boards of Nursing, Inc.: *Model nursing practice act and model administrative rules,* Chicago, 2006, Author.

states. For example, you work in Illinois and Iowa. You must know the laws and rules of both states.

State laws and rules limit nursing assistant functions. Your job description reflects those laws and rules. An agency can further limit what you can do. So can a nurse based on the person's needs. However, no agency or nurse can expand your range of functions beyond what your state's laws and rules allow.

See *Focus on Long-Term Care and Home Care: Roles and Responsibilities.*

Nursing Assistant Standards

OBRA defines the basic range of functions for nursing assistants. All NATCEPs include those functions (p. 23). Some states allow other functions. NATCEPs also prepare nursing assistants to meet the standards listed in Box 3-4.

Job Description

The *job description is a document describing what the agency expects you to do* (Fig. 3-2, pp. 28-29). It also states educational requirements.

Always obtain a written job description when you apply for a job. Ask questions about it during your job interview. Before accepting a job, tell the employer about:

- Functions you did not learn
- Functions you cannot do for moral or religious reasons

Clearly understand what is expected before taking a job. Do not take a job that requires you to:

- Act beyond the legal limits of your role.
- Function beyond your training limits.
- Perform acts that are against your morals or religion.

No one can force you to do something beyond the legal limits of your role. Sometimes jobs are threatened for refusing to follow a nurse's orders. Often staff obey out of fear. That is why you must understand:

- Your roles and responsibilities
- What you can safely do
- The things you should never do
- Your job description
- The ethical and legal aspects of your role (Chapter 4)

See *Focus on Communication: Job Description.*

DELEGATION

Nurse practice acts give nurses certain responsibilities. They also give them the legal authority to perform nursing actions. A *responsibility is the duty or obligation to perform some act or function.* For example, RNs are responsible for supervising LPNs/LVNs and nursing assistants. Only RNs can carry out this responsibility.

Delegate means to authorize another person to perform a nursing task in a certain situation. The person must be competent to perform the task in a given situation. For example, you know how to give a bed bath. However, Mr. Jones is a new resident. The RN wants to spend time with him and assess his nursing needs. You do not assess. Therefore the RN gives the bath.

Who Can Delegate

RNs can delegate nursing tasks to LPNs/LVNs and nursing assistants. In some states, LPNs/LVNs can delegate tasks to nursing assistants. Nurses can only delegate tasks within their scope of practice. And they can only delegate the tasks in your job description.

Delegation decisions must protect the person's health and safety. The delegating nurse is legally accountable for the nursing task. *Accountable means to be responsible for one's actions and the actions of others who performed the delegated tasks. It also involves answering questions about and explaining one's actions and the actions of others.*

FOCUS ON COMMUNICATION

Job Description

Your training prepares you to perform certain nursing tasks. The agency may not let you do everything you learned. Other agencies may want you to do things that you did not learn. Use your job description if you need to discuss these issues with the nurse.

For example, Mr. Wey is in the bathroom when the nurse brings a drug to him. The nurse tells you to give him the drug when he comes out of the bathroom. If you give the drug, you are performing a task and responsibility outside the limits of your role. With respect, you must firmly refuse to follow the nurse's direction. You can say: "I'm sorry, but I cannot give Mr. Wey that drug. I was not trained to give drugs, and that task is not in my job description. I'll let you know when Mr. Wey comes out of the bathroom."

The delegating nurse must make sure that the task was completed safely and correctly. If the RN delegates, the RN is responsible for the delegated task. If the LPN/LVN delegates, he or she is responsible for the delegated task. The RN also supervises LPNs/LVNs. Therefore the RN is legally accountable for the tasks that LPNs/LVNs delegate to nursing assistants. The RN is accountable for all nursing care.

Nursing assistants cannot delegate. You cannot delegate any task to other nursing assistants or to any other worker. You can ask someone to help you. But you cannot ask or tell someone to do your work.

Delegation Process

To make delegation decisions, the nurse follows a process. The person's needs, the nursing task, and the staff member doing the task must fit. The nurse decides if the task will be delegated to you. The person's needs and the task may require a nurse's knowledge, judgment, and skill. You may be asked to assist.

Do not get offended or angry if a task is not delegated to you. The nurse decides what is best for the person at the time. That decision is also best for you at that time. You must not do something that requires a nurse's judgment. For example, you always care for Mrs. Mills. Now she is weak and not eating well. The nurse wants to observe and evaluate the changes in her condition. The nurse gives needed care. At this time Mrs. Mills needs the nurse's knowledge and judgment.

The person's circumstances are central factors in delegation decisions. Delegation decisions must result in the best care for the person. Otherwise the person's health and safety are at risk. Also, the nurse may face serious legal problems. If you perform a task that places the person at risk, you may face serious legal problems.

Text continued on p. 30

POSITION DESCRIPTION/PERFORMANCE EVALUATION

Job Title: LTC Certified Nursing Assistant (CNA)

Supervised by: CNA Coordinator, Charge Nurse

Prepared by: _____

Approved by: _____

Date: _____

Date: _____

Job Summary: Provides direct and indirect resident care activities under the direction of an RN or LPN/LVN. Assists residents with activities of daily living, provides for personal care, comfort and assists in the maintenance of a safe and clean environment for an assigned group or residents.

DUTIES AND RESPONSIBILITIES:

3 = Exceeds Performance   2 = Expected Performance   1 = Needs Improvement

Demonstrates Competency in the Following Areas:

	3	2	1
Assists in the preparation for admission of residents.	3	2	1
Assists in and accompanies residents in the admission, transfer and discharge procedures.	3	2	1
Provides morning care, which may include bed bath, shower or whirlpool, oral hygiene, combing hair, back care, dressing residents, changing bed linen, cleaning overbed table and bedside stand, straightening room and other general care as necessary throughout the day.	3	2	1
Provides evening care which includes hands/face washing as needed, oral hygiene, backrubs, peri-care, freshening linen, cleaning overbed tables, straightening room and other general care as needed.	3	2	1
Notifies appropriate licensed staff when resident complains of pain.	3	2	1
Provides postmortem care and assists in transporting bodies to the morgue.	3	2	1
Assists LPN/LVN in treatment procedures.	3	2	1
Provides general nursing care such as positioning residents, lifting and turning residents, applying/utilizing special equipment, assisting in use of bedpan or commode and ambulating the residents.	3	2	1
Performs all aspects of resident care in an environment that optimizes resident safety and reduces the likelihood of medical/health care errors.	3	2	1
Takes and records temperature, pulse, respiration, weight, blood pressure and intake-output.	3	2	1
Makes rounds with outgoing shift; knows whereabouts of assigned residents.	3	2	1
Makes rounds with oncoming shift to ensure the unit is left in good condition.	3	2	1
Adheres to policies and procedures of the facility and the Nursing Department.	3	2	1
Participates in socialization activities on the unit.	3	2	1
Turns and positions residents as ordered and/or as needed, making sure no rough surfaces are in direct contact with the body. Lifts and turns with proper and safe body mechanics and with available resources.	3	2	1
Checks for reddened areas or skin breakdown and reports to RN or LPN/LVN.	3	2	1
Ensures residents are dressed properly and assists, as necessary. Ensures that used clothing is properly stored in bedside stand or on hangers in closet. Ensures that all residents are clean and dry at all times.	3	2	1
Checks unit for adequate linen. Folds neatly and arranges linen in linen closet. Cleans linen cart. Provides clean linen and clothing. Makes beds.	3	2	1
Treats residents and their families with respect and dignity.	3	2	1
Restrains residents properly, when ordered.	3	2	1
Accompanies residents to appointments, as directed.	3	2	1
Provides reality orientation in daily care.	3	2	1
Prepares residents for meals; serves and removes food trays and assists with meals or feeds residents, if necessary.	3	2	1
Distributes drinking water and other nourishments to residents.	3	2	1
Performs general care activities for residents in isolation.	3	2	1
Answers residents' call lights, anticipates residents' needs and makes rounds to assigned residents.	3	2	1
Assists residents with handling and care of clothing and other personal property (including dentures, glasses, contact lenses, hearing aids and prosthetic devices).	3	2	1
Transports residents to and from various departments, as requested.	3	2	1
Reports and, when appropriate, records any changes observed in condition or behavior of residents and unusual incidents.	3	2	1
Participates in and contributes to interdisciplinary care conferences.	3	2	1
Must be able to follow directions, both oral and written, and work cooperatively with other staff members.	3	2	1

Fig. 3-2 A sample nursing assistant job description. Note that the job description is also a performance evaluation.

POSITION DESCRIPTION/PERFORMANCE EVALUATION—cont'd

Must have the ability to acquire knowledge of and develop skills in basic nursing procedures and simple charting.	3	2	1
Establishes and maintains interpersonal relationship with residents, family members and other facility staff while assuring confidentiality of resident information.	3	2	1
Attends inservice education programs, as assigned, to learn new treatments, procedures, developmental skills, etc.	3	2	1
Practices careful, efficient and nonwasteful use of supplies and linen and follows established charge procedure for resident charge items.	3	2	1
Maintains personal health in order to prevent absence from work due to health problems.	3	2	1
Possesses a genuine interest and concern for geriatric and disabled persons.	3	2	1

Professional Requirements:

Adheres to dress code, appearance is neat and clean.	3	2	1
Completes annual education requirements.	3	2	1
Maintains regulatory requirements.	3	2	1
Maintains resident confidentiality at all times.	3	2	1
Reports to work on time and as scheduled, completes work within designated time.	3	2	1
Wears identification while on duty, uses computerized punch time system correctly.	3	2	1
Completes inservices and returns in a timely fashion.	3	2	1
Attends annual review and department inservices, as scheduled.	3	2	1
Attends at least _____ staff meetings annually, reads and returns all monthly staff meeting minutes.	3	2	1
Represents the organization in a positive and professional manner.	3	2	1
Actively participates in performance improvement and continuous quality improvement (CQI) activities.	3	2	1
Complies with all organizational policies regarding ethical business practices.	3	2	1
Communicates the mission, ethics and goals of the facility.	3	2	1

TOTAL POINTS _____ _____ _____

Regulatory Requirements:
- High School graduate or equivalent.
- Current Certified Nursing Assistant (CNA) certification in State of _____ for Long Term Care Facilities.
- Current Basic Cardiac Life Support certification within three (3) months of hire date.

Language Skills:
- Able to communicate effectively in English, both verbally and in writing.
- Additional languages preferred.

Skills:
- Basic computer knowledge.

Physical Demands:
- For physical demands of position, including vision, hearing, repetitive motion and environment, see following description.

  Reasonable accommodations may be made to enable individuals with disabilities to perform the essential functions of the position without compromising patient care.

I have received, read and understand the Position Description/Performance Evaluation above.

_____   _____

Name/Signature   Date Signed

Fig. 3-2, cont'd For legend see facing page.

The NCSBN describes the delegation process in four steps.

Step 1—Assess and Plan. Step 1 is done by the nurse. To safely delegate, the nurse needs to understand the person's needs. And the nurse needs to know your knowledge, skills, and job description.

When assessing the person's needs, the nurse answers these questions:

- What is the nature of the person's needs? How complex are they? How can they vary? How urgent are the care needs?
- What are the most important long-term needs? What are the most important short-term needs?
- How much judgment is needed to meet the person's needs and give care?
- How predictable is the person's health status? How does the person respond to health care?
- What problems might arise from the nursing task? How severe might they be?
- What actions are needed if a problem arises? How complex are those actions?
- What emergencies or incidents might arise? How likely might they occur?
- How involved is the person in health care decisions? How involved is the family?
- How will delegating the nursing task help the person? What are the risks to the person?

To assess your knowledge and skills, the nurse answers these questions:

- What knowledge and skills are needed to safely perform the nursing task?
- What is your role in the agency? What is in your job description?
- What are the conditions under which the nursing task will be performed?
- What is expected after the nursing task is performed?
- What problems can arise from the nursing task? What problems might the person develop during the nursing task?

The nurse then decides if it is safe to delegate the nursing task. It must be safe for the person and safe for you. If unsafe, the nurse stops the delegation process. If it is safe for the person and you, the nurse moves to step 2.

Step 2—Communication. This step involves the nurse and you. The nurse must provide clear and complete directions about:

- How to perform and complete the task.
- What observations to report and record.
- When to report observations.
- What specific patient and resident concerns to report at once.
- Priorities for nursing tasks.
- What to do if the person's condition changes or needs change.

The nurse must make sure that you understand the directions to give safe care. The nurse asks you questions to make sure you understand. He or she may ask you to explain what you are going to do. Do not be insulted by such questions. The intent is to protect the person and you.

Before performing a delegated task, it is important that you discuss the task with the nurse. Make sure that you:

- Ask questions about the delegated task.
- Ask questions about what you are expected to do.
- Tell the nurse if you have not done the task before or not often.
- Ask for needed training or supervision.
- Re-state what is expected of you.
- Re-state what specific patient and resident concerns to report to the nurse.
- Explain how and when you will report your progress in completing the task.
- Know how to contact the nurse for an emergency.
- Know what the nurse wants you to do during an emergency.

After completing a delegated task, you report and record the care given. You also report and record your observations. See "Reporting and Recording" in Chapter 6.

See *Focus on Long-Term Care and Home Care: Step 2—Communication.*

Step 3—Surveillance and Supervision. *Surveillance* means to keep a close watch over someone or something. *Supervise* means to oversee, direct, or manage. In this step, the nurse:

- Observes the care you give.
- Makes sure that you complete the task correctly.
- Observes the person's condition and response to your care.

How often the nurse makes observations depends on:

- The person's health status and needs.
- If the person's condition is stable or unstable.
- If the nurse can predict the person's responses and risks to care.
- The setting where the task occurs.
- The resources and support available.
- If the task is simple or complex.

The nurse must follow up on any problems or concerns. For example, the nurse takes action if:

- You did not complete the task in a timely manner.
- The task did not meet expectations.
- There is an unexpected change in the person's condition.

FOCUS ON LONG-TERM CARE AND HOME CARE

Step 2—Communication

Home Care

The delegating nurse is not with you during home care. The nurse may be at the agency or in another home. The nurse and you must decide how to communicate with each other. You must know how to get help at once if you need it. Work out a communication plan with the nurse before you leave the agency.

The nurse is alert for signs and symptoms that signal a possible change in the person's condition. This way the nurse, with your help, can take action before the person's condition changes in a major way.

Sometimes problems arise during a nursing task. By supervising you, the nurse can detect and solve problems early. This helps you complete the task safely and on time.

After you complete the task, the nurse may review and discuss what happened with you. This helps you learn. If a similar situation happens in the future, you have ideas about how to adjust.

Step 4—Evaluation and Feedback. This step is done by the nurse. *Evaluate* means to judge. The nurse decides if the delegation was successful. The nurse answers these questions:

- Was the task done correctly?
- Did the person respond to the task as expected?
- Was the outcome (the result) as desired? Was it a good or bad result?
- Was communication between you and the nurse timely and effective?
- What went well? What were the problems?
- Does the care plan need to change (Chapter 7)? Or can the plan stay the same?
- Did the task present ways for the nurse or you to learn?
- Did the nurse give you the right feedback? *Feedback* means *to respond*. The nurse tells you what you did correctly. If you did something wrong, the nurse tells you that too. Feedback is another way for you to learn and improve the care you give.
- Did the nurse thank you for completing the task?

The Five Rights of Delegation

The NCSBN's *Five Rights of Delegation* is another way to view the delegation process. To use the "five rights," the nurse answers the questions listed in the four steps described above. The *Five Rights of Delegation* are:

- *The right task.* Can the task be delegated? Is the nurse allowed to delegate the task? Is the task in your job description?
- *The right circumstances.* What are the person's physical, mental, emotional, and spiritual needs at this time?
- *The right person.* Do you have the training and experience to safely perform the task for this person?
- *The right directions and communication.* The nurse must give clear directions. The nurse tells you what to do and when to do it. The nurse tells you what observations to make and when to report back. The nurse allows questions and helps you set priorities.
- *The right supervision.* In this step, the nurse:
  - Guides, directs, and evaluates the care you give.

- Demonstrates tasks as necessary and is available to answer questions. The less experience you have with a task, the more supervision you need. Complex tasks require more supervision than do basic tasks. Also, the person's circumstances affect how much supervision you need.
- Assesses how the task affected the person and how well you performed the task.
- Tells you what you did well and how to improve your work. This helps you learn and give better care.

Your Role in Delegation

You perform delegated tasks for or on *a person*. You must protect the person from harm. You have two choices when a task is delegated to you. You either *agree* or *refuse* to do the task. Use the *Five Rights of Delegation* in Box 3-5, p. 32.

Accepting a Task. When you agree to perform a task, you are responsible for your own actions. What you do or fail to do can harm the person. *You must complete the task safely.* Ask for help when you are unsure or have questions about a task. Report to the nurse what you did and the observations you made.

Refusing a Task. You have the right to say "no." Sometimes refusing to follow the nurse's directions is your right and duty. You should refuse to perform a task when:

- The task is beyond the legal limits of your role.
- The task is not in your job description.
- You were not prepared to perform the task.
- The task could harm the person.
- The person's condition has changed.
- You do not know how to use the supplies or equipment.
- Directions are not ethical or legal.
- Directions are against agency policies.
- Directions are not clear or not complete.
- A nurse is not available for supervision.

Use common sense. This protects you and the person. Ask yourself if what you are doing is safe for the person.

Never ignore an order or a request to do something. Tell the nurse about your concerns. If the task is within the legal limits of your role and in your job description, the nurse can help increase your comfort with the task. The nurse can:

- Answer your questions.
- Demonstrate the task.
- Show you how to use supplies and equipment.
- Help you as needed.
- Observe you performing the task.
- Check on you often.
- Arrange for needed training.

Do not refuse a task because you do not like it or do not want to do it. You must have sound reasons. Otherwise, you place the person at risk for harm. You also could lose your job.

See *Focus on Communication: Refusing a Task*, p. 32.

BOX 3-5   THE *FIVE RIGHTS OF DELEGATION* FOR NURSING ASSISTANTS

The Right Task
- Does your state allow you to perform the task?
- Were you trained to do the task?
- Do you have experience performing the task?
- Is the task in your job description?

The Right Circumstances
- Do you have experience with the task given the person's condition and needs?
- Do you understand the purposes of the task for the person?
- Can you perform the task safely under the current circumstances?
- Do you have the equipment and supplies to safely complete the task?
- Do you know how to use the equipment and supplies?

The Right Person
- Are you comfortable performing the task?
- Do you have concerns about performing the task?

The Right Directions and Communication
- Did the nurse give clear directions and instructions?
- Did you review the task with the nurse?
- Do you understand what the nurse expects?

The Right Supervision
- Is a nurse available to answer questions?
- Is a nurse available if the person's condition changes or if problems occur?

Modified from the National Council of State Boards of Nursing, Inc.: *The five rights of delegation,* Chicago, 1997, Author.

FOCUS ON COMMUNICATION

Refusing a Task

A nurse may delegate a task that you did not learn in your training program. The task is in your job description. You can say: "I know this task is in my job description, but I did not learn it in school. Can you show me what to do and then observe me doing it? That would really help me."

A nurse may ask you to do something that is not in your job description. With respect, you must firmly refuse the nurse's request. You can say: "I'm sorry. That task is not in my job description. Can I help you with something else?"

FOCUS ON PRIDE

The Person, Family, and Yourself

Personal and Professional Responsibility

Health care is constantly changing. New opportunities are common. For example, some states have higher levels of nursing assistants. Medication Assistant-Certified (MA-C) is an example. MA-Cs are nursing assistants with extra training. Supervised by a licensed nurse, they give drugs as allowed by state law.

Continuing education increases your skills and knowledge and helps you provide safe, quality care. Agency in-services, staff meetings, and conferences offer learning opportunities. Continuing to learn is a personal and professional responsibility.

Your current training is just the start of a life-time of learning and possibilities. Find out about options available in your state and agency. Take advantage of them. Be proud of your training. And never stop learning!

Rights and Respect

Most training programs involve practice in a real clinical setting. Sometimes a patient or resident refuses to have a student. Or the person refuses to allow a student to watch a procedure. The person has the right to do so. The person's request must be respected.

When this happens, the student often feels disappointed and rejected. Or the student feels as if he or she did something wrong. If this happens to you, kindly accept the person's request. Try not to be ashamed or upset. Tell your instructor. Do not speak badly about the patient or resident. The person may have had a bad experience in the past. This had nothing to do with you. Respect the person's right to choose who is involved in his or her care.

Independence and Social Interaction

As a nursing assistant, you will interact with many people daily. Some are family and friends. Work relationships differ from social ones. Make sure your actions and conversations are appropriate. Patients, residents, and families notice what you do and say. Always show good judgment.

Delegation and Teamwork

You may be delegated several tasks at a time. Or multiple nurses delegate tasks to you. At times, you may have a long list of tasks to do. This can be overwhelming. For example, you have been asked to:
- Take Mr. Austin's temperature.
- Get Ms. Sams a glass of water.
- Empty Mr. Walter's catheter bag.
- Turn and re-position Mr. Mason.
- Assist Mrs. Phillips to the bathroom.

When delegated several tasks, remember to stay calm. Keep a positive attitude. Communicate with the nurse. Ask the nurse to help you set priorities. Also, good teamwork is needed. The nursing team must work together to provide care. When you know others have many delegated tasks, offer to help. Thank others when they help you.

Ethics and Laws

Some nursing assistants work in more than one setting. Some are also emergency medical technicians (EMTs). EMTs give emergency care outside of health care settings. These settings are called "in the field." EMTs work under the direction of doctors in hospital emergency departments.

State laws and rules for EMTs and nursing assistants differ. For example, Joan Woods is an EMT for a fire department. When off duty, she is a nursing assistant at Deer Valley Hospital. Her state allows EMTs to start intravenous (IV) infusions in the field. However, nursing assistants do not start IVs. Ms. Woods cannot start IVs when working at the hospital as a nursing assistant.

The situation is the same for former medics or corpsmen in military service. They can suture wounds. Nursing assistants cannot do so. When working as nursing assistants, medics and corpsmen must follow their state's laws and rules for nursing assistants. As with EMTs, the ability to do something does not give them the right to do so in all settings.

There are legal limits to your role. Be proud of the advanced skills and training you may have. But when working as a nursing assistant, follow your state's laws and rules for nursing assistants.

REVIEW QUESTIONS

Circle the BEST answer.

1 Nursing practice is regulated by
   a The National Council of State Boards of Nursing
   b Nurse practice acts
   c Medicare
   d Medicaid
2 What state law affects what nursing assistants can do?
   a Standards for nursing assistants
   b OBRA
   c Nurse practice act
   d Medicaid
3 Your nursing assistant certification can be revoked for
   a Refusing a nursing task
   b Asking the nurse questions
   c Performing acts beyond your role
   d Keeping the person's information confidential
4 Which requires a training and competency evaluation program for nursing assistants?
   a Medicare
   b Medicaid
   c NCSBN
   d OBRA
5 As a nursing assistant, you
   a Must perform all tasks as directed by the nurse
   b Make decisions about a person's care
   c Need a written job description before employment
   d Give a drug when a nurse tells you to
6 As a nursing assistant, you
   a Can take verbal or phone orders from doctors
   b Are responsible for your own actions
   c Can remove tubes from the person's body
   d Can ignore a nursing task if it is not in your job description

7 Which statement is *false*?
   a You are accountable for your actions.
   b You must be honest when performing nursing tasks.
   c You can use the person's property for your own needs.
   d A law can require you to share the person's confidential information.
8 Who assigns and supervises your work?
   a Other nursing assistants
   b The health team
   c Nurses
   d Doctors
9 You are responsible for
   a Supervising other nursing assistants
   b Delegation decisions
   c Completing delegated tasks safely
   d Deciding what treatments are needed
10 You perform a task not allowed by your state. Which is *true*?
   a If a nurse delegated the task, there is no legal problem.
   b You could be practicing nursing without a license.
   c You can perform the task if it is in your job description.
   d If you complete the task safely, there is no legal problem.
11 These statements are about delegation. Which is *false*?
   a Nurses can delegate their responsibilities to you.
   b A delegated task must be safe for the person.
   c The delegated task must be in your job description.
   d The delegating nurse is responsible for the safe completion of the task.
12 A task is in your job description. Which is *false*?
   a The nurse must delegate the task to you.
   b The nurse can delegate the task if the person's circumstances are right.
   c You must have the necessary education and training to complete the task.
   d You must have clear directions before you perform the task.
13 A nurse delegates a task to you. You must
   a Complete the task
   b Decide to accept or refuse the task
   c Delegate the task if you are busy
   d Ignore the request if you do not know what to do
14 You can refuse to perform a task for these reasons *except*
   a The task is beyond the legal limits of your role
   b The task is not in your job description
   c You do not like the task
   d A nurse is not available to supervise you
15 You decide to refuse a task. What should you do?
   a Delegate the task to a nursing assistant.
   b Communicate your concerns to the nurse.
   c Ignore the request.
   d Talk to the director of nursing.

Answers to these questions are on p. 832.

4 Ethics and Laws

OBJECTIVES

- Define the key terms and key abbreviations listed in this chapter.
- Describe ethical conduct.
- Describe the rules of conduct for nursing assistants.
- Explain how to maintain professional boundaries.
- Explain how to prevent negligent acts.
- Give examples of false imprisonment, defamation, assault, battery, and fraud.
- Describe how to protect the right to privacy.
- Explain the purpose of informed consent.
- Explain your role in relation to wills.
- Describe elder, child, and domestic abuse.
- Explain how to promote PRIDE in the person, the family, and yourself.

KEY TERMS

abuse The willful infliction of injury, unreasonable confinement, intimidation, or punishment that results in physical harm, pain, or mental anguish; depriving the person (or the person's caregiver) of the goods or services needed to attain or maintain well-being

assault Intentionally attempting or threatening to touch a person's body without the person's consent

battery Touching a person's body without his or her consent

boundary crossing A brief act or behavior outside of the helpful zone

boundary sign An act, behavior, or thought that warns of a boundary crossing or violation

boundary violation An act or behavior that meets your needs, not the person's

civil law Laws concerned with relationships between people

crime An act that violates a criminal law

criminal law Laws concerned with offenses against the public and society in general

defamation Injuring a person's name and reputation by making false statements to a third person

elder abuse Any knowing, intentional, or negligent act by a caregiver or any other person to an older adult; the act causes harm or serious risk of harm

ethics Knowledge of what is right conduct and wrong conduct

false imprisonment Unlawful restraint or restriction of a person's freedom of movement

fraud Saying or doing something to trick, fool, or deceive a person

invasion of privacy Violating a person's right not to have his or her name, photo, or private affairs exposed or made public without giving consent

law A rule of conduct made by a government body

libel Making false statements in print, writing, or through pictures or drawings

malpractice Negligence by a professional person

neglect Failure to provide the person with the goods or services needed to avoid physical harm, mental anguish, or mental illness

negligence An unintentional wrong in which a person did not act in a reasonable and careful manner and a person or the person's property was harmed

professional boundary That which separates helpful behaviors from behaviors that are not helpful

professional sexual misconduct An act, behavior, or comment that is sexual in nature

protected health information Identifying information and information about the person's health care that is maintained or sent in any form (paper, electronic, oral)

self-neglect A person's behaviors and way of living that threaten his or her health, safety, and well-being

slander Making false statements orally

standard of care The skills, care, and judgments required by a health team member under similar conditions

tort A wrong committed against a person or the person's property

vulnerable adult A person 18 years old or older who has a disability or condition that makes him or her at risk to be wounded, attacked, or damaged

will A legal document of how a person wants property distributed after death

KEY ABBREVIATIONS

HIPAA	Health Insurance Portability and Accountability Act of 1996	**OBRA**	Omnibus Budget Reconciliation Act of 1987

Nurse practice acts, your training and job description, and safe delegation serve to protect patients and residents from harm (Chapter 3). Protecting them from harm also involves a complex set of rules and standards of conduct. They form the ethical and legal aspects of care.

ETHICAL ASPECTS

Ethics is knowledge of what is right conduct and wrong conduct. Morals are involved. It also deals with choices or judgments about what should or should not be done. An ethical person behaves and acts in the right way. He or she does not cause a person harm.

Ethical behavior also involves not being *prejudiced* or *biased*. To be prejudiced or biased means making judgments and having views before knowing the facts. Judgments and views usually are based on one's values and standards. They are based on the person's culture, religion, education, and experiences. The person's situation may be very different from your own. For example:

* Children think their mother needs nursing home care. In your culture, children care for older parents at home.
* A person has many tattoos and body piercings. You do not like tattoos or body piercings.
* An older man does not want life-saving measures. You believe that everything must be done to save a life.

Do not judge the person by your values and standards. Do not avoid persons whose standards and values differ from your own.

Ethical problems involve making choices. What is the right thing to do? For example:

* A co-worker is in an empty room drinking from a cup. You smell alcohol on her breath. She asks you not to tell anyone.
* A resident has bruises all over her body. She told the nurse that she fell. She tells you that her son is very mean to her. She asks you not to tell the nurse.

Professional groups have codes of ethics. The code has rules, or standards of conduct, for group members to follow. The American Nurses Association (ANA) has a code of ethics for registered nurses (RNs). The National Federation of Licensed Practical Nurses (NFLPN) has one for licensed practical nurses/licensed vocational nurses (LPNs/LVNs). The rules of conduct in Box 4-1 can guide your thinking and behavior. See Chapter 5 for ethics in the workplace.

Boundaries

A *boundary* limits or separates something. For example, a fence forms a boundary. You stay inside or outside of the fenced area. As a nursing assistant, you help patients, residents, and families. Therefore you enter into a helping relationship with them. The helping relationship has professional boundaries.

BOX 4-1	CODE OF CONDUCT FOR NURSING ASSISTANTS

* Respect each person as an individual.
* Know the limits of your role and knowledge.
* Perform only those tasks that are within the legal limits of your role.
* Perform only those tasks that you have been prepared to do.
* Perform no act that will harm the person.
* Take drugs only if prescribed and supervised by your doctor.
* Follow the directions and instructions of the nurse to your best possible ability.
* Follow the agency's policies and procedures.
* Complete each task safely.
* Be loyal to your employer and co-workers.
* Act as a responsible citizen at all times.
* Keep the person's information confidential.
* Protect the person's privacy.
* Protect the person's property.
* Consider the person's needs to be more important than your own.
* Report errors and incidents at once.
* Be accountable for your actions.

PROFESSIONAL BOUNDARIES

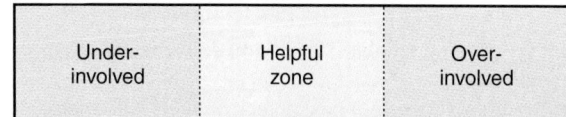

Under-involved	Helpful zone	Over-involved

Fig. 4-1 Professional boundaries.

Professional boundaries separate helpful behaviors from behaviors that are not helpful (Fig. 4-1). The boundaries create a helpful zone. If your behaviors are outside of the helpful zone, you are over-involved with the person or under-involved. The following can occur:

* *Boundary crossing is a brief act or behavior outside of the helpful zone.* The act or behavior may be thoughtless or something you did not mean to do. Or it could have purpose if it meets the person's needs. For example, you give a crying patient a hug. The hug meets the person's needs at that time. If giving a hug meets your needs, the act is wrong. Also, it is wrong to hug the person every time you see him or her.
* *Boundary violation is an act or behavior that meets your needs, not the person's.* The act or behavior is not ethical. It violates the code of conduct in Box 4-1. The person could be harmed. Boundary violations include:
  * Abuse (p. 39).
  * Giving a lot of information about yourself. You tell a person about your personal relationships or problems.
  * Keeping secrets with the person.
* *Professional sexual misconduct is an act, behavior, or comment that is sexual in nature.* It is sexual misconduct even if the person consents or makes the first move.

Some boundary violations and some types of professional sexual misconduct also are crimes. To maintain professional boundaries, follow the rules in Box 4-2. Be alert to boundary signs. *Boundary signs are acts, behaviors, or thoughts that warn of a boundary crossing or violation* (Box 4-3).

See *Focus on Communication: Professional Boundaries.*

BOX 4-2 **RULES FOR MAINTAINING PROFESSIONAL BOUNDARIES**

- Follow the code of conduct listed in Box 4-1.
- Talk to the nurse if you sense a boundary sign, crossing, or violation.
- Avoid caring for family, friends, and people with whom you do business. This may be hard to do in a small community. Always tell the nurse if you know the person. The nurse may change your assignment.
- Do not make sexual comments or jokes.
- Do not use offensive language.
- Use touch correctly (Chapter 8). Touch or handle sexual and genital areas only when necessary to give care. Such areas include the breasts, nipples, perineum, buttocks, and anus.
- Do not visit or spend extra time with a patient or resident who is not part of your assignment.
- The following apply to patients, residents, and family members:
  - Do not date, flirt with, kiss, or have a sexual relationship with them.
  - Do not discuss your sexual relationships with them.
  - Do not say or write things that could suggest a romantic or sexual relationship with them.
  - Do not accept gifts, loans, money, credit cards, or other valuables from them.
  - Do not give gifts, loans, money, credit cards, or other valuables to them.
  - Do not borrow from them. This includes money, personal items, and transportation.
  - Maintain a professional relationship at all times. Do not develop any personal relationship or friendship with them.
  - Do not share personal or financial information with them.
  - Do not help them with their finances.
  - Do not take a person home with you. This includes for holidays or other events.
- Ask these questions before you date or marry a person whom you cared for. Be aware of the risk for professional sexual misconduct.
  - How long ago did you assist with the person's care?
  - Was the person's care short-term or long-term?
  - What kind and how much information do you have about the person? How will that information affect your relationship with the person?
  - Will the person need more care in the future?
  - Does dating or marrying the person place the person at risk for harm?

BOX 4-3 **BOUNDARY SIGNS**

- You think about the person when you are not at work.
- You organize your work and provide other care around the person's needs.
- You spend free time with the person. You visit with the person during breaks, meal times, when off duty, and so on.
- You trade assignments with other staff so you can provide the person's care.
- You give more care or attention to the person at the expense of others.
- You believe that you are the only person who understands the person and his or her needs.
- The person gives you gifts or money.
- You give the person gifts or money.
- You share information about yourself with the person.
- You talk about your work situation with the person.
- You flirt with the person.
- You make comments that have a sexual message.
- You tell the person "off-color" jokes.
- You notice more touch between you and the person.
- You use foul, vulgar, or offensive language when talking to the person.
- You and the person have secrets.
- You choose the person's side when he or she disagrees with other staff or the family.
- You select what you report and record. You do not give complete information.
- You do not like questions about the care you give or your relationship with the person.
- You change how you dress or your appearance when you will work with the person.
- You receive gifts from the person after he or she leaves the agency.
- You have contact with the person after he or she leaves the agency.

FOCUS ON COMMUNICATION
Professional Boundaries

Some patients, residents, and families want to thank the staff for the care given. Some send thank-you cards and letters. Some offer gifts—candy, cookies, money, gift certificates, flowers, and so on. Accepting gifts is a boundary violation. When offered a gift, you can say:
- "Thank you so much for thinking of me. It's very kind of you. However, it is against center policy to accept gifts of any kind. I do appreciate your offer."
- "Thank you for wanting me to have the flowers from your friend. They are lovely. However, it is against hospital policy to receive gifts. Let me help you find a way to take them home."

LEGAL ASPECTS

Ethics is about what you *should or should not do*. Laws tell you what you *can and cannot do*. A *law is a rule of conduct made by a government body*. The U.S. Congress and state legislatures make laws. Enforced by the government, laws protect the public welfare.

Criminal laws are concerned with offenses against the public and society in general. An act that violates a criminal law is called a crime. A person found guilty of a crime is fined or sent to prison. Murder, robbery, rape, kidnapping, and abuse (p. 39) are crimes.

Civil laws are concerned with relationships between people. Examples of civil laws are those that involve contracts and nursing practice. A person found guilty of breaking a civil law usually has to pay a sum of money to the injured person.

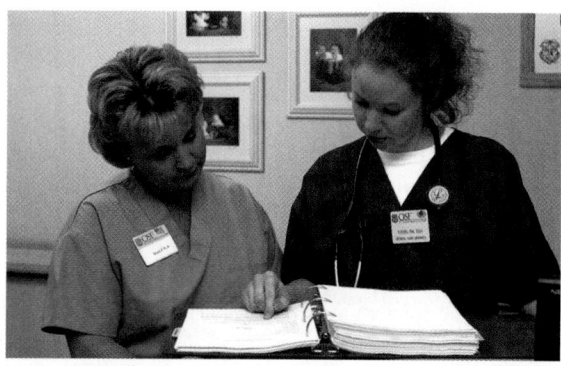

Fig. 4-2   A nurse and nursing assistant review the policy and procedure manual. It is kept at the nurses' station.

Torts

Tort comes from the French word meaning wrong. Torts are part of civil law. A *tort is a wrong committed against a person or the person's property*. Some torts are *unintentional*. Harm was not intended. Some torts are *intentional*. Harm was intended.

Unintentional Torts. *Negligence is an unintentional wrong. The negligent person did not act in a reasonable and careful manner. As a result, a person or the person's property was harmed.* The person causing the harm did not intend or mean to cause harm. The person failed to do what a reasonable and careful person *would have done*. Or he or she did what a reasonable and careful person *would not have done*. The negligent person may have to pay damages (a sum of money) to the one injured.

Malpractice is negligence by a professional person. A person has professional status because of training and the service provided. Nurses, doctors, dentists, and pharmacists are examples.

What you do or do not do can lead to a lawsuit if harm results to the person or property of another. *Standard of care refers to the skills, care, and judgments required by a health team member under similar conditions.* Standards of care come from:

- Laws, including nurse practice acts and those relating to nursing assistants.
- Textbooks.
- Agency policy and procedure manuals (Fig. 4-2). These explain how to perform certain procedures.
- Manufacturer instructions for equipment and supplies.
- Job descriptions.
- Approval and accrediting agency standards.
- Standards and guidelines from government agencies.

The following actions could lead to charges of negligence:

- A nurse asks you to apply a hot soak. You fail to test the water temperature. The water is too hot. The person is burned.

- Mrs. Parks needs help getting to the bathroom. You do not answer her signal light promptly. She gets up without help. She falls and breaks an arm.
- You use a mechanical lift to transfer Mr. Brown from bed to a chair. You do not follow the manufacturer's instructions for using the lift. Mr. Brown slips out of the lift and falls to the floor. He fractures a hip.
- Mrs. Clark complains of chest pain. You do not tell the nurse. Mrs. Clark has a heart attack and dies.
- Two residents have the same last name. You do not identify the person before a procedure. You perform the procedure on the wrong person. Both residents are harmed. One had a procedure that was not ordered. The other did not have a needed procedure.

You are legally responsible *(liable)* for your own actions. The nurse is liable as your supervisor. However, you have personal liability. Remember, sometimes refusing to follow the nurse's directions is your right and duty (Chapter 3).

Intentional Torts. Intentional torts are acts meant to be harmful. The act is done on purpose.

Defamation. *Defamation is injuring a person's name and reputation by making false statements to a third person.*

- *Libel is making false statements in print, writing, or through pictures or drawings.*
- *Slander is making false statements orally.*

Never make false statements about a patient, resident, family member, co-worker, or any other person. Examples of defamation include:

- Implying or suggesting that a person uses drugs
- Saying that a person is insane or mentally ill
- Implying or suggesting that a person steals money from the staff

False imprisonment. *False imprisonment is the unlawful restraint or restriction of a person's freedom of movement.* It involves:

- Threatening to restrain a person
- Restraining a person
- Preventing a person from leaving the agency

Invasion of privacy. *Invasion of privacy is violating a person's right not to have his or her name, photo, or private affairs exposed or made public without giving consent.* You must treat the person with respect and ensure privacy. Only staff involved in the person's care should see, handle, or examine his or her body. See Box 4-4 for measures to protect privacy.

The Health Insurance Portability and Accountability Act of 1996 (HIPAA) protects the privacy and security of a person's health information. *Protected health information refers to identifying information and information about the person's health care that is maintained or sent in any form (paper, electronic, oral).* Failure to follow HIPAA rules can result in fines, penalties, and criminal action including jail time. Always follow agency policies and procedures. Direct any questions about the person or the person's care to the nurse. Also follow the rules for using computers and other electronic devices (Chapter 6).

BOX 4-4   PROTECTING THE RIGHT TO PRIVACY

- Keep all information about the person confidential.
- Cover the person when he or she is being moved in hallways.
- Screen the person. Close the privacy curtain as in Figure 4-3. Close the door when giving care. Also close window coverings.
- Expose only the body part involved in a task.
- Do not discuss the person or the person's treatment with anyone except the nurse supervising your work. "Shop talk" is a common cause of invasion of privacy.
- Ask visitors to leave the room when care is given.
- Do not open the person's mail.
- Allow the person to visit with others in private.
- Allow the person to use the phone in private.
- Follow agency policies and procedures required to protect privacy.

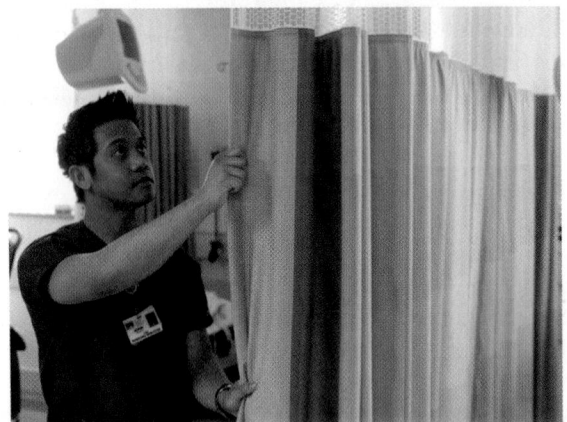

Fig. 4-3 Pulling the privacy curtain around the bed helps protect the person's privacy.

Fraud. *Fraud is saying or doing something to trick, fool, or deceive a person.* The act is fraud if it does or could harm a person or the person's property. Telling a person or family that you are a nurse is fraud. So is giving wrong or incomplete information on a job application.

Assault and battery. Assault and battery may result in both civil and criminal charges. *Assault is intentionally attempting or threatening to touch a person's body without the person's consent.* The person fears bodily harm. Threatening to "tie down" a person is an example of assault. *Battery is touching a person's body without his or her consent.* Consent is the important factor in assault and battery. The person must consent to any procedure, treatment, or other act that involves touching the body. The person has the right to withdraw consent at any time.

Protect yourself from being accused of assault and battery. Explain to the person what you are going to do and get the person's consent. Consent may be verbal—"yes" or "okay." Or it can be a gesture—a nod, turning over for a back rub, or holding out an arm for you to take a pulse.

Informed Consent

A person has the right to decide what will be done to his or her body and who can touch his or her body. The doctor is responsible for informing the person about all aspects of treatment. Consent is informed when the person clearly understands:

- The reason for a treatment, procedure, or care measure
- What will be done
- How it will be done
- Who will do it
- The expected outcomes
- Other treatment, procedure, or care options
- The effects of not having the treatment, procedure, or care measure

Persons under legal age (usually 18 years) cannot give consent. Nor can persons who are mentally incompetent. Such persons are unconscious, sedated, or confused. Or they have certain mental health problems. Informed consent is given by a responsible party—a wife, husband, parent, daughter, son, or legal representative.

Consent is given when the person enters the agency. A form is signed giving general consent to treatment. Special consent forms are required before admission to a secured Alzheimer's unit (Chapter 46). Certain procedures performed by the doctor require special consents. The doctor informs the person about all aspects of the procedure. The nurse may be given this responsibility.

You are never responsible for obtaining written consent. In some agencies, you can witness the signing of a consent. When a witness, you are present when the person signs the consent.

See *Focus on Communication: Informed Consent.*

FOCUS ON COMMUNICATION

Informed Consent

There are different ways to give consent:
- *Written consent*. The person signs a form agreeing to a treatment or procedure. You are not responsible for obtaining written consent.
- *Verbal consent*. The person says aloud that he or she consents. "Yes" and "okay" are examples.
- *Implied consent*. For example, you ask Mr. Jones if you can check his blood pressure. He extends his arm. His movement implies consent.

Before any procedure, explain the steps to the person. This is how you obtain verbal or implied consent. Also explain each step during a procedure. This allows the person the chance to refuse at any time.

FOCUS ON COMMUNICATION

Reporting Abuse

Persons being abused may confide in you. They may ask you to keep it a secret. For example, a person says: "If I tell you something, will you promise not to tell anyone?" Never promise to keep abuse a secret. You must also be honest. Do not tell the person you will keep a secret and then report it to the nurse. You can say: "For your safety, some things I must tell the nurse. What did you want to tell me?" If the person refuses to tell you, notify the nurse.

If you suspect abuse, tell the nurse what you observed. Give as much detail as you can. For example: "I am concerned about Ms. Sloan. She has been very quiet today. When I asked about her afternoon out with her niece yesterday, she didn't respond. She refused her bath. And when I helped her to the bathroom, I noticed bruises on her back."

Wills

A *will is a legal document of how a person wants property distributed after death.* You can ethically and legally witness a will signing. Or you can refuse to do so without fear of legal action.

A person may ask you to prepare a will. You must politely refuse. Explain that you do not have the legal knowledge or ability to prepare a will. Report the request to the nurse. The nurse will speak to the person or family member about contacting a lawyer.

Do not witness a will signing if you are named in the will. To do so prevents you from getting what was left to you. As a witness, be prepared to testify that:
- The person was of sound mind when the will was signed.
- The person stated that the document was his or her last will.

Many agencies do not let staff witness wills. Know your agency's policy before you agree to witness a will. If you have questions, ask the nurse. If you witness a will, tell the nurse.

REPORTING ABUSE

Some persons are mistreated or harmed on purpose. This is abuse. *Abuse is:*
- *The willful infliction of injury, unreasonable confinement, intimidation, or punishment that results in physical harm, pain, or mental anguish. Intimidation* means to make afraid with threats of force or violence.
- *Depriving the person (or the person's caregiver) of the goods or services needed to attain or maintain well-being.*

Abuse also includes involuntary seclusion (Chapter 2). Abuse is a crime. It can occur at home or in a health care agency. All persons must be protected from abuse. This includes persons in a coma.

The abuser is usually a family member or caregiver—spouse, partner, adult child, and others. The abuser can be a friend, neighbor, landlord, or other person. Both men and women are abusers. Both men and women are abused.

State laws, accrediting agencies, and the Omnibus Budget Reconciliation Act of 1987 (OBRA) do not allow agencies to employ persons who were convicted of abuse, neglect, or mistreatment. Before hiring, the agency must thoroughly check the applicant's work history. All references are checked. Efforts must be made to find out about any criminal records.

The agency also checks the nursing assistant registry for findings of abuse, neglect, or mistreatment. It also is checked for mis-using or stealing a person's property.

See *Focus on Communication: Reporting Abuse.*

Vulnerable Adults

Vulnerable comes from the Latin word *vulnerare*, which means *to wound. Vulnerable adults are persons 18 years old or older who have disabilities or conditions that make them at risk to be wounded, attacked, or damaged.* They have problems caring for or protecting themselves due to:
- A mental, emotional, physical, or developmental disability. See Chapter 47 for "Developmental Disabilities."
- Brain damage.
- Changes from aging.

All patients and residents, regardless of age, are vulnerable. Older persons and children are at risk for abuse.

See *Focus on Long-Term Care and Home Care: Vulnerable Adults*, p. 40.

FOCUS ON LONG-TERM CARE AND HOME CARE
Vulnerable Adults

Home Care

Some persons have *behaviors and ways of living that threaten their health, safety, and well-being* (**self-neglect**). Causes include declining health and chronic disease. Other causes are disorders that impair judgment or memory—Alzheimer's disease, dementia, depression, and drug or alcohol abuse. Some persons refuse care.

Persons at risk for self-neglect include those who:
- Live alone.
- Are women. More women live alone than men.
- Are depressed.
- Are confused.
- Are older.
- Have alcohol or drug problems.
- Have a history of poor hygiene or living conditions.

The person has the right to personal choice, to make decisions for himself or herself, and to be independent. However, report warning signs of self-neglect to the nurse:
- Hoarding—saving, hiding, or storing things. For example, the person saves newspapers, magazines, food containers, shopping bags, and so on. The hoarding can present fire, pest (mice, rats, insects), and other safety hazards.
- Not eating enough food.
- Absence of food, water, heat, and other necessities.
- Failing to take needed drugs.
- Refusing to seek medical treatment for serious illnesses.
- Dehydration—poor urinary output, dry skin, dry mouth, confusion.
- Weight loss.
- Leaving a stove or oven unattended.
- Poor hygiene. The person has dirty hair, nails, or skin. He or she smells of urine or feces.
- Skin rashes.
- Pressure ulcers (Chapter 34).
- Not wearing the correct clothing for the weather. Or wearing dirty or torn clothing.
- Not having dentures, eyeglasses, hearing aids, walkers, wheelchairs, commodes, or other needed devices.
- Confusion, disorientation, hallucinations, or delusions (Chapter 46).
- Not attending to or not being able to attend to housekeeping.
- Safety hazards in the home (Chapter 12).
- Mis-using drugs or alcohol.
- The person's condition seems worse.
- The person has untreated health problems.

Elder Abuse

Elder abuse is any knowing, intentional, or negligent act by a caregiver or any other person to an older adult. The act causes harm or serious risk of harm. Elder abuse can take these forms:

- *Physical abuse.* This involves inflicting, or threatening to inflict, physical pain or injury. Grabbing, hitting, slapping, kicking, pinching, hair-pulling, or beating are examples. It also includes *corporal punishment*—punishment inflicted directly on the body. Beatings, lashings, and whippings are examples. Depriving the person of a basic need also is physical abuse.
- *Neglect. Failure to provide the person with the goods or services needed to avoid physical harm, mental anguish, or mental illness is called neglect.* This includes failure to provide health care or treatment, food, clothing, hygiene, shelter, or other needs. In health care, neglect includes but is not limited to:
  - Leaving persons lying or sitting in urine or feces
  - Keeping persons alone in their rooms or other areas
  - Failing to answer signal lights
- *Verbal abuse.* Verbal abuse is using oral or written words or statements that speak badly of, sneer at, criticize, or condemn the person. It includes unkind gestures, threats of harm, or saying things to frighten the person. For example, a person is told that he or she will never see family members again.
- *Involuntary seclusion.* This involves confining the person to a certain area. People have been locked in closets, basements, attics, bathrooms, and other spaces.
- *Financial exploitation or misappropriation.* To *exploit* means *to use unjustly. Misappropriate* means *to dishonestly, unfairly, or wrongly take for one's own use.* The older person's resources (money, property, assets) are mis-used by another person. Or the resources are used for the other person's profit or benefit. The person's money is stolen or used by another person. It is also mis-using a person's property. For example, children sell their mother's house without her consent.
- *Emotional or mental abuse.* This involves inflicting mental pain, anguish, or distress through verbal or nonverbal acts. Humiliation, harassment, ridicule, and threats of punishment are examples. It includes being deprived of needs such as food, clothing, care, a home, or a place to sleep.
- *Sexual abuse.* The person is harassed about sex or is attacked sexually. The person may be forced to perform sexual acts out of fear of punishment or physical harm.
- *Abandonment. Abandon* means *to leave or desert someone.* The person is deserted by someone who is supposed to give his or her care. Abandonment occurs when you:
  - Accept an assignment to care for a person or group of persons.
  - Accept the assignment for a certain time period.
  - Remove yourself from the care setting—home, hospital, nursing center, or other agency.
  - Do not report off to a staff member who will assume responsibility for care.

Examples of abandonment include:

- You leave the agency before your shift ends. You did not tell anyone that you were leaving.
- You do not report to a home care assignment. You are the only one providing care.
- You leave without completing a home care assignment.
- You sleep on the job. You are not available to provide care.

There are many signs of elder abuse. The abused person may show only some of the signs in Box 4-5.

Federal and state laws require the reporting of elder abuse. If abuse is suspected, it must be reported. Where and how to report abuse varies among states. You may suspect abuse. If so, discuss the matter and your observations with the nurse. Give as many details as possible. The nurse contacts health team members as needed.

The nurse also contacts community agencies that investigate elder abuse. They act at once if the problem is life-threatening. Sometimes the police or courts are involved.

Helping abused older persons is not always easy or possible. Some abuse is not reported or recognized. Or the investigating agency cannot gain access to the person. Sometimes older persons are abused by a spouse or adult child. A victim may want to protect the spouse or child. Some victims are embarrassed or believe abuse is deserved. A victim may fear what will happen. He or she may think that the present situation is better than no care at all. Some people fear not being believed if they report the abuse themselves.

Box 4-6 lists some severe cases of elder abuse. The abusers were convicted of crimes. The examples of abuse on p. 42 are more common. However, such abuse is still wrong. It will be investigated. You can lose your job. Your

---

BOX 4-5 SIGNS OF ELDER ABUSE

- Living conditions are unsafe, unclean, or inadequate.
- Personal hygiene is lacking. The person is not clean. Clothes are dirty.
- Weight loss—there are signs of poor nutrition and poor fluid intake.
- Assistive devices are missing or broken—eyeglasses, hearing aids, dentures, cane, walker, and so on.
- Medical needs are not met.
- Frequent injuries—conditions behind the injuries are strange or seem impossible.
- Old and new injuries—bruises, pressure marks, welts, scars, fractures, punctures, and so on.
- Complaints of pain or itching in the genital area.
- Bleeding and bruising around the breasts or in the genital area.
- Burns on the feet, hands, buttocks, or other parts of the body. Cigarettes and cigars cause small circle-like burns.
- Pressure ulcers (Chapter 34) or contractures (Chapter 27).
- The person seems very quiet or withdrawn.
- Unexplained withdrawal from normal activities.
- The person seems fearful, anxious, or agitated.
- Sudden change in alertness.
- Depression.
- Sudden changes in finances.
- The person does not seem to want to talk or answer questions.
- The person is restrained. Or the person is locked in a certain area for long periods.
- The person cannot reach toilet facilities, food, water, and other needed items.
- Private conversations are not allowed. The caregiver is present during all conversations.
- Strained or tense relationships with a caregiver.
- Frequent arguments with a caregiver.
- The person seems anxious to please the caregiver.
- Drugs are not taken properly. Drugs are not bought. Or too much or too little of the drug is taken.
- Emergency room visits may be frequent.
- The person may change doctors often. Some people do not have a doctor.

BOX 4-6 PROSECUTED CASES OF ELDER ABUSE

- A resident was complaining of pain while being cleaned. To stop him from complaining, a nursing assistant stuck a rag down his throat.
- A patient was screaming. To stop the patient from screaming, a nurse poured water down her throat.
- A nursing assistant beat and kicked a 92-year-old man who was lying on the floor.
- A nursing assistant stepped on a resident's face.
- A person was visiting his grandmother. While there, he sexually abused a patient with head injuries.
- A female patient in a wheelchair was dragged into a room by a nursing assistant. The nursing assistant forced the patient to have sex with him.
- A nursing assistant teased and taunted a resident with dementia.
- A health care worker repeatedly insulted an older woman because her son was gay.
- A nursing assistant forced a person to urinate in bed. Then the nursing assistant made fun of the person.
- Two older women lived in a board and care home. Both had Alzheimer's disease. They were left in a room with blood splattered on the walls. The carpet was caked with feces, vomitus, and urine. The women were partially dressed. One woman was tied to the bed with a sheet.
- A nursing assistant failed to feed a resident who could not feed herself. A video camera caught the nursing assistant dumping the person's food into trash cans.
- A resident could not talk. She totally depended on the staff for care. She did not have a bowel movement for 26 days. She was given a laxative every 3 days. No other treatment was given for her constipation.
- Caregivers willfully neglected to give drugs to residents.

From *Elder abuse and neglect: prosecution and prevention*, San Francisco, American Society on Aging.

state nursing assistant registry will be notified. Nursing assistants have lost their certification (license, registration) because of elder abuse.

- A person constantly crying out for help is taken to his room. He is left alone with the door closed.
- A person is told to be nice. Otherwise care will not be given.
- A person cannot control her bowels. She is called "dirty" and "disgusting."
- A person is turned in a rough and hurried manner.
- The nurse uses the person's phone to call a friend.
- A person lies in a wet and soiled bed all night.
- Money is taken from a person's wallet.
- A person uses the signal light a lot. It is taken away from the person.
- A person's mouth is forced open. Food is forced into the person's mouth.
- A person is told that her daughter does not visit because she is so mean.

See *Focus on Long-Term Care and Home Care: Elder Abuse.*

Child Abuse and Neglect

Child abuse and neglect involve the following:

- A child 18 years old or younger.
- Any recent act or failure to act on the part of a parent or caregiver.
- The act or failure to act results in death, serious physical or emotional harm, sexual abuse, or exploitation.
- The act or failure to act presents a likely or immediate risk for harm.

Child abuse and neglect occur at every social level. They occur in low-, middle-, and high-income families. The abuser's education level may be low to high. Often the abuser is a household member—parent, a parent's partner, brother or sister, nanny. Usually an abuser is someone the family knows. Risk factors for child abuse include:

- Stress
- Family crisis (divorce, unemployment, moving, poverty, crowded living conditions)
- Drug or alcohol abuse
- Abuser history of being abused as a child
- Discipline beliefs that include physical punishment
- Lack of emotional attachment to the child
- A child with birth defects or chronic illness
- A child with a personality or behaviors that the abuser considers "different" or not acceptable
- Unrealistic expectations for the child's behavior or performance
- Families that move often and do not have family or friends nearby

Types of Child Abuse and Neglect. Child abuse and neglect have many forms. Often more than one type is present.

- *Physical abuse* is injuring the child on purpose. It can cause death. Physical abuse includes striking, kicking, shaking, burning, or biting the child. Any action that physically impairs the child is physical abuse.
- *Neglect* can be physical or emotional. *Physical neglect* means to deprive the child of food, clothing, shelter, and medical care. *Emotional neglect* is not meeting the child's need for affection and attention.
- *Sexual abuse* is using, persuading, or forcing a child to engage in sexual conduct.
  - *Rape or sexual assault*—forced sexual acts with a person against his or her will.
  - *Molestation*—sexual advances toward a child. It includes kissing, touching, or fondling sexual areas. The abuser may kiss, touch, or fondle the child. Or the child is forced to kiss, touch, or fondle the abuser.
  - *Incest*—sexual activity between family members. The abuser may be a parent, brother or sister, aunt or uncle, cousin, or grandparent.
  - *Child pornography*—taking pictures or video-taping a child involved in sexual acts or poses.
  - *Child prostitution*—forcing a child to engage in sexual activity for money. Usually the child is forced to have many sexual partners.
- *Emotional abuse* is injuring the child mentally. The child has changes in behavior, emotional responses, thinking, reasoning, learning, and so on. The child may show anxiety, depression, withdrawal, or aggressive behaviors.

- *Substance abuse* is part of child abuse and neglect in some states. A *controlled substance* is a drug or chemical substance whose possession and use are controlled by law. Substance abuse involves:
  - Making a controlled substance in the presence of a child
  - Making a controlled substance on the premises occupied by a child
  - Allowing a child to be present where there are chemicals or equipment used to make or store a controlled substance
  - Selling, distributing, or giving drugs or alcohol to a child
  - Using a controlled substance (a caregiver) that impairs the caregiver's ability to adequately care for the child
  - Exposing the child to equipment and supplies for using, selling, or distributing drugs
  - Exposing the child to other drug-related activities
- *Abandonment* is when a parent's identity or whereabouts are unknown. The child is left by the parent in circumstances where the child suffers serious harm. Or the parent fails to maintain contact with the child or provide support for the child.

Box 4-7 lists the signs of child abuse and neglect. Report any changes in the child's body or behavior. Child and parent behaviors may signal that something is wrong. The child may be quiet and withdrawn. He or she may fear adults. Sometimes children are afraid to go home. Sudden behavior changes are common. Bed-wetting, thumb-sucking, loss of appetite, poor grades, and running away from home are examples. Some children attempt suicide.

Parents give different stories about what happened. Injuries are blamed on play accidents or other children. Frequent emergency room visits are common.

Child abuse is complex. Many more behaviors, signs, and symptoms are present than discussed here. You must be alert for signs and symptoms of child abuse. All states require the reporting of suspected child abuse. However, someone should not be falsely accused.

If you suspect child abuse, share your concerns with the nurse. Give as much detail as you can. The nurse contacts health team members and child protection agencies as needed.

Domestic Abuse

Domestic abuse—also called domestic violence, intimate partner abuse, partner abuse, and spousal abuse—occurs in relationships. One partner has power and control over the other through abuse. Fear and harm occur. Usually more than one type is present.

- *Physical abuse*—unwanted punching, slapping, grabbing, choking, poking, biting, pulling hair, twisting arms, or kicking. It may involve burns and weapons. Physical injuries occur. Death is a constant threat.
- *Sexual abuse*—unwanted sexual contact.

| **BOX 4-7** | **SIGNS AND SYMPTOMS OF CHILD ABUSE AND NEGLECT** |

Physical Abuse
- Bruises on the face (eyes, lips, mouth, cheeks), back, buttocks, abdomen, chest, and inner thighs.
- Welts on the face (lips, mouth, cheeks), back, buttocks, abdomen, chest, and inner thighs.
  - The shape of the object causing the welt may be seen. The shape may be of a belt, belt buckle, wooden spoon, chain, clothes hanger, rope, or other object.
- Burns and scalds on the feet, hands, back, buttocks, or other body parts.
  - Intentional burns leave a pattern from the item causing the burn. Cigarettes, irons, curling irons, ropes, stove burners, and radiators are examples.
  - In scalds, the area put in hot liquid is clearly marked. For example, a scald to the hand looks like a glove. A scald to the foot looks like a sock.
- Fractures of the nose, skull, arms, or legs.
- Bite marks.

Neglect
- Fails to gain weight.
- Shows great affection to others.
- Wants to eat large amounts of food.
- Steals food.
- Is dirty or has a severe body odor.
- Lacks the correct clothing for the weather.

Neglect—cont'd
- Abuses alcohol or drugs.
- States that no one is home.

Sexual Abuse
- Bleeding, cuts, and bruises of the genitalia, anus, breasts, or mouth.
- Stains or blood on underclothing.
- Painful urination.
- Signs and symptoms of urinary tract infection (Chapter 44).
- Vaginal discharge.
- Genital odor.
- Genital pain.
- Difficulty walking or sitting.
- Pregnancy.
- Fearful behaviors—nightmares, depression, unusual fears, attempts to run away.
- Sexual behavior that does not fit with one's age.

Emotional Abuse
- Sudden changes in self-confidence.
- Headaches.
- Stomach aches.
- Abnormal fears.
- Nightmares.
- Attempts to run away.

- *Verbal abuse*—unkind and hurtful remarks. They make the person feel unwhole, unattractive, and without value.
- *Economic abuse*—controlling money. Having or not having a job is controlled by the abuser. So are paychecks, money gifts from family and friends, and money for household expenses (food, clothing).
- *Social abuse*—controlling friendships and other relationships. The abuser controls phone calls, car use, leaving the home, and visits with family and friends.

Patients and residents can suffer from domestic abuse. For example, a husband slaps his wife during a visit. Or a wife uses her husband's money for herself rather than buying her husband's medicine.

Domestic abuse is a safety issue. Like child and elder abuse, domestic abuse is complex. The victim often hides the abuse. He or she may protect the abuser. State laws vary about reporting domestic abuse. However, the health team has an ethical duty to give information about safety and community resources. If you suspect domestic abuse, share your concerns with the nurse. The nurse gathers information to help the person.

See *Focus on Long-Term Care and Home Care: Domestic Abuse.*

FOCUS ON LONG-TERM CARE AND HOME CARE
Domestic Abuse

Long-Term Care
Under OBRA, the resident has the right to be free from abuse, mistreatment, and neglect. If a resident is abused by anyone, the abuse must be reported. This includes abuse by a partner.

FOCUS ON PRIDE
The Person, Family, and Yourself

Personal and Professional Responsibility
Negligence occurs when the person or the person's property is harmed. Events that harm or could harm a person are called *incidents* (Chapter 12). Agencies have procedures for reporting and recording incidents. An error may not cause harm. The error must still be reported.

You are responsible for your actions. If an error occurs, tell the nurse. Report and record the incident according to agency policy.

Rights and Respect
Patients and residents have the right to be free from abuse, mistreatment, and neglect. Health care agencies have procedures for investigating suspected abuse. Be alert for signs and symptoms of abuse. If you suspect that a person is being abused, tell the nurse. Share your observations with the nurse. Take pride in protecting persons from harm.

Independence and Social Interaction
You will interact closely with patients, residents, and families. You may begin to know them well. Social and professional relationships differ. To maintain professional boundaries:
- Follow the "Code of Conduct for Nursing Assistants" in Box 4-1.
- Obey the "Rules for Maintaining Professional Boundaries" in Box 4-2.
- Monitor for "Boundary Signs." See Box 4-3.
- Ask the nurse if you have a question about an interaction.

Use good judgment when interacting with patients, residents, and families. Take pride in being professional.

Delegation and Teamwork
Working within the limits of your role protects persons from harm. You must understand your roles and responsibilities to know when a task is outside these limits. For example, the nurse asks you to obtain a written consent for a procedure. You accept the task. As a result, the person is not given needed information about the procedure. The person suffers harm.

Sometimes refusing a delegated task is your right and duty. Accepting a task beyond the legal limits of your role can lead to negligence.

Ethics and Laws
Ethics and laws deal with right and wrong conduct. The following is a real account of an intentional tort committed by a nursing assistant:

A licensed nursing assistant (LNA) worked at a nursing center. She had her license suspended for using a resident's credit card. The card was used without the resident's knowledge or permission. The LNA signed the resident's name to the charges. The charges totaled about $1490. The LNA had also taken and used the credit card of a nurse employed at the center. Criminal charges of false impersonation were filed against the LNA.

The LNA was charged for:
- *Failing to comply with federal or state laws and rules*
- *Abusing or neglecting a patient*
- *Misappropriating patient property (p. 40)*
- *Being unfit or incompetent to function as a nursing assistant by reason of any cause*
- *Engaging in conduct of a character likely to deceive, defraud, or harm the public*

The LNA's license was suspended indefinitely. This means that the LNA:
- *Had to give her license to the Board.*
- *Could ask the Board to re-instate her license, but she had to prove that:*
  - *She posed no danger to the public or the practice of nursing.*
  - *She would safely and competently perform an LNA's duties.*
  - *She meets the requirements for license renewal and re-instatement.*

(State of Vermont Board of Nursing in regard to M. Willard, 2000.)

REVIEW QUESTIONS

Circle the BEST answer.

1 Ethics is
  a Making judgments before you have the facts
  b Knowledge of right and wrong conduct
  c A behavior that meets your needs, not the person's
  d A health team member's skills, care, and judgment

2 Which is ethical behavior?
  a Sharing information about a person with a friend
  b Accepting gifts from a resident's family
  c Reporting errors
  d Calling your family before answering a signal light

3 On your days off, you call the agency to check on a patient. This is a
  a Professional boundary   c Boundary violation
  b Boundary crossing   d Boundary sign

4 To maintain professional boundaries, your behaviors must
  a Help the person   c Be biased
  b Meet your needs   d Show that you care

5 You help with a friend's hospital care. This is a
  a Professional boundary   c Tort
  b Boundary crossing   d Crime

6 Which is *not* a crime?
  a Abuse   c Negligence
  b Murder   d Robbery

7 These statements are about negligence. Which is *false*?
  a It is an unintentional tort.
  b The negligent person did not act in a reasonable manner.
  c The person or the person's property was harmed.
  d A prison term is likely.

8 Threatening to touch the person's body without the person's consent is
  a Assault   c Defamation
  b Battery   d False imprisonment

9 Restraining a person's freedom of movement is
  a Assault   c Defamation
  b Battery   d False imprisonment

10 A person's photos are shown to others without consent. This is
  a Battery   c Invasion of privacy
  b Fraud   d Malpractice

11 You tell others that you are a nurse. This is
  a Negligence   c Libel
  b Fraud   d Slander

12 Informed consent is when the person
  a Fully understands all aspects of his or her treatment
  b Signs a consent form
  c Is admitted to the agency
  d Decides what to do with property after his or her death

13 Who is at risk for being wounded, attacked, or damaged?
  a Children
  b Older adults
  c Persons with disabilities
  d All patients and residents

14 Self-neglect is when
  a A caregiver harms a person
  b The person's behaviors put him or her at risk for harm
  c A person is deprived of food, clothing, hygiene, and shelter
  d The person does not receive attention or affection

15 You scold an older person for not eating lunch. This is
  a Physical abuse   c Battery
  b Neglect   d Verbal abuse

16 You leave a home care patient before completing your assignment. This is abuse by
  a Abandonment   c Involuntary seclusion
  b Neglect   d Control

17 You fall asleep at work. This is
  a Abandonment   c A boundary violation
  b Neglect   d Malpractice

18 Which is *not* a sign of elder abuse?
  a Stiff joints and joint pain
  b Old and new bruises
  c Poor personal hygiene
  d Frequent injuries

19 Depriving a child of food, clothing, and shelter is
  a Physical abuse   c Abandonment
  b Neglect   d Emotional abuse

20 A child has a black eye, bruises on the face, and bite marks on the arms. These are signs of
  a Physical abuse   c Neglect
  b Sexual abuse   d Substance abuse

21 A child is dirty and has a body odor. These are signs of
  a Physical abuse   c Neglect
  b Sexual abuse   d Substance abuse

22 Blood stains on a child's underpants are a sign of
  a Physical abuse   c Neglect
  b Sexual abuse   d Substance abuse

23 These statements are about domestic abuse. Which is *true*?
  a It always involves physical harm.
  b It always involves violence.
  c One partner has control over the other partner.
  d Only one type of abuse is usually present.

24 You suspect a person was abused. What should you do?
  a Tell the family.
  b Call the police.
  c Tell the nurse.
  d Ask the person about the abuse.

Answers to these questions are on p. 832.

5 Work Ethics

OBJECTIVES

- Define the key terms and key abbreviations listed in this chapter.
- Identify good health and hygiene practices.
- Describe how to look professional.
- Describe the qualities and traits of a successful nursing assistant.
- Explain how to get a job.
- Explain how to plan for childcare and transportation.
- Describe ethical behavior on the job.
- Explain how to manage stress.
- Explain the aspects of harassment.
- Explain how to resign from a job.
- Identify the common reasons for losing a job.
- Explain the reasons for drug testing.
- Explain how to promote PRIDE in the person, the family, and yourself.

KEY TERMS

confidentiality Trusting others with personal and private information

courtesy A polite, considerate, or helpful comment or act

gossip To spread rumors or talk about the private matters of others

harassment To trouble, torment, offend, or worry a person by one's behavior or comments

mentor See "preceptor"

preceptor A staff member who guides another staff member; mentor

priority The most important thing at the time

professionalism Following laws, being ethical, having good work ethics, and having the skills to do your work

stress The response or change in the body caused by any emotional, physical, social, or economic factor

stressor The event or factor that causes stress

teamwork Staff members work together as a group; each person does his or her part to provide safe and effective care

work ethics Behavior in the workplace

KEY ABBREVIATIONS

NATCEP Nursing assistant training and competency evaluation program

OBRA Omnibus Budget Reconciliation Act of 1987

As a nursing assistant, you must act and function in a professional manner. *Professionalism involves following laws, being ethical, having good work ethics, and having the skills to do your work.* Laws and ethics are discussed in Chapter 4. *Laws* are rules of conduct made by government bodies. *Ethics* deals with right and wrong conduct. It involves choices and judgments about what to do or what not to do. An ethical person does the right thing. In the workplace, certain behaviors (conduct), choices, and judgments are expected. *Work ethics deals with behavior in the workplace.* Your conduct reflects your choices and judgments. Work ethics involves:

- How you look
- What you say
- How you behave
- How you treat others
- How you work with others

The *Employee Handbook* of OSF Saint Francis Medical Center (Peoria, Ill.) says it best:

You are what people see when they arrive here; yours are the eyes they look into when they're frightened and lonely. Yours are the voices people hear when they ride the elevators, when they try to sleep, and when they try to forget their problems. You are what they hear on their way to appointments which could affect their destinies, and what they hear after they leave those appointments. Yours are the comments people hear when you think they can't.

Yours is the intelligence and caring that people hope they'll find here. If you're noisy, so is the medical center. If you're rude, so is the medical center. And if you're wonderful, so is the medical center.

HEALTH, HYGIENE, AND APPEARANCE

Patients, residents, families, and visitors expect the health team to look and act healthy. For example, a person is told to stop smoking. Yet health team members are seen smoking. If you are not clean, people wonder if you give good care. You are part of the health team. Your health, appearance, and hygiene need careful attention.

Your Health

You must give safe and effective care. To do so, you must be physically and mentally healthy. Otherwise you cannot function at your best.

- *Diet.* You need a balanced diet (Chapter 24). Start your day with a good breakfast. To maintain your weight, balance the calories you take in with your energy needs. To lose weight, take in fewer calories than your energy needs. Avoid foods high in fat, oil, and sugar. Also avoid salty foods and "crash" diets.
- *Sleep and rest.* Most adults need 7 to 8 hours of sleep daily. Fatigue, lack of energy, and being irritable mean you need more rest and sleep.
- *Body mechanics.* You will bend; carry heavy objects; and handle, move, and turn persons. These tasks place stress and strain on your body. You need to use your muscles correctly (Chapter 16).
- *Exercise.* Exercise is needed for muscle tone, circulation, and weight loss. Walking, running, swimming, and biking are good forms of exercise. Regular exercise helps you feel better physically and mentally. Consult your doctor before starting a vigorous exercise program.
- *Your eyes.* You will read instructions and take measurements. Wrong readings can cause the person harm. Have your eyes checked. Wear needed eyeglasses or contact lenses. Provide enough light for reading and fine work.
- *Smoking.* Smoking causes lung, heart, and circulatory disorders. Smoke odors stay on your breath, hands, clothing, and hair. Hand washing and good personal hygiene are needed.
- *Drugs.* Some drugs affect thinking, feeling, behavior, and function. Working under the influence of drugs affects the person's safety. Take only those drugs ordered by your doctor. Take them in the prescribed way.
- *Alcohol.* Alcohol is a drug that depresses the brain. It affects thinking, balance, coordination, and mental alertness. Never report to work under the influence of alcohol. Do not drink alcohol while working. Like other drugs, alcohol affects the person's safety.

Your Hygiene

Personal hygiene needs careful attention. Bathe daily. Use a deodorant or antiperspirant to prevent body odors. Brush your teeth often—upon awakening, before and after meals, and at bedtime. Use a mouthwash to prevent breath odors. Shampoo often. Style hair in a simple, attractive way. Keep fingernails clean, short, and neatly shaped.

Menstrual hygiene is important. Change tampons or sanitary pads often, especially for heavy flow. Wash your genital area with soap and water at least twice a day. Also practice good hand washing.

Foot care prevents odors and infection. Wash your feet daily. Dry thoroughly between the toes. Cut toenails straight across after bathing or soaking them.

Your Appearance

Good health and hygiene practices help you look and feel well. Follow the practices in Box 5-1, p. 48. They help you look clean, neat, and professional (Fig. 5-1, p. 48).

GETTING A JOB

There are easy ways to find out about jobs and places to work:

- Newspaper ads
- Local state employment services
- Agencies you would like to work at
- Phone book yellow pages
- People you know—your instructor, family, and friends
- The Internet
- Your school's or college's job placement counselors
- Your clinical experience site

Your clinical experience site is an important source. The staff always looks at students as future employees. They look for good work ethics. They watch how students treat patients, residents, and co-workers. They look for the qualities and traits described in Box 5-2, p. 49. If that agency is not hiring, the staff may suggest other places to apply.

BOX 5-1	PRACTICES FOR A PROFESSIONAL APPEARANCE

- Practice good hygiene.
- Wear uniforms that fit well. They are modest in length and style. Follow the agency's dress code.
- Keep uniforms clean, pressed, and mended. Sew on buttons. Repair zippers, tears, and hems.
- Wear a clean uniform daily.
- Wear your name badge or photo ID at all times when on duty. Make sure it can be seen. Wear it according to agency policy. It is best to wear it above your waist. Agencies may use first names only or first and last names. The agency may let you decide what to have on your name badge. For security reasons, some staff choose the first name only option.
- Wear undergarments that are clean and fit properly. Change them daily.
- Wear undergarments in the correct color for your skin tone. Do not wear colored (red, pink, blue, and so on) ones. They can be seen through white and light-colored uniforms.
- Cover tattoos (body art). They may offend others.
- Follow the agency's dress code for jewelry. Wedding and engagement rings may be allowed. Rings and bracelets can scratch a person. Confused or combative persons can easily pull on jewelry (necklaces, dangling earrings). So can young children.
- Do not wear jewelry in pierced eyebrows, nose, lips, or tongue while on duty.
- Follow the agency's dress code for earrings. Usually small, simple earrings are allowed. For multiple ear piercings, usually only one set of earrings is allowed.
- Wear a wristwatch with a second (sweep) hand.
- Wear clean stockings and socks that fit well. Change them daily.
- Wear shoes that fit properly, are comfortable, give needed support, and have non-skid soles. Do not wear sandals or open-toed shoes.
- Clean and polish shoes often. Wash and replace laces as needed.
- Keep fingernails clean, short, and neatly shaped. Long nails can scratch a person. Nails must be natural.
- Do not wear nail polish. Chipped nail polish may provide a place for microbes to grow.
- Have a simple, attractive hairstyle. Hair is off your collar and away from your face. Use simple pins, combs, barrettes, and bands to keep long hair up and in place.
- Keep beards and mustaches clean and trimmed.
- Use make-up that is modest in amount and moderate in color. Avoid a painted and severe look.
- Do not wear perfume, cologne, or after-shave lotion. The scents may offend, nauseate, or cause breathing problems in patients and residents.

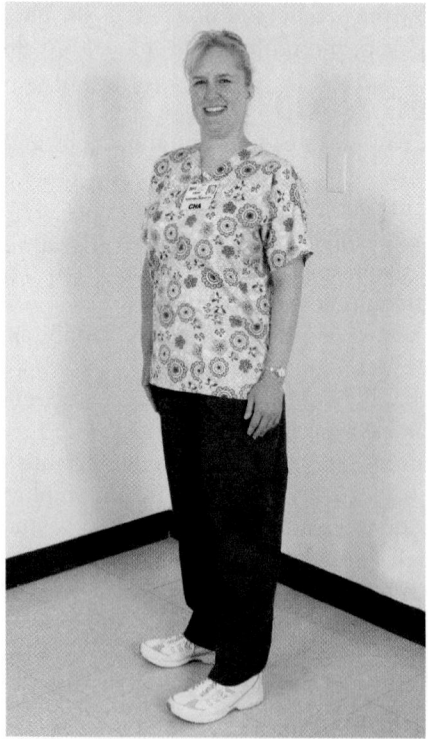

Fig. 5-1 This nursing assistant is well-groomed. Her uniform and shoes are clean. Her hair has a simple style. It is away from her face and off of her collar. She does not wear jewelry.

What Employers Look For

If you owned a business, who would you hire? Your answer helps you better understand the employer's point of view. Employers want people who:

- Are dependable.
- Are well-groomed.
- Have needed job skills and training.
- Have values and attitudes that fit with the agency.

Good work ethics involves the qualities and traits described in Box 5-2. They are necessary for you to function well (Fig. 5-2).

Applicants who look good communicate many things to the employer. You have one chance to make a good first impression. A well-groomed person will likely get the job. A sloppy person with wrinkled or dirty clothes may not get the job. Nor will someone with body or breath odors. See p. 52 for how to dress for an interview.

Being dependable is important. You must be at work on time and when scheduled. Undependable people cause everyone problems. Other staff take on extra work. Fewer people give care. Quality of care suffers. Supervisors spend time trying to find out if the person is coming to work. They also have to find someone to cover for the absent employee. You want co-workers to work when scheduled. Otherwise, you have extra work. You have less time to spend with patients and residents. Likewise, co-workers also expect you to work when scheduled.

See *Focus on Long-Term Care and Home Care: What Employers Look For.*

BOX 5-2 QUALITIES AND TRAITS FOR GOOD WORK ETHICS

- **Caring.** Have concern for the person. Help make the person's life happier, easier, or less painful.
- **Dependable.** Report to work on time and when scheduled. Perform delegated tasks. Keep obligations and promises.
- **Considerate.** Respect the person's physical and emotional feelings. Be gentle and kind toward patients, residents, families, and co-workers.
- **Cheerful.** Greet and talk to people in a pleasant manner. Do not be moody, bad-tempered, or unhappy while at work.
- **Empathetic.** Empathy is seeing things from the person's point of view—putting yourself in the person's place. How would you feel if you had the person's problems?
- **Trustworthy.** Patients, residents, families, and staff have confidence in you. They believe you will keep information confidential. They trust you not to gossip about patients, residents, families, or the health team.
- **Respectful.** Patients and residents have rights, values, beliefs, and feelings. They may differ from yours. Do not judge or condemn the person. Treat the person with respect and dignity at all times. Also show respect for the health team.
- **Courteous.** Be polite and courteous to patients, residents, families, visitors, and co-workers. See p. 57 for common courtesies in the workplace.
- **Conscientious.** Be careful, alert, and exact in following instructions. Give thorough care. Do not lose or damage the person's property.
- **Honest.** Accurately report the care given, your observations, and any errors.
- **Cooperative.** Willingly help and work with others. Also take that "extra step" during busy and stressful times.
- **Enthusiastic.** Be eager, interested, and excited about your work. Your work is important.
- **Self-aware.** Know your feelings, strengths, and weaknesses. You need to understand yourself before you can understand patients and residents.

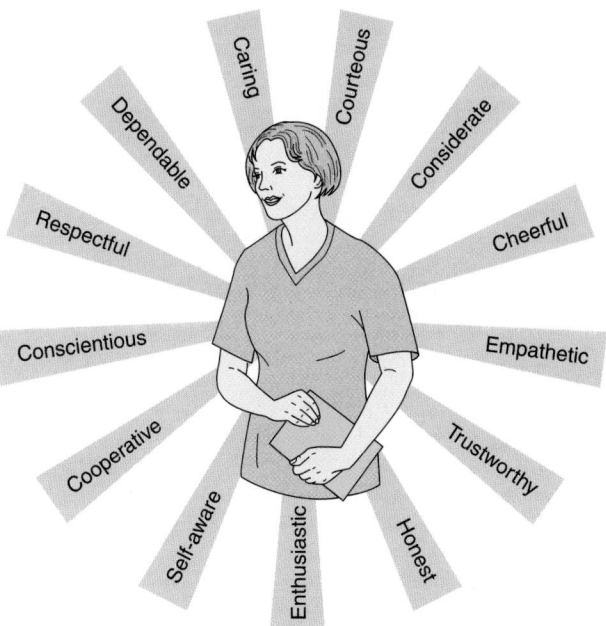

Fig. 5-2 Good work ethics involves these qualities and traits.

FOCUS ON LONG-TERM CARE AND HOME CARE
What Employers Look For

Home Care

Besides the qualities and traits listed in Box 5-2, home care requires:

- *The ability to work alone.* The nurse makes some home visits. Usually a nurse is not with you in the home. If problems occur, you can reach the nurse by phone. You must provide skillful and safe care.
- *Self-discipline.* You must arrive at homes on time. Plan activities so personal care needs and housekeeping tasks get done. Avoid temptations. This includes watching TV, talking on the phone, visiting, and stopping for a cup of coffee.
- *Honesty.* You might need to shop for the person. Be honest and thrifty with the person's money. Accurately report what you bought, the cost with receipts, amount spent, and amount of money returned.
- *Respect for the person's property.* You will handle valuables and personal property in health care settings. Access to the person's property is greater in the home. You use furnishings, appliances, linens, and household items to give care and for housekeeping. Treat personal and family property with respect. Prevent damage. Read the manufacturer's instructions before using any appliance. Clean the appliance after use.

Job Skills and Training. Employers need to know that you have the required job skills. The employer checks the nursing assistant registry and requests proof of training:
- A certificate of course completion
- A high school, college, or technical school transcript
- An official grade report (report card)

Give the employer a *copy* of your certificate, transcript, or grade report. Never give the original to anyone. Keep it in a safe place for future use. The employer may want a transcript sent directly from the school or college.

See *Focus on Long-Term Care and Home Care: Job Skills and Training.*

FOCUS ON LONG-TERM CARE AND HOME CARE
Job Skills and Training

Long-Term Care

To work in long-term care, you must complete a state-approved nursing assistant training and competency evaluation program (NATCEP). This is a requirement of the Omnibus Budget Reconciliation Act of 1987 (OBRA). The employer requests proof of training. The nursing assistant registry is checked. Nursing centers cannot hire persons convicted of abuse, neglect, or mistreatment. This also is an OBRA requirement.

Home Care

Home care agencies that receive Medicare funds must meet OBRA requirements. You must complete a NATCEP outlined by OBRA. Some states have additional training requirements for working in home care.

Job Applications

You get a job application from the *personnel office* or *human resources office* (Fig. 5-3). You can complete the application there. Or take it home for return by mail or in person. You must be well-groomed and behave pleasantly when seeking or returning a job application. It may be your first chance to make a good impression.

To complete a job application, follow the guidelines in Box 5-3, p. 52. How you fill out the application may mean getting or not getting the job. Often the application is your first chance to impress the employer. A neat, readable, and complete application gives a good image. A sloppy or incomplete one does not.

EMPLOYMENT APPLICATION

APPLICANT INSTRUCTIONS

If you need help filling out this application form or for any phase of the employment process, please notify the person that gave you this form and every effort will be made to accommodate your needs in a reasonable amount of time.

1. Please read "APPLICANT NOTE" below.
2. Complete both sides of this page.
3. If more space is needed to complete any question, use comments section at the bottom of this page.
4. Print clearly: incomplete or illegible applications will not be processed. PLEASE NOTE "NOT APPLICABLE" IF NOT ANSWERING A QUESTION.
5. Provide only requested information. Failure to do so may result in disqualification of your application.
6. Some packets may include an AFFIRMATIVE ACTION QUESTIONNAIRE. This information is being gathered for affirmative action under Section 503 of the Rehabilitation Act of 1973. The information requested is voluntary and will be kept confidential. An applicant will not be subject to any adverse treatment for refusing to complete the questionnaire.
7. DO NOT FILL OUT ANY OTHER ATTACHED FORMS OR PAGES UNTIL INSTRUCTED.

TODAY'S DATE: _____

NAME: _____
                LAST   FIRST   MI

SOCIAL SECURITY NUMBER: _____

HOME PHONE: _____ WORK PHONE: _____

CURRENT ADDRESS: _____
                 STREET

                 CITY   STATE   ZIP

PRIOR ADDRESS: _____
                 STREET

                 CITY   STATE   ZIP

APPLICANT NOTE

This application form is intended for use in evaluating your qualifications for employment. This is not an employment contract. Please answer all appropriate questions completely and accurately. False or misleading statements during the interview and on this form are grounds for terminating the application process or, if discovered after employment, terminating employment. All qualified applicants will receive consideration without discrimination based on sex, marital status, race, color, age, creed, national origin, sexual orientation, military reserve membership, ancestry, religion, height, weight, use of a guide or support animal because of blindness, deafness or physical handicap, or the presence of disabilities. A conviction will not necessarily bar an applicant from employment. Additional testing of job-related skills and for the presence of drugs in your body may be required prior to employment. After an offer of employment, and prior to reporting to work, you may be required to submit to a medical review. Depending on company policy and the needs of the job, you will be required to complete a medical history form and may be required to be examined by a medical professional designated by the company.

AVAILABILITY

For which position are you applying? _____

What date can you start? _____ What category would you prefer? ❏ Full time ❏ Part time ❏ Temporary ❏ Labor pool

For which schedules are you available?* ❏ Weekdays ❏ Weekends ❏ Evenings ❏ Nights ❏ Overtime ❏ Shift ❏ Other_____

*reasonable efforts will be made to accommodate sincerely held moral and ethical beliefs, (WI) religious beliefs and practices (All other States)

JOB-RELATED SKILLS

NOTE: Do not fill out any part of this section you believe to be non-job related.

❏ Yes   ❏ No   If the job requires, do you have the appropriate valid drivers license?
              Name on license _____ DL#_____ Type _____ State of Issue_____

❏ Yes   ❏ No   Have you had any moving violations within the last seven years? Please describe._____
              Please list any other skills, licenses or certificates that may be job-related or that you feel would be of value to this job or company. _____

❏ Yes   ❏ No   Have you been given a job description or had the essential functions of the job explained to you?

❏ Yes   ❏ No   Do you understand these essential functions?

❏ Yes   ❏ No   Can you perform the essential functions of this job with or without reasonable accommodation?

SECURITY

List states and counties of residence for the past seven years: _____

❏ Yes   ❏ No   Have you used any names or Social Security Numbers other than given above? If so, please list in comments, below.

❏ Yes   ❏ No   Have you been convicted of a crime in the past seven years? If so, please describe in the boxes below. (Conviction will not necessarily be a bar to employment. In accordance with company policy and applicable state and federal laws, factors such as age at time of the offense, remoteness of the offense, time since last conviction, nature of the job sought and rehabilitation effort will be reviewed.)

INCIDENT	CITY/STATE	CHARGE
1.		
2.		

COMMENTS

(ASK FOR AN ADDITIONAL PAGE IF NECESSARY) _____

_____

_____

_____

Fig. 5-3 A sample job application.

PREVIOUS EMPLOYERS

PLEASE NOTE: Your application will <u>not be</u> considered unless every question in this section is answered. Since we will make every effort to contact previous employers, the **correct telephone numbers of past employers are critical.** Ask for a phone book or call information if necessary. FOR EMPLOYERS OUTSIDE THE U.S., A CURRENT FAX NUMBER IS MANDATORY.

MOST RECENT EMPLOYER

❏ Yes ❏ No Are you currently working for this employer?
❏ Yes ❏ No If yes, may we contact?

PHONE (   )
FAX   (   )

COMPANY NAME   CITY   STATE

FROM   TO
DATES EMPLOYED   JOB TITLE   SUPERVISOR NAME

DUTIES

        PER
SALARY   (HOUR, WEEK, MONTH)   REASON FOR LEAVING

SECOND MOST RECENT EMPLOYER

PHONE (   )
FAX   (   )

COMPANY NAME   CITY   STATE

FROM   TO
DATES EMPLOYED   JOB TITLE   SUPERVISOR NAME

DUTIES

        PER
SALARY   (HOUR, WEEK, MONTH)   REASON FOR LEAVING

THIRD MOST RECENT EMPLOYER

PHONE (   )
FAX   (   )

COMPANY NAME   CITY   STATE

FROM   TO
DATES EMPLOYED   JOB TITLE   SUPERVISOR NAME

DUTIES

        PER
SALARY   (HOUR, WEEK, MONTH)   REASON FOR LEAVING

REFERENCES

Include only individuals familiar with your work ability. Do not include relatives.

NAME	ADDRESS/PHONE	YEARS KNOWN/RELATIONSHIP
1.		
2.		

EDUCATION

NOTE: Do not fill out any part of this section you believe to be non-job related.
Please circle highest grade completed.   7   8   9   10   11   12   13   14   15   16   16+

If your school records are under a different name than listed on page 1, please enter that name_____

NAME	CITY/STATE	GRADUATED	DEGREE?
HIGH SCHOOL			
COLLEGE			
OTHER			

CERTIFICATION AND RELEASE

I certify that I have read and understand the applicant note on page one of this form and that the answers given by me to the foregoing questions and the statements made by me are complete and true to the best of my knowledge and belief. I understand that any false information, omissions or misrepresentations of facts called for in this application, whether on this document or not, may result in rejection of my application or discharge at any time during my employment. I authorize the company and/or its agents, including consumer reporting bureaus, to verify any of this information. I authorize all former employers, persons, schools, companies and law enforcement authorities from any liability for any damage whatsoever for issuing this information. I also understand that the use of illegal drugs is prohibited during employment. If company policy requires, I am willing to submit to drug testing to detect the use of illegal drugs prior to and during employment.

SIGNATURE   DATE

© ADP SCREENING & SELECTION SERVICES 2002

Fig. 5-3, cont'd For legend see facing page.

BOX 5-3   GUIDELINES FOR COMPLETING A JOB APPLICATION

- Read and follow the directions. They may ask you to print using black ink. You must follow directions on the job. Employers look at job applications to see if you can follow directions.
- Write neatly. Writing must be readable. A messy application gives a bad image. Readable writing gives the correct information. The agency cannot contact you if unable to read your phone number. You may miss getting the job.
- Complete the entire form. Something may not apply to you. If so, write "N/A" for non-applicable. Or draw a line through the space. This shows that you read the section. It also shows that you did not skip the item on purpose.
- Report any felony arrests or convictions as directed. Write "no" or "none" as appropriate. Criminal background and fingerprint checks are common requirements.
- Give information about employment gaps. If you did not work for a time, the employer wonders why. Providing this information shows you are honest. Some reasons are an illness, going to school, raising your children, or caring for an ill or older family member.
- Tell why you left a job, if asked. Be brief, but honest. People leave jobs for one that pays better. Some leave for career advancement. Others leave for reasons given for employment gaps. If you were fired from a job, give an honest but positive response. Do not talk badly about a former employer.
- Provide references. Be prepared to give names, titles, addresses, and phone numbers of at least four non-family references. Have this information written down before completing an application. (Always ask references if an employer can contact them.) You may get the job faster if the employer can quickly check references. If they are missing or not complete, the employer waits for all the information. This wastes your time and the employer's time. Also, the employer wonders if you are hiding something with incomplete reference information.
- Be prepared to provide the following:
  - Social Security number
  - Proof of citizenship or legal residency
  - Proof of successful NATCEP completion
  - Identification—driver's license or government-issued ID card
- Give honest responses. Lying on an application is fraud. It is grounds for being fired.
- Keep a file of your education and work history.

Some agencies have job applications on-line. Follow the instructions for completing and sending an on-line application.

A job application is easier to complete if you have a file of your education and work history. The file should contain:

- A copy of your high school diploma or general equivalency diploma (GED).
- A copy of any grade reports, degrees, certificates, or military training.
- A copy of your NATCEP certificate of completion.
- Nursing assistant registry information for each state in which you are registered.
- Copies of communications with your state's nursing assistant registry agency.
- Copies of court records for criminal convictions.
- A copy of your Social Security card.
- Names, addresses, and phone numbers of references.
- Names, addresses, and phone numbers of current and past employers. Include:
  - Your job title
  - Dates employment started and ended
  - Your supervisor's name
  - Hourly salary
- Proof of in-services attended and continuing education units (CEUs).

The Job Interview

A job interview is when the employer gets to know and evaluate you. You also find out more about the agency.

The interview may be when you complete the job application. Some agencies schedule interviews after reviewing applications. Write down the interviewer's name and the interview date and time. If you need directions to the agency, ask for them at this time.

Preparing for the Interview. Box 5-4 lists common interview questions. Prepare your answers ahead of time. Also prepare a list of your skills. Give the list to the interviewer.

You must present a good image. You need to be neat, clean, and well-groomed (Fig. 5-4). How you dress is important. Follow the guidelines in Box 5-5.

Be on time. It shows you are dependable. Go to the agency some day before your interview. Note how long it takes to get there and where to park. Also find the personnel office. A *dry run* (practice run) gives an idea of how long it takes to get from your home to the personnel office.

When you arrive for the interview, turn off your wireless phone or pager. Tell the receptionist your name and why you are there. Also give the interviewer's name. Then sit quietly in the waiting area. Do not smoke, chew gum, or use your phone. While you wait, review your answers to the common interview questions. Waiting may be part of the interview. The interviewer may ask the receptionist about how you acted while waiting. Smile, and be polite and friendly.

During the Interview. Politely greet the interviewer. A firm hand-shake is correct for men and women. Address the interviewer as Miss, Mrs., Ms., Mr., or Doctor. Stand until asked to sit. Sit with good posture and in a professional way. If offered a beverage, you may accept. Be sure to thank the person.

Good eye contact is needed. Look directly at the interviewer when you answer or ask questions. Poor eye contact

BOX 5-4 COMMON INTERVIEW QUESTIONS

What the Interviewer May Ask You:
- Tell me about yourself.
- Tell me about your career goals.
- What are you doing to reach these goals?
- Describe what *professional* behavior means to you.
- Tell me about your last job. Why did you leave?
- What did you like the most about your last job? What did you like the least?
- What would your supervisor and co-workers tell me about you? Your dependability? Your skills? Your flexibility?
- Which functions are the hardest for you? How do you handle this difficulty?
- How do you set your priorities?
- How have your experiences prepared you for this job?
- What would you like to change about your last job?
- How do you handle problems with patients, residents, families, and co-workers?
- Why do you want to work here?
- Why should this agency hire you?

Questions You May Ask the Interviewer:
- Which job functions do you think are the most important?
- What employee qualities and traits are the most important to you?
- What nursing care pattern is used here (Chapter 1)?
- Who will I work with?
- When are performance evaluations done? Who does them? How are they done?

Questions You May Ask the Interviewer:—cont'd
- What performance factors are evaluated?
- How does the supervisor handle problems?
- What are the most common reasons that nursing assistants lose their jobs here?
- What are the most common reasons that nursing assistants resign from their jobs here?
- How do you see this job in the next year? In the next 5 years?
- What is the greatest reward from this job?
- What is the greatest challenge from this job?
- What do you like the most about nursing assistants who work here? What do you like the least?
- Why should I work here rather than in another agency?
- Why are you interested in hiring me?
- How much will I make an hour?
- What hours will I work?
- What uniforms are required?
- What benefits do you offer?
  - Health and disability insurance?
  - Continuing education?
  - Vacation time?
- Does the agency have a new employee orientation program? How long is it?
- May I have a tour of the agency and the unit I will work on? Will you introduce me to the nurse manager and unit staff?
- Can I have a few minutes to talk to the nurse manager?

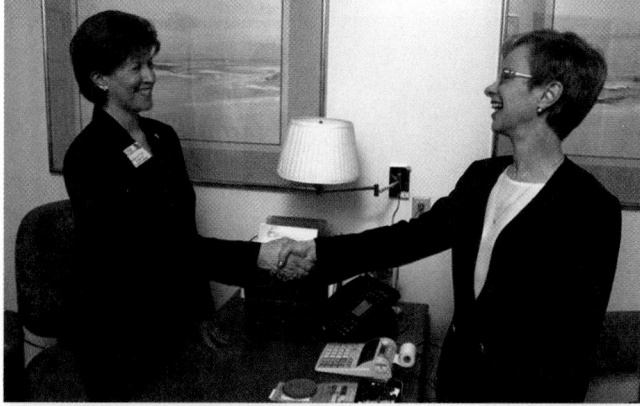

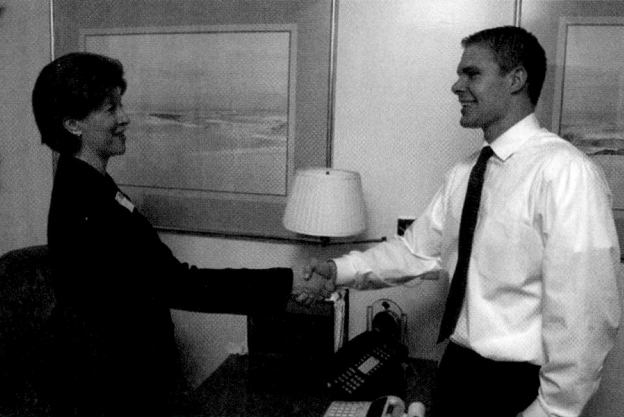

Fig. 5-4 A, A simple suit is worn for a job interview. **B,** This man wears slacks and a shirt and tie for his interview.

BOX 5-5 GROOMING AND DRESSING FOR AN INTERVIEW

- Bathe and brush your teeth. Wash your hair.
- Use deodorant or antiperspirant.
- Make sure your hands and fingernails are clean.
- Apply make-up in a simple, attractive manner.
- Style your hair in a neat and attractive way. Wear it as you would for work.
- Do not wear jeans, shorts, tank tops, halter tops, or other casual clothing.
- Iron clothing. Sew on loose buttons and mend garments as needed.
- Wear clothing that covers tattoos (body art).
- Wear a simple dress, skirt and blouse, or suit (women). Wear a suit or dark slacks and a shirt and tie (men). A jacket is optional. A long-sleeved white or light blue shirt is best.
- Wear socks (men and women) or hose (women). Hose should be free of runs and snags.
- Make sure shoes are clean and in good repair.
- Avoid heavy perfumes, colognes, and after-shave lotions. A light fragrance is okay.
- Wear only simple jewelry that complements your clothes. Avoid adornments in body piercings. If you have multiple ear piercings, wear only one set of earrings.
- Stop in the restroom when you arrive for the interview. Check your hair, make-up, and clothes.

sends negative information—being shy, insecure, dishonest, or lacking interest.

Watch your body language (Chapter 8). Body language involves facial expressions, gestures, posture, and body movements. What you say is important. However, how you use and move your body also tells a great deal. Avoid distracting habits—biting nails; playing with jewelry, clothing, or your hair; crossing your arms; and swinging legs back and forth. Focus on the interview. Do not touch or read things on the person's desk.

The interview lasts 15 to 45 minutes. Give complete and honest answers. Speak clearly and with confidence. Avoid short and long answers. "Yes" and "no" answers give little information. Briefly explain "yes" and "no" responses (Chapter 8).

The interviewer will ask about your skills. Share your skills list. You may be asked about a skill not on your list. Explain that you are willing to learn the skill if your state allows nursing assistants to perform the task.

Find the right job for you. An employer wants to hire someone who will be happy in the job and the agency. Box 5-4 lists some questions for you to ask at the end of the interview. The person's answers will help you decide if the job is right for you.

Review the job description with the interviewer. Ask any questions at this time. Advise the interviewer of functions you cannot perform because of training, legal, ethical, or religious reasons. Honesty now prevents problems later.

The interviewer signals the end of the interview. You may be offered a job at this time. Or you are told when to expect a call or letter. Follow-up is acceptable. Ask when you can check on your application. Before leaving, thank the interviewer. Say that you look forward to hearing from him or her. Shake the person's hand before you leave.

After the Interview.   A thank-you letter or note is advised (Fig. 5-5). Write this within 24 hours after the interview. Write neatly and clearly. Use a computer or typewriter if your writing is hard to read. The thank-you note should include:

- The date
- The interviewer's formal name using Miss, Mrs., Ms., Mr., or Dr.
- A statement thanking the person for the interview
- Comments about the interview, the agency, and your eagerness to hear about the job
- Your signature using your first and last names
  See *Focus on Long-Term Care and Home Care: The Job Interview.*

December 12

Dear Ms. O'Neal,

Thank you for the interview yesterday. I enjoyed meeting you and learning more about the nursing center. I was impressed by the friendliness of the staff and would enjoy working in that environment.

Again, thank you. I look forward to hearing from you soon.

Sincerely,
Alison M. Teal

Fig. 5-5 Sample thank-you note written after a job interview.

FOCUS ON LONG-TERM CARE AND HOME CARE
The Job Interview

Home Care
You need to ask more questions when interviewing with a home care agency:

- What part of the community does the agency serve?
- What neighborhoods will you go to?
- How far will you have to travel between homes?
- Do you use your own car or an agency car?
- If you use your own car, how are you paid for mileage?
- Will you use public transportation? If yes, who pays for bus or train fares? If the agency pays, are you given fare money beforehand or repaid later?

Accepting a Job

Accept the job that is best for you. You can apply many places and have many interviews. Think about all offers before accepting one. You might have more questions about an agency. Ask them before accepting the job. To help you decide, discuss the offer with a family member, friend, co-worker, or your instructor.

When you accept a job, agree on a starting date, pay rate, and work hours. Ask where to report on your first day. Ask for such information in writing. That way you and the agency have the same understanding of the job offer. Use the written offer later if questions arise. Also ask for the employee handbook and other agency information. Read everything before you start working.

New Employee Orientation

Agencies have orientation programs for new employees. The policy and procedure manual is reviewed. Your skills are checked. That is, the agency has you perform the procedures in your job description. This is to make sure that you do them safely and correctly. Also, you are shown how to use the agency's supplies and equipment.

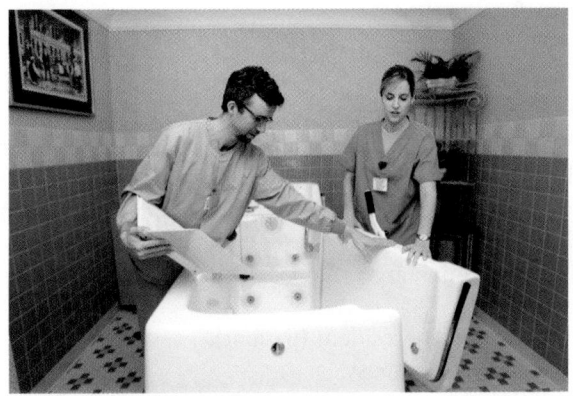

Fig. 5-6 A nurse preceptor shows a new nursing assistant how to use a whirlpool tub.

Preceptor programs are common. A *preceptor (mentor) is a staff member who guides another staff member* (Fig. 5-6). A nurse or nursing assistant:

- Helps you learn the agency's layout so you can find what you need.
- Introduces you to patients, residents, and staff.
- Helps you organize your work.
- Helps you feel comfortable as a part of the nursing team.
- Answers questions about the policy and procedure manual.

A nursing assistant preceptor is not your supervisor. Only nurses can supervise. A preceptor program usually lasts 2 to 4 weeks. Its purpose is to help you succeed in your role. It also helps ensure quality care. After the preceptor program, you should feel comfortable with the setting and your role. If not, ask for more orientation time.

PREPARING FOR WORK

You successfully completed a NATCEP. You had a successful job interview. To keep your job, you must function well and work well with others. You must:

- Work when scheduled.
- Get to work on time.
- Stay the entire shift.

Absences and tardiness (being late) are common reasons for losing a job. Childcare and transportation issues often interfere with getting to work. They need careful planning.

Childcare

Someone needs to care for your children when you leave for work, while you are at work, and before you get home. Also plan for emergencies:

- Your childcare provider is ill or cannot care for your children that day.
- A child becomes ill or injured while you are at work.
- You will be late getting home from work.

Transportation

Plan for getting to and from work. If you drive, keep your car in good working order. Keep enough gas in the car. Or leave early to get gas.

Carpooling is an option. Carpool members depend on each other. If the driver is late leaving, everyone is late for work. If one person is not ready when the driver arrives, everyone is late for work. Carpool with persons you trust to be ready and on time. When you drive, leave and pick up others on time. As a passenger, be ready to be picked up on time.

Know your bus or train schedule. Know what other bus or train to take if delays occur. Always carry enough money for fares to and from work.

Always have a back-up plan for getting to work. Your car may not start, the carpool driver may not go to work, or public transportation may not run.

TEAMWORK

Teamwork means that staff members work together as a group. Each person does his or her part to provide safe and effective care. Teamwork involves:

- Working when scheduled.
- Being cheerful and friendly.
- Performing delegated tasks.
- Being available to help others. Help willingly.
- Being kind to others.

You are an important member of the health team. Quality of care is affected by how you work with others and how you feel about your job.

Attendance

Report to work when scheduled and on time. The entire unit is affected when just one person is late. Call the agency if you will be late or cannot go to work. Follow the attendance policy in your employee handbook. Poor attendance can cause you to lose your job.

Be *ready to work* when your shift starts. Store your coat, purse, backpack, and other items before your shift starts. Use the restroom when you arrive at the agency. Arrive on your nursing unit a few minutes early. This gives you time to greet others and settle yourself.

Attendance also means staying the entire shift. Prepare for childcare emergencies. Watching the clock for when your shift ends gives a bad image. You may need to work over-time. Prepare to stay longer if necessary. When it is time to leave, report off duty to the nurse.

See *Focus on Communication: Attendance*, p. 56.
See *Teamwork and Time Management: Attendance*, p. 56.
See *Focus on Long-Term Care and Home Care: Attendance*, p. 56.

Your Attitude

You need a good attitude (see Box 5-2). Show that you enjoy your work. Listen to others. Be willing to learn. Stay busy, and use your time well.

Your work is very important. Nurses, patients, residents, and families rely on you for good care. They expect you to be pleasant and respectful. You must believe that you and your work have value.

Always think before you speak. These statements signal a bad attitude:

- "That's not my resident (patient)."
- "I can't. I'm too busy."
- "I didn't do it."
- "I don't feel like it."
- "It's not my fault."
- "Don't blame me."
- "It's not my turn. I did it yesterday."
- "Nobody told me."
- "That's not my job."
- "You didn't say that you needed it right away."
- "I work harder than anyone else."
- "No one appreciates what I do."
- "I'm tired of this place."
- "Is it time to leave yet?"
- "Good luck. I had a horrible day."

Gossip

To *gossip means to spread rumors or talk about the private matters of others.* Gossiping is unprofessional and hurtful. To avoid being a part of gossip:

- Remove yourself from a group or setting where people are gossiping.
- Do not make or repeat any comment that can hurt a person, family member, visitor, co-worker, or the agency.
- Do not make or repeat any comment that you do not know is true. Making or writing false statements about another person is defamation (Chapter 4).
- Do not talk about patients, residents, family members, visitors, co-workers, or the agency at home or in social settings, by email, instant messaging, text messages, or social networking sites (Twitter, Facebook, MySpace, and others).

Confidentiality

The person's information is private and personal. *Confidentiality means trusting others with personal and private information.* The person's information is shared only among the staff involved in his or her care. The person has the right to privacy and confidentiality. Agency, family, and co-worker information also is confidential.

FOCUS ON COMMUNICATION

Confidentiality

Your family and friends may ask you about people they know in the agency. They may ask about patients, residents, families, or employees. For example, your mother says: "Mrs. Drew goes to our church. I heard that she's in your nursing home. What's wrong with her?"

Do not share any information with your family and friends. Doing so violates the person's right to privacy and confidentiality (Chapters 2 and 4). You can say: "I'm sorry, but I can't tell you about anyone in the center. It is unprofessional and against center policies. And it violates the person's right to privacy and confidentiality. Please don't ask me about anyone in the center."

Share information only with the nurse. Avoid talking about patients, residents, families, the agency, or co-workers when others are present. Do not talk about them in hallways, elevators, dining areas, or outside the agency. Others may overhear you. Patients, residents, and visitors are very alert to comments. They think you are talking about them or their loved ones. This leads to wrong information and wrong impressions about the person's condition. You can easily upset the person or family. Be very careful about what, how, when, and where you say things.

Do not eavesdrop. To *eavesdrop* means to listen in or overhear what others are saying. It invades a person's privacy.

Many agencies have intercom systems. They allow for communication between the bedside and the nurses' station (Chapter 18). The person uses the intercom to signal when help is needed. Someone at the nurses' station answers the intercom. The nursing team also uses the intercom to communicate with each other. Be careful what you say over the intercom. It is like a loud speaker. Others nearby can hear what you are saying.

See *Focus on Communication: Confidentiality.*

Hygiene and Appearance

How you look affects the way people think about you and the agency. If the staff are clean and neat, people think the agency is clean and neat. They think the agency is unclean if the staff are messy and unkempt. People also wonder about the quality of care given.

Home and social attire is often improper at work. You cannot wear jeans, halter tops, tank tops, or short skirts. Clothing must not be tight, revealing, or sexual. Women cannot show cleavage, the tops of breasts, or upper thighs. Men must avoid tight pants and exposing their chests. Only the top shirt button is open. Follow the practices in Box 5-1.

Speech and Language

Your speech and language must be professional. Words used in home and social settings may be improper at work. Words used with family and friends may offend patients, residents, families, visitors, and co-workers. Remember the following:

- Do not swear or use foul, vulgar, or abusive language.
- Do not use slang.
- Control the volume and tone of your voice. Speak softly and gently.
- Speak clearly. The person may have a hearing problem (Chapter 39).
- Do not shout or yell.
- Do not fight or argue with a person, family member, visitor, or co-worker.

Courtesies

A *courtesy is a polite, considerate, or helpful comment or act.* Courtesies are easy. They take little time or energy. And they mean so much to people. Even the smallest kind act can brighten someone's day:

- Address others by Miss, Mrs., Ms., Mr., or Doctor. Use a first name only if the person asks you to do so.
- Say "please." Begin or end each request with "please."
- Say "thank you" whenever someone does something for you.
- Apologize. Say "I'm sorry" when you make a mistake or hurt someone. Even little things—like bumping someone in the hallway—need an apology.
- Be thoughtful. Compliment others. Wish others a happy birthday, a happy day or weekend off, or a happy holiday.
- Wish the person and family well when they leave the agency. "Stay well" or "stay healthy" are good phrases to use.
- Hold doors open for others. If you are at the door first, open the door and let others pass through. In business, men and women hold doors open for each other.
- Hold elevator doors open for others coming down the hallway.
- Let patients, residents, families, and visitors enter elevators first.
- Stand to greet visitors and families.
- Help others willingly when asked.
- Give praise. If you see a co-worker do or say something that impresses you, tell that person. Also tell your co-workers.
- Do not take credit for another person's deeds. Give the person credit for the action.

Personal Matters

You were hired to do a job. Personal matters cannot interfere with the job. Otherwise care is neglected. You could lose your job for tending to personal matters while at work. To keep personal matters out of the workplace:

- Make personal phone calls during meals and breaks. Use a pay phone or your wireless phone.
- Do not let family and friends visit you on the unit. If they must see you, have them meet you during a meal or break.
- Make appointments (doctor, dentist, lawyer, and others) for your days off.
- Do not use the agency's computers, printers, fax machines, copiers, or other equipment for your personal use.
- Do not take agency supplies (pens, paper, and others) for your personal use.
- Do not discuss personal problems.
- Control your emotions. If you need to cry or express anger, do so in a private place. Get yourself together quickly and return to your work.
- Do not borrow money from or lend it to co-workers. This includes meal money and bus or train fares. Borrowing and lending can lead to problems with co-workers.
- Do not sell things or engage in fund-raising. For example, do not sell your child's candy or raffle tickets to co-workers.
- Turn off personal pagers and wireless phones.
- Do not send or check text messages.

Meals and Breaks

Meal breaks are usually 30 minutes. Other breaks are usually 15 minutes. Meals and breaks are scheduled so some staff are always on the unit. Staff remaining on the unit cover for the staff on break.

Staff members depend on each other. Leave for and return from breaks on time. That way other staff can have their turn. Do not take longer than allowed. Tell the nurse when you leave and return to the unit.

Job Safety

You must protect patients, residents, families, visitors, co-workers, and yourself from harm. Everyone is responsible for safety. Negligent acts affect the safety of others (Chapter 4). Safety practices are presented throughout this book. These guidelines apply to everything you do:

- Understand the roles, functions, and responsibilities in your job description.
- Know the contents and policies in the employee handbook and policy and procedure manuals.
- Know what is right and wrong conduct.
- Know what you can and cannot do.
- Develop the desired qualities and traits in Box 5-2.
- Follow the nurse's directions and instructions.

- Question unclear directions and things you do not understand.
- Help others willingly when asked.
- Follow agency rules.
- Ask for any training that you might need.
- Report measurements, observations, the care given, the person's complaints, and any errors accurately (Chapters 6 and 12).
- Accept responsibility for your actions. Admit when you are wrong or make mistakes. Do not blame others. Do not make excuses for your actions. Learn what you did wrong and why. Always try to learn from your mistakes.
- Handle the person's property carefully and prevent damage.
- Follow the safety measures in Chapter 12 and throughout this book.

Planning Your Work

You will give care and perform routine tasks on the nursing unit. Some tasks are done at certain times. Others are done by the end of the shift.

The nurse, the Kardex, the care plan, and your assignment sheet help you decide what to do and when (Chapters 6 and 7). This is called *priority setting*. A *priority is the most important thing at the time*. Setting priorities involves deciding:

- Which person has the greatest or most life-threatening needs.
- What tasks the nurse or person needs done first.
- What tasks need to be done at a set time.
- What tasks need to be done when your shift starts.
- What tasks need to be done at the end of your shift.
- How much time it takes to complete a task.
- How much help you need to complete a task.
- Who can help you and when.

Priorities change as the person's needs change. A person's condition can improve or worsen. New patients and residents are admitted. Others are transferred to other nursing units or discharged. These and many other factors can change priorities.

Setting priorities is hard at first. It becomes easier as you gain experience. You can ask the nurse to help you set priorities. Plan your work to give safe, thorough care and to make good use of your time (Box 5-6).

MANAGING STRESS

Stress is the response or change in the body caused by any emotional, physical, social, or economic factor. Stress is normal. It occurs every minute of every day. It occurs in everything you do.

A *stressor is the event or factor that causes stress.* Many stressors are pleasant—watching a child play, planning a party, laughing with family and friends, enjoying a nice day. Some are not pleasant—illness, injury, family problems, death of loved ones, divorce, money concerns. Many parts of your job are stressful.

BOX 5-6 PLANNING YOUR WORK

- Discuss priorities with the nurse.
- Know the routine of your shift and nursing unit.
- Follow unit policies for shift reports.
- List tasks that are on a schedule. For example, some persons are turned or offered the bedpan every 2 hours.
- Judge how much time you need for each person and task.
- Identify the tasks to do while patients and residents are eating, visiting, or involved with activities or therapies.
- Plan care around meal times, visiting hours, and therapies. Also consider recreation and social activities.
- Identify when you will need help from a co-worker. Ask a co-worker to help you. Give the time when you will need help and for how long.
- Schedule equipment or rooms for the person's use. The shower room is an example.
- Review delegated tasks. Gather needed supplies ahead of time.
- Do not waste time. Stay focused on your work.
- Leave a clean work area. Make sure rooms are neat and orderly. Also clean utility areas.
- Be a self-starter. Have initiative. Ask others if they need help. Follow unit routines, stock supply areas, and clean utility rooms. Stay busy.

No matter the cause, stress affects the whole person:

- *Physically*—sweating, increased heart rate, faster and deeper breathing, increased blood pressure, dry mouth, and so on
- *Mentally*—anxiety, fear, anger, dread, depression, and using defense mechanisms (Chapter 45)
- *Socially*—changes in relationships, avoiding others, needing others, blaming others, and so on
- *Spiritually*—changes in beliefs and values and strengthening or questioning one's belief in God or a higher power

Prolonged or frequent stress can cause physical and mental health problems to occur. Some problems are minor—headaches, stomach upset, sleep problems, muscle tension, and so on. Others are life-threatening—high blood pressure, heart attack, stroke, ulcers, and so on.

Dealing with stress is important. If your job causes stress, it affects your family and friends. Stress in your personal life affects your work. Stress affects you, the care you give, the person's quality of life, and how you relate to co-workers. To reduce or cope with stress:

- Exercise regularly. It has physical and mental benefits— cardiovascular health, weight control, tension release, emotional well-being, and relaxation.
- Get enough rest and sleep.
- Eat healthy.
- Plan personal and quiet time for you. Read, take a hot bath, go for a walk, meditate, or listen to music. Do what makes you feel good.

- Use common sense about what you can do. Do not try to do everything that family and friends ask you to do. Consider the amount of time and energy that you have.
- Do one thing at a time. The demands on you may seem overwhelming. List each thing that you have to do. Set priorities.
- Do not judge yourself harshly. Do not try to be perfect or expect too much from yourself.
- Give yourself praise. You do good and wonderful things every day.
- Have a sense of humor. Laugh at yourself. Laugh with others. Spend time with those who make you laugh.
- Talk to the nurse if your work or a person is causing too much stress. The nurse can help you deal with the matter.

HARASSMENT

Harassment means to trouble, torment, offend, or worry a person by one's behavior or comments. Harassment can be sexual. Or it can involve age, race, ethnic background, religion, or disability. Respect others. Do not offend others by your gestures, remarks, or use of touch. Do not offend others with jokes, photos, or other pictures (drawings, cartoons, and so on).

See *Focus on Communication: Harassment.*

Sexual Harassment

Sexual harassment involves unwanted sexual behaviors by another. The behavior may be a sexual advance. Or it may be a request for a sexual favor. Some remarks, comments, and touching are sexual. The behavior affects the person's work and comfort. In extreme cases, the person's job is threatened if sexual favors are not granted.

Victims of sexual harassment may be men or women. Men harass women or men. Women harass men or women. You might feel that you are being harassed. If so, report the matter to the nurse and the human resources officer.

Be careful about what you say or do. Even innocent remarks and behaviors can be viewed as harassment. Employee orientation programs address harassment. You might not be sure about your own or another person's remarks or behaviors. If so, discuss the matter with the nurse. You cannot be too careful.

FOCUS ON COMMUNICATION

Harassment

You have the right to feel safe and not threatened. If someone's comments make you uncomfortable, you can say: "Please don't say things like that. It's unprofessional." If someone's actions make you uneasy, you can say: "Please don't do that. It's unprofessional." Leave the area. Report the person's statements or actions to the nurse.

BOX 5-7	**COMMON REASONS FOR LOSING A JOB**

- Poor attendance—not going to work or excessive tardiness (being late).
- Abandonment—leaving the job during your shift.
- Falsifying a record—job application or a person's record.
- Violent behavior in the workplace.
- Having weapons in the work setting—guns, knives, explosives, or other dangerous items.
- Having, using, or distributing alcohol in the work setting.
- Having, using, or distributing drugs in the work setting. This excludes taking drugs ordered by your doctor.
- Taking a person's drugs for your own use or giving them to others.
- Harassment (p. 59).
- Using offensive speech and language.
- Stealing the agency's or a person's property.
- Destroying the agency's or a person's property.
- Showing disrespect to patients, residents, families, visitors, co-workers, or supervisors.
- Abusing or neglecting a person.
- Invading a person's privacy.
- Failing to maintain patient, resident, family, agency, or co-worker confidentiality. This includes access to computer and other electronic information.
- Using the agency's supplies and equipment for your own use.
- Defamation—see Chapter 4 and "Gossip," p. 56.
- Abusing meal breaks and break periods.
- Sleeping on the job.
- Violating the agency's dress code.
- Violating any agency policy.
- Failing to follow agency care procedures.
- Tending to personal matters while on duty.

RESIGNING FROM A JOB

A job closer to home, better pay, or new opportunities may prompt you to leave your job. School, childcare, and illness are other reasons. Whatever the reason, tell your employer. Do one of the following:

- Give a written notice.
- Write a resignation letter.
- Complete a form in the human resources office.

A 2-week notice is a good practice. Do not leave a job without notice. Doing so can affect patient and resident care. Include the following in your notice:

- Reason for leaving
- The last date you will work
- Comments thanking the employer for the opportunity to work in the agency

An exit interview is common practice. You and the employer talk before you leave the agency. Or a survey may be sent to your home. The employer asks what you liked about the agency and your job. Often employees are asked how the agency can improve.

LOSING A JOB

A job is a privilege. You must perform your job well and protect patients and residents from harm. No pay raise or losing your job results from poor performance. Failure to follow agency policy is often grounds for termination. So is failure to get along with others. Box 5-7 lists the many reasons why you can lose your job. To protect your job, function at your best. Always practice good work ethics.

DRUG TESTING

Drug and alcohol use affects patient, resident, and staff safety. Quality of care suffers. Those who use drugs or alcohol are late to work or absent more often than staff who do not use such substances. Therefore drug testing policies are common. Review your agency's policy for when and how you might be tested.

FOCUS ON **PRIDE**

The Person, Family, and Yourself

Personal and Professional Responsibility

As a nursing assistant, you are responsible for following the ethical guidelines in this chapter. Patients, residents, families, visitors, and co-workers depend on you to give safe and effective care. They trust that you will:

- Work when scheduled.
- Arrive at work on time.
- Stay the entire shift.
- Complete your assignments.
- Work safely.
- Be pleasant and courteous.

Your job as a nursing assistant is important. You can help persons feel safe, secure, loved, and cared for. By practicing good work ethics, you can make others' lives happier, easier, and less painful. Take pride in your work ethics. Your work impacts quality of life.

Rights and Respect

Your attitude affects how you feel about your job. So do the attitudes of others. You will work with many different personalities. You may be more comfortable with some than with others. Your attitude and ability to work with others impact quality care.

Sometimes you may work without enough staff. Or you may work with a challenging person. It may be hard to keep a good attitude. Do not complain about or put down another staff member. For example, do not say: "She calls in sick all the time. You know she's not sick."

Every team member has value. Treat everyone with respect. Try to work well with everyone. Take pride in keeping a positive attitude.

Independence and Social Interaction

Social interaction is a vital part of your job. Employers look for good social skills. During an interview, smile, give a firm hand-shake, make eye contact, and answer questions confidently. At work, smile and greet patients and residents by name. Politely introduce yourself. Do not appear hurried. Display a caring and friendly manner all the time. Remain calm and helpful in stressful situations. These actions promote good relationships and reflect well on you and the agency.

Delegation and Teamwork

Your work ethics impacts the team. Greet co-workers pleasantly. Help others willingly when asked. Offer to help others if you can. After completing tasks, ask the nurse if you can help with anything else. Be available. Stay where you can easily be found. If you will be in one area for a while, tell the nurse. When you would like a break, ask the nurse. Return from breaks on time. Help others so they may take a break. Set a positive example with your behavior. Your actions help build a strong team.

Ethics and Laws

To be professional, you must be safe. You must follow federal, state, and agency laws and rules. Many agencies require a background check and drug testing before hiring. Show good judgment with your actions inside and outside the workplace. The following is a real example of a nursing assistant who did not follow ethical guidelines:

A certified nursing assistant (CNA) began working at an Arizona hospital. While employed, she received Employee Corrective Action reports for:
- *Poor communication with co-workers*
- *Arguing with an RN who gave her instructions*
- *Not being able to work in a team environment*
- *Excess time off the nursing unit for breaks*
- *Not taking the initiative in answering signal lights, collecting needed equipment, or transferring patients' belongings*
- *Excess socializing with staff in other departments*
- *Not meeting standards relating to customer service relations*

She was terminated from the hospital in January 2000.

Four years later she applied for a job at another Arizona hospital. A pre-employment urine drug screen was positive for benzodiazepine. The CNA reported the drug test to the Arizona Board of Nursing. The CNA reported that she had a headache the night before her interview at the hospital. She admitted taking a Valium (benzodiazepine) that was prescribed for her mother. The CNA explained that "she knew this was wrong, that this was a one time occurrence and that it would not happen again."

The Board requested that the CNA submit to a urine drug screen. It was positive for benzodiazepine. The CNA did not have a prescription for that drug.

The Board revoked the CNA's certificate for unprofessional conduct. The Arizona State Board of Nursing found that the CNA's actions violated these aspects of the state's Nurse Practice Act:
- *Conduct or practice that is or might be harmful or dangerous to the health of a patient or the public*
- *Committing an act that deceives, defrauds, or harms the public*

- *Obtaining, possessing, using, or selling any narcotic, controlled substance, or illegal drug in violation of any federal or state criminal law, or in violation of the policy of any employer*
- *Using violent or abusive behavior in any work setting*
- *Failing to cooperate with the Board during an investigation*
- *Practicing in any other manner that gives the Board reasonable cause to believe that the health of a patient or the public may be harmed*

(Arizona State Board of Nursing, November 16, 2005. Note: Names withheld by request of the Arizona State Board of Nursing.)

REVIEW QUESTIONS

Circle T if the statement is TRUE or F if it is FALSE.

1. T F You wear needed eyeglasses. This helps protect the person's safety.
2. T F Childcare requires planning before you go to work.
3. T F Being on time for work means arriving at the agency when your shift begins.
4. T F You share information about a person with a friend. This is grounds for losing your job.
5. T F You must be careful what you say over the intercom system.
6. T F You do not follow the agency's dress code. You could lose your job.
7. T F You can use the agency's computer for your homework.
8. T F You can keep your wireless phone turned on while at work.
9. T F You must know your agency's attendance policy.
10. T F Harassment is legal in the workplace.

Circle the BEST answer.

11. Which will *not* help you do your job well?
    a Enough rest and sleep
    b Regular exercise
    c Using drugs and alcohol
    d Good nutrition
12. Which is a good hygiene practice?
    a Bathing weekly
    b Wearing a strongly scented perfume or cologne
    c Brushing teeth after meals
    d Having long and polished fingernails
13. You are getting ready for work. Which is a good practice?
    a Styling hair up and off your collar
    b Wearing jewelry
    c Wearing your name badge at waist level
    d Applying heavy make-up
14. When should you ask questions about your job description?
    a After completing the job application
    b Before completing the job application
    c When your interview is scheduled
    d During the interview

Continued

REVIEW QUESTIONS—cont'd

15 Lying on a job application is
   a Negligence
   b Fraud
   c Libel
   d Defamation

16 You are completing a job application. You should do the following *except*
   a Write neatly and clearly
   b Provide references
   c Give information about employment gaps
   d Leave spaces blank that do not apply to you

17 Which of the following do employers look for the *most?*
   a Cooperation
   b Courtesy
   c Dependability
   d Empathy

18 Empathy is
   a Feeling sorry for a person
   b Seeing things from the other person's point of view
   c Being polite to others
   d Saying kind things

19 What should you wear to a job interview?
   a A uniform
   b Party clothes
   c A simple dress or suit
   d What is most comfortable

20 Which is a poor behavior during a job interview?
   a Good eye contact with the interviewer
   b Shaking hands with the interviewer
   c Asking the interviewer questions
   d Crossing your arms and legs

21 Which is the best response to an interview question?
   a "Yes" or "no"
   b Long answers
   c Brief explanations
   d A written response

22 Which statement reflects a good work attitude?
   a "It's not my fault."
   b "I'm sorry. I didn't know."
   c "That's not my job."
   d "I did it yesterday. It's your turn."

23 A co-worker says that a doctor and nurse are dating. This is
   a Gossip
   b Eavesdropping
   c Confidential information
   d Sexual harassment

24 Which is professional speech and language?
   a Speaking clearly
   b Using vulgar words
   c Shouting
   d Arguing

25 Which is *not* a courteous act?
   a Saying "please" and "thank you"
   b Wanting others to open doors for you
   c Saying "I'm sorry"
   d Complimenting others

26 You are on a meal break. Which is *true?*
   a You cannot make personal phone calls.
   b Family members cannot meet you.
   c You can take a few extra minutes if needed.
   d The nurse needs to know that you are off the unit.

27 You are planning your work. You should do the following *except*
   a Discuss priorities with the nurse
   b Ask others if they need help
   c Stay busy
   d Plan care so that you can watch the person's TV

28 These statements are about stress. Which is *false?*
   a Stress affects the whole person.
   b A stressor is an event that causes stress.
   c All stress is unpleasant.
   d Stress is normal.

29 Which helps to reduce stress?
   a Exercise, rest, and sleep
   b Blaming yourself for things you did not do
   c Putting off quiet time to get work done
   d Agreeing to do everything others ask

30 Which is *not* harassment?
   a Using touch to comfort a person
   b Joking about a person's religion
   c Asking for a sexual favor
   d Acting like a disabled person

31 A resignation letter should *not* include
   a Your reasons for leaving
   b The last day you will work
   c A thank-you to the employer
   d Problems you had during your work

32 Which is *not* a reason for losing your job?
   a Leaving the job during your shift
   b Using alcohol in the work setting
   c Sleeping on the job
   d Taking a meal break

Answers to these questions are on p. 832.

Communicating With the Health Team

6

OBJECTIVES

- Define the key terms and key abbreviations listed in this chapter.
- Explain why health team members need to communicate.
- Describe the rules for good communication.
- Explain the purpose, parts, and information found in the medical record.
- Describe the legal and ethical aspects of medical records.
- Describe the purpose of the Kardex.
- List the information you need to report to the nurse.
- List the rules for recording.
- Use the 24-hour clock, medical terminology, and abbreviations.
- Explain how computers and other electronic devices are used in health care.
- Explain how to protect the right to privacy when using computers and other electronic devices.
- Describe how to answer phones.
- Explain how to problem solve and deal with conflict.
- Explain how to promote PRIDE in the person, the family, and yourself.

KEY TERMS

abbreviation A shortened form of a word or phrase

anterior At or toward the front of the body or body part; ventral

chart See "medical record"

clinical record See "medical record"

communication The exchange of information—a message sent is received and correctly interpreted by the intended person

conflict A clash between opposing interests or ideas

distal The part farthest from the center or from the point of attachment

dorsal See "posterior"

end-of-shift report A report that the nurse gives at the end of the shift to the on-coming shift

Kardex A type of card file that summarizes information found in the medical record—drugs, treatments, diagnoses, routine care measures, equipment, and special needs

lateral Away from the mid-line; at the side of the body or body part

medial At or near the middle or mid-line of the body or body part

medical record A written or electronic account of a person's condition and response to treatment and care; chart or clinical record

posterior At or toward the back of the body or body part

prefix A word element placed before a root; it changes the meaning of the word

progress note Describes the care given and the person's response and progress

proximal The part nearest to the center or to the point of origin

recording The written account of care and observations; charting

reporting The oral account of care and observations

root A word element containing the basic meaning of the word

suffix A word element placed after a root; it changes the meaning of the word

ventral See "anterior"

word element A part of a word

KEY ABBREVIATIONS

ADL	Activities of daily living
EPHI; ePHI	Electronic protected health information
OBRA	Omnibus Budget Reconciliation Act of 1987

PHI	Protected health information

Health team members communicate with each other to give coordinated and effective care. They share information about:

- What was done for the person.
- What needs to be done for the person.
- The person's response to treatment.

For example, the doctor ordered a blood test for Mr. Bloom. Food and fluids affect the test results. Mr. Bloom must fast for 10 hours before the blood is drawn. A nurse tells the dietary department that Mr. Bloom will have breakfast later. She explains the breakfast delay to you and Mr. Bloom. A technician tells the nurse the blood sample was drawn. The nurse orders the meal. A dietary worker brings the tray to the nursing unit. You serve Mr. Bloom's tray. When he is done eating, you remove the tray and observe what he ate. You report your observations to the nurse. The nurse records your observations in Mr. Bloom's medical record.

Team members communicated with each other and Mr. Bloom. His care was coordinated and effective. He knew that he was not neglected or forgotten.

You need to understand the aspects and rules of communication. Then you can learn how to communicate with the nursing and health teams.

COMMUNICATION

Communication is the exchange of information—a message sent is received and correctly interpreted by the intended person. For good communication:

- Use words that mean the same thing to you and the message receiver. Avoid words with more than one meaning. What does "far" mean—10 feet, 50 feet, or 100 feet?
- Use familiar words. You will learn medical terms. If someone uses a strange term, ask what it means. Or use a dictionary. You must understand the message. Otherwise communication does not occur. Likewise, avoid terms that the person and family do not understand.
- Be brief and concise. Do not add unrelated or unnecessary information. Stay on the subject. Do not wander in thought or get wordy.
- Give information in a logical and orderly manner. Organize your thoughts. Present them step-by-step.
- Give facts and be specific. Give the receiver a clear picture of what you are saying. You report a pulse rate of 110. It is more specific and factual than saying the "pulse is fast."

THE MEDICAL RECORD

The *medical record (chart, clinical record) is a written or electronic account of a person's condition and response to treatment and care* (Fig. 6-1). The health team uses it to share information about the person. The record is permanent. Often it is used months or years later if the person's health history is needed. The record is a legal document. It can be used in court as legal evidence of the person's problems, treatment, and care.

The record has many forms organized into sections. Each page has the person's name, room and bed number, and other identifying information. This helps prevent errors and the wrong placement of records. The record includes the person's:

- Admission record
- Health history
- Physical examination results
- Doctor's orders
- Doctor's progress notes
- Progress notes (nursing team and health team)
- Graphic sheets
- Flow sheets
- Laboratory results
- X-ray reports
- IV (intravenous) therapy record
- Respiratory therapy record
- Consultation reports
- Assessments from nursing, social services, dietary services, and recreational therapy
- Special consents

The health team records on forms for their departments. Other team members read the information. It tells the care provided and the person's response.

Agencies have policies about medical records and who can see them. Policies address:

- Who records
- When to record
- Abbreviations
- Correcting errors
- Ink color
- Signing entries

Some agencies allow nursing assistants to record observations and care. Others do not. You must follow your agency's policies.

Professional staff involved in a person's care can review charts. Cooks and laundry, housekeeping, and office staff do not need to read charts. Some agencies let nursing assistants read charts. If not, the nurse shares needed information.

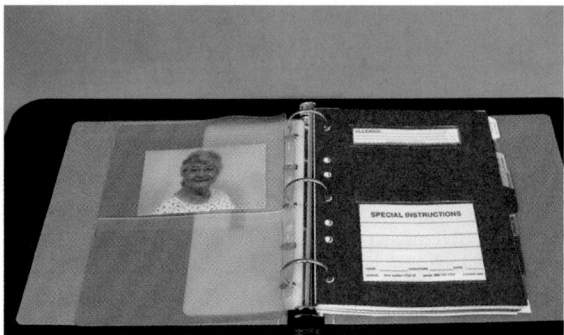

Fig. 6-1 A medical record.

You have an ethical and legal duty to keep the person's information confidential. You may know someone in the agency. If not involved in the person's care, you have no right to review the person's chart. Doing so is an invasion of privacy.

Patients and residents have the right to the information in their medical records. The person or the person's legal representative may ask you for the chart. Report the request to the nurse. The nurse deals with the request.

The following parts of the medical record relate to your work.

The Admission Record

The admission record is completed when the person is admitted to the agency. It has the person's identifying information—legal name, birth date, age, gender (male or female), address, and marital status. Nearest relative and legal representative names are included. Other information includes known allergies, diagnoses, date and time of admission, and doctor's name. Religion, place of worship, and employer are often included.

Each person receives an identification (ID) number. It is on the admission sheet and ID bracelet (Chapter 12). So is information about advance directives. An *advance directive* is a document stating a person's wishes about end-of-life care (Chapter 52).

Use the admission sheet to fill out forms needing the same information. That way the person does not have to answer the same question many times.

Health History

The health history (nursing history) is completed when the person is admitted. The nurse interviews the person. You can use the form to learn about the person's background and health history. It contains information about:

- The person's chief complaint—reason for seeking health care

- History of the current illness—sudden or gradual in onset, when it started, signs and symptoms, and so on
- Past health problems, surgeries, and injuries
- Childhood illnesses
- Allergies
- Current drugs
- Family health history
- Life-style—habits, diet, sleep, hobbies, and so on
- Wearing dentures, eyeglasses or contact lenses, and hearing aids
- Problems with activities of daily living (ADL)
- Education and occupation

The Graphic Sheet

The graphic sheet is used to record measurements and observations made daily, every shift, or 3 to 4 times a day (Fig. 6-2, p. 66). Information includes vital signs—blood pressure, temperature, pulse, respirations. It also includes weight, intake and output, bowel movements (feces), and doctor's visits.

Progress Notes

The *progress note describes the care given and the person's response and progress* (Fig. 6-3, p. 67). The nurse records:
- Signs and symptoms
- Information about treatments and drugs
- Information about teaching and counseling
- Procedures performed by the doctor
- Visits by other health team members
  See *Focus on Long-Term Care and Home Care: Progress Notes.*

FOCUS ON LONG-TERM CARE AND HOME CARE
Progress Notes

Long-Term Care
The nurse writes progress notes when there is an unusual event, a problem, or a change in the person's condition. The Omnibus Budget Reconciliation Act of 1987 (OBRA) requires that summaries of care be written at least every 3 months. They reflect the person's progress toward the goals set in the care plan (Chapter 7). They also reflect the person's response to care. Some centers require summaries more often.

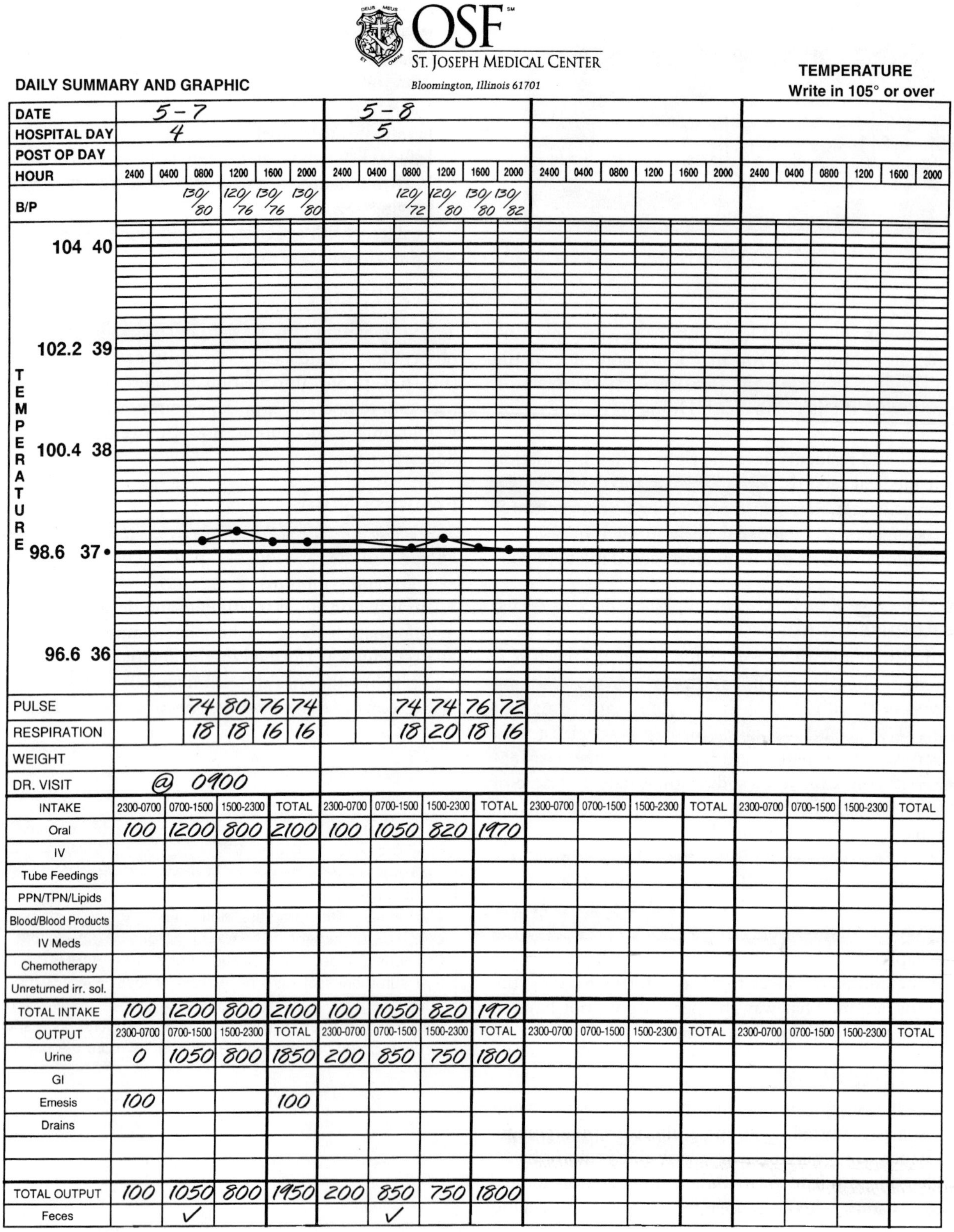

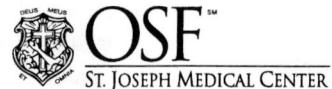

DAILY SUMMARY AND GRAPHIC

St. Joseph Medical Center
Bloomington, Illinois 61701

TEMPERATURE
Write in 105° or over

DATE	5 – 7						5 – 8																		
HOSPITAL DAY	4						5																		
POST OP DAY																										
HOUR	2400	0400	0800	1200	1600	2000	2400	0400	0800	1200	1600	2000	2400	0400	0800	1200	1600	2000	2400	0400	0800	1200	1600	2000
B/P			130/80	120/76	130/76	130/80			120/72	120/80	130/80	130/82												

TEMPERATURE	
104	40
102.2	39
100.4	38
98.6	37
96.6	36

PULSE			74	80	76	74			74	74	76	72												
RESPIRATION			18	18	16	16			18	20	18	16												
WEIGHT																								
DR. VISIT	@ 0900																							

INTAKE	2300-0700	0700-1500	1500-2300	TOTAL	2300-0700	0700-1500	1500-2300	TOTAL	2300-0700	0700-1500	1500-2300	TOTAL	2300-0700	0700-1500	1500-2300	TOTAL
Oral	100	1200	800	2100	100	1050	820	1970								
IV																
Tube Feedings																
PPN/TPN/Lipids																
Blood/Blood Products																
IV Meds																
Chemotherapy																
Unreturned irr. sol.																
TOTAL INTAKE	100	1200	800	2100	100	1050	820	1970								

OUTPUT	2300-0700	0700-1500	1500-2300	TOTAL	2300-0700	0700-1500	1500-2300	TOTAL	2300-0700	0700-1500	1500-2300	TOTAL	2300-0700	0700-1500	1500-2300	TOTAL
Urine	0	1050	800	1850	200	850	750	1800								
GI																
Emesis	100			100												
Drains																
TOTAL OUTPUT	100	1050	800	1950	200	850	750	1800								
Feces		✓				✓										

Fig. 6-2 Graphic sheet.

Date	Time	Nursing Margin / Other Depts Margin
3-19	1700	Out with family for dinner. Jane Doe, LPN
3-19	1930	Returned from outing accompanied by her son. States she had a pleasant time. Mary Smith, CNA
3-20	0900	In bed. Complains of headache. T 98.4 orally, radial pulse 72 and regular, respirations 18 and unlabored. BP 134/84 left arm lying down. Alice Jones, RN notified of resident complaint and vital signs. Ann Adams, CNA
3-20	0910	In bed resting. States she has had a headache for about 1/2 hour. Denies nausea and dizziness. No other complaints. PRN Tylenol given. Instructed resident to use signal light if headache worsens or other symptoms occur. Alice Jones, RN
3-20	0945	Resting quietly. Denies headache at this time. T 98.4 orally, radial pulse 70 and regular, respirations 18 and unlabored. BP 132/84 left arm lying down. Alice Jones, RN

Fig. 6-3 Progress notes. Note that other members of the health team also can record on this form.

FOCUS ON LONG-TERM CARE AND HOME CARE
Flow Sheets

Long-Term Care
An activities of daily living (ADL) flow sheet is used to record a person's ability to perform ADL (Fig. 6-4). This flow sheet addresses hygiene, food and fluids, elimination, rest and sleep, activities, and social interactions.

Home Care
In home care, a weekly record has boxes for each day and for care activities. You check the box for the day care was given. There are boxes for vital signs and weight. You record the measurements on the day they were done.

Flow Sheets

Flow sheets are used to record frequent measurements or observations. For example, a person's vital signs are measured every 30 minutes. A vital signs flow sheet is used. The bedside intake and output record is another flow sheet (Chapter 24).

See *Focus on Long-Term Care and Home Care: Flow Sheets.*

THE KARDEX

The *Kardex is a type of card file. It summarizes information in the medical record—drugs, treatments, diagnoses, routine care measures, equipment, and special needs.* The Kardex is a quick, easy source of information about the person (Fig. 6-5, p. 68).

REPORTING AND RECORDING

The health team communicates by reporting and recording. *Reporting is the oral account of care and observations. Recording (charting) is the written account of care and observations.*

Activities of Daily Living Flow Sheet

ORDER/INSTRUCTION	TIME	JAN 1	2	3	4	FEB 5	MAR 6	7	APR 8	9
Bowel Movements L = Large M = Medium S = Small IC = Incontinent	11-7	M								
	7-3		L							
	3-11									
Bladder Elimination I = Independent IC = Incontinent FC = Foley catheter	11-7	/	/	/	/					
	7-3	/	/	/	/					
	3-11	/	IC	/	/					
Weight Bearing Status TT = Toe touch AT = As tol. P = Partial F = Full NWB = No weight bearing	11-7	AT	AT	AT	AT					
	7-3	AT	AT	AT	AT					
	3-11	AT	AT	AT	AT					
Transfer Status ML = Mech lift SBA = Stand by assist; Assist of 1 or 2 (A-1, A-2)	11-7	SBA	SBA	SBA	SBA					
	7-3	SBA	SBA	SBA	SBA					
	3-11	SBA	SBA	SBA	A-1					
Activity A = Ambulate GC = Gerichair T = Turn every 2 hrs. W/C = Wheelchair	11-7	T	T	T	T					
	7-3	A	A	A	A					
	3-11	A	A	A	A					
Safety LT = Lap tray BR = Bed rails BA = Bed alarm SB = Seat belt	11-7									
	7-3									
	3-11									
Feeding Status I = Independent S = Set up F = Staff feed SP = Swallow precautions TL = Thickened liquids	Breakfast	S	S	S	S					
	Lunch	S	S	S	S					
	Supper	S	S	S	S					
Amount of food taken in %	Breakfast	75	100	100	75					
	Lunch	75	75	100	75					
	Supper	50	50	50	75					
Bath and Shampoo every Monday & Thursday on 7-3 shift T = Tub S = Shower B = Bed bath	11-7									
	7-3	T								
	3-11									
Oral Care Own/Dentures/No teeth I = Independent S = Set up A = Assist	11-7	S	S	S	S					
	7-3	S	S	S	S					
	3-11	S	S	S	S					
Dressing I = Independent S = Set up A = Assist T = Total care	11-7	A	A	S	S					
	7-3									
	3-11	A	A	A	A					
Grooming: Washing Face and Hands Combing Hair I = Independent S = Set up A = Assist T = Total care	11-7	A	A	A	A					
	7-3	A	A	A	A					
	3-11	A	A	A	A					
Trim Fingernails weekly Thursday	11-7									
	7-3		✓							
	3-11									
Lotion Arms and Legs twice daily	11-7									
	7-3	✓	✓	✓	✓					
	3-11	✓	✓	✓	✓					
Shave Men daily	11-7									
Shave Women every Monday & Thursday on 7-3 shift	7-3		✓							
	3-11									
Amount Between-Meal Nourishment taken in %	AM	100	75	100	50					
	PM	100	100	75	75					
	HS	50	75	75	75					
Intake and Output	11-7									
	7-3									
	3-11									
Vital Signs Every Thursday	11-7									
	7-3		✓							
	3-11									
Weight Every Thursday	11-7		✓							
	7-3									
	3-11									

Fig. 6-4 Some items on an activities of daily living flow sheet.

DIET	NOURISHMENT/SPECIAL FEEDING	INTAKE/OUTPUT			
Regular	Health shake at Bedtime	Encourage/Restrict Fluids _2000_ mL/24 Hr.			
Hold:		7-3 _1000_ 3-11 _800_ 11-7 _200_			

FUNCTIONAL STATUS						ACTIVITIES	ELIMINATION	VITALS
	SELF	ASSIST	TOTAL	OTHER	SPECIFY	Bedrest & BRP _____	Bladder - Cont. (Incont.)	Temp. _daily_
Feeding	☐	☒	☐	☐	_____	Bedside Commode _____	Catheter _____	Pulse _daily_
Bathing	☐	☒	☐	☐	_____	Up ad Lib __X__	Date Changed _____	Resp. _daily_
Toileting	☐	☒	☐	☐	_____	Chair _____	Irrigations _____	BP _daily_
Oral Care	☐	☒	☐	☐	_____	Ambulatory __X__		Weight _daily_
Positioning	☒	☐	☐	☐	_____	Ambulate & Assist _____	Bowel - (Cont.) Incont.	Other:
Transferring	☒	☐	☐	☐	_____	Turn _____	Ostomy _____	_Pulse OX_
Wheeling	☐	☐	☐	☐	_____	Dangle _____	Irrigations _____	_daily_
Walking	☒	☐	☐	☐	_____	Mode of Travel _____		
	☐	☐	☐	☐	_____			

COMMUNICATION DEFICITS	☐ None	SPECIAL CONDITIONS (Paralysis, Pressure Ulcers, Etc.)	RESPIRATORY THERAPY	OXYGEN
Hearing _Hard-of-hearing_			Aerosol	__2__ Liter/Minute
Vision _Impaired_			IPPB	☒ PRN ☐ Constant
Speech _____		**SAFETY/SUPPORTIVE MEASURES**	Ultrasonic	
Language _Impaired_		Bed rails: ☒ Nights Only ☐ Constant ☐ No Need		___ Tent ___ Catheter
PROSTHESIS	☐ None	Restraints: _____	Rx Med _____	___ Mask _X_ Cannula
Glasses __X__ Dentures __X__				
Contacts ___ Limb _____		Support Devices: ☐ PRN ☐ Constant		
Hearing Aid _L ear_				

SPECIAL EQUIPMENT/PROCEDURES/ANCILLARY SERVICES/ETC.		DATE	TREATMENTS
Speech therapy 3 times/wk.			

ORDERED	SCHEDULED	COMPLETED	X-RAY AND SPECIAL DIAGNOSTIC EXAMS
10-20	10-20	10-20	Chest x-ray

DATE	TIME	SCHEDULED MEDICATIONS	DATE	TIME	PRN MEDICATIONS
10-19		Lasix 40 mg PO daily			
10-19		Lanoxin 0.25 mg PO daily			
			MISCELLANEOUS		

ALLERGIES:	NURSING ALERTS:	EMERGENCY CONTACT:	
			Telephone No.
	fall prevention	Name: _Parker, Marie_	Home: _555-1212_
☒ None Known		Relationship: _Wife_	Bus: _____

ROOM	NAME	PHYSICIAN	ADMITTING DIAGNOSIS/PROBLEM	HOSP. NO.
310	Parker, Edwin	Dr. S Epstein	1. CHF 2. Dementia	1035B

Fig. 6-5 A sample Kardex.

Reporting and Recording Time

The 24-hour clock (military time or international time) has four digits (Fig. 6-6). The first two digits are for the hours: 0100 = 1:00 AM; 1300 = 1:00 PM. The last two digits are for minutes: 0110 = 1:10 AM. AM and PM are not used.

As Box 6-1 shows, the hour is the same for morning times, but AM is not used. For PM times add 12 to the hour. If it is 2:00 PM, add 12 and 2 for 1400. For 8:35 PM, add 12 and 8 for 2035. Some agencies use 0000 for midnight. Others use 2400. Follow agency policy.

See *Promoting Safety and Comfort: Reporting and Recording Time*, p. 70.

Reporting

You report care and observations to the nurse. Report to the nurse at these times:

- Whenever there is a change from normal or a change in the person's condition. Report these changes at once.
- When the nurse asks you to do so.
- When you leave the unit for meals, breaks, or for other reasons.
- Before the end-of-shift report.
  When reporting, follow the rules in Box 6-2.
  See *Teamwork and Time Management: Reporting*, p. 70.

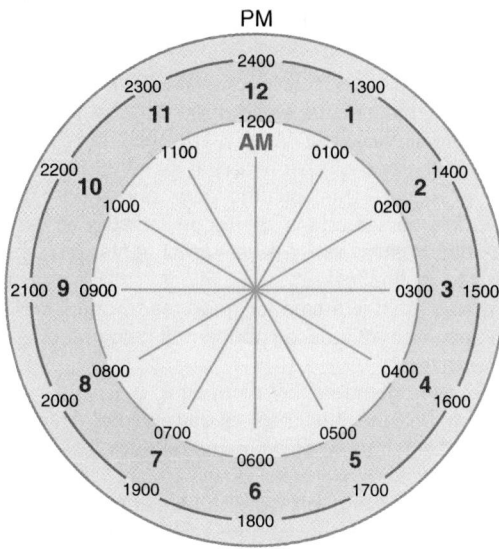

Fig. 6-6 The 24-hour clock.

AM		PM	
Conventional Time	24-Hour Time	Conventional Time	24-Hour Time
1:00 AM	0100	1:00 PM	1300
2:00 AM	0200	2:00 PM	1400
3:00 AM	0300	3:00 PM	1500
4:00 AM	0400	4:00 PM	1600
5:00 AM	0500	5:00 PM	1700
6:00 AM	0600	6:00 PM	1800
7:00 AM	0700	7:00 PM	1900
8:00 AM	0800	8:00 PM	2000
9:00 AM	0900	9:00 PM	2100
10:00 AM	1000	10:00 PM	2200
11:00 AM	1100	11:00 PM	2300
12:00 NOON	1200	12:00 MIDNIGHT	2400 or 0000

BOX 6-2 | RULES FOR REPORTING AND RECORDING

Reporting

- Be prompt, thorough, and accurate.
- Give the person's name and room and bed number.
- Give the time your observations were made or the care was given. Use conventional time (AM or PM) or 24-hour clock time according to agency policy.
- Report only what you observed or did yourself.
- Report care measures that you expect the person to need. For example, the person may need the bedpan during your meal break.
- Report expected changes in the person's condition. For example, the person may be tired after physical therapy.
- Give reports as often as the person's condition requires. Or give them when the nurse asks you to.
- Report any changes from normal or changes in the person's condition. Report these changes at once. See Chapter 7.
- Use your written notes to give a specific, concise, and clear report (Fig. 6-7, p. 70).

Recording

General Rules

- Follow agency policies and procedures for recording. Ask for needed training.
- Include the date and time for every recording. Use conventional time (AM or PM) or 24-hour clock time according to agency policy.
- Use only agency-approved abbreviations (p. 71).
- Use correct spelling, grammar, and punctuation.
- Do not use ditto marks.
- Sign all entries with your name and title as required by agency policy.
- Make sure each form has the person's name and other identifying information.
- Record only what you observed and did yourself. Do not record for another person.
- Never chart a procedure, treatment, or care measure until after it is completed.
- Be accurate, concise, and factual. Do not record judgments or interpretations.

Recording—cont'd

General Rules—cont'd

- Record in a logical and sequential manner.
- Be descriptive. Avoid terms with more than one meaning.
- Use the person's exact words whenever possible. Use quotation marks ("...") to show that the statement is a direct quote.
- Chart any changes from normal or changes in the person's condition. Also chart that you told the nurse (include the nurse's name), what you said, and the time you made the report.
- Do not omit information.
- Record safety measures. Examples include placing the signal light within reach, assisting a person when up, or reminding a person not to get out of bed.

Paper Charting

- Always use ink. Use the ink color required by the agency.
- Make sure writing is readable and neat.
- Never erase or use correction fluid. Draw a line through the incorrect part. Date and initial the line. Write "mistaken entry" over it if this is agency policy. Then re-write the part. Follow agency policy for correcting errors.
- Do not skip lines. Draw a line through the blank space of a partially completed line or to the end of the page. This prevents others from recording in a space with your signature.

Electronic Charting

- Log in using your username and password. Do not chart using another person's username.
- Check the time your entry is made. Make sure it is the right time.
- Check for accuracy. Review your entry before saving.
- Save your entries. Unsaved data will be lost.
- Follow the manufacturer's instructions for changing or uncharting a mistaken entry. Most electronic systems keep a record of an entry before a change was made. This works the same way as drawing a line through a mistaken entry in paper charting. The first entry is still visible.
- Log off when done charting. This prevents others from charting under your username.

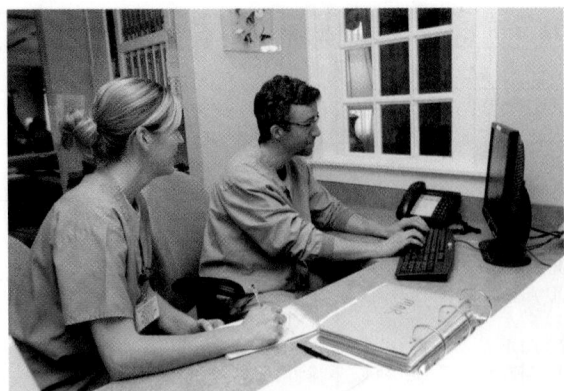

Fig. 6-7 The nursing assistant uses notes to report to the nurse.

PROMOTING SAFETY AND COMFORT
Reporting and Recording Time

Safety
Communication is better with the 24-hour clock. You must use AM and PM with conventional clock time. Someone may forget to use AM or PM. Writing may be unclear. This means that the correct time is not communicated. Harm to the person could result.

TEAMWORK AND TIME MANAGEMENT
Reporting

The nurse needs your full attention when reporting. If distracted, you could omit or forget to report important things.

Nurses must give their full attention when receiving reports. If someone is reporting to a nurse, do not interrupt unless the matter is urgent. You must not distract the nurse.

End-of-Shift Report. *The nurse gives a report at the end of the shift to the on-coming shift. This is called the end-of-shift report or change-of-shift report.* The nurse reports about:

- The care given
- The care to give during other shifts
- The person's current condition
- Likely changes in the person's condition

In some agencies, the entire nursing team hears the end-of-shift report as they come on duty. In other agencies, only nurses hear the report. After the report, information is shared with nursing assistants.

> See *Teamwork and Time Management: End-of-Shift Report.*
>
> See *Promoting Safety and Comfort: End-of-Shift Report.*

TEAMWORK AND TIME MANAGEMENT
End-of-Shift Report

Two staffs are present at the end of a shift—the staff going off duty and the staff coming on duty. The entire on-coming shift may attend the end-of-shift report. If so, staff going off duty answer all signal lights, provide care, and tend to routine tasks. If only nurses attend the report, nursing assistants of the on-coming shift also answer signal lights, provide care, and tend to routine tasks.

The end-of-shift is a time for good teamwork. Continue to do your job. Your attitude is important. If going off duty, avoid saying or thinking:

- "I'm ready to go home. Let them do it."
- "It's their turn. I've been here all day (evening or night)."
- "No one helped us when we came on duty."

Some agencies have clear duties for the two shifts. For example, those going off duty continue to answer signal lights. They know about changes in the person's condition and care plan and about new orders. They also know about the care needs of new patients or residents. The on-coming shift has yet to learn this information. The on-coming shift uses this time to perform routine tasks for the shift and to collect needed supplies and equipment.

PROMOTING SAFETY AND COMFORT
End-of-Shift Report

Safety
You may not hear the end-of-shift report as you come on duty. Yet you need to answer signal lights and give care before the nurse shares new information with you. To give safe care:

- Check the care plan and Kardex before granting a request. The person's condition or care plan may have changed. There may be new doctor's orders.
- Ask a nurse about the care needs of new patients or residents. If necessary, politely interrupt the end-of-shift report to ask your questions.
- Do not take directions or orders from another nursing assistant. Remember, nursing assistants cannot supervise or delegate to other nursing assistants.

Recording

When recording on the person's chart, you must communicate clearly and thoroughly. Follow the rules in Box 6-2. The charting sample in Figure 6-8 shows how the rules apply. Anyone who reads your charting should know:

- What you observed
- What you did
- The person's response

> See *Focus on Communication: Recording.*

Date	Time	Nursing Margin	Other Depts Margin
7/26	1045	Requested assistance to lie down. States, "I don't feel well. I have a little upset stomach."	
		Denies pain. VS taken. T-99 (O). P-76 regular rate and rhythm. R-18 unlabored.	
		BP 134/84 L arm lying down. Signal light within reach. Paula Jones, RN notified at 1040	
		of resident's complaint and VS. Mary Jensen, CNA	
7-26	1100	Asleep in bed. Appears to be resting comfortably. Color good. No signs of	
		discomfort or distress noted at this time. Paula Jones, RN	
7-26	1145	Refused to go to the dining room for lunch. Complains of nausea.	
		Denies abdominal pain. Has not had an emesis. Abdomen soft to	
		palpation. Good bowel sounds. VS taken. T-98.8 99.2. P-76 regular *(Mistaken entry 7-26, PJ)*	
		rate and rhythm. R-18 unlabored. BP-134/84. States she will try to	
		eat something. Full liquid room tray ordered. Paula Jones, RN	

Fig. 6-8 Charting sample.

FOCUS ON COMMUNICATION

Recording

"Small," "moderate," "large," "long," and "short" mean different things to different people. Is small the size of a dime? Or is it the size of a quarter? In health care, different meanings can cause serious problems. Give accurate descriptions and measurements. If you have a question, ask the nurse to look at what you are trying to describe.

MEDICAL TERMS AND ABBREVIATIONS

Medical terms and abbreviations are used in health care. Someone may use a word or phrase that you do not understand. If so, ask a nurse to explain its meaning. Otherwise, communication does not occur. A medical dictionary is useful for learning new words.

Like all words, medical terms are made up of *parts of words* or *word elements*—prefixes, roots, and suffixes (Box 6-3, pp. 72-73). Most are from Greek or Latin. They are combined to form medical terms. To translate a term, the word is separated into its elements.

Prefixes, Roots, and Suffixes

A *prefix is a word element placed before a root. It changes the meaning of the word.* The prefix *olig* (scant, small amount) is placed before the root *uria* (urine) to make *oliguria*. It means a scant amount of urine. Prefixes are always used with other word elements. They are never used alone.

The *root is the word element that contains the basic meaning of the word.* It is combined with another root, prefixes, and suffixes. A vowel (an *o* or an *i*) is added when two roots are combined or when a suffix is added to a root. The vowel makes the word easier to pronounce.

A *suffix is a word element placed after a root. It changes the meaning of the word.* Suffixes are not used alone. When translating medical terms, begin with the suffix. For example, *nephritis* means inflammation of the kidney. It was formed by combining *nephro* (kidney) and *itis* (inflammation).

Medical terms are formed by combining word elements. Remember, prefixes always come before roots. Suffixes always come after roots. A root can be combined with prefixes, roots, and suffixes. For example:

- The prefix *dys* (difficult) is combined with the root *pnea* (breathing). This forms *dyspnea*. It means difficulty breathing.
- The root *mast* (breast) combined with the suffix *ectomy* (excision or removal) forms *mastectomy*. It means the removal of a breast.
- Endocarditis has the prefix *endo* (inner), the root *card* (heart), and the suffix *itis* (inflammation). *Endocarditis* means inflammation of the inner part of the heart.

Abdominal Regions

The abdomen is divided into regions (Fig. 6-9, p. 73). They are used to describe the location of body structures, pain, or discomfort. The regions are:

- Right upper quadrant (RUQ)
- Left upper quadrant (LUQ)
- Right lower quadrant (RLQ)
- Left lower quadrant (LLQ)

Directional Terms

Certain terms describe the position of one body part in relation to another. These terms give the direction of the body part when a person is standing and facing forward (Fig. 6-10, p. 73):

- *Anterior (ventral)—at or toward the front of the body or body part*
- *Posterior (dorsal)—at or toward the back of the body or body part*
- *Proximal—the part nearest to the center or to the point of origin*
- *Distal—the part farthest from the center or from the point of attachment*
- *Lateral—away from the mid-line; at the side of the body or body part*
- *Medial—at or near the middle or mid-line of the body or body part*

BOX 6-3 MEDICAL TERMINOLOGY

Prefix	Meaning	Root (combining vowel)	Meaning
a-, an-	without, not, lack of	abdomin (o)	abdomen
ab-	away from	aden (o)	gland
ad-	to, toward, near	adren (o)	adrenal gland
ante-	before, forward, in front of	angi (o)	vessel
anti-	against	arterio	artery
auto-	self	athr (o)	joint
bi-	double, two, twice	broncho	bronchus, bronchi
brady-	slow	card, cardi (o)	heart
circum-	around	cephal (o)	head
contra-	against, opposite	chole, chol (o)	bile
de-	down, from	chondr (o)	cartilage
dia-	across, through, apart	colo	colon, large intestine
dis-	apart, free from	cost (o)	rib
dys-	bad, difficult, abnormal	crani (o)	skull
ecto-	outer, outside	cyan (o)	blue
en-	in, into, within	cyst (o)	bladder, cyst
endo-	inner, inside	cyt (o)	cell
epi-	over, on, upon	dent (o)	tooth
eryth-	red	derma	skin
eu-	normal, good, well, healthy	duoden (o)	duodenum
ex-	out, out of, from, away from	encephal (o)	brain
hemi-	half	enter (o)	intestines
hyper-	excessive, too much, high	fibr (o)	fiber, fibrous
hypo-	under, decreased, less than normal	gastr (o)	stomach
in-	in, into, within, not	gloss (o)	tongue
inter-	between	gluc (o)	sweetness, glucose
intra-	within	glyc (o)	sugar
intro-	into, within	gyn, gyne, gyneco	woman
leuk-	white	hem, hema, hemo, hemat (o)	blood
macro-	large		
mal-	bad, illness, disease	hepat (o)	liver
meg-	large	hydr (o)	water
micro-	small	hyster (o)	uterus
mono-	one, single	ile (o), ili (o)	ileum
neo-	new	laparo	abdomen, loin, flank
non-	not	laryng (o)	larynx
olig-	small, scant	lith (o)	stone
para-	beside, beyond, after	mamm (o)	breast, mammary gland
per-	by, through	mast (o)	mammary gland, breast
peri-	around	meno	menstruation
poly-	many, much	my (o)	muscle
post-	after, behind	myel (o)	spinal cord, bone marrow
pre-	before, in front of, prior to	necro	death
pro-	before, in front of	nephr (o)	kidney
re-	again, backward	neur (o)	nerve
retro-	backward, behind	ocul (o)	eye
semi-	half	oophor (o)	ovary
sub-	under, beneath	ophthalm (o)	eye
super-	above, over, excess	orth (o)	straight, normal, correct
supra-	above, over	oste (o)	bone
tachy-	fast, rapid	ot (o)	ear
trans-	across	ped (o)	child, foot
uni-	one	pharyng (o)	pharynx

BOX 6-3	MEDICAL TERMINOLOGY—cont'd

Root (combining vowel)	Meaning
phleb (o)	vein
pnea	breathing, respiration
pneum (o)	lung, air, gas
proct (o)	rectum
psych (o)	mind
pulmo	lung
py (o)	pus
rect (o)	rectum
rhin (o)	nose
salping (o)	eustachian tube, uterine tube
splen (o)	spleen
sten (o)	narrow, constriction
stern (o)	sternum
stomat (o)	mouth
therm (o)	heat
thoraco	chest
thromb (o)	clot, thrombus
thyr (o)	thyroid
toxic (o)	poison, poisonous
toxo	poison
trache (o)	trachea
urethr (o)	urethra
urin (o)	urine
uro	urine, urinary tract, urination
uter (o)	uterus
vas (o)	blood vessel, vas deferens
ven (o)	vein
vertebr (o)	spine, vertebrae

Suffix	Meaning
-algia	pain
-asis	condition, usually abnormal
-cele	hernia, herniation, pouching
-centesis	puncture and aspiration of
-cyte	cell
-ectasis	dilation, stretching
-ectomy	excision, removal of
-emia	blood condition
-genesis	development, production, creation
-genic	producing, causing
-gram	record
-graph	a diagram, a recording instrument
-graphy	making a recording
-iasis	condition of
-ism	a condition
-itis	inflammation
-logy	the study of
-lysis	destruction of, decomposition
-megaly	enlargement
-meter	measuring instrument
-oma	tumor
-osis	condition
-pathy	disease
-penia	lack, deficiency
-phagia	to eat or consume, swallowing
-phasia	speaking
-phobia	an exaggerated fear
-plasty	surgical repair or reshaping
-plegia	paralysis
-ptosis	falling, sagging, dropping down
-rrhage, -rrhagia	excessive flow
-rrhaphy	stitching, suturing
-rrhea	flow, discharge
-scope	examination instrument
-scopy	examination using a scope
-stasis	maintenance, maintaining a constant level
-stomy, -ostomy	creation of an opening
-tomy, -otomy	incision, cutting into
-uria	condition of the urine

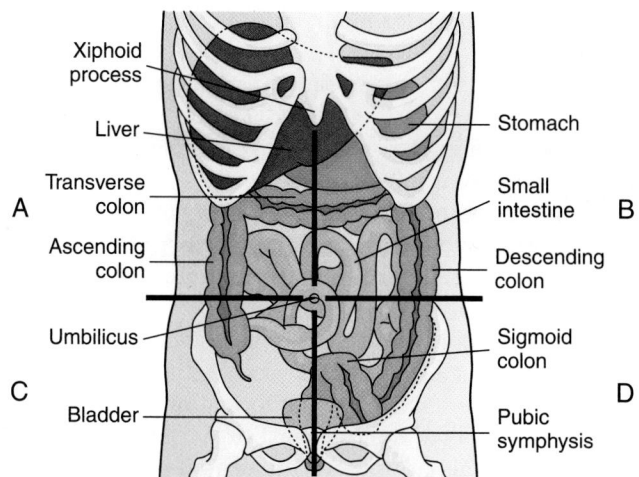

Fig. 6-9 The four abdominal regions. **A,** Right upper quadrant. **B,** Left upper quadrant. **C,** Right lower quadrant. **D,** Left lower quadrant.

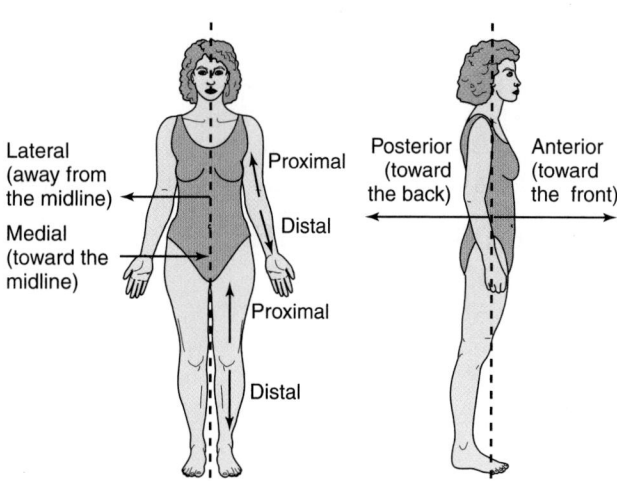

Fig. 6-10 Directional terms describe the position of one body part in relation to another.

BOX 6-4	COMMON HEALTH CARE TERMS AND PHRASES
activities of daily living (ADL)	The activities usually done during a normal day in a person's life
assistive device	Any item used by the person or staff to promote the person's function or safety (hand rails, grab bars, transfer lifts, canes, walkers, wheelchairs, and so on)
atrophy	The decrease in size or the wasting away of tissue
care plan	A written guide about the person's care
cognitive function	Involves memory, thinking, reasoning, understanding, judgment, and behavior
contracture	The lack of joint mobility caused by abnormal shortening of a muscle
dementia	The loss of cognitive and social function caused by changes in the brain; the loss of cognitive function
dysphagia	Difficulty (dys) swallowing (phagia)
dyspnea	Difficult, labored, or painful (dys) breathing (pnea)
feces	The semi-solid mass of waste products in the colon that are expelled through the anus
fever	Elevated body temperature
Fowler's position	A semi-sitting position; the head of the bed is raised between 45 and 60 degrees
incontinence	Not being able to control urination (urinary incontinence) or defecation (fecal incontinence)
pressure ulcer	A localized injury to the skin and/or underlying tissue usually over a bony prominence resulting from pressure or pressure in combination with shear; any lesion caused by unrelieved pressure that results in damage to underlying tissues
prone	Lying on the abdomen with the head turned to one side
semi-Fowler's position	The head of the bed is raised 30 degrees; or the head of the bed is raised 30 degrees and the knee portion is raised 15 degrees
signal light	Part of the call system allowing the person to signal the nurses' station for help
supine	The back-lying or dorsal recumbent position
vital signs	Temperature, pulse, respirations, and blood pressure (and pain in some agencies)
voiding	Urinating

Abbreviations

Abbreviations are shortened forms of words or phrases. They save time and space when recording. Each agency has a list of accepted abbreviations. Obtain the list when you are hired. Use only those on the list. If not sure about using an abbreviation, write the term out in full. This promotes accurate communication.

Common abbreviations are on the inside of the back book cover for easy use.

Common Terms and Phrases

Some terms and phrases apply to basic care and safety. Because they are used throughout this book, they are defined in Box 6-4. Many are key terms in other chapters.

COMPUTERS AND OTHER ELECTRONIC DEVICES

Computer systems collect, send, record, and store information (data). Data are retrieved when needed. Many agencies store charts and care plans (Chapter 7) on computers. Entering data on a computer or other electronic device is often easier and faster than paper charting.

Computers and faxes are used to send messages and reports to the nursing unit. This reduces clerical work and phone calls. And data are sent with greater speed and accuracy.

Computers are used for measurements such as blood pressures, temperatures, and heart rates. The computer senses normal and abnormal measurements. When the abnormal is sensed, an alarm alerts the nursing staff. Computer monitoring is common in hospitals and in skilled nursing units.

Computers and other electronic devices save time. Quality care and safety are increased. Fewer errors are made in recording. Records are more complete (Fig. 6-11). Staff are more efficient.

Each staff member using computers and other electronic devices is issued a username and password. They are used to access, send, receive, or store protected health information (PHI).

You must follow the agency's policies when using computers and other electronic devices. You must keep PHI and electronic protected health information (ePHI, EPHI) confidential. Follow the rules in Box 6-5 and the ethical and legal rules about privacy, confidentiality, and defamation (Chapter 4).

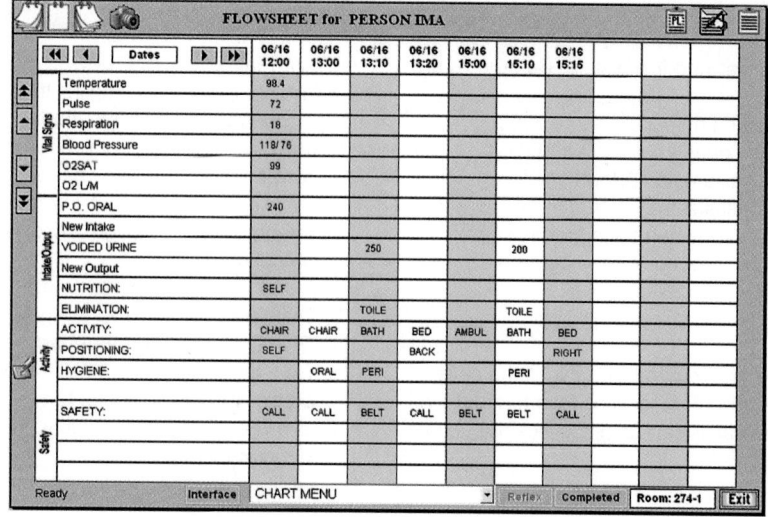

Fig. 6-11 Electronic charting sample.

BOX 6-5 USING THE AGENCY'S COMPUTER AND OTHER ELECTRONIC DEVICES

Computers

- Do not tell anyone your username or password. If someone has your information, he or she can access, record, send, receive, or store EPHI under your name. It will be hard to prove that someone else did so and not you.
- Do not write down, post, or expose your username or password. This is for your security. For example, do not write them on a notepad or post them at your work station.
- Change your password often. Follow agency policy.
- Do not use another person's username or password.
- Follow the rules for recording (see Box 6-2).
- Enter data carefully. Double-check your entries.
- Prevent others from seeing what is on the screen:
  - Position the monitor so the screen cannot be seen in the hallway or by others.
  - Be aware of anyone standing behind you.
  - Stand or sit with your back to the wall if recording on a mobile computer unit.
  - Do not leave the computer unattended.
- Log off after making an entry.
- Do not leave printouts where others can read them or pick them up.
- Shred or destroy computer-printed documents or worksheets. Follow agency policy.
- Send e-mail and messages only to those needing the information.
- Do not use e-mail for information or messages that require immediate reporting. Give the report in person. The person may not read the e-mail in a timely manner.
- Do not use e-mail or messages to report confidential information. This includes addresses, phone numbers, and Social Security numbers. The computer system may not be secure.
- Do not use the agency's computer for your personal use. Do not:
  - Send personal e-mail messages.
  - Send or receive e-mail or messages that are offensive, not legal, or sexual.

Computers—cont'd

- Send or receive e-mail or messages for illegal activities, jokes, politics, gambling (including football and other pools), chain letters, or other non-work activities.
- Post information, opinions, or comments on Internet message boards or social networking sites (Twitter, Facebook, MySpace, and others).
- Take part in Internet discussion groups.
- Upload, download, or send materials containing a copyright, trademark, or patent.
- Remember that any communication can be read or heard by someone other than the intended person.
- Remember that deleted communications can be retrieved by authorized staff.
- Remember that the agency has the right to monitor your use of computers or other electronic devices. This includes Internet use.
- Do not open another person's e-mail or messages.
- Follow agency policy for mis-directed e-mails.

Faxes

- Use the agency's approved "cover sheet." The sheet has instructions about:
  - The confidentiality of PHI (EPHI)
  - The receiver's responsibilities concerning PHI (EPHI)
  - The receiver's responsibilities if the fax is received in error (mis-directed fax)
- Complete the "cover sheet" according to agency policy. Usually the following information is required:
  - Name of the person to receive the fax
  - Receiver's fax number
  - Date
  - Number of pages being faxed
  - Department name
  - Name and phone number of the employee sending the fax
- Follow agency policy for a mis-directed fax.
- Do not leave sent or received faxes unattended in the fax machine or lying around.

BOX 6-6	**GUIDELINES FOR ANSWERING PHONES**

- Answer the call after the first ring if possible. Be sure to answer by the fourth ring.
- Do not answer the phone in a rushed or hasty manner.
- Give a courteous greeting. Identify the nursing unit, and give your name and title. For example: "Good morning. Three center. Mark Wills, nursing assistant."
- Write the following information when taking a message:
  - The caller's name and phone number (include area code and extension number)
  - The date and time
  - The message
- Repeat the message and phone number back to the caller.
- Ask the caller to "Please hold" if necessary. First find out who is calling. Then ask if the caller can hold. Do not put callers with an emergency on hold.
- Do not lay the phone down or cover the receiver with your hand when not speaking to the caller. The caller may overhear confidential conversations.
- Return to a caller on hold within 30 seconds. Ask if the caller can wait longer or if the call can be returned.
- Do not give confidential information to any caller. Patient, resident, and employee information is confidential. Refer such calls to a nurse.
- Transfer the call if appropriate:
  - Tell the caller that you are going to transfer the call.
  - Give the name of the department if appropriate.
  - Give the caller the phone number in case the call gets disconnected or the line is busy.
- End the conversation politely. Thank the person for calling, and say good-bye.
- Give the message to the appropriate person.

PHONE COMMUNICATIONS

You will answer phones at the nurses' station or in the person's room. You need good communication skills. The caller cannot see you. But you give much information by your tone of voice, how clearly you speak, and your attitude. Act as if speaking to someone face-to-face. Be professional and courteous. Also practice good work ethics. Follow the agency's policy and the guidelines in Box 6-6.

See *Focus on Long-Term Care and Home Care: Phone Communications.*

FOCUS ON LONG-TERM CARE AND HOME CARE
Phone Communications

Home Care

When answering phones in patients' homes, simply answer with "hello." This is for everyone's safety—the person, family, and you. The caller has too much information when you give the person's name ("Price residence") or your name and title.

People call homes for many reasons. Some make sales calls or to obtain donations. Others have criminal intent. They want to know who is there. Saying that you are a home health assistant tells that an ill, older, or disabled person is in the home. It is hard for these people to protect and defend themselves. They are easy prey for criminals.

Do not give your name or the person's name until you know who is calling and why. Make sure it is someone you want to talk to—the person's family or friend, your supervisor, or a caller expected by the person.

DEALING WITH CONFLICT

People bring their values, attitudes, opinions, experiences, and expectations to the work setting. Differences often lead to conflict. *Conflict is a clash between opposing interests or ideas.* People disagree and argue. There are misunderstandings and unrest.

Conflicts arise over issues or events. Work schedules, absences, and the amount and quality of work performed are examples. The problems must be worked out. Otherwise, unkind words or actions may occur. The work setting becomes unpleasant. Care is affected.

To resolve conflict, identify the real problem. This is part of *problem solving.* The problem solving process involves these steps:

- Step 1: Define the problem. *A nurse ignores me.*
- Step 2: Collect information about the problem. Do not include unrelated information. *The nurse does not look at me. The nurse does not talk to me. The nurse does not respond when I ask for help. The nurse does not ask me to help with tasks that require two people. The nurse talks to other staff members.*
- Step 3: Identify possible solutions. *Ignore the nurse. Talk to my supervisor. Talk to co-workers about the problem. Change jobs.*
- Step 4: Select the best solution. *Talk to my supervisor.*
- Step 5: Carry out the solution. *See below.*
- Step 6: Evaluate the results. *See below.*

Communication and good work ethics help prevent and resolve conflicts. Identify and solve problems before they become major issues. To deal with conflict:

- Ask your supervisor for some time to talk privately. Explain the problem. Give facts and specific examples. Ask for advice in solving the problem.
- Approach the person with whom you have the conflict. Ask to talk privately. Be polite and professional.
- Agree on a time and place to talk.

- Talk in a private setting. No one should hear you or the other person.
- Explain the problem and what is bothering you. Give facts and specific behaviors. Focus on the problem. Do not focus on the person.
- Listen to the person. Do not interrupt.
- Identify ways to solve the problem. Offer your thoughts. Ask for the co-worker's ideas.
- Set a date and time to review the matter.
- Thank the person for meeting with you.
- Carry out the solution.
- Review the matter as scheduled.

  See *Focus on Communication: Dealing With Conflict.*

FOCUS ON COMMUNICATION
Dealing With Conflict

You may find it hard to talk to someone with whom you have a conflict. This is hard for many people. However, letting the problem or issue continue only makes the matter worse. The following may help you start talking to the person:

- "You say 'no' when I ask you to help me. I help you when you ask me to. This really bothers me. Can we talk privately for a few minutes?"
- "I heard you tell John that you saw me sitting in Mrs. Gordon's room. You seemed angry when you said it. Can we talk privately? I want to explain why I was sitting and find out why that bothers you."
- "The new schedule shows me working every weekend this month. Please tell me why. The employee handbook says that we work every other weekend."

FOCUS ON PRIDE
The Person, Family, and Yourself

Personal and Professional Responsibility

Health team members must communicate for effective and coordinated care. Communication must be factual, concise, and understandable. This helps the team provide quality care.

You are responsible for the information you report and record. It must be accurate. False or incomplete information can harm the person. If your agency allows nursing assistants to chart:

- Chart what you do. If not charted, there is no proof that you completed a task.
- Never falsify charting. Never chart that something was done when it really was not.
- Only chart after completing a delegated task. If events change, your charting is wrong.
- Ask the nurse if you have questions about what or how to chart.

Rights and Respect

Conflict among co-workers will arise. Dealing with conflict can be hard. But, it must be addressed. Deal with conflict in a respectful and mature way. Do not gossip, put others down, or talk about people behind their backs. These are not professional behaviors.

Everyone, including you, deserves to be treated with respect. If you feel someone has wronged you, address the issue. Politely ask to talk to the person in private. Speak calmly and respectfully. Focus on the problem and the solution. Do not attack the person's character. For example, do not say: "You are so mean. I can't believe you were talking about me behind my back." Instead, you can say: "It bothers me that you didn't come to me about this. Next time could you talk to me first?" For good working relationships, identify and resolve conflict in a respectful and professional manner.

Independence and Social Interaction

Communication with the health team is not limited to reporting and recording. You also interact in the nurses' station, hallways, break room, cafeteria, parking lot, and so on. Your informal interactions carry over into working relationships. Treat co-workers with kindness and respect. Have a good attitude. Be someone others enjoy working with!

Delegation and Teamwork

You are responsible for your speech, actions, and charting. This is called being accountable. For example, you are delegated a task. You are responsible for completing the task and reporting or recording its completion. If you do not complete it, you are still held accountable. You must tell the nurse why it was not done. Or you must complete the task.

Do not be offended when asked if you completed a task or charted. This is part of accountability. The delegating nurse must know what was done and what was not done. Show you are accountable by:

- Completing tasks in a timely manner
- Recording accurately
- Reporting when you complete a task
- Telling the nurse if a task was not done and why

Ethics and Laws

Truthful recording is taken seriously. Legal action can be taken against persons who record false information. For example:

A licensed nursing assistant (LNA) worked at a home health and hospice agency. On November 9, 2001, she recorded on a time sheet that she was in a patient's home for about 30 minutes. However, the patient was in the hospital from November 8 through November 14, 2001.

The LNA admitted to unprofessional conduct. Her conduct violated Administrative Rules of the Board of Nursing for:

- *Making inaccurate or misleading entries*
- *Failing to comply with federal or state laws or rules*

  The LNA was given a reprimand by the Board.

  (State of Vermont Board of Nursing in regard to T. Brigham, 2003.)

A reprimand means that the Board considered her conduct to be improper. However, the Board did not limit her right to work as an LNA.

You are accountable for the information you record. Take pride in honest and accurate recording.

REVIEW QUESTIONS

Circle T if the statement is TRUE or F if it is FALSE.

1 T F You help with Mrs. Gordon's care. Reading her medical record violates her right to privacy.

2 T F You can access all medical records in the agency.

3 T F When using a computer, the person's privacy must be protected.

4 T F All employees have the same password for computer use.

5 T F You can give information about the person over the phone.

6 T F You should leave faxes in the fax machine for the nurse to read.

Circle the BEST answer.

7 To communicate, you should do the following *except*
   a Use terms with many meanings
   b Be brief and concise
   c Present information logically and in sequence
   d Give facts and be specific

8 A person is discharged from the agency. The medical record is
   a Destroyed
   b Sent home with the family
   c Permanent
   d Stored on a computer

9 These statements are about medical records. Which is *false*?
   a They are used to communicate information about patients and residents.
   b They are a written or electronic account of illness and response to treatment.
   c They can be used as evidence of the care given.
   d All agency staff can read them.

10 A person is weighed daily. The measurement is recorded on the
   a Graphic sheet
   b Kardex
   c Flow sheet
   d Progress notes

11 Where does the nurse describe the nursing care given?
   a Admission sheet
   b ADL flow sheet
   c Progress notes
   d Kardex

12 When recording, you do the following *except*
   a Use ink
   b Include the date and time
   c Erase errors
   d Sign all entries with your name and title

13 These statements are about recording. Which is *false*?
   a Use the person's exact words when possible.
   b Record only what you did and observed.
   c Sign your initials to a mistaken entry.
   d Chart a procedure before completing it.

14 In the evening the clock shows 9:26. In 24-hour clock time this is
   a 9:26 PM
   b 1926
   c 0926
   d 2126

15 A suffix is
   a Placed at the beginning of a word
   b Placed after a root
   c A shortened form of a word or phrase
   d The main meaning of the word

16 Which term relates to the side of the body?
   a Anterior
   b Lateral
   c Posterior
   d Proximal

17 These statements are about computers in health care. Which is *false*?
   a They are used to collect, send, record, and store data.
   b Computers link one department to another.
   c You should log off after making an entry.
   d You can use another person's username if yours does not work.

18 You have access to the agency's computer. Which is *true*?
   a E-mail and messages are sent only to those needing the information.
   b E-mail is used for reports the nurse needs at once.
   c You can open another person's e-mail.
   d You can use the computer for your personal needs.

19 You answer a person's phone in a nursing center. How should you answer?
   a "Good morning. Mrs. Park's room."
   b "Good morning. Third floor."
   c "Hello."
   d "Good morning. Tammy Brown, nursing assistant, speaking."

20 A co-worker is often late for work. This means extra work for you. To resolve the conflict you should do the following *except*
   a Explain the problem to your supervisor
   b Discuss the matter during the end-of-shift report
   c Give facts and specific behaviors
   d Suggest ways to solve the problem

Answers to these questions on p. 832.

Assisting With the Nursing Process

OBJECTIVES

- Define the key terms and key abbreviations listed in this chapter.
- Explain the purpose of the nursing process.
- Describe the steps of the nursing process.
- Explain your role in each step of the nursing process.
- Explain the difference between objective data and subjective data.
- Identify the observations that you need to report to the nurse.
- Explain the purpose of care conferences.
- Explain how to promote PRIDE in the person, the family, and yourself.

KEY TERMS

assessment Collecting information about the person; a step in the nursing process

evaluation To measure if goals in the planning step were met; a step in the nursing process

goal That which is desired for or by a person as a result of nursing care

implementation To perform or carry out nursing measures in the care plan; a step in the nursing process

medical diagnosis The identification of a disease or condition by a doctor

nursing care plan A written guide about the person's nursing care; care plan

nursing diagnosis Describes a health problem that can be treated by nursing measures; a step in the nursing process

nursing intervention An action or measure taken by the nursing team to help the person reach a goal

nursing process The method nurses use to plan and deliver nursing care; its five steps are assessment, nursing diagnosis, planning, implementation, and evaluation

objective data Information that is seen, heard, felt, or smelled by an observer; signs

observation Using the senses of sight, hearing, touch, and smell to collect information

planning Setting priorities and goals; a step in the nursing process

signs See "objective data"

subjective data Things a person tells you about that you cannot observe through your senses; symptoms

symptoms See "subjective data"

KEY ABBREVIATIONS

ADL	Activities of daily living
CAA	Care Area Assessment
IDCP	Interdisciplinary care planning
MDS	Minimum Data Set
NANDA-I	North American Nursing Diagnosis Association International
OASIS	Outcome and Assessment Information Set
OBRA	Omnibus Budget Reconciliation Act of 1987
RN	Registered nurse

Nurses communicate with each other about the person's strengths, problems, needs, and care. This information is shared through the nursing process. The *nursing process is the method nurses use to plan and deliver nursing care. It has five steps:*
* *Assessment*
* *Nursing diagnosis*
* *Planning*
* *Implementation*
* *Evaluation*

The nursing process focuses on the person's nursing needs. The person and nursing team need good communication.

Each step is important. If done in order with good communication, nursing care is organized and has purpose. All nursing team members do the same things for the person. They have the same goals. The person feels safe and secure with consistent care.

The nursing process is used in all health care settings and for all age-groups. It is on-going. New information is gathered and the person's needs may change. However, the steps are the same. You will see how the nursing process is continuous as each step is explained (Fig. 7-1).

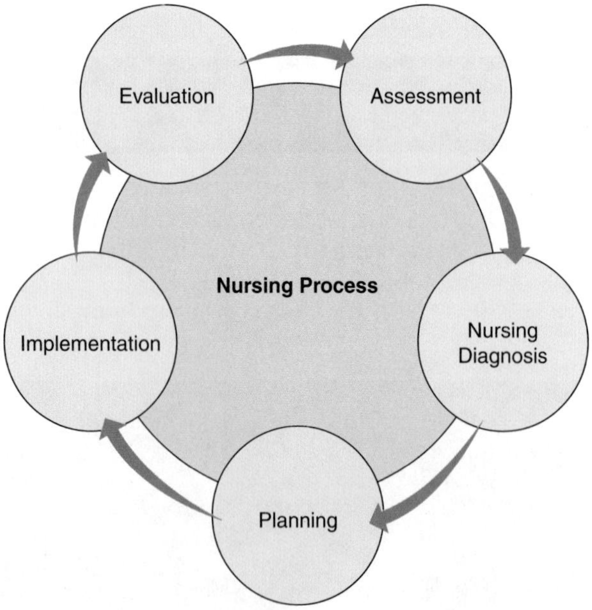

ASSESSMENT

Assessment involves collecting information about the person. Nurses use many sources. A health history is taken about current and past health problems. The family's health history is important. Many diseases are genetic. That is, the risk for certain diseases is inherited from parents. For example, a mother had breast cancer. Her daughters are at risk. Information from the doctor is reviewed. So are test results and past medical records.

An RN (registered nurse) assesses the person's body systems and mental status. You play a key role in assessment. You make many observations as you give care and talk to the person.

Observation is using the senses of sight, hearing, touch, and smell to collect information:
* You *see* how the person lies, sits, or walks. You see flushed or pale skin. You see red and swollen body areas.
* You *listen* to the person breathe, talk, and cough. You use a stethoscope to listen to the heartbeat and to measure blood pressure.
* Through *touch*, you feel if the skin is hot or cold, or moist or dry. You use touch to take the person's pulse.
* *Smell* is used to detect body, wound, and breath odors. You also smell odors from urine and bowel movements.

Objective data (signs) are seen, heard, felt, or smelled by an observer. You can feel a pulse. You can see urine color. *Subjective data (symptoms) are things a person tells you about that you cannot observe through your senses.* You cannot feel or see the person's pain, fear, or nausea.

Box 7-1 lists the observations to report at once. Box 7-2 lists the basic observations you need to make and report to the nurse. Make notes of your observations. Use them to report and record observations. Carry a note pad and pen in your pocket. Note your observations as you make them. The agency may provide electronic devices for this purpose (Fig. 7-2, p. 82).

The assessment step never ends. New information is collected with every patient or resident contact. New observations are made. The person shares more information. Often the family adds more information.

See *Focus on Long-Term Care and Home Care: Assessment,* p. 82.

Fig. 7-1 The nursing process is continuous.

BOX 7-1	OBSERVATIONS TO REPORT AT ONCE

* A change in the person's ability to respond
  * A responsive person no longer responds.
  * A non-responsive person now responds.
* A change in the person's mobility
  * The person cannot move a body part.
  * The person can now move a body part.
* Complaints of sudden, severe pain
* A sore or reddened area on the person's skin
* Complaints of a sudden change in vision
* Complaints of pain or difficulty breathing
* Abnormal respirations
* Complaints of or signs of difficulty swallowing
* Vomiting
* Bleeding
* Vital signs outside their normal ranges

BOX 7-2   BASIC OBSERVATIONS

Ability to Respond
- Is the person easy or hard to wake up?
- Can the person give his or her name, the time, and location when asked?
- Does the person identify others correctly?
- Does the person answer questions correctly?
- Does the person speak clearly?
- Are instructions followed correctly?
- Is the person calm, restless, or excited?
- Is the person conversing, quiet, or talking a lot?

Movement
- Can the person squeeze your fingers with each hand?
- Can the person move arms and legs?
- Are the person's movements shaky or jerky?
- Does the person complain of stiff or painful joints?

Pain or Discomfort
- Where is the pain located? (Ask the person to point to the pain.)
- Does the pain go anywhere else?
- How does the person rate the severity of the pain—mild, moderate, severe?
- How does the person rate the pain on a scale of 0 to 10 (Chapter 28)?
- When did the pain begin?
- What was the person doing when the pain began?
- How long does the pain last?
- How does the person describe the pain?
  - Sharp
  - Severe
  - Knife-like
  - Dull
  - Burning
  - Aching
  - Comes and goes
  - Depends on position
- Was a pain-relief drug given?
- Did the pain-relief drug relieve the pain? Is the pain still present?
- Is the person able to sleep and rest?
- What is the position of comfort?

Skin
- Is the skin pale or flushed?
- Is the skin cool, warm, or hot?
- Is the skin moist or dry?
- Does the skin appear mottled (blotchy, spotted with color)?
- What color are the lips and nail beds?
- Is the skin intact? Are there broken areas? If so, where?
- Are sores or reddened areas present?
- Are bruises present? Where are they located?
- Does the person complain of itching? If yes, where?

Eyes, Ears, Nose, and Mouth
- Is there drainage from the eyes? What color is the drainage?
- Are the eyelids closed? Do they stay open?
- Are the eyes reddened?
- Does the person complain of spots, flashes, or blurring?
- Is the person sensitive to bright lights?
- Is there drainage from the ears? What color is the drainage?
- Can the person hear? Is repeating necessary? Are questions answered appropriately?

Eyes, Ears, Nose, and Mouth—cont'd
- Is there drainage from the nose? What color is the drainage?
- Can the person breathe through the nose?
- Is there breath odor?
- Does the person complain of a bad taste in the mouth?
- Does the person complain of painful gums or teeth?

Respirations
- Do both sides of the person's chest rise and fall with respirations?
- Is breathing noisy?
- Does the person complain of pain or difficulty breathing?
- What is the amount and color of sputum?
- What is the frequency of the person's cough? Is it dry or productive?

Bowels and Bladder
- Is the abdomen firm or soft?
- Does the person complain of gas?
- Which does the person use: toilet, commode, bedpan, or urinal?
- What are the amount, color, and consistency of bowel movements?
- What is the frequency of bowel movements?
- Can the person control bowel movements?
- Does the person have pain or difficulty urinating?
- What is the amount of urine?
- What is the color of urine?
- Is the urine clear? Are there particles in the urine?
- Does urine have a foul smell?
- Can the person control the passage of urine?
- What is the frequency of urination?

Appetite
- Does the person like the food served?
- How much of the meal is eaten?
- What foods does the person like?
- Can the person chew food?
- What is the amount of fluid taken?
- What fluids does the person like?
- How often does the person drink fluids?
- Can the person swallow food and fluids?
- Does the person complain of nausea?
- What is the amount and color of vomitus?
- Does the person have hiccups?
- Is the person belching?
- Does the person cough when swallowing?

Activities of Daily Living
- Can the person perform personal care without help?
  - Bathing?
  - Brushing teeth?
  - Combing and brushing hair?
  - Shaving?
- Does the person feed himself or herself?
- Can the person walk?
- What amount and kind of help is needed?

Other
- Is the person bleeding from any body part? If yes, where and how much?

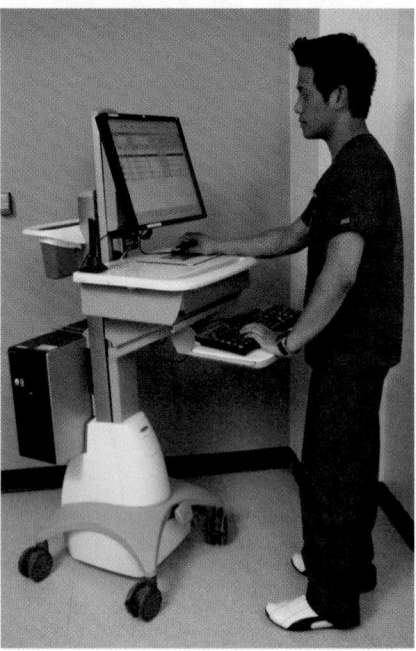

Fig 7-2 The nursing assistant uses an electronic device to note observations.

NURSING DIAGNOSIS

The RN uses assessment information to make a nursing diagnosis. A *nursing diagnosis describes a health problem that can be treated by nursing measures* (Box 7-3). The problem may exist or develop.

Nursing diagnoses and medical diagnoses are not the same. A *medical diagnosis is the identification of a disease or condition by a doctor.* Cancer, stroke, heart attack, infection, and diabetes are examples. Doctors order drugs, therapies, and surgery to cure or heal.

A person can have many nursing diagnoses. They deal with the total person—physical, emotional, social, and spiritual needs. They may change as assessment information changes. Or new nursing diagnoses are added. For example, "Acute pain" is added after surgery.

PLANNING

Planning involves setting priorities and goals. Nursing measures or actions are chosen to help the person meet the goals. The person, family, and health team help the RN plan care.

Priorities relate to what is most important for the person. Maslow's theory of basic needs is useful for setting priorities (Chapter 8). The needs are arranged in order of importance. Some needs are required for life and survival (oxygen, water, and food). They must be met before all other needs. They have priority and must be done first.

Goals are then set. A *goal is that which is desired for or by a person as a result of nursing care.* Goals are aimed at the person's highest level of well-being and function—physical, emotional, social, spiritual. Goals promote health and prevent health problems. They also promote rehabilitation.

- Activity Intolerance; Activity Intolerance, Risk for
- Activity Planning, Ineffective; Activity Planning, Ineffective, Risk for
- Adverse Reaction to Iodinated Contrast Media, Risk for
- Airway Clearance, Ineffective
- Allergy Response, Risk for
- Anxiety
- Aspiration, Risk for
- Attachment, Risk for Impaired
- Autonomic Dysreflexia; Autonomic Dysreflexia, Risk for
- Bathing Self-Care Deficit
- Bleeding, Risk for
- Body Image, Disturbed
- Body Temperature, Risk for Imbalanced
- Breastfeeding: Ineffective, Interrupted, Readiness for Enhanced
- Breast Milk, Insufficient
- Breathing Pattern, Ineffective
- Cardiac Output, Decreased
- Caregiver Role Strain; Caregiver Role Strain, Risk for
- Childbearing Process: Ineffective, Readiness for Enhanced, Risk for Ineffective
- Comfort: Impaired, Readiness for Enhanced
- Communication: Impaired Verbal, Readiness for Enhanced
- Community Coping: Ineffective, Readiness for Enhanced
- Confusion: Acute, Chronic, Risk for Acute
- Constipation; Constipation: Perceived, Risk for
- Contamination; Contamination, Risk for
- Coping: Defensive, Ineffective, Readiness for Enhanced
- Death Anxiety
- Decisional Conflict
- Decision Making, Readiness for Enhanced
- Denial, Ineffective
- Dentition, Impaired
- Development, Risk for Delayed
- Diarrhea
- Dignity, Human, Risk for Compromised
- Disuse Syndrome, Risk for
- Diversional Activity, Deficient
- Dressing Self-Care Deficit
- Dry Eye, Risk for
- Electrolyte Imbalance, Risk for
- Energy Field, Disturbed
- Environmental Interpretation Syndrome, Impaired
- Failure to Thrive, Adult
- Falls, Risk for
- Family Coping: Compromised, Disabled, Readiness for Enhanced
- Family Processes: Dysfunctional, Interrupted, Readiness for Enhanced
- Fatigue
- Fear
- Feeding Self-Care Deficit
- Fluid Balance, Readiness for Enhanced
- Fluid Volume: Deficient, Excess, Risk for Deficient, Risk for Imbalanced
- Gas Exchange, Impaired
- Glucose Level, Blood: Risk for Unstable
- Grieving; Grieving: Complicated, Risk for Complicated
- Growth and Development, Delayed

- Growth, Risk for Disproportionate
- Health Behavior, Risk-Prone
- Health, Deficient Community
- Health Maintenance, Ineffective
- Home Maintenance, Impaired
- Hope, Readiness for Enhanced
- Hopelessness
- Hyperthermia
- Hypothermia
- Immunization Status, Readiness for Enhanced
- Impulse Control, Ineffective
- Incontinence, Bowel
- Incontinence, Urinary: Functional; Overflow; Reflex; Stress; Urge; Urge, Risk for
- Infant Behavior: Disorganized; Organized, Readiness for Enhanced; Risk for Disorganized
- Infant Feeding Pattern, Ineffective
- Infection, Risk for
- Injury, Risk for
- Insomnia
- Intracranial Adaptive Capacity, Decreased
- Jaundice: Neonatal, Risk for Neonatal
- Knowledge: Deficient, Readiness for Enhanced
- Latex Allergy Response; Latex Allergy Response, Risk for
- Lifestyle, Sedentary
- Liver Function, Risk for Impaired
- Loneliness, Risk for
- Maternal/Fetal Dyad, Risk for Disturbed
- Memory, Impaired
- Mobility: Impaired Bed, Impaired Physical, Impaired Wheelchair
- Moral Distress
- Motility, Dysfunctional Gastro-intestinal; Motility, Dysfunctional Gastro-intestinal, Risk for
- Nausea
- Neglect: Self, Unilateral
- Noncompliance
- Nutrition, Imbalanced: Less Than Body Requirements; More Than Body Requirements; More Than Body Requirements, Risk for
- Nutrition, Readiness for Enhanced
- Oral Mucous Membrane, Impaired
- Pain: Acute, Chronic
- Parental Role Conflict
- Parenting: Impaired, Readiness for Enhanced, Risk for Impaired
- Perfusion: Ineffective Peripheral Tissue, Risk for Ineffective Peripheral Tissue, Risk for Decreased Cardiac Tissue, Risk for Ineffective Cerebral Tissue, Risk for Ineffective Gastro-intestinal, Risk for Ineffective Renal
- Perioperative-Positioning Injury, Risk for
- Peripheral Neurovascular Dysfunction, Risk for
- Personal Identity, Disturbed, Risk for Disturbed
- Poisoning, Risk for
- Post-Trauma Syndrome; Post-Trauma Syndrome, Risk for
- Powerlessness; Powerlessness, Risk for
- Power, Readiness for Enhanced
- Protection, Ineffective
- Rape-Trauma Syndrome

Continued

BOX 7-3	**NURSING DIAGNOSES APPROVED BY THE NORTH AMERICAN NURSING DIAGNOSIS ASSOCIATION INTERNATIONAL (NANDA-I)—cont'd**

- Relationship: Ineffective, Risk for Ineffective, Readiness for Enhanced
- Religiosity: Impaired, Readiness for Enhanced, Risk for Impaired
- Relocation Stress Syndrome; Relocation Stress Syndrome, Risk for
- Resilience: Impaired Individual, Readiness for Enhanced, Risk for Compromised
- Role Performance, Ineffective
- Self-Care, Readiness for Enhanced
- Self-Concept, Readiness for Enhanced
- Self-Esteem: Chronic Low; Chronic Low, Risk for; Situational Low; Situational Low, Risk for
- Self Health Management: Ineffective, Readiness for Enhanced
- Self-Mutilation; Self-Mutilation, Risk for
- Sexual Dysfunction
- Sexuality Pattern, Ineffective
- Shock, Risk for
- Skin Integrity: Impaired, Risk for Impaired
- Sleep Deprivation
- Sleep Pattern, Disturbed
- Sleep, Readiness for Enhanced
- Social Interaction, Impaired

- Social Isolation
- Sorrow, Chronic
- Spiritual Distress; Spiritual Distress, Risk for
- Spiritual Well-Being, Readiness for Enhanced
- Stress, Overload
- Sudden Infant Death Syndrome, Risk for
- Suffocation, Risk for
- Suicide, Risk for
- Surgical Recovery, Delayed
- Swallowing, Impaired
- Therapeutic Regimen Management, Ineffective Family
- Thermal Injury, Risk for
- Thermoregulation, Ineffective
- Tissue Integrity, Impaired
- Toileting Self-Care Deficit
- Transfer Ability, Impaired
- Trauma, Risk for; Trauma, Risk for Vascular
- Urinary Elimination: Impaired, Readiness for Enhanced
- Urinary Retention
- Ventilation, Impaired Spontaneous
- Ventilatory Weaning Response, Dysfunctional
- Violence: Risk for Other-Directed, Risk for Self-Directed
- Walking, Impaired
- Wandering

Nursing interventions are chosen after goals are set. An *intervention* is an action or measure. A *nursing intervention is an action or measure taken by the nursing team to help the person reach a goal.* Nursing intervention, nursing action, and nursing measure mean the same thing. A nursing intervention does not need a doctor's order. However, some nursing measures come from a doctor's order. For example, a doctor orders that Mrs. Lange walk 50 yards 2 times a day. The nurse includes this order in the care plan.

The *nursing care plan (care plan) is a written guide about the person's nursing care.* It has the person's nursing diagnoses and goals. It also has measures or actions for each goal. The care plan is a communication tool. Nursing staff use it to see what care to give. The care plan helps ensure that nursing team members give the same care.

Each agency has a care plan form. It is found in the medical record, on the Kardex, or on a computer (Fig. 7-3).

Care Conferences

The RN may conduct a care conference to share information and ideas about the person's care. The purpose is to develop or revise the person's nursing care plan. Effective care is the goal. Nursing assistants usually take part in the conference.

FOCUS ON COMMUNICATION
Care Conferences

You spend a lot of time with the patients and residents. You see what they like and do not like. You see what they can and cannot do. Patients and residents talk to you. They tell you about their families and interests. You make observations every time you are with them. Share this information during care conferences. Also share ideas about the person's care. Your sharing can improve the person's quality of life. For example, you can say:

- "Mr. Antonio never eats his squash. He says that he misses the fresh green beans and broccoli from his garden. Can he have those more often?"
- "Mrs. Clark can use her feet to propel her wheelchair. Why do we have to push her wheelchair?"
- "Miss Walsh never talks when her family visits. She just sits there. Yet she talks to her roommate all the time."

The plan is carried out. It may change as the person's nursing diagnoses change.

See *Focus on Communication: Care Conferences.*

See *Focus on Long-Term Care and Home Care: Care Conferences.*

Nursing Diagnosis	Goal	Intervention
Constipation related to lack of privacy as evidenced by no BM for 5 days.	Patient will have regular bowel movements by 6/30.	Ask patient to use signal light when urge to have bowel movement is felt. Answer signal light promptly. Assist patient to bathroom. Close bathroom door for privacy. Leave the room if the patient can be alone; tell the patient you are leaving and that you will return when the signal light is on.
Insomnia related to noisy environment as evidenced by patient complaints of noise and lack of sleep.	Patient will report a restful sleep by 6/29.	Perform any necessary care measures before bedtime. Close the door to the patient's room. Turn off television or radio or keep volume low if patient prefers. Ask staff to avoid unnecessary talking outside the patient's room. Ask staff to speak in low voices. Turn off unneeded equipment.

Fig. 7-3 Nursing care plan. Each nursing diagnosis has a goal. There are nursing interventions (measures) for each goal.

FOCUS ON LONG-TERM CARE AND HOME CARE

Care Conferences

Long-Term Care

OBRA requires two types of resident care conferences:

- *Interdisciplinary care planning (IDCP) conference.* This is held regularly to review and update care plans. It also is held to develop care plans for new residents. The RN, doctor, and other health team members attend.
- *Problem-focused conference.* This is used when one problem affects a person's care. Only staff involved with the problem attend.

The person has the right to take part in planning conferences. Sometimes the family is involved. The person may refuse actions suggested by the health team.

Problems identified on the MDS give *triggers* (clues) for the Care Area Assessments (CAAs) (Appendix B, p. 837).

OBRA requires a *comprehensive care plan*. Like the nursing care plan, it is a written guide about the person's care.

Developed by the health team, the resident and family give input. The care plan includes nursing diagnoses and goals. It has the person's problems, goals for care, and actions to take to help the person.

For example, Mr. Woo is weak from illness and no exercise. The MDS shows that he cannot do activities of daily living (ADL). This triggers the CAAs. A care plan is developed to solve the problem. The goal is for Mr. Woo to do his own ADL. Actions to help Mr. Woo reach the goal are:

- Occupational therapy to work with Mr. Woo on ADL daily
- Physical therapy to work with Mr. Woo on exercises daily
- Nursing staff to walk Mr. Woo 20 yards twice daily

The care plan also states the person's strengths. For example, Mr. Woo can feed himself. This strength increases his independence. The health team helps Mr. Woo continue to feed himself.

IMPLEMENTATION

To *implement* means to perform or carry out. The *implementation step is performing or carrying out nursing measures (interventions) in the care plan.* Care is given in this step.

Nursing care ranges from simple to complex. The nurse delegates tasks within your legal limits and job description. The nurse may ask you to assist with complex measures.

You report the care given to the nurse. In some agencies, you record the care given. Report and record *after* giving care, not before. Also report and record your observations. Observing is part of assessment. New observations may change the nursing diagnoses. If so, care plan changes are made. To give correct care, you must know about any changes in the care plan.

Assignment Sheets

The nurse communicates delegated tasks to you. An assignment sheet is used for this purpose (Fig. 7-4). The assignment sheet tells you about:

- Each person's care.
- What measures and tasks need to be done.
- Which nursing unit tasks to do. Cleaning kitchenettes and utility rooms and stocking shower rooms are examples.

Talk to the nurse about an unclear assignment. Also check the care plan and Kardex if you need more information.

See *Focus on Communication: Assignment Sheets.*

See *Teamwork and Time Management: Assignment Sheets.*

EVALUATION

Evaluation means to measure. The *evaluation step involves measuring if the goals in the planning step were met.* Progress is evaluated. Goals may be met totally, in part, or not at all. Assessment information is used for this step. Changes in nursing diagnoses, goals, and the care plan may result.

YOUR ROLE

The nursing process never ends. Nurses constantly collect information about the person. Nursing diagnoses, goals, and the care plan may change as the person's needs change.

You have a key role in the nursing process. Your observations are used for nursing diagnoses and planning. You may help develop the care plan. In the implementation step, you perform tasks in the care plan. Your assignment sheet tells you what to do. Your observations are used for the evaluation step.

Assignment Sheet

Date: 9–10
Shift: Day
Nursing assistant: John Reed
Supervisor: Mary Adams, RN

Breaks: 1000   1400
Lunch: 1230
Unit Tasks: *Pass ice water at 0900*
Clean utility room at 1430

***Check the care plan for other care measures and information**

Room # 501A Name: Mrs. Ann Lopez ID Number: S1514491530 Date of birth: 11/04/1925 VS: Daily at 0700 T _____ P _____ R _____ BP _____ Wt: Weekly (Monday at 0700) _____ Intake _____ Output _____ BM _____ Bath: Portable tub Shampoo Bed rails	**Functional status/other care measures and procedures** Total assist with ADL Stand-pivot transfers Uses w/c Incontinent of bowel and bladder – uses briefs Bilateral passive ROM exercises to extremities twice daily Turn and re-position q2h when in bed Wears eyeglasses and dentures Diet: High fiber (Total Assist)
Room # 510B Name: Mr. Mark Lee ID Number: D4468947762 Date of birth: 12/29/1926 VS: 2 times daily, at 0700 and 1500 0700: T _____ P _____ R _____ BP _____ 1500: T _____ P _____ R _____ BP _____ Wt: Daily at 0700 _____ Intake _____ Output _____ BM _____ Bath: Shower	**Functional status/other care measures and procedures** Independent with ADL Independent with ambulation Attends exercise group every morning Continent of bowel and bladder – q4h bathroom schedule to maintain continence Wears eyeglasses Coughing and deep breathing exercises q4h Diet: Sodium-controlled (Independent)

Fig 7-4 Sample assignment sheet. Note: This assignment sheet is a computer printout.

FOCUS ON COMMUNICATION
Assignment Sheets

Assignment sheets provide a summary of the information you need to care for your patients or residents. The sheets communicate information clearly and in an organized manner. See Figure 7-4. Use your assignment sheets when receiving a report from the nurse. Add any new information. Ask the nurse any questions you may have. For example: "I have a question about Mr. Lee. My assignment sheet does not mention any assistive devices. Last week physical therapy was helping him transfer from a walker to a cane. Which is he using now?"

TEAMWORK AND TIME MANAGEMENT
Assignment Sheets

Use your assignment sheet to organize your work and to set priorities:

* What do you need to do first?
* What can be done while the person is having a meal?
* What can you do when the person is at a therapy (physical, occupational, and so on) or an activity?
* Do you need to reserve a room (shower room, tub room) or equipment (portable tub, shower chair)?
* What do you need help with?
* How many co-workers are needed to complete tasks such as turning and transferring a person?
* Ask a co-worker to help you. Tell what you need help with, when you need the help, and how long the task will take.
* Check off tasks as you complete them.

FOCUS ON PRIDE
The Person, Family, and Yourself

Personal and Professional Responsibility

In Chapter 26, you will learn how to measure vital signs—temperature, pulse, respirations, and blood pressure. Chapter 27 is about positioning and assisting with range-of-motion exercises and walking. And Chapter 31 shows you how to collect specimens. These are only some of the ways that you will assist in the nursing process.

How you perform these actions affects the person's care. You are responsible for doing these skills correctly. You will practice skills in your training. Practice them until you feel comfortable. Ask your instructor if you have questions about a skill. Take pride in learning to do your job well. Take your skills training seriously.

Rights and Respect

The person has the right to take part in care planning. The person also has the right to refuse actions suggested by the health team. The team works with the person to agree upon a plan of care that meets the person's needs and preferences.

For example, the health team suggests applying elastic stockings (Chapter 32) on Mr. Barton's legs to prevent blood clots. Mr. Barton says he wore the stockings 2 years ago, and they were "too tight" and "uncomfortable." He refuses to wear them. The nurse speaks with Mr. Barton about trying a sequential compression device (Chapter 32) instead. The nurse explains that adjustable sleeves are placed on the lower legs. The sleeves attach to a pump. The pump inflates and deflates one sleeve at a time. Mr. Barton agrees to try the device.

Independence and Social Interaction

Patients and residents often feel a loss of independence. Involving persons in care planning can help them feel in control of their care. Care planning begins when the person is admitted to the agency. The plan is focused on the person's specific needs. The plan is modified as needs change. It is an on-going process. The person remains involved the whole time.

To help the person feel involved in his or her care, you can:

* Listen to the person's needs and concerns.
* Ask about the person's preferences.
* Tell the nurse about your observations and ideas to improve care.

Delegation and Teamwork

Assignment sheets are used to communicate the care and unit tasks delegated to you. Do not trade assignments and unit tasks among nursing assistants without the nurse's approval. If you have a problem with an assignment or task, politely speak to the nurse about it. Do not complain. Give the reason. Not liking an assignment or task is not a good reason. The nurse will decide if a change is needed.

Ethics and Laws

Assignment sheets contain confidential information. Keep your sheets with you at all times. Do not leave them lying around for others to find. This violates the Health Insurance Portability and Accountability Act of 1996 (Chapter 4). Before leaving work, place your assignment sheets in a wastebasket marked CONFIDENTIAL INFORMATION for shredding. Take pride in protecting the privacy and security of protected health information.

REVIEW QUESTIONS

Circle the BEST answer.

1 Which is *not* a step in the nursing process?
a Observation
b Assessment
c Planning
d Implementation

2 The nursing process
a Involves guidelines for care plans
b Is a care conference
c Involves triggers
d Is the method nurses use to plan and deliver nursing care

3 What happens during assessment?
a Goals are set.
b Information is collected.
c Nursing measures are carried out.
d Progress is evaluated.

4 Which is a symptom?
a Redness
b Vomiting
c Pain
d Pulse rate of 78

5 Which is a sign?
a Nausea
b Headache
c Dizziness
d Dry skin

6 Which should you report at once?
a The person had a bowel movement.
b The person complains of sudden, severe pain.
c The person does not like the food served for lunch.
d The person complains of stiff, painful joints.

7 Which should you report at once?
a The person can no longer move a body part.
b The person answers questions correctly.
c The person has a breath odor.
d The person walked to the dining room.

8 Measures in the nursing care plan are carried out. This is
a A nursing diagnosis
b Planning
c Implementation
d Evaluation

9 Which statement about the nursing process is *true*?
a It is done without the person's input.
b You are responsible for it.
c It is used to communicate the person's care.
d Steps can be done in any order.

10 The care plan is
a Written by the doctor
b The measures to help the person
c The same for all persons
d Also called the Kardex

11 What is used to communicate the nursing tasks delegated to you?
a The care plan
b The Kardex
c An assignment sheet
d Care conferences

12 Which is a nursing diagnosis?
a Cancer
b Heart attack
c Kidney failure
d Chronic pain

Answers to these questions are on p. 832.

Understanding the Person

OBJECTIVES

- Define the key terms listed in this chapter.
- Identify the parts that make up the whole person.
- Explain Abraham Maslow's theory of basic needs.
- Explain how culture and religion influence health and illness.
- Identify the emotional and social effects of illness.
- Describe persons cared for in health care agencies.
- Identify the elements needed for good communication.
- Describe how to use verbal and nonverbal communication.
- Explain the methods and barriers to good communication.
- Explain how to communicate with persons who have behavior problems.
- Explain how to communicate with persons who have disabilities or who are comatose.
- Explain why family and visitors are important to the person.
- Identify the courtesies given to the person, family, and friends.
- Explain how to promote PRIDE in the person, the family, and yourself.

KEY TERMS

bariatrics The field of medicine focused on the treatment and control of obesity

body language Messages sent through facial expressions, gestures, posture, hand and body movements, gait, eye contact, and appearance

comatose Being unable to respond to stimuli

culture The characteristics of a group of people—language, values, beliefs, habits, likes, dislikes, customs—passed from one generation to the next

disability Any lost, absent, or impaired physical or mental function

esteem The worth, value, or opinion one has of a person

geriatrics The branch of medicine concerned with the problems and diseases of old age and older persons

holism A concept that considers the whole person; the whole person has physical, social, psychological, and spiritual parts that are woven together and cannot be separated

morbid obesity The person weighs 100 pounds or more over his or her normal weight

need Something necessary or desired for maintaining life and mental well-being

nonverbal communication Communication that does not use words

obesity Having an excess amount of total body fat; a person is said to be obese when his or her weight is 20% or more above what is considered normal for that person's height and age

obstetrics The branch of medicine concerned with the care of women during pregnancy, labor, and childbirth and for 6 to 8 weeks after birth

optimal level of function A person's highest potential for mental and physical performance

paraphrasing Restating the person's message in your own words

pediatrics The branch of medicine concerned with the growth, development, and care of children; they range in age from newborns to teenagers

psychiatry The branch of medicine concerned with mental health problems

religion Spiritual beliefs, needs, and practices

self-actualization Experiencing one's potential

self-esteem Thinking well of oneself and seeing oneself as useful and having value

verbal communication Communication that uses written or spoken words

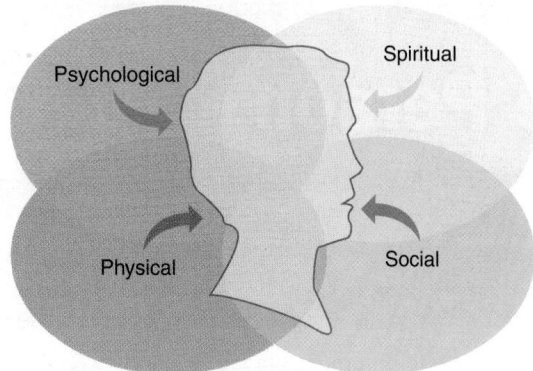

Fig. 8-1 A person is a physical, psychological, social, and spiritual being. The parts overlap and cannot be separated.

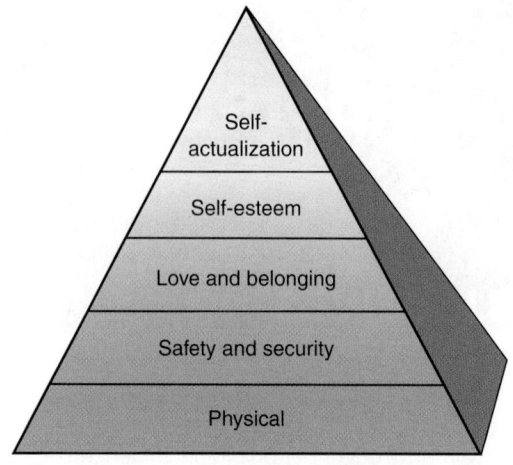

Fig. 8-2 Basic needs for life as described by Maslow.

The patient or resident is the most important person in the agency. Age, religion, and nationality make each person unique. So do culture, education, occupation, and life-style. Each person is important and special. Each has value. The person is treated as someone who thinks, acts, feels, and makes decisions.

CARING FOR THE PERSON

For effective care, you must consider the whole person. Holism means *whole*. *Holism is a concept that considers the whole person. The whole person has physical, social, psychological, and spiritual parts. These parts are woven together and cannot be separated* (Fig. 8-1).

Each part relates to and depends on the others. As a social being, a person speaks and communicates with others. Physically, the brain, mouth, tongue, lips, and throat structures must function for speech. Communication is also psychological. It involves thinking and reasoning.

To consider only the physical part is to ignore the person's ability to think, make decisions, and interact with others. It also ignores the person's experiences, life-style, culture, religion, joys, sorrows, and needs.

Disability and illness affect the whole person. For example, Mrs. Beal had a stroke. She needs help with physical needs. She had to leave her home. Relationships with her husband and children are changed. She is angry with God for letting this happen to her. The health team plans care to help her deal with her problems.

Addressing the Person

You must know and respect the whole person for effective, quality care. Too often a person is referred to as a room number. For example: "12A needs the bedpan," rather than "Mrs. Brown in 12A needs the bedpan." This strips the person of his or her identity. It reduces the person to a thing.

Patients and residents are not things. They are not your family or children. They are complex, adult human beings. To address patients and residents with dignity and respect:
- Use their titles—Mrs. Jones, Mr. Smith, Miss Turner, or Dr. Gonzalez.
- Do not call them by their first names unless they ask you to.
- Do not call them by any other name unless they ask you to.
- Do not call them Grandma, Papa, Sweetheart, Honey, or other names.

BASIC NEEDS

A *need is something necessary or desired for maintaining life and mental well-being.* According to Abraham Maslow, a famous psychologist, basic needs must be met for a person to survive and function. In this theory, needs are arranged in order of importance (Fig. 8-2). Lower-level needs must be met before the higher-level needs. Basic needs, from the lowest level to the highest level, are:
- Physical needs
- Safety and security needs
- Love and belonging needs
- Self-esteem needs
- The need for self-actualization

People normally meet their own needs. When they cannot, it is usually because of disease, illness, injury, or advanced age. The ill or injured usually seek health care.

Physical Needs

Oxygen, food, water, elimination, rest, and shelter are needed for life and to survive. A person dies within minutes without oxygen. Without food or water, a person feels weak and ill within a few hours. The kidneys and intestines must function. Otherwise, poisonous wastes build up in the blood and can cause death. Without enough rest and sleep, a person becomes very tired. Without shelter, the person is exposed to extremes of heat and cold.

Safety and Security Needs

Safety and security needs relate to feeling safe from harm, danger, and fear. Many people are afraid of health care agencies. Some care involves strange equipment. Some care causes pain or discomfort. People feel safer and more secure if they know what will happen. For every task, even a simple bath, the person should know:

- Why it is needed
- Who will do it
- How it will be done
- What sensations or feelings to expect
  See *Focus on Long-Term Care and Home Care: Safety and Security Needs.*

Love and Belonging Needs

Love and belonging needs relate to love, closeness, and affection. They also involve meaningful relationships with others. There are cases in which people became weaker or died from the lack of love and belonging. This is seen in children and in older persons who have out-lived family and friends. Family, friends, and the health team can meet love and belonging needs.

Self-Esteem Needs

Esteem is the worth, value, or opinion one has of a person. Self-esteem means to think well of oneself and to see oneself as useful and having value. People often lack self-esteem when ill, injured, older, or disabled. For example:

- An older man once built his own home and worked a farm. He supported and raised a family. Now he cannot dress or feed himself.
- Cancer treatments caused a woman to lose her hair. She does not feel attractive or whole.
- A person has a slow, crippling disease.
- A person had a leg amputated.

You must treat all persons with respect. Although it takes more time, encourage them to do as much for themselves as possible. This helps increase self-esteem.

The Need for Self-Actualization

Self-actualization means experiencing one's potential. It involves learning, understanding, and creating to the limit of a person's capacity. This is the highest need. Rarely, if ever, is it totally met. Most people constantly try to learn and understand more. This need can be postponed, and life will continue.

CULTURE AND RELIGION

Culture is the characteristics of a group of people—language, values, beliefs, habits, likes, dislikes, and customs. They are passed from one generation to the next. The person's culture influences health beliefs and practices. Culture also affects thinking and behavior during illness and when in a hospital or nursing center.

People come from many cultures, races, and nationalities. Their family practices and food choices may differ from yours. So might their hygiene habits and clothing styles. Some speak a foreign language. Some cultures have beliefs about what causes and cures illness. (See *Caring About Culture: Health Care Beliefs.*) They may perform rituals to rid the body of disease. (See *Caring About Culture: Sick Care Practices.*) Many have beliefs and rituals about dying and death (Chapter 52). Culture also is a factor in communication.

Religion relates to spiritual beliefs, needs, and practices. A person's religion influences health and illness practices. Religions may have beliefs and practices about daily living, behaviors, relationships with others, diet, healing, days of worship, birth and birth control, drugs, and death.

Many people find comfort and strength from religion during illness. They may want to pray and observe religious practices. Hospitals and nursing centers offer religious services. Many have chapels or meditation areas for prayer. Assist the person to attend services as needed (Fig. 8-3). Some residents leave nursing centers to worship.

A person may want to see a spiritual leader or advisor. If so, tell the nurse. Make sure the room is neat and orderly. Have a chair ready for the cleric. Provide privacy during the visit.

The nursing process reflects the person's culture and religion. The care plan includes the person's cultural and religious practices.

You must respect and accept the person's culture and religion. You will meet people from other cultures and religions. Learn about their beliefs and practices. This helps you understand the person and give better care.

A person may not follow all beliefs and practices of his or her culture or religion. Some people do not practice a religion. Each person is unique. Do not judge the person by your standards. And do not force your ideas on the person.

See *Focus on Communication: Culture and Religion.*

See *Focus on Long-Term Care and Home Care: Culture and Religion.*

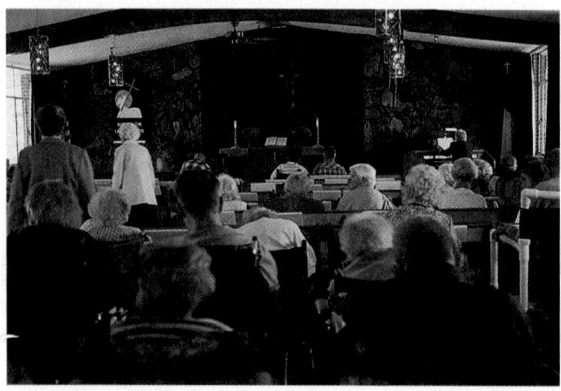

Fig. 8-3 Residents attend a religious service at a nursing center.

FOCUS ON COMMUNICATION
Culture and Religion

Hospitals and nursing centers ask about culture and religion upon admission. The care plan communicates practices to include in the person's care. Check the care plan for the person's preferences. You can also ask: "Do you have any cultural or religious practices that should be included in your care?"

FOCUS ON LONG-TERM CARE AND HOME CARE
Culture and Religion

Home Care
Culture is reflected in the home. Homes vary in size, cleanliness, and furnishings. Some are expensive. Others reflect poverty. Whether rich or poor, treat each person and family with respect, kindness, and dignity. Do not judge the person's life-style, habits, religion, or culture.

EFFECTS OF ILLNESS AND DISABILITY

People do not choose sickness or injury. Physical, psychological, and social effects occur. Some result in disabilities. A *disability is any lost, absent, or impaired physical or mental function.* It may be temporary or permanent.

Normal activities—work, driving, fixing meals, yard work, hobbies—may be hard or impossible. Daily activities bring pleasure, worth, and contact with others. People often feel angry, upset, and useless when unable to perform them. These feelings may increase if the person needs help with routine functions.

Fears of death, disability, chronic illness, and loss of function are common. Some people explain why they are afraid. Others do not share feelings. Some fear being laughed at for being afraid. A person with a broken leg may fear having a limp or not walking again. Persons having surgery may fear cancer. These feelings are normal and expected. You need to understand the effects of illness and disability. How would you feel and react if you had the person's problems?

Sick people are expected to behave in a certain way. They need to see a doctor, rest, and have others provide care and comfort. Sometimes recovery is delayed or does not occur. Then the psychological and social effects of illness or disability become greater.

Anger is a common response to illness and disability. Persons who need nursing center care are often angry. The person may direct anger at you. However, the person is usually angry at the situation. You might have problems dealing with the person's anger. If so, ask the nurse for help.

You can help the person feel safe, secure, and loved. Take an extra minute to "visit," to hold a hand, or to give a hug. (Remember to maintain professional boundaries. See Chapter 4.) Show that you are willing to help with personal needs. Respond promptly. Treat each person with respect and dignity.

See *Focus on Long-Term Care and Home Care: Effects of Illness and Disability.*

Optimal Level of Function

Patients and residents are helped to maintain their *optimal level of function. This is the person's highest potential for mental and physical performance.* Encourage the person to be as independent as possible. Always focus on the person's abilities. Do not focus on disabilities.

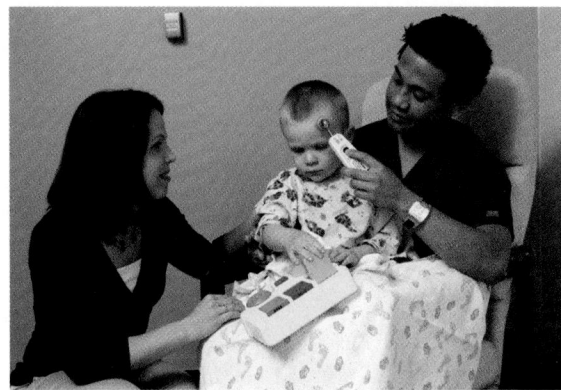

Fig. 8-4 The nursing assistant gives care to a sick child.

Hospital patients are often treated as sick, dependent people. Promoting this "sick role" in a nursing center reduces quality of life. The health team focuses on improving the person's quality of life. You must help each person regain or maintain as much physical and mental function as possible.

PERSONS YOU WILL CARE FOR

People are grouped in health care agencies by their problems, needs, and age. Doctors and nurses have special knowledge and skills to care for these groups.

- *Mothers and newborns. Obstetrics is the branch of medicine concerned with the care of women during pregnancy, labor, and childbirth and for 6 to 8 weeks after birth.* They are seen in clinics or doctors' offices during pregnancy. When labor begins, mothers usually go to a hospital. They are admitted to the obstetric (maternity) department. Pregnancy, labor, and childbirth are normal and natural events. However, problems can occur during and after pregnancy and childbirth.

- *Children. Pediatrics is the branch of medicine concerned with the growth, development, and care of children. They range in age from newborns to teenagers* (usually to age 16). Pediatric units are designed and equipped to meet the needs of children and parents. The nursing staff meets the child's physical, safety, and emotional needs (Fig. 8-4).

- *Adults with medical problems.* Medical problems are illnesses, diseases, and injuries that do not need surgery. There are acute, chronic, and terminal illnesses. Examples are infections, strokes, and heart attacks.

- *Persons having surgery.* Surgical patients need care before and after surgery. Surgeries range from simple to very complex. Appendix removal (appendectomy) is a simple surgery. Heart and brain surgeries are complex. Before surgery, the person is prepared for the surgery and for what happens after it. This includes addressing the person's fears and concerns. Needs after surgery relate to relieving pain, preventing complications, and adjusting to body changes.

- *Persons with mental health problems. Psychiatry is the branch of medicine concerned with mental health problems.* Problems vary from mild to severe mental and emotional disorders (Chapter 45). Some persons need help making decisions or coping with life stresses. Others are severely disturbed. They cannot do simple things—eat, bathe, or get dressed. Some persons present dangers to themselves or others. They need special care and treatment.

- *Persons needing bariatric care. Bariatrics is the field of medicine focused on the treatment and control of obesity. Obesity is having an excess amount of total body fat. A person is said to be obese when his or her weight is 20% or more above what is considered normal for that person's height and age.* Some people are morbidly obese. (*Morbid means diseased.*) *Morbid obesity means that the person weighs 100 pounds or more over his or her normal weight.* Bariatric patients and residents are at risk for many serious health problems. Such problems include heart disease, high blood pressure, stroke, cancer, diabetes, skin problems, and depression. The person has many physical and emotional needs.

- *Persons in special care units.* Some people are seriously ill or injured. Special care units are designed and equipped to treat and prevent life-threatening problems. They include emergency departments, and intensive care, coronary care, burn, and kidney dialysis units (Fig. 8-5, p. 94).

- *Persons needing subacute care or rehabilitation.* Some persons need more time to recover than hospital care allows. Others need rehabilitation (Chapter 38). They need to regain functions lost from surgery, illness, or accidents.

- *Older persons. Geriatrics is the branch of medicine concerned with the problems and diseases of old age and older persons.* Aging is a normal process (Chapter 11). It is not an illness or disease. Many older people enjoy good health. Others have acute or chronic illnesses. Some have diseases common in older persons. Body changes normally occur with aging. Social and psychological changes also occur. (See *Focus on Long-Term Care and Home Care: Persons You Will Care For*, p. 94.)

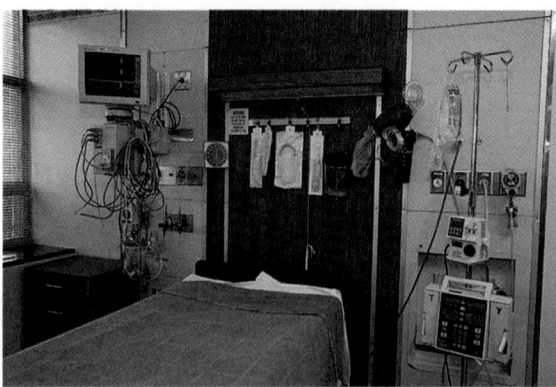

Fig. 8-5 A room in an intensive care unit.

FOCUS ON LONG-TERM CARE AND HOME CARE

Persons You Will Care For

Long-Term Care

Most residents are older. Their problems and care needs vary.

- *Alert, oriented persons.* They know who they are and where they are. They have physical problems. Some are paralyzed from a stroke, injury, or birth defect. Others are disabled from arthritis or multiple sclerosis. Still others have chronic heart, liver, kidney, or respiratory diseases. The amount of care required depends on the degree of disability.
- *Confused and disoriented persons.* These persons are mildly to severely confused and disoriented. Sometimes the problem is temporary. This is especially true for new residents. Some persons have Alzheimer's disease and other dementias. Confusion and disorientation are permanent and become worse (Chapter 46).
- *Persons needing complete care.* They are very disabled, confused, or disoriented. They need total assistance with all activities of daily living (ADL). They cannot meet any of their own needs. Some cannot say what they need or want.
- *Short-term residents.* These people need to recover from fractures, acute illness or surgery, and other injuries. Often they are younger than most residents. Some may need tube feedings, wound care, rehabilitation, or other treatments. Others need therapy programs: physical, occupational, speech and language, or respiratory. The goal is to regain their optimal level of function to return home.
- *Persons needing respite care.* Some people cared for at home go to nursing centers for short stays. This is *respite care. Respite* means *rest* or *relief.* The caregiver can take a vacation, tend to business, or simply rest. Respite care may be from a few days to several weeks.
- *Life-long residents.* Birth defects and childhood injuries and diseases can cause disabilities. A disability occurring before 22 years of age is called a developmental disability (Chapter 47). It may be a physical impairment, intellectual impairment, or both. The person needs life-long assistance, support, and special devices.
- *Residents who are mentally ill.* Behavior and function are affected. In severe cases, self-care and independent living are impaired. Some persons have physical and mental illnesses.
- *Terminally ill residents.* Terminally ill persons are dying (Chapter 52). The goal is to provide quality end-of-life care to persons who are dying (Chapter 52).

COMMUNICATING WITH THE PERSON

You communicate with patients and residents every time you give care. You give information to the person. The person gives information to you. Your body sends messages all the time—at the bedside, in hallways, at the nurses' station, in the dining room, and elsewhere. The person and family are aware of what you say and what you do. Good work ethics and understanding the person are needed for good communication. What you say and do also is important.

Effective Communication

For effective communication between you and the person, you must:

- Follow the rules of communication (Chapter 6):
  - Use words that have the same meaning for you and the person.
  - Avoid medical terms and words not familiar to the person.
  - Communicate in a logical and orderly manner. Do not wander in thought.
  - Give facts and be specific.
  - Be brief and concise.
- Understand and respect the patient or resident as a person.
- View the person as a physical, psychological, social, and spiritual human being.
- Appreciate the person's problems and frustrations.
- Respect the person's rights.
- Respect the person's religion and culture.
- Give the person time to understand the information that you give.
- Repeat information as often as needed. Repeat what you said. Use the exact same words. Do not give the person a new message to process. If the person does not seem to understand after repeating, try re-phrasing the message. This is very important for persons with hearing problems.
- Ask questions to see if the person understood you.
- Be patient. People with memory problems may ask the same question many times. Do not say that you are repeating information. Accept the memory loss as a disability.
- Include the person in conversations when others are present. This includes when a co-worker is assisting you with care.

See *Focus on Communication: Effective Communication.*

Verbal Communication

Verbal communication uses written or spoken words. You talk to the person. You share information and find out how the person feels. Most verbal communication involves the spoken word. Follow these rules:
- Face the person. Look directly at the person.
- Position yourself at the person's eye level. Sit or squat by the person as needed.
- Control the loudness and tone of your voice.
- Speak clearly, slowly, and distinctly.
- Do not use slang or vulgar words.
- Repeat information as needed.
- Ask one question at a time. Wait for an answer.
- Do not shout, whisper, or mumble.
- Be kind, courteous, and friendly.

You use the written word when the person cannot speak or hear but can read. The nurse and care plan tell you how to communicate with the person. The devices shown in Figure 8-6 are often used. The person also may have poor vision. When writing messages:
- Keep them simple and brief.
- Use a black felt pen on white paper.
- Print in large letters.

Some persons cannot speak or read. Ask questions that have "yes" or "no" answers. The person can nod, blink, or use other gestures for "yes" and "no." Follow the care plan. A picture board may be helpful (Fig. 8-7, p. 97).

Persons who are deaf may use sign language. See Chapter 39.

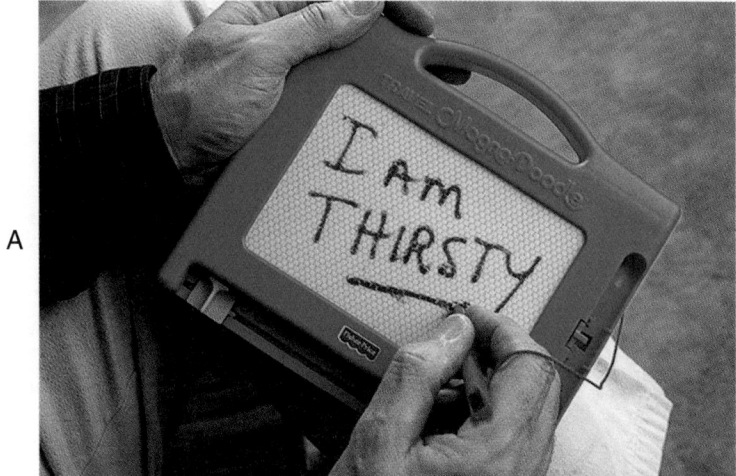

Fig. 8-6 Communication aids. **A,** Magic Slate. *Continued*

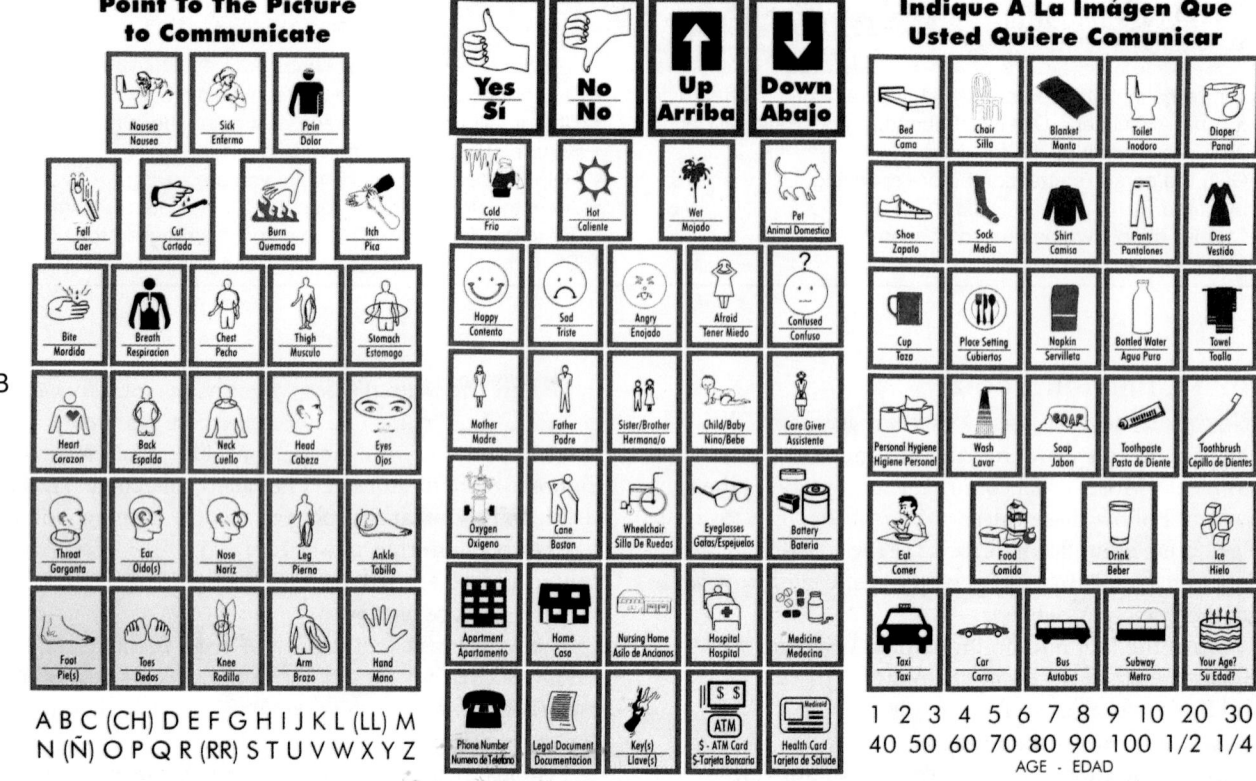

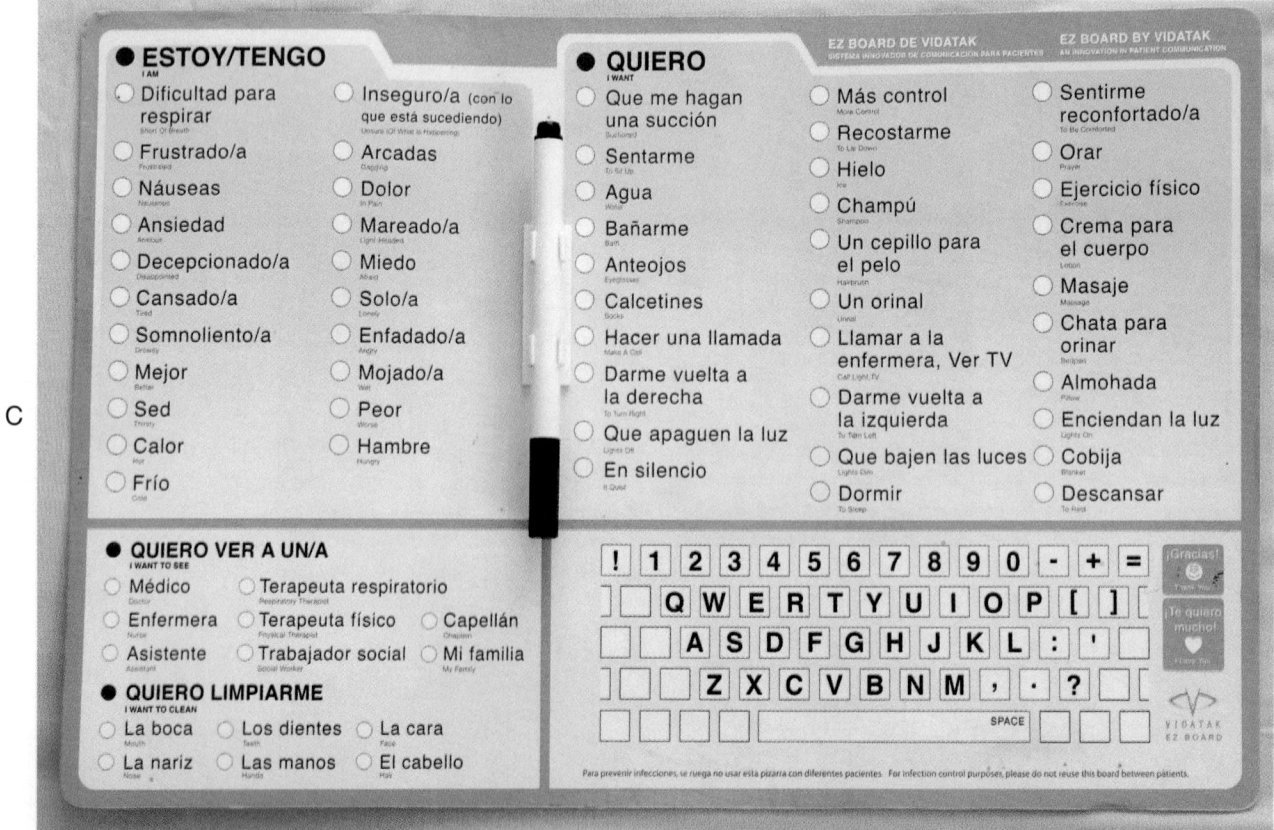

Fig. 8-6, cont'd Communication aids. **B,** Picture board in English and Spanish. **C,** Communication board in Spanish.

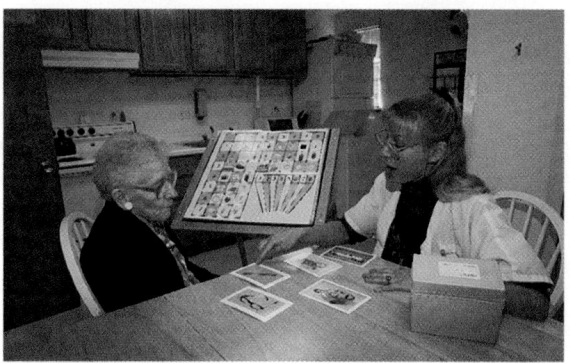

Fig. 8-7 A therapist helps a resident use a picture board and picture cards to communicate.

Nonverbal Communication

Nonverbal communication does not use words. Messages are sent with gestures, facial expressions, posture, body movements, touch, and smell. Nonverbal messages more accurately reflect a person's feelings than words do. They are usually involuntary and hard to control. A person may say one thing but act another way. Watch the person's eyes, hand movements, gestures, posture, and other actions. Sometimes they tell you more than words.

Touch. Touch is a very important form of nonverbal communication. It conveys comfort, caring, love, affection, interest, trust, concern, and reassurance. Touch means different things to different people. The meaning depends on age, gender (male or female), experiences, and culture.

Cultural groups have rules or practices about touch. They relate to who can touch, when it can occur, and where to touch the body. (See *Caring About Culture: Touch Practices.*)

Some people do not like being touched. However, touch can show caring and warmth. Stroking or holding a hand can comfort a person. Touch should be gentle. It should not be hurried, rough, or sexual. To use touch, follow the person's care plan. Remember to maintain professional boundaries.

See *Focus on Children and Older Persons: Touch.*

Body Language. People send messages through their *body language:*

* *Facial expressions* (See *Caring About Culture: Facial Expressions,* p. 98.)
* *Gestures*
* *Posture*
* *Hand and body movements*
* *Gait*
* *Eye contact*
* *Appearance* (dress, hygiene, jewelry, perfume, cosmetics, body art and piercings, and so on)

Slumped posture may mean the person is not happy or not feeling well. A person may deny pain. However, he or she protects the affected body part by standing, lying, or sitting in a certain way. Many messages are sent through body language.

Your actions, movements, and facial expressions send messages. So do how you stand, sit, walk, and look at the person. Your body language should show interest and enthusiasm. It should show caring and respect for the person. Often you will need to control your body language. Control reactions to odors from body fluids, secretions, excretions, or the person's body. Many odors are beyond the person's control. Embarrassment and humiliation increase if you react to odors.

CARING ABOUT CULTURE
Touch Practices

Touch practices vary among cultural groups. Touch is a friendly gesture in the *Philippine* culture. Touch is used often in *Mexico*. Some people believe that using touch while complimenting a person is important. It is thought to neutralize the power of the evil eye *(mal de ojo).*

Persons from the *United Kingdom* tend to reserve touch for persons they know well. Within limits, touch is acceptable in *Poland.* Its use depends on age, gender, and the relationship.

In *India,* men shake hands with other men but not with women. For women, they place their palms together and bow slightly. As a sign of respect or to seek a blessing, people touch the feet of older adults.

In *Vietnam,* a person's head is not touched by others. It is considered the center of the soul. Men do not touch women they do not know. Men commonly shake hands with men.

People from *China* do not like touching by strangers. A nod or slight bow is given during introductions. Health care workers of the same gender are preferred.

In *Ireland,* a firm handshake is preferred. Only family and close friends are embraced.

Modified from D'Avanzo CE, Geissler EM: *Pocket guide to cultural health assessment,* ed 4, St Louis, 2008, Mosby.

✿ CARING ABOUT CULTURE
Facial Expressions

Through facial expressions, *Americans* communicate:
- *Coldness*—there is a constant stare. Face muscles do not move.
- *Fear*—eyes are open wide. Eyebrows are raised. The mouth is tense with the lips drawn back.
- *Anger*—eyes are fixed in a hard stare. Upper lids are lowered. Eyebrows are drawn down. Lips are tightly compressed.
- *Tiredness*—eyes are rolled upward.
- *Disapproval*—eyes are rolled upward.
- *Disgust*—narrowed eyes. The upper lip is curled. There are nose movements.
- *Embarrassment*—eyes are turned away or down. The face is flushed. The person pretends to smile. He or she rubs the eyes, nose, or face. He or she twitches the hair, beard, or mustache.
- *Surprise*—direct gaze with raised eyebrows.

Italian, Jewish, African-American, and *Hispanic* persons smile readily. They use many facial expressions and gestures for happiness, pain, or displeasure. *Irish, English,* and *Northern European* persons tend to have less facial expression.

In some cultures, facial expressions mean the opposite of what the person is feeling. For example, *Asians* may conceal negative emotions with a smile.

Modified from Giger JN, Davidhizar RE: *Transcultural nursing: assessment and intervention,* ed 5, St Louis, 2008, Mosby.

✿ CARING ABOUT CULTURE
Eye Contact Practices

In the *American* culture, eye contact signals a good self-concept. It also shows openness, interest in others, attention, honesty, and warmth. Lack of eye contact can mean:
- Shyness
- Lack of interest
- Humility
- Guilt
- Embarrassment
- Low self-esteem
- Rudeness
- Dishonesty

For some *Asian* and *American Indian* cultures, eye contact is impolite. It is an invasion of privacy. In certain *Indian* cultures, eye contact is avoided with persons of higher or lower socio-economic class. It is also given a special sexual meaning.

In *Iraq,* men and women avoid direct eye contact. Long, direct eye contact is rude in *Mexico.* In rural parts of *Vietnam,* it is not respectful to look at another person while talking. Blinking means that a message is received. In the *United Kingdom,* looking directly at a speaker means the listener is paying attention.

Modified from Giger JN, Davidhizar RE: *Transcultural nursing: assessment and intervention,* ed 5, St Louis, 2008, Mosby. Modified from D'Avanzo CE, Geissler EM: *Pocket guide to cultural health assessment,* ed 4, St Louis, 2008, Mosby.

Communication Methods

Certain methods help you communicate with others. They result in better relationships. More information is gained for the nursing process.

Listening. Listening means to focus on verbal and nonverbal communication. You use sight, hearing, touch, and smell. You focus on what the person is saying. You observe nonverbal clues. They can support what the person says. Or they can show other feelings. For example, Mrs. Hays says, "I want to stay here. That way my son won't have to care for me." You see tears, and she looks away from you. Her verbal says *happy.* Her nonverbal shows *sadness.*

Listening requires that you care and have interest. Follow these guidelines:
- Face the person.
- Have good eye contact with the person. See *Caring About Culture: Eye Contact Practices.*
- Lean toward the person (Fig. 8-8). Do not sit back with your arms crossed.
- Respond to the person. Nod your head. Say "uh huh," "mmm," and "I see." Repeat what the person says. Ask questions.
- Avoid communication barriers.

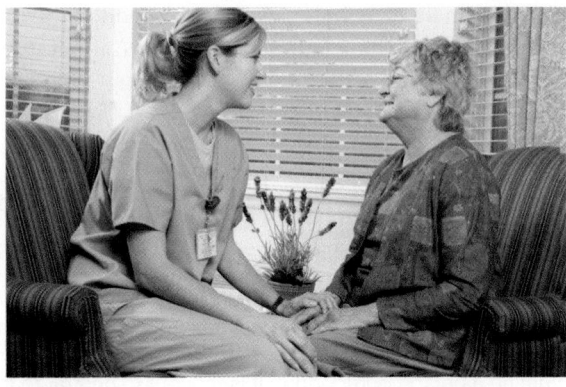

Fig. 8-8 Listen by facing the person. Have good eye contact. Lean toward the person.

Paraphrasing. *Paraphrasing is restating the person's message in your own words.* You use fewer words than the person did. Paraphrasing:
- Shows you are listening.
- Lets the person see if you understand the message.
- Promotes further communication.

The person usually responds to your statement. For example:

Mrs. Hays: My son was crying after he spoke with the doctor. I don't know what they talked about.

You: You don't know why your son was crying.

Mrs. Hays: The doctor must have said that I have a tumor.

Direct Questions. Direct questions focus on certain information. You ask the person something you need to know. Some direct questions have "yes" or "no" answers. Others require more information. For example:

You: Mrs. Hays, do you want to shower this morning?

Mrs. Hays: Yes.

You: Mrs. Hays, when would you like to do that?

Mrs. Hays: Could we start in 15 minutes? I'd like to call my son first.

You: Yes, we can start in 15 minutes. Did you have a bowel movement today?

Mrs. Hays: No.

You: You said you didn't eat well this morning. Can you tell me what you ate?

Mrs. Hays: I only had toast and coffee. I just don't feel like eating this morning.

Open-Ended Questions. Open-ended questions lead or invite the person to share thoughts, feelings, or ideas. The person chooses what to talk about. He or she controls the topic and the information given. Answers require more than a "yes" or "no." For example:

- "What do you like about living with your son?"
- "What was your husband like?"
- "What do you like about being retired?"

The person chooses how to answer. Responses to open-ended questions are longer. They give more information than do responses to direct questions.

Clarifying. Clarifying lets you make sure that you understand the message. You can ask the person to repeat the message, say you do not understand, or restate the message. For example:

- "Could you say that again?"
- "I'm sorry, Mrs. Hays. I don't understand what you mean."
- "Are you saying that you want to go home?"

Focusing. Focusing is dealing with a certain topic. It is useful when a person rambles or wanders in thought. For example, Mrs. Hays talks at length about food and places to eat. You need to know why she did not eat much breakfast. To focus on breakfast you say: "Let's talk about breakfast. You said you don't feel like eating."

Silence. Silence is a very powerful way to communicate. Sometimes you do not need to say anything. This is true during sad times. Just being there shows you care. At other times, silence gives time to think, organize thoughts, or choose words. Silence is useful when making decisions. It also helps when the person is upset and needs to gain control. Silence on your part shows caring and respect for the person's situation and feelings.

Sometimes pauses or long silences are uncomfortable. You do not need to talk when the person is silent. The person may need silence. Dealing with silence gets easier as you gain experience in your role.

See *Caring About Culture: The Meaning of Silence.*

⚜ CARING ABOUT CULTURE

The Meaning of Silence

In the *English* and *Arabic* cultures, silence is used for privacy. Among *Russian, French,* and *Spanish* cultures, silence means agreement between parties. In some *Asian* cultures, silence is a sign of respect, particularly to an older person.

Modified from Giger JN, Davidhizar RE: *Transcultural nursing: assessment and intervention,* ed 5, St Louis, 2008, Mosby.

Communication Barriers

Communication barriers prevent the sending and receiving of messages. Communication fails. You must avoid these barriers:

- *Using unfamiliar language.* You and the person must use and understand the same language. If not, messages are not accurately interpreted. See *Mosby's Nursing Assistant Companion CD,* included with this textbook, for useful Spanish words and phrases.
- *Cultural differences.* The person may attach different meanings to verbal and nonverbal communication. See *Caring About Culture: Communicating With Persons From Other Cultures,* p. 100.
- *Changing the subject.* Someone changes the subject when the topic is uncomfortable. Avoid changing the subject whenever possible.
- *Giving your opinion.* Opinions involve judging values, behaviors, or feelings. Let others express feelings and concerns without adding your opinion. Do not make judgments or jump to conclusions.
- *Talking a lot when others are silent.* Talking too much is usually because of nervousness and discomfort with silence. Silences have meaning. They show acceptance, rejection, and fear. They also show the need for quiet and time to think.
- *Failure to listen.* Do not pretend to listen. It shows lack of interest and caring. This causes poor responses. You miss complaints of pain, discomfort, or other symptoms that you must report to the nurse.
- *Pat answers.* "Don't worry." "Everything will be okay." "Your doctor knows best." These make the person feel that you do not care about his or her concerns, feelings, and fears.
- *Illness and disability.* Some illnesses, injuries, and birth defects affect speech, hearing, vision, cognitive function, and body movements. Verbal and nonverbal communication are affected.
- *Age.* Values and communication styles vary among age-groups.

⚙ **CARING ABOUT CULTURE**
Communicating With Persons From Other Cultures

To communicate with persons from other cultures:

- Ask the nurse about the beliefs and values of the person's culture. You can also ask the person and family. Learn as much as you can about the person's culture.
- Do not judge the person by your own attitudes, values, beliefs, and ideas.
- Follow the person's care plan. It includes the person's cultural beliefs and customs.
- Do the following when communicating with foreign-speaking persons:
  - Convey comfort by your tone of voice and body language.
  - Do not speak loudly or shout. It will not help the person understand English.
  - Speak slowly and distinctly.
  - Keep messages short and simple.
  - Be alert for words the person seems to understand.
  - Use gestures and pictures.
  - Repeat the message in other ways.
  - Avoid using medical terms and abbreviations.
  - Be alert for signs the person is pretending to understand. Nodding and answering "yes" to all questions are signs that the person does not understand what you are saying.

Modified from Giger JN, Davidhizar RE: *Transcultural nursing: assessment and intervention,* ed 5, St Louis, 2008, Mosby.

| **BOX 8-1** | **DISABILITY ETIQUETTE** |

- Extend the same courtesies to the person as you would to anyone else.
- Allow the person privacy.
- Do not hang on or lean on a person's wheelchair.
- Treat adults as adults. Do not use the person's first name unless he or she asks you to do so.
- Do not pat a person who is in a wheelchair on the head.
- Speak directly to the person. Do not address questions intended for the person to his or her companion.
- Do not be embarrassed if you use words that relate to a disability. For example, you say, "Did you see that?" to a person with a vision problem.
- Sit or squat to talk to a person in a wheelchair or chair. This puts you and the person at eye level.
- Ask the person if he or she needs help before acting. If the person says "no," respect the person's wishes. If the person wants help, ask the person what to do and how to do it.
- Think before giving directions to a person in a wheelchair. Think about distance, weather conditions, stairs, curbs, steep hills, and other obstacles.
- Allow the person extra time to say or do things. Let the person set the pace in walking, talking, or other activities.

Modified from Easter Seals, *Disability etiquette,* 2010.

PERSONS WITH DISABILITIES

A person may acquire a disability any time from birth through old age. Disease and injury are common causes. For example, children can develop hearing problems from ear infections. Head injuries from accidents can impair cognitive function. Spinal cord injuries can affect movements. And loud noise (music, machines) is linked to hearing loss. The cause or the age of onset does not matter. The person does not choose to have a disability. The person has to adjust to the disability. For many people, this can be long and hard (Chapter 38).

You will care for many people with disabilities. Your attitude is important for effective communication. People with disabilities have the same basic needs as you and everyone else. They feel joy, sorrow, happiness, sadness, and other emotions just like you and everyone else. They laugh, cry, have families, go to school, work, get married, and pay bills just like you and everyone else. And they have the right to dignity and respect just like you and everyone else.

To communicate with persons who have certain disabilities, see persons:

- Who have speech impairments—Chapter 39
- Who are hard-of-hearing—Chapter 39
- Who are blind—Chapter 39
- Who are confused—Chapter 46
- With Alzheimer's disease and other dementias—Chapter 46

Common courtesies and manners *(etiquette)* apply to any person with a disability. See Box 8-1 for disability etiquette.

The Person Who Is Comatose

Comatose means being unable to respond to stimuli. The person who is comatose is unconscious. The person cannot respond to others. Often the person can hear and can feel touch and pain. Often pain may be shown by grimacing or groaning. Assume that the person hears and understands you. Use touch and give care gently. Practice these measures:

- Knock before entering the person's room.
- Tell the person your name, the time, and the place every time you enter the room.
- Give care on the same schedule every day.
- Explain what you are going to do. Explain care measures step-by-step as you do them.
- Tell the person when you are finishing care.
- Use touch to communicate care, concern, and comfort.
- Tell the person what time you will be back to check on him or her.
- Tell the person when you are leaving the room.

FAMILY AND FRIENDS

Family and friends help meet safety and security, love and belonging, and self-esteem needs. They offer support and comfort. They lessen loneliness. Some also help with the person's care. This helps both the person and family. The family knows they are doing something to help the person. And the person's physical and emotional needs are met. The presence or absence of family or friends affects the person's quality of life.

The person has the right to visit with family and friends in private and without unnecessary interruptions. You may need to give care when visitors are there. Protect the right to privacy. Do not expose the person's body in front of them. Politely ask them to leave the room. Show them where to wait. Promptly tell them when they can return. A partner or family member may want to help you. If the patient or resident consents, you may allow the person to stay.

Treat family and friends with courtesy and respect. They have concerns about the person's condition and care. They need support and understanding. However, do not discuss the person's condition with them. Refer their questions to the nurse.

Visiting rules depend on agency policy and the person's condition. Parents can visit children as often and as long as they want. Dying persons usually can have family members present all the time. This is policy for hospice units. Know your agency's visiting policies and what is allowed for the person.

Visitors may have questions about the chapel, gift shop, lounge, dining room, or business office. Know the location, special rules, and hours of these areas.

A visitor may upset or tire a person. Report your observations to the nurse. The nurse will speak with the visitor about the person's needs.

See *Caring About Culture: Family Roles in Sick Care.*

See *Focus on Children and Older Persons: Family and Friends.*

See *Focus on Long-Term Care and Home Care: Family and Friends.*

⊛ CARING ABOUT CULTURE

Family Roles in Sick Care

In *Vietnam,* family members are involved in the person's hospital care. They stay at the bedside and sleep in the person's bed or on straw mats. In *Vietnam* and *China,* family members provide food, hygiene, and comfort.

In *Pakistan,* hospitals have different sections for females and males. Adult family members of the opposite sex are not allowed to stay overnight.

Modified from D'Avanzo CE, Geissler EM: *Pocket guide to cultural health assessment,* ed 4, St Louis, 2008, Mosby.

FOCUS ON CHILDREN AND OLDER PERSONS

Family and Friends

Older Persons

Sometimes older brothers, sisters, and cousins live together. They provide companionship and share living expenses. They care for each other during illness or disability.

Some older people live with their children. The older parent may be healthy, need some supervision, or be ill or disabled. The older parent moves in with the child. Or the child moves into the parent's home. Living with a child can help the older person feel safe and secure. Often the adult child gives care to an ill or disabled parent.

Adult children often need to work even though the parent cannot be left alone. Adult day-care centers provide meals, supervision, and supervised activities for older persons. Cards, board games, movies, crafts, dancing, walks, and lectures are common. Some provide bowling and swimming. Help is given as needed. Some provide transportation from home to the center.

Living with an adult child is a social change. The parent, child, and the child's family need to adjust. The child's family needs time alone. Other family members may help give care. Respite care provides a break for the family. The parent enters a nursing center for a few days or weeks. Caregivers can rest, go on vacation, or take a break from care-giving stresses. Church and community groups may have volunteers who help with care.

FOCUS ON LONG-TERM CARE AND HOME CARE

Family and Friends

Home Care

Family personalities and attitudes affect the mood in the home. Many families are happy and supportive. Others have poor relationships. Mental or physical illness, drug or alcohol abuse, unemployment, and delinquency may affect the family. Some families have problems coping with or accepting the person's illness or disability.

Your supervisor explains family problems to you. Do not get involved. Be professional and have empathy. Do not give advice, take sides, or make judgments about family conflicts. Maintain professional boundaries at all times.

BEHAVIOR ISSUES

Many people accept illness, injury, and disability. Others do not adjust well. They have some of the following behaviors. These behaviors are new for some people. For others, they are life-long. They are part of one's personality.

- *Anger.* Anger is a common emotion. Causes include fear, pain, and dying and death. Loss of function and loss of control over health and life are causes. Anger is a symptom of some diseases that affect thinking and behavior. Some people are generally angry. Anger is communicated verbally and nonverbally. Verbal outbursts, shouting, raised voices, and rapid speech are common. Some people are silent. Others are not cooperative. They may refuse to answer questions. Nonverbal signs include rapid movements, pacing, clenched fists, and a red face. Glaring and getting close to you when speaking are other signs. Violent behaviors can occur.
- *Demanding behavior.* Nothing seems to please the person. The person is critical of others. He or she wants care given at a certain time and in a certain way. Loss of independence, loss of health, and loss of control of life are causes. So are unmet needs.
- *Self-centered behavior.* The person cares only about his or her own needs. The needs of others are ignored. The person demands the time and attention of others. The person becomes impatient if needs are not met.
- *Aggressive behavior.* The person may swear, bite, hit, pinch, scratch, or kick. Fear, anger, pain, and dementia (Chapter 46) are causes. Protect the person, others, and yourself from harm (Chapter 12).
- *Withdrawal.* The person has little or no contact with family, friends, and staff. He or she spends time alone and does not take part in social or group events. This may signal physical illness or depression. Some people are not social. They prefer to be alone.
- *Inappropriate sexual behavior.* Some people make inappropriate sexual remarks. Or they touch others in the wrong way. Some disrobe or masturbate in public. These behaviors may be on purpose. Or they are caused by disease, confusion, dementia, or drug side effects.

Some behaviors are not pleasant. You cannot avoid the person or lose control. Good communication is needed. Behaviors are addressed in the care plan. The care plan may include some of the guidelines in Box 8-2.

See *Focus on Communication: Behavior Issues.*

See *Teamwork and Time Management: Behavior Issues.*

BOX 8-2   DEALING WITH BEHAVIOR ISSUES

- Recognize frustrating and frightening situations. Put yourself in the person's situation. How would you feel? How would you want to be treated?
- Treat the person with dignity and respect.
- Answer questions clearly and thoroughly. Ask the nurse to answer questions you cannot answer.
- Keep the person informed. Tell the person what you are going to do and when.
- Do not keep the person waiting. Answer signal lights promptly. If you tell the person that you will do something for him or her, do it promptly.
- Explain the reason for long waits. Ask if you can get or do something to increase the person's comfort.
- Stay calm and professional, especially if the person is angry or hostile. Often the person is not angry at you. He or she is angry at another person or situation.
- Do not argue with the person.
- Listen and use silence (p. 99). The person may feel better if able to express his or her feelings.
- Protect yourself from violent behaviors (Chapter 12).
- Report the person's behavior to the nurse. Discuss how to deal with the person.

FOCUS ON COMMUNICATION
Behavior Issues

Anger is a common response to illness and disability. Patients and residents may be angry with their situation. A person may direct anger at you. You might have problems dealing with the person's anger. You must continue to act in a professional manner. Remain calm. Do not yell at or insult the person. Listen to his or her concerns. Provide needed care. Try not to take his or her statements personally. If a person says hurtful things, you can kindly say: "Please don't say those things. I'm trying to help you." Tell the nurse about the person's behavior.

Caring for demanding or angry persons can be hard. Ask the nurse or co-workers to help if needed.

TEAMWORK AND TIME MANAGEMENT
Behavior Issues

Persons who are demanding can take a lot of time. A simple task such as filling a water pitcher can take several minutes. The pitcher may be too full or not full enough. The water may be too warm or too cold. Or the person may have a list of other care needs.

This may happen to you or to co-workers. Learn to recognize these situations. Offer to help co-workers with the person or other tasks. Hopefully they also will help you.

FOCUS ON PRIDE

The Person, Family, and Yourself

Personal and Professional Responsibility

Improving communication is an on-going process. Do not feel bad if you are uncomfortable with patient or resident interactions at first. You will have many chances to develop better communication. You are responsible for taking advantage of these opportunities. To improve your communication:

- Use methods such as listening and clarifying.
- Pay attention to the nonverbal messages you may be sending.
- Avoid communication barriers.
- Know where your agency keeps resources to aid with communication. These may include devices like those shown in Figure 8-6 or translation lists with useful words or phrases (*Mosby's Nursing Assistant Companion CD*).
- Learn from your mistakes.

With practice, you will communicate more effectively. This is a valuable skill.

Rights and Respect

You will care for many kinds of people. You may care for young and old persons, ill and disabled persons, obese persons, and those with mental health problems. Each person is different. Each has his or her own needs and concerns.

Avoid labeling the person or making assumptions. For example, a person is obese. That does not mean the person is lazy or lacks control. Or a person has a mental health problem. That does not mean the person is unstable or "crazy." Or a person is elderly. Myths about older persons are common. See Chapter 11.

Each person is unique and has value. Try to understand the person. Listen and use good communication. Treat the person with dignity and respect.

Independence and Social Interaction

Fear and anxiety are common emotions for persons in a nursing center or hospital. Nursing center residents may feel lonely or abandoned by their families and friends. Patients may fear loss of function that will have social effects. For example, a stroke can cause a person to lose function on one side of the body. The person may lose the ability to work, live at home, perform daily activities, walk, drive a car, and so on. Feeling abandoned or worthless harms a person's self-esteem. Such feelings affect a person's over-all health.

To promote a sense of identity, worth, and belonging:

- Greet each person by name.
- Talk to the person while providing care.
- Take an extra minute to visit or just listen.
- Treat each person with respect and dignity.
- Encourage as much independence as possible.
- Focus on the person's abilities, not his or her disabilities.
- Allow private time with visitors.

Delegation and Teamwork

Caring for persons with behavior issues requires great teamwork. Staff members may become frustrated. But the person's quality of care must not be lowered. The health team must work together to manage such persons. Care assignments may rotate to allow breaks. When not assigned to the person, assist your co-worker with the person or other tasks. When you interact with the person, be respectful. Treat the person as nicely as you treat other persons. Often when treated kindly, the person's behavior will improve. A supportive and encouraging team makes caring for difficult persons easier.

Ethics and Laws

You will care for persons with different ideas, values, and lifestyles. These shape the person's character and identity. It is not ethical to:

- Force your views and beliefs on another person.
- Make negative comments or insult the person's customs.
- Argue with a person about health care or religious beliefs.

Respect the person as a whole. This includes his or her cultural and religious practices.

REVIEW QUESTIONS

Circle the BEST answer.

1 You work in a health care agency. You focus on
   a The person's care plan
   b The person's physical, safety and security, and self-esteem needs
   c The person as a physical, psychological, social, and spiritual being
   d The person's cultural and spiritual needs

2 Which basic need is the *most* essential?
   a Self-actualization
   b Self-esteem
   c Love and belonging
   d Safety and security

3 A person says, "What are they doing to me?" Which basic needs are *not* being met?
   a Physical needs
   b Safety and security needs
   c Love and belonging needs
   d Self-esteem needs

4 A person has a garden behind the nursing center. This relates to
   a Self-actualization
   b Self-esteem
   c Love and belonging
   d Safety and security

5 Which is *false*?
   a Culture influences health and illness practices.
   b Culture and religion influence food practices.
   c Cultural and religious practices are allowed in nursing centers.
   d A person must follow all beliefs and practices of his or her culture or religion.

Continued

REVIEW QUESTIONS—cont'd

6 Which is *true?*
  a Mental health problems are the focus of psychiatry.
  b Sick children are the focus of pediatrics.
  c The diseases of aging are the focus of obstetrics.
  d Childbirth is the focus of geriatrics.

7 These statements are about illness and disability. Which is *false?*
  a They are matters of personal choice.
  b They affect normal activities.
  c Anger is a common response.
  d A goal is for the person to maintain optimal level of function.

8 Alert and oriented residents need nursing center care because they
  a Are very disabled and confused
  b Have trouble remembering things
  c Have physical problems
  d Need surgery

9 Which is *false?*
  a Verbal communication uses the written or spoken word.
  b Verbal communication is the truest reflection of a person's feelings.
  c Messages are sent by facial expressions, gestures, posture, and body movements.
  d Touch means different things to different people.

10 To communicate with a person you should
  a Use medical words and phrases
  b Change the subject often
  c Give your opinions
  d Be quiet when the person is silent

11 Which might mean that you are *not* listening?
  a You sit facing the person.
  b You have good eye contact with the person.
  c You sit with your arms crossed.
  d You ask questions.

12 Which is a direct question?
  a "Do you feel better now?"
  b "What are your plans for home?"
  c "What will you do at home?"
  d "Why can't you sleep?"

13 A person wants to take a shower. You say, "You would like to take a shower." This is
  a A communication barrier
  b Direct question
  c Paraphrasing
  d An open-ended question

14 Focusing is useful when
  a A person is rambling
  b You want to make sure you understand the message
  c You want the person to share thoughts and feelings
  d A person is silent

15 Which promotes communication?
  a "Don't worry."
  b "Everything will be just fine."
  c "This is a good nursing center."
  d "Why are you crying?"

16 Which is *not* a barrier to communication?
  a Using silence
  b Giving your opinions
  c Changing the subject
  d Illness

17 A person uses a wheelchair. For effective communication, you should
  a Lean on the wheelchair
  b Pat the person on the head
  c Direct questions to the companion
  d Sit or squat next to the person

18 A person is comatose. Which action is *not* correct?
  a Assume that the person can hear and can feel touch.
  b Explain what you are going to do.
  c Use listening and silence to communicate.
  d Tell the person when you are leaving the room.

19 A person has many visitors. Which is *false?*
  a They can help meet basic needs.
  b Privacy should be allowed.
  c The nurse answers their questions about the person's care.
  d Visitors can stay in the room when care is given.

20 A visitor seems to tire a person. What should you do?
  a Ask the person to leave.
  b Tell the nurse.
  c Stay in the room to observe the person and visitor.
  d Find out the visitor's relationship to the person.

21 A person wants care given at a certain time and in a certain way. Nothing seems to please the person. The person is most likely demonstrating
  a Angry behavior
  b Demanding behavior
  c Withdrawn behavior
  d Aggressive behavior

22 A person is demonstrating problem behavior. You should do the following *except*
  a Put yourself in the person's situation
  b Tell the person what you are going to do and when
  c Ask the person to be nicer
  d Listen and use silence

Answers to these questions are on p. 832.

Body Structure and Function

OBJECTIVES

- Define the key terms and key abbreviations listed in this chapter.
- Identify the basic structures of the cell.
- Explain how cells divide.
- Describe four types of tissue.

- Identify the structures of each body system.
- Identify the functions of each body system.
- Explain how to promote PRIDE in the person, the family, and yourself.

KEY TERMS

artery A blood vessel that carries blood away from the heart

capillary A tiny blood vessel; food, oxygen, and other substances pass from the capillaries into the cells

cell The basic unit of body structure

digestion The process that breaks down food physically and chemically so that it can be absorbed for use by the cells

hemoglobin The substance in red blood cells that carries oxygen and gives blood its red color

hormone A chemical substance secreted by the endocrine glands into the bloodstream

immunity Protection against a disease or condition; the person will not get or be affected by the disease

menstruation The process in which the lining of the uterus (endometrium) breaks up and is discharged from the body through the vagina

metabolism The burning of food for heat and energy by the cells

organ Groups of tissues with the same function

peristalsis Involuntary muscle contractions in the digestive system that move food down the esophagus through the alimentary canal

respiration The process of supplying the cells with oxygen and removing carbon dioxide from them

system Organs that work together to perform special functions

tissue A group of cells with similar functions

vein A blood vessel that returns blood to the heart

KEY ABBREVIATIONS

CNS	Central nervous system	**RBC**	Red blood cell
GI	Gastro-intestinal	**WBC**	White blood cell
mL	Milliliter		

Ideally, the human body is in a steady state called *homeostasis*. (*Homeo* means sameness. *Stasis* means standing still.) Various body functions and processes work to promote health and survival. Homeostasis is affected by illness, disease, and injury.

You help residents meet their basic needs. Your care promotes comfort, healing, and recovery. Therefore you need to know the body's normal structure (*anatomy*) and function (*physiology*). It will help you understand signs, symptoms, and the reasons for care and procedures. You will give safe and more efficient care.

See Chapter 11 for changes in body structure and function that occur with aging.

CELLS, TISSUES, AND ORGANS

The basic unit of body structure is the cell. Cells have the same basic structure. Function, size, and shape may differ. Cells are very small. You need a microscope to see them. Cells need food, water, and oxygen to live and function.

Figure 9-1 shows the cell and its structures. The *cell membrane* is the outer covering. It encloses the cell and helps it hold its shape. The *nucleus* is the control center of the cell. It directs the cell's activities. The nucleus is in the center of the cell. The *cytoplasm* surrounds the nucleus. Cytoplasm contains smaller structures that perform cell functions. *Protoplasm* means "living substance." It refers to all structures, substances, and water within the cell. Protoplasm is a semi-liquid substance much like an egg white.

Chromosomes are thread-like structures in the nucleus. Each cell has 46 chromosomes. Chromosomes contain *genes*. Genes control the traits children inherit from their parents. Height, eye color, and skin color are examples.

The nucleus controls cell reproduction. Cells reproduce by dividing in half. The process of cell division is called *mitosis*. It is needed for tissue growth and repair. During mitosis, the 46 chromosomes arrange themselves in 23 pairs. As the cell divides, the 23 pairs are pulled in half. The two new cells are identical. Each has 46 chromosomes (Fig. 9-2).

Cells are the body's building blocks. *Groups of cells with similar functions combine to form tissues:*

- *Epithelial tissue* covers internal and external body surfaces. Tissue lining the nose, mouth, respiratory tract, stomach, and intestines is epithelial tissue. So are the skin, hair, nails, and glands.
- *Connective tissue* anchors, connects, and supports other tissues. It is in every part of the body. Bones, tendons, ligaments, and cartilage are connective tissue. Blood is a form of connective tissue.
- *Muscle tissue* stretches and contracts to let the body move.
- *Nerve tissue* receives and carries impulses to the brain and back to body parts.

Groups of tissue with the same function form organs. An organ has one or more functions. Examples of organs are the heart, brain, liver, lungs, and kidneys. *Systems are formed by organs that work together to perform special functions* (Fig. 9-3).

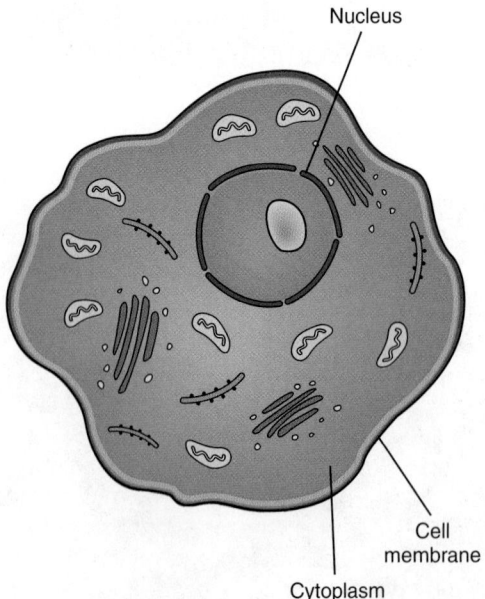

Nucleus

Cell membrane

Cytoplasm

Fig. 9-1 Parts of a cell.

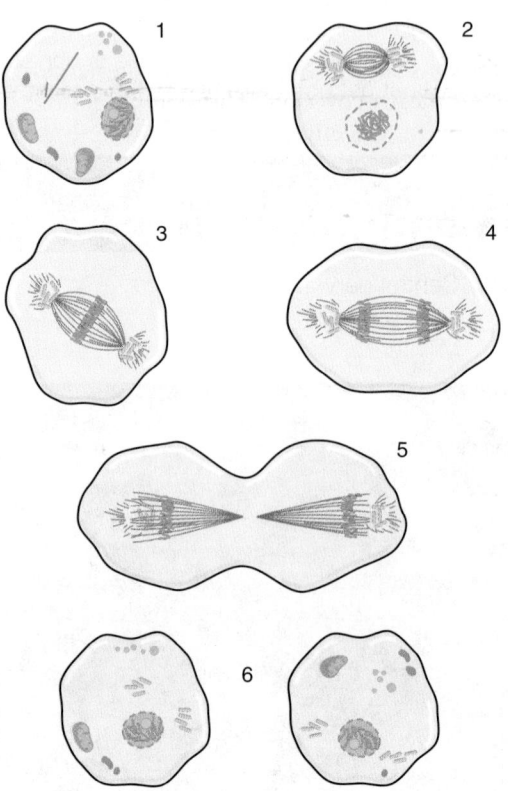

Fig. 9-2 Cell division.

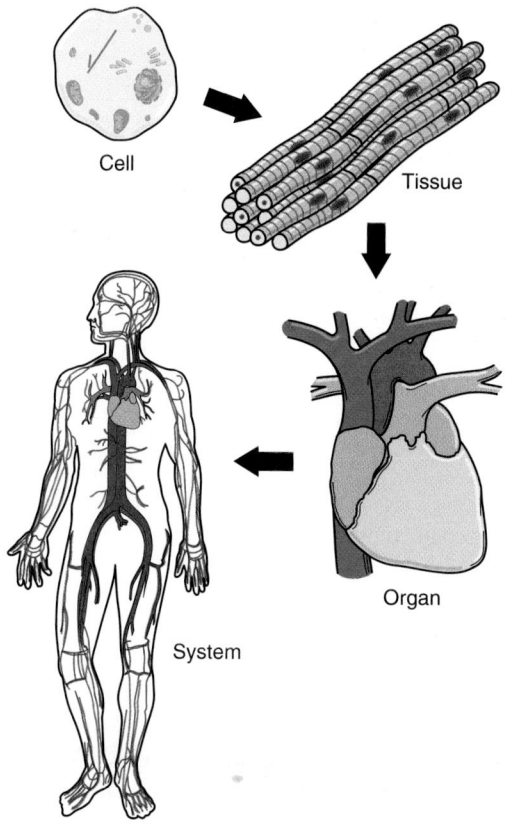

Fig. 9-3 Organization of the body.

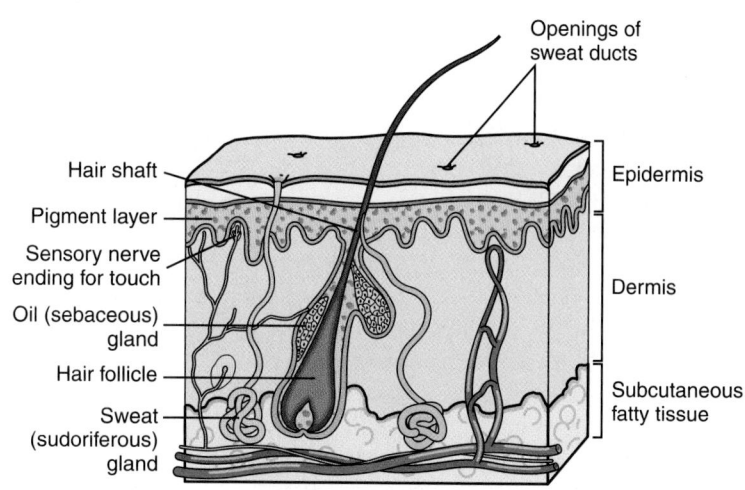

Fig. 9-4 Layers of the skin.

THE INTEGUMENTARY SYSTEM

The *integumentary system*, or *skin*, is the largest system. *Integument* means covering. The skin covers the body. It has epithelial, connective, and nerve tissue. It also has oil glands and sweat glands. There are two skin layers (Fig. 9-4):

* The *epidermis* is the outer layer. It has living cells and dead cells. The dead cells were once deeper in the epidermis. They were pushed upward as the cells divided. Dead cells constantly flake off. They are replaced by living cells. Living cells also die and flake off. Living cells of the epidermis contain *pigment*. Pigment gives skin its color. The epidermis has no blood vessels and few nerve endings.
* The *dermis* is the inner layer. It is made up of connective tissue. Blood vessels, nerves, sweat glands, and oil glands are found in the dermis. So are hair roots.

The epidermis and dermis are supported by *subcutaneous tissue*. The subcutaneous tissue is a thick layer of fat and connective tissue.

Oil glands and *sweat glands*, *hair*, and *nails* are skin appendages:

* Hair—covers the entire body, except the palms of the hands and the soles of the feet. Hair in the nose and ears and around the eyes protects these organs from dust, insects, and other foreign objects.
* Nails—protect the tips of the fingers and toes. Nails help fingers pick up and handle small objects.
* Sweat glands (sudoriferous glands)—help the body regulate temperature. Sweat consists of water, salt, and a small amount of wastes. Sweat is secreted through pores in the skin. The body is cooled as sweat evaporates.
* Oil glands (sebaceous glands)—lie near the hair shafts. They secrete an oily substance into the space near the hair shaft. Oil travels to the skin surface. This helps keep the hair and skin soft and shiny.

The skin has many functions:

* It is the body's protective covering.
* It prevents microorganisms and other substances from entering the body.
* It prevents excess amounts of water from leaving the body.
* It protects organs from injury.
* Nerve endings in the skin sense both pleasant and unpleasant stimulation. Nerve endings are over the entire body. They sense cold, pain, touch, and pressure to protect the body from injury.
* It helps regulate body temperature. Blood vessels dilate (widen) when temperature outside the body is high. More blood is brought to the body surface for cooling during evaporation. When blood vessels constrict (narrow), the body retains heat. This is because less blood reaches the skin.
* It stores fats and water.

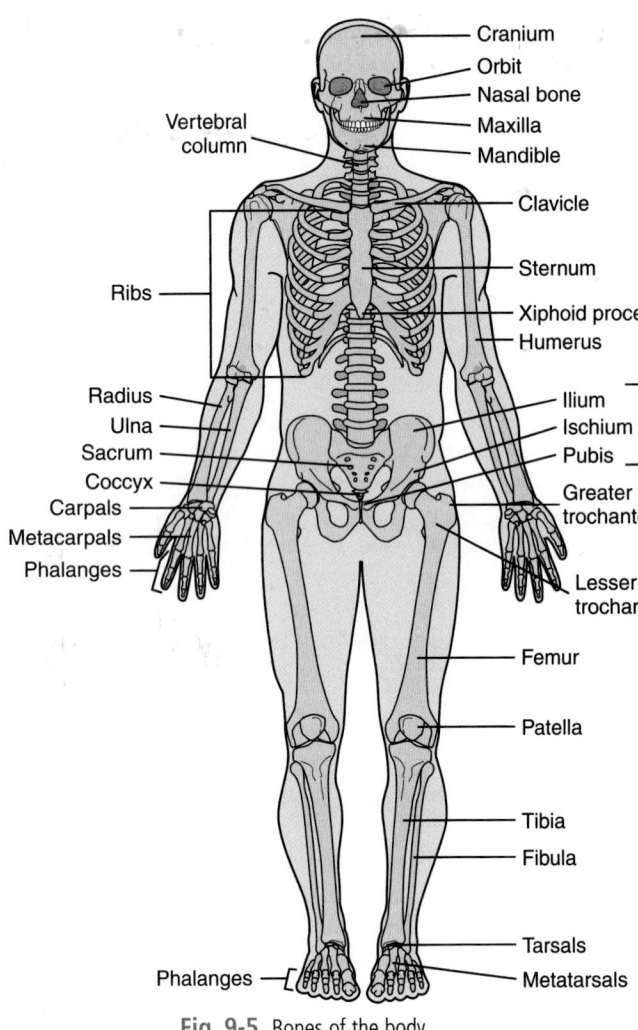

Fig. 9-5 Bones of the body.

cells with oxygen and food. Inside the hollow centers of the bones is a substance called *bone marrow*. Blood cells are formed in the bone marrow.

Joints

A *joint* is the point at which two or more bones meet. Joints allow movement (Chapter 27). *Cartilage* is the connective tissue at the end of the long bones. It cushions the joint so that the bone ends do not rub together. The *synovial membrane* lines the joints. It secretes *synovial fluid*. Synovial fluid acts as a lubricant so the joint can move smoothly. Bones are held together at the joint by strong bands of connective tissue called *ligaments*.

There are three major types of joints (Fig. 9-6):

- *Ball-and-socket joint* allows movement in all directions. It is made up of the rounded end of one bone and the hollow end of another bone. The rounded end of one fits into the hollow end of the other. The joints of the hips and shoulders are ball-and-socket joints.
- *Hinge joint* allows movement in one direction. The elbow is a hinge joint.
- *Pivot joint* allows turning from side to side. A pivot joint connects the skull to the spine.

Some joints are immovable. They connect the bones of the skull.

Muscles

The human body has more than *500 muscles* (Figs. 9-7 and 9-8). Some are voluntary. Others are involuntary.

- *Voluntary muscles* can be consciously controlled. Muscles attached to bones *(skeletal muscles)* are voluntary. Arm muscles do not work unless you move your arm; likewise for leg muscles. Skeletal muscles are *striated*. That is, they look striped or streaked.

THE MUSCULO-SKELETAL SYSTEM

The musculo-skeletal system provides the framework for the body. It lets the body move. This system also protects internal organs and gives the body shape.

Bones

The human body has *206 bones* (Fig. 9-5). There are four types of bones:

- *Long bones* bear the body's weight. Leg bones are long bones.
- *Short bones* allow skill and ease in movement. Bones in the wrists, fingers, ankles, and toes are short bones.
- *Flat bones* protect the organs. They include the ribs, skull, pelvic bones, and shoulder blades.
- *Irregular bones* are the vertebrae in the spinal column. They allow various degrees of movement and flexibility.

Bones are hard, rigid structures. They are made up of living cells. Calcium and phosphorus are needed for bone formation and strength. Bones store these minerals for use by the body. Bones are covered by a membrane called *periosteum*. Periosteum contains blood vessels that supply bone

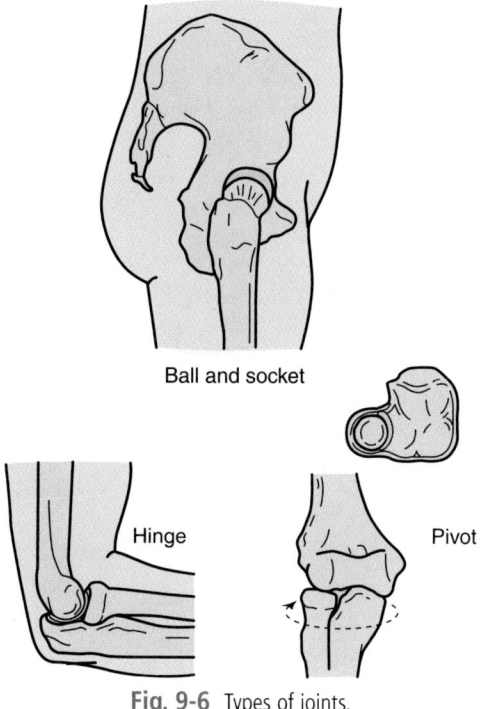

Fig. 9-6 Types of joints.

- *Involuntary muscles* work automatically. You cannot control them. They control the action of the stomach, intestines, blood vessels, and other body organs. Involuntary muscles also are called *smooth muscles.* They look smooth, not streaked or striped.
- *Cardiac muscle* is in the heart. It is an involuntary muscle. However, it appears striated like skeletal muscle. Muscles have three functions:
- Movement of body parts
- Maintenance of posture or muscle tone
- Production of body heat

Strong, tough connective tissues called *tendons* connect muscles to bones. When muscles contract (shorten), tendons at each end of the muscle cause the bone to move. The body has many tendons. See the Achilles tendon in Figure 9-8. Some muscles constantly contract to maintain the body's posture. When muscles contract, they burn food for energy. Heat is produced. The more muscle activity, the greater the amount of heat produced. Shivering is how the body produces heat when exposed to cold. Shivering is from rapid, general muscle contractions.

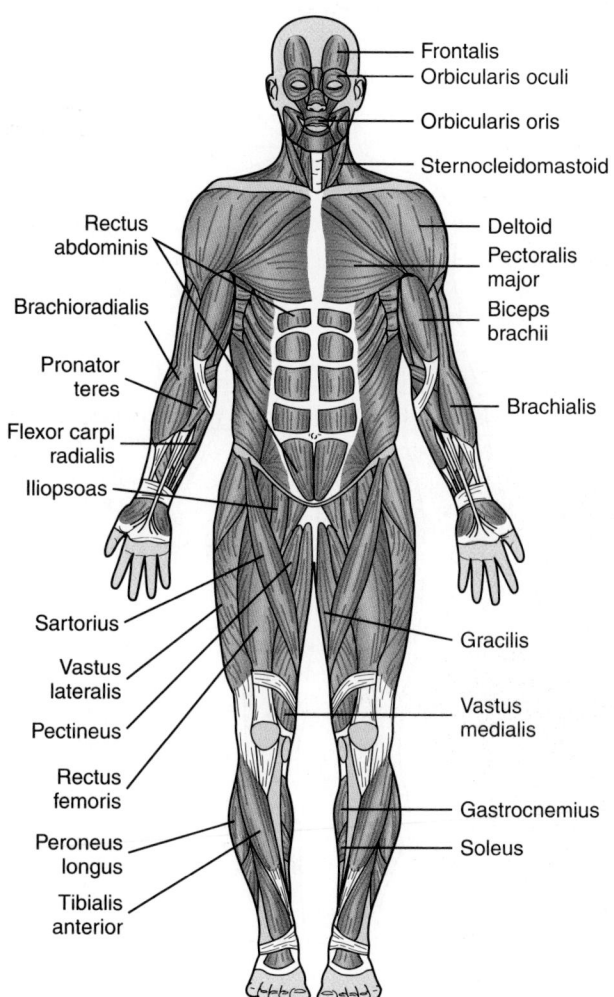

Fig. 9-7 Anterior view of the muscles of the body.

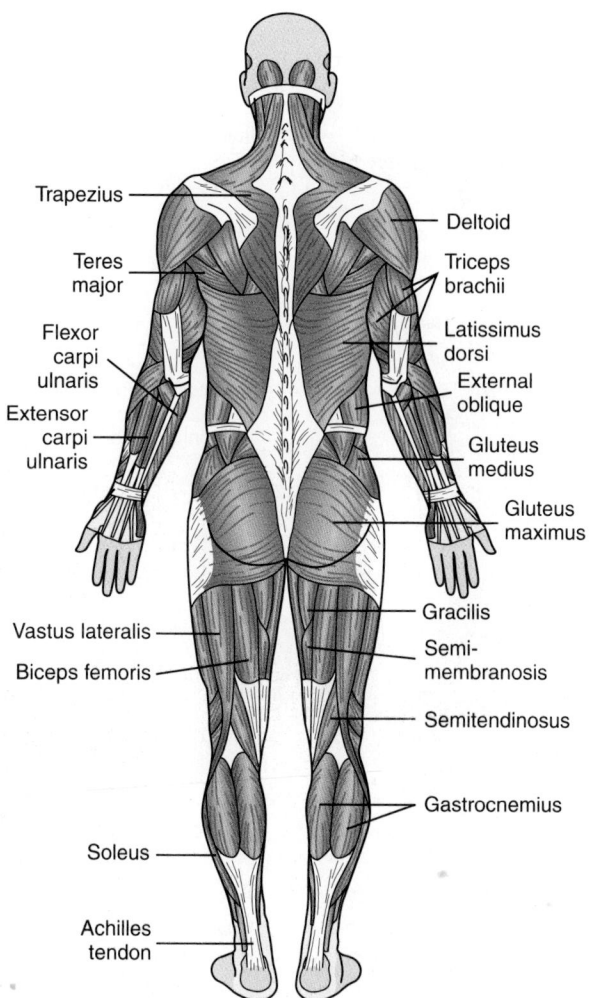

Fig. 9-8 Posterior view of the muscles of the body.

Sphincters are circular bands of muscle fibers. They constrict (narrow) a passage. Or they close a natural body opening. For example:

- The *pyloric sphincter* (Fig. 9-9) is an opening from the stomach into the small intestine. Closed, it holds food in the stomach for partial digestion. It opens to allow partially digested food to enter the small intestine.
- The *anal sphincter* keeps the anus closed. It opens for a bowel movement.
- Urethral sphincters seal off the bladder. This allows urine to collect in the bladder. The sphincters open for urination.

THE NERVOUS SYSTEM

The nervous system controls, directs, and coordinates body functions. Its two main divisions are:

- The *central nervous system* (CNS). It consists of the brain and spinal cord (Fig. 9-10).
- The *peripheral nervous system*. It involves the *nerves* throughout the body (Fig. 9-11).

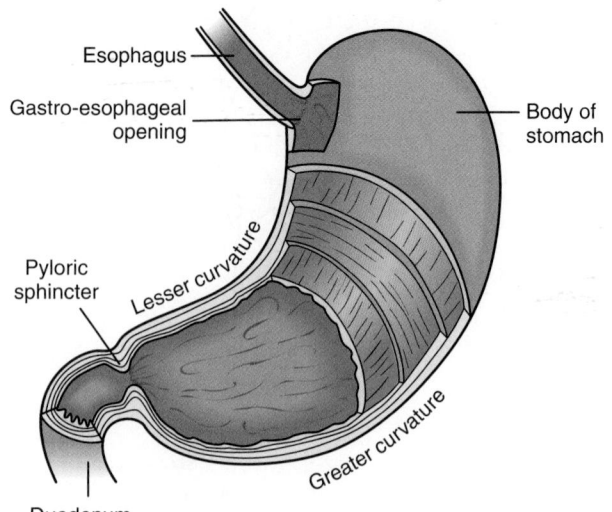

Fig. 9-9 Pyloric sphincter.

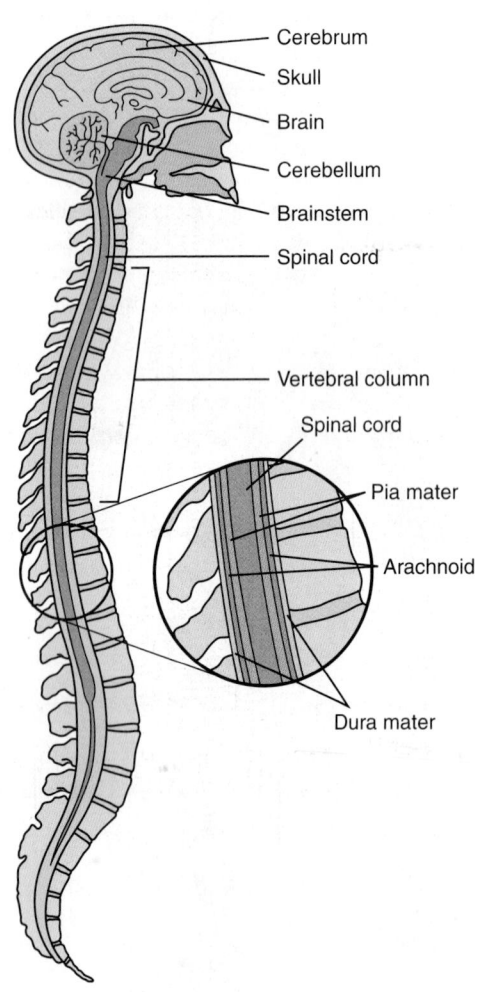

Fig. 9-10 Central nervous system.

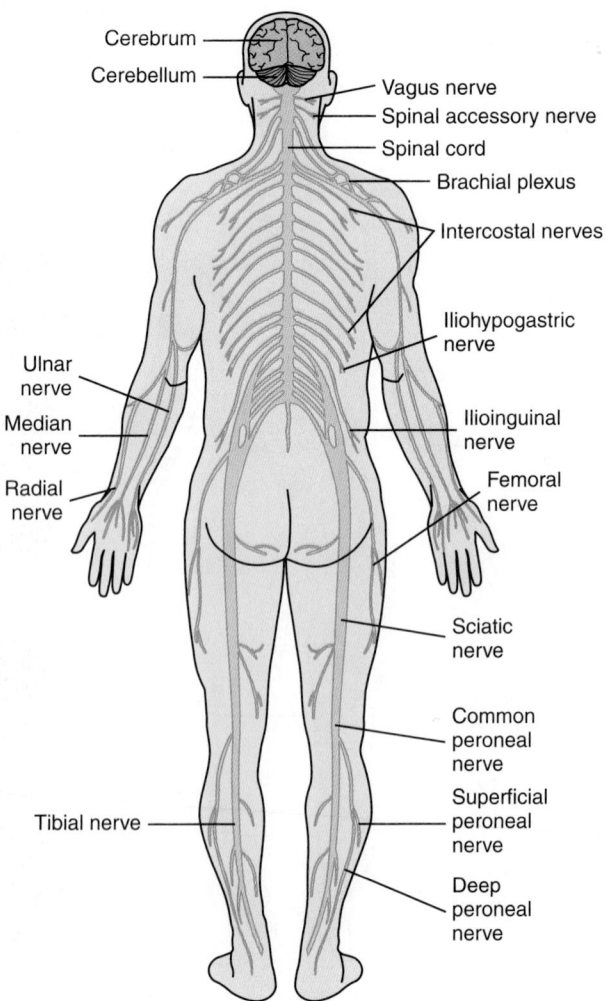

Fig. 9-11 Peripheral nervous system.

Nerves connect to the spinal cord. Nerves carry messages or impulses to and from the brain. A stimulus causes a nerve impulse. A *stimulus* is anything that excites or causes a body part to function, become active, or respond. A *reflex* is the body's response (functioning or movement) to a stimulus. Reflexes are involuntary, unconscious, and immediate. The person cannot control reflexes.

Nerves are easily damaged and take a long time to heal. Some nerve fibers have a protective covering called a *myelin sheath*. The myelin sheath also insulates the nerve fiber. Nerve fibers covered with myelin conduct impulses faster than those fibers without it.

The Central Nervous System

The *brain* and *spinal cord* make up the central nervous system. The brain is covered by the skull. The three main parts of the brain are the *cerebrum*, the *cerebellum*, and the *brainstem* (Fig. 9-12).

The cerebrum is the largest part of the brain. It is the center of thought and intelligence. The cerebrum is divided into two halves called the *right* and *left hemispheres*. The right hemisphere controls movement and activities on the body's left side. The left hemisphere controls the right side.

The outside of the cerebrum is called the *cerebral cortex*. It controls the highest functions of the brain. These include reasoning, memory, consciousness, speech, voluntary muscle movement, vision, hearing, sensation, and other activities.

The cerebellum regulates and coordinates body movements. It controls balance and the smooth movements of voluntary muscles. Injury to the cerebellum results in jerky movements, loss of coordination, and muscle weakness.

The brainstem connects the cerebrum to the spinal cord. The brainstem contains the *midbrain, pons,* and *medulla*. The midbrain and pons relay messages between the medulla and the cerebrum. The medulla is below the pons. The medulla controls heart rate, breathing, blood vessel size, swallowing, coughing, and vomiting. The brain connects to the spinal cord at the lower end of the medulla.

The spinal cord lies within the spinal column. The cord is 17 to 18 inches long. It contains pathways that conduct messages to and from the brain.

The brain and spinal cord are covered and protected by three layers of connective tissue called meninges:
* The outer layer lies next to the skull. It is a tough covering call the *dura mater.*
* The middle layer is the *arachnoid.*
* The inner layer is the *pia mater.*

The space between the middle layer (arachnoid) and inner layer (pia mater) is the *arachnoid space*. The space is filled with *cerebrospinal fluid*. It circulates around the brain and spinal cord. Cerebrospinal fluid protects the central nervous system. It cushions shocks that could easily injure brain and spinal cord structures.

The Peripheral Nervous System

The peripheral nervous system has 12 pairs of *cranial nerves* and 31 pairs of *spinal nerves*. Cranial nerves conduct impulses between the brain and the head, neck, chest, and abdomen. They conduct impulses for smell, vision, hearing, pain, touch, temperature, and pressure. They also conduct impulses for voluntary and involuntary muscles. Spinal nerves carry impulses from the skin, extremities, and internal structures not supplied by cranial nerves.

Some peripheral nerves form the *autonomic nervous system*. This system controls involuntary muscles and certain body functions. The functions include the heartbeat, blood pressure, intestinal contractions, and glandular secretions. These functions occur automatically.

The autonomic nervous system is divided into the *sympathetic nervous system* and the *parasympathetic nervous system*. They balance each other. The sympathetic nervous system speeds up functions. The parasympathetic nervous system slows functions. When you are angry, scared, excited, or exercising, the sympathetic nervous system is stimulated. The parasympathetic system is activated when you relax or when the sympathetic system is stimulated for too long.

The Sense Organs

The five senses are *sight, hearing, taste, smell,* and *touch*. Receptors for taste are in the tongue. They are called *taste buds*. Receptors for smell are in the nose. Touch receptors are in the dermis, especially in the toes and fingertips.

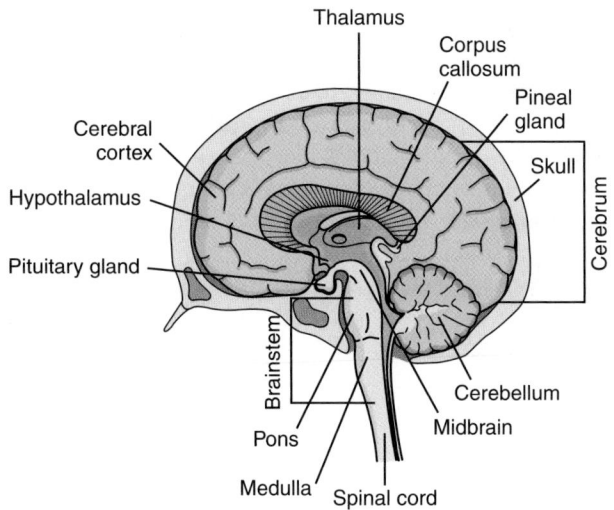

Thalamus

Corpus callosum

Pineal gland

Cerebral cortex

Skull

Hypothalamus

Cerebrum

Pituitary gland

Brainstem

Cerebellum

Midbrain

Pons

Medulla

Spinal cord

Fig. 9-12 The brain.

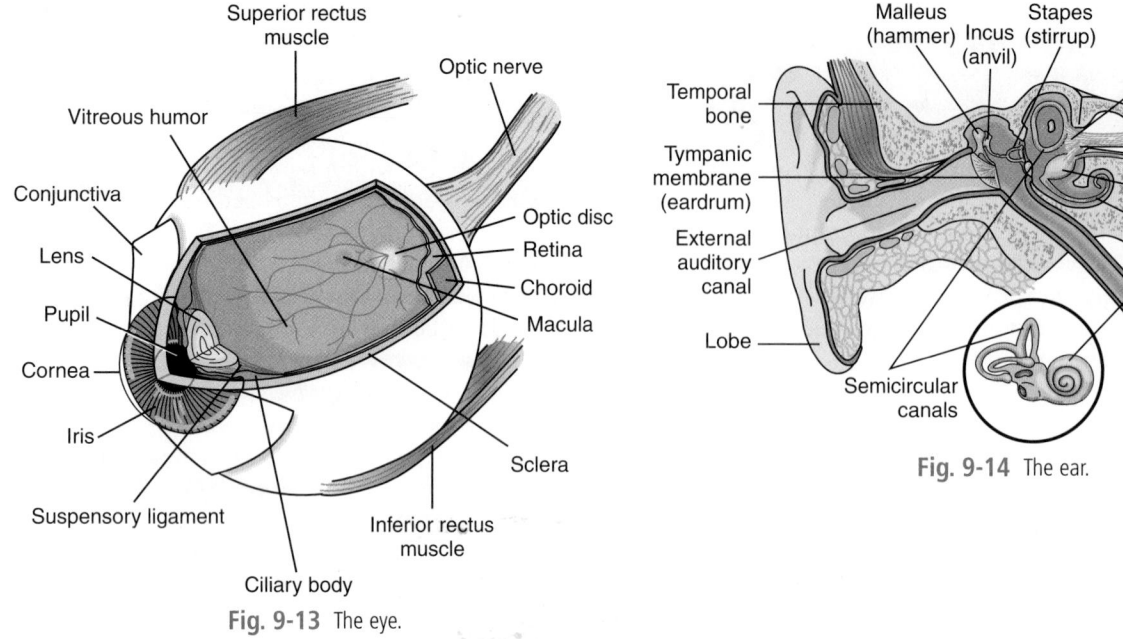

Fig. 9-13 The eye.

Fig. 9-14 The ear.

The Eye. Receptors for vision are in the *eyes* (Fig. 9-13). The eye is easily injured. Bones of the skull, eyelids and eyelashes, and tears protect the eyes from injury. The eye has three layers:

- The *sclera*, the white of the eye, is the outer layer. It is made of tough connective tissue.
- The *choroid* is the second layer. Blood vessels, the *ciliary muscle*, and the *iris* make up the choroid. The iris gives the eye its color. The opening in the middle of the iris is the *pupil*. Pupil size varies with the amount of light entering the eye. The pupil constricts (narrows) in bright light. It dilates (widens) in dim or dark places.
- The *retina* is the inner layer. It has receptors for vision and the nerve fibers of the *optic nerve*.

Light enters the eye through the *cornea*. It is the transparent part of the outer layer that lies over the eye. Light rays pass to the *lens*, which lies behind the pupil. The light is then reflected to the retina. Light is carried to the brain by the optic nerve.

The *aqueous chamber* separates the cornea from the lens. The chamber is filled with a fluid called *aqueous humor*. The fluid helps the cornea keep its shape and position. The *vitreous humor* is behind the lens. It is a gelatin-like substance that supports the retina and maintains the eye's shape.

The Ear. The *ear* is a sense organ (Fig. 9-14). It functions in hearing and balance. It has three parts: the *external ear, middle ear,* and *inner ear.*

The external ear (outer part) is called the *pinna* or *auricle.* Sound waves are guided through the external ear into the *auditory canal.* Glands in the auditory canal secrete a waxy substance called *cerumen.* The auditory canal extends about 1 inch to the *eardrum.* The eardrum *(tympanic membrane)* separates the external and middle ear.

The middle ear is a small space. It contains the *eustachian tube* and three small bones called *ossicles.* The eustachian tube connects the middle ear and the throat. Air enters the eustachian tube so that there is equal pressure on both sides of the eardrum. The ossicles amplify sound received from the eardrum and transmit the sound to the inner ear. The three ossicles are:

- The *malleus.* It looks like a hammer.
- The *incus.* It looks like an anvil.
- The *stapes.* It is shaped like a stirrup.

The inner ear consists of *semicircular canals* and the *cochlea.* The cochlea looks like a snail shell. It contains fluid. The fluid carries sound waves from the middle ear to the *acoustic nerve.* The acoustic nerve then carries the message to the brain.

The three semicircular canals are involved with balance. They sense the head's position and changes in position. They send messages to the brain.

THE CIRCULATORY SYSTEM

The circulatory system is made up of the *blood, heart,* and *blood vessels*. The heart pumps blood through the blood vessels. The circulatory system has many functions:

- Blood carries food, hormones, and other substances to the cells.
- Blood transports (carries) the gases of respiration (p. 115). It brings oxygen to the cells and removes carbon dioxide from the cells.
- Blood removes waste products from cells.
- Blood plays a role in maintaining the body's fluid balance.
- Blood and blood vessels help regulate body temperature. The blood carries heat from muscle activity to other body parts. Blood vessels in the skin dilate to cool the body. They constrict to retain heat.
- The system produces and carries cells that defend the body from microbes that cause disease.

The Blood

The blood consists of blood cells and *plasma*. Plasma is mostly water. It carries blood cells to other body cells. Plasma also carries substances that cells need to function. This includes food (proteins, fats, and carbohydrates), hormones (p. 119), and chemicals.

Red blood cells (RBCs) are called *erythrocytes. Hemoglobin is a substance in RBCs that carries oxygen and gives blood its red color.* As RBCs circulate through the lungs, hemoglobin picks up oxygen. Hemoglobin carries oxygen to the cells. When blood is bright red, hemoglobin in the RBCs is saturated (filled) with oxygen. As blood circulates through the body, oxygen is given to the cells. Cells release carbon dioxide (a waste product). It is picked up by the hemoglobin. RBCs saturated with carbon dioxide make the blood look dark red.

The body has about 25 trillion (25,000,000,000,000) RBCs. About 4½ to 5 million cells are in a cubic millimeter of blood (the size of a tiny drop). RBCs live for 3 or 4 months. They are destroyed by the liver and spleen as they wear out. New RBCs are formed in the bone marrow. About 1 million RBCs are produced every second.

White blood cells (WBCs) are called *leukocytes*. They have no color. They protect the body against infection. There are about 5,000 to 10,000 WBCs in a cubic millimeter of blood. At the first sign of infection, WBCs rush to the infection site. There they multiply rapidly. The number of WBCs increases when there is an infection. WBCs are formed by the bone marrow. They live about 9 days.

Platelets (thrombocytes) are needed for blood clotting. They are formed by the bone marrow. There are about 200,000 to 400,000 platelets in a cubic millimeter of blood. A platelet lives about 4 days.

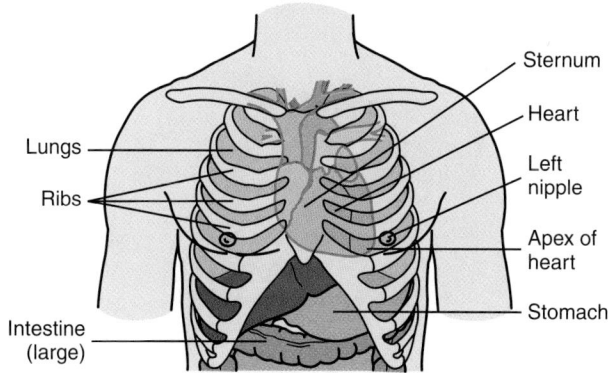

Fig. 9-15 Location of the heart in the chest cavity.

The Heart

The heart is a muscle. It pumps blood through the blood vessels to the tissues and cells. The heart lies in the middle to lower part of the chest cavity toward the left side (Fig. 9-15). The heart is hollow and has three layers (Fig. 9-16, p. 114):

- The *pericardium* is the outer layer. It is a thin sac covering the heart.
- The *myocardium* is the second layer. It is the thick, muscular part of the heart.
- The *endocardium* is the inner layer. A membrane, it lines the inner surface of the heart.

The heart has four chambers (see Fig. 9-16, p. 114). Upper chambers receive blood and are called *atria*. The *right atrium* receives blood from body tissues. The *left atrium* receives blood from the lungs. Lower chambers are called *ventricles*. Ventricles pump blood. The *right ventricle* pumps blood to the lungs for oxygen. The *left ventricle* pumps blood to all parts of the body.

Valves are between the atria and ventricles. The valves allow blood flow in one direction. They prevent blood from flowing back into the atria from the ventricles. The *tricuspid valve* is between the right atrium and the right ventricle. The *mitral valve (bicuspid valve)* is between the left atrium and left ventricle.

Heart action has two phases:

- *Diastole*. It is the resting phase. Heart chambers fill with blood.
- *Systole*. It is the working phase. The heart contracts. Blood is pumped through the blood vessels when the heart contracts.

The Blood Vessels

Blood flows to body tissues and cells through the blood vessels. There are three groups of blood vessels: arteries, capillaries, and veins.

Arteries carry blood away from the heart. Arterial blood is rich in oxygen. The *aorta* is the largest artery. It receives blood directly from the left ventricle. The aorta branches into other arteries that carry blood to all parts of the body (Fig. 9-17, p. 114). These arteries branch into smaller parts within the tissues. The smallest branch of an artery is an *arteriole*.

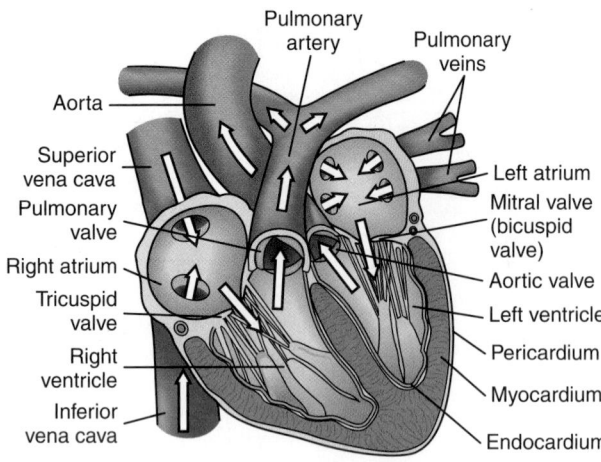

Fig. 9-16 Structures of the heart.

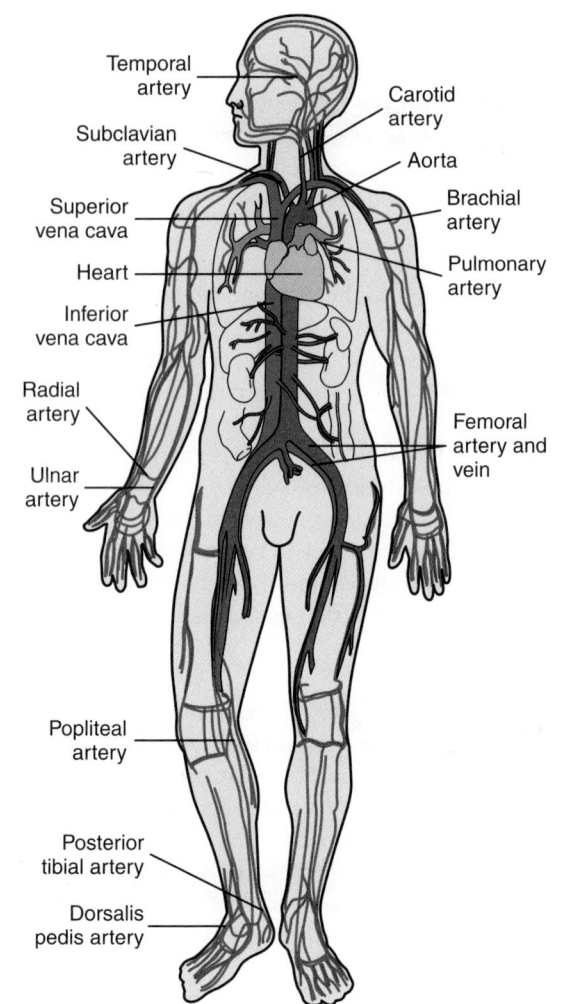

Fig. 9-17 Arterial and venous systems. Arterial system is red. Venous system is blue.

Arterioles connect to capillaries. *Capillaries are very tiny blood vessels. Food, oxygen, and other substances pass from capillaries into the cells.* The capillaries pick up waste products (including carbon dioxide) from the cells. Veins carry waste products back to the heart.

Veins return blood to the heart. They connect to the capillaries by *venules.* Venules are small veins. Venules branch together to form veins. The many veins also branch together as they near the heart to form two main veins (see Fig. 9-17). The two main veins are the *inferior vena cava* and the *superior vena cava.* Both empty into the right atrium. The inferior vena cava carries blood from the legs and trunk. The superior vena cava carries blood from the head and arms. Venous blood is dark red. It has little oxygen and a lot of carbon dioxide.

Blood flow through the circulatory system is shown in Fig. 9-16. The path of blood flow is as follows:

- Venous blood, poor in oxygen, empties into the right atrium.
- Blood flows through the tricuspid valve into the right ventricle.
- The right ventricle pumps blood into the lungs to pick up oxygen.
- Oxygen-rich blood from the lungs enters the left atrium.
- Blood from the left atrium passes through the mitral valve into the left ventricle.
- The left ventricle pumps the blood to the aorta. It branches off to form other arteries.
- Arterial blood is carried to the tissues by arterioles and to the cells by capillaries.
- Cells and capillaries exchange oxygen and nutrients for carbon dioxide and waste products.
- Capillaries connect with venules. Venules carry blood that has carbon dioxide and waste products.
- Venules form veins.
- Veins return blood to the heart.

THE LYMPHATIC SYSTEM

The lymphatic (lymph) system is a complex network that transports lymph throughout the body (Fig. 9-18). *Lymph is a clear, thin, watery fluid.* Lymph contains proteins and fats from the intestines. Lymph also contains white blood cells.

The lymphatic system:

- Collects extra lymph from the tissues and returns it to the blood. This helps maintain fluid balance. Water, proteins, and other substances normally leak out of the capillaries into surrounding tissues. The lymphatic system drains the extra fluid from the tissues. Otherwise, the tissues swell.
- Defends the body against infection by producing lymphocytes. Lymphocytes are a type of white blood cell that defends the body against microorganisms that cause infection (Chapter 15).
- Absorbs fats from the intestines and transports them to the blood.

Lymph is formed in the tissues. Lymph is transported by *lymphatic vessels*—lymphatic capillaries to lymphatic

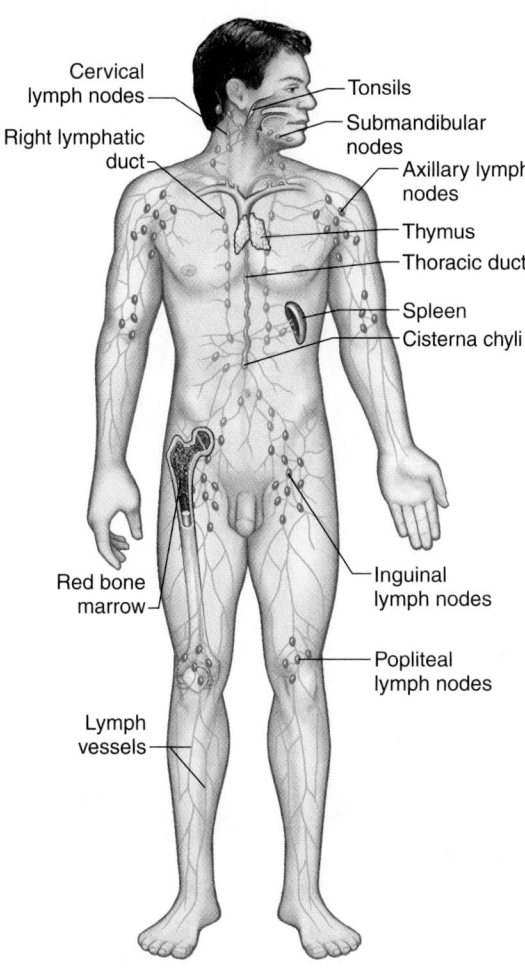

Fig. 9-18 The lymphatic system.

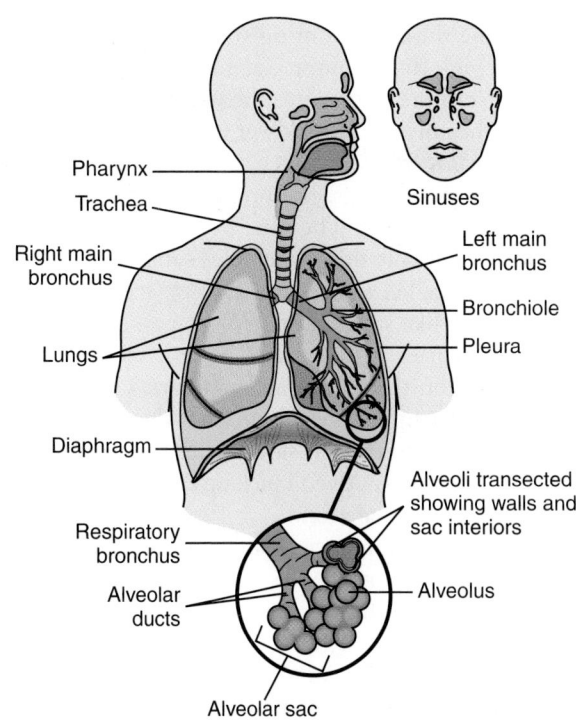

Fig. 9-19 Respiratory system.

replaced by fat and connective tissue. By age 80, it is usually gone.

The *tonsils* are in the back of the throat. *Adenoids* are behind the nose. These structures trap microorganisms in the mouth and nose to help prevent infection.

The *spleen* is the largest structure in the lymphatic system. It is about the size of a fist. The spleen has a rich blood supply—about 500 milliliters (mL) (1 pint) of blood. The spleen:

* Filters and removes bacteria and other substances.
* Destroys old RBCs.
* Saves the iron found in hemoglobin when RBCs are destroyed.
* Stores blood. When needed, the blood is returned to the circulatory system.

THE RESPIRATORY SYSTEM

Oxygen is needed to live. Every cell needs oxygen. Air contains about 21% oxygen. This meets the body's needs under normal conditions. The respiratory system (Fig. 9-19) brings oxygen into the lungs and removes carbon dioxide. *Respiration is the process of supplying the cells with oxygen and removing carbon dioxide from them.* Respiration involves *inhalation* (breathing in) and *exhalation* (breathing out). The terms *inspiration* (breathing in) and *expiration* (breathing out) also are used.

Air enters the body through the *nose*. The air then passes into the *pharynx* (throat). It is a tube-shaped passageway for air and food. Air passes from the pharynx into the *larynx* (voice box). A piece of cartilage, the *epiglottis*, acts like a lid over the larynx. The epiglottis prevents food

venules to the right lymphatic duct and the thoracic duct. Lymph then enters the blood in veins near the neck.

* The *right lymphatic duct* collects lymph from the right arm and from the right side of the head, neck, and chest. It empties into a vein on the right side of the neck.
* The *thoracic duct* collects lymph from the pelvis, abdomen, lower chest, and rest of the body. It empties into a vein on the left side of the neck.

Lymph nodes are shaped like beans. They range from the size of a pinhead to as large as a lima bean. They are found in the neck, underarm, groin area, chest, abdomen, and pelvis. Usually, you cannot see or feel lymph nodes. They swell when producing more lymphocytes to fight infection.

Lymph enters lymph nodes through the lymphatic vessels. The lymph nodes filter bacteria, cancer cells, and damaged cells from the lymph. This prevents such substances from entering the blood and circulating throughout the body.

See Figure 9-18 for the location of the *thymus (thymus gland)*. Certain lymphocytes—T lymphocytes (T cells) develop in the thymus. Such lymphocytes are important for immune system function (p. 120). The thymus reaches full growth at puberty. Then thymus tissue is slowly

from entering the airway during swallowing. During inhalation the epiglottis lifts up to let air pass over the larynx. Air passes from the larynx into the *trachea* (windpipe).

The trachea divides at its lower end into the *right bronchus* and the *left bronchus.* Each bronchus enters a lung. Upon entering the lungs, the bronchi divide many times into smaller branches. The smaller branches are called *bronchioles.* Eventually the bronchioles subdivide. They end up in tiny one-celled air sacs called *alveoli.*

Alveoli look like small clusters of grapes. They are supplied by capillaries. Oxygen and carbon dioxide are exchanged between the alveoli and capillaries. Blood in the capillaries picks up oxygen from the alveoli. Then the blood is returned to the left side of the heart and pumped to the rest of the body. Alveoli pick up carbon dioxide from the capillaries for exhalation.

The lungs are spongy tissues. They are filled with alveoli, blood vessels, and nerves. Each lung is divided into lobes. The right lung has three lobes; the left lung has two. The lungs are separated from the abdominal cavity by a muscle called the *diaphragm.*

Each lung is covered by a two-layered sac called the *pleura.* One layer is attached to the lung and the other to the chest wall. The pleura secretes a very thin fluid that fills the space between the layers. The fluid prevents the layers from rubbing together during inhalation and exhalation. A bony framework made up of the ribs, sternum, and vertebrae protects the lungs.

THE DIGESTIVE SYSTEM

Digestion is the process that breaks down food physically and chemically so it can be absorbed for use by the cells. The digestive system is also called the *gastro-intestinal (GI) system.* The system also removes solid wastes from the body.

The digestive system involves the *alimentary canal (GI tract)* and the accessory organs of digestion (Fig. 9-20). The alimentary canal is a long tube. It extends from the mouth to the anus. Its major parts are the mouth, pharynx, esophagus, stomach, small intestine, and large intestine. Accessory organs are the teeth, tongue, salivary glands, liver, gallbladder, and pancreas.

Digestion begins in the *mouth.* The mouth also is called the *oral cavity.* It receives food and prepares it for digestion. Using chewing motions, the *teeth* cut, chop, and grind food into small particles for digestion and swallowing. The *tongue* aids in chewing and swallowing. Taste buds on the tongue's surface contain nerve endings. Taste buds allow sweet, sour, bitter, and salty tastes to be sensed. *Salivary glands* in the mouth secrete *saliva.* Saliva moistens food particles to ease swallowing and begin digestion. During swallowing, the tongue pushes food into the *pharynx.*

The pharynx (throat) is a muscular tube. Swallowing continues as the pharynx contracts. Contraction of the pharynx pushes food into the *esophagus.* The esophagus is a muscular tube about 10 inches long. It extends from

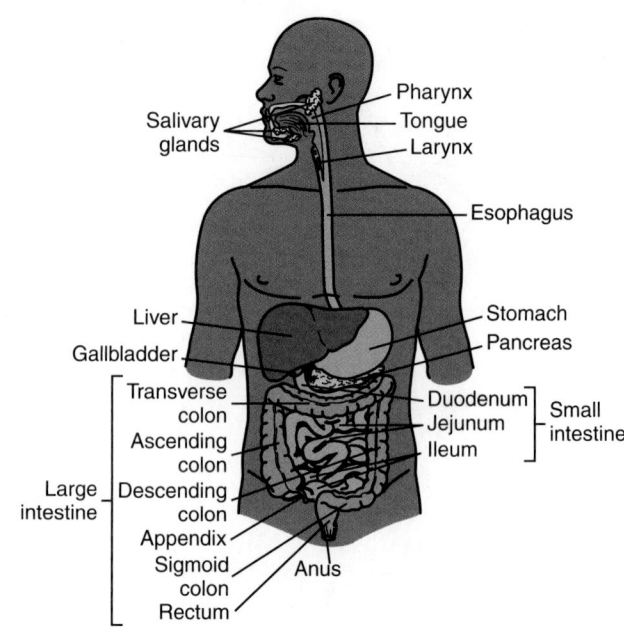

Fig. 9-20 Digestive system.

the pharynx to the *stomach. Involuntary muscle contractions move food down the esophagus through the alimentary canal (peristalsis).*

The stomach is a muscular, pouch-like sac. It is in the upper left part of the abdominal cavity. Strong stomach muscles stir and churn food to break it up into even smaller particles. A mucous membrane lines the stomach. It contains glands that secrete *gastric juices.* Food is mixed and churned with the gastric juices to form a semi-liquid substance called *chyme.* Through peristalsis, the chyme is pushed from the stomach into the small intestine.

The *small intestine* is about 20 feet long. It has three parts. The first part is the *duodenum.* There more digestive juices are added to the chyme. One is called *bile.* Bile is a greenish liquid made in the *liver.* Bile is stored in the *gallbladder.* Juices from the *pancreas* and small intestine are added to the chyme. Digestive juices chemically break down food so it can be absorbed.

Peristalsis moves the chyme through the two other parts of the small intestine: the *jejunum* and the *ileum.* Tiny projections called *villi* line the small intestine. Villi absorb the digested food into the capillaries. Most food absorption takes place in the jejunum and the ileum.

Some chyme is not digested. Undigested chyme passes from the small intestine into the *large intestine (large bowel* or *colon).* The colon absorbs most of the water from the chyme. The remaining semi-solid material is called *feces.* Feces contain a small amount of water, solid wastes, and some mucus and germs. These are the waste products of digestion. Feces pass through the colon into the *rectum* by peristalsis. Feces pass out of the body through the *anus.*

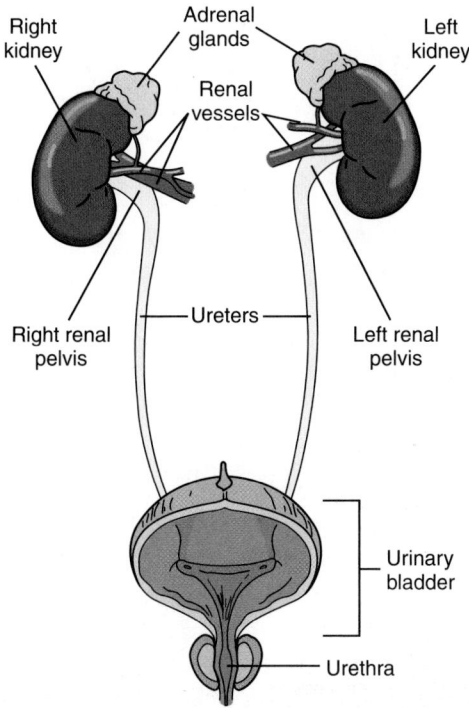

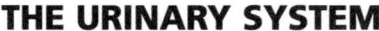

Fig. 9-21 Urinary system.

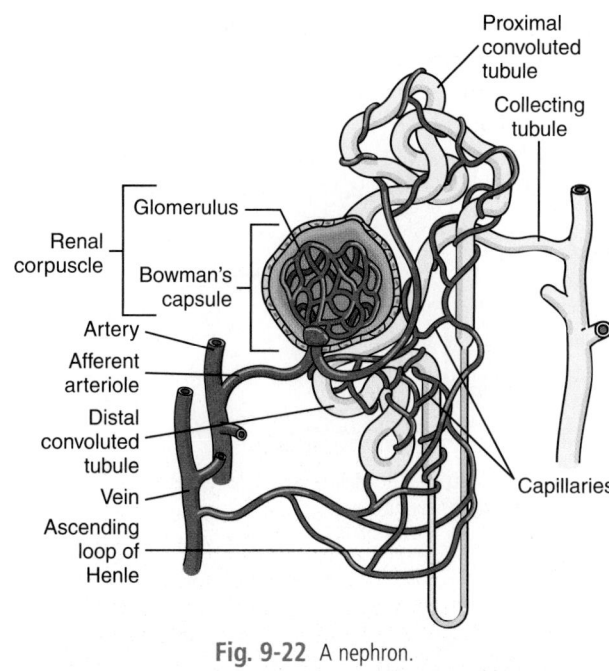

Fig. 9-22 A nephron.

THE URINARY SYSTEM

The digestive system rids the body of solid wastes. The lungs rid the body of carbon dioxide. Water and other substances leave the body through sweat. There are other waste products in the blood from cells burning food for energy. The urinary system (Fig. 9-21):

- Removes waste products from the blood.
- Maintains water balance within the body.
- Maintains electrolyte balance. *Electrolytes* are substances that dissolve in water—sodium, potassium, and calcium.
  - Sodium is needed for fluid balance. The body retains water if sodium levels are high. Loss of sodium (through vomiting, diarrhea, some drugs, and so on) can result in dehydration.
  - Potassium and calcium are needed for the proper function of skeletal and cardiac muscles.
- Maintains acid-base balance. A pH scale measures if a substance is acidic, neutral, or basic. A pH of 7 is neutral. Anything below 7 is acidic. Anything above 7 is basic. The blood must remain within a certain pH range (7.35-7.45) for the body to function normally.

The *kidneys* are two bean-shaped organs in the upper abdomen. They lie against the back muscles on each side of the spine. They are protected by the lower edge of the rib cage.

Each kidney has over a million tiny *nephrons* (Fig. 9-22). Each nephron is the basic working unit of the kidney. Each nephron has a *convoluted tubule*, which is a tiny coiled tubule. Each convoluted tubule has a *Bowman's capsule* at one end. The capsule partly surrounds a cluster of capillaries called a *glomerulus*. Blood passes through

the glomerulus and is filtered by the capillaries. The fluid part of the blood is squeezed into the Bowman's capsule. The fluid then passes into the tubule. Most of the water and other needed substances are reabsorbed by the blood. The rest of the fluid and the waste products form *urine* in the tubule. Urine flows through the tubule to a *collecting tubule*. All collecting tubules drain into the *renal pelvis* in the kidney.

A tube, called the *ureter*, is attached to the renal pelvis of the kidney. Each ureter is about 10 to 12 inches long. The ureters carry urine from the kidneys to the *bladder*. The bladder is a hollow, muscular sac. It lies toward the front in the lower part of the abdominal cavity.

Urine is stored in the bladder until the need to urinate is felt. This usually occurs when there is about a half pint (250 mL) of urine in the bladder. Urine passes from the bladder through the *urethra*. The opening at the end of the urethra is the *meatus*. Urine passes from the body through the meatus. Urine is a clear, yellowish fluid.

THE REPRODUCTIVE SYSTEM

Human reproduction results from the union of a male sex cell and a female sex cell. The male and female reproductive systems are different. This allows for the process of reproduction.

The Male Reproductive System

The male reproductive system is shown in Figure 9-23, p. 118. The *testes (testicles)* are the male sex glands. Sex glands also are called *gonads*. The two testes are oval or almond-shaped glands. Male sex cells are produced in the testes. Male sex cells are called *sperm* cells.

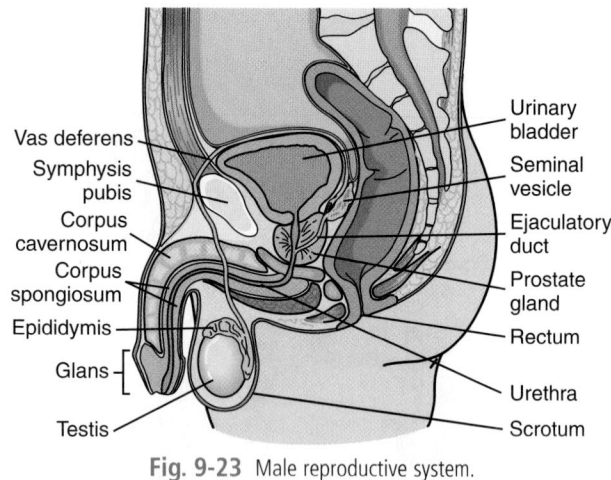

Fig. 9-23 Male reproductive system.

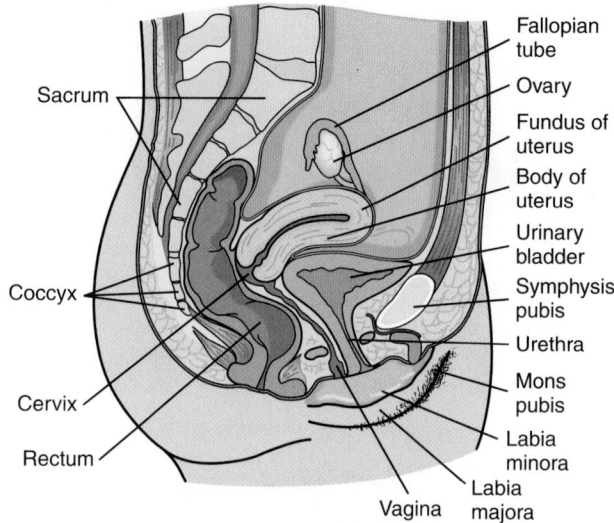

Fig. 9-24 Female reproductive system.

Testosterone, the male hormone, is produced in the testes. This hormone is needed for reproductive organ function. It also is needed for the development of the male secondary sex characteristics. There is facial hair; pubic and axillary (underarm) hair; and hair on the arms, chest, and legs. Neck and shoulder sizes increase.

The testes are suspended between the thighs in a sac called the *scrotum*. The scrotum is made of skin and muscle.

Sperm travel from a testis to the *epididymis*. The epididymis is a coiled tube on top and to the side of the testis. From the epididymis, sperm travel through a tube called the *vas deferens*. Each vas deferens joins a *seminal vesicle*. The two seminal vesicles store sperm and produce *semen*. Semen is a fluid that carries sperm from the male reproductive tract. The ducts of the seminal vesicles unite to form the *ejaculatory duct*. It passes through the *prostate gland*.

The prostate gland lies just below the bladder. It is shaped like a donut. The gland secretes fluid into the semen. As the ejaculatory ducts leave the prostate, they join the *urethra*. The urethra runs through the prostate gland. The urethra is the outlet for urine and semen. The urethra is contained within the *penis*.

The penis is outside of the body. The *glans* is at the end of the penis. The urethra opens at the end of the glans. A fold of skin (*prepuce* or *foreskin*) is at the end of the penis (Chapters 20 and 22).

The penis has *erectile* tissue. When a man is sexually excited, blood fills the erectile tissue. The penis enlarges and becomes hard and erect. The erect penis can enter a female's vagina. *Cowper's glands* are two pea-sized glands under the prostate. They produce a clear, colorless fluid before ejaculation (release of semen). The fluid cleanses the urethra, protects sperm from damage, and provides some lubrication for intercourse. With ejaculation, semen—containing sperm—is released into the vagina.

The Female Reproductive System

Figure 9-24 shows the female reproductive system. The female gonads are two almond-shaped glands called *ovaries*. An ovary is on each side of the uterus in the abdominal cavity.

The ovaries contain *ova* or eggs. Ova are the female sex cells. One ovum (egg) is released monthly during the woman's reproductive years. Release of an ovum is called *ovulation*.

The ovaries secrete the female hormones *estrogen* and *progesterone*. These hormones are needed for reproductive system function. They also are needed for the development of secondary sex characteristics in the female. These include increased breast size, pubic and axillary (underarm) hair, slight deepening of the voice, and widening and rounding of the hips.

When an ovum is released from an ovary, it travels through a *fallopian tube*. There are two fallopian tubes, one on each side. The tubes are attached at one end to the uterus. The ovum travels through the fallopian tube to the *uterus*.

The *uterus* is a hollow, muscular organ shaped like a pear. It is in the center of the pelvic cavity behind the bladder and in front of the rectum. The main part of the uterus is the *fundus*. The neck or narrow section of the uterus is the *cervix*. Tissue lining the uterus is called the *endometrium*. The endometrium has many blood vessels. If sex cells from the male and female unite into one cell, that cell implants into the endometrium. There the cell grows into a baby. The uterus serves as a place for the *fetus* (unborn baby) to grow and receive nourishment.

The cervix of the uterus projects into a muscular canal called the *vagina*. The vagina opens to the outside of the body. It is just behind the urethra. The vagina receives the penis during intercourse. It also is part of the birth canal. Glands in the vaginal wall keep it moistened with secretions.

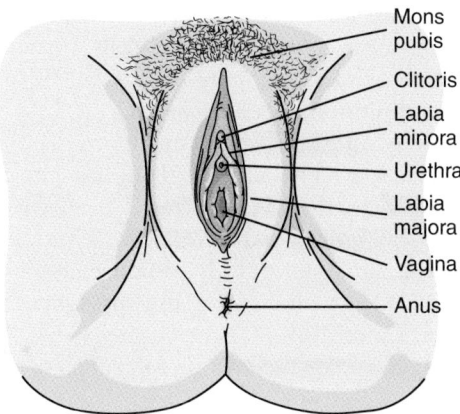

Fig. 9-25 External female genitalia.

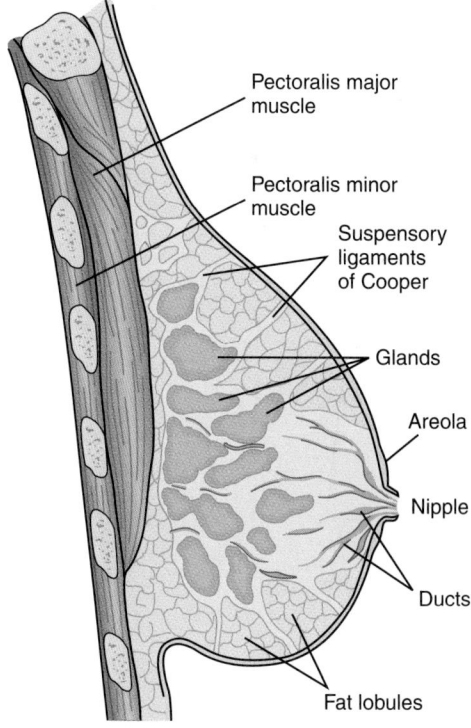

Fig. 9-26 The female breast.

The Bartholin's glands are examples. In young girls, the external vaginal opening is partially closed by a membrane called the *hymen*. The hymen ruptures when the female has intercourse for the first time.

The external female genitalia are called the *vulva* (Fig. 9-25):

- The *mons pubis* is a rounded, fatty pad over a bone called the *symphysis pubis*. The mons pubis is covered with hair in the adult female.
- The *labia majora* and *labia minora* are two folds of tissue on each side of the vaginal opening.
- The *clitoris* is a small organ composed of erectile tissue. It becomes hard when sexually stimulated.

The *mammary glands (breasts)* secrete milk after childbirth. The glands are on the outside of the chest. They are made up of glandular tissue and fat (Fig. 9-26). The milk drains into ducts that open onto the *nipple*.

Menstruation. The endometrium is rich in blood to nourish the cell that grows into a fetus. If pregnancy does not occur, menstruation begins. *Menstruation is the process in which the lining of the uterus (endometrium) breaks up and is discharged from the body through the vagina.* It occurs about every 28 days. Therefore it is called the *menstrual cycle*.

The first day of the menstrual cycle begins with menstruation. Blood flows from the uterus through the vaginal opening. Menstrual flow usually lasts 3 to 7 days. Ovulation occurs during the next phase. An ovum matures in an ovary and is released. Ovulation usually occurs on or about day 14 of the cycle.

Meanwhile, estrogen and progesterone (the female hormones) are secreted by the ovaries. These hormones cause the endometrium to thicken for pregnancy. If pregnancy does not occur, the hormones decrease in amount. This causes the blood supply to the endometrium to decrease. The endometrium breaks up. It is discharged through the vagina. Another menstrual cycle begins.

Fertilization

To reproduce, a male sex cell (sperm) must unite with a female sex cell (ovum). The uniting of the sperm and ovum into one cell is called *fertilization*. A sperm has 23 chromosomes. An ovum has 23 chromosomes. When the two cells unite, the fertilized cell has 46 chromosomes.

During intercourse, millions of sperm are deposited into the vagina. Sperm travel up the cervix, through the uterus, and into the fallopian tubes. If a sperm and an ovum unite in a fallopian tube, fertilization results. Pregnancy occurs. The fertilized cell travels down the fallopian tube to the uterus. After a short time, the fertilized cell implants in the thick endometrium and grows during pregnancy.

THE ENDOCRINE SYSTEM

The endocrine system is made up of glands called the *endocrine glands* (Fig. 9-27, p. 120). *The endocrine glands secrete chemical substances called hormones into the bloodstream.* Hormones regulate the activities of other organs and glands in the body.

The *pituitary gland* is called the *master gland*. About the size of a cherry, it is at the base of the brain behind the eyes. The pituitary gland is divided into the *anterior pituitary lobe* and the *posterior pituitary lobe*. The anterior pituitary lobe secretes:

- *Growth hormone (GH)*—needed for growth of muscles, bones, and other organs. It is needed throughout life to maintain normal-size bones and muscles. Growth is stunted if a baby is born with deficient amounts of growth hormone. Too much of the hormone causes excessive growth.

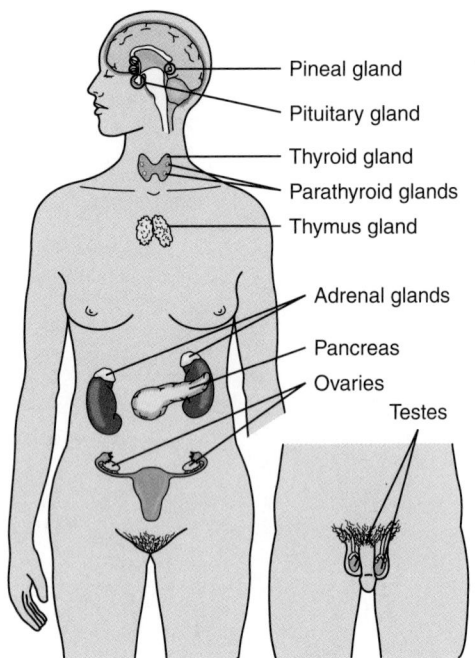

Fig. 9-27 Endocrine system.

- Pineal gland
- Pituitary gland
- Thyroid gland
- Parathyroid glands
- Thymus gland
- Adrenal glands
- Pancreas
- Ovaries
- Testes

- *Thyroid-stimulating hormone (TSH)*—needed for thyroid gland function.
- *Adrenocorticotropic hormone (ACTH)*—stimulates the adrenal glands.

The anterior lobe also secretes hormones that regulate growth, development, and function of the male and female reproductive systems.

The posterior pituitary lobe secretes *antidiuretic hormone (ADH)* and *oxytocin*. ADH prevents the kidneys from excreting excessive amounts of water. Oxytocin causes uterine muscles to contract during childbirth.

The *thyroid gland*, shaped like a butterfly, is in the neck in front of the larynx. *Thyroid hormone (TH, thyroxine)* is secreted by the thyroid gland. It regulates metabolism. *Metabolism is the burning of food for heat and energy by the cells.* Too little TH results in slowed body processes, slowed movements, and weight gain. Too much TH causes increased metabolism, excess energy, and weight loss. Some babies are born with deficient amounts of TH. Their physical growth and mental growth are stunted.

The four *parathyroid glands* secrete *parathormone*. Two lie on each side of the thyroid gland. Parathormone regulates calcium use. Calcium is needed for nerve and muscle function. Insufficient amounts of calcium cause *tetany*. Tetany is a state of severe muscle contraction and spasm. If untreated, tetany can cause death.

The *thymus* secretes the hormone *thymosin*. This hormone is important for the development and function of the immune system.

The *pancreas* secretes *insulin*. Insulin regulates the amount of sugar in the blood available for use by the cells.

Insulin is needed for sugar to enter the cells. If there is too little insulin, sugar cannot enter the cells. If sugar cannot enter the cells, excess amounts of sugar build up in the blood. This condition is called *diabetes*.

There are two *adrenal glands*. An adrenal gland is on the top of each kidney. The adrenal gland has two parts: the *adrenal medulla* and the *adrenal cortex*. The adrenal medulla secretes *epinephrine* and *norepinephrine*. These hormones stimulate the body to quickly produce energy during emergencies. Heart rate, blood pressure, muscle power, and energy all increase.

The adrenal cortex secretes three groups of hormones needed for life:
- *Glucocorticoids*—regulate the metabolism of carbohydrates. They also control the body's response to stress and inflammation.
- *Mineralocorticoids*—regulate the amount of salt and water that is absorbed and lost by the kidneys.
- Small amounts of male and female sex hormones.

The *gonads* are the glands of human reproduction. Male sex glands (testes) secrete *testosterone*. Female sex glands (ovaries) secrete *estrogen* and *progesterone*.

THE IMMUNE SYSTEM

The immune system protects the body from disease and infection. Abnormal body cells can grow into tumors. Sometimes the body produces substances that cause the body to attack itself. Microorganisms (bacteria, viruses, and other germs) can cause an infection. The immune system defends against threats inside and outside the body.

The immune system gives the body immunity. *Immunity means that a person has protection against a disease or condition. The person will not get or be affected by the disease.*
- *Specific immunity* is the body's reaction to a certain threat.
- *Nonspecific immunity* is the body's reaction to anything it does not recognize as a normal body substance.

Special cells and substances function to produce immunity:
- *Antibodies*—normal body substances that recognize other substances. They are involved in destroying abnormal or unwanted substances.
- *Antigens*—substances that cause an immune response. Antibodies recognize and bind with unwanted antigens. This leads to the destruction of unwanted substances and the production of more antibodies.
- *Phagocytes*—white blood cells that digest and destroy microorganisms and other unwanted substances (Fig. 9-28).
- *Lymphocytes*—white blood cells that produce antibodies. Lymphocyte production increases as the body responds to an infection.

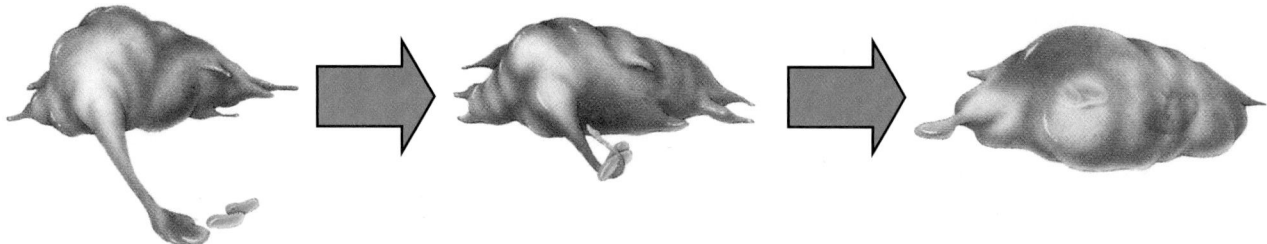

Fig. 9-28 A phagocyte digests and destroys a microorganism.

- *B lymphocytes (B cells)*—cause the production of antibodies that circulate in the plasma. The antibodies react to specific antigens.
- *T lymphocytes (T cells)*—cells that destroy invading cells. *Killer T cells* produce poisons near the invading cells. Some T cells attract other cells. The other cells destroy the invaders.

When the body senses an antigen from an unwanted substance, the immune system acts. Phagocyte and lymphocyte production increases. Phagocytes destroy the invaders through digestion. The lymphocytes produce antibodies that identify and destroy the unwanted substances.

FOCUS ON PRIDE

The Person, Family, and Yourself

Personal and Professional Responsibility

To function, you must care for your body. A healthy diet (Chapter 24), exercise, and rest are needed for over-all health. See your doctor for a check-up at least once a year. Or do so sooner if you have a concern. Take prescription or over the counter drugs as instructed. Keep your immunizations up to date. For example, get a tetanus booster every 10 years. Protect your bones and muscles from injury by using good body mechanics (Chapter 16). Follow Standard Precautions to protect yourself from infection (Chapter 15). Also practice good hand hygiene (Chapter 15). Taking care of yourself is a personal and professional responsibility. To care for others, you need a strong and healthy body.

Rights and Respect

Patients and residents have the right to make decisions about their bodies. You may not agree with those decisions. But you must respect the person's choice. If the decision will cause no harm, comply with the request. For example, Mr. Ferris does not want to wear his hearing aid today. He says: "I don't need that thing." His request will not harm him. Respect his choice. Tell the nurse.

If the person's decision may cause harm, tell the nurse at once. For example, Ms. Lane's kidneys do not function. She goes to dialysis 3 times a week. (Dialysis is the process of artificially removing wastes from the blood when the kidneys do not function.) Ms. Lane tells you that she does not want to go today. She says: "I just can't sit there for that long." You know the importance of the urinary system. Without dialysis, she will become very sick. You tell the nurse. Ms. Lane cannot be forced to go to dialysis. But the nurse can talk with Ms. Lane about her decision, the consequences, and possible solutions.

Independence and Social Interaction

The body does not always work right. People become ill or injured. Some illnesses cannot be cured. Sometimes the health team cannot prevent loss of function. However, patients and residents are helped to maintain their optimal level of function. This is the person's highest potential for mental and physical performance.

To help maintain the person's optimal level of function:
- Do not treat the person as a sick, dependent person. This reduces quality of life.
- Encourage the person to be as independent as possible.
- Always focus on the person's abilities, not disabilities.
- Tell the person when you notice progress.
- Promote social interaction. This improves mental performance.

Take pride in helping each person regain or maintain the highest level of functioning possible.

Delegation and Teamwork

The body works like a team. Each system has independent functions. But all systems interact and depend on each other. They work together to keep the body functioning. When a person has a problem with one body system, other systems are affected. Understanding each system and how the systems interact helps you provide better care.

Ethics and Laws

Sometimes a person is not able to make decisions about his or her own body. For example, the person has dementia. Or the person is unconscious or under the influence of drugs or alcohol. Maybe the person is thinking of harming himself or herself. Or the person may be a child. Ethical issues may arise over who makes decisions for such persons.

Spouses, parents, family members, or legal guardians may make decisions. Some persons have a durable power of attorney (Chapter 52). This is someone assigned to make decisions for that person if he or she is unable to do so. Some fill out a legal document called an advance directive (Chapter 52). This document states a person's wishes about health care when that person is unable to make his or her own decisions. In cases such as drug and alcohol abuse or attempts to harm oneself, the person's safety is the priority. Sometimes the court appoints a guardian for a short time. Finally, the agency's ethics committee may address complex issues. In all cases, the person's safety and best interests guide the care given.

REVIEW QUESTIONS

Circle the BEST answer.

1 The basic unit of body structure is the
   a Cell
   b Neuron
   c Nephron
   d Ovum

2 The outer layer of the skin is called the
   a Dermis
   b Epidermis
   c Integument
   d Myelin

3 Which is *not* a function of the skin?
   a Provides the protective covering for the body.
   b Regulates body temperature.
   c Senses cold, pain, touch, and pressure.
   d Provides the shape and framework for the body.

4 Which allows movement?
   a Bone marrow
   b Synovial membrane
   c Joints
   d Ligaments

5 Skeletal muscles
   a Are under involuntary control
   b Appear smooth
   c Are under voluntary control
   d Appear striped and smooth

6 The highest functions in the brain take place in the
   a Cerebral cortex
   b Medulla
   c Brainstem
   d Spinal nerves

7 The ear is involved with
   a Regulating body movements
   b Balance
   c Smoothness of body movements
   d Controlling involuntary muscles

8 The liquid part of the blood is the
   a Hemoglobin
   b Red blood cell
   c Plasma
   d White blood cell

9 Which part of the heart pumps blood to the body?
   a Right atrium
   b Left atrium
   c Right ventricle
   d Left ventricle

10 Which carry blood away from the heart?
   a Capillaries
   b Veins
   c Venules
   d Arteries

11 Oxygen and carbon dioxide are exchanged
   a In the bronchi
   b Between the alveoli and capillaries
   c Between the lungs and pleura
   d In the trachea

12 Digestion begins in the
   a Mouth
   b Stomach
   c Small intestine
   d Colon

13 Most food absorption takes place in the
   a Stomach
   b Small intestine
   c Colon
   d Large intestine

14 Urine is formed by the
   a Jejunum
   b Kidneys
   c Bladder
   d Liver

15 Urine passes from the body through the
   a Ureters
   b Urethra
   c Anus
   d Nephrons

16 The male sex gland is called the
   a Penis
   b Semen
   c Testis
   d Scrotum

17 The male sex cell is the
   a Semen
   b Ovum
   c Gonad
   d Sperm

18 The female sex gland is the
   a Ovary
   b Cervix
   c Uterus
   d Vagina

19 The discharge of the lining of the uterus is called
   a The endometrium
   b Ovulation
   c Fertilization
   d Menstruation

20 The endocrine glands secrete
   a Hormones
   b Mucus
   c Semen
   d Insulin

21 The immune system protects the body from
   a Low blood sugar
   b Disease and infection
   c Loss of fluid
   d Stunted growth

Answers to these questions are on p. 832.

Growth and Development

OBJECTIVES

- Define the key terms listed in this chapter.
- Explain the principles of growth and development.
- Identify the stages of growth and development.
- Identify the developmental tasks for each age-group.
- Describe the normal growth and development for each age-group.
- Explain how to promote PRIDE in the person, the family, and yourself.

KEY TERMS

adolescence The time between puberty and adulthood; a time of rapid growth and physical, sexual, emotional, and social changes

development Changes in mental, emotional, and social function

developmental task A skill that must be completed during a stage of development

ejaculation The release of semen

growth The physical changes that are measured and that occur in a steady, orderly manner

infancy The first year of life

menarche The first menstruation and the start of menstrual cycles

menopause The time when menstruation stops and menstrual cycles end

peer A person of the same age-group and background

primary caregiver The person mainly responsible for providing or assisting with the child's basic needs

puberty The period when reproductive organs begin to function and secondary sex characteristics appear

reflex An involuntary movement

sexual orientation Sexual arousal or romantic attraction to persons of the other gender (heterosexual), the same gender (homosexual), or both genders (bisexual)

You care for people of all ages. They are in different stages of growth and development. Understanding growth and development helps you give better care. The person's needs are easier to understand. This chapter presents the basic changes that occur in normal, healthy persons from birth until death.

Growth and development are presented in stages. Age ranges and normal characteristics are given for each stage. The stages overlap. It is hard to see the start and end of each stage. Also, the rate of growth and development varies with each person.

Growth and development theories usually involve the two-parent family. However, single-parent households are common. A relative may care for children while the parent works or is in school. In this chapter, *primary caregiver* is used in place of *mother*, *father*, or *parent*. The *primary caregiver is the person mainly responsible for providing or assisting with the child's basic needs.* A mother, father, grandparent, sister, brother, aunt, uncle, or court-appointed guardian may have this role. *Parent* and *parents* are sometimes used here. However, another primary caregiver may have the parent role.

Age ranges for each stage vary among growth and development experts. The groupings and content in this chapter are broad and general.

PRINCIPLES

Growth is the physical changes that are measured and that occur in a steady and orderly manner. Growth is measured in weight, height, and changes in appearance and body functions (Fig. 10-1, p. 124).

Development relates to changes in mental, emotional, and social function. A person behaves and thinks in certain ways in each stage of development. A 2-year-old thinks in simple terms. A primary caregiver is needed for basic needs. A 40-year-old thinks in complex ways. Most basic needs are met without help.

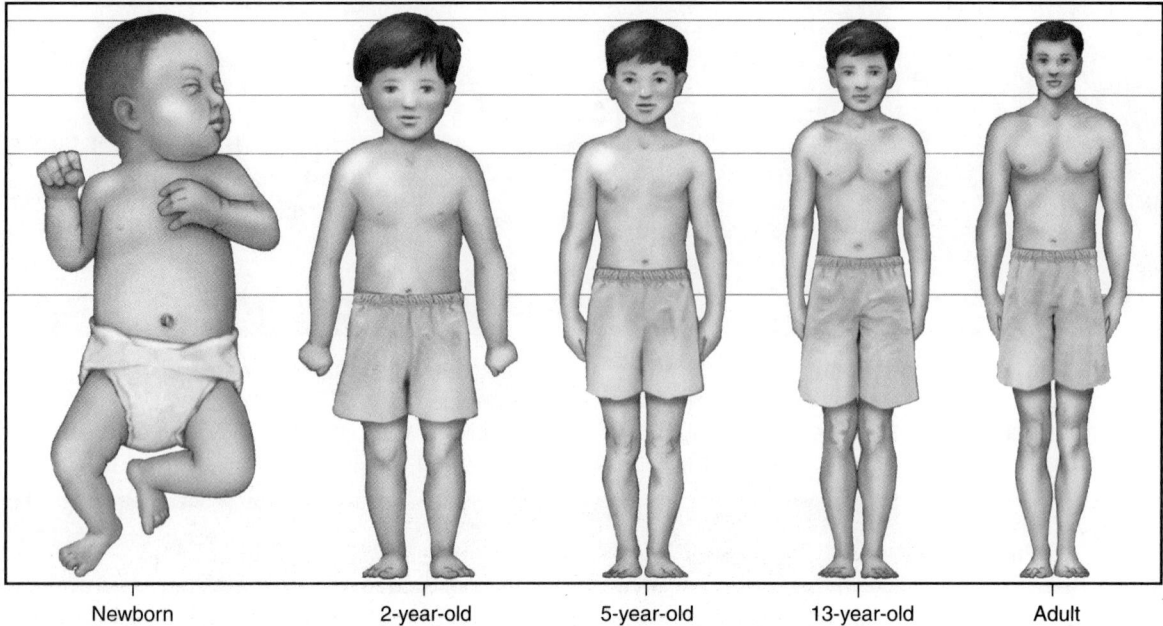

| Newborn | 2-year-old | 5-year-old | 13-year-old | Adult |

Fig. 10-1 Changes in appearance from birth to maturity.

The entire person is affected. Although they differ, growth and development:
- Overlap
- Depend on each other
- Occur at the same time

For example, an infant cannot coo or babble (development) until the physical structures for speech are strong enough (growth). Basic principles of growth and development are:
- The process starts at fertilization and continues until death.
- The process proceeds from the simple to the complex. A baby sits before standing, stands before walking, and walks before running.
- The process occurs in certain directions:
  - From head to the foot. Babies hold up their heads before they sit; they sit before they stand.
  - From the center of the body outward. Babies control shoulder movements before they control hand movements.
- The process occurs in a sequence, order, and pattern. Certain skills must be completed during each stage. A *developmental task is a skill that must be completed during a stage of development*. A stage cannot be skipped. Each stage is the basis for the next stage.
- The rate of the process is uneven. It is not at a set pace. Growth is rapid during infancy. Children have growth spurts. Some children develop fast. Others develop slowly.
- Each stage has its own characteristics and developmental tasks.

INFANCY (BIRTH TO 1 YEAR)

Infancy is the first year of life. Growth and development are rapid during this time. The developmental tasks of infancy are:
- Learning to walk
- Learning to eat solid foods
- Beginning to talk and communicate with others
- Learning to trust
- Beginning to have emotional relationships with parents, brothers, and sisters
- Developing stable sleep and feeding patterns

The Newborn (Birth to 1 Month)

The neonatal period of infancy is from birth to 1 month. A baby is called a *neonate* or *newborn* at this time.

The average newborn weighs 6 to 9 pounds. Birth weight doubles by 5 to 6 months of age. At 6 months, the baby weighs an average of 16 pounds. Birth weight triples by 1 year of age. The average 1-year-old weighs 21½ pounds.

The average newborn is 19 to 21 inches long. Length increases in spurts. At 6 months, the average length is 25½ inches. The average 1-year-old is 29 inches.

The newborn's head is large compared with the rest of the body. The trunk is long. The abdomen is large, round, and soft. The newborn has fat, pudgy cheeks, a flat nose, and a receding chin (Fig. 10-2).

The skin is smooth. It is bright red at birth in light-skinned babies but turns to pink a few days later. Dark-skinned newborns may appear pinkish to yellowish brown. The skin turns to its natural color in a few days. Eyes are a

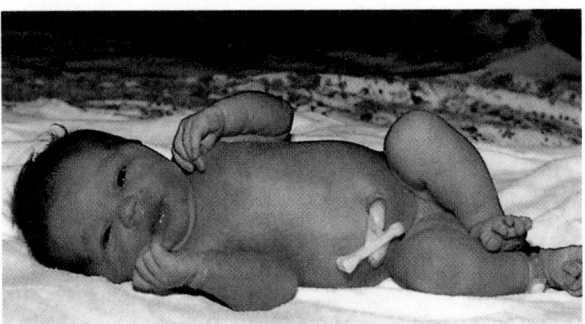

Fig. 10-2 A newborn.

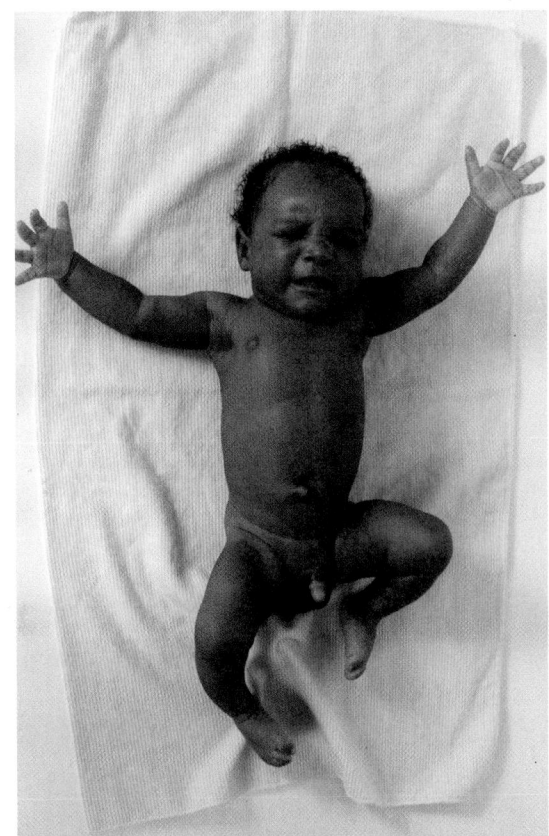

Fig. 10-3 Moro reflex.

deep blue in light-skinned babies. Dark-skinned babies have brown eyes.

The newborn's central nervous system is not well developed. Movements lack purpose and are uncoordinated. Newborns can see clearly up to about 8 inches. They see in color preferring yellow, green, and pink colors. Newborns hear well. Loud sounds startle them. Soft sounds soothe them. They know the mother's voice. They react to touch and pain. They can taste and smell.

Newborns have certain *reflexes (involuntary movements)*. These reflexes decline and then disappear as the central nervous system develops.

- *Moro reflex (startle reflex)*—occurs when a baby is startled by a loud noise, a sudden movement, or the head falling back. The arms are thrown apart. The legs extend and then flex. A brief cry is common. See Figure 10-3.
- *Rooting reflex*—occurs when the cheek is touched near the mouth (Fig. 10-4). The mouth opens, and the head turns toward the touch. This reflex is necessary for feeding. It guides the baby's mouth to the nipple.
- *Sucking reflex*—occurs when the lips are touched.
- *Grasp (palmar) reflex*—occurs when the palm is stroked. The fingers close firmly around the object (Fig. 10-5, p. 126).
- *Step (dance) reflex*—occurs when the baby is held upright and the feet touch a surface. The feet move up and down and in stepping motions (Fig. 10-6, p. 126).

Specific, voluntary, and coordinated movements occur as the nervous and muscular systems develop. Newborns cannot hold their heads up. They turn their heads from side to side.

Newborns sleep 16 to 18 hours a day. They awaken when hungry and fall asleep right after a feeding. Bottle-fed infants feed every 2½ to 4 hours. Breast-fed infants are hungry more often—every 2 to 3 hours. The time between feedings lengthens as infants grow and develop. They also stay awake more and sleep less.

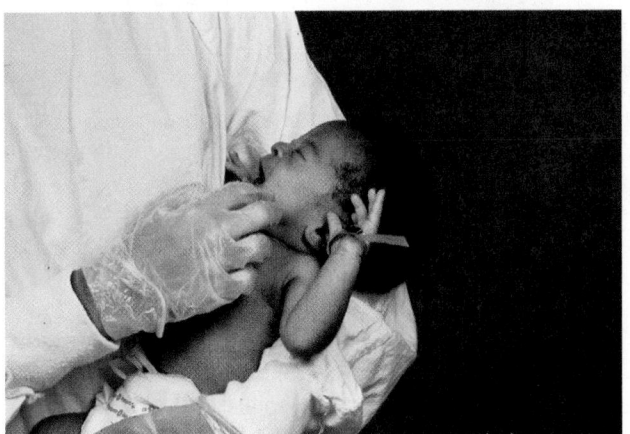

Fig. 10-4 Rooting reflex.

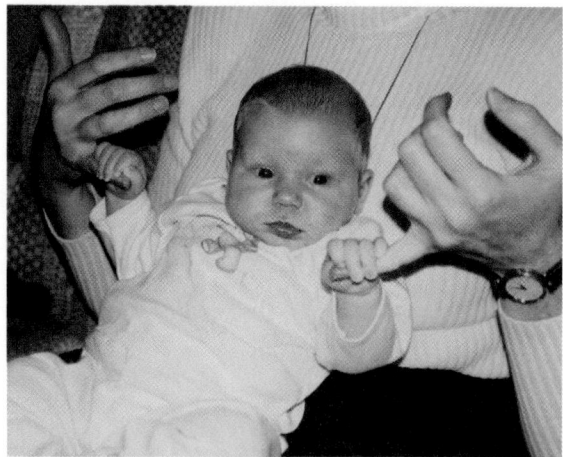

Fig. 10-5 The grasp reflex.

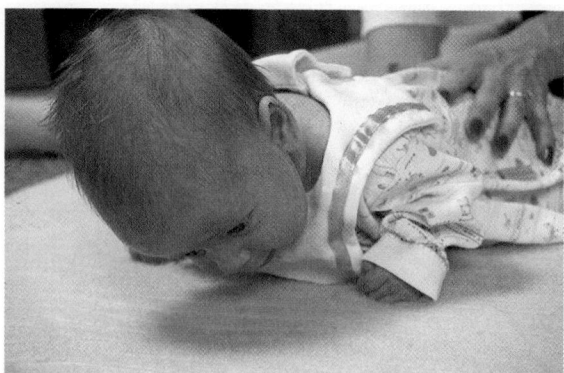

Fig. 10-7 The 1-month-old can briefly lift her head when lying on her stomach.

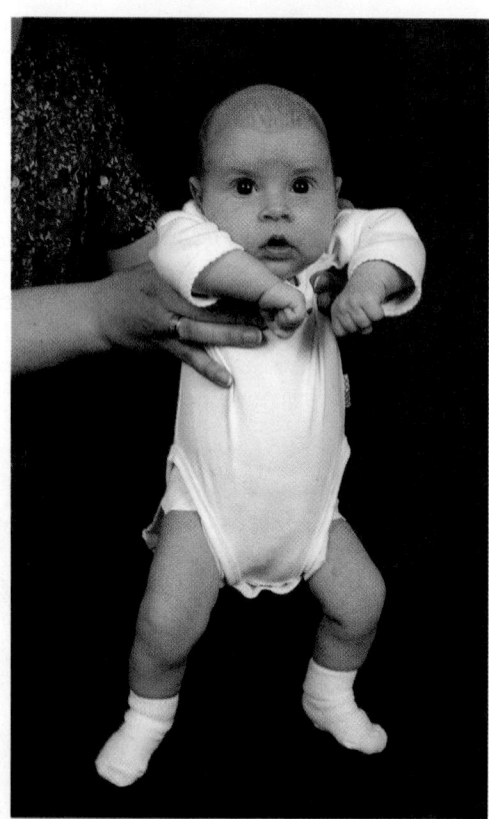

Fig. 10-6 Step (dance) reflex.

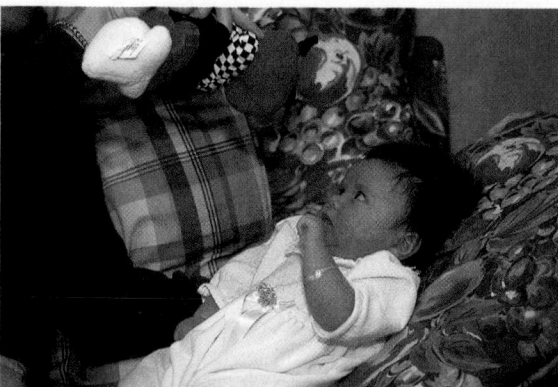

Fig. 10-8 A 2-month-old child follows an object with her eyes.

angled position. They have tears and can follow objects with their eyes (Fig. 10-8). They smile when responding to others.

Infants 3 to 4 months of age can hold their heads up (Fig. 10-9). They reach for objects. Pleasure causes squealing. They babble, coo, gurgle, and laugh out loud. The Moro, rooting, and grasp reflexes disappear.

By 4 to 5 months, infants can roll from front to back. They roll from back to front by 5 to 6 months. They also can sit by leaning forward on their hands (Fig. 10-10). Teething may begin with the bottom front teeth. They sleep all night. They can play "peak-a-boo."

Solid foods are given at 4 to 6 months. Rice cereal mixed with milk is given first with an infant spoon. Fruits, vegetables, and meats are introduced slowly. These foods are thin in consistency at first. Thicker and chunkier foods are given as more teeth erupt and chewing and swallowing skills increase.

Infants have more skills at 6 months. They can bear weight when pulled up into a standing position. They sit with support and move around by rolling. Some start to drink from a cup. They smile at themselves in a mirror. They respond to their names.

Infants (1 Month to 1 Year)

When lying on their stomachs, 1-month-old infants can lift their heads up briefly (Fig. 10-7). They also can turn their heads. They smile.

Two-month-old infants can hold their heads up when held upright. When on their stomachs, they can turn their heads from side to side. They need support to sit in an

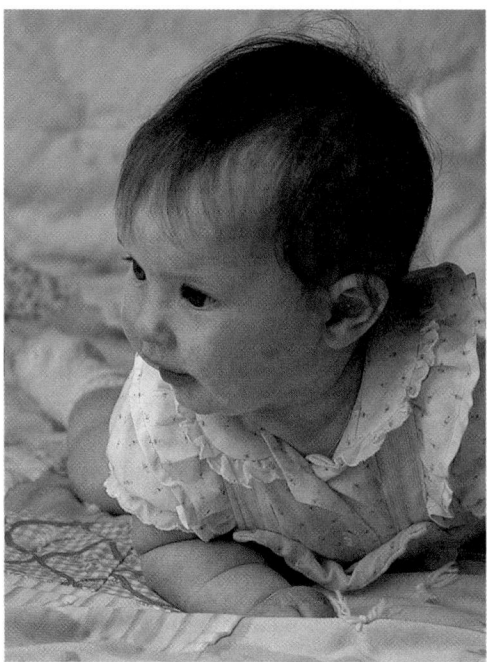

Fig. 10-9 The 3-month-old child can raise the head and shoulders.

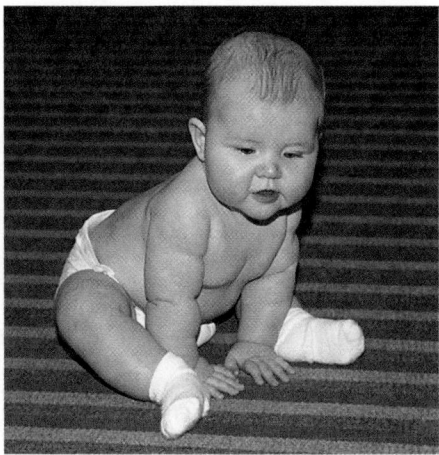

Fig. 10-10 A 6-month-old sits forward leaning on the hands.

Some infants start to crawl at 7 months. They can stand while holding on for support. They make sounds in response to caregivers.

Eight-month-old infants can sit for long periods. They also can change from lying to sitting and from sitting to lying positions. The pincer grasp develops—they can hold small objects with the thumb and index finger. They can pick up small finger foods. They learn to drink from a cup with handles. Language skills increase. They can say "mama" and "dada."

When holding on to something, 9-month-olds can pull up into a standing position. They can hold a bottle, play "pat-a-cake," and drink from a cup or glass. They understand their names and "no." They point and use gestures to communicate.

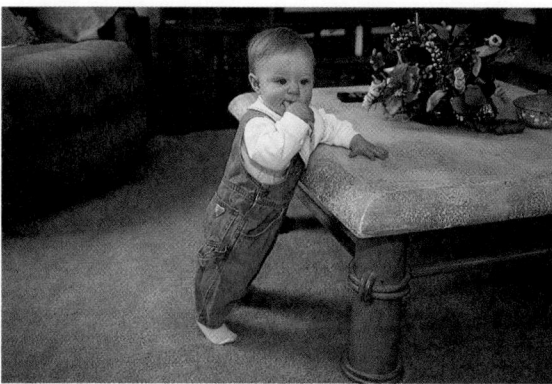

Fig. 10-11 A 10-month-old infant can walk while holding on to furniture.

At 10 months, infants can stand alone. They may walk with help or while holding on to something (Fig. 10-11). They also may crawl up stairs. At 11 months, they may walk alone and use push toys.

At 12 months, walking skills increase. They can climb onto furniture. They can turn book pages and put objects into a container. They can say a few words. Bottle weaning may begin.

The infant must develop a sense of trust. If successful, the infant trusts himself or herself and others. Trust develops when care is consistent. The infant's physical and safety needs are met—feeding, comfort, warmth, touch, stimulation, and caring.

TODDLERHOOD (1 TO 3 YEARS)
The growth rate is slower than during infancy. Developmental tasks are:
* Tolerating separation from the primary caregiver
* Gaining control of bowel and bladder function
* Using words to communicate
* Becoming less dependent on the primary caregiver

Toddlers need to assert independence. Therefore this time is called the "terrible twos." Toddlers learn to walk well. They are curious. They get into everything and anything. They touch, smell, and taste everything within reach. They climb on tables, chairs, counters, and other high places. With these new skills, toddlers can explore their settings. They venture farther away from primary caregivers. They learn to do some things without a primary caregiver. By the age of 3, they can run, jump, climb, ride a tricycle, and walk up and down stairs.

Hand coordination increases. They learn to feed themselves. They progress from eating with fingers to using a spoon (Fig. 10-12, p. 128). Toddlers can drink from cups. They can scribble, build towers with blocks, and string beads. Right- or left-handedness is seen during the second year.

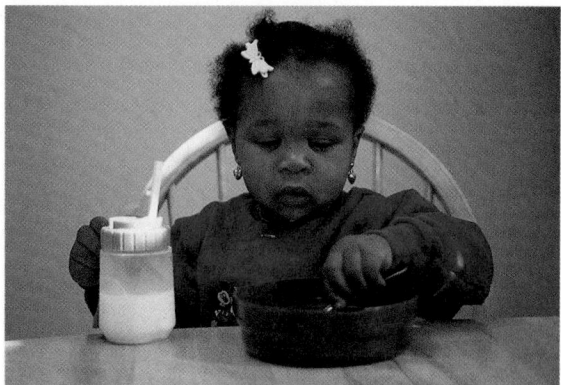

Fig. 10-12 A toddler uses a spoon.

Toilet training is a major task for toddlers. Bowel and bladder control is related to central nervous system development. Children must be mentally and physically ready for toilet training. Some children are ready at age 2 years. Others are ready at 2½ to 3 years of age. The process starts with bowel control. Bladder control during the day occurs before bladder control at night.

Speech and language skills increase. Speech is clearer. Toddlers imitate others to learn words. They understand more words than they say. An 18-month-old knows 6 to 18 words. By age 2 years, the child knows about 300 words. "Me" and "mine" are used often.

Play skills increase. The child plays alongside other children but not with them. Toddlers do not share toys. They are very possessive and do not understand sharing.

Temper tantrums and saying "no" are common during this stage. Toddlers express anger and frustration by kicking and screaming. That is how they object to having independence challenged. Using "no" can frustrate primary caregivers. Almost every request may be answered "no," even if the child follows the request.

Another task is tolerating separation from the primary caregiver. As toddlers start to explore, they move away from the primary caregiver. With discomfort, frustration, or injury, they quickly return to primary caregivers or cry for their attention. If primary caregivers are consistently present when needed, children learn to feel secure. They learn to tolerate brief periods of separation.

PRESCHOOL (3 TO 6 YEARS)
The preschool years are from the ages of 3 to 6 years. Children grow 2 to 3 inches per year. They gain about 5 pounds per year. Preschoolers are thinner, more coordinated, and more graceful than toddlers.

Developmental tasks include:
- Increasing the ability to communicate and understand others
- Performing self-care
- Learning gender differences and developing sexual modesty

- Learning right from wrong and good from bad
- Learning to play with others
- Developing family relationships

The 3-Year-Old
Three-year-olds become more coordinated. They can walk on tiptoe and balance on one foot for a few seconds. They run, jump, kick a ball, and climb with ease.

Personal care skills increase. They can put on clothes and shoes, manage buttons, wash their hands, and brush their teeth (Fig. 10-13). They can feed themselves, pour from a bottle, and help set the table without breaking dishes. Hand skills also include drawing circles and crosses.

Language skills increase. Three-year-olds know about 900 words. They talk and ask questions ("how" and "why") constantly. They can name body parts, family members, and friends. They like talking toys and musical toys.

Play is important. They play with 2 or 3 other children and can share. They play simple games and learn simple rules. Imaginary friends and imitating adults are common. They enjoy crayons, cutting paper, pasting, painting, and playing "house" and "dress-up" (Fig. 10-14). They also like wagons, tricycles, and other riding toys.

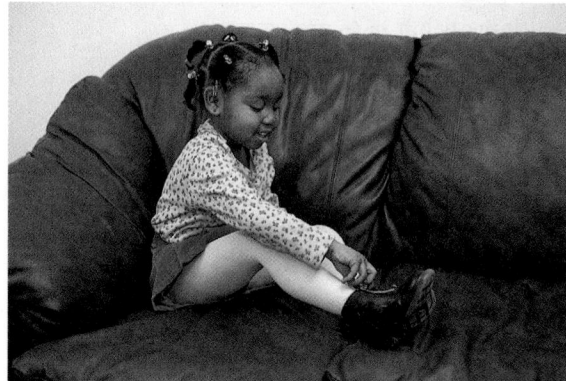

Fig. 10-13 A 3-year-old has increased coordination.

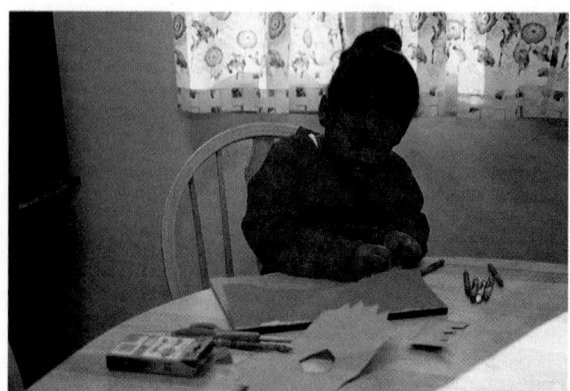

Fig. 10-14 This 3-year-old enjoys cutting paper.

Three-year-olds know that there are two sexes. They know that male and female bodies differ. They also know their own sex. Little girls may wonder how the penis works and why they don't have one. Little boys may wonder how girls can urinate without a penis.

The concept of time develops. Three-year-olds may speak of the past, present, and future. "Yesterday" and "to-morrow" are confusing. Children may fear the dark and need night-lights in bedrooms. Nightmares are common.

Three-year-olds are less fearful of strangers. They can be away from primary caregivers for short periods. They are less jealous than toddlers of a new baby. They try to please primary caregivers.

The 4-Year-Old

Four-year-olds can hop, skip, and throw and catch a ball. They can lace shoes, draw faces, and copy a square. They try to print letters. With help, they can bathe and tend to toileting needs.

They know about 1500 words. They ask many questions and tend to exaggerate stories. They can sing simple songs, repeat four numbers, count to five, and name a few colors.

Four-year-olds tend to tease, tattle, and tell fibs. When bad, they may blame an imaginary friend. Bragging, telling tales about family members, and showing off are common. They can play with other children. They are proud of accomplishments but have mood swings.

These children enjoy playing "dress-up," wearing costumes, and telling and hearing stories. They like to draw and make things. Imagination, drama, and imitating adults are part of play. They play in groups of 2 or 3 and tend to be bossy. Playing "doctor and nurse" is common as curiosity about the other sex continues (Fig. 10-15).

Four-year-olds prefer the primary caregiver of the other sex. Rivalries with brothers and sisters are seen, especially when a younger child takes the 4-year-old's things. Rivalries also occur when older children have more and different privileges. The family is often the focus of the child's frustrations and aggressive behavior. A 4-year-old may try to run away from home.

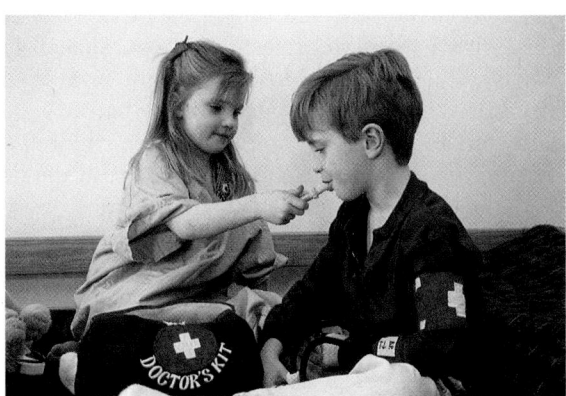

Fig. 10-15 Four-year-olds play "doctor and nurse."

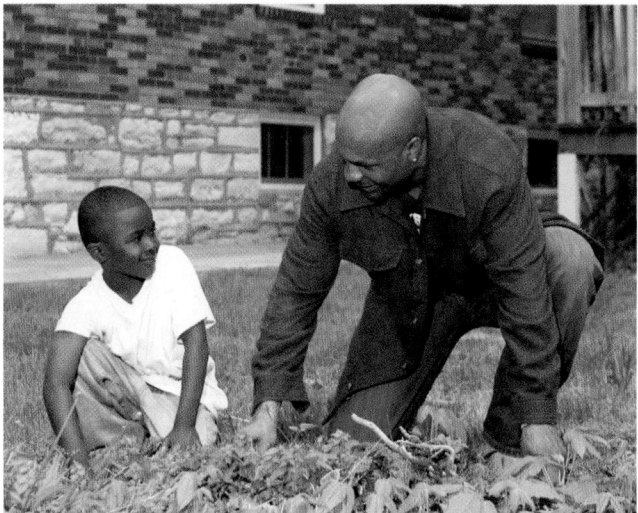

Fig. 10-16 This 5-year-old does yard work with his father.

The 5-Year-Old

Coordination increases. Five-year-olds can jump rope, skate, tie shoelaces, dress, and bathe. They can use a pencil well and copy diamond and triangle shapes. They can print a few letters, numbers, and their first names. Drawings of people include body parts.

Communication skills increase. They speak in full sentences. Questions are fewer than before but have more meaning. They want words defined and take part in conversations. They can name colors, coins, days, and the months. They specify and describe drawings.

Five-year-olds are more responsible and truthful. They quarrel less than before. They are more aware of rules and are eager to do things correctly. They have manners, are independent, and can be trusted within limits. Fears are fewer, but nightmares and dreams are common. They are proud of accomplishments.

These children like books about animals and other children. They like board games and try to follow rules. They imitate adults during play and are interested in TV. They also enjoy doing things with the primary caregiver of the same sex (Fig. 10-16). These include cooking, housekeeping, shopping, yard work, and sports.

Younger children are considered a nuisance. However, 5-year-olds usually protect them. They tolerate brothers and sisters well.

SCHOOL AGE (6 TO 9 OR 10 YEARS)

School-age children enter the world of peer groups, games, and learning. They grow 2 to 3 inches a year. They gain 4½ to 6½ pounds a year. Their developmental tasks are:

- Developing the social and physical skills needed for playing games
- Learning to get along with *persons of the same age and background (peers)*
- Learning gender-appropriate behaviors and attitudes
- Learning basic reading, writing, and math skills
- Developing a conscience and morals
- Developing a good feeling and attitude about oneself

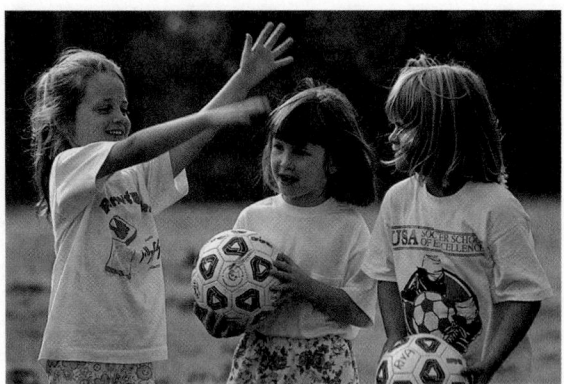

Fig. 10-17 These 6-year-old girls enjoy soccer.

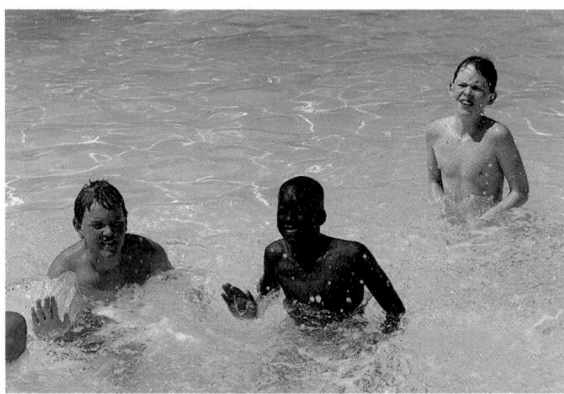

Fig. 10-18 Belonging to a peer group is important to school-age children.

Baby teeth are lost and permanent teeth erupt. This starts around age 6 years.

Children are very active. They can run, jump, skip, hop, and ride a two-wheeled bike. They can swim, skate, dance, and jump rope. These children can take part in team sports. Soccer, T-ball, baseball, football, and volleyball are examples (Fig. 10-17). Children learn to play in groups. They learn teamwork and sportsmanship and follow rules. Quiet play involves collections, board games, computer and video games, and crafts.

Language skills increase rapidly. Reading, writing, grammar, and math skills develop. They learn to print first. Printing is followed by cursive writing. Sentences are longer and more complex. As reading skills increase, so do language skills. Children like to read and be read to.

Play activities have purpose and involve "work." Children in this age-group like household tasks (cleaning, cooking, yard work). They also like crafts, building things, and scout groups. Rewards are important—good grades, trophies, payment for chores, scouting badges.

At about age 7, boys prefer playing with boys. Girls prefer playing with girls. From 8 to 9 years, they play with children of their own sex. Some play involves boys and girls. Interest in boy-girl relationships starts at about 8 to 9 years. However, children may deny such interest.

School-age children are concerned about being well liked. A peer group is important for love, belonging, and self-esteem needs. These children get along well with and need adults. However, they prefer peer group fads, opinions, and activities (Fig. 10-18).

LATE CHILDHOOD (9 OR 10 TO 12 YEARS)

Late childhood (pre-adolescence) is the time between childhood and adolescence. Developmental tasks are like those for school-age children. Pre-adolescents are expected to show more refinement and maturity in achieving these tasks:

- Becoming independent of adults and learning to depend on oneself

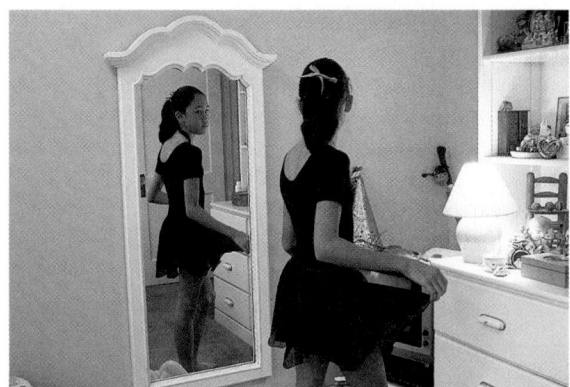

Fig. 10-19 Movements are smooth and graceful in late childhood.

- Developing and keeping friendships with peers
- Understanding the physical, psychological, and social roles of one's sex
- Developing moral and ethical behavior
- Developing greater muscular strength, coordination, and balance
- Learning how to study

Many permanent teeth erupt. Girls have a growth spurt. By age 12 years, they are taller and heavier than boys. Both boys and girls have more graceful and coordinated body movements (Fig. 10-19). Muscle strength and physical skills increase. Skill in team sports is important.

Math and language skills increase. These children read to find information and for pleasure. They read the news. They enjoy books and stories about romance, mystery, adventure, and science fiction.

The onset of puberty nears. *Puberty is the period when reproductive organs begin to function and secondary sex characteristics appear.* In girls, the hips widen and breast buds appear. Some 9-, 10-, and 11-year-old girls begin puberty. Boys show fewer signs of maturing sexually. Genital organs begin to grow.

These children need factual sex education. Friends share information about sex. It is often not complete and not accurate. Parents and children may be uncomfortable discussing sex with each other. They may avoid the subject. When children ask questions, answers must be honest and complete. They must be given in terms that children understand.

Peer groups are the center of activities. The group affects the child's attitudes and behavior. Children prefer friends of the same sex. Friends are loyal and share problems. A "best friend" is common. Interest in the other sex begins.

These children are aware of the mistakes and faults of adults. They do not accept adult standards and rules without question. It is common to rebel against adults and test limits. Parents and children disagree. However, parents are needed for the child's development.

ADOLESCENCE (12 TO 18 YEARS)

Adolescence is the time between puberty and adulthood. There is rapid growth and physical, sexual, emotional, and social changes. The stage begins with puberty. Girls reach puberty between the ages of 9 and 16 years. Boys reach puberty between the ages of 13 and 15 years.

Developmental tasks include:
* Accepting changes in the body and appearance
* Developing appropriate relationships with males and females of the same age
* Accepting the male or female role appropriate for one's age
* Becoming independent from parents and adults
* Preparing for marriage and family life
* Preparing for a career
* Developing morals, attitudes, and values needed to function in society

Both boys and girls have a growth spurt. Both gain height and weight. They need about 9½ hours of sleep a night because of such rapid growth. Girls usually complete physical development by age 17. Boys usually stop growing between the ages of 18 and 21 years.

Oil glands are more active, leading to acne. Sweat glands are more active. Good hygiene is important. Deodorants or antiperspirants are needed to prevent body odors.

Menarche marks the onset of puberty in girls. *Menarche is the first menstruation and the start of menstrual cycles* (Chapter 9). *Pregnancy can occur with the onset of menarche.* Secondary sex characteristics appear. These include:
* Increase in breast size
* Pubic, axillary (underarm), and leg hair
* Slight deepening of the voice
* Widening and rounding of the hips

Ejaculation (the release of semen) signals the onset of puberty in boys. *Nocturnal emissions* ("wet dreams") occur. During sleep *(nocturnal)* the penis becomes erect. Semen is

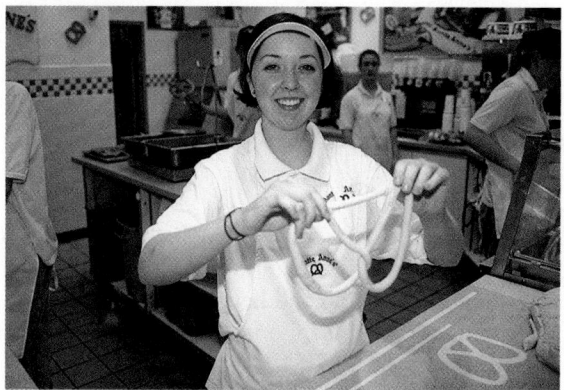
Fig. 10-20 This teenager has a part-time job.

released *(emission). The male can father children.* Other secondary sex characteristics include:
* Facial, pubic, and axillary (underarm) hair
* Hair on the chest, arms, and legs
* Deepening of the voice
* Increases in neck and shoulder sizes

Movements often seem awkward and clumsy. Muscle and bone growth is uneven. Coordination and graceful movements develop as muscle and bone growth even out.

Accepting body changes and appearance occurs over time. Girls worry about weight gain. Breast development can embarrass girls, especially if breasts are very large or small. Some do not like wearing a bra. Others wear clothes that show off the breasts. Boys may worry about genital size. Height is a problem for both genders. Being small limits play in some sports. Boys do not like being shorter than their peers. Tall girls may feel embarrassed about being taller than other girls and boys.

Mood swings occur. Emotional reactions vary from high to low. They can be happy one moment and sad the next. It is hard to predict their reaction to a comment or event. They control emotions better later in this stage. Fourteen- to 18-year-olds are sometimes sad and depressed. However, they have more control over the time and place of emotional reactions.

Adolescents need to become independent of adults, especially parents. They must learn to function, make decisions, and act responsibly without adult supervision. Many teenagers have part-time jobs or babysit (Fig. 10-20). They go to dances and parties, shop without an adult, and stay home alone. Many take part in school clubs and organizations.

Judgment and reasoning are not always sound. They still need guidance, discipline, and emotional and financial support from parents. The child and parents often disagree about behavior and activity restrictions and limits. Teenagers prefer being with peers rather than doing things with their families. They tend to confide in and seek advice from adults other than their parents.

Interests and activities also reflect the need to develop intimate relationships and to act like males or females. Adolescents may begin to feel or show a sexual orientation (Chapter 48). *Sexual orientation is sexual arousal or romantic attraction to persons of the other gender (heterosexual), the same gender (homosexual), or both genders (bisexual).*

Both sexes like parties, dances, and other social events. Appearance is important (clothing, hairstyles). Teenagers experiment with make-up and hairstyles. They spend time talking to friends on the phone, listening to music, and reading teen magazines.

The age for dating varies. At first, dating involves school events, such as a dance or football game. Group dating is common. The same group of girls just happens to be with the same group of boys. Pairing off as a couple replaces group dating. Couples may be sexual partners.

Many hard choices and conflicts result as teens mature physically, mentally, emotionally, and socially. Parents and teens often disagree about dating. Parents worry about sexual activities, pregnancy, and sexually transmitted diseases. Teens usually do not understand or appreciate these concerns. Dating helps meet security, love and belonging, and self-esteem needs. Teens may have problems controlling sexual urges and considering the results of sexual activity.

Adolescents begin to think about careers and what to do after high school. Interests, skills, talents, and money are some factors that influence the choice of college or getting a job.

Teens also need to develop morals, values, and attitudes for living in society. They need to develop a sense about good and bad, right and wrong, and the important and unimportant. Parents, peers, culture, religion, the media, and school are some influencing factors. Substance abuse, unwanted pregnancy, criminal acts, and suicide are risks for troubled teens.

YOUNG ADULTHOOD (18 TO 40 YEARS)

Mental and social development continue during young adulthood. There is little physical growth. Adult height has been reached. Body systems are fully developed. Developmental tasks include:

- Choosing education and a career
- Selecting a partner
- Learning to live with a partner
- Becoming a parent and raising children
- Developing a satisfactory sex life

Education and career are closely related. Most jobs require certain knowledge and skills. The education needed depends on career choice. Education usually increases job choices. Employment is needed for economic independence and to support a family.

Most adults marry at least once. Others choose to remain single. They may live alone or with friends of the

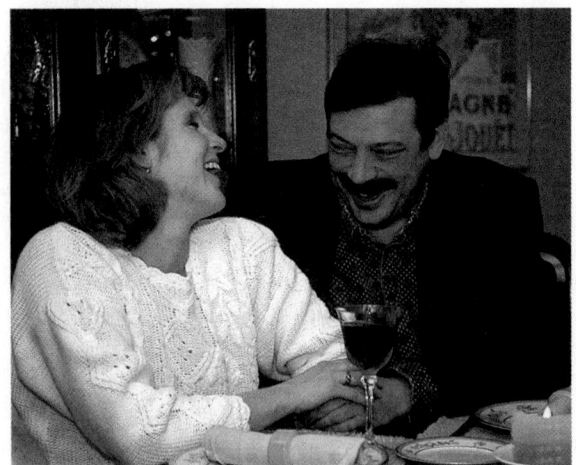
Fig. 10-21 Communication is needed for a successful partnership.

same or other gender. Gay and lesbian persons may commit to a partner.

People marry for many reasons. They include love, emotional security, wanting a family, and sex. Some want to leave an unhappy home life. Some marry for social status, money, and companionship. Some marry to feel wanted, needed, and desirable.

Many factors affect partner selection. They include age, religion, interests, education, race, personality, and love. Some marriages or partnerships are happy and successful. Others are not. That a relationship will work is not certain. Therefore partners must work together to build a relationship based on trust, respect, caring, and friendship.

Partners must learn to live together. Habits, routines, meals, and pastimes are changed or adjusted to "fit" the other person's needs. They must learn to solve problems and make decisions together. They need to work toward the same goals. Open and honest communication is needed for a successful partnership (Fig. 10-21).

Adults need to develop a satisfactory sex life. Sexual frequency, desires, practices, and preferences vary. For a satisfying and intimate relationship, a partner must understand and accept the other's needs.

With modern birth control methods, couples can plan when to have children and how many to have. Some pregnancies are not planned. Some couples decide not to have children. The man or woman may have physical problems that interfere with or prevent pregnancy.

Most couples have a child early in their marriage. Some wait several years to start a family. Parents must agree on child-rearing practices and discipline methods. They need to adjust to the child and to the child's needs for parental time, energy, and attention.

MIDDLE ADULTHOOD (40 TO 65 YEARS)

This stage is more stable and comfortable. Children are usually grown and have moved away. Partners have time

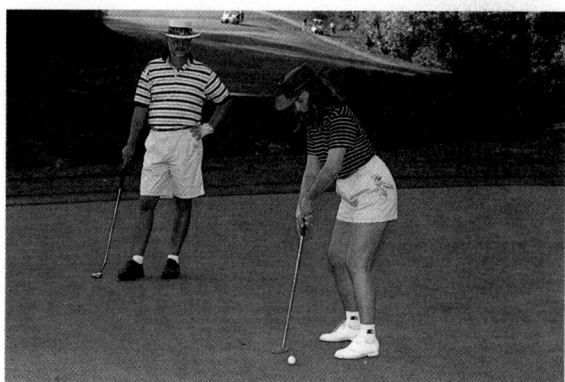

Fig. 10-22 Middle-age adults usually have more time for leisure activities.

together. Worries about children and money are fewer. Developmental tasks relate to:

- Adjusting to physical changes
- Having grown children
- Developing leisure-time activities
- Adjusting to aging parents

Several physical changes occur. Many are gradual and are not noticed. Others are seen early. Energy and endurance begin to slow down. So do metabolism and physical activities. Therefore weight control becomes a problem. Facial wrinkles and gray hair appear. Needing eyeglasses is common. Hearing loss may begin. *Menstruation stops, and menstrual cycles end (menopause).* It occurs between the ages of 45 and 55 years. Ovaries stop secreting hormones. The woman cannot have children.

Many diseases and illnesses can develop. The disorders become chronic and threaten life.

Children leave home for college, marry, move to their own homes, and start families. Adults have to cope with letting children go and being in-laws and grandparents. Parents must let children lead their own lives. However, they provide emotional support when needed.

Spare time increases as the demands of parenthood decrease. Hobbies and pastimes bring pleasure. They include gardening, fishing, painting, golfing, volunteer work, and being part of clubs and organizations (Fig. 10-22). These activities are even more important after retirement and during late adulthood.

Some middle-age adults have parents who are aging and in poor health. Responsibility for aging parents may begin during this stage. Many middle-age adults deal with the death of parents.

LATE ADULTHOOD (65 YEARS AND OLDER)

Chapter 11 describes the many changes that occur in older persons. Developmental tasks are:

- Adjusting to decreased strength and loss of health
- Adjusting to retirement and reduced income
- Coping with a partner's death
- Developing new friends and relationships
- Preparing for one's own death

FOCUS ON P R I D E

The Person, Family, and Yourself

Personal and Professional Responsibility

Growth and development affect the care you give. Care measures and procedures change. Safety concerns differ. The person's level of trust and fears vary. These affect your interactions. For example, you are caring for a 1-year-old. You need to use your stethoscope to check an apical pulse (Chapter 26). You know a developmental task for this age is learning to trust. The child may be afraid of you and your stethoscope. To gain the child's trust:

- Ask the parent to hold the child.
- Show the child the procedure on the parent.
- Let the child play with the stethoscope.
- Talk in a kind, playful voice.

You are responsible for knowing how growth and development affect the care you give. Throughout this book, read the *Focus on Children and Older Persons* boxes. They explain how to adjust your care for persons in different stages of growth and development.

Rights and Respect

Some family situations may bother you. For example, two men raise a child. Or an adolescent does so. Or a child's family is not around much. Show respect to all persons. Do not gossip about them. Be kind. Treat them as you treat others. Take pride in not allowing your personal opinions to affect the care you give.

Independence and Social Interaction

Nursing assistants often work in areas with certain patient or resident groups. You may care for children, the elderly, or persons with developmental delays. You may see the same patients or residents daily. It is easy to develop close relationships with them.

Social and professional relationships differ. Avoid crossing professional boundaries (Chapter 4). For example, sharing too much personal information is not professional. Bringing the person gifts or food from home crosses boundaries. And taking pictures of yourself with a patient or resident violates the right to privacy and confidentiality. Plus the person must give written consent for photography. Take pride in protecting the person and yourself by maintaining professional boundaries.

Delegation and Teamwork

When caring for children, the primary caregiver is an important part of the health care team. The nurse teaches the caregiver how to be involved in the care. For example, an infant is bottle-fed. The mother is taught her role in measuring intake and output (Chapter 24). The nurse instructs her to save the bottles and report intake to the nursing staff. She is also taught to save the diapers to be weighed for output.

When interacting with caregivers:

- Be polite. Treat them with kindness and respect.
- Thank them for helping with their child's care.
- Praise actions that are done well.
- Remind them of care measures taught by the nurse.
- Tell the nurse about any questions or concerns.
- Inform the nurse if you notice that they need more teaching.

Continued

FOCUS ON P R I D E—cont'd

Ethics and Laws

Development affects a person's ability to make health care decisions. A child does not have the reasoning and judgment to make decisions. As one develops, he or she gains independence and the ability to function in society.

State laws determine the age of adulthood for making legal and health care decisions. This age varies, but age 18 is common. *Minors* are under the age to legally make decisions. A parent or legal guardian makes decisions for a minor. An *emancipated minor* is under the legal age but is able to make his or her own decisions. This can occur by marriage, by joining the armed forces, or by a court ruling. In some states, pregnancy and having children are other ways. Agencies often have individuals or groups responsible for handling questions of emancipation. Risk management nurses and ethics committees are examples.

REVIEW QUESTIONS

Circle the BEST answer.

1   Changes in mental, emotional, and social function are called
   a   Growth
   b   Development
   c   A reflex
   d   A stage

2   These statements are about growth and development. Which is *false?*
   a   They occur from the simple to the complex.
   b   They occur in an orderly pattern.
   c   They occur at a set pace.
   d   Each stage has its own characteristics.

3   Which reflexes does the infant need for feeding?
   a   The Moro and startle reflexes
   b   The rooting and sucking reflexes
   c   The grasping and Moro reflexes
   d   The rooting and grasping reflexes

4   Which occurs first in infants?
   a   Holding the head up
   b   Rolling from front to back
   c   Rolling from back to front
   d   The pincer grasp

5   An infant can stand alone at about
   a   9 months   c   11 months
   b   10 months   d   12 months

6   Infants point and use gestures to communicate at around
   a   5 months   c   9 months
   b   7 months   d   11 months

7   Toilet training begins
   a   During infancy
   b   During the toddler years
   c   When the primary caregiver is ready
   d   At the age of 3 years

8   The toddler can
   a   Use a spoon and cup
   b   Ride a bike
   c   Help set the table
   d   Name parts of the body

9   Playing with other children begins during
   a   Infancy
   b   The toddler years
   c   The preschool years
   d   Middle childhood

10   Losing baby teeth usually begins at the age of
   a   4 years
   b   5 years
   c   6 years
   d   7 years

11   Peer groups become important to
   a   Toddlers
   b   Preschool children
   c   School-age children
   d   Adolescents

12   Reproductive organs being to function. Secondary sex characteristics appear. This is called
   a   Late childhood
   b   Adolescence
   c   Puberty
   d   Adulthood

13   Which is *false?*
   a   Boys reach puberty earlier than girls.
   b   Girls reach puberty between the ages of 9 and 16 years.
   c   Menarche marks the onset of puberty in girls.
   d   A growth spurt occurs during adolescence.

14   Dating usually begins
   a   During late childhood
   b   With group dating
   c   With "pairing off"
   d   During late adolescence

15   Adolescence is a time when parents and children
   a   Talk openly about sex
   b   Express love and affection
   c   Disagree
   d   Do things as a family

16   Which is *not* a development task of young adulthood?
   a   Adjusting to changes in the body and appearance
   b   Selecting a partner
   c   Choosing a career
   d   Becoming a parent

17   Middle adulthood is from about
   a   25 to 35 years
   b   30 to 40 years
   c   40 to 60 years
   d   40 to 65 years

18   Middle adulthood is a time when
   a   Families are started
   b   Physical energy and free time increase
   c   Children are grown and leave home
   d   People need to prepare for death

Answers to these questions are on p. 832.

Care of the Older Person

OBJECTIVES

- Define the key terms and key abbreviations listed in this chapter.
- Identify the psychological and social changes common in older adulthood.
- Describe the physical changes from aging and the care required.
- Describe housing options for older persons.
- Explain how to promote PRIDE in the person, the family, and yourself.

KEY TERMS

atrophy Shrink
geriatrics The care of aging people

gerontology The study of the aging process

KEY ABBREVIATIONS

CCRC Continuing care retirement community
CMS Centers for Medicare & Medicaid Services

OBRA Omnibus Budget Reconciliation Act of 1987

People live longer than ever before. They are healthier and more active. Late adulthood ranges from 65 years of age and older. The oldest-old are 85 years of age and older. U.S. Government 2010 Census reports show the following:

- There were nearly 40,300,000 people age 65 and older.
- There were about 17,300,000 men age 65 and older. There were about 22,900,000 women age 65 and older.
- There were more older men who were married than older women.
- There were about 5,500,000 people age 85 and older. The number of older people over age 65 is expected to increase to 54,800,000 in 2020.

Chronic illness is common in older persons. Disability often results. Many older persons have at least one disability. Disabilities increase and become more severe with aging. They can interfere with:

- Self-care—bathing, dressing, eating, elimination
- Mobility and getting around one's home setting
- Fixing meals
- Shopping
- Managing money
- Using a phone
- Doing housework
- Taking drugs
- Leisure and recreational activities

Still, most older people live in a family setting. They live with a partner, children, brothers or sisters, or other family. Some live alone or with friends. Still others live in assisted living residences or nursing centers. The need for nursing center care increases with aging.

Gerontology is the study of the aging process. Geriatrics is the care of aging people. Aging is normal. It is not a disease. Normal changes occur in body structure and function. They increase the risk for illness, injury, and disability. Psychological and social changes also occur. Often changes are slow. Most people adjust well to these changes. They lead happy, meaningful lives.

There are many myths about aging and older persons. A *myth* is a widely believed story that is not true. To provide good care, you need to know the facts about older persons and aging. See Box 11-1, p. 136 for some common myths and facts.

BOX 11-1	MYTHS AND FACTS ABOUT AGING
Myth	**Fact**
All old people are the same.	Each person is unique. People age in different ways. Culture, religion, education, income, and life experiences affect aging. People develop throughout life.
Aging means illness and disability.	Older persons are at risk for health problems and disabilities. However, most are healthy. Not smoking, good nutrition, and exercise can reverse or slow many changes blamed on aging.
Older persons lose interest in sex.	Aging does not mean that sexual activity and expression must end. Many older people enjoy a fulfilling sex life. Sexuality is important throughout life. Intimacy, love, and companionship are needed.
Older people are lonely and isolated.	Most older people have frequent contact with their children. Most see a child at least once a week and take part in family activities. Regular contact with sisters and brothers is common. They can provide support and companionship. Many older persons have jobs, do volunteer work, and enjoy hobbies.
Mental function declines with age.	Older persons may receive and process information more slowly than younger people. However, people learn until very late in life. Many 90-year-olds have high levels of mental function.
Most older persons live in nursing centers.	In 2010 only about 1,600,000 (4.1%) of the people 65 years and older lived in nursing centers or other care settings.
Old people are crabby and rude.	Some old people are crabby and rude. So are people of all ages. Older persons who are crabby and rude were probably crabby and rude when younger.

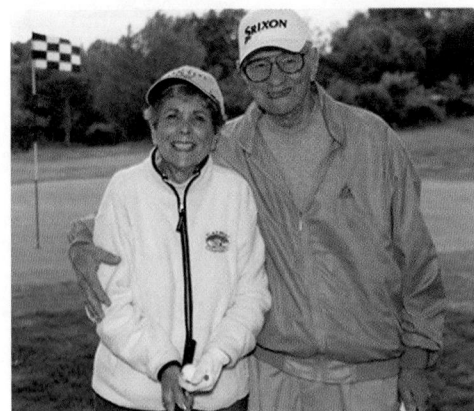

Fig. 11-1 A retired couple enjoys golf as a leisure time activity.

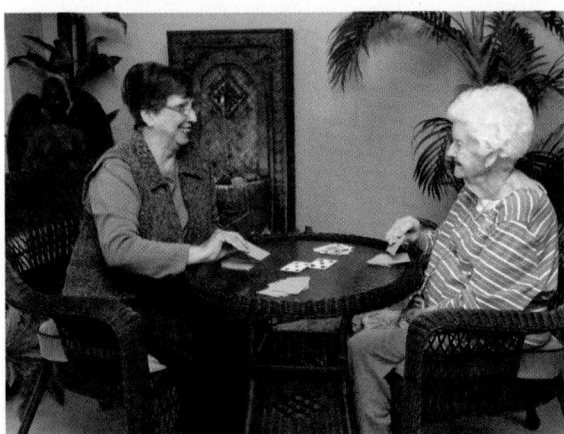

Fig. 11-2 This retired woman is a nursing center volunteer.

PSYCHOLOGICAL AND SOCIAL CHANGES

Graying hair, wrinkles, and slow movements are physical reminders of growing old. These changes threaten self-esteem, self-image, and feelings of self-worth. They also threaten independence.

Social roles also change. A parent may rely on an adult child for care. Retirees need activities to replace the work role. Adjusting to the death of a partner, family members, and friends is common. The person faces his or her own death.

People cope with aging in their own way. How they cope depends on:

- Health status
- Life experiences
- Finances
- Education
- Social support systems

Retirement

Age 65 is the usual retirement age. Some retire earlier. Others work into their 70s. Retirement is a reward for a life-time of work. The person can relax and enjoy life (Fig. 11-1). Travel, leisure, and doing what one wants to are retirement "benefits." Many people enjoy retirement. Others are not so lucky. They are ill or disabled. Poor health and medical bills can make retirement very hard.

Work helps meet love, belonging, and self-esteem needs. The person feels fulfilled and useful. Friendships form. Co-workers share daily events. Leisure time, recreation, and companionship often involve co-workers. Some retired people want to work. They have part-time jobs or do volunteer work (Fig. 11-2).

Reduced Income. Retirement often means reduced income. Social Security may provide the only income.

The retired person still has expenses. Rent or house payments continue. Food, clothing, utility bills, and taxes are other expenses. Car expenses, home repairs, drugs, and health care are other costs. So are entertainment and gifts.

Reduced income may force life-style changes. Examples include:

- Limiting social and leisure events
- Buying cheaper food, clothes, and household items
- Moving to cheaper housing
- Living with children or other family
- Avoiding health care or needed drugs
- Relying on children or other family for money or needed items

Severe money problems can result. Some people plan for retirement with savings, investments, retirement plans, and insurance. They are financially comfortable during retirement.

Social Relationships

Social relationships change throughout life. (See *Caring About Culture: Foreign-Born Persons*.) Children grow up, leave home, and have their own families. Some live far away from parents. Older family members and friends die, move away, or are disabled. Yet most older people have regular contact with children, grandchildren, family, and friends. Others are lonely. Separation from children is a common cause. So is lack of companionship with people their own age (Fig. 11-3).

Many older people adjust to these changes. Hobbies, religious and community events, and new friends help prevent loneliness. Some community groups sponsor bus trips to ball games, shopping, plays, and concerts.

Grandchildren can bring great love and joy (Fig. 11-4). Family times help prevent loneliness. They help the older person feel useful and wanted (Fig. 11-5).

See *Focus on Communication: Social Relationships*.

FOCUS ON COMMUNICATION

Social Relationships

The social changes of aging can cause loneliness. With nursing center care, the loneliness can seem even greater. The person is in a building with other people. However, those people do not replace family and friends. To help the person feel less lonely, you can:

- Suggest that the person call a family member or friend. Offer to help with phone numbers and dialing.
- Keep the phone within the person's reach. He or she can place or answer calls with greater ease.
- Suggest that the person read cards and letters. Offer to assist.
- Visit with the person a few times during your shift.
- Introduce new residents to other residents and staff.

CARING ABOUT CULTURE

Foreign-Born Persons

Some older persons speak and understand a foreign language. Communication occurs with family and friends who speak the same language. They also share cultural values and practices. Family and friends may move away or die. The person may not have anyone to talk to. He or she may not be understood by others. The person feels greater loneliness and isolation.

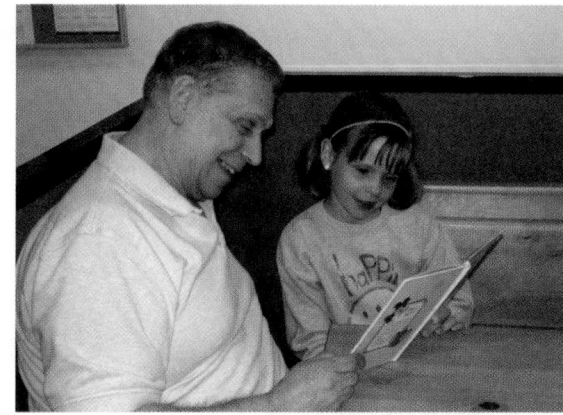

Fig. 11-4 An older man reads to his grandchild.

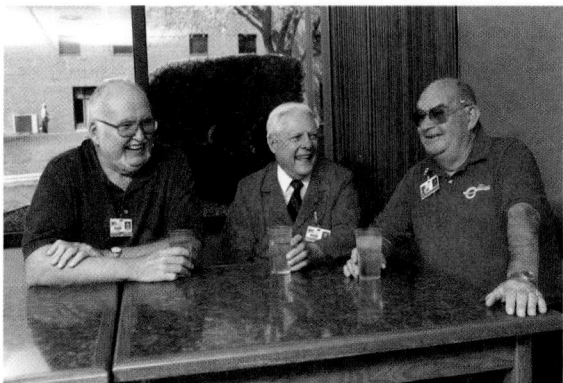

Fig. 11-3 Older people enjoy being with others of their own age.

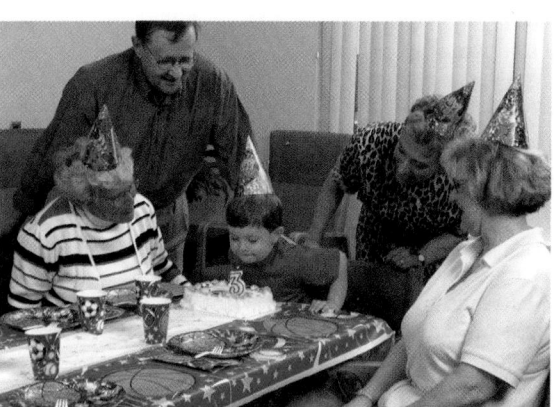

Fig. 11-5 An older couple takes part in family activities.

Children as Caregivers

Some children care for older parents. Parents and children change roles. The child cares for the parent. Some older persons feel more secure. Others feel unwanted, in the way, and useless. Some lose dignity and self-respect. Tensions may occur among the child, parent, and other household members. Lack of privacy is a cause. So are disagreements and criticisms about housekeeping, raising children, cooking, and friends.

Death of a Partner

As couples age, chances increase that a partner will die. Women usually live longer than men. Therefore many women become widows.

A person may try to prepare for a partner's death. When death occurs, the loss is crushing. No amount of preparation is ever enough for the emptiness and changes that result. The person loses a lover, friend, companion, and confidant. Grief may be very great. The person's life will likely change. Serious physical and mental health problems may result. Some lose the will to live. Some attempt suicide.

PHYSICAL CHANGES

Physical changes occur with aging (Box 11-2). They happen to everyone. Body processes slow down. Energy level and body efficiency decline. The rate and degree of change vary with each person. They depend on diet, health, exercise, stress, environment, heredity, and other factors. Changes are slow over many years. Often they are not seen for a long time.

Normal aging does not mean loss of health. Quality of life does not have to decline. The person can adjust to many of the changes.

The Integumentary System

The skin loses its elasticity, strength, and fatty tissue layer. The skin thins and sags. Wrinkles appear. Secretions from oil and sweat glands decrease. Dry skin and itching occur. The skin is fragile and easily injured. The skin's blood vessels are fragile, increasing the risk for:

- Skin breakdown
- Skin tears (Chapter 33)
- Pressure ulcers (Chapter 34)
- Bruising
- Delayed healing

Brown spots appear on sun-exposed areas. They are called "age spots" or "liver spots." They are common on the wrists and hands.

Loss of the skin's fatty tissue layer affects body temperature. The person is more sensitive to cold. Protect the person from drafts and cold. Sweaters, lap blankets, socks, and extra blankets are helpful. So are higher thermostat settings.

Dry skin causes itching. It is easily damaged. A shower or bath twice a week is enough for hygiene. Partial baths are taken at other times. Mild soaps or soap substitutes are used to clean the underarms, genitals, and under the breasts. Often soap is not used on the arms, legs, back, chest, and abdomen. Lotions and creams prevent drying and itching. Deodorants may not be needed because sweat gland secretion is decreased. See Chapter 20 for hygiene.

BOX 11-2	COMMON PHYSICAL CHANGES DURING THE AGING PROCESS

Integumentary System
- Skin becomes less elastic
- Skin loses strength
- Brown spots ("age spots" or "liver spots") on the wrists and hands
- Fewer nerve endings
- Fewer blood vessels
- Fatty tissue layer is lost
- Skin thins and sags
- Skin is fragile and easily injured
- Folds, lines, and wrinkles appear
- Blood vessels in the dermis become more fragile
- Decreased secretion of oil and sweat glands
- Dry skin
- Itching
- Increased sensitivity to heat and cold
- Decreased sensitivity to pain
- Nails become thick and tough
- Whitening or graying hair
- Facial hair in some women
- Loss or thinning of hair
- Drier hair

Musculo-Skeletal System
- Muscles atrophy
- Strength, tone, and contractility decrease
- Bone mass decreases
- Bones become weaker
- Bones become brittle; can break easily
- Vertebrae shorten
- Joints become stiff and painful
- Hip and knee joints become flexed
- Gradual loss of height; trunk becomes shorter
- Decreased mobility

Nervous System
- Brain and spinal cord lose nerve cells
- Nerve cells send messages at a slower rate
- Reflexes slow
- Reduced blood flow to the brain
- Abnormal structures can form in the brain
- Brain tissue may atrophy
- Changes in brain cells
- Shorter memory
- Forgetfulness

| **BOX 11-2** | **COMMON PHYSICAL CHANGES DURING THE AGING PROCESS—cont'd** |

Nervous System—cont'd
- Slower ability to respond
- Confusion
- Dizziness
- Sleep patterns change (harder/less)
- Reduced sensitivity to touch
- Reduced sensitivity to pain
- Smell and taste decrease
- Eyelids thin and wrinkle
- Less tear secretion
- Pupils less responsive to light
- Decreased vision at night or in dark rooms
- Problems seeing green and blue colors
- Poor vision
- Changes in acoustic nerve
- Eardrums atrophy
- High-pitched sounds are not heard
- Decreased earwax secretion
- Hearing loss

Circulatory System
- Heart pumps with less force
- Heart valves thicken and become stiff
- Heart rate may slow
- Abnormal heart rhythms may occur
- Heart may enlarge slightly
- Heart walls thicken
- Arteries narrow and become stiffer
- Less blood flows through narrowed arteries
- Weakened heart works harder to pump blood through narrowed vessels
- Number of red blood cells decreases

Respiratory System
- Respiratory muscles weaken
- Some lung tissue is lost
- Lung tissue becomes less elastic
- Chest is less able to stretch to breathe
- Difficulty breathing (dyspnea)
- Decreased strength for coughing and clearing the airway

Digestive System
- Decreased saliva production
- Difficulty swallowing (dysphagia)
- Decreased appetite
- Decreased secretion of digestive juices
- Difficulty digesting fried and fatty foods
- Indigestion
- Loss of teeth
- Decreased peristalsis causing flatulence and constipation

Urinary System
- Kidney function decreases
- Reduced blood supply to kidneys
- Kidneys atrophy
- Bladder tissue less able to stretch
- Bladder muscles weaken
- Bladder may not empty completely when urinating
- Urinary frequency
- Urinary urgency may occur
- Urinary incontinence may occur
- Night-time urination may occur

Reproductive System
- Men
  - Testosterone decreases slightly
  - Erections take longer
  - Longer phase between erection and orgasm
  - Less forceful orgasms
  - Erections lost quickly
  - Longer time between erections
- Women
  - Menopause
  - Estrogen and progesterone decrease
  - Uterus, vagina, and genitalia atrophy
  - Thinning of vaginal walls
  - Vaginal dryness
  - Arousal takes longer
  - Less intense orgasms
  - Quicker return to pre-excitement state

Nails become thick and tough. Feet usually have poor circulation. A nick or cut can lead to a serious infection. See Chapter 21 for nail and foot care.

The skin has fewer nerve endings. This affects sensing heat, cold, pressure, and pain. Burns are great risks. Fragile skin, poor circulation, and decreased sensing of heat and cold increase the risk of burns. Older persons often complain of cold feet. Socks provide warmth. Do not use hot water bottles and heating pads because of the risk for burns.

White or gray hair is common. Hair loss occurs in men. Hair thins on men and women. Thinning occurs on the head, in the pubic area, and under the arms. Women and men may choose to wear wigs. Some color hair to cover graying. Facial hair (lip and chin) may occur in women.

Hair is drier from decreases in scalp oils. Brushing promotes circulation and oil production. Shampoo frequency depends on personal choice. Usually it decreases with age. It is done as needed for hygiene and comfort.

Skin disorders increase with age. They rarely cause death if treated early. The risk of skin cancers increases with age. Prolonged sun exposure is a cause.

Skin changes can be seen. Gray hair, hair loss, brown spots, wrinkles, and sagging skin are some examples. These changes can affect self-esteem and body image.

The Musculo-Skeletal System
Muscle cells decrease in number. Muscles *atrophy (shrink)*. They decrease in strength.

Bones lose minerals, especially calcium. Bones lose strength. They become brittle and break easily. Sometimes just turning in bed can cause fractures (broken bones).

Vertebrae shorten. Joints become stiff and painful. Hip and knee joints flex (bend) slightly. These changes cause gradual loss of height and strength. Mobility also decreases.

Older persons need to stay active. Activity, exercise, and diet help prevent bone loss and loss of muscle strength. Walking is good exercise. Exercise groups and range-of-motion exercises are helpful (Chapter 27). A diet high in protein, calcium, and vitamins is needed.

Bones can break easily. Protect the person from injury and falls (Chapters 12 and 13). Turn and move the person gently and carefully (Chapter 17). Some persons need help and support getting out of bed. Some need help walking.

The Nervous System

Nerve cells are lost. Nerve conduction and reflexes slow. Responses are slower. For example, an older person slips. The message telling the brain of the slip travels slowly. The message from the brain to prevent the fall also travels slowly. The person falls.

Blood flow to the brain is reduced. Dizziness may occur. It increases the risk for falls. Practice measures to prevent falls (Chapter 13). Remind the person to get up slowly from bed or chair. This helps prevent dizziness (Chapter 27).

Changes occur in brain cells. This affects personality and mental function. So does reduced blood flow to the brain. Memory is shorter. Forgetfulness increases. Responses slow. Confusion, dizziness, and fatigue may occur. Older persons often remember events from long ago better than recent ones. Many older people are mentally active and involved in current events. They show fewer personality and mental changes. (See Chapter 46 for confusion and dementia.)

Sleep patterns change. Falling asleep is harder for older persons. Sleep periods are shorter. They wake often at night and have less deep sleep. Less sleep is needed. Loss of energy and decreased blood flow may cause fatigue. They may rest or nap during the day. They may go to bed early and get up early.

The Senses. Aging affects touch, smell, taste, sight, and hearing.

Touch. Touch and sensitivity to pain and pressure are reduced. So is sensing heat and cold. These changes increase the risk for injury. The person may not notice painful injuries or diseases. Or the person feels minor pain. You need to:
- Protect older persons from injury (Chapters 12 and 13).
- Follow safety measures for heat and cold (Chapter 35).
- Check for signs of skin breakdown (Chapters 20, 33, and 34).
- Give good skin care (Chapter 20).
- Prevent skin tears (Chapter 33) and pressure ulcers (Chapter 34).

Taste and smell. Taste and smell dull. Appetite decreases. Taste buds decrease in number. The tongue senses sweet, salty, bitter, and sour tastes. Sweet and salty tastes are lost first. Older people often complain that food has no taste or tastes bitter. They like more salt and sugar on food.

The eye. Eyelids thin and wrinkle. Tear secretion is less. Dust and pollutants can irritate the eyes.

The pupil becomes smaller and responds less to light. Vision is poor at night or in dark rooms. The eye takes longer to adjust to lighting changes, causing vision problems when:
- Going from a dark to a bright room
- Going from a bright to a dark room

Clear vision is reduced. Eyeglasses are often needed. The lens of the eye yellows, making greens and blues harder to see.

Older persons become more farsighted. This is called *presbyopia.* (*Presby* relates to *aging. Opia* means *eye.*) The lens becomes more rigid with age. It is harder for the eye to shift from far to near vision and from near to far vision. These changes increase the risk of falls and accidents. The risk is greater on stairs and where lighting is poor. Eyeglasses are worn as needed. Keep rooms well-lit. Nightlights help at night.

The ear. Changes occur in the acoustic nerve. Eardrums atrophy. High-pitched sounds are hard to hear. Severe hearing loss occurs if these changes progress. A hearing aid may be needed. It must be clean and correctly placed in the ear.

Wax secretion decreases. Wax becomes harder and thicker. It is easily impacted (wedged in the ear). This can cause hearing loss. A doctor or nurse removes the wax.

The Circulatory System

The heart muscle weakens. It pumps blood with less force. Problems may not occur at rest. Activity, exercise, excitement, and illness increase the body's need for oxygen and nutrients. A damaged or weak heart cannot meet these needs.

Arteries narrow and are less elastic. Less blood flows through them. Poor circulation occurs in many body parts. A weak heart works harder to pump blood through narrowed vessels.

Exercise helps maintain health and well-being. Many older persons exercise daily. They walk, jog, golf, and bicycle. They also hike, ski, play tennis, swim, and play other sports. Older persons need to be as active as possible.

Sometimes circulatory changes are severe. Rest is needed during the day. Over-exertion is avoided. The person should not walk far, climb many stairs, or carry heavy things. Personal care items, TV, phone, and other needed items are kept nearby. Some exercise helps circulation. It also prevents blood clots in leg veins. Some persons need to stay in bed. They need range-of-motion exercises (Chapter 27). Doctors may order certain exercises and activity limits.

The Respiratory System

Respiratory muscles weaken. Lung tissue becomes less elastic. Often lung changes are not noted at rest. Difficult, labored, or painful breathing *(dyspnea)* may occur with activity. *(Dys* means *difficult. Pnea* means *breathing.)* The person may lack strength to cough and clear the airway of secretions. Respiratory infections and diseases may develop. These can threaten life.

Normal breathing is promoted. Avoid heavy bed linens over the chest. They prevent normal chest expansion. Turning, re-positioning, and deep breathing are important. They help prevent respiratory complications from bedrest. Breathing usually is easier in semi-Fowler's position (Chapter 18). The person should be as active as possible.

The Digestive System

Salivary glands produce less saliva. This can cause difficulty swallowing *(dysphagia). (Dys* means *difficult. Phagia* means *swallowing.)* Dry foods may be hard to swallow. Taste and smell dull. This decreases appetite.

Secretion of digestive juices decreases. This makes fried and fatty foods hard to digest. They may cause indigestion.

Loss of teeth and ill-fitting dentures cause chewing problems. This causes digestion problems. Hard-to-chew foods are avoided. Ground or chopped meat is easier to chew and swallow.

Dry, fried, and fatty foods are avoided. This helps swallowing and digestion problems. Oral hygiene and denture care improve taste. Some people do not have teeth or dentures. Their food is pureed or ground.

Peristalsis decreases. The stomach and colon empty slower. Flatulence and constipation can occur (Chapter 23). High-fiber foods help prevent constipation. However, they are hard to chew and can irritate the intestines. They include apricots, celery, and fruits and vegetables with skins and seeds. Persons with chewing problems or constipation often need foods that provide soft bulk. They include whole-grain cereals and cooked fruits and vegetables.

Fewer calories are needed. Energy and activity levels decline. More fluids are needed for chewing, swallowing, digestion, and kidney function. Foods are needed to prevent constipation and bone changes. High-protein foods are needed for tissue growth and repair. However, some older persons lack protein in their diets. High-protein foods (meat and fish) are costly.

The Urinary System

Kidney function decreases. The kidneys shrink. Blood flow to the kidneys is reduced. Waste removal is less efficient.

The ureters, bladder, and urethra lose tone and elasticity. Bladder muscles weaken. Bladder size decreases, storing less urine. Urinary frequency or urgency may occur. Many older persons have to urinate (void) during the night. Urinary incontinence (the loss of bladder control) may occur (Chapter 22).

In men, the prostate gland enlarges. This puts pressure on the urethra. Difficulty voiding or frequent urination occurs.

Urinary tract infections are risks. Adequate fluids are needed. The person needs water, juices, milk, and gelatin. Provide fluids according to the care plan. Remind the person to drink. Offer fluids often to those who need help. Most fluids should be taken before 1700 (5:00 PM). This reduces the need to void during the night.

Persons with incontinence may need bladder training programs. Sometimes catheters are needed (Chapter 22).

The Reproductive System

Reproductive organs change with aging. For the effects of aging on sexuality, see Chapter 48.

- *Men.* The hormone *testosterone* decreases slightly. It affects strength, sperm production, and reproductive tissues. These changes affect sexual activity. An erection takes longer. The phase between erection and orgasm also is longer. Orgasm is less forceful than when younger. Erections are lost quickly. The time between erections also is longer. Older men may need the penis stimulated for arousal. Fatigue, over-eating, and drinking too much alcohol affect erections. Some men fear performance problems. They may avoid closeness.
- *Women. Menopause* is when menstruation stops and there has been at least 1 year without a menstrual period. The woman can no longer have children. This occurs between 45 and 55 years of age. Female hormones *(estrogen* and *progesterone)* decrease. The uterus, vagina, and genitalia atrophy. Vaginal walls thin. There is vaginal dryness. These make intercourse uncomfortable or painful. Arousal takes longer. Orgasm is less intense. The pre-excitement state returns more quickly.

HOUSING OPTIONS

A person's home is more than a place to live. A home has family memories. It is a link to neighbors and the community. It brings pride and self-esteem. Aging can lead to changes in a person's home setting.

Most older people live in their own homes. Many function without help. Others need help from family, home care, or community-based services for activities of daily living (Box 11-3, p. 142). Bathing, dressing, meals, housekeeping, shopping, and transportation are examples. Many services also provide social contact.

Some older persons choose smaller homes when children are gone. Some retire to warmer climates or move closer to children and family. Still others must give up their homes. Reduced income, taxes, home repairs, and yard work are factors. Some people cannot care for themselves.

Many housing options meet the needs of older people. A new home setting could maintain or improve the person's quality of life.

See *Focus on Long-Term Care and Home Care: Housing Options,* p. 142.

BOX 11-3   IN-HOME AND COMMUNITY-BASED SERVICES

- *Adult day-care services.* Provide social and some rehabilitation activities in supervised group settings for those who cannot be alone during the day.
- *Case management.* A case manager assesses the needs of the older person and family. Needed services are arranged.
- *Meal programs.* Meals are provided in-home or in a senior center. Home delivery programs are often called *Meals-on-Wheels.*
- *Financial counseling.* Help is given with checking accounts, paying bills, income taxes, and insurance forms and claims.
- *Companionship services.* A volunteer visits the older person at home. Supervision and support services are provided as needed.
- *Home health care.* Nursing and physical, occupational, and speech therapies are provided. The person may need help with such things as taking drugs, changing dressings, or catheter care.
- *Homemaker services.* Help is given with household tasks. Cleaning, laundry, shopping, and preparing meals are examples. Some people need help with personal care.
- *Respite care.* This service relieves caregivers of daily care for a short time.
- *Hospice care.* See Chapters 1 and 52. Nursing, comfort, and homemaker services are provided.
- *Personal care.* Help is given with eating, bathing, oral care, grooming, and dressing.

- *Rehabilitation.* Therapies are given to assist the person to regain or maintain his or her highest level of functioning.
- *Senior centers.* These centers offer many social and recreational activities. Classes, day trips, travel groups, performing arts, and nature activities are examples. Services also include meals, counseling, legal help, health screenings, and transportation.
- *Telephone reassurance.* Regular phone contact is provided. The person is called at various times. If the person does not answer, someone is sent to the person's home. Also, the older person can call the service when help is needed.
- *Medical alert services.* The person wears a necklace or bracelet with a button to push if help is needed. The person pushes the button in case of a fall or an emergency. He or she is connected to an operator who will send help.
- *Transportation.* Older persons are given rides to and from doctor visits, appointments, shopping, religious services, and other places.
- *Wellness programs.* Blood pressure, blood sugar, and other tests are done to promote health. Sessions are held about fitness, nutrition, and other health topics.
- *Home repair and improvement.* Such services often include roofing, building ramps, and installing insulation.

FOCUS ON LONG-TERM CARE AND HOME CARE
Housing Options

Home Care
Simple changes can make a home safe and easy to use. The nurse discusses needed changes with the patient and family.

The Bathroom
- Non-slick flooring
- Grab bars by showers, tubs, and toilets
- Non-skid surfaces in showers and tubs (bath mat, non-skid bath decals)
- Rugs with non-slip backing outside the tub and shower and in front of the toilet
- Hand-held shower nozzle or adjustable shower head
- Shower chair for shower or bathtub
- Transfer bench
- Lever-handle faucets
- Water controls close to the shower or tub entrance
- Anti-scald devices on faucets and showerheads
- Towel bars or hooks raised or lowered for the person's reach
- Raised toilet seat or a toilet seat riser
- Chair placed in front of the sink so the person can sit
- Knee space under the sink for the person who sits
- Bright, non-glare lighting

The Bedroom
- Closet rods that adjust for height
- Lower shelves or pull-down shelves
- Pull-out drawers, bins, and baskets in closets
- A commode chair near the bed for night-time use (Chapter 22)

The Kitchen
- Appliances within reach—side-by-side refrigerator/freezer, cook-top range, wall-mounted oven, dishwasher raised off the floor
- Stove controls on the front of the stove
- Stove controls easily marked and easy to see
- Lowered shelves or pull-down shelves
- Pull-out drawers, bins, and baskets
- Height of sink and countertops adjusted for the person's needs (lowered for the person who uses a wheelchair; raised for the person who cannot bend easily)
- Anti-scald devices on faucets
- Lever-handle faucets
- Spray attachment to the sink—the person can fill pots after placing them on the stove

FOCUS ON LONG-TERM CARE AND HOME CARE
Housing Options—cont'd

Other

- Lever door handles on all doors
- Easy-to-grasp cabinet and drawer handles
- Hand rails on both sides of stairways and outside steps
- Keyless locking system
- Security system
- Shelves near outside doors—the person can set items down to open the door
- Bright lights inside and outside entryways
- Motion-activated entrance lights
- Slip-free walkways and entryways
- House numbers that are easy to see from the street
- Automatic garage door opener
- Rocker light switches that turn on and off with a push
- Electrical outlets 18 inches above the floor
- Peepholes or view panels in doors at the correct height for the person
- Washer and dryer on the main floor
- Wall-mounted, fold down ironing board
- Stair or platform lifts
- No scatter or throw rugs
- Thick carpeting replaced with low pile carpeting
- Furniture arranged to allow wheelchair use

Other—cont'd

- Phones in all rooms including the bathroom
- Cordless phone or wireless phone
- More chairs throughout the home so the person can sit when tired, weak, dizzy, and so on
- Smoke detectors as required by local fire code
- For poor eyesight
  - Water controls that are color-coded or have large words
  - Light bulbs with increased wattage
  - Lights in closets and stairways
  - Outside lights by sidewalks, stairs, and doors
  - Task lighting under cabinets and over counters
  - Night-lights in bedrooms, bathrooms, and hallways
  - Phones with large keypads
- For hearing loss
  - Phone volume increased
  - Smoke detectors with strobe lights
  - Text teletypewriters (TTYs) or Telecommunications Devices for the Deaf (TDDs) (Fig. 11-6)
  - Amplified phone handset—increases sound and makes the caller's voice louder
  - Extension bells that make the phone ring louder
  - Doorbells that can be heard throughout the house

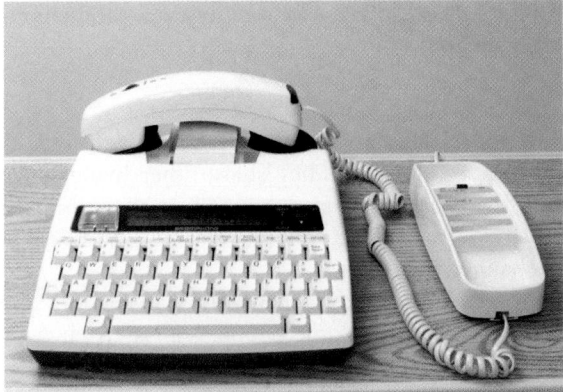

Fig. 11-6 The Americans With Disabilities Act of 1990 requires that every state must provide access to Telecommunications Relay Services (TRS). A communications assistant relays messages between the caller and the hard-of-hearing person. Messages are typed by the hard-of-hearing person. They are relayed orally to the caller. The communications assistant must relay everything that is said and maintain the confidentiality of all conversations.

Living With Family

Sometimes older brothers, sisters, and cousins live together. They:
- Provide companionship.
- Share living expenses.
- Provide care during illness or disability.

Living with children is an option. The older parent (or parents) moves in with the child. Or the child moves to the parent's home. The parent may be healthy, may need some help, or may be ill or disabled. Some adult children give care to avoid nursing center care.

Living with an adult child is a social change. Everyone in the home must adjust. Sleeping plans may change if there is no spare bedroom. The parent may need a hospital bed. It can go in a family or living room, dining room, den, or bedroom.

The adult child's family needs time alone. Other family members may help give care. Respite care is an option for weekends and vacations. (*Respite* means *a short period of rest or relief.*) The person goes to a nursing center for a short time. This gives the family relief from the demands of the person's care.) Home care agencies can provide nurses or home health care aides. Many community and church groups have volunteers who help give care.

Adult Day Care. Many children need to work even though the parent cannot stay alone. Adult day-care centers provide meals, supervision, and activities. Some provide rides to and from the center. Some provide rehabilitation and serve persons with dementia (Chapter 46).

Requirements vary. Some require that the person be able to walk. A cane or walker is used as needed. Others allow wheelchairs. Most require that the person perform some self-care.

Many activities are offered. Cards, board games, movies, crafts, dancing, walks, exercise groups, and lectures are common (Fig. 11-7, p. 144). Some provide bowling and swimming. All activities are supervised. Needed help is given.

Some areas have inter-generational day-care centers. Children and older persons are in the same center. They

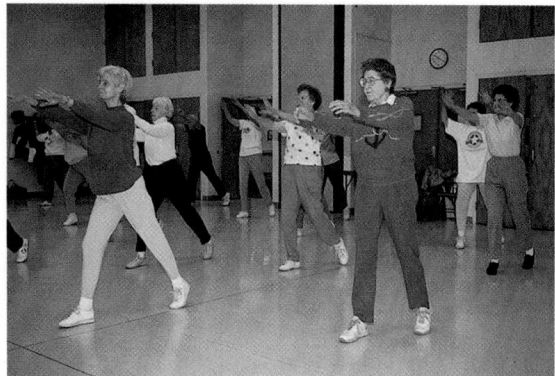

Fig. 11-7 An adult day-care center.

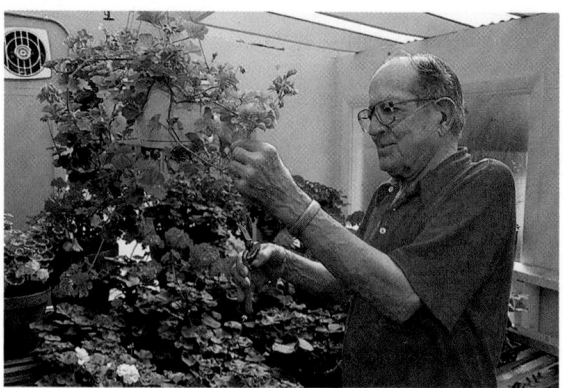

Fig. 11-8 This man enjoys gardening.

work together on some activities. They eat and play together. Young children bring much joy to older persons. They give older persons purpose, love, and affection. In turn, children learn about aging. They also receive love and affection from older persons.

Elder Cottage Housing Opportunity

Elder Cottage Housing Opportunity (ECHO) homes are small homes designed for older and disabled persons. The portable home is placed in the yard of a single-family home. The older person lives independently but near family or friends.

Apartments

Some older persons live in apartments. They pay rent and utility bills. The owner provides maintenance, yard work, snow removal, and appliance repair. Older persons remain independent. They can keep personal items. Many older persons like to garden or do yard work (Fig. 11-8). Apartment living may not provide such activities.

An *accessory dwelling unit (ADU)* is a separate living area in a home. It has a kitchen, bedroom, and bathroom. Some have a small living room. The older person lives independently near other people. Some children have these apartments for their parents. Or the older person's home may have an apartment. ADUs are also called an "in-law apartment," an "accessory apartment," and a "second unit."

Residential Hotels

Some cities have residential hotels. Private rooms or small apartments are rented. Food services may include a dining room, cafeteria, or room service. Some provide recreational activities and emergency medical services. Most hotels are close to shopping, places of worship, and other civic services.

Congregate Housing

Congregate means *a group, gathering, or cluster.* In congregate housing, apartments are for older people. Buildings have wheelchair access, hand rails, elevators, and other safety features. Apartments are designed to meet the needs of older persons. Some are furnished.

Services are many. A doctor or nurse is on call. Someone checks on the person daily. A dining room is common. Rides are provided to places of worship, the doctor, or shopping areas. Tenants pay monthly rent.

Senior Citizen Housing. In many areas, state and federal funds support apartment complexes for older and disabled persons. Such persons have low to moderate incomes. Monthly rents are lower. The rent depends on the person's monthly income.

Home-Sharing

Two or more people share a house or apartment. Each person has a bedroom. They share other living spaces—kitchen, bathroom, living room. They share household chores and expenses. Or cooking, cleaning, and yard work are exchanged for rent.

Shared housing is a way to avoid living alone. It provides companionship. Some people feel safer when living with another person.

Assisted Living Residences

Assisted living residences are for persons who need help with daily living (Chapters 1 and 50). The person has social contact with others in a home-like setting. Health care and 24-hour over-sight are provided.

Board and Care Homes

Board and care homes (group homes) provide a room, meals, laundry, and supervision. Some homes are for older persons. Others are for people with certain problems. Dementia, mental health problems, and developmental disabilities are examples.

Homes vary in size—from housing 4 to 30 people or more. The care provided and rules vary from state to state. The person pays monthly rent. Some board and care homes receive government funds.

Adult Foster Care

Adult foster care can take two forms:
- An older person lives with a family.
- A single family home serves 4 to 5 persons with special needs. They may be older, disabled, or mentally ill.

The person receives help with daily living. A room, meals, and laundry are provided. Help is given with shopping and transportation. The person receives needed health care.

Continuing Care Retirement Communities

Continuing care retirement communities (CCRCs) offer many services. They range from independent living units to 24-hour nursing care. A CCRC has housing, activity, and health care services. It meets the changing needs of older persons living alone or with a partner. CCRCs usually provide:
- Nursing care and other health care services
- Meals (including special diets)
- Housekeeping
- Transportation
- Personal assistance
- Recreational and educational activities

Independent living units are small apartments. Residents perform self-care and take their own drugs. Food service is provided. Help is nearby if needed. Many people have their own cars. They travel or drive about as desired. Rides are provided for those who need them.

Services are added as the person's needs change. Over time, some persons need nursing center care. They move into the nursing center within the CCRC. Many older couples find comfort in this plan. One partner needs nursing care. The other is close by and can visit often.

The person signs a contract with the CCRC. The contract is for a certain time or for the person's life-time. The contract lists services provided and the required fees.

Nursing Centers

Some older persons cannot care for themselves. Nursing centers are options for them (Chapter 1). Some people stay in nursing centers until death. Others stay until they can return home. The nursing center is the person's temporary or permanent home. The setting is as home-like as possible (Fig. 11-9).

The person needing nursing center care may suffer some or all of these losses:
- Loss of identity as a productive member of a family and community
- Loss of possessions—home, household items, car, and so on
- Loss of independence
- Loss of real-world experiences—shopping, traveling, cooking, driving, hobbies, and so on
- Loss of health and mobility

The person may feel useless, powerless, and hopeless. The health team helps the person cope with loss and improve quality of life. Treat the person with dignity and respect. Also practice good communication skills. Follow the care plan.

Nursing centers serve to meet the needs of older and disabled persons. Physical changes of aging are considered in the center's design. So are safety needs. Programs and services meet the person's basic needs. Box 11-4, p. 146 lists the features of a quality nursing center.

Most nursing centers receive Medicare or Medicaid funds. They must meet requirements of the Omnibus Budget Reconciliation Act of 1987 (OBRA). OBRA protects the person's rights and promotes quality of life. The Centers for Medicare & Medicaid Services (CMS) has rules and regulations for OBRA. See Box 11-5, p. 147.

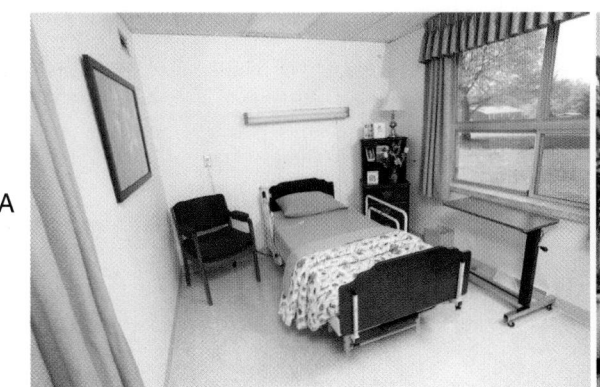
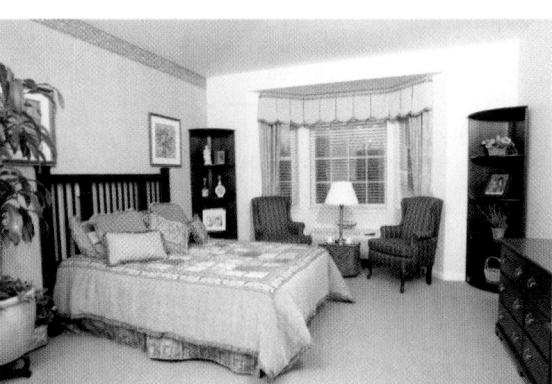

Fig. 11-9 A, A nursing center is as home-like as possible. **B,** Some centers allow residents to bring their own bed and furniture from home.

BOX 11-4   FEATURES OF A QUALITY NURSING CENTER

Basic Information
- The center is Medicare-certified.
- The center is Medicaid-certified.
- The center provides the level of care needed. Rehabilitation, dementia, and ventilator services are examples.
- The center is located close enough for family and friends to visit.

Resident Appearance
- Residents are clean and well-groomed.
- Residents are dressed appropriately for the season or time of day.

Living Spaces
- The center is free from overwhelming, unpleasant odors.
- The center appears clean and well-kept.
- The temperature is comfortable for the residents.
- The center has good lighting.
- Noise levels in the dining room are comfortable.
- Noise levels in common areas are comfortable.
- Smoking is not allowed. If allowed, it is restricted to certain areas.
- Furnishings are sturdy, comfortable, and attractive.

Staff
- The relationship between the staff and residents appears to be warm, polite, and respectful.
- All staff wear name tags.
- Staff knock on the person's door before entering the room.
- Staff refer to residents by name.
- The center offers a training and continuing education program for all staff.
- The center does background checks on all staff.
- The center has licensed nurses 24 hours a day. An RN is present at least 8 hours a day, 7 days a week.
- The same nursing team (including nursing assistants) works with the same resident 4 to 5 days a week.
- Nursing assistants work with a reasonable number of residents.
- Nursing assistants take part in care planning meetings.
- The center has a full-time social worker on staff.
- A licensed doctor is on staff. He or she is there daily and can be reached at all times.
- The center's management team has worked together for at least 1 year. This includes the administrator and director of nursing.

Residents' Rooms
- Residents may have personal belongings in their rooms.
- Residents may have personal furniture in their rooms.

Residents' Rooms—cont'd
- Each resident has storage space (closet and drawers) in his or her room.
- Each resident has a window in his or her room.
- Residents have access to a personal telephone.
- Residents have access to a personal TV.
- Residents have a choice of roommates.
- The resident can reach his or her water pitcher.
- The center has policies and procedures to protect residents' belongings.

Hallways, Stairs, Lounges, and Bathrooms
- Exits are clearly marked.
- The center has quiet areas where residents can visit with family and friends.
- The center has smoke detectors and sprinklers.
- All common areas, resident rooms, and doorways are designed for wheelchair use.
- The center has hand rails in the hallways.
- The center has grab bars in bathrooms.

Menus and Food
- Residents have a choice of food items at each meal.
- The person's favorite foods are served.
- Nutritious snacks are available upon request.
- Staff help residents eat and drink if help is needed.

Activities
- Residents may choose to take part in a variety of activities. This includes residents who cannot leave their rooms.
- The center has outdoor areas for resident use. Staff help residents to go outside.
- The center has an active volunteer program.

Safety and Care
- The center has an emergency evacuation plan.
- Regular fire drills are held. Residents, including bed-bound residents, are moved to safety.
- Residents receive preventive care to stay healthy. Yearly flu shots are an example.
- Residents may see their personal doctors.
- The center has an arrangement with a nearby hospital for emergencies.
- Care plan meetings are held with residents and family members.
- The center has corrected all problems on its last state inspection report.

Modified from Centers for Medicare & Medicaid Services: *Guide to choosing a nursing home,* Baltimore, revised May 2011, U.S. Department of Health and Human Services.

BOX 11-5   ENVIRONMENT REQUIREMENTS

- The person's care equipment is clean and properly stored. This includes toothbrushes, dentures, denture cups, water pitchers and cups, emesis basins, hair brushes and combs, bedpans, urinals, feeding tubes, leg bags and catheter bags, pads, and positioning devices.
- Bed linens are clean and in good condition.
- There are clean towels and washcloths for each person.
- The person has closet space with shelves. The person can reach the shelves.
- Lighting levels are comfortable and adequate.
- Temperature levels are comfortable and safe. The temperature is between 71°F and 81°F (Fahrenheit).
- Sound levels are comfortable. Sound levels allow for hearing, privacy, and social interaction.
- Safety precautions are followed for persons who smoke. See Chapter 12.
- Hand rails, assistive devices, and other surfaces are in good repair. They are free from sharp edges or other hazards.
- Furniture is appropriate for the residents.
- The person's setting is as free from accident hazards as possible.
  - Resident care equipment is used following the manufacturer's instructions.
  - Safety measures are practiced for hazardous substances (Chapter 12).
  - Safety measures are practiced to prevent burns from hot water temperatures (Chapter 12).
  - Safety measures are practiced to prevent equipment accidents (Chapter 12). This includes electrical safety.
  - Safety measures are practiced to prevent accidents from assistive devices and equipment. This includes canes, walkers, wheelchairs, mechanical lifts, restraints, bed rails, mattresses, and so on.

Modified from Centers for Medicare & Medicaid Services: *State operations manual*, Baltimore, 2009, U.S. Department of Health and Human Services.

FOCUS ON PRIDE

The Person, Family, and Yourself

Personal and Professional Responsibility

Myths about aging are common. Some believe that all older persons have decreased mental and physical function. For example, they are hard-of-hearing, confused, or move slowly. Others think the elderly cannot care for themselves. Or they lose interest in activities.

Your beliefs about others affect the care you give. You may struggle with a myth. Review the facts about aging in Box 11-1. Each person is unique. Treat each person as an individual. This is a personal and professional responsibility.

Rights and Respect

A nursing center provides a temporary or permanent residence for some persons. This setting must promote quality of life. It must be clean, safe, comfortable, and as home-like as possible. Give care that reflects these principles. To do so:

- Make sure the person, clothes, and linens are clean and dry.
- Keep the person's room clean and orderly.
- Place soiled linens in the correct containers. Empty the containers often. Do not let them overflow.
- Clean up your work area and the bathroom after giving care.
- Help the person display personal items if asked. Do not touch the person's items without permission.
- Treat the person as if you were in his or her home.
- Respect the person and his or her setting.

Independence and Social Interaction

Older persons may feel lonely and isolated. Loss of friends and loved ones, a new home setting, reduced income, and physical changes are causes. To promote social interaction:

- Encourage the person to talk about friends and family.
- Ask about the person's hobbies or interests.
- Use touch to show caring. For example, gently place your hand on the person's shoulder or arm. Remember to maintain professional boundaries.
- Take time to listen. Avoid seeming rushed.

Some persons prefer quiet and privacy. They may avoid social contacts. Respect their wishes for privacy. Take pride in considering their social needs.

Delegation and Teamwork

Team members often work together to assist older persons. For example, two nursing assistants help an older woman to the bathroom. Or team members work close by with groups of older persons. For example, two Russian-speaking nursing assistants sit near each other when feeding residents. When working this way, they may be tempted to talk to each other in their native language.

Co-workers may be closer to your age, share your interests, relate to your work, share your native language, and so on. You must not ignore the patient, resident, or group or speak in a foreign language. Talk with the person or group. Focus on them, not on others. This promotes a sense of belonging and self-worth.

Ethics and Laws

The CMS is a federal agency. It has the power to issue standards, rules, and regulations. These are called agency-made laws. Employers and employees must comply with them. Unannounced surveys are conducted for agency compliance. If requirements are not met, funding is lost. A survey team will:

- Review policies, procedures, and medical records.
- Interview staff, patients and residents, and families.
- Check for cleanliness and safety.
- Make sure staff meets state requirements.
- Observe how care is given.

You may be observed or asked questions during a survey. You must provide safe, quality care and protect the person's rights. Also, you must help keep the agency clean and follow agency policies and procedures. Answer survey questions completely and honestly. Act professionally and use good work ethics (Chapter 5).

You may be tempted to act differently when surveyors are present. This is wrong. Your conduct and care must reflect a normal day. Provide the same quality care every day.

REVIEW QUESTIONS

Circle the BEST answer.

1 People age 85 and older are
   a The young-old
   b Old
   c The oldest-old
   d Elderly

2 The study of the aging process is called
   a Geriatrics
   b Dysphagia
   c Gerontology
   d Dyspnea

3 Retirement usually means
   a Lowered income
   b Changes from aging
   c Less free time
   d Financial security

4 Which does *not* cause loneliness in older persons?
   a Children moving away
   b The death of family and friends
   c Problems communicating with others
   d Contact with other older persons

5 Older persons living with their children often feel
   a Independent
   b Wanted and a part of things
   c Useless
   d Dignified

6 These statements are about a partner's death. Which is *false*?
   a The person loses a lover, friend, and companion.
   b Preparing for the event lessens grief.
   c The survivor may develop health problems.
   d The survivor's life will likely change.

7 Skin changes occur with aging. Care should include the following *except*
   a Providing for warmth
   b Applying lotion
   c A daily bath with soap
   d Providing good skin care

8 An older person complains of cold feet. You should
   a Provide socks
   b Apply a hot water bottle
   c Soak the feet in hot water
   d Apply a heating pad

9 Aging causes changes in the musculo-skeletal system. Which is *false*?
   a Bones become brittle. They can break easily.
   b Bedrest is needed for loss of strength.
   c Joints become stiff and painful.
   d Exercise slows musculo-skeletal changes.

10 Changes occur in the nervous system. Which is *true*?
   a Less sleep is needed than when younger.
   b The person forgets events from long ago.
   c Sensitivity to pain increases.
   d Confusion occurs in all older persons.

11 Changes occur in the eye. Which is *false*?
   a Night vision decreases.
   b Blue and green colors are easy to see.
   c Eyelids thin and wrinkle.
   d The eye is easily irritated by dust.

12 Which is *not* a common cause of hearing loss in older persons?
   a Changes in the acoustic nerve
   b Atrophy of the eardrums
   c Impacted earwax
   d Ear infections

13 Arteries narrow and lose their elasticity. These changes result in
   a A slower heart rate
   b Lower blood pressure
   c Poor circulation to many body parts
   d Less blood in the body

14 An older person has cardiovascular changes. Care includes the following *except*
   a Placing needed items nearby
   b A moderate amount of daily exercise
   c Avoiding exertion
   d Long walks

15 Respiratory changes occur with aging. Which is *false*?
   a Heavy bed linens are avoided.
   b The person is turned often if on bedrest.
   c The side-lying position is best for breathing.
   d The person should be as active as possible.

16 Older persons should avoid dry foods because of
   a Decreases in saliva
   b Loss of teeth or ill-fitting dentures
   c Decreased amounts of digestive juices
   d Decreased peristalsis

17 Changes occur in the digestive system. Older persons should eat
   a Fruits and vegetables with skins and seeds
   b Dry and fatty foods
   c Raw apricots and celery
   d Protein foods

18 Changes occur in the urinary system. Which is *true*?
   a Kidneys increase in size.
   b Fluids are needed for kidney function.
   c The bladder becomes larger.
   d Blood flow to the kidneys increases.

19 The doctor orders increased fluid intake for an older person. You should
   a Give most of the fluid before 1700 (5:00 PM)
   b Provide mostly water
   c Start a bladder training program
   d Insert a catheter

20 Most older people live
   a In nursing centers
   b In a family setting
   c With children
   d In senior citizen housing

21 These statements are about adult day-care centers. Which is *false*?
   a They provide meals, supervision, and activities.
   b Usually the person must do some self-care.
   c All activities are supervised.
   d Personal care is provided.

22 Which housing option provides lodging, meals, and some help with personal care?
   a Apartments
   b Senior citizen housing
   c Board and care homes
   d Residential hotels

23 A continuing care retirement community provides the following *except*
   a Independent living units
   b A nursing center
   c Adult foster care
   d Meals, transportation, and recreational activities

24 A quality nursing center
   a Is Medicare and Medicaid certified
   b Is owned by doctors and nurses
   c Has independent living units
   d Provides adult and child day care

Answers to these questions are on p. 832.

OBJECTIVES

- Define the key terms and key abbreviations listed in this chapter.
- Describe accident risk factors.
- Identify safety measures for infants and children.
- Explain why you identify a person before giving care.
- Explain how to correctly identify a person.
- Describe the safety measures to prevent burns, poisoning, and suffocation.
- Identify the signs and causes of choking.
- Explain how to prevent equipment accidents.
- Explain how to handle hazardous substances.
- Describe safety measures for fire prevention and oxygen use.
- Explain what to do during a fire.
- Give examples of natural and human-made disasters.
- Explain how to report accidents and errors.
- Explain how to protect yourself from workplace violence.
- Describe your role in risk management.
- Perform the procedures described in this chapter.
- Explain how to promote PRIDE in the person, the family, and yourself.

KEY TERMS

coma A state of being unaware of one's setting and being unable to react or respond to people, places, or things

dementia The loss of cognitive and social function caused by changes in the brain

disaster A sudden catastrophic event in which people are injured and killed and property is destroyed

electrical shock When electrical current passes through the body

ground That which carries leaking electricity to the earth and away from an electrical item

hazard Any thing in the person's setting that may cause injury or illness

hazardous substance Any chemical in the workplace that can cause harm

hemiplegia Paralysis (*plegia*) on one side (*hemi*) of the body

incident Any event that has harmed or could harm a patient, resident, visitor, or staff member

paralysis Loss of muscle function, sensation, or both

paraplegia Paralysis in the legs and lower trunk (*para* means *beyond; plegia* means *paralysis*)

poison Any substance harmful to the body when ingested, inhaled, injected, or absorbed through the skin

quadriplegia Paralysis in the arms, legs, and trunk (*quad* means *four; plegia* means *paralysis*); tetraplegia

suffocation When breathing stops from the lack of oxygen

tetraplegia See "quadriplegia" (*tetra* means *four; plegia* means *paralysis*)

workplace violence Violent acts (including assault and threat of assault) directed toward persons at work or while on duty

KEY ABBREVIATIONS

AED	Automated external defibrillator
C	Centigrade
CDC	Centers for Disease Control and Prevention
CO	Carbon monoxide
CPR	Cardiopulmonary resuscitation
EMS	Emergency Medical Services
F	Fahrenheit
FBAO	Foreign-body airway obstruction
ID	Identification
MSDS	Material safety data sheet
OSHA	Occupational Safety and Health Administration
PASS	*Pull* the safety pin, *aim* low, *squeeze* the lever, *sweep* back and forth
RACE	Rescue, alarm, confine, extinguish
RRT	Rapid Response Team

Safety is a basic need. Patients and residents are at great risk for accidents and falls. (See Chapter 13 for falls.) Some accidents and injuries cause death.

The health team must provide for safety. This includes you. Common sense and simple safety measures can prevent most accidents. Sometimes extraordinary measures are needed. You must protect patients, residents, visitors, co-workers, and yourself. The safety measures in this chapter apply to all health care agencies and everyday life.

The goal is to decrease the person's risk of accidents and injuries without limiting mobility and independence. The care plan lists other safety measures needed by the person. Measures to promote safety must not interfere with the person's rights (Chapter 2).

A SAFE SETTING

In a safe setting, a person has little risk of illness or injury. The person's setting is free of hazards to the extent possible. *A hazard is any thing in the person's setting that may cause injury or illness.*

The person feels safe and secure physically and mentally. The risk of infection, falls, burns, poisoning, and other injuries is low. Temperature and noise levels are comfortable. Smells are pleasant. There is enough room and light to move about safely. The person and the person's property are safe from fire and intruders. The person is not afraid and has few worries and concerns.

The person must receive the right care and treatment. To protect the person from harm, follow the person's care plan. Also practice the safety measures in this chapter.

See *Teamwork and Time Management: A Safe Setting.*

ACCIDENT RISK FACTORS

Some people cannot protect themselves. They present dangers to themselves and others. They rely on others for safety. Know the factors that increase a person's risk of accidents and injuries. Follow the person's care plan.

- *Age.* Children and older persons are at risk for injuries. See *Focus on Children and Older Persons: Accident Risk Factors (Age).*
- *Awareness of surroundings.* People need to know their surroundings to protect themselves from injury. *Coma is a state of being unaware of one's setting and being unable to react or respond to people, places, or things.* A coma can occur from illness or injury. The person in a coma relies on others for protection. Confused and disoriented persons may not understand what is happening to and around them.

- *Agitated and aggressive behaviors.* Pain can cause these behaviors. So can confusion, decreased awareness of surroundings, and fear of what may happen.
- *Vision loss.* Persons with poor vision have problems seeing things. They can fall or trip over toys, rugs, equipment, furniture, and cords. Some cannot read labels on containers. Poisoning can result. It also can result from taking the wrong drug or the wrong dose.
- *Hearing loss.* Persons with hearing loss have problems hearing explanations and instructions. They may not hear warning signals or fire alarms. Some cannot hear approaching meal carts, drug carts, stretchers, or people in wheelchairs. They do not know to move to safety.
- *Impaired smell and touch.* Illness and aging affect smell and touch. The person may not detect smoke or gas odors. Burns are a risk from impaired touch. The person has problems sensing heat and cold. Some people have a decreased pain sense. They may be unaware of injury. For example, Mrs. Parks does not feel a blister from her shoes. She has poor circulation in her legs and feet. The blister can become a serious wound.
- *Impaired mobility.* Some diseases and injuries affect mobility. A person may know there is danger but cannot move to safety. Some persons cannot walk or propel wheelchairs. Some persons are paralyzed.
  - *Paralysis means loss of muscle function, sensation, or both.*
  - *Paraplegia is paralysis in the legs and lower trunk. (Para* means *beyond. Plegia* means *paralysis.)*
  - *Quadriplegia (tetraplegia) is paralysis in the arms, legs, and trunk. (Quad* and *tetra* mean *four. Plegia* means *paralysis.)*
  - *Hemiplegia is paralysis* (plegia) *on one side* (hemi) *of the body.*
- *Drugs.* Drugs have side effects. They include loss of balance, drowsiness, and lack of coordination. Reduced awareness, confusion, and disorientation can occur. The person may be fearful and uncooperative. Report behavior changes and the person's complaints to the nurse.

Text continued on p. 156

TEAMWORK AND TIME MANAGEMENT
A Safe Setting

You may see something unsafe. Correct the matter right away if it is something you can do. For example:

- Wipe up water spills right away. Do so even if you did not cause the spill.
- A person is sliding out of a wheelchair. Position the person correctly in the chair. Do so even if a co-worker is responsible for the person's care.
- A person is having problems holding a cup of coffee. Offer to help the person.
- Food is left unattended in an oven. Turn off the device. Then tell your co-worker the reason for your action.
- A grab bar is loose in the bathroom. Tell the nurse. Report the problem following agency policy.

You cannot correct some safety issues. Follow agency policy for reporting such problems. They include:

- Electrical outlets or switches coming out of the wall
- Electrical outlets that do not work
- Water leaks from windows, doors, ceilings, pipes, faucets, tubs, showers, toilets, water heaters, and other sources
- Toilets that do not work properly
- Water from faucets that does not warm up or that is very hot
- Broken windows
- Windows and doors that do not work properly
- Knobs and handles that are broken or do not work properly
- Hand rails and grab bars that are loose or need repair
- Odd smells, odors, and sounds
- Signs of rodents, flies, or other pests
- Broken or damaged furniture
- Lights and lamps that do not work or have burnt-out bulbs
- Flooring (carpeting, tiles) in need of repair

FOCUS ON CHILDREN AND OLDER PERSONS
Accident Risk Factors (Age)

Children

Infants are helpless. Young children have not learned the difference between safety and danger. They explore their settings, put objects in their mouths, and touch and feel new things. Falls, poisoning, choking, burns, and other accidents are risks. Practice the safety measures in Box 12-1.

Older Persons

Changes from aging increase the risk for falls and other injuries. Many older persons have decreased strength and move slowly. Some are unsteady. Often balance is affected. These changes prevent quick and sudden movements to avoid dangers and prevent falls. Older persons also are less sensitive to heat and cold. They have poor vision, hearing problems, and a dulled sense of smell. Confusion, poor judgment, memory problems, and disorientation may occur (Chapter 46).

Some persons suffer from dementia. *Dementia is the loss of cognitive and social function caused by changes in the brain* (Chapter 46). Memory and the ability to think and reason are lost. Dementia is caused by diseases and injuries.

Persons with dementia are confused and disoriented. Their awareness of surroundings is reduced. They may not understand what is happening to and around them. Judgment is poor. They no longer know what is safe and what are dangers. They may access closets, cupboards, or other unsafe and unlocked areas. They may eat or drink cleaning products, drugs, or poisons. Accidents and injuries are great risks.

BOX 12-1   SAFETY MEASURES FOR INFANTS AND CHILDREN

General Safety

- Do not leave infants and children unattended. Supervise them at all times.
- Do not leave any child alone on or near balconies, decks, and open windows.
- Use childproof locks or door knob covers (Fig. 12-1, p. 154) leading to the outside, garage, attic, basement, and non-childproof areas.
- Install finger-pinch guards on doors.
- Make sure used items have not been recalled for safety reasons. This includes toys, cribs, furniture, strollers, car seats, and other items.
- Avoid baby walkers on wheels.
- Use the safety strap to fasten a child in a highchair or infant carrier seat.
- Lock the highchair tray after putting the child in the chair.
- Keep highchairs away from stoves, tables, and counters.
- Do not hang items with strings, cords, or elastic cords around cribs or playpens.
- Keep child-resistant caps on drugs and other harmful substances.
- Store knives (including kitchen knives), razor blades, matches, guns, tools, and other harmful items where children cannot reach them. Keep them in locked storage areas.

General Safety—cont'd

- Keep glassware, knives, dishes, appliance cords, and other objects away from counter and table edges.
- Do not prop baby bottles on a rolled towel or blanket. Hold the baby and bottle during feedings.
- Use safety gates at the top and bottom of stairs. They prevent small children from climbing up and down stairs. Make sure the child cannot get caught in the gate slats.
- Use safety guards on rails and banisters. They prevent the child from getting caught in the slats.
- Supervise children on stairs. Hold the child's hand when he or she is going up or down stairs.
- Keep stairs free of toys, cords, and other items.
- Keep one hand on a child lying in a crib or on a scale, bed, table, or other surface or furniture (Fig. 12-2, p. 154).
- Read all package and label instructions. Follow the manufacturer's instructions.
- Use shopping carts safely:
  - Use the safety harness or belt to restrain a child in a cart.
  - Do not let a child stand up in a cart.
  - Do not let a child push a cart.
  - Stay close to the shopping cart.
- Remove heavy items from low tables and shelves. Also remove items that can break.

Modified from http://keepkidshealthy.com and www.safekids.org.

Continued

BOX 12-1   SAFETY MEASURES FOR INFANTS AND CHILDREN—cont'd

General Safety—cont'd

- Supervise children carefully when animals are present.
- Place a plastic cover over electronic devices (TV, computer, and so on). This prevents the child from touching controls and buttons.
- Do not let children near appliances that pose entrapment hazards. Refrigerators, washers, dryers, and dishwashers are examples.
- Keep emergency numbers near the phone.
- Keep a phone nearby in case of an emergency.

Bedroom Safety

- Check infants often when in cribs.
- Check that the crib meets federal safety standards. Drop-side cribs do *not* meet current safety standards. In December 2010, the United States government banned the manufacture and sale of drop-side cribs. If a crib has drop-sides, keep crib rails up and locked.
- Do not use a crib with loose, broken, or missing parts. This includes screws, nuts, and bolts.
- Remove mobiles from the crib when the child can stand. Also remove them from playpens.
- See Chapters 19 and 49 for other crib safety measures.
- Promote bunk bed safety:
  - Make sure the beds are fastened and supported properly.
  - Do not let children younger than 6 years sleep on the top bunk.
  - Make sure guard-rails are firmly attached to the bed with screws or bolts.
  - Check guard-rails. The space between the bed frame and bottom of the guard-rail is no more than 3.5 inches. Spaces between the slats are less than 3.5 inches. Guard-rails raise at least 5 inches above the mattress.
  - Make sure openings on the upper and lower bunks are small enough to prevent the child's head, torso, arm, or leg from passing through the opening.
  - Use guard-rails on both sides of the upper bunk.
  - Make sure the ladder is secure to the bed frame.
  - Have the child use the ladder for getting in and out of the upper bunk.
  - Use a night-light so children can see when using the ladder during the night.
- Keep bedroom doors closed. Bedrooms of parents and older children may contain perfumes, toys, and other items that present hazards to young children. Choking, poisoning, burns, and suffocation are risks.

Electrical Safety

- Keep electrical items away from sinks, tubs, toilets, and other water sources.
- Unplug electrical items when not in use.
- Tie appliance cords up and out of reach.
- Place safety covers over electrical outlets (Fig. 12-3, p. 155). They prevent children from sticking their fingers into the outlet.
- Keep electrical cords, electrical strips, surge protectors, and electrical items out of the reach of children.
- Use safety plugs with caution (Fig. 12-4, p. 155). A choking hazard, children can remove them from electrical outlets, electrical strips, and surge protectors. When removed, children can stick their fingers or small objects into the openings.

Window Safety

- Install safety guards on windows.
- Keep cords for window coverings out of the reach of children. Tie the cords up or use a cord wind-up device.
- Remove loops from blinds and other window coverings.
- Do not place a crib, playpen, bed, or other furniture near a window. This prevents children from climbing from furniture onto a window seat or sill.
- Keep children away from open windows. Do not let them sit on window sills. Window screens are not strong enough to prevent children from falling out of windows.
- Open windows from the top down.

Water Safety

- Supervise any child who is in or near water. This includes when using tubs, toilets, sinks, buckets and containers, wading pools, swimming pools, hot tubs, spas, and whirlpools.
- Be aware of small bodies of water than can present dangers. Examples include fountains, fish ponds, ditches, rain barrels, and watering cans.
- Do not rely on bathtub seats, water wings, inner tubes, air mattresses, or other flotation devices to keep a child afloat. Never leave the child alone even if he or she is wearing a flotation device.
- Keep bathroom doors closed to prevent drowning in toilets or bathtubs. Also close laundry room doors.
- Keep sinks, tubs, and basins empty when not in use.
- Keep buckets, pails, containers, and wading pools empty and upside down when not in use.
- Keep toilet lids down. Use toilet safety locks.
- Keep diaper pails locked.
- Make sure door, window, and pool alarms are on. They alert you if a child wanders into an unsafe area.
- Fence in pools, spas, hot tubs, and whirlpools. Fences are at least 4 feet high. Gates are self-closing and self-latching.
- Keep locked safety covers on spas, hot tubs, and whirlpools when not in use.
- Remove pool, spa, hot tub, and whirlpool covers before use. The cover must be completely off. If not, the child can get trapped under the cover.
- Remove steps to above-ground pools when not in use.
- Keep tables and chairs away from pool fences. This prevents children from climbing over the fence into the pool area.
- Keep toys away from the pool, spa, hot tub, or whirlpool. Children playing with such toys could fall into the water.
- Have a phone by the pool, spa, hot tub, and whirlpool.
- Keep rescue equipment near pools.
- Promote safe swimming and diving:
  - Teach water survival when a child can crawl or walk to a pool.
  - Make sure children older than 4 years learn how to swim.
  - Do not let children swim alone.
  - Do not let children swim in areas where there are boats, fishermen, and large waves.
  - Allow children to swim at beaches only if lifeguards are present.
  - Do not let children dive into above-ground pools. They are too shallow. For safe diving, water must be 9 feet deep or greater.

Modified from http://keepkidshealthy.com and www.safekids.org.

BOX 12-1   SAFETY MEASURES FOR INFANTS AND CHILDREN—cont'd

Water Safety—cont'd

- Have children enter pools feet first.
- Teach safe diving. Children should dive only from the diving board. They should dive with their hands in front of them.
- Have children slide down a pool slide feet first—not head first. Head injuries can occur.
- Prevent hair entanglement or body part entrapment in pools, spas, hot tubs, and whirlpools. They can occur in suction and drain covers. If hair is caught, the head is kept underwater. Trapped body parts can keep the person underwater or cause serious injury.
  - Have suction and drain covers installed that meet current safety standards. Replace missing or broken covers.
  - Do not let children play near drain or suction covers.
  - Have children pin-up long hair or wear a swimming cap.
- Know where to find the power cut-off switch for pools, spas, hot tubs, or whirlpools. Quickly turn off the electricity in an emergency.
- Keep hot tub, spa, and whirlpool temperatures no higher than 104°F. Higher temperatures can cause drowsiness which can lead to drowning. Heat stroke and death are risks.

Vehicle Safety

- Lock vehicle doors and the trunk. Keep keys where children cannot see or reach them. They can open a door or trunk with a remote control key.
- Show children how to find and use the emergency trunk release mechanism.
- Do not let children play in vehicles. They like to play hide-and-seek in cars and trunks. They can easily suffocate and die from high temperatures in the car or trunk.
- Keep any access to the trunk closed. Some vehicles have fold-down seats that give more trunk space. Children can get into the trunk from inside the car. Keep fold-down seats closed.
- Do not leave children alone in any vehicle, even if the windows are down. They can develop heat-related illness, suffocate, and die very quickly from high temperatures in the vehicle. It only takes a few minutes.
- Make sure all children leave the vehicle when you arrive at your destination.
- Use car safety seats correctly:
  - Use federally approved safety seats that fit the child's size and weight (Fig. 12-5, p. 155). Follow the manufacturer's instructions.
  - Do not use a car safety seat that does not have the manufacturer's instructions.
  - Use a car safety seat that is labeled with the manufacturer's name, model number, and the date it was made.
  - Install infant car safety seats rear-facing only (Fig. 12-6, p. 155). Children ride rear-facing as long as possible or until they reach the weight or height limit set by the seat's manufacturer.
  - Do not use a rear-facing car seat or convertible seat in the front seat of a vehicle with an air bag.
  - Do not use a car safety seat that is more than 6 years old. Check the label for the date it was made.
  - Do not use a car safety seat that was involved in a crash.
  - Do not use a car safety seat that has cracks, missing parts, or torn or loose harnesses and buckles.

Vehicle Safety—cont'd

- Use booster seats for children between the ages of 4 and 8 years (about 40 and 80 pounds). Secure them with lap and shoulder belts according to the manufacturer's instructions.
- Have children younger than 12 years ride in the back seat.
- Make sure regular seat belts fit correctly. Children weighing about 80 pounds and who are about 4 feet 9 inches tall should be able to use regular seat belts.
- Follow seat-belt laws.
- Never allow anyone to ride in the cargo bed of a pickup truck.
- Do not let children ride as passengers on tractors, mowers, mini-bikes, or all-terrain vehicles.

Clothing Safety

- Do not use pins on children's clothing.
- Remove drawstrings, ribbons, and cords from jackets, coats, sweaters, swimsuits, and other clothing (Fig. 12-7, p. 155). This includes drawstrings, ribbons, and cords on hoods, purses, scarves, helmets, and backpacks; at the neckline; and at the waist. Drawstrings, ribbons, and cords can get entangled or caught in play equipment, furniture, hand rails, car or bus doors, elevators, escalators, and other moving devices.
- Do not dress children in loose clothing or clothing with drawstrings, ribbons, cords, fringe, strings, or ties if they will use playground equipment. The clothing can get caught.
- Do not dress children in long clothing that touches or drags on the floor.
- Do not let children wear necklaces, strings, cords, ribbons, or other items around the neck. These can get caught on furniture, door knobs, and playground equipment.
- Warn children to check for hanging or dangling items from clothing and backpacks. Examples include key rings, scarves, ribbons, belt and backpack buckles, and loose clothing. They can catch on doors, hand rails, playground equipment, furniture, and other things.
- Make sure children wear safety shoes.
- Make sure shoelaces are tied.

Toy and Play Safety

- Do not let children play in driveways or on streets, parking lots, or curbs. Do not let children play behind parked cars.
- Do not let children play in piles of leaves or snow near streets.
- Keep children away from exercise bikes and equipment.
- Read all warning labels on toys.
- Check the age range on toys. Give children age-appropriate toys.
- Check toys and other play equipment regularly. Look for cracks, chips, breaks, sharp edges, loose parts, and other damage. This includes playground equipment.
- Do not let children play with toys that:
  - Have sharp points or edges.
  - Shoot objects into the air.
  - Make loud, sharp, or shrill noises.
  - Have long strings, straps, or cords. Strings, straps, and cords should be less than 7 inches long.
- Keep older children's toys away from infants and younger children.

Continued

BOX 12-1 **SAFETY MEASURES FOR INFANTS AND CHILDREN—cont'd**

Toy and Play Safety—cont'd

- Keep small toys away from children. Make sure toys are too large to fit into the child's mouth. Objects should have a diameter of 1.75 inches or more. This includes marbles, balls, and games with balls.
- Do not let children use riding toys near stairs, pools, or traffic.
- Have children put away toys when done playing with them.
- Practice safety measures for bicycles, skateboards, scooters, in-line skates, and other devices with wheels:
  - Perform a safety inspection—reflectors, brakes, gears, tires, spokes, and so on.
  - Make sure children wear safety gear. This includes a helmet, elbow and knee pads, wrist guards, goggles, and reflective shoes and clothing.
  - Do not let children wear loose or long clothing.
  - Do not let children use such items in the dark or around cars.
- Make sure bike helmets are removed before children use playground equipment.
- Do not allow pushing, shoving, or crowding on playground equipment.
- Do not let children under 6 years of age play on trampolines. Death or injury (sprains, fractures, cuts, bruises, and so on) can result from falling off, landing wrong, falling on the trampoline parts, or colliding with another person.
- Supervise any child playing on a trampoline. Also:
  - Place the trampoline away from buildings and play areas.
  - Allow 1 person at a time on the trampoline.
  - Do not allow somersaults.
  - Cover springs, hooks, and the frame with shock-absorbent padding.
  - Use a trampoline enclosure to prevent injuries from falls.
  - Place padded material on the ground around the trampoline. The material should be shock-absorbent.

Furniture Safety

- Prevent furniture from tipping over. Injuries and deaths can occur from children falling on, leaning on, climbing on, pulling on, sitting on, or trying to move poorly secured furniture. TV carts, bookcases, stands, chests-of-drawers, and tables present dangers.
- Prevent bookcases, shelving, and chests-of-drawers from being top heavy. If top heavy, they can tip and fall. Store heavier items on the lower shelves and in lower drawers.

Furniture Safety—cont'd

- Do not let children climb on furniture. This includes using drawers and shelves as steps.
- Place furniture away from windows.
- Do not place toys or things that attract children on the top of furniture.
- Make sure TVs, microwave ovens, and fish tanks are placed on low stands and are as far back on the stand as possible. Do not use carts or stands that could easily tip over.
- Remove furniture with sharp edges. Or use soft guards on rough edges.
- Make sure that angle-braces or anchors are used to secure furniture to walls.
- Do not use tablecloths and placemats. This prevents infants and young children from pulling things off the table and onto themselves. Centerpieces, items on the table, and hot food and liquids can injure the child.
- Do not use toy chests with free-falling lids. The lid can fall on the child's head or neck. The lid should have a spring-loaded lid-support or sliding panels. Toy chests with no lids are best.

Gun Safety

- Store guns unloaded.
- Store guns locked up and out of the reach of children.
- Store ammunition in a separate, locked location.
- Use quality gun locks, lock boxes, or gun safes for each firearm.
- Keep gun storage keys and lock combinations hidden in a separate location.
- Teach children to never touch or play with a gun.
- Teach children to tell an adult if they find a gun.
- Teach children to call 911 if they find a gun when no adult is present.
- Do not let children visit or play in homes where gun safety is not practiced.

Other

- Protect the child from falls (Chapter 13).
- Protect the child from burns (p. 157).
- Protect the child from poisoning (p. 158).
- Protect the child from choking and suffocating (p. 163).
- See Chapter 49 for other infant safety measures.

Modified from http://keepkidshealthy.com and www.safekids.org.

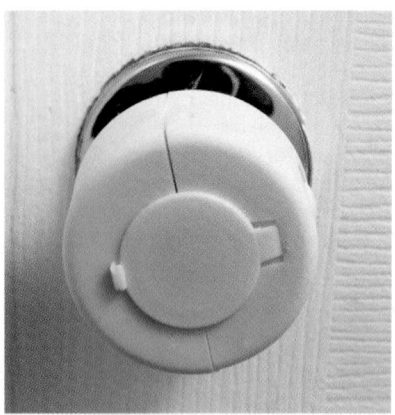

Fig. 12-1 Door knob cover.

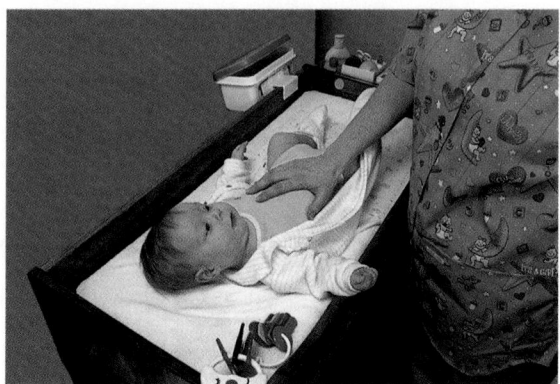

Fig. 12-2 Keep one hand on a child lying in a crib or on a scale, bed, table, or other surface or furniture.

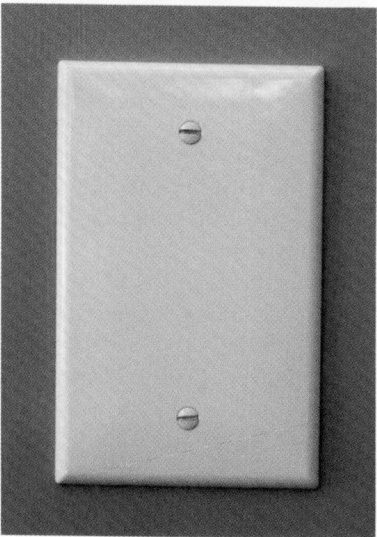

Fig. 12-3 Outlet cover.

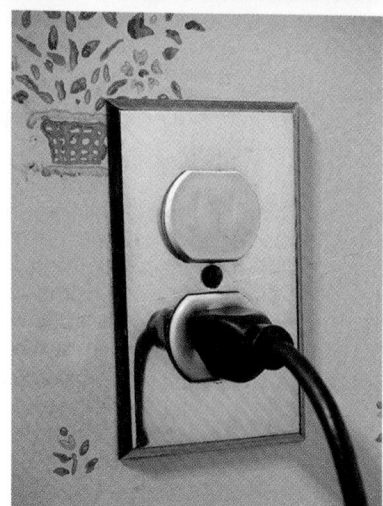

Fig. 12-4 Safety plug in an outlet.

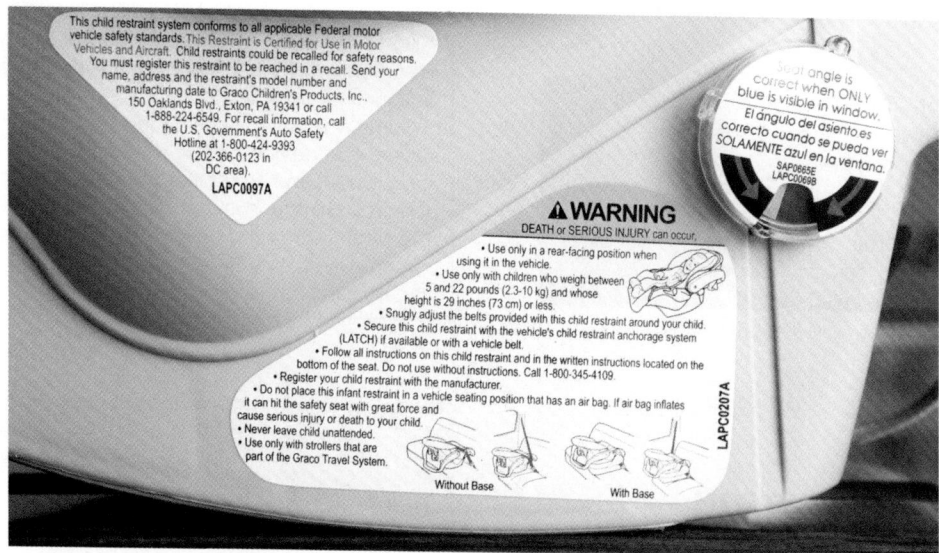

Fig. 12-5 Federally approved car safety seats carry this label.

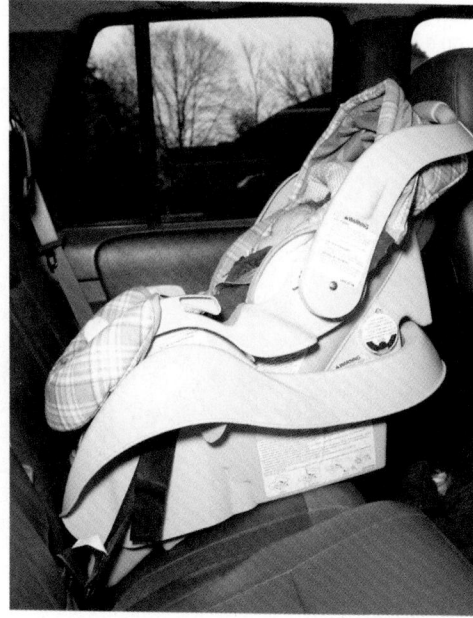

Fig. 12-6 Car safety seat that is rear-facing.

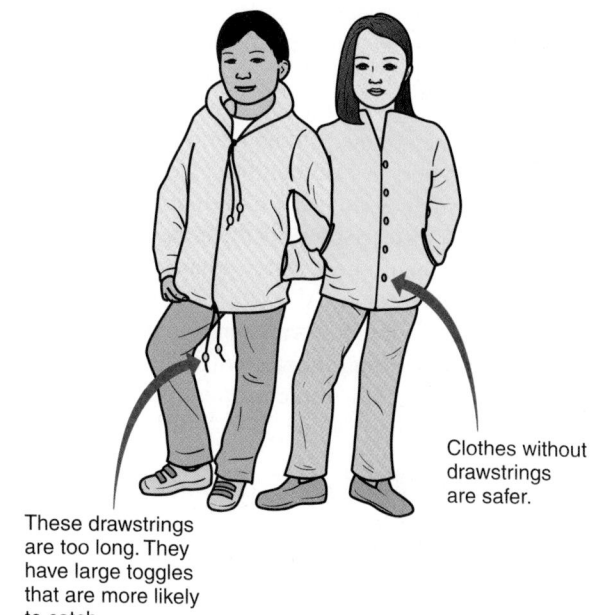

Clothes without drawstrings are safer.

These drawstrings are too long. They have large toggles that are more likely to catch.

Fig. 12-7 Drawstrings, ribbons, and cords can get caught in many things and strangle the child.

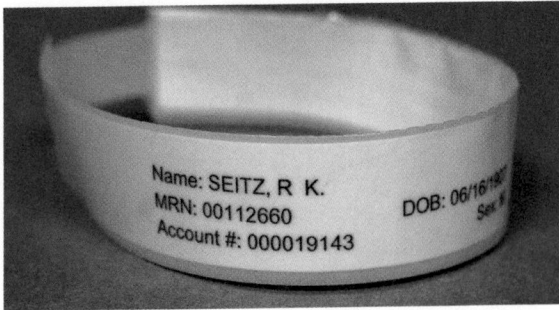

Fig. 12-8 ID bracelet.

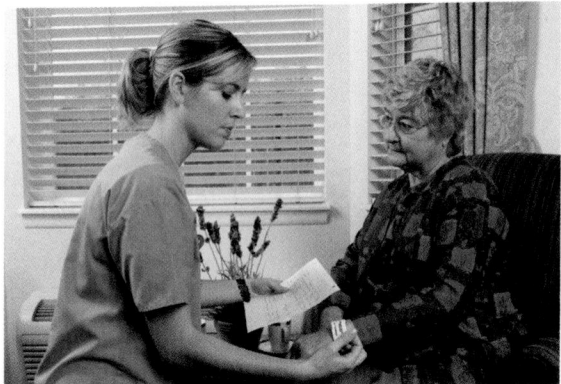

Fig. 12-9 The ID bracelet is checked against the assignment sheet to accurately identify the person.

IDENTIFYING THE PERSON

You will care for many people. Each has different treatments, therapies, and activity limits. You must give the right care to the right person. Life and health are threatened if the wrong care is given.

The person may receive an identification (ID) bracelet when admitted to the agency (Fig. 12-8). The bracelet has the person's name, room and bed number, birth date, age, doctor, and agency name. Other identifying information may include the person's ID number given by the agency. Some agencies include the person's religion.

You use the bracelet to identify the person before giving care. The assignment sheet states what care to give. To identify the person:

- Compare identifying information on the assignment sheet with that on the ID bracelet (Fig. 12-9). Carefully check the information. Some people have the same first and last names. For example, John Smith is a very common name.
- Use at least 2 identifiers. An identifier cannot be the person's room or bed number. Some agencies require that the person state and spell his or her name and give his or her birth date. Others require using the person's ID number. Always follow agency policy.

- Call the person by name when checking the ID bracelet. This is a courtesy given as you touch the person and before giving care. Just calling the person by name is not enough to identify him or her. Confused, disoriented, drowsy, hard-of-hearing, or distracted persons may answer to any name.

See *Focus on Communication: Identifying the Person.*

See *Focus on Long-Term Care and Home Care: Identifying the Person.*

See *Promoting Safety and Comfort: Identifying the Person.*

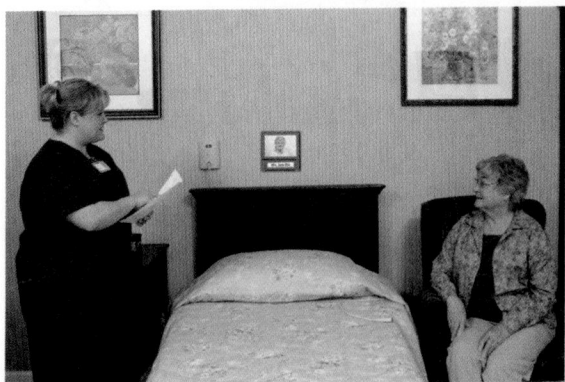

Fig. 12-10 The person's photo is at the head-board. Her name is under the photo. The nursing assistant is using the photo to identify the person.

Safety

Always identify the person before you begin a task or procedure. Do not identify the person and then leave the room to collect supplies and equipment. You could go to the wrong room and give care to the wrong person. And the person for whom the care was intended would not receive it. This too could cause harm.

Sometimes ID bracelets become damaged from water, spilled food and fluids, and everyday wear and tear. Make sure you can read the information on the ID bracelet. If you cannot, tell the nurse. The nurse can have a new bracelet made for the person.

Comfort

Make sure the person's ID bracelet is not too loose or too tight. You should be able to slide 1 or 2 fingers under the bracelet. If it is too loose or too tight, tell the nurse.

TABLE 12-1	WATER TEMPERATURE AND LENGTH OF EXPOSURE FOR A THIRD DEGREE BURN	
Fahrenheit (F)	Centigrade (C)	Time Required for a Third Degree Burn to Occur
155°F	68°C	1 second
148°F	64°C	2 seconds
140°F	60°C	5 seconds
133°F	56°C	15 seconds
127°F	52°C	1 minute
124°F	51°C	3 minutes
120°F	48°C	5 minutes
100°F	37°C	Usually a safe temperature for bathing

Modified from Centers for Medicare & Medicaid Services, *State operations manual,* Baltimore, 2009, U.S. Department of Health and Human Services.

PREVENTING BURNS

Burns are a leading cause of death among children and older persons. Smoking, spilled hot liquids, children playing with matches, barbecue grills, fireplaces, and stoves are common causes. Burns also occur from electrical items and very hot water (hand sinks, tubs, showers).

Burn severity (Chapter 51) depends on water temperature and length of exposure (Table 12-1). The person's condition also is a factor.

- *Superficial (first degree) burn*—involves the epidermis (top layer of skin). Sunburn is an example. The skin is red and painful to touch. There may be mild swelling.
- *Partial-thickness (second degree) burn*—involves the epidermis and dermis. The skin appears deep red. The person has pain and blisters. The skin may appear glossy from leaking fluid.
- *Full-thickness (third degree) burn*—the epidermis and dermis, fat, muscle, and bone may be injured or destroyed. These burns are not painful. Nerve endings are destroyed. The skin appears charred or has white, brown, or black patches.

The safety measures in Box 12-2 can prevent burns.

See *Focus on Children and Older Persons: Preventing Burns,* p. 158.

BOX 12-2	SAFETY MEASURES TO PREVENT BURNS

Children

- Do not leave children home alone.
- Supervise young children at all times.
- Do not leave children alone in the kitchen, bathroom, or a room with a fireplace.
- Secure fireplaces with door guards or gates that are heat-resistant.
- Install barriers around fireplaces, ovens, and furnaces.
- Store matches, lighters, lamp oils, or other flammable materials where children cannot reach them.
- Do not let children near stoves, space heaters, fireplaces, barbecue grills, radiators, registers, oil lamps, candles, curling irons, and other heat sources.
- Keep space heaters and materials that can catch fire away from children.

Children—cont'd

- Teach children fire safety and fire prevention measures. Also teach the dangers of fire.
- Check metal playground equipment before children play. Metal surfaces exposed to sunlight can heat to high temperatures. They can burn the face, hands, arms, legs, and buttocks.
- Check car seats, seat belts, and seat-belt buckles. If hot, they can burn children.
- Cover car seats with towels if you park in the sun. Also use a sun visor for the windshield.
- Do not let children play with fireworks.
- Protect children from sun exposure:
  - Use a sunscreen.
  - Cover exposed areas.
  - Limit time in the sun.

Continued

BOX 12-2	SAFETY MEASURES TO PREVENT BURNS—cont'd

Cooking

- Do not let children help you cook at the stove, in a microwave oven, or on a barbecue grill.
- Use the back burners of stoves when cooking.
- Point pot and pan handles inward. They point away from where people stand and walk.
- Do not leave cooking utensils in pots and pans.
- Do not wear clothing with long sleeves or that is loose-fitting when cooking.
- Keep things that can catch fire away from stoves. This includes paper towels, dish towels, food packages, wooden spoons, oven mitts, curtains, and so on.
- Do not put wet food into frying pans or deep-fryers. The water causes the oil to splatter.
- Use dry oven mitts and pot-holders. Water conducts heat.
- Stay near the stove, oven, microwave oven, and barbecue grill when cooking. Do not leave them unattended.
- Keep hot food and liquids away from counter and table edges. Use the center of the counter or table.
- Turn the oven and stove burners off when not in use.
- Do not pour hot liquids near a child or older person.

Eating and Drinking

- Assist with eating and drinking as needed. Spilled hot food or fluids can cause burns.
- Be careful when carrying hot foods and fluids especially when near children and older persons.

Water

- Set the hot water heater temperature no higher than 120°F.
- Turn on cold water first, then hot water. Turn off hot water first, then cold water.

Water—cont'd

- Measure bath or shower water temperature (Chapter 20). Check it before a person gets into the tub or shower.
- Check for "hot spots" in bath water. Move your hand back and forth.

Appliances

- See "Preventing Equipment Accidents" (p. 167).
- Do not allow the use of space heaters.
- Do not let the person sleep with a heating pad.
- Do not let the person use an electric blanket.
- Turn off curling irons, electric rollers, and hair dryers when not in use.

Smoking

- Be sure patients and residents smoke only in smoking areas.
- Do not leave smoking materials at the bedside. They are only left at the bedside if the person is trusted to smoke alone in smoking areas. Follow the care plan.
- Supervise the smoking of persons who cannot protect themselves.
- Do not allow smoking in bed.
- Do not allow smoking where oxygen is used or stored (Chapter 36).
- Be alert to ashes that may fall onto an older person.

Other

- Follow safety guidelines when applying heat and cold (Chapter 35).

FOCUS ON CHILDREN AND OLDER PERSONS

Preventing Burns

Older Persons

Older persons are at risk for burns. Risk factors include decreased skin thickness, decreased sensitivity to heat, reduced reaction time, decreased mobility, communication problems, confusion, and dementia. Many of the measures in Box 12-2 for children apply to persons who are confused or have dementia.

PREVENTING POISONING

A *poison is any substance harmful to the body when ingested, inhaled, injected, or absorbed through the skin.* If enough is taken, any substance can be poisonous. Poisonings are intentional or unintentional:

- *Unintentional*—the person takes or gives a substance without intending to cause harm. This includes drugs or chemicals used in excessive amounts—an "overdose."
- *Intentional*—the person takes (suicide) or gives (assault or homicide) a substance with the intent to cause harm.

Poisoning is a health hazard and a major cause of death. Children and older persons are at risk. Drugs and household products are common poisons. Poisoning in adults may be from carelessness, confusion, or poor vision when reading labels. As a result, a person may take too much of a drug.

Common poisons include:

- Drugs (legal and illegal) and vitamins
- Household products—detergents, soaps, sprays, furniture polish, window cleaners, bleach, paint, paint thinner, toilet bowl and other cleaners, gasoline, kerosene, glue, and so on
- Personal care products—soaps, shampoos, hair conditioners, bath oils, powders, lotions, nail polish removers, sprays, make-up, perfumes, after-shave lotions, deodorants, mouthwashes, and so on
- Fertilizers, insecticides, bug sprays, and so on
- Lead (p. 160)
- House plants
- Wild mushrooms
- Alcohol
- Carbon monoxide (p. 161)

The measures in Box 12-3 can prevent poisoning.

See *Focus on Long-Term Care and Home Care: Preventing Poisoning*, p. 160.

See *Promoting Safety and Comfort: Preventing Poisoning*, p. 160.

BOX 12-3 SAFETY MEASURES TO PREVENT POISONING

All Ages

- Keep harmful products in high, locked areas (Fig. 12-11). Children and confused persons cannot see or reach them.
- Buy products with child-resistant packaging.
- Keep child-resistant caps on all harmful products. Do not store them in food containers.
- Keep harmful products in their original containers.
- Leave the original label on harmful products (p. 170).
- Store personal care items according to agency policy. Soap, mouthwash, lotion, deodorant, and shampoo are examples. These items could cause harm when swallowed.
- Use and store harmful products according to the manufacturer's instructions (p. 170).
- Do not leave harmful products unattended when in use.
- Do not mix cleaning products.
- Read all labels carefully before using the product. Have good lighting.
- Do not store harmful products near food.
- Discard harmful products that are outdated (p. 170).
- Use safety latches on kitchen, bathroom, utility, garage, basement, and workshop cabinets and drawers.
- Discard poisonous household plants. Or place them where persons at risk cannot reach them.
- Keep emergency numbers by the telephone: Poison Control Center (1-800-222-1222), police, ambulance, hospital, and doctor.
- Prevent carbon monoxide poisoning (p. 161).

Children

- Keep children in your sight when using a harmful product.
- Teach children not to eat plants and unknown foods. Teach them not to eat leaves, stems, seeds, berries, nuts, or bark.
- Do not leave lamp oil, lamps with lamp oil, or candles containing lamp oil where children can reach them. Lamp oil is very harmful if ingested.
- Do not take drugs in front of children.
- Do not call drugs or vitamins "candy."
- Place warning stickers ("Mr. Yuk") on harmful substances (Fig. 12-12).
- Do not let children have access to purses, handbags, briefcases, or similar items. Many people have drugs in such items. This includes family and friends.
- Supervise children when visiting family and friends. Look for harmful products in and on counters, tables, bathrooms, and other areas and surfaces.
- Prevent lead poisoning (p. 160).

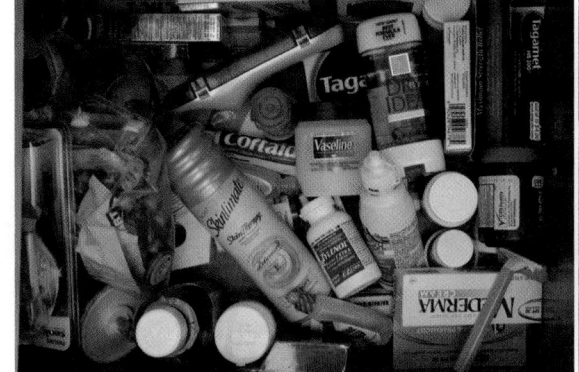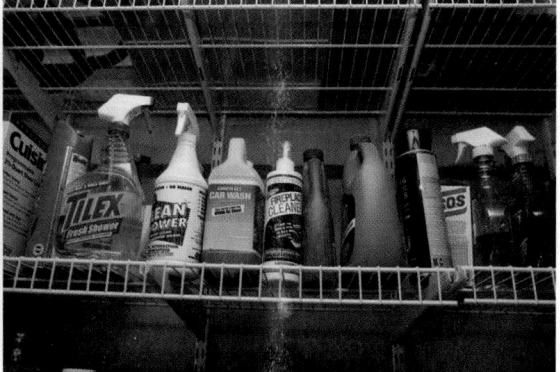

Fig. 12-11 Harmful products must be kept in locked areas and out of the reach of children. **A,** Bathroom drawers and cabinets hold many harmful products. **B,** Household cleaners must be kept out of reach.

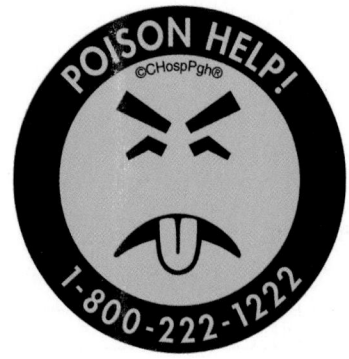

Fig. 12-12 The "Mr. Yuk" warning sticker is placed on harmful products.

Preventing Poisoning

Home Care
Provide good lighting when patients are taking their drugs. Make sure they read prescription labels correctly and are taking the correct drug and dosage (Chapter 50).

Bathroom medicine cabinets, drawers, and counters need to be checked for outdated products and drugs. Also check for such items in kitchens and bedrooms. To safely dispose of outdated products and drugs:
- Obtain permission from the person and the nurse.
- Follow agency policy for disposal.

Preventing Poisoning

Safety
The Poison Control Center number is 1-800-222-1222. If you need to call the Poison Control Center, give the following information:
- The person's age
- The person's weight
- The person's condition and health problems
- The substance, containers, or bottles involved
- How the substance entered the body:
  - Swallowed
  - Inhaled or smelled
  - Injected
  - Skin contact
  - Splashed into the eyes
- When the substance entered the body
- First aid given
- If the person has vomited
- Your location, name, and phone number
- Distance to the nearest hospital

Lead Poisoning

Lead is a metal. When in the body, it affects normal body functions. It can injure the brain, nervous system, red blood cells, kidneys, liver, teeth, and bones. It can lower intelligence and cause learning problems and behavior problems.

Lead is found in batteries, pipes, pottery glazes, printing inks, industrial paints, plastics, crystal, and dirt. The use of lead in household paint was banned in the 1970s. However, many older homes still have lead paint on walls and other surfaces. Old pipes and old painted furniture are other sources of lead. So are toys made outside of the United States.

Lead enters the body through:
- *Inhalation.* Dust in the air may contain lead. Windows may have lead-based paint. When widows are open and closed, dust is created. Dust from soil may contain lead.
- *Ingestion.* Young children can eat, chew, and suck on non-food items that may contain lead. Toys and lead-painted surfaces—window sills and railings—are examples. They may eat paint chips. Water is a source of lead if plumbing materials contain lead.

Children between the ages of 6 months and 6 years are at risk for lead poisoning. Lead can affect almost every body system. Signs and symptoms are gradual in onset. They are not always obvious. See Box 12-4.

See *Focus on Long-Term Care and Home Care: Lead Poisoning.*

BOX 12-4   LEAD POISONING

Signs and Symptoms of Lead Poisoning in Children
- Abdominal pain
- Activity: decreased
- Appetite: poor
- Behavior problems
- Constipation
- Coordination: poor
- Diarrhea
- Fatigue
- Growth: decreased
- Headaches
- Hearing loss
- Hyperactivity
- Irritability
- Language problems
- Learning problems
- Memory problems
- Muscle weakness
- Pallor

Signs and Symptoms of Lead Poisoning in Children—cont'd
- Reflexes: slow
- Seizures
- Sleep: increased
- Sluggishness
- Speech problems
- Vomiting
- Weight loss

Safety Measures to Prevent Lead Poisoning
- Prevent or discourage children from eating, chewing, or sucking on non-food items. They include:
  - Toys and furniture painted before 1978
  - Painted toys and decorations made outside the United States
  - Paint chips
  - Dirt
  - Keys
  - Pewter and lead-based figurines
  - Fishing sinkers

Modified from www.keepkidshealthy.com.

BOX 12-4 LEAD POISONING—cont'd

Safety Measures to Prevent Lead Poisoning—cont'd
- Do not let children play in dirt. Have them play in grassy or sandy areas.
- Assist the child with hand washing before eating, after playing outside, and before going to bed.
- Wash toys often.
- Rinse pacifiers, baby bottles, and other items that fall to the floor.
- Prevent exposure to lead-based plumbing:
  - Let cold water run for 1 to 2 minutes before drinking water or using it for coffee or cooking. This helps flush the lead out of the plumbing.
  - Do not use hot tap water to make baby formula.
  - Do not use hot tap water for cooking or drinking.
- Prevent exposure to lead-based paint:
  - Keep children away from paint chips.
  - Keep children away from dust contaminated with lead paint.
  - Do not sweep or vacuum lead-based paint dust or paint chips.
  - Use a wet mop and wet cloths to clean up dust and paint chips.
  - Use a wet mop and wet cloths to clean furniture, window sills, and dusty surfaces.
  - Use duct tape to cover peeling or chipping paint. This is only a temporary measure. Peeling and chipping paint must be removed.

Safety Measures to Prevent Lead Poisoning—cont'd
- Do not bump into walls or furniture that may contain lead-based paint. This prevents dust and paint chips.
- Do not open and close windows that have lead-based paint. This prevents dust and paint chips.
- Prevent exposure to food contaminated with lead:
  - Do not use glazed pottery to cook food.
  - Do not eat foods that are stored or served in glazed pottery.
  - Do not eat foods that are canned outside the United States.
  - Wash fruits and vegetables before eating or serving them. They may have been grown in soil that contains lead.
- Prevent children from having contact with work or hobby materials that may contain lead. Welding, pottery, home building and repair, and automotive repair products and supplies are examples. So are children's paint sets and art supplies.
  - Store lead-based products where children cannot see or reach them.
  - Take shoes off before entering the home.
  - Shower and change clothes before having contact with children.
  - Wash and store clothes contaminated with lead separately from others.
- Do not let children handle or play with old newspapers, magazines, or comic books. The ink may contain lead.

FOCUS ON LONG-TERM CARE AND HOME CARE
Lead Poisoning

Home Care
Household dust is a major source of lead. Window sills and window wells contain high levels of leaded dust. The Centers for Disease Control and Prevention (CDC) recommends cleaning floors, window sills, window wells, and other surfaces every 2 to 3 weeks. For cleaning, the CDC recommends using a wet mop for floors and wet-wiping other surfaces.

The CDC also recommends keeping windows shut to avoid chipping painted surfaces. If windows are to be opened, the CDC suggests opening them from the top.

FOCUS ON CHILDREN AND OLDER PERSONS
Carbon Monoxide Poisoning

Older Persons
According to the CDC, more than 400 people die each year from unintentional CO poisoning. The death rate is highest among persons 65 years and older.

Carbon Monoxide Poisoning

Carbon monoxide (CO) is a colorless, odorless, and tasteless gas. It is produced by the burning of fuel—gas, oil, kerosene, wood, charcoal. Motor vehicles, furnaces, gas water heaters, gas stoves, lanterns, and gas clothes dryers use fuel. These devices must be in good working order and must be used correctly. Otherwise, dangerous levels of CO can build up in closed or semi-closed areas. Instead of breathing in oxygen, the person breathes in air filled with CO. Red blood cells pick up CO faster than oxygen. Oxygen does not get into the body. CO can damage tissues and cause sudden illness and death.

People and animals are at risk for CO poisoning. Those who are sleeping or intoxicated can die before having symptoms. CO poisoning may be unintentional or intentional as a suicide attempt. See Box 12-5, p. 162 for the signs and symptoms of CO poisoning and related safety measures.

See *Focus on Children and Older Persons: Carbon Monoxide Poisoning.*

BOX 12-5 CARBON MONOXIDE POISONING

Signs and Symptoms
- Breathing problems
- Cherry-pink skin
- Chest pain
- Confusion
- Dizziness
- Fainting
- Headache
- Nausea
- Sleepiness
- Slurred speech
- Vomiting
- Weakness

Safety Measures to Prevent Carbon Monoxide Poisoning
- Have CO detectors installed in each sleeping area.
- Have vehicle exhaust systems checked regularly.
- Have fuel-burning appliances checked regularly. This includes furnaces, gas water heaters, gas stoves and ovens, gas clothes dryers, gas or kerosene space heaters, fireplaces, and wood stoves.
- Follow the manufacturer's instructions when using fuel-burning devices.

Safety Measures to Prevent Carbon Monoxide Poisoning—cont'd
- Use the correct fuel when using fuel-burning devices.
- Do not idle a vehicle, lawn mower, snow blower, weed trimmer, or other device in an open or closed area or garage. Fumes can leak into the house.
- Have fuel-burning devices and chimneys checked when people in the same building show signs and symptoms.
- If you or others have signs and symptoms:
  - Open doors and windows.
  - Turn off appliances.
  - Leave the home.
  - Go to an emergency room.
- Open doors and windows if you notice gas odors. Turn off appliances, and leave the home.
- Have gas odors checked by trained professionals.
- Do not use a gas stove or oven to heat a home or room. Do not use a gas stove or oven to dry clothing or other items.
- Do not use charcoal grills, barbecue grills, and gas camp stoves indoors or in a garage.
- Never burn charcoal indoors.
- Do not use a generator indoors, in a basement, in a garage, or by a window, door, or vent.

BOX 12-6 SAFETY MEASURES TO PREVENT SUFFOCATION

All Age-Groups
- Cut food into small, bite-sized pieces for persons who cannot do so themselves.
- Make sure dentures fit properly and are in place.
- Make sure the person can chew and swallow the food served.
- Report loose teeth or dentures.
- Check the care plan for swallowing problems before serving food (including snacks) or fluids. The person may ask for something that he or she cannot swallow.
- Tell the nurse at once if the person has swallowing problems.
- Do not give oral food or fluids to persons with feeding tubes (Chapter 25).
- Follow aspiration precautions (Chapter 24).
- Do not leave a person unattended in a bathtub or shower.
- Remove the key for a gas fireplace. Store it out of reach.
- Move all persons from the area if you smell smoke.
- Position the person in bed properly (Chapter 16).
- Use bed rails correctly (Chapter 13).
- Use restraints correctly (Chapter 14).
- Prevent entrapment in the bed system (Chapter 18).
- Do not use power strips for care equipment.
- See "Preventing Equipment Accidents" (p. 167).

Children
- Keep plastic bags, covers, and dry-cleaning bags away from children.
- Tie large plastic bags and garment bags in knots. Then discard them.
- Place childproof covers on outlets. This includes electrical strips and surge protectors.
- Use safety plugs in outlets with caution. Children can remove and choke on them. And they can be misplaced when removed to use the outlet.
- Keep electrical cords and electrical items out of the reach of children.
- Position infants on their backs for sleep. (See Chapter 49.)
- Do not use pillows to position infants.
- Do not use pillows to prevent infants from falling off of beds and furniture.
- Remove pillows, loose sheets or blankets, comforters, quilts, sheepskin, stuffed toys, crib bumpers, sleep positioners, and other soft items from the crib when the baby is sleeping.
- Have babies wear sleep sacks to keep them warm when sleeping. A sleep sack is a wearable blanket.

BOX 12-6	SAFETY MEASURES TO PREVENT SUFFOCATION—cont'd

Children—cont'd

- Do not let toddlers sleep on soft surfaces. This includes couches, chairs, and regular beds.
- Do not feed an infant while he or she is lying down.
- Have children sit when they eat. They should not eat or suck on anything while lying down or playing.
- Do not give infants and young children small, round, or hard foods. This includes hot dogs, peanuts, popcorn, nuts, grapes, raisins, hard candy, jellybeans, gum, raw vegetables, raw and unpeeled fruit slices, dried fruits, and chunks of meat.
- Cut foods into small pieces.
- Give infants soft foods that do not require chewing.
- Practice balloon safety:
  - Use Mylar balloons instead of latex ones.
  - Store latex balloons where children cannot see or reach them.
  - Do not let children inflate or deflate latex balloons.
  - Deflate and discard latex balloons after use.
  - Pick up and discard broken balloon pieces at once. Do not let children near them.

Children—cont'd

- Check floors for small objects—buttons, coins, beads, marbles, pins, tacks, nails, screws, jewelry, and so on. Keep them out of a child's reach. Pick up and store or discard such objects. Children can choke on them. When checking floors, it is best to get on the floor on your hands and knees—the child's eye level.
- Check toys for removable parts.
- Do not string or hang any object on or near a crib. This includes a mobile, toy, or diaper bag. The child could get caught in it and strangle.
- Never tie pacifiers or teethers around a child's neck.
- Do not use bibs that tie around the baby's neck.
- Remove bibs and necklaces whenever the child is put in a crib or playpen.
- Keep appliance doors closed—ovens, refrigerators, clothes dryers, washing machines, refrigerators, freezers, dishwashers, coolers, and so on.
- Remove rubber knobs or tips from door stops.

PREVENTING SUFFOCATION

Suffocation is when breathing stops from the lack of oxygen. Death occurs if the person does not start breathing. Common causes include choking, drowning, inhaling gas or smoke, strangulation, and electrical shock (p. 167).

Measures to prevent suffocation are listed in Box 12-6. Clear the airway if the person is choking.

Choking

Foreign bodies can obstruct the airway. This is called *choking* or *foreign-body airway obstruction (FBAO)*. Air cannot pass through the airways into the lungs. The body does not get enough oxygen. It can lead to cardiac arrest. *Cardiac arrest* is when the heart stops suddenly and without warning (Chapter 51).

Choking often occurs during eating. A large, poorly chewed piece of meat is the most common cause. Laughing and talking while eating also are common causes. So is excessive alcohol intake.

Unconscious persons can choke. Common causes are aspiration of vomitus and the tongue falling back into the airway. These also occur during cardiac arrest.

Foreign bodies can cause mild or severe airway obstruction. With *mild airway obstruction*, some air moves in and out of the lungs. The person is conscious and usually can speak. Often forceful coughing can remove the object. Breathing may sound like wheezing between coughs. For mild airway obstruction:

- Stay with the person.
- Encourage the person to keep coughing to expel the object.
- Do not interrupt the person's efforts to clear the airway. If the person is breathing and coughing, abdominal thrusts are not needed.
- If the obstruction persists, call for help.

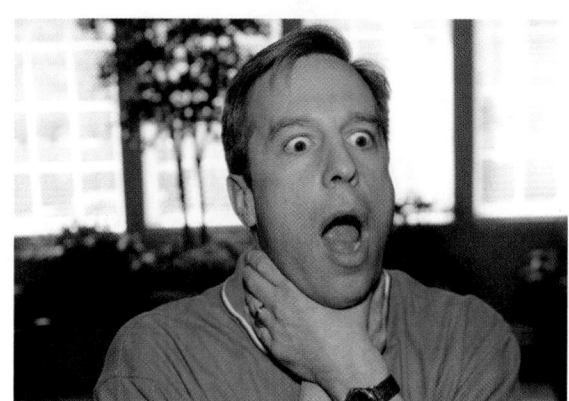

Fig. 12-13 A choking person clutches at the throat.

A person with *severe airway obstruction* has difficulty breathing. Air does not move in and out of the lungs. The person may not be able to breathe, speak, or cough. If able to cough, the cough is of poor quality. Infants cannot cry. When the person tries to inhale, there is no noise or a high-pitched noise. The person may appear pale and cyanotic (bluish color).

The conscious person clutches at the throat (Fig. 12-13). Clutching at the throat is often called the "universal sign of choking." The conscious person is very frightened. If the obstruction is not removed, the person will die. Severe airway obstruction is an emergency.

Relieving Choking. Abdominal thrusts are used to relieve severe airway obstruction. Abdominal thrusts are quick, upward thrusts to the abdomen. They force air out of the lungs and create an artificial cough. They are done to try to expel the foreign body from the airway.

Abdominal thrusts are not used for very obese persons or pregnant women. Chest thrusts are used (Box 12-7 and Fig. 12-14, p. 164).

BOX 12-7	CHOKING–CHEST THRUSTS FOR OBESE OR PREGNANT PERSONS

1 Stand behind the person.
2 Place your arms under the person's underarms. Wrap your arms around the person's chest.
3 Make a fist. Place the thumb side of the fist on the middle of the sternum (breastbone).
4 Grasp the fist with your other hand.
5 Give chest thrusts until the object is expelled or the person becomes unresponsive.
6 If the person becomes unresponsive, activate the Emergency Medical Services (EMS) system or the agency's Rapid Response Team (RRT). This team quickly responds to give care in life-threatening situations. Start cardiopulmonary resuscitation (CPR). See Chapter 51.

You may observe a person choking. And you may perform emergency measures to relieve choking. Relief of choking occurs when the foreign body is removed. Or it occurs when you feel air move and see the chest rise and fall when giving rescue breaths. The person may still be unresponsive.

If you assist a choking person, report and record what happened. Include what you did and the person's response. See Figure 12-15.

See *Focus on Children and Older Persons: Choking.*

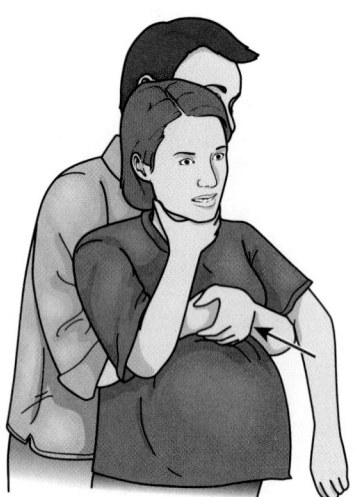

Fig. 12-14 Chest thrusts to relieve choking in a pregnant woman.

FOCUS ON CHILDREN AND OLDER PERSONS
Choking

Children
Children can choke on small objects. Pieces of hot dogs, marbles, hard candy, peanuts, apples, and grapes are examples. Peanut butter and popcorn also can cause choking. So can coins and small toys and toy parts. FBAO in children is marked by the *sudden* onset of symptoms.

Respiratory infections can cause airway obstruction in infants and children. Airway structures become swollen. The airway narrows or becomes completely obstructed. Air cannot enter the airway. The child needs emergency care at once.

The procedures that follow will not relieve airway obstruction caused by an infection. Do not try them if the child has a fever, rash, congestion, hoarseness, or other signs and symptoms of respiratory infection. You will waste precious time. Activate the EMS system or the agency's RRT. Give rescue breaths if the child is not breathing but has a pulse. Start CPR if the child is not responding, not breathing or not breathing normally (gasping), and has no pulse. See Chapter 51.

Abdominal thrusts are not given to infants. They can damage the liver and other organs. Back slaps (back blows) and chest thrusts are used for infants. See the procedure *Relieving Choking—In the Infant (Less Than 1 Year of Age)* (p. 166).

Older Persons
Older persons are at risk for choking. Weakness, dentures that fit poorly, dysphagia (difficulty swallowing), and chronic illness are common causes.

Date	Time	Nursing Margin	Other Depts Margin
9-10	1215	While eating lunch, Mrs. Rand began coughing and clutching at her throat. Her	
		tablemate shouted "she's choking." I went to Mrs. Rand's table. She mouthed the words	
		"I can't breathe." I performed abdominal thrusts with Mrs. Rand sitting in her	
		chair. After three abdominal thrusts, she coughed out a piece of meat. She then	
		began breathing. Mary Jones, RN arrived and took over the care of Mrs. Rand.	
		Ben Armes, CNA.	

Fig. 12-15 Charting sample for choking.

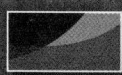

RELIEVING CHOKING—ADULT OR CHILD (OVER 1 YEAR OF AGE)

PROCEDURE

1 Ask the person if he or she is choking. Help the person if he or she nods "yes" and cannot talk.

2 Have someone call for help:

  a *In a public area*, have someone activate the EMS system by calling 911. Send someone to get an automated external defibrillator (AED). See Chapter 51.

  b *In an agency*, have someone call the RRT. Send someone to get the AED.

3 *If the person is standing or sitting*, give abdominal thrusts:

  a Stand or kneel behind the person.

  b Wrap your arms around the person's waist.

  c Make a fist with one hand.

  d Place the thumb side of the fist against the abdomen. The fist is slightly above the navel in the middle of the abdomen and well below the end of the sternum (breastbone). See Figure 12-16, A.

  e Grasp the fist with your other hand (Fig. 12-16, B).

  f Press your fist into the person's abdomen with a quick, upward thrust (Fig. 12-17, p. 166).

  g Repeat thrusts until the object is expelled or the person becomes unresponsive.

4 *If the person is lying down but responsive*, give abdominal thrusts (Fig. 12-18, p. 166):

  a Straddle the person's thighs.

  b Place the heel of one hand against the abdomen. It is in the middle slightly above the navel and well below the end of the sternum (breastbone).

  c Place your second hand on top of your first hand.

  d Press both hands into the abdomen with a quick, upward thrust.

  e Repeat thrusts until the object is expelled or the person becomes unresponsive.

5 *If the object is dislodged,* encourage the person to go to the hospital. Injuries can occur from abdominal thrusts.

6 *If the person becomes unresponsive,* lower the person to the floor or ground. Position the person supine (lying flat on the back). Make sure EMS or the RRT was called (step 2). If alone, provide 5 cycles (2 minutes) of CPR first. Then call EMS or the RRT.

7 Start CPR. See Chapter 51.

  a Do not check for a pulse. Begin with compressions. Give 30 compressions. Chest compressions help dislodge an obstruction. (See Chapter 51 for 2-rescuer child CPR.)

  b Use the head tilt-chin lift method to open the airway (Fig. 12-19, p. 166). Open the person's mouth. The mouth should be wide open. Look for an object. Remove the object if you see it and can remove it easily. Use your fingers.

  c Give 2 breaths.

  d Continue cycles of 30 compressions and 2 breaths. Look for an object every time you open the airway for rescue breaths.

8 *If you relieve choking in an unresponsive person:*

  a Check for a response, breathing, and a pulse.

    1 *If no response, normal breathing, or pulse*— continue CPR. Attach an AED (Chapter 51).

    2 *If no response and no normal breathing but there is a pulse*—give rescue breaths. For an adult, give 1 breath every 5 to 6 seconds (10 to 12 breaths per minute). For a child, give 1 breath every 3 to 5 seconds (12 to 20 breaths per minute). Check for a pulse every 2 minutes. If no pulse, begin CPR.

    3 *If the person has normal breathing and a pulse*— place the person in the recovery position if there is no response (Chapter 51). Continue to check the person until help arrives. Encourage the person to go to the hospital if the person responds.

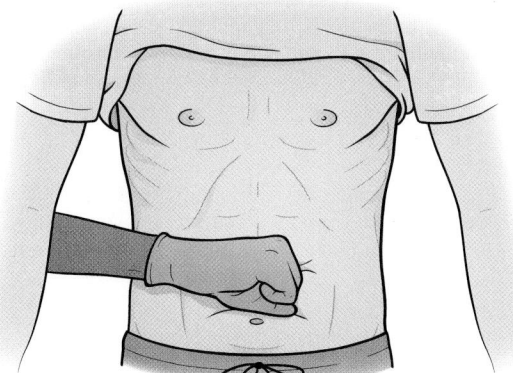
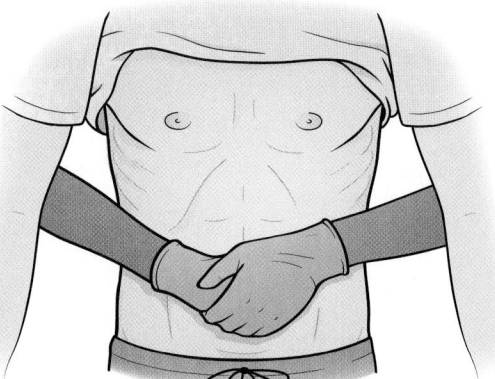

Fig. 12-16 Hand positioning for abdominal thrusts. **A,** The fist is slightly above the navel in the midline of the abdomen. **B,** The other hand clasps the fist.

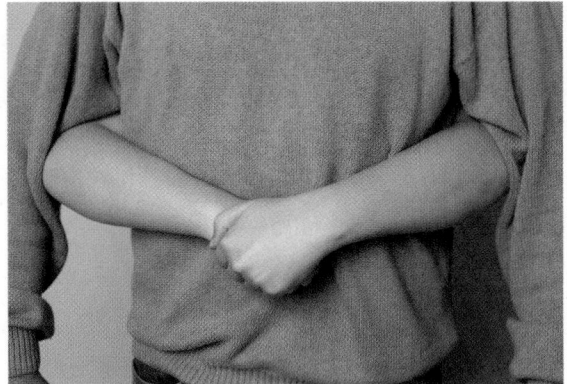

Fig. 12-17 Abdominal thrusts with the person standing.

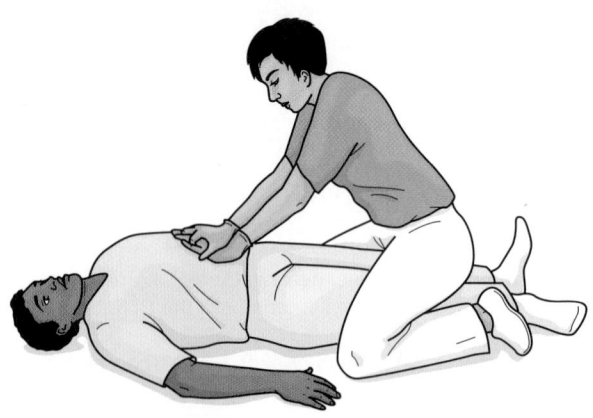

Fig. 12-18 Abdominal thrusts with the person lying down.

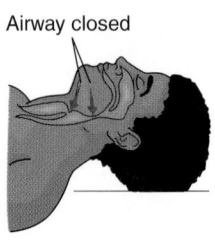

Airway closed

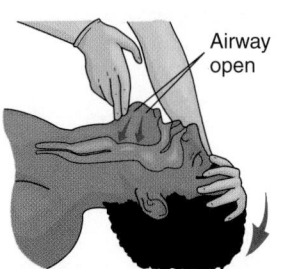

Airway open

Fig. 12-19 The head tilt–chin lift method opens the airway. One hand is on the person's forehead. Pressure is applied to lift the head back. The chin is lifted with the fingers of the other hand.

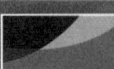

RELIEVING CHOKING—IN THE INFANT (LESS THAN 1 YEAR OF AGE)

PROCEDURE

1 Have someone call for help:
 a *In a public area*, have someone activate the EMS system by calling 911. Send someone to get an AED. See Chapter 51.
 b *In an agency*, have someone call the agency's RRT and get a defibrillator (AED).
2 Kneel next to the infant. Or sit with the infant in your lap.
3 Expose the infant's chest and back. Perform this step only if it can be done easily.
4 Hold the infant facedown over your forearm. (Support your arm on your thigh or lap.) The infant's head is lower than the chest. Support the head and jaw with your hand.
5 Give up to 5 forceful back slaps (back blows) (Fig. 12-20). Use the heel of your hand. Give the back slaps between the shoulder blades. (Stop the back slaps if the object is expelled.)
6 Turn the infant as a unit:
 a Continue to support the infant's face, jaw, head, neck, and chest with one hand.
 b Support the back and the back of the infant's head with your other hand. Your palm supports the back of the head.
 c Turn the infant as a unit. The infant is in a back-lying position on your forearm. Your forearm rests on your thigh. The infant's head is lower than the chest.

7 Give up to 5 chest thrusts (Fig. 12-21). The chest thrusts are quick and downward.
 a Locate hand position as for chest compressions (Chapter 51). The location is just below the nipple line in the center of the chest.
 b Give chest thrusts at a rate of about 1 every second.
 c Stop chest thrusts if the object is expelled.
8 Continue giving 5 back slaps followed by 5 chest thrusts until:
 a The object is expelled.
 b The infant becomes unresponsive.
9 *If the infant becomes unresponsive:*
 a Send someone to activate the EMS system or the RRT if not already done (step 1). If alone, do so after 2 minutes of CPR.
 b Place the infant on a firm, flat surface.
 c Start CPR (Chapter 51). Begin with compressions. Give 30 compressions. (See Chapter 51 for infant CPR.)
 d Open the airway. Use the head tilt-chin lift method. Open the infant's mouth. Look for an object. Remove the object if you see it and can remove it easily. Use your fingers.
 e Give 2 breaths.
 f Continue cycles of 30 compressions and 2 breaths. Look for an object each time you open the airway.
 g Continue CPR until help arrives or until choking is relieved.

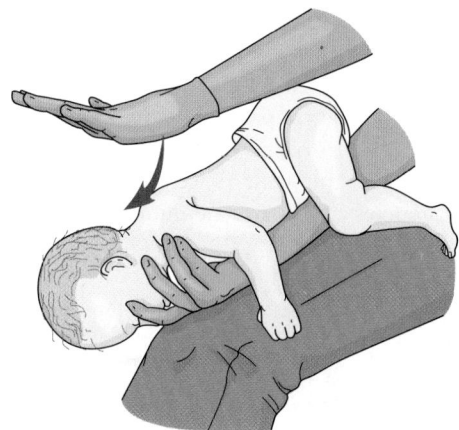

Fig. 12-20 Back slaps (back blows). The infant is held face down and supported with one hand. The rescuer's forearm is supported on his or her thigh. Back slaps are given between the shoulder blades with the heel of one hand.

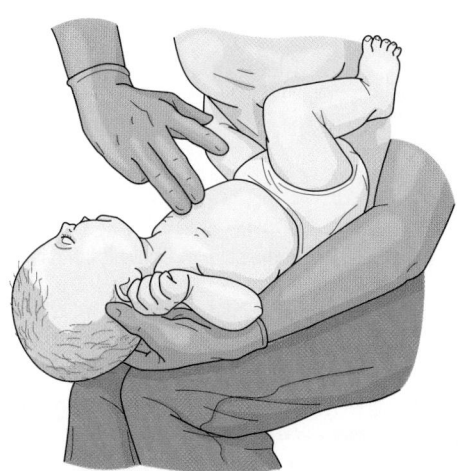

Fig. 12-21 Chest thrusts. The infant is in the back-lying position. Hand position for chest thrusts is the same as for chest compressions (Chapter 51).

Self-administered abdominal thrusts. You may choke when by yourself. Perform abdominal thrusts to relieve the obstructed airway.

1 Make a fist with one hand.
2 Place the thumb side of the fist above your navel and below the lower end of the sternum.
3 Grasp your fist with your other hand.
4 Press inward and upward quickly.
5 Press the upper abdomen against a hard surface if the thrust did not relieve the obstruction. Use the back of a chair, a table, or a railing.
6 Use as many thrusts as needed.

The unresponsive adult. You may find an adult who is unresponsive. You did not see the person lose consciousness, and you do not know the cause. Do not assume the cause is choking. Check to see if the person is responding. If not, start CPR (Chapter 51).

PREVENTING EQUIPMENT ACCIDENTS

All equipment is unsafe if broken, not used correctly, or not working properly. This includes hospital beds. Inspect all equipment before use. Check glass and plastic items for cracks, chips, and sharp or rough edges. They can cause cuts, stabs, or scratches. Follow the Bloodborne Pathogen Standard (Chapter 15).

Electrical Equipment

Electrical items must work properly and be in good repair. Frayed cords (Fig. 12-22) and over-loaded electrical outlets (Fig. 12-23) can cause fires, burns, and electrical shocks. *Electrical shock is when electrical current passes through the body.* It can burn the skin, muscles, nerves, and other tissues. It can affect the heart and cause death.

Three-pronged plugs (Fig. 12-24) are used on all electrical items. Two prongs carry electrical current. The third

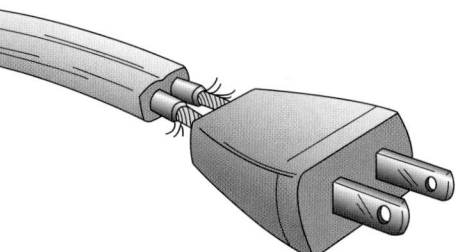

Fig. 12-22 A frayed electrical cord.

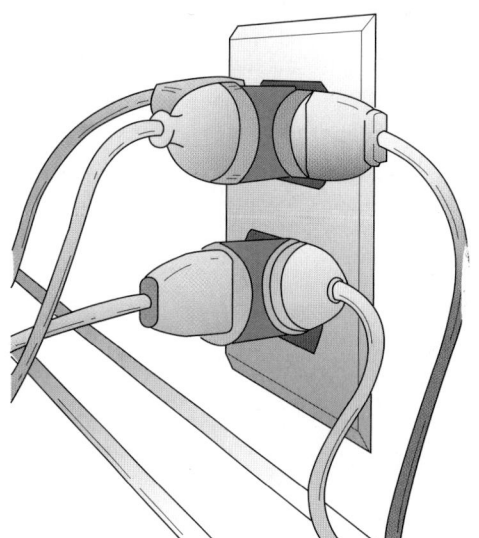

Fig. 12-23 An over-loaded electrical outlet.

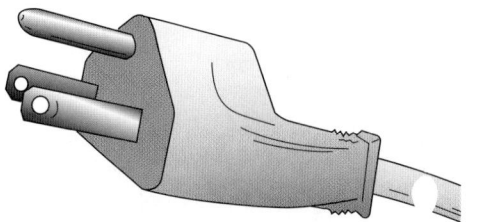

Fig. 12-24 A three-pronged plug.

prong is the ground. *A ground carries leaking electricity to the earth and away from an electrical item.* If a ground is not used, leaking electricity can be conducted to the person. It can cause electrical shocks and possible death. If you receive a shock, report it at once. Do not use the item.

Warning signs of a faulty electrical item include:
- Shocks
- Loss of power or a power outage
- Dimming or flickering lights
- Sparks
- Sizzling or buzzing sounds
- Burning odor
- Loose plugs

Do not use or give damaged items to patients or residents. Take the item to the nurse. The nurse will have you do one of the following:
- Discard the item following agency policy.
- Tag the item and send it for repair following agency policy.

Practice the safety measures in Box 12-8 when using equipment. An incident report (p. 181) is completed if a patient, resident, visitor, or staff member has an equipment-related accident. The Safe Medical Devices Act requires that agencies report equipment-related illnesses, injuries, and deaths.

Bariatric-Safe Equipment

Beds, chairs, wheelchairs, stretchers, toilets, commodes, and other equipment usually have a weight capacity of 250 to 350 pounds. Bariatric patients and residents can weigh from 250 pounds to over 1000 pounds. The equipment used must support the person's weight.

Many agencies have bariatric equipment. Such equipment is labeled with:
- "EC" for "expanded capacity"
- The weight limit suggested by the manufacturer

You must know the weight capacity of the equipment and the person's weight. Do not use the item if the person's weight is greater than the weight capacity. Follow the nurse's directions and the care plan.

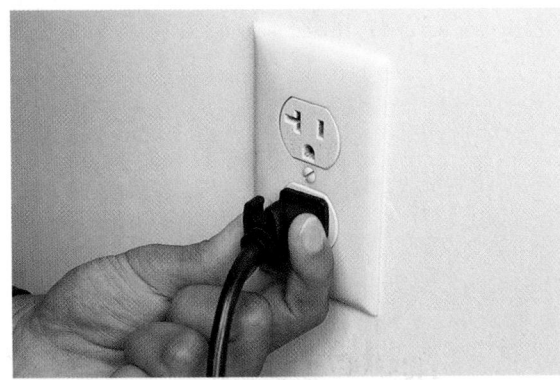

Fig. 12-25 Hold on to the plug to remove it from an outlet.

BOX 12-8 SAFETY MEASURES TO PREVENT EQUIPMENT ACCIDENTS

General Safety
- Follow agency policies and procedures.
- Follow the manufacturer's instructions. Use equipment correctly.
- Read all caution and warning labels.
- Do not use an unfamiliar item. Ask for needed training. Also ask a nurse to supervise you the first time you use an item.
- Use an item only for its intended purpose.
- Make sure the item works before you begin.
- Make sure you have all needed equipment. For example, you need to plug in an item. There must be an outlet.
- Show a broken or damaged item to the nurse. Follow the nurse's instructions and agency policies for discarding items or sending them for repair.
- Do not try to repair broken or damaged items.
- Do not use broken or damaged items.

Electrical Safety
- Inspect electrical cords and appliances for damage. Make sure they are in good repair.
- Use three-pronged plugs on all electrical devices.
- Avoid using extension cords. If one is needed, use it for only one device. This prevents over-loading a circuit.
- Do not use power strips for care equipment.
- Do not cover any electrical cord with rugs, carpets, linens, or other materials. Do not run power cords under rugs.

Electrical Safety—cont'd
- Connect a bed power cord directly to a wall outlet. Do not connect a bed power cord to an extension cord or outlet strip.
- Do not use electrical items owned by the person until they are safety checked. The maintenance staff does this.
- Keep electrical items away from water.
- Keep work areas clean and dry. Wipe up spills right away.
- Do not touch electrical items if you are wet, if your hands are wet, or if you are standing in water.
- Do not put a finger or any item into an outlet.
- Turn off equipment before unplugging it. Sparks occur when electrical items are unplugged while turned on.
- Hold on to the plug (not the cord) when removing it from an outlet (Fig. 12-25).
- Do not give showers or tub baths during electrical storms. Lightning can travel through pipes.
- Do not use electrical items or phones during storms.
- Do not use water to put out an electrical fire. If possible, turn off or unplug the item.
- Do not touch a person who is having an electrical shock. If possible, turn off or unplug the item. Call for help at once.
- Keep electrical cords away from heating vents and other heat sources.
- Turn off the device when done using the item.
- Unplug all devices when not in use.

WHEELCHAIR AND STRETCHER SAFETY

Some people cannot walk or they have severe problems walking. A wheelchair may be useful (Fig. 12-26). If able, the person propels the chair using the hand rims. Some use their feet to move the chair. Other wheelchairs are propelled by motors. The person moves the chair with hand, chin, mouth, or other controls. If the person cannot propel the wheelchair, another person pushes it using the hand grips/push handles.

Stretchers are used to transport persons who cannot use wheelchairs. They cannot sit up or must lie down.

Follow the safety measures in Box 12-9 when using wheelchairs and stretchers. The person can fall from the wheelchair or stretcher. Or the person can fall during transfers to and from the wheelchair or stretcher.

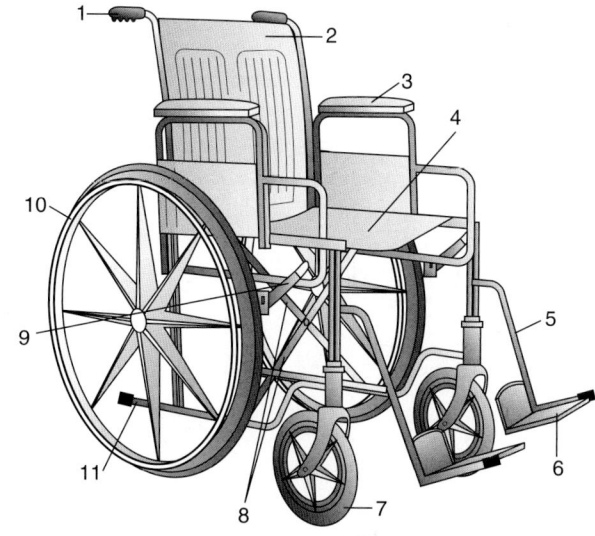

1 Hand grip/push handle	7 Caster
2 Back upholstery	8 Crossbrace
3 Armrest	9 Wheel lock/brake
4 Seat upholstery	10 Wheel and hand rim
5 Front rigging	11 Tipping lever
6 Footplate	

Fig. 12-26 Parts of a wheelchair.

BOX 12-9 | WHEELCHAIR AND STRETCHER SAFETY

Wheelchair Safety

- Check the wheel locks (brakes). Make sure you can lock and unlock them.
- Check for flat or loose tires. A wheel lock will not work on a flat or loose tire.
- Make sure the wheel spokes are intact. Damaged, broken, or loose spokes can interfere with moving the wheelchair or locking the wheels.
- Make sure the casters point forward. This keeps the wheelchair balanced and stable.
- Position the person's feet on the footplates.
- Make sure the person's feet are on the footplates before moving the chair. The person's feet must not touch or drag on the floor when the chair is moving.
- Push the chair forward when transporting the person. Do not pull the chair backward unless going through a doorway or down a steep ramp or incline.
- Follow the care plan and agency policy for the number of staff needed to transport the person. As many as 4 staff members may be needed. This depends on:
  - The person's weight
  - If the person is cooperative
  - If the wheelchair is powered
- Lock both wheels before you transfer a person to or from the wheelchair.
- Follow the care plan for keeping the wheels locked when not moving the wheelchair. Locking the wheels prevents the chair from moving if the person wants to move to or from the chair. (Locking the wheelchair may be viewed as a restraint. See Chapter 14.)
- Do not let the person stand on the footplates.
- Do not let the footplates fall back onto the person's legs.

Wheelchair Safety—cont'd

- Make sure the person has needed wheelchair accessories—safety belt, pouch, tray, lapboard, cushion.
- Remove the armrests (if removable) when the person transfers to the bed, toilet, commode, tub, or car (Chapter 17).
- Swing front rigging out of the way for transfers to and from the wheelchair. Some front riggings detach for transfers.
- Clean the wheelchair according to agency policy.
- Ask a nurse or physical therapist to show you how to propel wheelchairs up steps and ramps and over curbs.
- Follow the safety measures to prevent equipment accidents (p. 167).

Stretcher Safety

- Ask 2 or more co-workers to help you transfer the person to or from the stretcher (Chapter 17).
- Lock the stretcher wheels before the transfer.
- Fasten the safety straps when the person is properly positioned on the stretcher.
- Follow the care plan and agency policy for the number of staff needed to transport the person. As many as 4 staff members may be needed. This depends on:
  - The person's weight
  - If the person is cooperative
- Raise the side rails. Keep them up during the transport.
- Make sure the person's arms, hands, legs, and feet do not dangle through the side rail bars.
- Stand at the head of the stretcher. Your co-worker stands at the foot of the stretcher.
- Move the stretcher feet first (Fig. 12-27, p. 170).
- Do not leave the person alone.
- Follow the safety measures to prevent equipment accidents (p. 167).

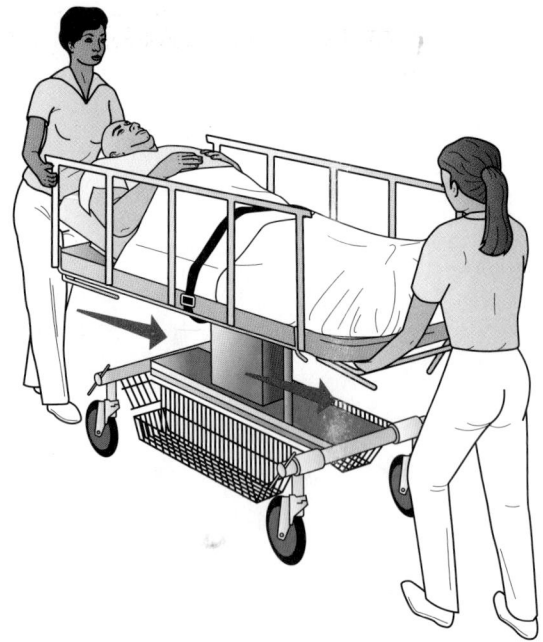

Fig. 12-27 A person is transported by stretcher. The stretcher is moved feet first.

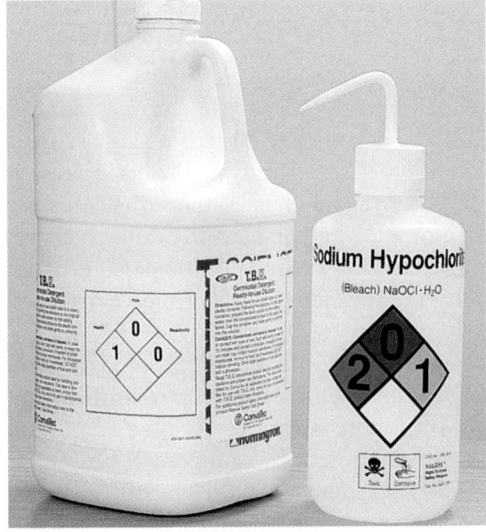

Fig. 12-28 Warning labels on hazardous substances.

HANDLING HAZARDOUS SUBSTANCES

A *hazardous substance is any chemical in the workplace that can cause harm.* The Occupational Safety and Health Administration (OSHA) requires that health care employees:

* Understand the risks of hazardous substances.
* Know how to safely handle them.

Physical hazards can cause fires or explosions. *Health hazards* are chemicals that can cause acute or chronic health problems. Acute problems occur rapidly and last a short time. They usually are from short-term exposure. Chronic problems usually result from long-term exposure. They occur over a long time.

Health hazards can:

* Cause cancer.
* Affect blood cell formation and function.
* Damage the kidneys, nervous system, lungs, skin, eyes, or mucous membranes.
* Cause birth defects, miscarriages, and fertility problems from reproductive system damage.

Exposure to hazardous substances can occur under normal working conditions. It also can happen during certain emergencies. Examples include equipment failures, container ruptures, or the uncontrolled release of a hazard into the workplace. Hazardous substances include:

* Drugs used in cancer therapy (chemotherapy, anticancer drugs). See Chapter 40.
* Anesthesia gases.
* Gases used to sterilize equipment.
* Oxygen.
* Disinfectants and cleaning agents.
* Radiation used for x-rays and cancer treatments. See Chapter 40.
* Mercury (found in thermometers and blood pressure devices). See Chapter 26.

OSHA requires a hazard communication program. The program includes container labeling, material safety data sheets (MSDS), and employee training. The agency also provides eyewash and total body wash stations in areas where hazardous substances are used.

Labeling

Hazardous substance containers include bags, barrels, bottles, boxes, cans, cylinders, drums, and storage tanks. All need warning labels (Fig. 12-28). The manufacturer supplies all labels. Warning labels identify:

* Physical and health hazards. Health hazards include the organs affected and potential health problems.
* Precaution measures. For example, "Do not use near open flame." Or "Avoid skin contact."
* What personal protective equipment to wear—gown, mask, gloves, goggles, and so on.
* How to use the substance safely.
* Storage and disposal information.

Words, pictures, and symbols communicate the warnings. A container must have a label. If a warning label is removed or damaged, do not use the substance. Take the container to the nurse, and explain the problem. Do not leave the container unattended.

Material Safety Data Sheets

Every hazardous substance has an MSDS. It provides detailed information about the substance:

* The chemical name and any common names
* The ingredients in the substance

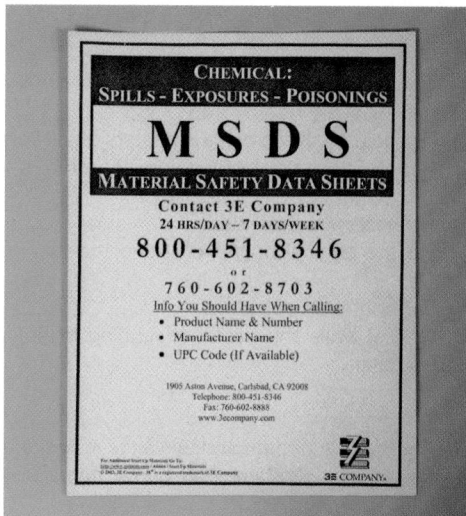

Fig. 12-29 The MSDS is accessed with an 800 hotline number.

- Physical and chemical characteristics (appearance, color, odor, boiling point, and others)
- Potential physical effects (fire, explosion)
- Conditions that could cause a chemical reaction
- How the chemical enters the body (inhalation, ingestion, skin contact, or absorption)
- Health hazards, including signs and symptoms
- Protective measures (how to use, handle, and store the substance)
- Emergency and first aid procedures
- Explosion information and fire-fighting measures (including what type of fire extinguisher to use [p. 174])
- How to clean up a spill or leak
- Personal protective equipment needed during clean-up
- How to dispose of the hazardous substance
- Manufacturer information (name, address, and phone number for more information)

Employees must have ready access to the MSDS. Know where to find them on your nursing unit (Fig. 12-29). Check the MSDS before using a hazardous substance, cleaning up a leak or spill, or disposing of the substance. Tell the nurse about a leak or spill right away. Do not leave a leak or spill unattended.

Employee Training

Your employer provides hazardous substance training. You are told about hazards, exposure risks, and protection measures. You learn to read and use warning labels and the MSDS.

Each hazardous substance requires certain protection measures. Box 12-10 lists general rules to safely handle hazardous substances.

BOX 12-10	SAFETY MEASURES FOR HAZARDOUS SUBSTANCES

- Read all warning labels.
- Follow the safety measures on the warning label and MSDS.
- Make sure each container has a warning label that is not damaged.
- Use a leak-proof container to carry or transport a hazardous substance.
- Wear personal protective equipment to clean spills and leaks. The warning label or MSDS tells you what to wear (mask, gown, gloves, eye protection, safety boots).
- Clean up spills at once. Work from clean areas to dirty areas using circular motions.
- Dispose of hazardous waste in sealed bags or containers.
- Stand behind a lead shield during x-ray or radiation therapy procedures.
- Do not enter a room while a person is having x-rays or radiation therapy.
- Wash your hands after handling hazardous substances.
- Work in well-ventilated areas to avoid inhaling gases.
- Use cleaning products safely:
  - Read and follow warnings and label directions.
  - Keep all products in their original containers.
  - Make sure the area is well-ventilated.
  - Do not mix products. Mixing products can cause dangerous gases. For example, do not mix ammonia and bleach.
  - Close containers properly.
  - Put cleaning products away after use.
  - Do not store cleaning products near food.
  - Empty buckets, pails, basins, and other containers with cleaning solutions.
  - Do not use an empty container for other purposes or things.
- Store a hazardous substance according to the MSDS.

FIRE SAFETY

Fire is a constant danger. Faulty electrical equipment and wiring, over-loaded electrical circuits, and smoking are major causes of fires. The entire health team must prevent fires. They must act quickly and responsibly during a fire.

See *Focus on Long-Term Care and Home Care: Fire Safety*, p. 172.

Fire and the Use of Oxygen

Three things are needed for a fire:
- A spark or flame
- A material that will burn
- Oxygen

FOCUS ON LONG-TERM CARE AND HOME CARE
Fire Safety

Home Care
Fire and the Use of Oxygen
Home care patients may need oxygen therapy. Remind the patient, family, and visitors about safety measures. See Chapter 36.

Preventing Fires
Smoke detectors save lives, prevent injuries, and lessen property damage. Always locate them in a patient's home. They should be outside every sleeping area, in every bedroom, and on every floor. Make sure they are working. Tell the nurse, patient, and family if a smoke detector does not work.

Cooking equipment is the leading cause of home fires. Practice the safety measures to prevent burns (p. 157).

Space heaters present fire hazards. Electric and fuel-burning heaters are common. Practice these safety measures:
- Follow the manufacturer's instructions. Use the correct fuel.
- Light a gas space heater correctly:
  - Strike the match first.
  - Then turn on the gas.
- Do not use extension cords with space heaters.
- Keep heaters at least 3 feet away from window coverings, furniture, and anything that will burn.
- Do not place heaters on stairs, in doorways, or where people walk.
- Protect yourself and others from burns. Heaters are hot. Do not touch them. Keep them away from children and persons who cannot protect themselves.

Preventing Fires—cont'd
- Prevent electrocution. Keep electric heaters away from water. (Water conducts electricity.) Make sure the cord is in good repair.
- Do not leave heaters unattended.
- Store fuel in the original container. Keep the fuel container outside.
- Refill the fuel container outside.
- Do not add fuel while the heater is running or hot. Do not over-fill the heater.

What To Do During a Fire
Know two exits from each room and two exits from the building. Keep exits clear. Keep furniture and heavy items away from doors and windows.

If a fire occurs, get the patient, family, and yourself out as fast as possible. Do not use elevators. In an apartment building, alert others to the fire. Use the fire alarm system and yell "FIRE" in the hallways. Call 911 or the fire department when out of the building. Do not go back into the building.

Using a Fire Extinguisher
Locate fire extinguishers in the patient's home. Read the manufacturer's instructions. Make sure the device works. Tell the nurse, patient, and family if a fire extinguisher does not work.

Air has some oxygen. However, some people need extra oxygen (Chapter 36). Safety measures are needed where oxygen is used and stored:
- NO SMOKING signs are placed on the door and near the bed.
- The person and visitors are reminded not to smoke in the room.
- Smoking materials (cigarettes, cigars, and pipes), matches, and lighters are removed from the room.
- Electrical items are turned off *before* being unplugged.
- Wool blankets and synthetic fabrics that cause static electricity are removed from the person's room.
- The person wears a cotton gown or pajamas.
- Electrical items are in good working order. This includes electric shavers, TVs, radios, computers, and other electronic devices.
- Lit candles, incense, and other open flames are not allowed.
- Materials that ignite easily are removed from the room. They include oil, grease, nail polish remover, and so on.

Agencies have no-smoking policies and smoke-free areas. No smoking is allowed inside the buildings. Signs are posted on all entry doors. Some people ignore such rules. Remind them about the no-smoking rules.

See *Focus on Communication: Fire and the Use of Oxygen.*

FOCUS ON COMMUNICATION
Fire and the Use of Oxygen
You may have to remind a patient, resident, or visitor not to smoke inside the agency. You can simply say:
- "Mrs. Murphy, this is a smoke-free area. Here is an ashtray to put out your cigarette. If you want to smoke, I'll be happy to show you the smoking area outside."
- "Mr. Garcia, please don't smoke inside the center. We have a smoking area outside the back entrance on hallway 2. I'll be happy to show you the way."

Tell the nurse what happened, what you said, and what you did. The nurse may need to speak with the person about not smoking.

Preventing Fires

Fire prevention measures were described in relation to burns, equipment accidents, and oxygen use. Other fire safety measures are listed in Box 12-11.

BOX 12-11 FIRE PREVENTION MEASURES

- Follow the safety measures for oxygen use.
- Smoke only where allowed to do so. Do not smoke in patients' homes.
- Empty ashtrays only when sure that all ashes, cigars, cigarettes, and other smoking materials are out.
- Empty ashtrays into a metal container partially filled with sand or water. Do not empty ashtrays into plastic containers or wastebaskets lined with paper or plastic bags.
- Provide ashtrays for persons who are allowed to smoke. Deep, wide ashtrays on a sturdy table are best.
- Supervise persons who smoke. This is very important for persons who are confused, disoriented, or sedated.
- Follow safety practices when using electrical items.
- Keep matches, lighters, and flammable liquids and materials away from children and confused or disoriented persons.
- Light matches carefully.
  - Be alert for sparks when lighting a match. The sparks can ignite materials that can burn.
  - Keep your hair, clothing, and anything that will burn away from the match and flame.
- Do not leave cooking unattended on stoves, in ovens, in microwave ovens, or on grills.
- Practice these safety measures for candles:
  - Do not leave candles unattended.
  - Blow out candles when you leave the room or go to bed.
  - Avoid using candles in bedrooms or other sleeping areas.

- Keep candles at least 12 inches away from anything that can burn.
- Use sturdy candle holders.
- Place candle holders on a sturdy, clutter-free surface.
- Do not use candles during power outages. Use flashlights and battery-operated lighting.
- Keep candles and incense away from flammable liquids and materials.
- Store flammable liquids outside in their original containers. Keep the containers where children and confused or disoriented persons cannot reach them.
- Keep materials that will burn away from space heaters, fireplaces, radiators, registers, candles, incense, oil lamps, and other heat sources. Stacked newspapers, magazines, books, and paint rags are examples.
- Do not smoke or light matches or lighters around flammable liquids or materials.
- Use clothes dryers safely:
  - Clean the lint filter before and after each use.
  - Use the correct plug and outlet.
  - Turn the dryer off when you leave the home.
  - Do not run clothes dryers when people are sleeping.
- Follow the safety measures to prevent equipment accidents (p. 167).
- Follow the safety measures to prevent burns (p. 157).

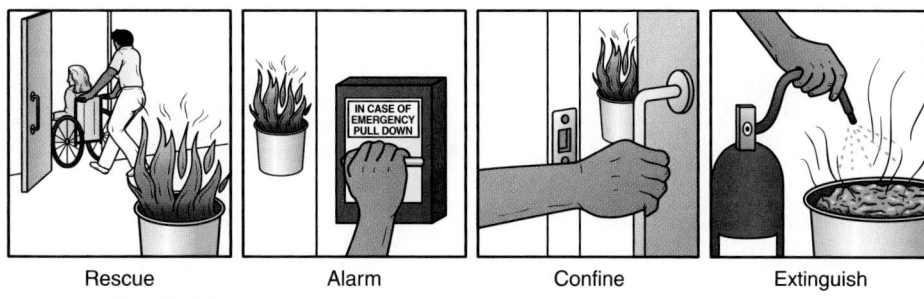

Rescue   Alarm   Confine   Extinguish

Fig. 12-30 During a fire, remember RACE: Rescue, Alarm, Confine, and Extinguish.

What To Do During a Fire

Know your agency's policies and procedures for fire emergencies. Know where to find fire alarms, fire extinguishers, and emergency exits. Fire drills are held to practice emergency fire procedures. Remember the word *RACE* (Fig. 12-30):

- *R*—for *rescue*. Rescue persons in immediate danger. Move them to a safe place.
- *A*—for *alarm*. Sound the nearest fire alarm. Notify the operator.

- *C*—for *confine*. Close doors and windows to confine the fire. Turn off oxygen or electrical items used in the general area of the fire.
- *E*—for *extinguish*. Use a fire extinguisher on a small fire that has not spread to a larger area.

Clear equipment from all normal and emergency exits.

Do not use elevators if there is a fire.

See *Promoting Safety and Comfort: What To Do During a Fire*, p. 174.

PROMOTING SAFETY AND COMFORT
What To Do During a Fire

Safety

Touch doors before opening them. Do not open a hot door. Use another way out of the room or building.

If your clothing is on fire, do not run. Drop to the floor or ground. Cover your face. Roll to smother flames. If another person's clothing is on fire, get the person to the floor or ground. Roll the person, or cover the person with a blanket, bedspread, or coat. This smothers the flames.

If smoke is present, cover your nose and mouth with a damp cloth. Do the same for patients, residents, visitors, and other staff. Have everyone crawl to the nearest exit.

Do the following if you cannot get out of the building because of flames or smoke:

- Call 911 or the fire department. Tell the operator where you are. Give exact information: agency name or the home care patient's name, address, phone number, and where you are in the building or home.
- Cover your nose and mouth with a damp cloth. Do the same for patients, residents, visitors, and other staff.
- Move away from the fire. Go to a room with a window. Close the room door. Stuff wet towels, blankets, sheets, or bedspreads at the bottom of the door.
- Open the window.
- Hang something from the window (towel, sheet, blanket, clothing). This helps firefighters find you.

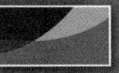 **Using a Fire Extinguisher.** Agencies may require that all employees demonstrate use of a fire extinguisher. Different extinguishers are used for different kinds of fires:

- Oil and grease fires
- Electrical fires
- Paper and wood fires

A general procedure for using a fire extinguisher follows. Remember the word *PASS* used by the National Fire Protection Association:

- P—for *pull the safety pin.* Doing so unlocks the handle on many types of fire extinguishers.
- A—for *aim low.* Direct the hose or nozzle at the base of the fire. Do not try to spray the tops of the flames.
- S—for *squeeze the lever.* Squeeze or push down on the lever, handle, or button to start the stream. Release the lever, handle, or button to stop the stream.
- S—for *sweep back and forth.* Sweep the stream back and forth (side to side) at the base of the fire.

Evacuating. Agencies have evacuation policies and procedures. If evacuation is necessary, patients and residents closest to the fire go out first. Those who can walk are given blankets to wrap around themselves. A staff member takes them to a safe place. Figures 12-32 and 12-33, p. 176 show how to rescue persons who cannot walk. Once firefighters arrive, they direct rescue efforts.

USING A FIRE EXTINGUISHER

PROCEDURE

1 Pull the fire alarm.
2 Get the nearest fire extinguisher.
3 Carry it upright.
4 Take it to the fire.
5 Follow the word *PASS:*
   a P—for *pull the safety pin* (Fig. 12-31, A). This unlocks the handle.
   b A—for *aim low* (Fig. 12-31, B). Direct the hose or nozzle at the base of the fire. Do not try to spray the tops of the flames.
   c S—for *squeeze the lever* (Fig. 12-31, C). Squeeze or push down on the lever, handle, or button to start the stream. Release the lever, handle, or button to stop the stream.
   d S—for *sweep back and forth* (Fig. 12-31, D). Sweep the stream back and forth (side to side) at the base of the fire.

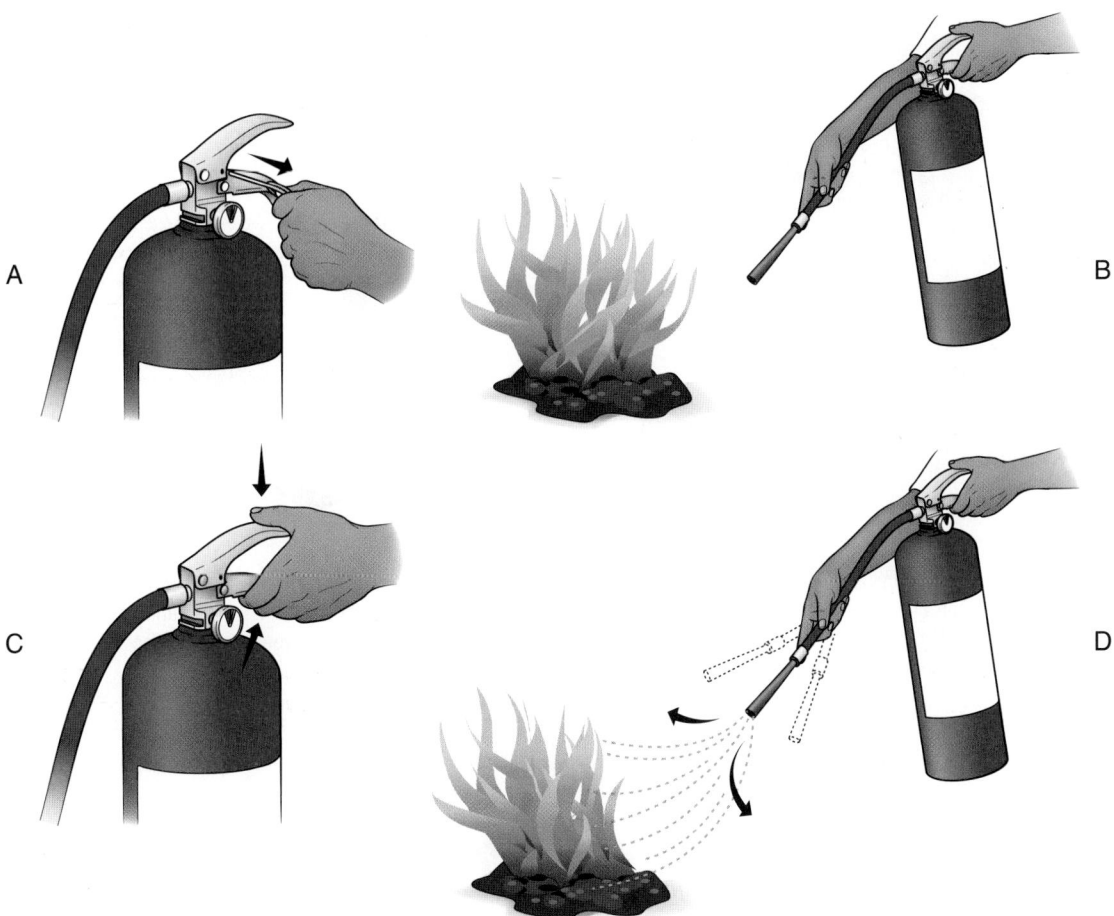

A
B
C
D

Fig. 12-31 Using a fire extinguisher. **A,** *Pull* the safety pin. **B,** *Aim* the hose at the base of the fire. **C,** *Squeeze* the top handle down. **D,** *Sweep* back and forth.

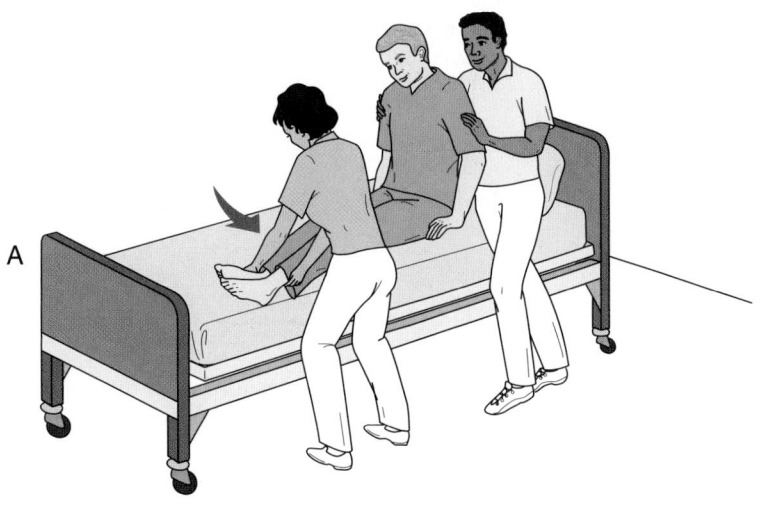
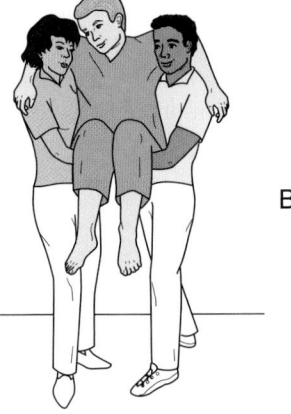

A
B

Fig. 12-32 Swing-carry technique. **A,** Assist the person to a sitting position. A co-worker grasps the person's ankles as you both turn the person so that he sits on the side of the bed. **B,** Pull the person's arm over your shoulder. With one arm, reach across the person's back to your co-worker's shoulder. Reach under the person's knees and grasp your co-worker's arm. Your co-worker does the same.

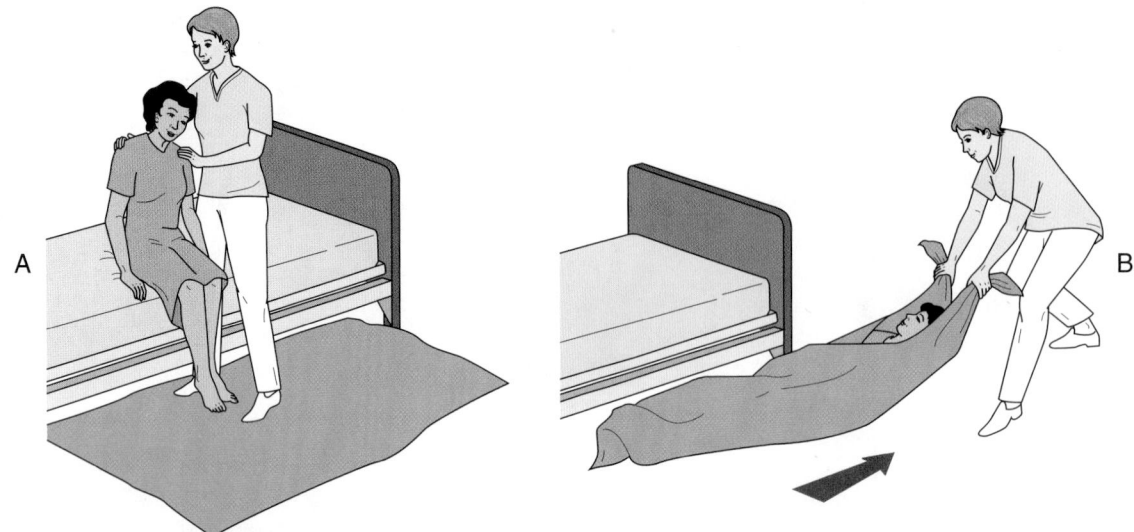

Fig. 12-33 One-rescuer carry. **A,** Spread a blanket on the floor. Make sure the blanket will extend beyond the person's head. Assist the person to sit on the side of the bed. Grasp the person under the arms, and cross your hands over her chest. Lower the person to the floor by sliding her down one of your legs. **B,** Wrap the blanket around the person. Grasp the blanket over the head area. Pull the person to a safe area.

DISASTERS

A *disaster is a sudden catastrophic event. People are injured and killed. Property is destroyed.* Natural disasters include tornadoes, hurricanes, blizzards, earthquakes, volcanic eruptions, floods, and some fires. Human-made disasters include auto, bus, train, and airplane accidents. They also include fires, bombings, nuclear power plant accidents, riots, gas or chemical leaks, explosions, and wars.

The agency has procedures for disasters that could occur in your area. Follow them to keep patients, residents, visitors, staff, and yourself safe.

Communities, fire and police departments, and health care agencies have disaster plans. They include procedures to deal with the people needing treatment. The plan generally provides for:

- Discharging persons who can go home
- Assigning staff and equipment to an emergency area
- Assigning staff to transport persons from treatment areas
- Calling off-duty staff to work

A disaster may damage the agency. The disaster plan includes evacuation procedures.

See *Focus on Long-Term Care and Home Care: Disasters.*

FOCUS ON LONG-TERM CARE AND HOME CARE
Disasters

Home Care

A severe storm may develop when you are in a patient's home. For safety:

- Stay informed through local TV and radio stations. With satellite TV service, you may not have signal with heavy storm clouds.
- Keep a flashlight with you in case the power goes out.
- Move the patient, family, and yourself to a "safe room:"
  - Basement
  - Room on the ground floor
  - Interior room away from outside wall, windows, and doors
  - Center hallway
  - Bathroom
  - Closet

Bomb Threats

Agencies have procedures for bomb threats. You must follow them if a caller makes a bomb threat or if you find an item that looks or sounds strange. Bomb threats can be sent by phone, mail, e-mail, messenger, or other means. Or the person can leave a bomb in the agency. If you see a stranger in the agency, tell the nurse at once. You cannot be too safe.

WORKPLACE VIOLENCE

Workplace violence is violent acts (including assault or threat of assault) directed toward persons at work or while on duty. It includes:

- Murders
- Beatings, stabbings, and shootings
- Rapes and sexual assaults
- Use of weapons—firearms, bombs, knives, and so on
- Kidnapping
- Robbery
- Threats—obscene phone calls; threatening oral, written, or body language; and harassment of any nature (being followed, sworn at, or shouted at)

Workplace violence can occur in any place where staff perform work-related duties. It can be a permanent or temporary place. This includes buildings, parking lots, field sites, homes, and travel to and from work assignments. Workplace violence can occur anywhere in the agency. However, common settings are mental health units, emergency departments, waiting rooms, and geriatric units.

According to OSHA, more assaults occur in health care settings than in other industries. Nurses and nursing assistants are at risk. They have the most contact with patients, residents, and visitors. Risk factors include:

- People with weapons.
- Police holds—persons arrested or convicted of crimes.
- Acutely disturbed and violent persons seeking health care.
- Alcohol and drug abuse.
- Mentally ill persons who do not take needed drugs, do not have follow-up care, and are not in hospitals unless they are an immediate threat to themselves or others.
- Pharmacies have drugs and are a target for robberies.
- Gang members and substance abusers are patients, residents, or visitors.
- Upset, agitated, and disturbed family and visitors.
- Long waits for emergency care or other services.
- Being alone with the person during care or transport to other areas.
- Low staff levels during meals, emergencies, and at night.
- Poor lighting in hallways, rooms, parking lots, and other areas.
- Lack of training in recognizing and managing potentially violent situations.

OSHA has guidelines for violence prevention programs. The goal is to prevent or reduce employee exposure to situations that can cause death or injury. Work-site hazards are identified. Prevention measures are developed and followed. Also, staff receive safety and health training. You need to:

- Understand and follow your agency's workplace violence prevention program.
- Understand and follow safety and security measures.
- Voice safety and security concerns.
- Report strange or suspicious persons right away.
- Report violent incidents promptly and accurately.
- Serve on health and safety committees that review workplace violence.
- Attend training programs that help you recognize and manage agitation, assaultive behavior, and criminal intent.

Box 12-12 lists some measures to prevent or control workplace violence. Box 12-13, p. 179 lists personal safety practices. Follow them all the time. Complete an incident report (p. 181), as needed, for workplace violence.

The nurse assesses the behavior and the behavioral history of new and transferred patients and residents. Restraints may be ordered if persons are a threat to themselves or others (Chapter 14). Persons with mental health problems are supervised as they move throughout the agency. Aggressive and agitated persons are treated in open areas. Privacy and confidentiality are maintained. Security officers deal with agitated, aggressive, or disruptive persons.

See *Focus on Long-Term Care and Home Care: Workplace Violence*, p. 180.

Text continued on p. 180

BOX 12-12   MEASURES TO PREVENT OR CONTROL WORKPLACE VIOLENCE

Agitated or Aggressive Persons

- Stand away from the person. Judge the length of the person's arms and legs. Stand far enough away so that the person cannot hit or kick you.
- Stand close to the door. Do not become trapped in the room.
- Be aware of items in the room that can be used as weapons. Move away from such objects. Examples include vases, phones, radios, letter openers, paper weights, and belts.
- Know where to find panic buttons, signal lights, alarms, closed-circuit monitors, and other security devices.
- Keep your hands free.

Agitated or Aggressive Persons—cont'd

- Stay calm. Talk to the person in a calm manner. Do not raise your voice or argue, scold, or interrupt the person.
- Be aware of your body language. Do not point a finger or glare at the person. Do not put your hands on your hips.
- Do not touch the person.
- Tell the person that you will get the nurse to speak to him or her.
- Leave the room as soon as you can. Make sure the person is safe.
- Tell the nurse or security officer about the matter at once. Report items in the room that can be used as weapons.

Continued

BOX 12-12 | MEASURES TO PREVENT OR CONTROL WORKPLACE VIOLENCE—cont'd

Safety Devices

- Alarm systems, closed-circuit video monitoring, panic buttons, hand-held alarms, wireless phones, two-way radios, and phone systems are installed (Fig. 12-34). These systems have a direct line to security staff or the police.
- Metal detectors are at entrances to identify guns, knives, or other weapons.
- Curved mirrors are at hallway intersections and hard-to-see areas.
- Bullet-resistant, shatter-proof glass is at nurses' stations.
- Door alarms remain on.
- Staff do not share security codes with anyone.

Weapons

- Jewelry and scarves that can serve as weapons are not worn. For example, a person can grab earrings and bracelets. Or a person can strangle someone with a necklace or scarf.
- Long hair is worn up and off the collar (Chapter 5). A person can pull long hair and cause head injuries.
- Keys, scissors, pens, or other items that can serve as weapons are not visible.
- Pictures, vases, and other items that can serve as weapons are few in number.
- Tools or items left by maintenance staff or visitors are removed if they can serve as weapons.

Family and Visitors

- Visitors sign in and receive a pass to access patient and resident areas.
- Visiting hours and policies are enforced.
- A list of "restricted visitors" is made for patients and residents with a history of violence or who are victims of violence.

Family and Visitors—cont'd

- Waiting rooms and lounges are comfortable and reduce stress.
- Family and visitors are informed in a timely manner.

Building Safety and Security

- Unused doors are locked.
- Bright lights are inside and outside buildings.
- Broken lights, windows, and door locks are replaced or repaired.
- Staff restrooms lock and prevent access to visitors.
- Access to the pharmacy and drug storage areas is controlled.
- Furniture is placed to prevent entrapment. This includes furniture in patient and resident rooms and in therapy areas, dining rooms, and lounges.
- Keys are always attended and secure.

Staff Safety Measures

- Staff are not alone when caring for persons with agitated or aggressive behaviors.
- Staff wear ID badges that prove employment.
- Staff use a "buddy system" when using elevators, stairways, restrooms, and low traffic areas.
- Uniforms fit well. Tight uniforms limit running. An attacker can grab loose uniforms.
- Shoes have good soles. Shoes that cause slipping limit running.
- Vehicles are locked and in good repair.
- Security escort services are used for walking to vehicles, bus stops, or train stations.

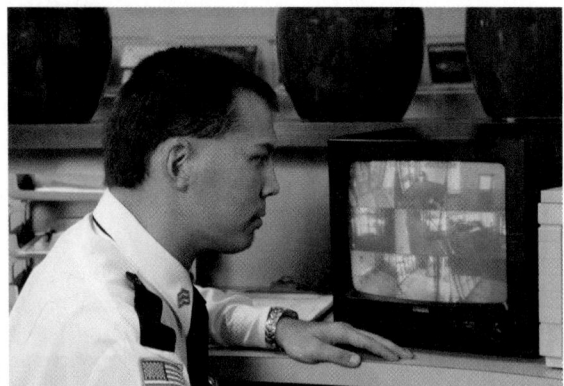

Fig. 12-34 People entering and leaving the agency are monitored on closed-circuit TV.

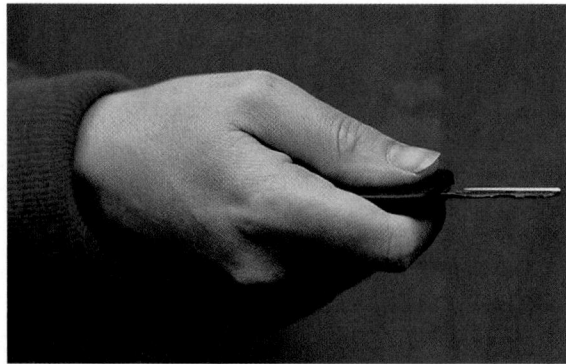

Fig. 12-35 A car key is used as a weapon.

BOX 12-13 PERSONAL SAFETY PRACTICES

General Measures

- Know the area where you are going. Ask questions about the area.
- Make a "dry run" of the area. Know the way in advance. The shortest way is not always the safest.
- Let someone know where you are at all times. Tell someone when you leave and when you arrive at your destination. If you do not call in when expected, the person knows something is wrong.
- Make it known that you do not carry drugs, needles, or syringes.
- Do not carry large amounts of money or valuables. Leave them at home or in the locked car trunk. If someone wants what you have, give it. The only thing of value is *you*.
- Carry wallets, purses, and backpacks safely. Men should carry wallets in an inside coat pocket or in a side pant pocket. Never carry a wallet in the rear pocket. Keep a firm grip on a purse. Keep it close to your body.
- Keep your wireless phone in your hand.
- Carry a whistle or shriek alarm.
- Avoid ATM machines at night.
- Be careful when getting on elevators and when entering stairways.
- Do not approach a stranger or someone acting in a strange way. Report the matter right away.

Home Settings

- Keep doors and windows to the home locked at all times.
- Do not open doors to strangers. Ask for identification.
- Do not let a stranger into the home to use a phone or bathroom. Offer to call the police if the person needs help.
- Do not give personal information to callers or people at the door.

Car Safety

- Have plenty of gas in your car.
- Keep your car in good working order.
- Keep these in your car—local map, flashlight with working batteries, flares, a fire extinguisher, and a first aid kit.
- Raise the hood and use the flares if the car breaks down. Stay in the car. Call the police if you have a wireless phone. If someone stops by to help, ask that person to call the police.
- Lock your car. Sometimes you may want to leave it unlocked. If you need to get in the car fast, you do not want to fumble with keys. Use your judgment. Do not leave anything in the car if you leave it unlocked.
- Have your car key ready so you can get into the car quickly. Do not fumble for keys on the way to or at the car.
- Check under the car as you approach it. A person hiding under the car can grab your ankle or leg. Leave at once if someone is under the car. The person under the car may be working with a buddy who is waiting to attack you while you are being held or injured at the leg or ankle.
- Check the back seat before getting into the car. Make sure no one is in the car. Leave at once if someone is in the car.
- Lock car doors when you get in the car. Keep windows rolled up.

Car Safety—cont'd

- Do not open the car door or window to talk to a person approaching your car.
- Do not get out of the car to remove something from the windshield.
- Keep purses, backpacks, and other valuables under the seat or near your side. Do not leave them on the seat. They are easy targets for smash-and-grab robbers.
- Do not hitchhike or pick up hitchhikers.

Parking Your Car

- Check for places to park. Choose a well-lit area. In a parking garage, park near entrances, exits, and on the lower level. Try to get close to the attendant if possible. The closest space to your destination is not always the safest for parking.
- Park so you can leave quickly and easily. Park at street corners so no one can park in front of you. In parking lots, back in. You see more from the front windshield than from the back window.

Walking

- Do not wear headphones or earbuds. You cannot hear cars and people around you.
- Use well-lit and busy streets. Avoid vacant lots, alleys, wooded areas, and construction sites. The shortest way is not always the safest.
- Walk near the curb. Stay away from doorways, shrubs, and bushes.
- Know where to find phone booths. And carry a wireless phone. Know your location, and keep phone calls simple.
- Go to a police or fire station or a store if you think someone is following you.

Public Transportation

- Carry money for phone calls and for bus, train, or taxi fares. Have money in your pocket to avoid fumbling with a purse or wallet.
- Stand with others and near the ticket booth.
- Sit near the driver or conductor.
- Keep your wireless phone in your hand.

If You Are Threatened or Attacked

- Scream as loud and as long as you can. Keep screaming. Men and women should scream.
- Yell "FIRE," not "help." Most people will respond to "FIRE."
- Use your car keys as a weapon. Carry them in your strong hand. Have one key extended (Fig. 12-35). Hold the key firmly. If you are attacked, go for the person's face. Slash the person's face with the key. Do not use poking motions. Do not try for a certain target because you might miss. Do not be shy—your attacker will not be.
- Remember, you have two arms, two hands, two feet, and two knees. You can attack from more than one direction at once. Do not be shy—your attacker will not be. Push, pull, yank, and so on. You can attack a man's or woman's genitals.
- Use your thumbs as weapons. Go for the eyes and push hard.
- Carry a travel size can of aerosol hair spray. Go for the face.

RISK MANAGEMENT

Risk management involves identifying and controlling risks and safety hazards affecting the agency. The intent is to:
- Protect everyone in the agency—patients, residents, visitors, and staff.
- Protect agency property from harm or danger.
- Protect the person's valuables.
- Prevent accidents and injuries.

Risk management deals with these and other safety issues:
- Accident and fire prevention
- Negligence and malpractice
- Abuse
- Workplace violence
- Federal and state requirements

Risk managers work with all agency departments. They look for patterns and trends in incident reports, complaints (patients, residents, staff), and accident and injury investigations. Risk managers look for and correct unsafe situations. They also make procedure changes and training recommendations as needed.

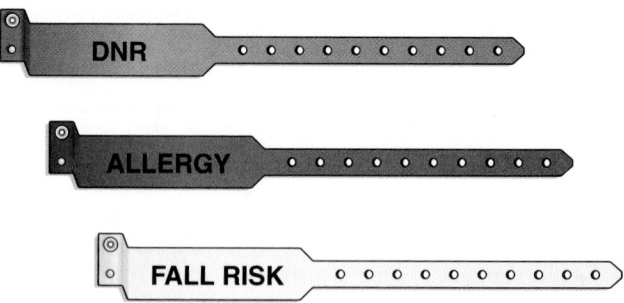

Fig. 12-36 Color-coded wristbands. The alert is printed on the band.

Color-Coded Wristbands

Color-coded wristbands promote the person's safety and prevent harm. They quickly communicate an alert or warning (Fig. 12-36). The type of alert is printed on the band. The printing is useful in dim lighting and for persons who are color blind. Many states use these three colors:
- Red—for an "allergy alert." Red is a warning to "stop." A red wristband warns of allergies to food, drugs, treatment supplies such as tape or latex gloves, dust, plants, grass, and so on. Allergies are not listed on the wristband.
- Yellow—for a "fall risk." Yellow implies "caution." The person is at risk for falling. Yellow wristbands are used for persons with a history of falls. Or they are used for persons at risk for falls because of dizziness, balance problems, confusion, and so on.
- Purple—for a "do not resuscitate" (DNR) order. See Chapter 52.

Some agencies use other colors for other alerts. For example pink is for a "limb alert." This means that an arm or leg is not used for blood pressure measurements, blood draws, or intravenous infusions. To safely use color-coded wristbands:
- Know the wristband colors used in your agency. Colors may vary among agencies.
- Check the care plan and your assignment sheet when you see a color-coded wristband. You need to know the reason for the wristband and the care measures needed. Ask the nurse if you have questions.
- Do not confuse "social cause" bands with your agency's color-coded wristbands. "Live Strong" is an example.
- Check for wristbands on persons transferred from another agency. That agency may use different colors. Or the meanings may differ from those in your agency. The nurse needs to remove wristbands from another agency.
- Tell the nurse if you think a person needs a color-coded wristband.

Personal Belongings

The person's belongings must be kept safe. Often they are sent home with the family. A personal belongings list is completed. Each item is listed and described. The staff member and person sign the completed list.

A valuables envelope is used for jewelry and money. Each jewelry item is listed and described on the envelope. Describe what you see. For example, describe a ring as having a white stone with six prongs in a yellow setting. Do not assume the stone is a diamond in a gold setting. For valuables:

- Count money with the person.
- Put money and each jewelry item in the envelope. Have the person watch. Seal and sign the envelope like a personal belongings list.
- Give the envelope to the nurse. The nurse takes it to the safe or sends it home with the family.

Dentures, eyeglasses, hearing aids, watches, some jewelry, radios, computers, and other electronic devices are kept at the bedside. Items kept at the bedside are listed in the person's record. Some people keep money for newspapers and personal items. The amount kept is noted in the person's record.

See *Focus on Long-Term Care and Home Care: Personal Belongings.*

Reporting Incidents

An *incident is any event that has harmed or could harm a patient, resident, visitor, or staff member.* It includes accidents and errors in giving care.

Report accidents and errors at once. This includes:

- Accidents involving patients, residents, visitors, or staff.
- Errors in care. This includes giving the wrong care, giving care to the wrong person, or not giving care.
- Broken or lost items owned by the person. Dentures, hearing aids, and eyeglasses are examples.
- Lost money or clothing.
- Hazardous substance incidents.
- Workplace violence incidents.

An *incident report* is completed as soon as possible after the incident. The following information is required:

- Names of those involved
- Date and time of the accident or error
- Location of the accident or error
- A complete description of what happened
- Names of witnesses
- Any other requested information

Not part of the medical record, incident reports are reviewed by risk management and a committee of health care workers. They look for patterns and trends in accidents or errors. For example, are falls occurring on the same shift and on the same unit? Are lost or missing items being reported on the same shift or same unit? Are residents being injured on the same shift or same unit? There may be new policies and procedures to prevent future incidents.

FOCUS ON PRIDE

The Person, Family, and Yourself

Personal and Professional Responsibility

Accidents happen. Errors occur. No matter how much you try, mistakes are made. Do not lie or try to hide the incident. This is wrong. You must:

- Be honest.
- Tell the nurse.
- Fill out an incident report.

Incident reports are used to improve systems and promote safety, not for punishment. Information gained signals areas for improvement. Processes may be changed to make mistakes more difficult. Or they are changed to make it easier to do the right thing.

Always do your best to give safe care. When errors or accidents happen, take responsibility. Be accountable. Take pride in doing the right thing by honest reporting.

Rights and Respect

Patients and residents have the right to the care and security of personal items. Treat the person's items with respect. The items may not have value to you but are important to the person. Label a person's belongings with his or her name. Put valuables in a secure place until a family member can take them home. Follow agency policies for charting and storing personal items.

Protect yourself and the agency from being accused of stealing. Do not go through a person's belongings without consent. Sometimes the nurse wants a person's items inspected for safety reasons. If so, make sure the nurse and the person or legal representative are present. Do not search on your own. The nurse charts the details of the search in the person's record.

Independence and Social Interaction

Children and older persons are at increased risk for injury. Children often try to show independence before they are able to judge safety. Older persons cannot do some things they used to do. They still may try. To promote safety:

- Know who you need to protect.
- Know common safety hazards and the causes of accidents.
- Practice safety measures to prevent accidents and injuries.
- Talk to children about safety. Explain the reasons for safety measures.
- Respect the desire of older persons to maintain independence. Listen to them. Discuss letting them try a task with help. Let them do as much as they safely can. Kindly communicate safety limits.

Continued

FOCUS ON PRIDE—cont'd

Delegation and Teamwork

Staff come and go from health care agencies at all hours. Work as a team to ensure the safety of all staff arriving and leaving the agency.

- Wait for a person finishing work a few minutes late. Ask if you can help the person.
- Walk with others to and from the parking area.
- Walk in well-lit areas at night.
- Do not leave the parking area until all of your co-workers are safely in their vehicles.
- Offer to call security escort services for a co-worker going a different direction. For example, a person is walking to a bus stop.

Take pride in caring about the safety of all team members.

Ethics and Laws

Some persons are at risk for choking. Persons with developmental disabilities (Chapter 47), young children, and older persons are examples. Safety measures must be taken to avoid harm. The following case shows what can occur when safety measures are neglected.

A 32-year-old man was a patient at a developmental center. He was retarded and had a history of epilepsy. He was a patient at the center since the age of 25.

According to the facts reported in the court case, the following occurred:

- *He had a dinner of braised beef and noodles. The pieces of beef were about ½ inch wide and ¾ inch long.*
- *While eating dinner, he stood up, coughed out his milk, reached for his throat, and collapsed.*
- *Efforts were made to revive him.*
- *He was transported to the hospital where he died a short while later.*
- *His death was caused by "meat mass inhalation . . . associated with mental retardation with chronic seizure disorder. . . ."*

The lawsuit claimed negligence because:

- *His swallowing was affected by the dosage of a drug.*
- *He was not given a soft diet.*
- *He was not properly supervised at meal time.*

In the Court's opinion, negligent care resulted in the patient's death.

(B. Szydelko v The Department of Mental Health of the State of Illinois, 1984.)

You can help prevent such incidents. Know which persons are at risk for choking. Ask the nurse or check the care plan. Monitor those persons closely. Check that they have the right diet. See Chapter 24 for more precautions.

REVIEW QUESTIONS

Circle the BEST answer.

1 Who provides a safe setting for the person?
  a The health team
  b The family
  c The administrator
  d The risk manager

2 Which of the following is safe?
  a Needing eyeglasses
  b Hearing problems
  c Memory problems
  d Oriented to person, time, and place

3 A person in a coma
  a Has suffered an electrical shock
  b Has dementia
  c Is unaware of surroundings
  d Has stopped breathing

4 A person with dementia
  a Cannot think and reason
  b Is not aware of his or her surroundings
  c Is paralyzed
  d Has suffered an electrical shock

5 A person with dementia
  a Is at high risk for accidents and injuries
  b Knows what is safe
  c Knows when to move away from danger
  d Is agitated and aggressive

6 You are caring for infants. Which is *not* safe?
  a Checking them in cribs often
  b Laying them on their backs to sleep
  c Propping a baby bottle on a rolled towel
  d Keeping plastic bags away from them

7 Which is safe for children?
  a Bicycle helmets
  b Clothes with drawstrings
  c Dangling items from backpacks
  d Necklaces

8 Which is a safety hazard for children?
  a Toilet with the lid down
  b Empty bucket
  c A crib away from the window
  d An open diaper pail

9 A person with quadriplegia is paralyzed
  a From the waist down
  b From the neck down
  c On the right side of the body
  d On the left side of the body

10 To identify a person, you
  a Call the person by name
  b Ask the person his or her name
  c Compare information on the ID bracelet against your assignment sheet
  d Ask both roommates their names

11 Which does *not* cause burns?
  a Smoking
  b Spilled hot liquids
  c Very hot bath water
  d Oxygen

12 Which does *not* prevent poisoning?
  a Keeping harmful products in low storage areas
  b Keeping child-resistant caps on harmful products
  c Making sure all harmful products have labels
  d Storing harmful products away from food

13 Which signals a poison?
  a The "Mr. Yuk" sticker   c RACE
  b The MSDS   d PASS

14 Who has the greatest risk of lead poisoning?
  a Newborns
  b Infants between the ages of 1 and 6 months
  c Children between the ages of 6 months and 6 years
  d Older persons

15 A home has lead-based plumbing. You should
  a Use hot tap water for cooking and drinking
  b Use hot tap water to make baby formula
  c Let cold water run for 1 to 2 minutes before using it for cooking or drinking
  d Be alert for signs and symptoms of carbon monoxide poisoning

16 Which can cause suffocation?
  a Reporting loose teeth or dentures
  b Using electrical items that are in good repair
  c Cutting food into small, bite-size pieces
  d Restraints

17 The most common cause of choking in adults is
  a A loose denture
  b Meat
  c Marbles
  d Candy

18 If severe airway obstruction occurs, the person usually
  a Clutches at the throat
  b Can speak, cough, and breathe
  c Is calm
  d Has a seizure

19 These statements are about relieving FBAO. Which is *false?*
  a Abdominal thrusts can be self-administered.
  b A person is pregnant. Give abdominal thrusts.
  c Injuries can occur from abdominal or chest thrusts.
  d CPR is started if the responsive victim loses consciousness.

20 You need to shave a new resident. Before using the person's electric shaver
  a You need to inspect it
  b The maintenance staff must do a safety check
  c You need to check for a frayed cord
  d You need an electrical outlet

21 You are using equipment. Which measure is *not* safe?
  a Following the manufacturer's instructions
  b Keeping electrical items away from water and spills
  c Pulling on the cord to remove a plug from an outlet
  d Turning off electrical items after using them

22 A person uses a wheelchair. Which measure is *not* safe?
  a The wheels are locked for transfers.
  b The chair is pulled backward to transport the person.
  c The feet are positioned on the footplates.
  d The casters point forward.

23 Stretcher safety involves the following *except*
  a Locking the wheels for transfers
  b Fastening the safety straps
  c Raising the side rails
  d Moving the stretcher head first

24 You spilled a hazardous substance. You should do the following *except*
  a Read the material safety data sheet
  b Cover the spill and go tell the nurse
  c Wear personal protective equipment to clean up the spill
  d Complete an incident report

25 The fire alarm sounds. The following is done *except*
  a Turning off oxygen
  b Using elevators
  c Closing doors and windows
  d Moving residents to a safe place

26 Your clothing is on fire. You should do the following *except*
  a Run to get help
  b Drop to the floor or ground
  c Cover your face
  d Roll to smother the flames

27 You work in a nursing center. What should you do for a severe weather alert?
  a Take cover.
  b Follow the center's disaster plan.
  c Make sure your family is safe.
  d Pull the fire alarm.

28 A person is agitated and aggressive. Which is *not* safe?
  a Standing away from the person
  b Standing close to the door
  c Using touch to show you care
  d Talking to the person without raising your voice

29 A person has a yellow wristband. This means that the person
  a Is at risk for bleeding
  b Has an allergy
  c Is at risk for falling
  d Has an acute illness

30 You work the night shift. Which is *not* safe?
  a Parking in a well-lit area
  b Locking your car
  c Finding your keys after getting into the car
  d Checking under the car and in your back seat

31 A resident brought a radio from home. Which helps prevent property loss?
  a Completing a personal belongings list
  b Labeling the item with the person's name
  c Putting the item in a safe
  d Using a wheelchair pouch for the item

32 You gave a person the wrong treatment. Which is *true?*
  a Report the error at the end of the shift.
  b Take action only if the person was injured.
  c You are guilty of negligence.
  d You must complete an incident report.

Answers to these questions are on p. 832.

13 Preventing Falls

OBJECTIVES

- Define the key terms listed in this chapter.
- Identify the causes and risk factors for falls.
- Describe the safety measures that prevent falls.
- Explain how to use bed rails safely.
- Explain the purpose of hand rails and grab bars.
- Explain how to use wheel locks safely.
- Describe how to use transfer/gait belts.
- Explain how to help the person who is falling.
- Perform the procedures described in this chapter.
- Explain how to promote PRIDE in the person, the family, and yourself.

KEY TERMS

bed rail A device that serves as a guard or barrier along the side of the bed; side rail

gait belt See "transfer belt"

transfer belt A device used to support a person who is unsteady or disabled; gait belt

---

The risk of falling increases with age. Persons older than 65 years are at risk. A history of falls increases the risk of falling again. Falls are the most common accidents in nursing centers.

According to the Centers for Disease Control and Prevention (CDC):

- Falls are the main cause of injury-related deaths in older adults.
- In the United States, over one third of adults 65 years old and older fall each year.
- About 1800 nursing center residents die each year from falls.
- Falls can cause serious injury including fractures. Fractures of the spine, hip, forearm, leg, ankle, pelvis, upper arm, and hand are the most common. Hip fractures and head trauma increase the risk of death.
- Falls result in disability, decline in function, and reduced quality of life.
- Fear of falling can cause further loss of function, depression, feelings of helplessness, and social isolation. This may increase the person's risk of falling again.

CAUSES AND RISK FACTORS FOR FALLS

Most falls occur in patient and resident rooms and in bathrooms. Poor lighting, cluttered floors, throw rugs, and out-of-place furniture are causes. So are wet and slippery floors, bathtubs, and showers. Needing to use the bathroom, usually to urinate, is a major cause of falls. For example, Mrs. Hines has an urgent need to urinate. She falls trying to get to the bathroom.

Most falls occur between 1600 (4:00 PM) and 2000 (8:00 PM). Falls also are more likely during shift changes. During shift changes, staff are busy going off and coming on duty. Confusion can occur about who gives care and answers signal lights. Shift changes vary among agencies. They often occur between these hours:

- 0600 (6:00 AM) and 0800 (8:00 AM)
- 1400 (2:00 PM) and 1600 (4:00 PM)
- 2200 (10:00 PM) and 2400 (midnight)

The accident risk factors described in Chapter 12 can lead to falls. The problems listed in Box 13-1 also increase a person's risk of falling.

See *Focus on Long-Term Care and Home Care: Causes and Risk Factors for Falls.*

See *Teamwork and Time Management: Causes and Risk Factors for Falls.*

BOX 13-1	FACTORS INCREASING THE RISK OF FALLS

Care Setting
- Care equipment: IV (intravenous) poles, drainage tubes and bags, and others
- Cluttered floors
- Furniture out-of-place
- Lighting: poor
- Setting: strange and unfamiliar
- Throw rugs
- Wet and slippery floors, bathtubs, and showers
- Wheelchairs, walkers, canes, and crutches: improper use or fit

The Person
- Alcohol: over-use
- Balance problems
- Blood pressure: low or high
- Confusion
- Depression
- Disorientation
- Dizziness; dizziness on standing
- Drug side effects
  - Low blood pressure when standing or sitting
  - Drowsiness
  - Fainting
  - Dizziness
  - Coordination: poor
  - Unsteadiness
  - Urination: frequent
  - Diarrhea
  - Confusion and disorientation
- Elimination needs
- Falls: history of
- Foot problems
- Incontinence: urinary or fecal
- Joint pain and stiffness
- Judgment: poor
- Light-headedness
- Memory problems
- Mobility: decreased
- Muscle weakness
- Reaction time: slow
- Shoes that fit poorly
- Vision problems
- Weakness

FOCUS ON LONG-TERM CARE AND HOME CARE
Causes and Risk Factors for Falls

Home Care
In the home care setting, many factors increase the risk for falls. Hazards include:
- Cluttered rooms and hallways
- Objects on the floor—wires, cords, shoes, books, magazines, blankets, and so on
- Throw rugs
- Pets
- Flooring problems—loose tiles and floor boards, raised linoleum, frayed carpet
- Slippery bathtub or shower floors
- Wet floors
- Ice or snow on driveways, steps, and sidewalks
- Loose or missing hand rails and grab bars (p. 190)
- Poor lighting
- No footwear or unsafe footwear—slippers, shoes without non-skid surfaces, and shoes with long shoelaces
- Assistive devices that need repair—walkers, canes, wheelchairs
- Having to climb or reach for objects

TEAMWORK AND TIME MANAGEMENT
Causes and Risk Factors for Falls

The entire health team must protect the person from harm. If you see something unsafe, tell the nurse at once. Do not assume the nurse knows or that someone is tending to the matter.

Answer all signal lights promptly. This includes the signal lights of patients and residents assigned to co-workers.

Know your role during shift changes. Nursing staff going off duty and those of the on-coming shift must work together to prevent falls.

FALL PREVENTION PROGRAMS

Agencies have fall prevention programs. The measures listed in Box 13-2, p. 186 are part of the program and the person's care plan. Many measures also apply to home settings. The care plan also lists measures for the person's specific risk factors.

Common sense and simple safety measures can prevent many falls. The health team works with the person and family to reduce the risk of falls. The goal is to prevent falls without decreasing the person's quality of life.

See *Focus on Communication: Fall Prevention Programs*, p. 188.

See *Focus on Long-Term Care and Home Care: Fall Prevention Programs*, p. 188.

See *Promoting Safety and Comfort: Fall Prevention Programs*, p. 188.

Text continued on p. 188

BOX 13-2   SAFETY MEASURES TO PREVENT FALLS

Basic Needs

- Fluid needs are met.
- Eyeglasses and hearing aids are worn as needed. Reading glasses are not worn when up and about.
- Tasks are explained before and while performing them.
- Help is given with elimination needs. It is given at regular times and whenever requested. Assist the person to the bathroom. Or provide the bedpan, urinal, or commode.
- The bedpan, urinal, or commode is kept within easy reach if the person can use the device without help.
- A warm drink, soft lights, or a back massage is used to calm the person who is agitated.
- Barriers are used to prevent wandering (Fig. 13-1).
- The person is properly positioned when in bed, a chair, or a wheelchair. Use pillows, wedge pads, or seats as the nurse and care plan direct (Chapter 16).
- Correct procedures are used for transfers (Chapter 17).
- The person is involved in meaningful activities.
- Exercise programs are followed. They help improve balance, strength, walking, and physical function.

Bathrooms and Shower/Tub Rooms

- Tubs and showers have non-slip surfaces or non-slip bath mats.
- Grab bars (safety bars) are in showers. They also are by tubs and toilets.
- Bathrooms have grab bars.
- Shower chairs are used (Chapter 20).
- Safety measures for tub baths and showers are followed (Chapter 20).

Floors

- Carpeting (if used) is wall-to-wall or tacked down.
- Scatter, area, and throw rugs are not used.
- Floor covers are one color. Bold designs can cause dizziness in older persons.
- Floors have non-glare, non-slip surfaces.
- Non-skid wax is used on hardwood, tiled, or linoleum floors.
- Loose floor boards and tiles are reported. So are frayed rugs and carpets.
- Floors and stairs are free of clutter, cords, and other items that can cause tripping.
- Floors are free of spills. Wipe up spills at once. Put a WET FLOOR sign by the wet area.
- Floors are free of excess furniture and equipment.
- Electrical and extension cords are out of the way. This includes power strips.
- Equipment and supplies are kept on one side of the hallway.

Furniture

- Furniture is placed for easy movement.
- Furniture is kept in place. It is not re-arranged.
- Chairs have armrests. Armrests give support when standing or sitting.
- A phone, lamp, and personal belongings are within the person's reach.

Beds and Other Equipment

- The bed is at the correct height for the person.
- The bed is in the lowest horizontal position, except when giving bedside care. The distance from the bed to the floor is reduced if the person falls or gets out of bed.

Beds and Other Equipment—cont'd

- Bed rails are used according to the care plan (p. 188).
- A mattress, special mat, or floor cushion is placed on the floor beside the bed (Fig. 13-2). This reduces the chance of injury if the person falls or gets out of bed.
- Wheelchairs, walkers, canes, and crutches fit properly. They are in good repair. Another person's equipment is not used.
- Crutches, canes, and walkers have non-skid tips.
- Correct equipment is used for transfers (Chapter 17). Follow the care plan.
- Positioning devices are used as directed (Chapter 16).
- Wheelchair and stretcher safety is followed (Chapter 12).
- Wheel locks on beds (p. 190), wheelchairs, and stretchers are in working order.
- Bed and wheelchair or stretcher wheels are locked for transfers.
- Linens are checked for sharp objects and for the person's property (dentures, eyeglasses, hearing aids, and so on).

Lighting

- Rooms, hallways, and stairways have good lighting. So do bathrooms and shower/tub rooms.
- Light switches (including those in bathrooms) are within reach and easy to find.
- Night-lights are in bedrooms, hallways, and bathrooms.

Shoes and Clothing

- Non-skid footwear is worn. Socks, bedroom slippers, and long shoelaces are avoided.
- Shoes fit well. They should not slip up and down on the person's feet. All shoelaces and straps are fastened.
- Clothing fits properly. Clothing is not loose. It does not drag on the floor. Belts are tied or secured in place.

Signal Lights and Alarms

- The person is taught how to use the signal light (Chapter 18).
- The signal light is always within the person's reach. This includes when sitting in the chair, on the commode, and when in the bathroom and tub/shower room.
- The person is asked to call for assistance when help is needed:
  - When getting out of bed or a chair
  - With walking
  - With getting to or from the bathroom or commode
  - With getting on or off the bedpan
- Signal lights are answered promptly. The person may need help right away. He or she may not wait for help.
- Bed, chair, door, floor mat, and belt alarms are used. They sense when the person tries to get up, get out of bed, or open a door (Fig. 13-3).
- Alarms are responded to at once.

Other

- Color-coded alerts are used to warn of a fall risk. Yellow is the common color for a fall alert. Besides wristbands (Chapter 12), some agencies also use color-coded blankets, non-skid footwear, socks, and magnets or stickers to place on room doors.
- The person is checked often. This may be every 15 minutes or as required by the care plan. Careful and frequent observation is important.
- Frequent checks are made on persons with poor judgment or memory. This may be every 15 minutes or as required by the care plan.
- Persons at risk for falling are close to the nurses' station.

BOX 13-2	SAFETY MEASURES TO PREVENT FALLS—cont'd

Other—cont'd

- Hand rails are on both sides of stairs and hallways.
- The person uses hand rails when walking or using stairs.
- The person uses grab bars in bathrooms and shower/tub rooms.
- Family and friends are asked to visit during busy times. Meal times and shift changes are examples. They are also asked to visit during the evening and night shifts.
- Companions are provided. Sitters, companions, or volunteers are with the person.
- Non-slip strips are on the floor next to the bed and in the bathroom. They are intact.

Other—cont'd

- Caution is used when turning corners, entering corridor intersections, and going through doors. You could injure a person coming from the other direction.
- Pull (do not push) wheelchairs, stretchers, carts, and other wheeled equipment through doorways. This allows you to lead the way and to see where you are going.
- A safety check is made of the room after visitors leave. (See the inside of the front book cover.) They may have lowered a bed rail, removed a signal light, or moved a walker out of reach. Or they may have brought an item that could harm the person.

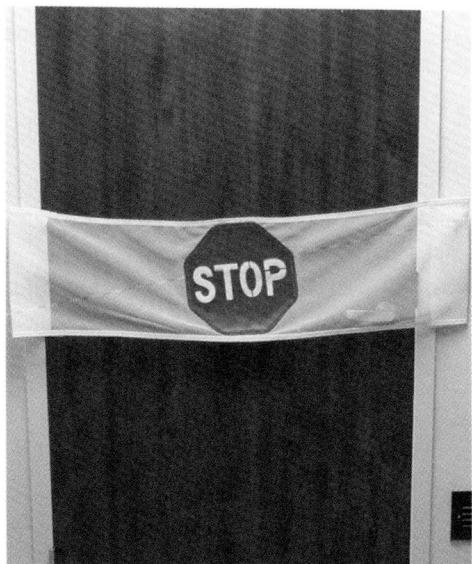

Fig. 13-1 Barriers are used to prevent wandering.

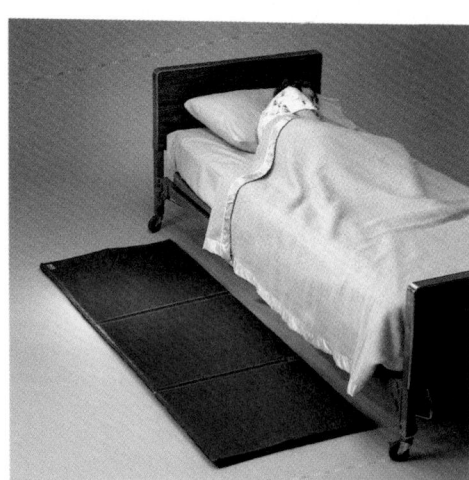

Fig. 13-2 Floor cushion.

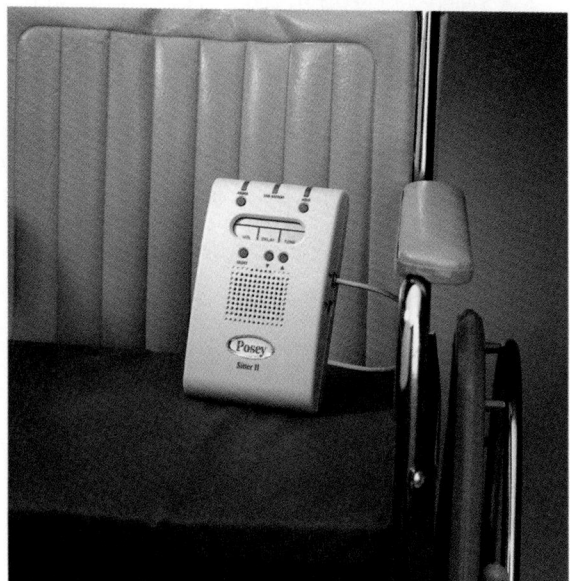

A

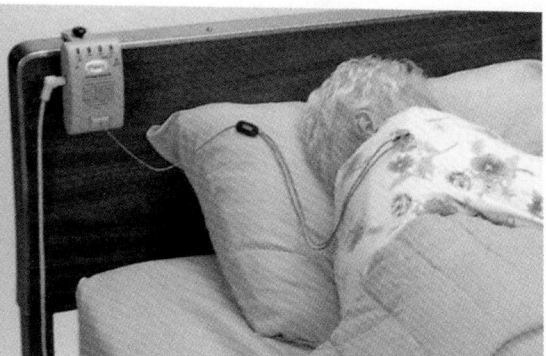

B

Fig. 13-3 Alarms. **A,** Chair alarm. **B,** Bed alarm.

Bed Rails

A *bed rail (side rail) is a device that serves as a guard or barrier along the side of the bed.* Bed rails are raised and lowered (Fig. 13-4). They lock in place with levers, latches, or buttons. Bed rails are half, three quarters, or the full length of the bed. When half-length rails are used, each side may have two rails. One is for the upper part of the bed, the other for the lower part.

The nurse and care plan tell you when to raise bed rails. They are needed by persons who are unconscious or sedated with drugs. Some confused or disoriented people need them. If a person needs bed rails, keep them up at all times except when giving bedside nursing care.

Bed rails present hazards. The person can fall when trying to climb over them, or the person cannot get out of bed or use the bathroom. *Entrapment* is a risk (Chapter 18). That is, the person can get caught, trapped, entangled, or strangled.

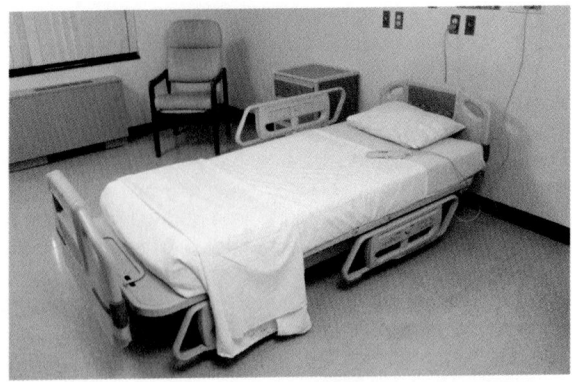

Fig. 13-4 Bed rails. The far bed rail is raised. The near bed rail is lowered.

Bed rails prevent the person from getting out of bed. They are considered restraints (Chapter 14) by the Omnibus Budget Reconciliation Act of 1987 (OBRA) and the Centers for Medicare & Medicaid Services (CMS) if:

- The person cannot get out of bed.
- The person cannot lower them without help.

Bed rails cannot be used unless needed to treat a person's medical symptoms. Some people feel safer with bed rails up. Others use them to change positions in bed. The person or legal representative must give consent for raised bed rails. The need for bed rails is carefully noted in the person's medical record and the care plan.

Accrediting agency standards and federal and state laws affect bed rail use. They are allowed when the person's condition requires them. Bed rails must be in the person's best interests.

The procedures in this book include using bed rails. This helps you learn to use them correctly. The nurse, the care plan, and your assignment sheet tell you which people use bed rails. If a person does not use them, omit the "raise bed rails" and "lower bed rails" steps.

Check the person often. Report to the nurse that you checked the person. If you are allowed to chart, record when you check the person and your observations (Fig. 13-5).

See *Focus on Children and Older Persons: Bed Rails.*
See *Focus on Long-Term Care and Home Care: Bed Rails.*
See *Promoting Safety and Comfort: Bed Rails.*

Date	Time	Nursing Margin	Other Depts Margin
11/10	0900	I turned Mr. Adams from his back to his L side. One pillow placed under his head, one against his back, and one supporting his R leg. Full bed rails raised according to the care plan. Bed lowered to its lowest position. Water pitcher and filled water cup c̄ straw placed on the overbed table within Mr. Adams' reach. Phone and box of tissue on the bedside table within reach. Urinal hung on the bed rail per Mr. Adams' request. Signal light attached to the bed rail within reach. Mr. Adams states he is comfortable and that needed items are within his reach. I told him that I would be checking on him every 15 minutes and that he should use the signal light if he needed anything. Gwen Rider, CNA.	

Fig. 13-5 Charting sample.

FOCUS ON CHILDREN AND OLDER PERSONS
Bed Rails

Children
Check that the crib meets federal safety standards. Drop-side cribs do *not* meet current safety standards. In December 2010, the United States government banned the manufacture and sale of drop-side cribs. If a crib has drop-sides, keep crib rails up and locked.

Crib rails must be safe. The space between crib rail slats must be no more than 2⅜ inches. If the space is larger, the baby's head can get caught between the slats. The baby can suffocate.

For toddlers and older children, rails may be placed on beds. Entrapment is a risk (Chapter 18). Rails must fit the child's bed and be installed according to the manufacturer's instructions.

FOCUS ON LONG-TERM CARE AND HOME CARE
Bed Rails

Long-Term Care
Not all persons in nursing centers use bed rails. The person's condition determines their use. You need to know who does and does not use bed rails. Consult the nurse and the person's care plan.

Home Care
Bed rails may also be used in home care settings. The same risks and safety measures apply. Check the safety of bed rails installed by the family. Look for loose or poor fitting rails. Tell the nurse if you suspect a problem.

PROMOTING SAFETY AND COMFORT
Bed Rails

Safety
You raise the bed to give care. Follow these safety measures to prevent the person from falling:
- *For a person who uses bed rails.* Always raise the far bed rail if you are working alone. Raise both bed rails if you need to leave the bedside for any reason.
- *For the person who does not use bed rails.* Ask a co-worker to help you. The co-worker stands on the far side of the bed. This protects the person from falling.
- Never leave the person alone when the bed is raised.
- Always lower the bed to its lowest position when you are done giving care.

Comfort
The person has to reach over raised bed rails for items on the bedside stand and overbed table. Such items include the water pitcher and cup, tissues, phone, and TV and light controls. Adjust the overbed table so it is within the person's reach. Ask if the person wants other items nearby. Place them on the overbed table too. Always make sure needed items, including the signal light, are within the person's reach.

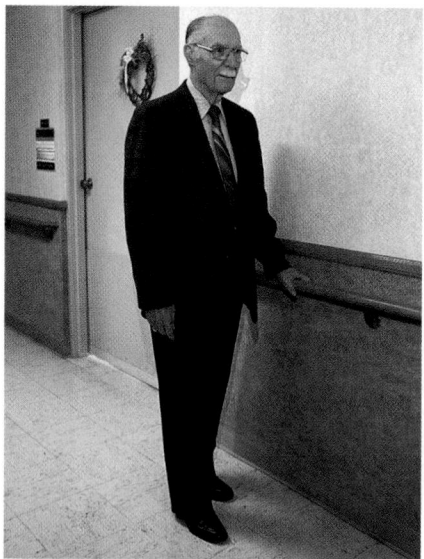

Fig. 13-6 Hand rails provide support when walking.

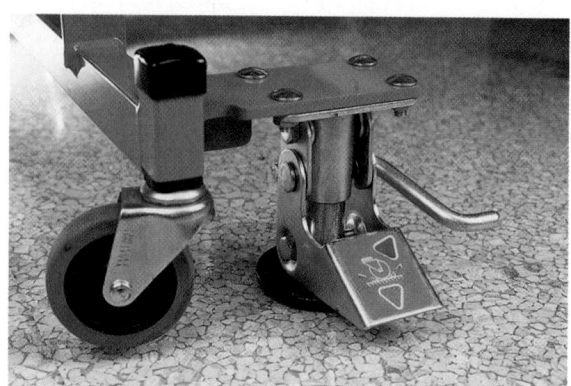

Fig. 13-8 Lock on a bed wheel.

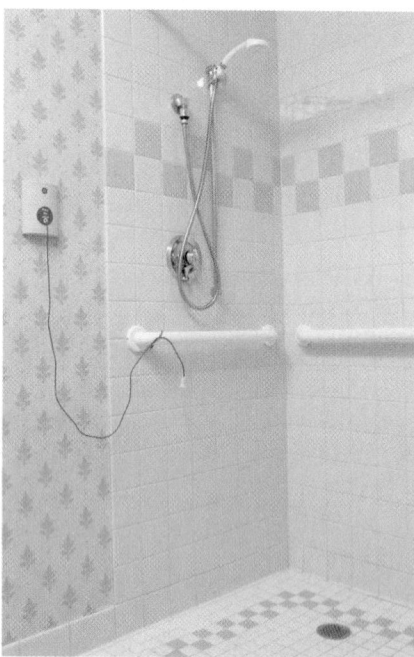

Fig. 13-7 Grab bars in a shower.

Hand Rails and Grab Bars

Hand rails are in hallways and stairways (Fig. 13-6). They give support to persons who are weak or unsteady when walking.

Grab bars are in bathrooms and in shower/tub rooms (Fig. 13-7). They provide support for sitting down or getting up from a toilet. They also are used for getting in and out of the shower or tub.

Wheel Locks

Bed legs have wheels. They let the bed move easily. Wheels have locks to prevent the bed from moving (Fig. 13-8). Wheels are locked at all times except when moving the bed. Make sure bed wheels are locked:

* When giving bedside care
* When you transfer a person to and from the bed

Wheelchair and stretcher wheels also are locked during transfers (Chapter 17). You or the person can be injured if the bed, wheelchair, or stretcher moves.

◼ TRANSFER/GAIT BELTS

A *transfer belt (gait belt) is a device used to support a person who is unsteady or disabled* (Fig. 13-9). It helps prevent falls and injuries. When used to transfer a person (Chapter 17), it is called a *transfer belt*. When used to help a person walk, it is called a *gait belt*.

The belt goes around the person's waist. Grasp under the belt to support the person during the transfer or when assisting the person to walk. If the belt has handles, grasp the belt by the handles (Fig. 13-10).

The standard-size transfer/gait belt fits waist sizes up to 51 inches. Bariatric-size belts fit waist sizes up to 71 inches. The nurse and care plan tell you what size to use. If the person's waist size is greater than 71 inches, follow the nurse's directions and the care plan.

See *Focus on Communication: Transfer/Gait Belts.*

See *Promoting Safety and Comfort: Transfer/Gait Belts.*

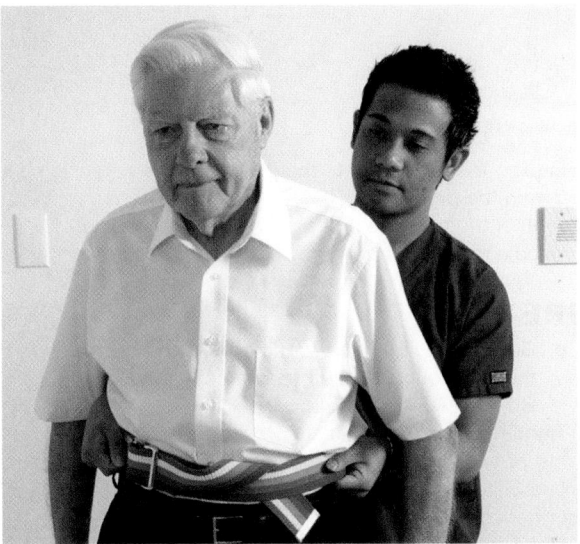

Fig. 13-9 Transfer/gait belt. The belt buckle is positioned off-center. The buckle is not over the spine. Excess strap is tucked into the belt. The nursing assistant grasps the belt from underneath.

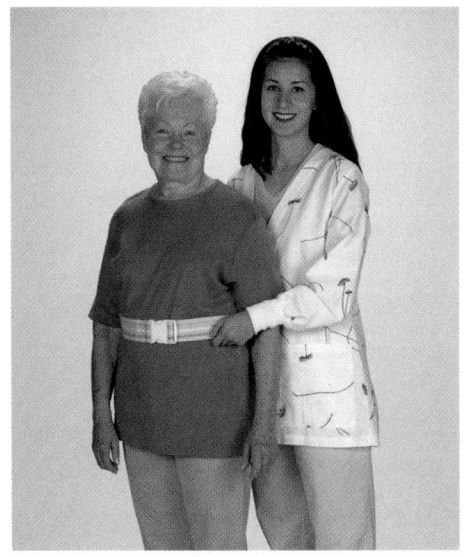

Fig. 13-11 A transfer/gait belt with a quick-release buckle.

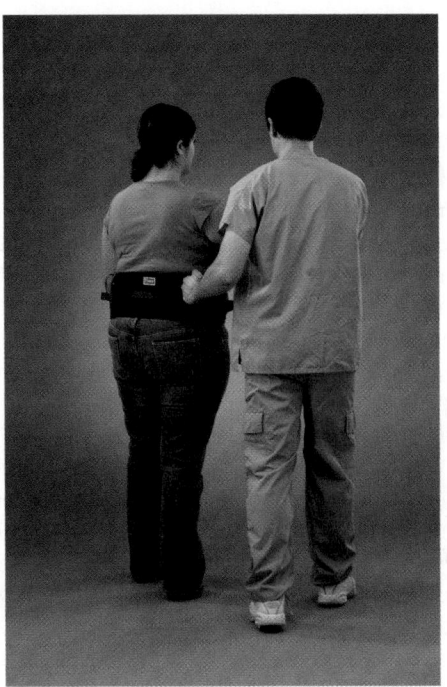

Fig. 13-10 A transfer/gait belt with handles. The nursing assistant grasps the belt by the handles.

FOCUS ON COMMUNICATION
Transfer/Gait Belts

When applying a transfer/gait belt, ask the person about his or her comfort. You can say: "How does that feel? Is the belt too loose? Is it too tight?" Adjust the belt as needed for the person's comfort and safety.

PROMOTING SAFETY AND COMFORT
Transfer/Gait Belts

Safety

Transfer/gait belts are routinely used in nursing centers. If the person needs help, a belt is required. To use one safely, always follow the manufacturer's instructions.

Some transfer/gait belts have a quick-release buckle (Fig. 13-11). Position the quick-release buckle at the person's back where he or she cannot reach it. This prevents the person from releasing the buckle during the procedure. Injury could result if the buckle is released.

Do not leave excess strap dangling. Tuck the excess strap into the belt (see Fig. 13-9).

Remove the belt after the procedure. Do not leave the person alone while he or she is wearing a transfer/gait belt.

Using a transfer/gait belt is unsafe for some persons. The belt could cause pressure or rub against care equipment. Check with the nurse and the care plan before using a transfer/gait belt if the person has:

- An ostomy—colostomy, ileostomy, urostomy (Chapters 23 and 44)
- A gastrostomy tube (Chapter 25)
- Chronic obstructive pulmonary disease (Chapter 42)
- An abdominal wound, incision, or drainage tube
- A chest wound, incision, or drainage tube
- Monitoring equipment
- A hernia (part of an organ that protrudes or projects through an opening in a muscle wall. Hernias often involve a loop of bowel or the stomach.)
- Other conditions or care equipment involving the chest or abdomen

Comfort

A transfer/gait belt is always applied over clothing. It is never applied over bare skin. Also, it is applied under the breasts. Breasts must not be caught under the belt. The belt buckle is never positioned over the person's spine.

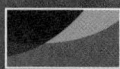 **APPLYING A TRANSFER/GAIT BELT**

QUALITY OF LIFE

Remember to:
- Knock before entering the person's room.
- Address the person by name.
- Introduce yourself by name and title.

- Explain the procedure to the person before beginning and during the procedure.
- Protect the person's rights during the procedure.
- Handle the person gently during the procedure.

PROCEDURE

1 See *Promoting Safety and Comfort: Transfer/Gait Belts,* p. 191.
2 Practice hand hygiene.
3 Identify the person. Check the identification (ID) bracelet against the assignment sheet. Also call the person by name.
4 Provide for privacy.
5 Assist the person to a sitting position.
6 Apply the belt:
   a Wrap the belt around the person's waist. Apply the belt over clothing. Do not apply it over bare skin.
   b Insert the belt's metal tip into the buckle. Pass the belt through the side with the teeth first (Fig. 13-12, A).

   c Bring the belt tip across the front of the buckle. Insert the tip through the buckle's smooth side (Fig. 13-12, B).
7 Tighten the belt so it is snug. It should not cause discomfort or impair breathing. You should be able to slide your open, flat hand under the belt. Ask the person about his or her comfort.
8 Make sure that a woman's breasts are not caught under the belt.
9 Place the buckle off-center in the front or off-center in the back for the person's comfort (Fig. 13-12, C). The buckle is not over the spine.
10 Tuck any excess strap into the belt (see Fig. 13-12, C).

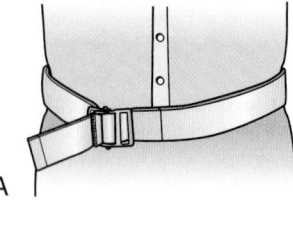

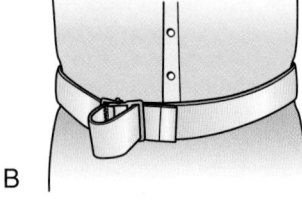

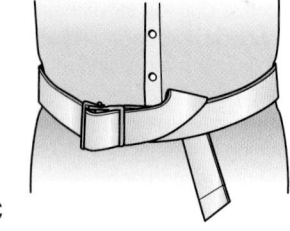

Fig. 13-12 Applying a transfer/gait belt at the waist. **A,** The belt is inserted into the buckle. The belt goes through the side with the teeth first. **B,** The belt is inserted into the buckle's smooth side. **C,** The buckle is in the front. The excess strap is tucked into the belt.

THE FALLING PERSON

A person may start to fall when standing or walking. The person may be weak, light-headed, or dizzy. Fainting may occur. Falling may be caused by slipping or sliding on spills, waxed floors, throw rugs, or improper shoes. See p. 184 for the causes and risk factors for falls.

Do not try to prevent the fall. You could injure yourself and the person while twisting and straining to prevent the fall. Balance is lost as the person falls. If you try to prevent the fall, you could lose your balance. Thus both you and the person could fall or cause the other person to fall. Head, wrist, arm, hip, knee and back injuries could occur.

If a person starts to fall, ease him or her to the floor. This lets you control the direction of the fall. You can also protect the person's head. Do not let the person move or get up before the nurse checks for injuries. Calmly explain that the nurse will check for injuries such as broken bones.

If you find a person on the floor, do not move the person. Stay with the person, and call for the nurse.

An incident report is completed after all falls. The nurse may ask you to help with the report.

See *Focus on Children and Older Persons: The Falling Person.*

See *Promoting Safety and Comfort: The Falling Person.*

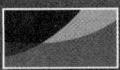

HELPING THE FALLING PERSON

PROCEDURE

1. Stand behind the person with your feet apart. Keep your back straight.
2. Bring the person close to your body as fast as possible (Fig. 13-13, A). Use the transfer/gait belt. Or wrap your arms around the person's waist. If necessary, you can also hold the person under the arms.
3. Move your leg so the person's buttocks rest on it (Fig. 13-13, B). Move the leg near the person.
4. Lower the person to the floor. The person slides down your leg to the floor (Fig. 13-13, C). Bend at your hips and knees as you lower the person.
5. Call a nurse to check the person. Stay with the person.
6. Help the nurse return the person to bed. Ask other staff to help if needed.

POST-PROCEDURE

7. Provide for comfort. (See the inside of the front book cover.)
8. Place the signal light within reach.
9. Raise or lower bed rails. Follow the care plan.
10. Complete a safety check of the room. (See the inside of the front book cover.)
11. Practice hand hygiene.
12. Report and record the following:
    - How the fall occurred
    - How far the person walked
    - How activity was tolerated before the fall
    - Complaints before the fall
    - How much help the person needed while walking
13. Complete an incident report.

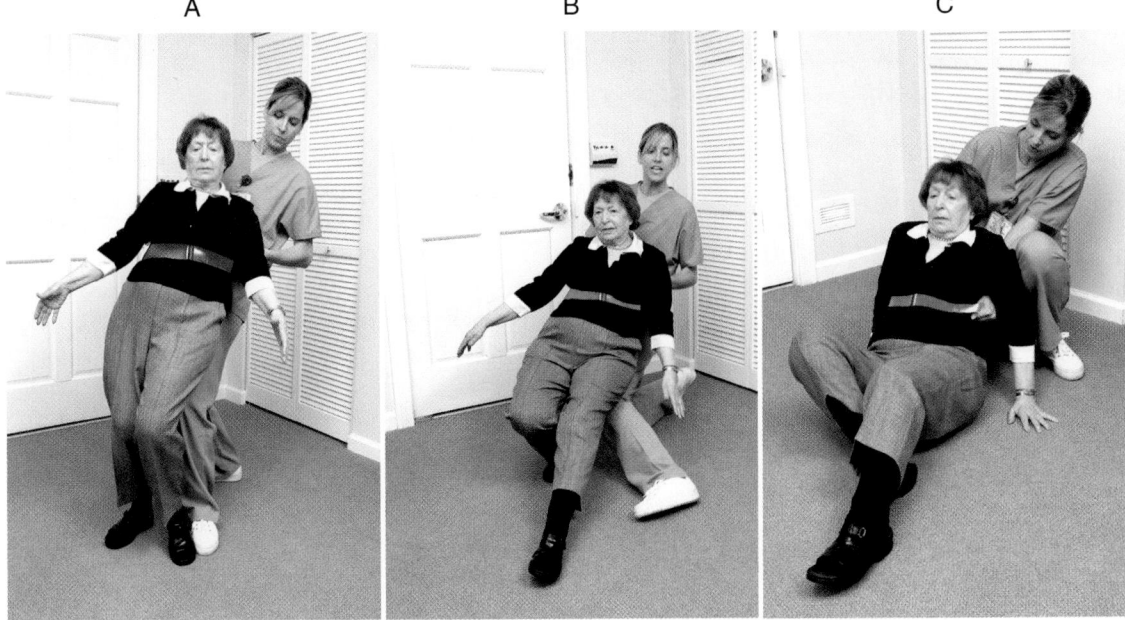

Fig. 13-13 The falling person. **A,** The falling person is supported with the gait belt. **B,** The person's buttocks rest on the nursing assistant's leg. **C,** The person is eased to the floor on the nursing assistant's leg.

FOCUS ON PRIDE

The Person, Family, and Yourself

Personal and Professional Responsibility

Safety measures can be time consuming. Perhaps you cannot find a transfer belt. Or you need to get a walker. Or you must put on the person's shoes. Resist the urge to take short cuts. Take the time to:

- Find and use assistive devices.
- Put proper footwear on the person.
- Raise or lower the bed and side rails as appropriate.
- Lock wheels on beds, stretchers, and wheelchairs.
- Ask others to help if needed.

You are responsible for providing safe care. This includes taking measures to prevent falls. See Box 13-2. Hurrying is never an acceptable excuse for causing harm. Take time for safety. Take pride in doing the right thing by providing safe care.

Rights and Respect

Patients and residents have the right to feel safe. Safety and security are not only rights, but basic needs (Chapter 8). Fear of falling does not make a person feel safe. Before moving a person, explain what you are going to do and what he or she needs to do. Also give step-by-step instructions as you progress. Do not move the person without telling him or her first. These measures help increase the person's comfort. See Chapter 17 for how to safely move and transfer the person. Good communication promotes comfort. It supports the person's right to safety and security.

Independence and Social Interaction

Some persons feel restricted by the use of safety devices. They may feel it limits independence. For example, Ms. Mills does not like having her bed rails up. She says: "I feel trapped. Do those have to be up?" Ms. Mills has fallen out of bed at night. The care plan includes having bed rails up while she is in bed.

Listen to the person's concerns. Kindly explain the reason for the safety device. If the person still refuses, tell the nurse. Do not let the person talk you out of performing a safety measure or using a safety device. Safety is always a priority.

Delegation and Teamwork

Helping co-workers with their patients or residents is an important part of teamwork. However, you may not be familiar with the person and his or her care plan. You must promote safety. Communication is essential. When assisting with the transfer of a co-worker's patient or resident, you must have information about the person. Ask the nurse or co-worker:

- Is the person at risk for falls?
- Is the person weak? Can he or she bear weight?
- Are there any activity limits?
- How many persons are needed for the transfer?
- Are any assistive devices needed? A cane, transfer belt, wheelchair, and walker are examples.
- Is any other equipment needed? Oxygen and braces are examples.

Ethics and Laws

Falls are a serious matter. Failing to take measures to prevent falls can result in legal action. The following is a case in which the nursing staff neglected to use safety measures to prevent a fall:

A hospital patient fell and injured her right shoulder 6 days after knee surgery. The patient claimed that the nursing staff did not follow orders to assist with ambulation to and from the bathroom. According to the patient:

- *She asked for help to raise herself from a commode to a standing position.*
- *She was not given assistance.*
- *She fell when the commode (with wheels) shifted while she tried to stand.*

According to the hospital's lawyers, the staff did not use a transfer belt. Failure to use the belt violated hospital policy.

The case settled for $25,000.

(N. Martinez and M. Martinez v St. Catherine's Hospital, Sentry Insurance and Wisconsin Patient Compensation Fund, 1998, Wisconsin.)

You must help prevent falls. Follow the safety measures presented in this chapter. Take pride in protecting yourself, the agency, and most importantly the person.

REVIEW QUESTIONS

Circle the BEST answer.

1 Most falls occur in
  a Patient and resident rooms and bathrooms
  b Dining rooms
  c Lounges
  d Hallways

2 Most falls occur
  a In the morning
  b At lunch time
  c In the afternoon
  d During the evening

3 A person's care plan includes fall prevention measures. Which should you question?
  a Assist with elimination needs.
  b Keep phone, lamp, and TV controls within reach.
  c Check the person every 2 hours.
  d Complete a safety check after visitors leave the room.

4 You observe the following in the person's room. Which is *not* safe?
  a The lamp cord is by the chair.
  b The chair has armrests.
  c The night-light works.
  d The bed is in the lowest horizontal position.

5 You note the following after a person got dressed. Which is safe?
  a The person is wearing non-skid shoes.
  b Pant cuffs are dragging on the floor.
  c The belt is not fastened.
  d The shirt is too big.

6 A co-worker is helping Mr. Polk today. His chair alarm goes off. What should you do?
  a Find your co-worker.
  b Tell the nurse.
  c Assist Mr. Polk.
  d Wait for someone to respond to the alarm.

7 To help prevent falls, you need to report
  a Equipment and supplies being on one side of the hallway
  b A mattress on the floor beside the bed
  c A co-worker pulling a wheelchair through a doorway
  d Clutter on stairways

8 Bed rails are used
  a When you think they are needed
  b When the bed is raised
  c According to the care plan
  d To support persons who are weak or unsteady

9 You are going to transfer a person from the bed to a chair. Bed wheels must be locked.
  a True
  b False

10 A transfer/gait belt is applied
  a To the skin
  b Over clothing at the waist
  c Over the breasts
  d Under the robe

11 To safely use a transfer/gait belt, you must
  a Follow the manufacturer's instructions
  b Be able to slide a closed fist under the belt
  c Leave the belt on if the person is left alone
  d Position the buckle over the person's spine

12 You apply a transfer/gait belt. What should you do with the excess strap?
  a Cut it off.
  b Wrap it around the person's waist.
  c Tuck it into the belt.
  d Let it dangle.

13 A person starts to fall. Your first action is to
  a Try to prevent the fall
  b Call for help
  c Bring the person close to your body as fast as possible
  d Lower the person to the floor

14 You found a person lying on the floor. What should you do?
  a Call for the nurse.
  b Help the person back to bed.
  c Apply a transfer belt.
  d Lock the bed wheels.

Answers to these questions are on p. 832.

14 Restraint Alternatives and Safe Restraint Use

OBJECTIVES

- Define the key terms and key abbreviations listed in this chapter.
- Describe the purpose of restraints.
- Identify the risks related to restraint use.
- Identify restraint alternatives.

- Explain the legal aspects of restraint use.
- Explain how to use restraints safely.
- Perform the procedure described in this chapter.
- Explain how to promote PRIDE in the person, the family, and yourself.

KEY TERMS

chemical restraint Any drug that is used for discipline or convenience and not required to treat medical symptoms

enabler A device that limits freedom of movement but is used to promote independence, comfort, or safety

freedom of movement Any change in place or position of the body or any part of the body that the person is able to control

medical symptom An indication or characteristic of a physical or psychological condition

physical restraint Any manual method or physical or mechanical device, material, or equipment attached to or near the person's body that he or she cannot remove easily and that restricts freedom of movement or normal access to one's body

remove easily The manual method, device, material, or equipment used to restrain the person that can be removed intentionally by the person in the same manner it was applied by the staff

KEY ABBREVIATIONS

CMS	Centers for Medicare & Medicaid Services	**OBRA**	Omnibus Budget Reconciliation Act of 1987
FDA	Food and Drug Administration	**TJC**	The Joint Commission

Chapters 12 and 13 have many safety measures. However, some persons need extra protection. They may present dangers to themselves or others (including staff).

The Centers for Medicare & Medicaid Services (CMS) have rules for using restraints. The rules apply to agencies receiving Medicare and Medicaid funds—hospitals, nursing centers, rehabilitation centers, and centers for the treatment of alcohol abuse, drug dependence, or mental health problems.

Like the Omnibus Budget Reconciliation Act of 1987 (OBRA), CMS rules protect the person's rights and safety. This includes the right to be free from restraint. Restraints may be used only to treat a medical symptom or for the immediate physical safety of the person or others. Restraints may be used only when less restrictive measures fail to protect the person or others. They must be discontinued at the earliest possible time.

The CMS uses these terms:

- *Physical restraint—any manual method or physical or mechanical device, material, or equipment attached to or near the person's body that he or she cannot remove easily and that restricts freedom of movement or normal access to one's body.*
- *Chemical restraint—any drug used for discipline or convenience and not required to treat medical symptoms.* The drug or dosage is not a standard treatment for the person's condition.
- *Freedom of movement—any change in place or position of the body or any part of the body that the person is able to control.*
- *Remove easily—the manual method, device, material, or equipment used to restrain the person that can be removed intentionally by the person in the same manner it was applied by the staff.* For example, the person can put bed rails down, untie a knot, or unclasp a buckle.

HISTORY OF RESTRAINT USE

Restraints were once thought to *prevent* falls. Research shows that restraints *cause* falls. Falls occur when persons try to get free of the restraints. Injuries are more serious from falls in restrained persons than in those not restrained.

Restraints also were used to prevent wandering or interfering with treatment. They were often used for persons who showed confusion, poor judgment, or behavior problems. Older persons were restrained more often than younger persons were. Restraints were viewed as necessary devices to protect a person. However, they can cause serious harm, even death (Box 14-1).

Besides the CMS, the Food and Drug Administration (FDA), state agencies, and The Joint Commission (TJC–an accrediting agency) have guidelines for restraint use. They do not forbid the use of restraints. However, *they require considering or trying all other appropriate alternatives first.*

Every agency has policies and procedures about restraints. They include identifying persons at risk for harm, harmful behaviors, restraint alternatives, and proper restraint use. Staff training is required.

BOX 14-1   RISKS OF RESTRAINT USE

- Agitation
- Anger
- Constipation
- Contractures (Chapter 27)
- Cuts and bruises
- Decline in physical function (ability to walk, muscle condition)
- Dehydration
- Delirium
- Depression
- Dignity: loss of
- Embarrassment and humiliation
- Falls
- Fractures
- Head trauma
- Incontinence
- Infections: pneumonia and urinary tract
- Mistrust
- Nerve injuries
- Pressure ulcers
- Self-respect: loss of
- Social contact: reduced
- Strangulation
- Withdrawal

RESTRAINT ALTERNATIVES

Often there are causes and reasons for harmful behaviors. Knowing and treating the cause can prevent restraint use. The nurse tries to find out what the behavior means. This is very important for persons with speech or cognitive problems. The focus is on these questions:

- Is the person in pain, ill, or injured?
- Is the person short of breath? Are cells getting enough oxygen (Chapter 36)?
- Is the person afraid in a new setting?
- Does the person need to use the bathroom?
- Is a dressing tight or causing other discomfort (Chapter 33)?
- Is clothing tight or causing other discomfort?
- Is the person's position uncomfortable?
- Are body fluids, secretions, or excretions causing skin irritation?
- Is the person too hot or too cold?
- Is the person hungry or thirsty?
- What are the person's life-long habits at this time of day?
- Does the person have problems communicating?
- Is the person seeing, hearing, or feeling things that are not real (Chapter 45)?
- Is the person confused or disoriented (Chapter 46)?
- Are drugs causing the behaviors?

Restraint alternatives for the person are identified (Box 14-2, p. 198). They become part of the care plan. Care plan changes are made as needed. Restraint alternatives may not protect the person. The doctor may need to order restraints.

SAFE RESTRAINT USE

Restraints can cause serious injury and even death. CMS, OBRA, FDA, and TJC guidelines are followed. So are state laws. They are part of the agency's policies and procedures for restraint use.

Restraints are not used to discipline a person. They are not used for staff convenience. *Discipline* is any action that punishes or penalizes a person. *Convenience* is any action that:

- Controls or manages the person's behavior.
- Requires less effort by the agency.
- Is not in the person's best interests.

Restraints are used only when necessary to treat a person's medical symptoms. The CMS defines a *medical symptom as an indication or characteristic of a physical or psychological condition.* Symptoms may relate to physical, emotional, or behavioral problems. Sometimes restraints are needed to protect the person or others. That is, a person may have violent or aggressive behaviors that are harmful to self or others.

BOX 14-2 ALTERNATIVES TO RESTRAINT USE

- Diversion is provided—TV, videos, music, games, relaxation tapes, and so on.
- Life-long habits and routines are in the care plan. For example, showers before breakfast; reads in the bathroom; walks outside before lunch; watches TV after lunch; and so on.
- Family and friends make videos of themselves for the person to watch.
- Videos are made of visits with family and friends for the person to watch.
- Time is spent in supervised areas (dining room, lounge, near the nurses' station).
- Pillows, wedge cushions, and posture and positioning aids are used.
- The signal light is within reach.
- Signal lights are answered promptly.
- Food, fluid, hygiene, and elimination needs are met.
- The bedpan, urinal, or commode is within the person's reach.
- Back massages are given.
- Family, friends, and volunteers visit.
- The person has companions or sitters.
- Time is spent with the person.
- Extra time is spent with a person who is restless.
- Reminiscing is done with the person.
- A calm, quiet setting is provided.
- The person wanders in safe areas.
- The entire staff is aware of persons who tend to wander. This includes staff in housekeeping, maintenance, the business office, dietary, and so on.

- Exercise programs are provided.
- Outdoor time is planned during nice weather.
- The person does jobs or tasks he or she consents to.
- Knob guards are used on doors.
- Padded hip protectors are worn under clothing (Fig. 14-1).
- Floor cushions are placed next to beds (Chapter 13).
- Roll guards are attached to the bed frame (Fig. 14-2).
- Falls are prevented (Chapter 13).
- Warning devices are used on beds, chairs, and doors (Fig. 14-3).
- The person's furniture meets his or her needs (lower bed, reclining chair, rocking chair).
- Walls and furniture corners are padded.
- Observations and visits are made at least every 15 minutes. Or as often as noted in the care plan.
- The person is moved to a room close to the nurses' station.
- Procedures and care measures are explained.
- Frequent explanations are given about equipment or devices.
- Confused persons are oriented to person, time, and place. Calendars and clocks are provided.
- Light is adjusted to meet the person's basic needs and preferences.
- Staff assignments are consistent.
- Sleep is not interrupted.
- Noise levels are reduced.

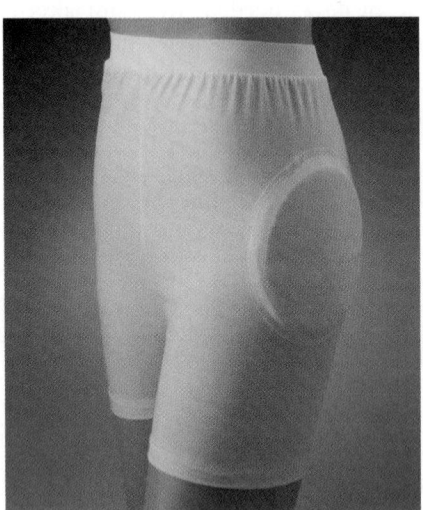

Fig. 14-1 Hip protector.

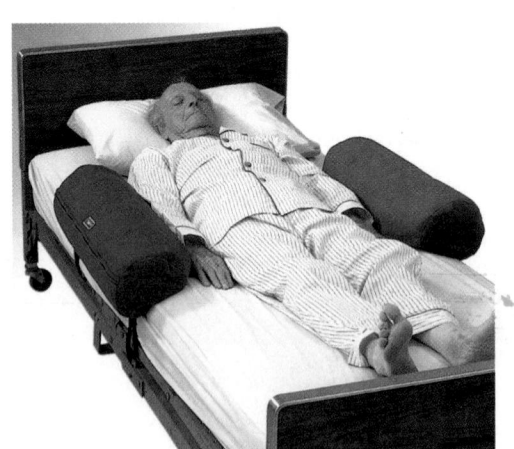

Fig. 14-2 Roll guard.

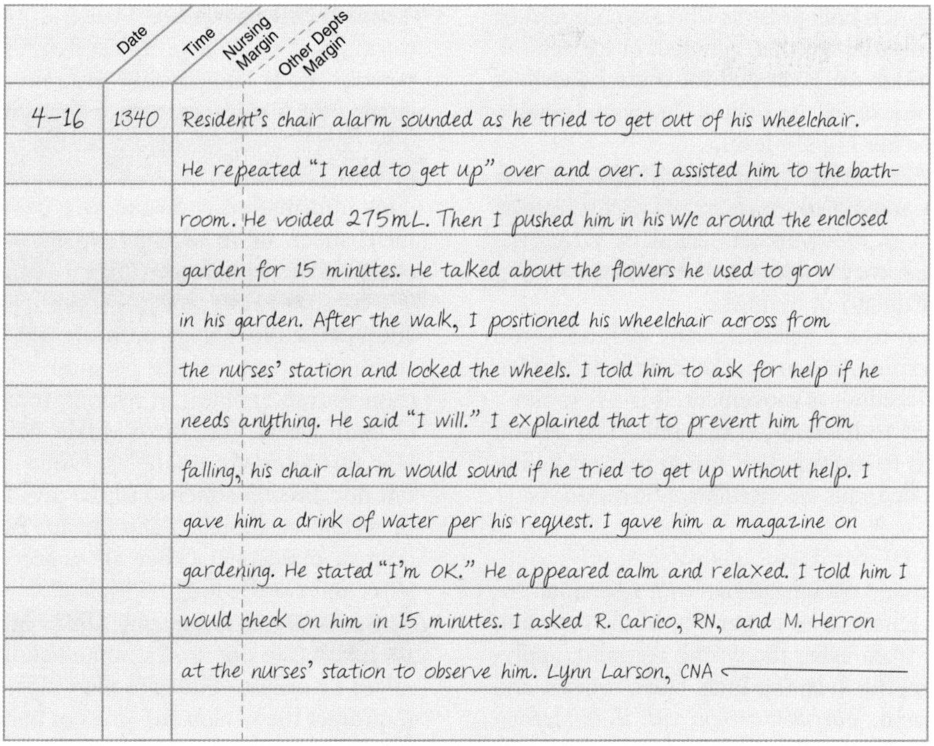

Date	Time	Nursing Margin	Other Depts Margin
4-16	1340	Resident's chair alarm sounded as he tried to get out of his wheelchair.	
		He repeated "I need to get up" over and over. I assisted him to the bath-	
		room. He voided 275 mL. Then I pushed him in his w/c around the enclosed	
		garden for 15 minutes. He talked about the flowers he used to grow	
		in his garden. After the walk, I positioned his wheelchair across from	
		the nurses' station and locked the wheels. I told him to ask for help if he	
		needs anything. He said "I will." I explained that to prevent him from	
		falling, his chair alarm would sound if he tried to get up without help. I	
		gave him a drink of water per his request. I gave him a magazine on	
		gardening. He stated "I'm OK." He appeared calm and relaxed. I told him I	
		would check on him in 15 minutes. I asked R. Carico, RN, and M. Herron	
		at the nurses' station to observe him. Lynn Larson, CNA	

Fig. 14-3 Charting sample.

Physical and Chemical Restraints

According to the CMS, *physical restraints* include these points:

- May be any manual method, physical or mechanical device, material, or equipment
- Is attached to or next to the person's body
- Cannot be easily removed by the person
- Restricts freedom of movement or normal access to one's body

Physical restraints are applied to the chest, waist, elbows, wrists, hands, or ankles. They confine the person to a bed or chair. Or they prevent movement of a body part. Some furniture or barriers also prevent freedom of movement:

- A device used with a chair that the person cannot remove easily. The device prevents the person from rising. Trays, tables, bars, and belts are examples (Fig. 14-4).
- Any chair that prevents the person from rising.
- Any bed or chair placed so close to the wall that the person cannot get out of the bed or chair.
- Bed rails (Chapter 13) that prevent the person from getting out of bed. For example, four half-length bed rails are raised. They are restraints if the person cannot lower them.
- Tucking in or using Velcro to hold a sheet, fabric, or clothing so tightly that freedom of movement is restricted.

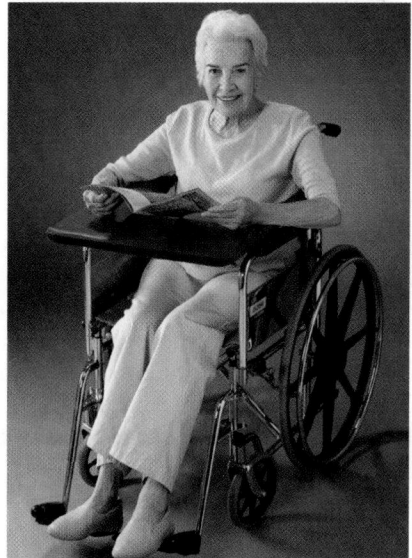

Fig. 14-4 This lap-top tray is a restraint alternative. It is a restraint when used to prevent freedom of movement.

Drugs or drug dosages are *chemical restraints* if they:

- Control behavior or restrict movement.
- Are not standard treatment for the person's condition.

Drugs cannot be used for discipline or staff convenience. They cannot be used if they affect physical or mental function.

Sometimes drugs can help persons who are confused or disoriented. They may be anxious, agitated, or aggressive. The doctor may order drugs to control these behaviors. The drugs should not make the person sleepy and unable to function at his or her highest level.

Enablers. An *enabler is a device that limits freedom of movement but is used to promote independence, comfort, or safety.* Some devices are both restraints and enablers. When the person can easily remove the device and it helps the person function, it is an enabler. For example:

- When the person uses a geriatric chair with a lap-top tray for meals, writing, and so on, the chair is an enabler. If used to limit freedom of movement, it is a restraint.
- A person chooses to have raised bed rails. The person uses the bed rails to move in bed and to prevent falling out of bed. The bed rails are enablers, not restraints.

Complications of Restraint Use

Box 14-1 lists the many complications from restraints. Injuries occur as the person tries to get free of the restraint. Injuries also occur from using the wrong restraint, applying it wrong, or keeping it on too long. Cuts, bruises, and fractures are common. *The most serious risk is death from strangulation.*

There are also mental effects. Restraints affect dignity and self-esteem. See Box 14-1.

Restraints are medical devices. The Safe Medical Devices Act applies if a restraint causes illness, injury, or death. Also, CMS requires the reporting of any death that occurs:

- While a person is in a restraint.
- Within 24 hours after a restraint was removed.
- Within 1 week after a restraint was removed. This is done if the restraint may have contributed directly or indirectly to the person's death.

Legal Aspects

Laws applying to restraint use are followed. Remember:

- *Restraints must protect the person.* They are not used for staff convenience or to discipline a person. Using restraints is not easier than properly supervising and observing the person. A restrained person requires more staff time for care, supervision, and observation. A restraint is used only when it is the best safety measure for the person. Restraints are not used to punish or penalize uncooperative persons.

- *A doctor's order is required.* OBRA, CMS, state laws, FDA warnings, TJC, and other accrediting agencies protect persons from unnecessary restraint. If restraints are needed for medical reasons, a doctor's order is required. The doctor gives the reason for the restraint, what body part to restrain, what to use, and how long to use it. This information is on the care plan and your assignment sheet. In an emergency, the nurse can decide to apply restraints before getting a doctor's order.

- *The least restrictive method is used.* It allows the greatest amount of movement or body access possible. Some restraints attach to the person's body and to a fixed (non-movable) object. It restricts freedom of movement or body access. Vest, jacket, ankle, wrist, hand, and some belt restraints are examples. Other restraints are near but not directly attached to the person's body (bed rails or wedge cushions). They do not totally restrict freedom of movement. They allow access to certain body parts and are the least restrictive.

- *Restraints are used only after other measures fail to protect the person* (see Box 14-2). Some people can harm themselves or others. The care plan must include measures to protect the person and prevent harm to others. Many fall prevention measures are restraint alternatives (Chapter 13).

- *Unnecessary restraint is false imprisonment* (Chapter 4). You must clearly understand the reason for the restraint and its risk. If not, politely ask about its use. If you apply an unneeded restraint, you could face false imprisonment charges.

- *Informed consent is required.* The person must understand the reason for the restraint. The person is told how the restraint will help the planned medical treatment. The person is told about the risks of restraint use. If the person cannot give consent, his or her legal representative is given the information. Either the person or his or her representative must give consent before a restraint can be used. The doctor or nurse provides needed information and obtains the consent.

See *Focus on Communication: Legal Aspects.*

FOCUS ON COMMUNICATION
Legal Aspects

You may not know the reason for a restraint. If so, politely ask the nurse why it is needed. For example:
- "Why does Mr. Reed need a restraint?"
- "I don't understand. Why did the doctor order the restraint?"

Safety Guidelines

The restrained person must be kept safe. Follow the safety measures in Box 14-3. Also remember these key points:

- *Observe for increased confusion and agitation.* Restraints can increase confusion and agitation. Whether confused or alert, people are aware of restricted movements. They may try to get out of the restraint or struggle or pull at it. Some restrained persons beg others to free or to help release them. These behaviors often are viewed as signs of confusion. Some people become more confused because they do not understand what is happening to them. Restrained persons need repeated explanations and reassurance. Spending time with them has a calming effect.

- *Protect the person's quality of life.* Restraints are used for as short a time as possible. The care plan must show how to reduce restraint use. The person's needs are met with as little restraint as possible. You must meet the person's physical, emotional, and social needs. Visit with the person and explain the reason for the restraints.

- *Follow the manufacturer's instructions.* They explain how to safely apply and secure the restraint. The restraint must be snug and firm, but not tight. Tight restraints affect circulation and breathing. The person must be comfortable and able to move the restrained part to a limited and safe extent. You could be negligent if you do not apply or secure a restraint properly.

- *Apply restraints with enough help to protect the person and staff from injury.* Persons in immediate danger of harming themselves or others are restrained quickly. Combative and agitated people can hurt themselves and the staff when restraints are applied. Enough staff members are needed to complete the task safely and quickly.

- *Observe the person at least every 15 minutes or as often as noted in the care plan.* Restraints are dangerous. Injuries and deaths can result from improper restraint use and poor observation. Prevent complications. Interferences with breathing and circulation are examples.

- *Remove or release the restraint, re-position the person, and meet basic needs at least every 2 hours or as often as noted in the care plan.* The restraint is removed or released for at least 10 minutes. Provide for food, fluid, comfort, safety, hygiene, and elimination needs and give skin care. Perform range-of-motion exercises or help the person walk (Chapter 27). Follow the care plan.

See *Focus on Communication: Safety Guidelines.*
See *Teamwork and Time Management: Safety Guidelines.*

Text continued on p. 205

FOCUS ON COMMUNICATION
Safety Guidelines

Restraints can increase confusion. Remind the person why the restraint is necessary and to call for help when it is needed. Repeat the following as often as needed:

- "Dr. Monroe ordered this restraint so you don't hurt yourself. If you need to get up, please call for help. I'll check on you every 15 minutes. Other staff will check on you too."
- "How does the restraint feel? Is it too tight? Is it too loose?"
- "Please put your signal light on. I want to make sure that you can reach and use it with the restraint on."
- "Please call for help right away if the restraint is too tight."
- "Please call for help right away if you feel pain in your fingers or hands. Also call for me if you feel numbness or tingling."
- "Please call for help right away if you are having problems breathing."

TEAMWORK AND TIME MANAGEMENT
Safety Guidelines

You may not be assigned to a restrained person. However, make sure you know who is restrained on your unit. Every time you walk past the person or the person's room, check to see if the person is safe and comfortable. Answer the person's signal light promptly.

BOX 14-3 | SAFETY MEASURES FOR USING RESTRAINTS

Before Applying Restraints

- Do not use sheets, towels, tape, rope, straps, bandages, Velcro, or other items to restrain a person.
- Apply a restraint only after being instructed about its proper use.
- Demonstrate proper application of the restraint before applying it.
- Use the restraint noted in the care plan. Use the correct size. Small restraints are tight. They cause discomfort and agitation. They also restrict breathing and circulation. Strangulation is a risk from big or loose restraints.
- Use only restraints that have manufacturer instructions and warning labels.

Before Applying Restraints—cont'd

- Read the manufacturer's warning labels. Note the front and back of the restraint.
- Follow the manufacturer's instructions. Some restraints are safe for bed, chair, and wheelchair use. Others are used only with certain equipment.
- Use intact restraints. Look for broken stitches, tears, cuts, or frayed fabric or straps. Look for missing or loose buckles, locks, hooks, loops, or straps or other damage. The restraint must hold securely.
- Test zippers, buckles, locks, hooks, loops, and other fasteners. The device must fasten securely.
- Do not use a restraint near a fire, a flame, or smoking materials.

Continued

BOX 14-3   SAFETY MEASURES FOR USING RESTRAINTS—cont'd

Applying Restraints

- Do not use restraints to position a person on a toilet.
- Do not use restraints to position a person on furniture that does not allow for correct application. Follow the manufacturer's instructions.
- Follow agency policies and procedures.
- Position the person in good alignment before applying the restraint (Chapter 16).
- Pad bony areas and the skin as instructed by the nurse. This prevents pressure and injury from the restraint.
- Apply the device following the manufacturer's instructions. A restraint applied incorrectly or backwards may result in serious injury or death. Death may occur from suffocation or strangulation.
  - For a vest restraint, the "V" neck is in front (Fig. 14-5).
  - For a jacket restraint, the opening is in the back.
- Do not criss-cross straps in the back unless required by the manufacturer's instructions (Fig. 14-6). Straps may loosen when the person moves and cause serious injury.
- Secure the restraint. It should be snug but allow some movement of the restrained part. Follow the manufacturer's instructions to check for snugness. For example:
  - If applied to the chest or waist—Make sure that the person can breathe easily. A flat hand should slide between the restraint and the person's body (Fig. 14-7). Check with the nurse if you have very small or very large hands. Small or large hands could cause the restraint to be too tight or too loose.
  - For wrist and mitt restraints—You should be able to slide 1 finger under the restraint. Check with the nurse if you have very small or very large fingers. Small or large fingers could cause the restraint to be too tight or too loose.
- Buckle or tie restraints according to agency policy. The policy should follow the manufacturer's instructions and allow for quick release in an emergency. Quick-release buckles or airline-type buckles are used (Fig. 14-8). So are quick-release ties (Fig. 14-9).
- Secure straps out of the person's reach.
- Leave 1 to 2 inches of slack in the straps (if directed to do so by the nurse). This allows some movement of the part.
- Secure the restraint to the movable part of the bed frame (Fig. 14-10, p. 204). The restraint will not tighten or loosen when the head or foot of the bed is raised or lowered. For chairs, secure straps under the seat of the wheelchair or chair (Fig. 14-11, p. 204).
- Make sure the straps cannot tighten, loosen, slip, or cause too much slack.
- Make sure that straps will not slide in any direction. If straps slide, they change the restraint's position. The person can get suspended off the mattress or chair (Figs. 14-12 and 14-13, p. 204). Strangulation can result.
- Never secure restraints to the bed rails. The person can reach bed rails to release knots or buckles. Also, injury to the person is likely when raising or lowering bed rails.
- Use bed rail covers or gap protectors as instructed by the nurse (Fig. 14-14, p. 205). They prevent entrapment between the rails or the bed rail bars (see Fig. 14-12). Entrapment can occur between:
  - The bars of a bed rail
  - The space between half-length (split) bed rails
  - The bed rail and mattress
  - The head-board or foot-board and mattress

Applying Restraints—cont'd

- Position the person as the nurse directs. This is usually semi-Fowler's position (Chapter 18) when using a vest, jacket, or belt restraint.
- Position the person in a chair so the hips are well to the back of the chair.
- Apply a belt restraint at a 45-degree angle over the thighs (Fig. 14-15, p. 205).

After Applying Restraints

- Keep full bed rails up when using a vest, jacket, or belt restraint. Also use bed rail covers or gap protectors. Otherwise the person could fall off the bed and strangle on the restraint. If half-length bed rails are used, the person can get caught between them.
- Do not use back cushions when a person is restrained in a chair. If the cushion moves out of place, slack occurs in the straps. Strangulation could result if the person slides forward or down from the extra slack (see Fig. 14-13).
- Do not cover the person with a sheet, blanket, bedspread, or other covering. The restraint must be within plain view at all times.
- Check the person at least every 15 minutes for safety, comfort, and signs of injury.
- Check the person's circulation at least every 15 minutes if mitt, wrist, or ankle restraints are applied. You should feel a pulse at a pulse site below the restraint. Fingers or toes should be warm and pink. Tell the nurse at once if:
  - You cannot feel a pulse.
  - Fingers or toes are cold, pale, or blue in color.
  - The person complains of pain, numbness, or tingling in the restrained part.
  - The skin is red or damaged.
- Check the person at least every 15 minutes if a belt, jacket, or vest restraint is used. The person should be able to breathe easily. Also check the position of the restraint, especially in the front and back.
- Monitor persons in the supine (back-lying) position constantly. They are at great risk for aspiration if vomiting occurs (Chapter 24). Call for the nurse at once.
- Keep scissors in your pocket. In an emergency, cutting the tie may be faster than untying a knot. Never leave scissors at the bedside where the person can reach them. Make sure the person cannot reach the scissors in your pocket.
- Remove or release the restraint and re-position the person every 2 hours or as often as noted in the care plan. The restraint is removed or released for at least 10 minutes. Meet the person's basic needs. You need to:
  - Measure vital signs.
  - Meet elimination needs.
  - Offer food and fluids.
  - Meet hygiene needs.
  - Give skin care.
  - Perform range-of-motion exercises or help the person walk. Follow the care plan.
  - Provide for physical and emotional comfort. (See the inside of the front book cover.)
- Keep the signal light within the person's reach. Chart that this was done.
- Complete a safety check before leaving the room. (See the inside of the front book cover.)
- Report to the nurse every time you checked the person and removed or released the restraint. Report your observations and the care given. Follow agency policy for recording.

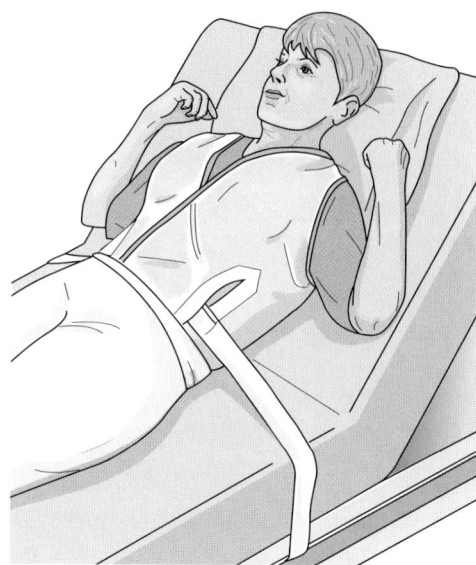

Fig. 14-5 The vest restraint criss-crosses in front. (NOTE: The bed rails are raised after the restraint is applied.)

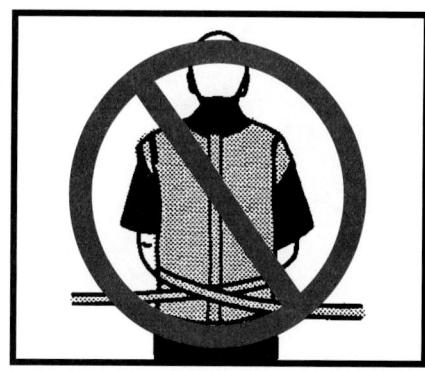

Fig. 14-6 Never criss-cross vest or jacket straps in the back.

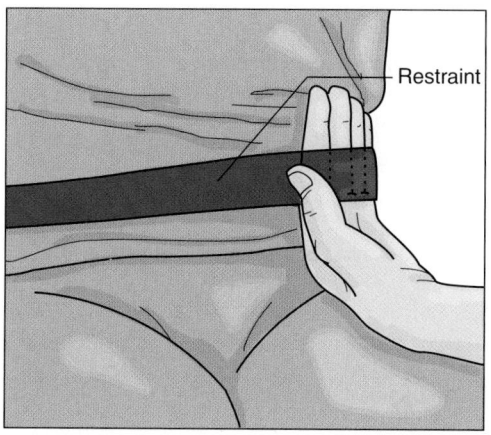

Fig. 14-7 A flat hand slides between the restraint and the person.

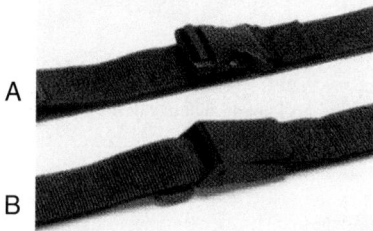

Fig. 14-8 **A,** Quick-release buckle. **B,** Airline-type buckle.

How to Tie the Posey Quick-Release Tie

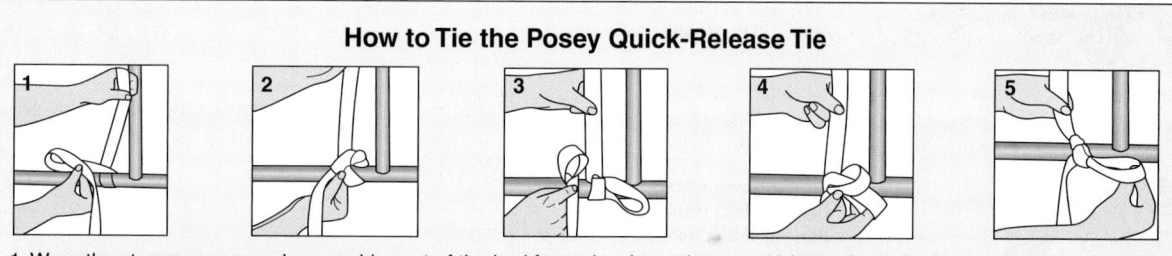

1. Wrap the strap once around a movable part of the bed frame leaving at least an 8" (20 cm) tail. Fold the loose end in half to create a loop and cross it over the other end.
2. Insert the folded strap where the straps cross over each other, as if tying a shoelace. Pull on the loop to tighten.
3. Fold the loose end in half to create a second loop.
4. Insert the second loop into the first loop.
5. Pull on the loop to tighten. Test to make sure strap is secure and will not slide in any direction.
6. Repeat on other side. Practice quick-release ties to ensure the knot releases with one pull on the loose end of the strap.

Fig. 14-9 The Posey quick-release tie.

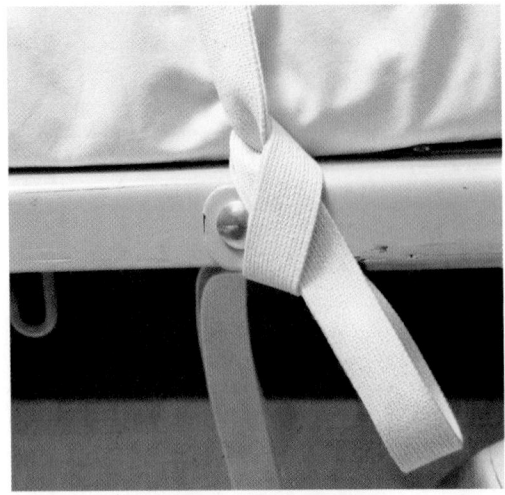

Fig. 14-10 The restraint is secured to the movable part of the bed frame.

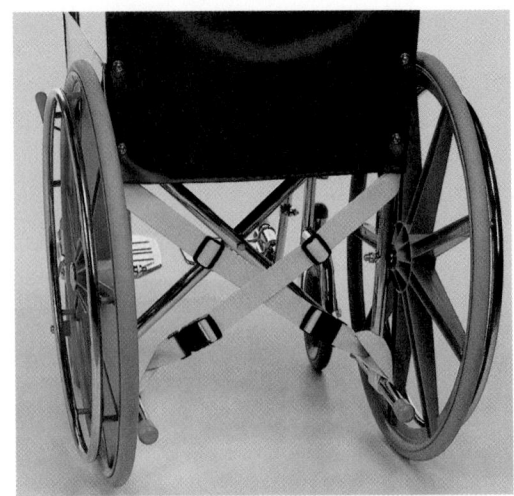

Fig. 14-11 The restraint straps are secured to the wheelchair frame.

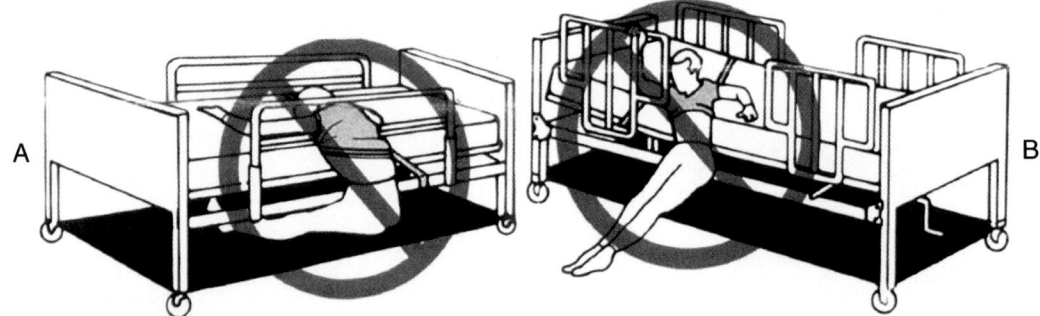

Fig. 14-12 **A,** A person can get suspended and caught between bed rail bars. **B,** The person can get suspended and caught between half-length bed rails.

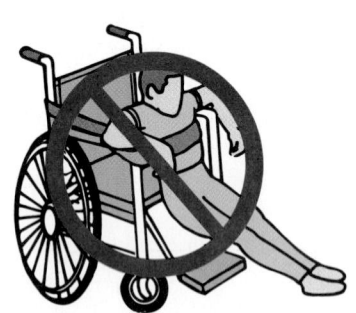

Straps to prevent sliding should always be over the thighs—NOT around the waist or chest. Straps should be at a 45° angle and secured to the chair under the seat, not behind the back. They should be snug but comfortable and not restrict breathing. If a belt or vest is too loose or applied around the waist, the person may slide partially off the seat—resulting in possible suffocation and death.

Fig. 14-13 Strangulation could result if the person slides forward or down in the chair because of extra slack in the restraint.

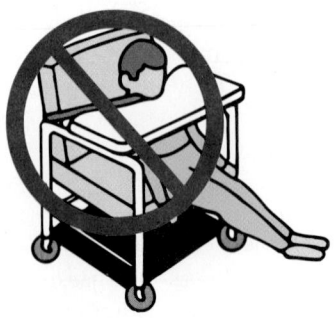

Tray tables (with or without a belt or vest) pose potential danger if the person should slide partly under the table and become caught. This could result in suffocation and death. Make sure the person's hips are positioned at the back of the chair—this may necessitate the use of an anti-slide material (Posey Grip), a pommel cushion, or a restrictive device if the person shows any tendency to slide forward.

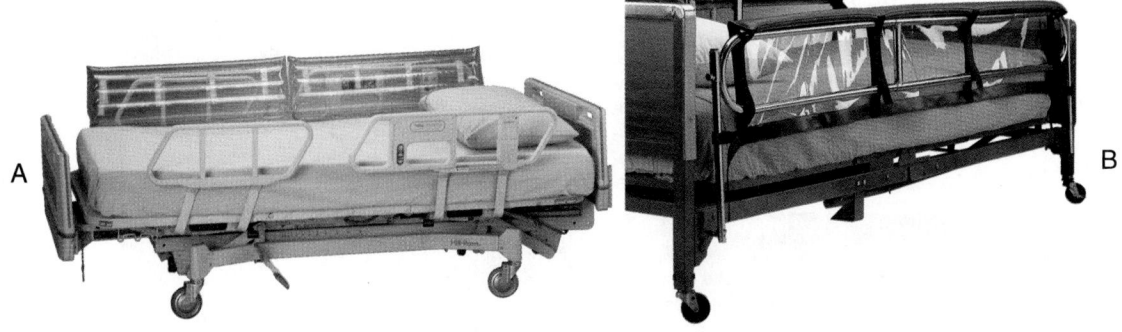

Fig. 14-14 A, Bed rail protector. **B,** Guard-rail pads.

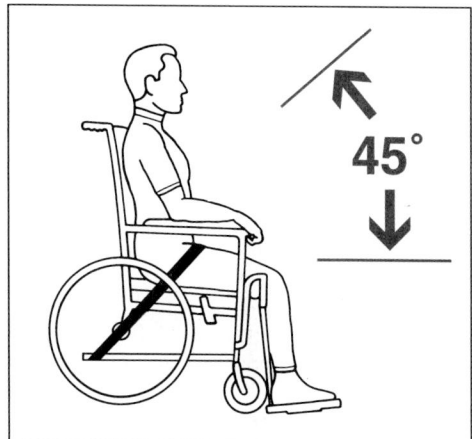

Fig. 14-15 The safety belt is at a 45-degree angle over the thighs.

Reporting and Recording

Information about restraints is recorded in the person's medical record (Fig. 14-16, p. 206). You might apply restraints or care for a restrained person. Report and record the following:

- The type of restraint applied.
- The body part or parts restrained.
- The reason for the application.
- Safety measures taken (for example, bed rails padded and up, signal light within reach).
- The time you applied the restraint.
- The time you removed or released the restraint and for how long.
- The person's vital signs.
- The care given when the restraint was removed or released.
- Skin color and condition.
- Condition of the limbs.
- The pulse felt in the restrained part.
- Changes in the person's behavior.
- Complaints of discomfort; a tight restraint; difficulty breathing; or pain, numbness, or tingling in the restrained part. Report these complaints to the nurse at once.

Applying Restraints

Restraints are made of cloth or leather. Cloth restraints (soft restraints) are mitts, belts, straps, jackets, and vests. They are applied to the wrists, ankles, hands, waist, and chest. Leather restraints are applied to the wrists and ankles. Leather restraints are used for extreme agitation and combativeness.

Wrist Restraints. Wrist restraints (limb holders) limit arm movement (Fig. 14-17, p. 206). They may be used when the person:

- Is at risk for pulling out tubes used for life-saving treatment (intravenous [IV] infusion, feeding tube).
- Is at risk for pulling at devices used to monitor vital signs.
- Scratches at, pulls at, or peels the skin, a wound, or a dressing. This can damage the skin or the wound.

Mitt Restraints. Hands are placed in mitt restraints. They prevent finger use. They allow hand, wrist, and arm movements. They are used for the same reasons as wrist restraints. Most mitts are padded (Fig. 14-18, p. 206).

Belt Restraints. The belt restraint (Fig. 14-19, p. 206) is used when injuries from falls are risks or for positioning during a medical treatment. The person cannot get out of bed or out of a chair. However, a roll belt allows the person to turn from side to side or sit up in bed.

The belt is applied around the waist and secured to the bed or chair (lap belt). It is applied over a garment. The person can release the quick-release type. It is less restrictive than those that only staff members can release.

Vest Restraints and Jacket Restraints. Vest and jacket restraints are applied to the chest. They may be used to prevent injuries from falls. And they may be used for persons who need positioning for a medical treatment. The person cannot turn in bed or get out of a chair.

A jacket restraint is applied with the opening in the back. For a vest restraint, the "V neck" is in front and the vest crosses in front (see Fig. 14-5). Vest and jacket restraints are never worn backward. Strangulation or other injury could occur if the person slides down in the bed or chair. The restraint is always applied over a garment.

RESTRAINT RELEASE RECORD
(Reference tag: F221)

PLEASE NOTE: Restrained individuals must be checked at least every 15 minutes. In addition, restraints must be released for the purpose of exercise, toileting, etc. for at least 10 minutes at least every two hours.

REASON FOR RESTRAINT	RESTRAINT ORDERED (Circle)		REMOVAL REASON CODES	
Is non-weight bearing and attempts to rise when in W/C.	Waist Pelvic Siderails Wrist (Belt) 2 Full Geri Chair Vest 1 Full Ankle Bar 2 Half Other_____ 1 Half		A- Supervised meals B- Supervised group activities C- Care provided by CNA D- One-to-one with volunteer E- One-to-one with social worker	F- 2-3 hrs. with periodic evaluation G- Total elimination of restraint H- _off when in bed_ I- _____ J- _____

DATE	15 MINUTE CHECK WHEN RESTRAINED			RELEASE EVERY TWO HOURS FOR PERSONAL CARE			TOTAL HOURS RELEASED PER SHIFT AND REASONS (USE REASON CODES ABOVE)			COMMENTS/ RESIDENT'S RESPONSE (Negative or Positive)
7/18	**Shift Initials**			**Shift Initials**						
Month/Year	11-7	7-3	3-11	11-7	7-3	3-11	11-7	7-3	3-11	
1	Lg	BG	MM	Lg	BG	MM	8(H)	4(A,B, C,H)	5(A,C, D,H)	No agitation – no falls no attempts to rise Joan Grieg, RN
2	Lg	BG	MM	Lg	BG	MM	8(H)	5(A,B, C,F,H)	6(A,C, F,H)	Doing well – no falls – Joan Grieg, RN
3	DL	RD	DL	ML	RD	ML	8(H)	6(A,B, C,F,H)	8(A,C, F,H)	No falls – Resident wants belt removed Ray Lopez, RN
4										
5										
6										

Fig. 14-16 Charting sample.

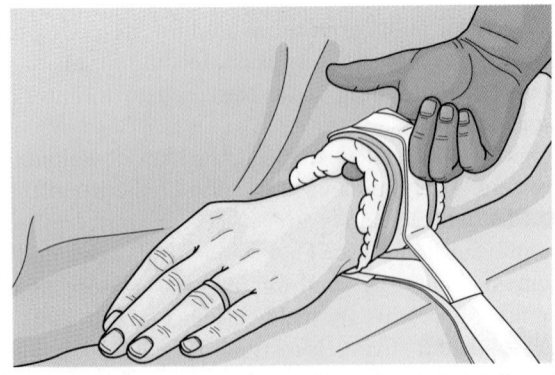

Fig. 14-17 Wrist restraint. The soft part is toward the skin. Note that 1 finger fits between the restraint and the wrist.

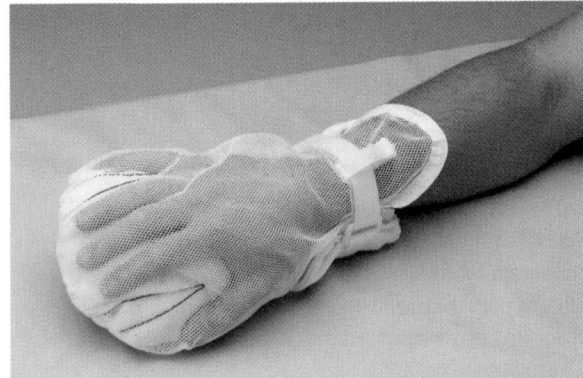

Fig. 14-18 Mitt restraint.

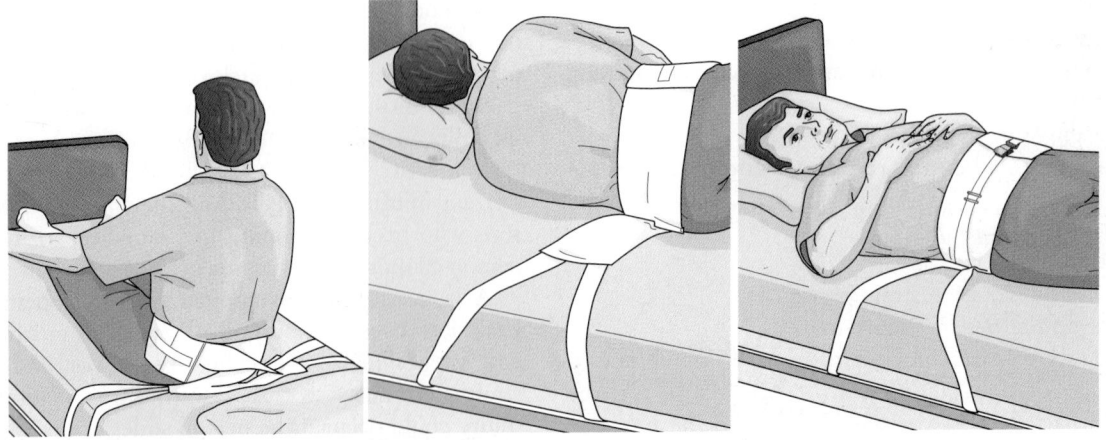

Fig. 14-19 Belt restraint. (NOTE: The bed rails are raised after the restraint is applied.)

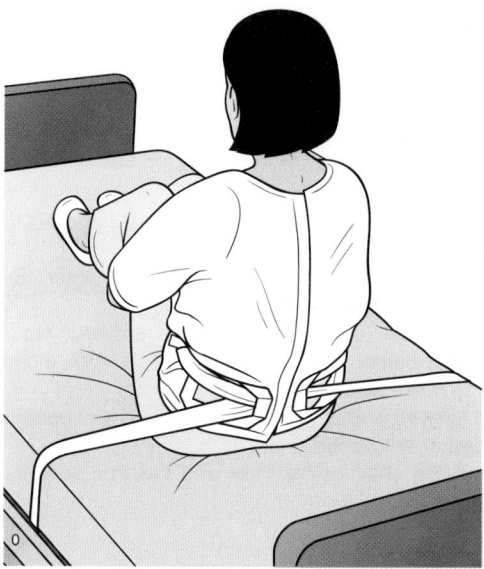

Fig. 14-20 Jacket restraint. (NOTE: The bed rails are raised after the restraint is applied.)

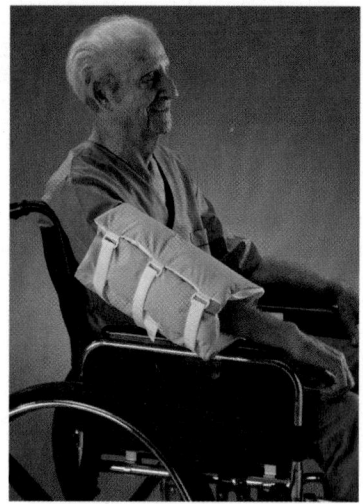

Fig. 14-21 Elbow restraint.

(Note: The straps of vest and jacket restraints cross in the front. A vest or jacket restraint may have a positioning slot in the back [Fig. 14-20]. Criss-cross straps following the manufacturer's instructions.)

Vest and jacket restraints have life-threatening risks. Death can occur from strangulation. If the person gets caught in the restraint, it can become so tight that the person's chest cannot expand to inhale air. The person quickly suffocates and dies. Correctly applying vest and jacket restraints is critical. You are advised to only assist the nurse in applying them. The nurse should assume full responsibility for applying a vest or jacket restraint.

See *Focus on Children and Older Persons: Applying Restraints.*

See *Focus on Communication: Applying Restraints.*

See *Delegation Guidelines: Applying Restraints.*

See *Promoting Safety and Comfort: Applying Restraints,* p. 208.

FOCUS ON CHILDREN AND OLDER PERSONS
Applying Restraints

Older Persons
Restraints may increase confusion and agitation in persons with dementia. They do not understand what you are doing. They may resist your efforts to apply a restraint. They may actively try to get free from the restraint. Serious injury and death are risks.

Never use force to apply a restraint. If a person is confused or agitated, ask a co-worker to help apply the restraint. Report problems to the nurse at once.

Children
Elbow restraints (elbow splints) limit arm movements. They prevent infants and children from bending their elbows (Fig. 14-21). They are used to prevent scratching and touching incisions or pulling out tubes. Both arms are restrained to achieve the desired effect.

FOCUS ON COMMUNICATION
Applying Restraints

The nurse may ask you to apply a restraint you have not used before. If you do not know how to apply a certain restraint, do not do so. Tell the nurse. Ask him or her to show you the correct application. You can say: "I've never applied a restraint like this before. Would you please show me how and then watch me apply it?" Then thank the nurse for helping you.

When applying a restraint, explain to the person what you are going to do. Then tell the person what you are doing step-by-step. Always check for safety and comfort. You can ask: "How does the restraint feel? Is it too tight? Is it too loose?"

Make sure the person can communicate with you after you leave the room. Place the signal light in reach. Make sure the person can use it with the restraint on. Remind the person to call if he or she becomes uncomfortable or if anything is needed.

DELEGATION GUIDELINES
Applying Restraints

Before applying a restraint, you need this information from the nurse and the care plan:
- Why the doctor ordered the restraint
- What type and size to use
- Where to apply the restraint
- How to safely apply the restraint (Have the nurse show you how to apply it. Then show correct application back to the nurse.)
- How to correctly position the person
- What bony areas to pad and how to pad them
- If bed rail covers or gap protectors are needed
- If bed rails are up or down
- What special equipment is needed
- If the person needs to be checked more often than every 15 minutes
- When to apply and release the restraint
- What observations to report and record (p. 205)
- When to report observations
- What patient or resident concerns to report at once

PROMOTING SAFETY AND COMFORT
Applying Restraints

Safety

Restraints can cause serious harm, even death. Always follow the manufacturer's instructions. Manufacturers have many types of restraints. The instructions for one type may not apply to another. Also, the manufacturer may have instructions for applying restraints on persons who are agitated.

Never use force to apply a restraint. Ask a co-worker to help if a person is confused and agitated. Report problems to the nurse at once.

Check the person at least every 15 minutes or more often as instructed by the nurse and the care plan. Make sure the signal light is within reach. Ask the person to use the signal light at the first sign of problems or discomfort.

Never use a restraint as a seat belt in a car or other vehicle.

Mitt Restraints

Mitt restraints prevent finger use. Often they are not secured to the bed or chair. Therefore, the person can raise the mitt to his or her mouth. Observe the person closely to make sure that he or she does not:
- Use the teeth to remove or damage the device.
- Ingest any mitt material.

Persons with mitt restraints may be out of bed and able to walk about. Falls are a risk. Practice safety measures to prevent falls (Chapter 13).

Belt, Vest, and Jacket Restraints

These restraints are not used if the person has:
- A colostomy or ileostomy (Chapter 23)
- A gastrostomy tube (Chapter 25)
- Drainage tubes after surgery (Chapters 33 and 37)
- Incisions (Chapter 33)
- Chronic obstructive pulmonary disease (Chapter 42)
- Devices to monitor vital signs

If a belt, vest, or jacket restraint is ordered, remind the nurse of the person's condition and needs. Also monitor the person to make sure that he or she cannot:
- Slide forward or down in the chair or bed and become suspended or entrapped.
- Fall off the chair or mattress and become suspended or entrapped.

Comfort

The person's comfort is always important. It is more so when restraints are used. Remember, restraints limit movement. This affects position changes and reaching needed items. Position the person in good alignment before applying a restraint (Chapter 16). Also make sure the person can reach needed items—signal light, water, tissues, phone, bed controls, and so on.

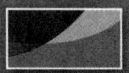 **APPLYING RESTRAINTS**

QUALITY OF LIFE

Remember to
- Knock before entering the person's room.
- Address the person by name.
- Introduce yourself by name and title.

- Explain the procedure to the person before beginning and during the procedure.
- Protect the person's rights during the procedure.
- Handle the person gently during the procedure.

PRE-PROCEDURE

1 Follow *Delegation Guidelines: Applying Restraints*, p. 207. See *Promoting Safety and Comfort: Applying Restraints*,.
2 Collect the following as instructed by the nurse:
- Correct type and size of restraints
- Padding for skin and bony areas
- Bed rail pads or gap protectors (if needed)

3 Practice hand hygiene.
4 Identify the person. Check the ID (identification) bracelet against the assignment sheet. Also call the person by name.
5 Provide for privacy.

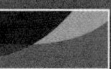 **APPLYING RESTRAINTS—cont'd**

PROCEDURE

6 Make sure the person is comfortable and in good alignment.

7 Put the bed rail pads or gap protectors (if needed) on the bed if the person is in bed. Follow the manufacturer's instructions.

8 Pad bony areas. Follow the nurse's instructions and the care plan.

9 Read the manufacturer's instructions. Note the front and back of the restraint.

10 *For wrist restraints:*
   a Apply the restraint following the manufacturer's instructions. Place the soft or foam part toward the skin.
   b Secure the restraint so it is snug but not tight. Make sure you can slide 1 finger under the restraint (see Fig. 14-17). Follow the manufacturer's instructions. Adjust the straps if the restraint is too loose or too tight. Check for snugness again.
   c Secure the straps to the movable part of the bed frame out of the person's reach. Use the buckle or a quick-release tie.
   d Repeat steps 10 a, b, and c for the other wrist.

11 *For mitt restraints:*
   a Make sure the person's hands are clean and dry.
   b Insert the person's hand into the restraint with the palm down. Follow the manufacturer's instructions.
   c Secure the restraint to the bed if directed to do so by the nurse. Secure the straps to the movable part of the bed frame. Use the buckle or a quick-release tie.
   d Make sure the restraint is snug. Slide 1 finger between the restraint and the wrist. Follow the manufacturer's instructions. Adjust the straps if the restraint is too loose or too tight. Check for snugness again.
   e Repeat steps 11 b, c, and d for the other hand.

12 *For a belt restraint:*
   a Assist the person to a sitting position.
   b Apply the restraint following the manufacturer's instructions.
   c Remove wrinkles or creases from the front and back of the restraint.
   d Bring the ties through the slots in the belt.
   e Position the straps at a 45-degree angle between the wheelchair seat and sides (see Fig. 14-15, p. 205). Or help the person lie down if he or she is in bed.
   f Make sure the person is comfortable and in good alignment.
   g Secure the straps to the movable part of the bed frame. Use the buckle or a quick-release tie. The buckle or tie is out of the person's reach. For a wheelchair, criss-cross and secure the straps as in Figure 14-11.
   h Make sure the belt is snug. Slide an open hand between the restraint and the person. Adjust the restraint if it is too loose or too tight. Check for snugness again.

13 *For a vest restraint:*
   a Assist the person to a sitting position. If the person is in a wheelchair:
      (1) Position him or her as far back in the wheelchair as possible.
      (2) Make sure the buttocks are against the chair back.
   b Apply the restraint following the manufacturer's instructions. The "V" part of the vest crosses in front.
   c Bring the straps through the slots.
   d Position the straps at a 45-degree angle between the wheelchair seat and sides. (Omit this step if the person is in bed.)
   e Make sure the vest is free of wrinkles in the front and back.
   f Help the person lie down if he or she is in bed.
   g Make sure the person is comfortable and in good alignment.
   h Secure the straps to the movable part of the bed frame at waist level. Use the buckle or a quick-release tie. The buckle or tie is out of the person's reach. For a wheelchair, criss-cross and secure the straps as in Figure 14-11.

14 *For a jacket restraint:*
   a Assist the person to a sitting position. If the person is in a wheelchair:
      (1) Position him or her as far back in the wheelchair as possible.
      (2) Make sure the buttocks are against the chair back.
   b Apply the restraint following the manufacturer's instructions. The jacket opening goes in the back.
   c Close the back with the zipper, ties, or hook and loop closures.
   d Make sure the side seams are under the arms. Remove any wrinkles in the front and back.
   e Position the straps at a 45-degree angle between the wheelchair seat and sides. Or help the person lie down if he or she is in bed.
   f Make sure the person is comfortable and in good alignment.
   g Secure the straps to the movable part of the bed frame at waist level. Use the buckle or a quick-release tie. The buckle or tie is out of the person's reach. For a wheelchair, criss-cross and secure the straps as in Figure 14-11.
   h Make sure the jacket is snug. Slide an open hand between the restraint and the person. Adjust the restraint if it is too loose or too tight. Check for snugness again.

Continued

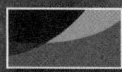

APPLYING RESTRAINTS—cont'd

POST-PROCEDURE

15 Position the person as the nurse directs.

16 Provide for comfort. (See the inside of the front book cover.)

17 Place the signal light within the person's reach.

18 Raise or lower bed rails. Follow the care plan and the manufacturer's instructions for the restraint.

19 Unscreen the person.

20 Complete a safety check of the room. (See the inside of the front book cover.)

21 Practice hand hygiene.

22 Check the person and the restraint at least every 15 minutes. Report and record your observations:

   a For wrist, mitt, or elbow restraints: check the pulse, color, and temperature of the restrained parts.

   b For a vest, jacket, or belt restraint: check the person's breathing. *Call for the nurse at once if the person is not breathing or is having problems breathing.* Make sure the restraint is properly positioned in the front and back.

23 Do the following at least every 2 hours for at least 10 minutes:

   a Remove or release the restraint.

   b Measure vital signs.

   c Re-position the person.

   d Meet food, fluid, hygiene, and elimination needs.

   e Give skin care.

   f Perform range-of-motion exercises or help the person walk. Follow the care plan.

   g Provide for physical and emotional comfort. (See the inside of the front book cover.)

   h Re-apply the restraints.

24 Complete a safety check of the room. (See the inside of the front book cover.)

25 Practice hand hygiene.

26 Report and record your observations and the care given.

FOCUS ON PRIDE

The Person, Family, and Yourself

Personal and Professional Responsibility

Restraints have many risks. See Box 14-1. Therefore restraint use brings many responsibilities for you. You must:

- Monitor the person for safety.
- Apply the restraint properly.
- Promote comfort.
- Supervise the person closely.
- Meet basic needs.
- Report any concerns to the nurse.

If you do not know how to apply a restraint, do not do so. Ask the nurse to show you. Always monitor restrained persons closely. To use restraints safely and responsibly, follow the guidelines in Box 14-3.

Rights and Respect

Every person has the right to freedom from restraint. Restraints are used only as a last resort to protect the person or others from harm. Other methods must be tried before restraints are used. You may be asked to assist with an alternative method (see Box 14-2). Make a genuine effort. Be honest. Do not tell the nurse you tried if you really did not. Do your best to allow the person the right to freedom from restraint.

Independence and Social Interaction

All restraint forms limit movement. Independence is restricted. You can promote independence even when restraints are used. To do so:

- Place the signal light within reach at all times. Make sure the person can use it. Tell the person to signal for you if anything is needed. Answer the signal light and meet the person's needs promptly.
- Make sure needed items are within reach. This is most important with restraints that allow hand and arm use. Belt, vest, and jacket restraints are examples.
- Check on the person at least every 15 minutes.
- Remove or release the restraint at least every 2 hours.
- Meet food, fluid, hygiene, and elimination needs.
- Assist the person with walks or range-of-motion exercises.
- Allow choice. For example, let the person choose where to walk or what to eat and drink.
- Let the person do as much for himself or herself as safely possible.

Personal choice and freedom of movement promote independence, dignity, and self-esteem. Provide care that gives restrained persons the independence they deserve.

Delegation and Teamwork

Agencies hold patient or resident care conferences to meet the person's safety needs. The health team reviews and updates the person's care plan. Every attempt is made to protect the person without using restraints.

You are an important member of the team. Your input has value. Share your observations and ideas. For example, you notice that Mrs. Garner does not try to get out of her chair when she looks through her photo albums or reads a book. You share this with the team. They include diversion activities in her care plan.

Ethics and Laws

Imagine the following:

- Your nose itches. But your hands are restrained. You cannot scratch your nose.
- You need to use the bathroom. Your arms and legs are restrained. You cannot get up. You cannot reach your signal light. You soil yourself with urine or a bowel movement.

- Your phone is ringing. You cannot answer it.
- You are not wearing your eyeglasses. You are wearing mitt restraints. You cannot reach your glasses or put them on. You cannot see who is coming into and going out of your room. And you cannot speak because of a stroke.
- You are uncomfortable. You have a vest restraint. You cannot move or turn in bed.
- You are thirsty. The water cup is within your reach but your hands and arms are restrained.
- You hear the fire alarm. You have on a restraint. You cannot get up to move to a safe place. You must wait until someone rescues you.

What would you do? Would you calmly lie or sit there? Would you try to get free from the restraint? Would you yell for help? What would the nursing staff think? Would they think that you are uncomfortable? Or would they think that you are agitated and uncooperative? Would you feel angry, embarrassed, or humiliated?

Ethics deals with how others are treated. Restraints lessen the person's dignity and freedom. A person should not be treated in this way. That is why restraints are a last resort. When caring for a restrained person, put yourself in his or her situation. Then you can better understand how the person feels. Treat the person like you would want to be treated—with kindness, caring, respect, and dignity.

REVIEW QUESTIONS

Circle T if the statement is TRUE or F if it is FALSE.

1. T F Restraint alternatives fail to protect a person. You can apply a restraint.
2. T F A restraint restricts a person's freedom of movement.
3. T F Some drugs are restraints.
4. T F Restraints can be used for staff convenience.
5. T F A device is a restraint only if it is attached to the person's body.
6. T F Bed rails are restraints if the person cannot lower them.
7. T F Restraints are used only for a person's specific medical symptom.
8. T F Unnecessary restraint is false imprisonment.
9. T F You can apply restraints when you think they are needed.
10. T F You can use a vest restraint to position a person on the toilet.
11. T F Restraints are removed or released at least every 2 hours.
12. T F Restraints are tied to bed rails.
13. T F Wrist restraints are used to prevent falls.
14. T F A vest restraint crosses in front.
15. T F Bed rails are left down when vest restraints are used.

Circle the BEST answer.

16. Which is *not* a restraint alternative?
    a Positioning the person's chair close to the wall
    b Answering signal lights promptly
    c Taking the person outside in nice weather
    d Padding walls and corners of furniture
17. Physical restraints
    a Can be removed easily by the person
    b Are not allowed by OBRA
    c Restrict freedom of movement
    d Are safer than chemical restraints
18. The following can occur because of restraints. Which is the *most* serious?
    a Fractures
    b Strangulation
    c Pressure ulcers
    d Urinary tract infections
19. A belt restraint is applied to a person in bed. Where should you secure the straps?
    a To the bed rails
    b To the head-board
    c To the movable part of the bed frame
    d To the foot-board
20. A person has a restraint. You should check the person and the position of the restraint at least every
    a 15 minutes
    b 30 minutes
    c Hour
    d 2 hours
21. A person has mitt restraints. Which of these is especially important to report to the nurse?
    a The heart rate
    b The respiratory rate
    c Why the restraints were applied
    d If you felt a pulse in the restrained extremities
22. The doctor ordered mitt restraints for a person. You need the following information from the nurse *except*
    a What size to use
    b What other equipment is needed
    c What drugs the person is taking
    d When to apply and release the restraints
23. A person has a vest restraint. It is not too tight or too loose if you can slide
    a A fist between the vest and the person
    b One finger between the vest and the person
    c An open hand between the vest and the person
    d Two fingers between the vest and the person
24. The correct way to apply any restraint is to follow the
    a Nurse's directions
    b Doctor's orders
    c Care plan
    d Manufacturer's instructions

Answers to these questions are on p. 832.

15 Preventing Infection

OBJECTIVES

- Define the key terms and key abbreviations listed in this chapter.
- Identify what microbes need to live and grow.
- List the signs and symptoms of infection.
- Explain the chain of infection.
- Describe healthcare-associated infections and the persons at risk.
- Describe the practices of medical asepsis.
- Describe disinfection and sterilization methods.

- Explain how to care for equipment and supplies.
- Describe Standard Precautions and Transmission-Based Precautions.
- Explain the Bloodborne Pathogen Standard.
- Explain the principles and practices of surgical asepsis.
- Perform the procedures described in this chapter.
- Explain how to promote PRIDE in the person, the family, and yourself.

KEY TERMS

antibiotic A drug that kills certain microbes that cause infections

asepsis Being free of disease-producing microbes

biohazardous waste Items contaminated with blood, body fluids, secretions, or excretions; *bio* means *life,* and *hazardous* means *dangerous* or *harmful*

carrier A human or animal that is a reservoir for microbes but does not develop the infection

clean technique See "medical asepsis"

communicable disease A disease caused by pathogens that spread easily; a contagious disease

contagious disease See "communicable disease"

contamination The process of becoming unclean

disinfection The process of destroying pathogens

healthcare-associated infection (HAI) An infection that develops in a person cared for in any setting where health care is given; the infection is related to receiving health care

immunity Protection against a certain disease

infection A disease state resulting from the invasion and growth of microbes in the body

infection control Practices and procedures that prevent the spread of infection

medical asepsis Practices used to remove or destroy pathogens and to prevent their spread from one person or place to another person or place; clean technique

microbe See "microorganism"

microorganism A small *(micro)* living thing *(organism)* seen only with a microscope; a microbe

non-pathogen A microbe that does not usually cause an infection

normal flora Microbes that live and grow in a certain area

pathogen A microbe that is harmful and can cause an infection

reservoir The environment in which a microbe lives and grows; host

spore A bacterium protected by a hard shell

sterile The absence of *all* microbes

sterile field A work area free of *all* pathogens and non-pathogens (including spores)

sterile technique See "surgical asepsis"

sterilization The process of destroying *all* microbes

surgical asepsis The practices that keep items free of *all* microbes; sterile technique

vaccination Giving a vaccine to produce immunity against an infectious disease

vaccine A preparation containing dead or weakened microbes

vector A carrier (animal, insect) that transmits disease

vehicle Any substance that transmits microbes

KEY ABBREVIATIONS

AIDS	Acquired immunodeficiency syndrome	**MRSA**	Methicillin-resistant *Staphylococcus aureus*
AIIR	Airborne infection isolation room	**MSDS**	Material safety data sheet
CDC	Centers for Disease Control and Prevention	**OPIM**	Other potentially infectious materials
cm	Centimeter	**OSHA**	Occupational Safety and Health Administration
EPA	Environmental Protection Agency		
GI	Gastro-intestinal	**PPE**	Personal protective equipment
HAI	Healthcare-associated infection	**SARS**	Severe acute respiratory syndrome
HBV	Hepatitis B virus	**TB**	Tuberculosis
HIV	Human immunodeficiency virus	**VRE**	Vancomycin-resistant *Enterococci*
MDRO	Multidrug-resistant organism		

An *infection is a disease state resulting from the invasion and growth of microbes in the body.* Infection is a major safety and health hazard. Minor infections cause short illnesses. Some infections are serious and can cause death. Infants, older persons, and disabled persons are at risk. The health team follows certain *practices and procedures to prevent the spread of infection (infection control).* The goal is to protect patients, residents, visitors, and staff from infection.

MICROORGANISMS

A *microorganism (microbe) is a small* (micro) *living thing* (organism). *It is seen only with a microscope.* Microbes are everywhere—in the mouth, nose, respiratory tract, stomach, and intestines. They are on the skin and in the air, soil, water, and food. They are on animals, clothing, and furniture.

Microbes that are harmful and can cause infections are called pathogens. Non-pathogens are microbes that do not usually cause an infection.

Types of Microbes

There are five types of microbes:

- *Bacteria*—are one-celled organisms that multiply rapidly. Often called *germs*, they can cause an infection in any body system.
- *Fungi*—are plant-like organisms that live on other plants or animals. Mushrooms, yeasts, and molds are common fungi. Fungi can infect the mouth, vagina, skin, feet, and other body areas.
- *Protozoa*—are one-celled animals. They can infect the blood, brain, intestines, and other body areas.
- *Rickettsiae*—are found in fleas, lice, ticks, and other insects. They are spread to humans by insect bites. Rocky Mountain spotted fever is an example. The person has fever, chills, headache, and rash.
- *Viruses*—grow in living cells. They cause many diseases. The common cold, herpes, acquired immunodeficiency syndrome (AIDS), and hepatitis are examples.

Requirements of Microbes

Microbes need a reservoir to live and grow. The *reservoir (host) is the environment in which a microbe lives and grows.* People, plants, animals, the soil, food, and water are common reservoirs. Microbes need *water* and *nourishment* from the reservoir. Most need *oxygen* to live. A *warm* and *dark* environment is needed. Most grow best at body temperature. They are destroyed by heat and light.

Normal Flora

Normal flora are microbes that live and grow in a certain area. Certain microbes are in the respiratory tract, in the intestines, and on the skin. They are non-pathogens when in or on a natural reservoir. When a non-pathogen is transmitted from its natural site to another site or host, it becomes a pathogen. For example, *Escherichia coli (E. coli)* is normally found in the colon. If it enters the urinary system, it can cause an infection.

Multidrug-Resistant Organisms

Multidrug-resistant organisms (MDROs) are microbes that can resist the effects of antibiotics. *Antibiotics are drugs that kill certain microbes that cause infections.* Some microbes can change their structures. This makes them harder to kill. They can survive in the presence of antibiotics. Therefore the infections they cause are hard to treat.

MDROs are caused by prescribing antibiotics when they are not needed (over-prescribing). Not taking antibiotics for the length of time prescribed is another cause. Two common MDROs are:

- *Methicillin-resistant Staphylococcus aureus (MRSA). Staphylococcus aureus* ("staph") is a bacterium normally found in the nose and on the skin. MRSA is resistant to antibiotics often used for "staph" infections. MRSA can cause serious wound and bloodstream infections and pneumonia.
- *Vancomycin-resistant Enterococci (VRE). Enterococcus* is a bacterium normally found in the intestines and in feces. It can be transmitted to others by contaminated hands, toilet seats, care equipment, and other items that the hands touch. When not in their natural site (the intestines), enterococci can cause urinary tract, wound, pelvic, and other infections. Vancomycin is an antibiotic often used to treat such infections. Enterococci resistant to Vancomycin are called Vancomycin-resistant enterococci (VRE).

INFECTION

A *local infection* is in a body part. A *systemic infection* involves the whole body. (*Systemic* means entire.) The person has some or all of the signs and symptoms listed in Box 15-1.

See *Focus on Children and Older Persons: Infection.*

The Chain of Infection

The chain of infection (Fig. 15-1) is a process involving a:

- Source
- Reservoir
- Portal of exit
- Method of transmission
- Portal of entry
- Susceptible host

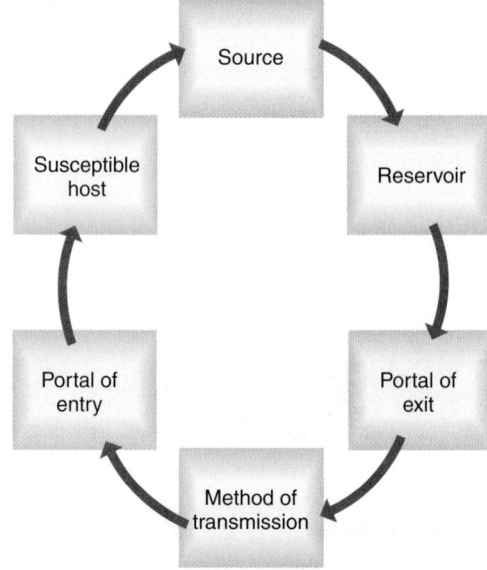

Fig. 15-1 The chain of infection.

BOX 15-1	SIGNS AND SYMPTOMS OF INFECTION

- Fever (elevated body temperature)
- Chills
- Pulse rate: increased
- Respiratory rate: increased
- Pain or tenderness
- Fatigue and loss of energy
- Appetite: loss of (anorexia)
- Nausea
- Vomiting
- Diarrhea
- Rash
- Sores on mucous membranes
- Redness and swelling of a body part
- Discharge or drainage from the infected area
- Heat or warmth in a body part
- Limited use of a body part
- Headache
- Muscle aches
- Joint pain
- Confusion

FOCUS ON CHILDREN AND OLDER PERSONS
Infection

Older Persons

The immune system protects the body from disease and infection (Chapter 9). Like other body systems, changes occur in the immune system with aging. Therefore older persons are at risk for infection.

During an infection, an older person may not show the signs and symptoms listed in Box 15-1. The person may have only a slight fever or no fever at all. Redness and swelling may be very slight. The person may not complain of pain. Confusion and delirium may occur (Chapter 46).

An infection can become life-threatening before the older person has obvious signs and symptoms. Be alert to the most minor changes in the person's behavior or condition. Report any concerns to the nurse at once.

Healing takes longer than when younger. Therefore an infection can prolong the rehabilitation process. Independence and quality of life are affected.

The *source* is a pathogen. It must have a *reservoir* where it can grow and multiply. Humans, animals, and objects are reservoirs. A *carrier is a human or animal that is a reservoir for microbes but does not develop the infection.* Carriers can pass pathogens to others. A *vector is a carrier (animal, insect) that transmits disease.* Common vectors are:

- Dogs, which carry rabies
- Mosquitoes, which carry malaria
- Ticks, which carry Rocky Mountain spotted fever
- Mites, which cause scabies (Chapter 21)

To leave the reservoir, the pathogen needs a *portal of exit.* Exits are the respiratory, gastro-intestinal (GI), urinary, and reproductive tracts; breaks in the skin; and the blood.

After leaving the reservoir, the pathogen must be *transmitted* to another host (Fig. 15-2). A *vehicle is any substance that transmits microbes.* The pathogen enters the body through a *portal of entry.* Portals of entry and exit are the same—the respiratory, GI, urinary, and reproductive tracts; breaks in the skin; and the blood. A *susceptible host* is needed for the microbe to grow and multiply. Susceptible hosts are persons at risk for infection.

Susceptible Hosts. Susceptible hosts include persons who:

- Are very young or who are older.
- Are ill.
- Were exposed to the pathogen.
- Do not follow practices to prevent infection.

The human body can protect itself from infection. The ability to resist infection relates to age, nutrition, stress, fatigue, and health. Drugs, disease, and injury also are factors.

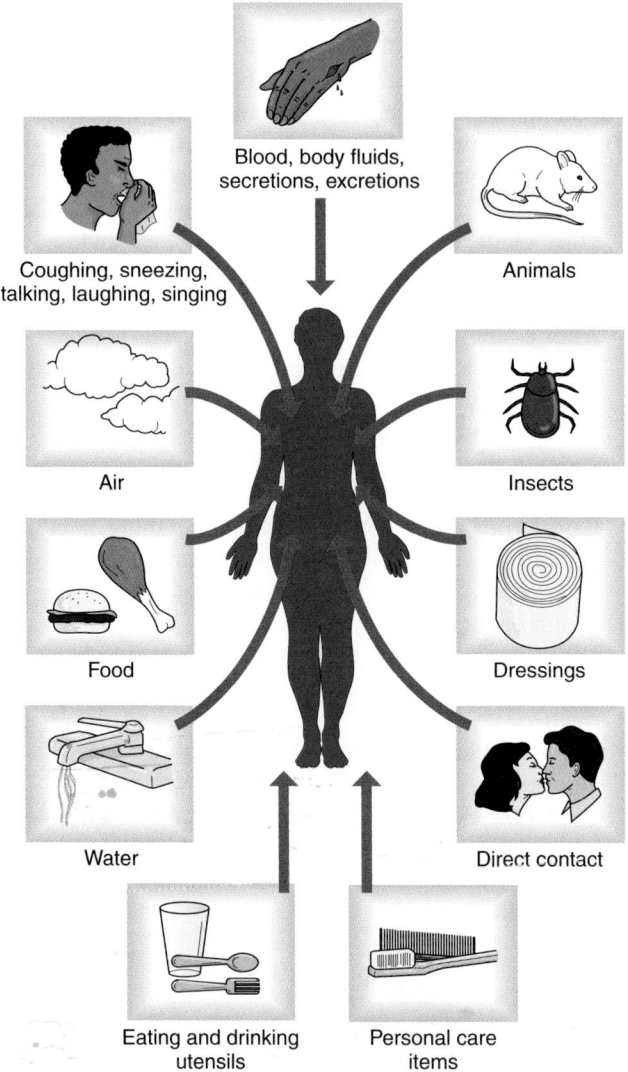

Fig. 15-2 Methods of transmitting microbes.

Coughing, sneezing, talking, laughing, singing

Blood, body fluids, secretions, excretions

Animals

Air

Insects

Food

Dressings

Water

Direct contact

Eating and drinking utensils

Personal care items

Some persons are at great risk for infection. Burn, transplant, and chemotherapy patients are examples. Severe infections can be deadly for these persons.

- *Burn patients.* The skin is the body's protective covering. It prevents microbes from entering the body. When burns destroy the skin, the wound is a portal of entry for microbes. Sources of microbes are from the person's normal flora (skin, respiratory tract, GI tract), the health care environment, and the health team. MRSA and VRE are of particular concern. Also, burns affect the body's immune system (Chapter 9) and the ability to fight infection.

- *Transplant patients.* A *transplant* involves transferring an organ or tissue from one person to another person or from one body part to another part. Kidney, liver, heart, lung, bone, tendon, blood vessel, and skin are examples. The immune system recognizes the new organ or tissue as a foreign object. The body's normal immune response is to attack (reject) the new organ or tissue. Therefore, drugs are given to prevent rejection. Such drugs suppress (prevent) the immune system from producing antibodies. Antibodies are needed to fight infection.

- *Chemotherapy patients.* Some types of chemotherapy affect the bone marrow's ability to produce white blood cells (WBCs). Fewer WBCs are produced. WBCs are needed to fight infection.

Healthcare-Associated Infection

A *healthcare-associated infection (HAI) is an infection that develops in a person cared for in any setting where health care is given* (Box 15-2). *The infection is related to receiving health care.* Hospitals, nursing centers, clinics, and home care settings are examples. HAIs also are called *nosocomial infections.* (*Nosocomial* comes from the Greek word for *hospital.*)

HAIs are caused by normal flora. Or they are caused by microbes transmitted to the person from other sources. For example, *E. coli* is normally in the colon. Feces contain *E. coli.* Poor wiping after bowel movements can cause *E. coli* to enter the urinary system. The hands can transmit *E. coli* to other body areas. With poor hand washing, *E. coli* spreads to any body part or anything the hands touch. It also can be transmitted to other people.

BOX 15-2	**POSSIBLE HEALTHCARE-ASSOCIATED INFECTIONS**

- *Clostridium difficile*—Chapter 23
- Gastro-intestinal infections
- Hepatitis A, B, and C—Chapter 43
- Human immunodeficiency virus—Chapter 40
- Influenza—Chapter 42
- Methicillin-resistant *Staphylococcus aureus*—p. 213
- Tuberculosis—Chapter 42
- Vancomycin-resistant enterococci—p. 213

Modified from Centers for Disease Control and Prevention: *Health-care associated infections (HAIs)*, Atlanta, March 25, 2011.

Microbes can enter the body through equipment used in treatments, therapies, and tests. Such items must be free of microbes. Staff can transfer microbes from one person to another and from themselves to others. Common sites for HAIs are:

- The urinary system
- The respiratory system
- Wounds
- The bloodstream

Patients and residents are weak from disease or injury. Some have wounds or open skin areas. Infants and older persons have a hard time fighting infections. The health team must prevent infection by:

- Medical asepsis. This includes hand hygiene.
- Surgical asepsis.
- Standard Precautions, p. 223.
- Transmission-Based Precautions, p. 225.
- The Bloodborne Pathogen Standard, p. 235.
  See *Focus on Long-Term Care and Home Care: Healthcare-Associated Infection.*

MEDICAL ASEPSIS

Asepsis is being free of disease-producing microbes. Microbes are everywhere. Measures are needed to achieve asepsis. *Medical asepsis (clean technique) is the practices used to:*

- *Remove or destroy pathogens.* The number of pathogens is reduced.
- *Prevent pathogens from spreading from one person or place to another person or place.*

Microbes cannot be present during surgery or when instruments are inserted into the body. Open wounds (cuts, burns, incisions) require the absence of microbes. They are portals of entry for microbes. *Surgical asepsis (sterile technique) is the practices that keep items free of all microbes. Sterile means the absence of all microbes*—pathogens and non-pathogens. *Sterilization is the process of destroying all microbes (pathogens and non-pathogens).*

Contamination is the process of becoming unclean. In medical asepsis, an item or area is "clean" when it is free of pathogens. The item or area is "contaminated" when pathogens are present. A sterile item or area is "contaminated" when pathogens or non-pathogens are present.

Common Aseptic Practices

Aseptic practices break the chain of infection. To prevent the spread of microbes, wash your hands:

- After urinating or having a bowel movement.
- After changing tampons or sanitary pads.
- After contact with your own or another person's blood, body fluids, secretions, or excretions. This includes saliva, vomitus, urine, feces, vaginal discharge, mucus, semen, wound drainage, pus, and respiratory secretions.
- After coughing, sneezing, or blowing your nose.
- Before and after handling, preparing, or eating food.
- After smoking a cigarette, cigar, or pipe.
  Also do the following:
- Provide all persons with their own linens and personal care items.
- Cover your nose and mouth when coughing, sneezing, or blowing your nose. If tissues are not available, cough or sneeze into your upper arm (Fig. 15-3). Do not cough or sneeze into your hands.
- Bathe, wash hair, and brush your teeth regularly.
- Wash fruits and raw vegetables before eating or serving them.
- Wash cooking and eating utensils with soap and water after use.
  See *Focus on Children and Older Persons: Common Aseptic Practices.*
  See *Focus on Long-Term Care and Home Care: Common Aseptic Practices.*

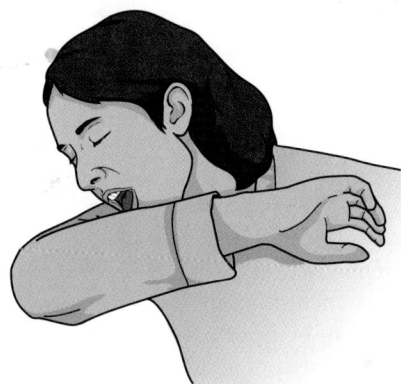

Fig. 15-3 Sneezing into the upper arm.

FOCUS ON LONG-TERM CARE AND HOME CARE
Common Aseptic Practices

Home Care

You must prevent the spread of microbes in home settings. Also, protect the person from microbes brought into the home. The measures described on p. 216 and others are needed. Also protect the person from foodborne illnesses (Chapter 24).

Microbes easily grow and spread in bathrooms. The entire family must help keep the bathroom clean. Aseptic measures are needed whenever the bathroom is used.
- Flush the toilet after each use.
- Rinse the sink after washing, shaving, or oral hygiene.
- Wipe out the tub or shower after each use.
- Remove and dispose of hair from the sink, tub, or shower.
- Hang towels out to dry. Or place them in a hamper.
- Wipe up water spills.

Your job may include cleaning bathrooms every day. Wear utility gloves for this task. Use a disinfectant or water and detergent to clean all surfaces:
- Toilet surfaces—bowl, seat, and all outside areas
- The floor
- The sides, walls, and curtain or door of the shower or tub
- Towel racks
- Toilet tissue, toothbrush, and soap holders

- The mirror (use a glass cleaner)
- The sink
- Window sills

For bathroom cleaning, you also need to:
- Mop uncarpeted floors. Vacuum carpeted floors.
- Empty wastebaskets.
- Put out clean towels and washcloths.
- Open bathroom windows for a short time and use air fresheners. These actions help reduce odors and give the bathroom a fresh smell.
- Wash bath mats, the wastebasket, and the laundry hamper weekly.
- Replace toilet and facial tissue as needed.

The care plan and assignment sheet tell you when to clean other areas of the home. For general housekeeping:
- Wipe up spills right away.
- Dust furniture and blinds.
- Vacuum or mop floors. Damp-mop uncarpeted floors at least weekly.
- Use a dust mop to sweep. Use a dustpan to collect dust, crumbs, and other things swept up. Sweep daily or more often if needed.
- Wash clothes and linens.

Hand Hygiene

Hand hygiene is the easiest and most important way to prevent the spread of infection. Your hands are used for almost everything. They are easily contaminated. They can spread microbes to other persons or items. *Practice hand hygiene before and after giving care.* See Box 15-3 for the rules of hand hygiene.

See *Promoting Safety and Comfort: Hand Hygiene*, p. 219.

Text continued on p. 221

BOX 15-3 | RULES OF HAND HYGIENE

- Wash your hands (with soap and water):
  - When they are visibly dirty or soiled with blood, body fluids, secretions, or excretions
  - Before eating and after using a restroom
  - If exposure to the anthrax spore is suspected or proven
  - If an alcohol-based hand rub is not available
- Use an alcohol-based hand rub to practice hand hygiene if they are not visibly soiled. Follow this rule:
  - Before direct contact with a person.
  - After contact with the person's intact skin. After taking a pulse or blood pressure or after moving a person are examples.
  - After contact with body fluids or excretions, mucous membranes, non-intact skin, and wound dressings if hands are not visibly soiled.
  - When moving from a contaminated body site to a clean body site during care activities.
  - After contact with objects (including equipment) in the person's care setting.
  - After removing gloves.

- Follow these rules for washing your hands with soap and water. See procedure: *Hand Washing*, p. 219.
  - Wash your hands under warm running water. Do not use hot water.
  - Stand away from the sink. Do not let your hands, body, or uniform touch the sink. The sink is contaminated. See Figure 15-4, p. 218.
  - Do not touch the inside of the sink at any time.
  - Keep your hands and forearms lower than your elbows. Your hands are dirtier than your elbows and forearms. If you hold your hands and forearms up, dirty water runs from your hands to your elbows. Those areas become contaminated.
  - Rub your palms together (Fig. 15-5, p. 218) and interlace your fingers (Fig. 15-6, p. 218) to work up a good lather. The rubbing action helps remove microbes and dirt.
  - Pay attention to areas often missed during hand washing—thumbs, knuckles, sides of the hands, little fingers, and under the nails.

Modified from Centers for Disease Control and Prevention: Guideline for hand hygiene in health-care settings, *Morbidity and Mortality Weekly Report* 51 (RR-16), October 2002.

Continued

BOX 15-3	RULES OF HAND HYGIENE—cont'd

- Clean fingernails by rubbing the fingertips against your palms (Fig. 15-7).
- Use a nail file or orangewood stick to clean under fingernails (Fig. 15-8). Microbes easily grow under the fingernails.
- Wash your hands for at least 20 seconds. Wash your hands longer if they are dirty or soiled with blood, body fluids, secretions, or excretions. Use your judgment and follow agency policy.
- Use clean, dry paper towels to dry your hands.
- Dry your hands starting at the fingertips. Work up to your forearms. You will dry the cleanest area first.
- Use a clean, dry paper towel for each faucet to turn the water off (Fig. 15-9). Faucets are contaminated. The paper towels prevent you from contaminating your clean hands.

- Follow these rules when decontaminating your hands with an alcohol-based hand rub. See procedure: *Using an Alcohol-Based Hand Rub*, p. 220.
  - Apply the product to the palm of one hand. Follow the manufacturer's instructions for the amount to use.
  - Rub your hands together.
  - Make sure you cover all surfaces of your hands and fingers.
  - Continue rubbing your hands together until your hands are dry.
- Apply hand lotion or cream after hand hygiene. This prevents the skin from chapping and drying. Skin breaks can occur in chapped and dry skin. Skin breaks are portals of entry for microbes.

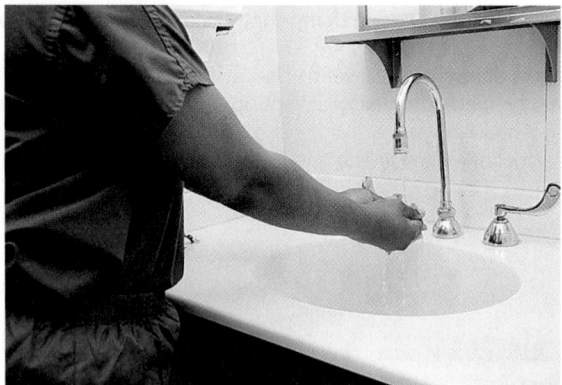

Fig. 15-4 The uniform does not touch the sink. Soap and water are within reach. Hands are lower than the elbows. Hands do not touch the inside of the sink.

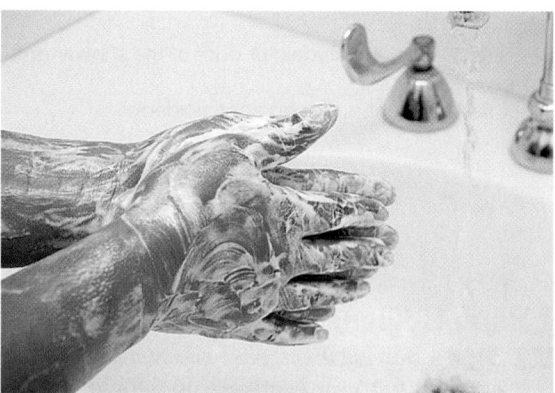

Fig. 15-5 The palms are rubbed together to work up a good lather.

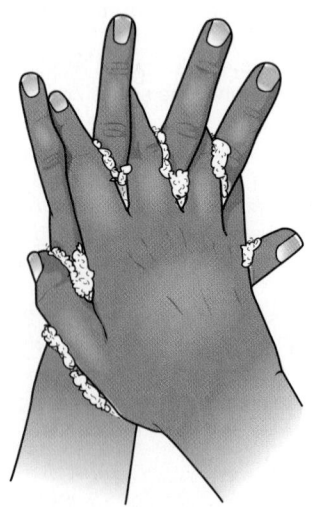

Fig. 15-6 The fingers are interlaced to work up a good lather.

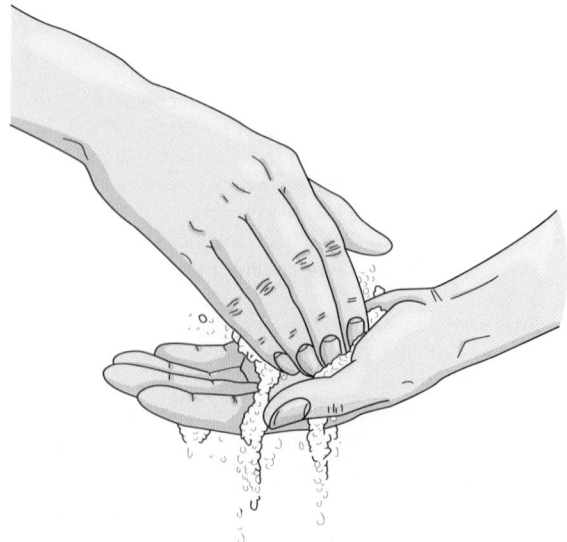

Fig. 15-7 The fingertips are rubbed against the palms to clean under the fingernails.

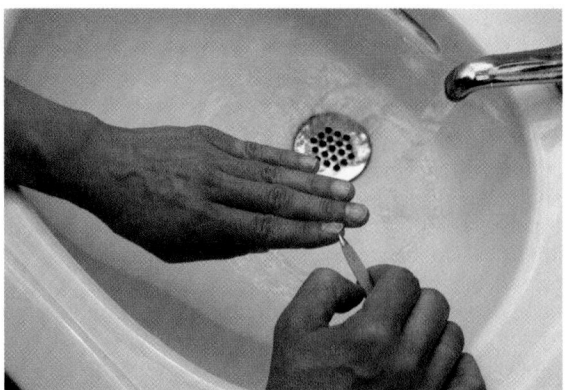

Fig. 15-8 A nail file is used to clean under the fingernails.

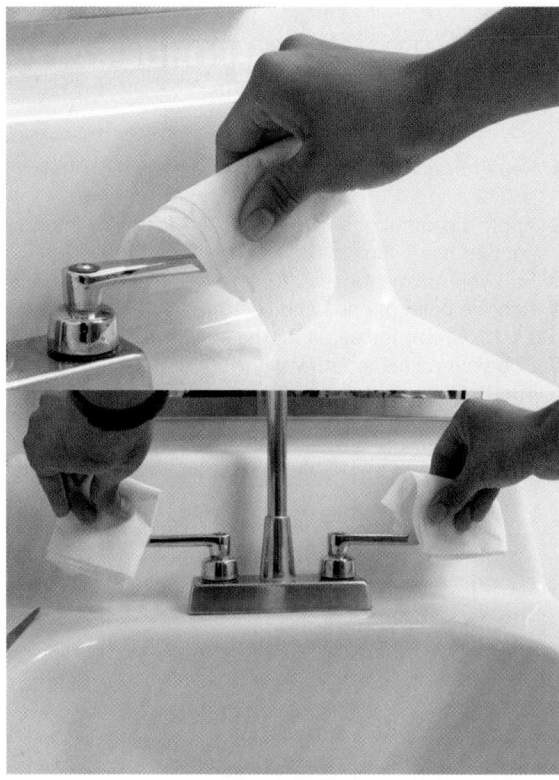

Fig. 15-9 A paper towel is used to turn off each faucet.

PROMOTING SAFETY AND COMFORT
Hand Hygiene

Safety

You use your hands for almost every task. They can pick up microbes from a person, place, or thing. Your hands transfer them to other people, places, and things. That is why hand hygiene is so very important. Always practice hand hygiene before and after giving care.

Comfort

You will practice hand hygiene very often during your shift. Hand lotions and hand creams help prevent chapping and dry skin. Apply hand lotion or cream as often as needed. Use an agency-approved lotion or cream.

HAND WASHING

 VIDEO VIDEO CLIP NNAAP® Skill

PROCEDURE

1 See *Promoting Safety and Comfort: Hand Hygiene*.
2 Make sure you have soap, paper towels, an orangewood stick or nail file, and a wastebasket. Collect missing items.
3 Push your watch up your arm 4 to 5 inches. If your uniform sleeves are long, push them up too.
4 Stand away from the sink so your clothes do not touch the sink. Stand so the soap and faucet are easy to reach (see Fig. 15-4). Do not touch the inside of the sink at any time.
5 Turn on and adjust the water until it feels warm.
6 Wet your wrists and hands. Keep your hands lower than your elbows. Be sure to wet the area 3 to 4 inches above your wrists.
7 Apply about 1 teaspoon of soap to your hands.
8 Rub your palms together and interlace your fingers to work up a good lather (see Fig. 15-5). Lather your wrists, hands, and fingers. Keep your hands lower than your elbows. This step should last at least 20 seconds.

9 Wash each hand and wrist thoroughly. Clean the back of your fingers and between your fingers (see Fig. 15-6).
10 Clean under the fingernails. Rub your fingertips against your palms (see Fig. 15-7).
11 Clean under the fingernails with a nail file or orangewood stick (see Fig. 15-8). This step is done for the first hand washing of the day and when your hands are highly soiled.
12 Rinse your wrists, hands, and fingers well. Water flows from the wrists to your fingertips.
13 Repeat steps 7 through 12, if needed.
14 Dry your wrists and hands with clean, dry paper towels. Pat dry starting at your fingertips.
15 Discard the paper towels into the wastebasket.
16 Turn off faucets with clean, dry paper towels. This prevents you from contaminating your hands (see Fig. 15-9). Use a clean paper towel for each faucet. Or use knee or foot controls to turn off the faucet.
17 Discard the paper towels into the wastebasket.

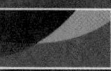**USING AN ALCOHOL-BASED HAND RUB** VIDEO | VIDEO CLIP

PROCEDURE

1 See *Promoting Safety and Comfort: Hand Hygiene,* p. 219.
2 Apply a palmful of an alcohol-based hand rub into a cupped hand (Fig. 15-10, A).
3 Rub your palms together (Fig. 15-10, B).
4 Rub the palm of one hand over the back of the other (Fig. 15-10, C). Do the same for the other hand.
5 Rub your palms together with your fingers interlaced (Fig. 15-10, D).

6 Interlock your fingers as in Figure 15-10, E. Rub your fingers back and forth.
7 Rub the thumb of one hand in the palm of the other (Fig. 15-10, F). Do the same for the other thumb.
8 Rub the fingers of one hand into the palm of the other hand (Fig. 15-10, G). Use a circular motion. Do the same for the fingers of the other hand.
9 Continue rubbing your hands until they are dry.

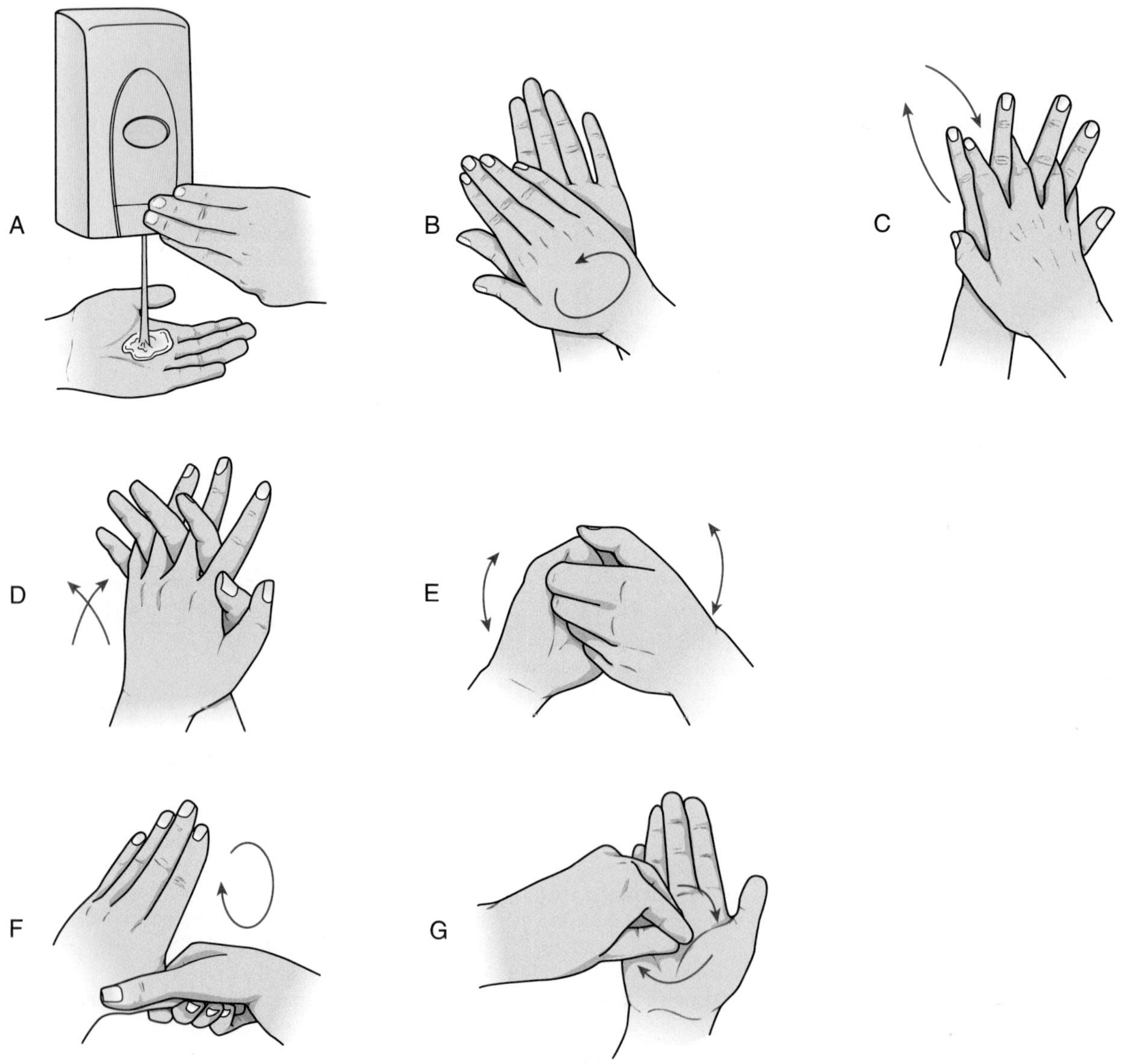

A B C

D E

F G

Fig. 15-10 Using an alcohol-based hand rub. **A,** A palmful of an alcohol-based hand rub is applied into a cupped hand. **B,** The palms are rubbed together. **C,** The palm of one hand is rubbed over the back of the other. **D,** The palms are rubbed together with the fingers interlaced. **E,** The fingers are interlocked and the fingers rubbed back and forth. **F,** The thumb of one hand is rubbed in the palm of the other. **G,** The fingers of one hand are rubbed into the palm of the other hand with circular motions.

Supplies and Equipment

Most health care supplies and equipment are disposable. They help prevent the spread of infection. You discard single-use items after use. A person uses multi-use items many times. They include bedpans, urinals, wash basins, and water pitchers and drinking cups. Do not "borrow" such items for another person.

Non-disposable items are cleaned and then disinfected. Then they are sterilized. This is usually done by the supply department.

Cleaning. Cleaning reduces the number of microbes present. It also removes organic matter such as blood, body fluids, secretions, and excretions. To clean equipment:

- Wear personal protective equipment (PPE) when cleaning items contaminated with blood, body fluids, secretions, or excretions. PPE includes gloves, a mask, a gown, and goggles or a face shield.
- Work from "clean" to "dirty" areas. If you work from a "dirty" to a "clean" area, the "clean" area becomes contaminated ("dirty").
- Rinse the item to remove organic matter. Use cold water. Heat makes organic matter thick, sticky, and hard to remove.
- Wash the item with soap and hot water.
- Scrub thoroughly. Use a brush if necessary.
- Rinse the item in warm water.
- Dry the item.
- Disinfect or sterilize the item.
- Disinfect equipment and the sink used in the cleaning procedure.
- Discard PPE.
- Practice hand hygiene.

Hospitals and nursing centers have "clean" and "dirty" utility rooms. Equipment is cleaned in the "dirty" utility room. Then it is disinfected or sterilized in the "clean" utility room.

Disinfection. *Disinfection is the process of destroying pathogens.* Spores are not destroyed. *Spores are bacteria protected by a hard shell.* Spores are killed by very high temperatures.

Chemical disinfectants are used to clean surfaces. Counters, tubs, and showers are examples. They also are used to clean re-usable items. Such items include:

- Blood pressure cuffs
- Commodes and metal bedpans
- Wheelchairs and stretchers
- Furniture

See *Focus on Long-Term Care and Home Care: Disinfection.*
See *Promoting Safety and Comfort: Disinfection.*

Sterilization. Sterilizing destroys all non-pathogens and pathogens, including spores. Very high temperatures are used. Heat destroys microbes.

Boiling water, radiation, liquid or gas chemicals, dry heat, and *steam under pressure* are sterilization methods. An *autoclave* (Fig. 15-11) is a pressure steam sterilizer. Glass, surgical items, and metal objects are autoclaved. High

---

Home Care

Detergent and hot water are used for cooking, eating, and drinking utensils and for linens. Many commercial products disinfect household surfaces—sinks, counters, floors, toilets, tubs, and showers. Use the products the family prefers or as the nurse instructs.

White vinegar and water is a good, cheap disinfectant. You can use it to clean bedpans, urinals, commodes, toilets, mirrors, bathroom tiles, and so on. To make a vinegar solution:
- Mix 1 cup of white vinegar with 3 cups of water.
- Label the container as a "vinegar solution: 1 cup white vinegar; 3 cups water."
- Include the date, time, and your name on the label.

PROMOTING SAFETY AND COMFORT
Disinfection

Safety

Chemical disinfectants can burn and irritate the skin. Wear utility gloves or rubber household gloves to prevent skin irritation. These gloves are *waterproof.* Do not wear disposable gloves.

Some chemical disinfectants have special measures for use and storage. Check the material safety data sheet (MSDS) before handling a disinfectant. See Chapter 12.

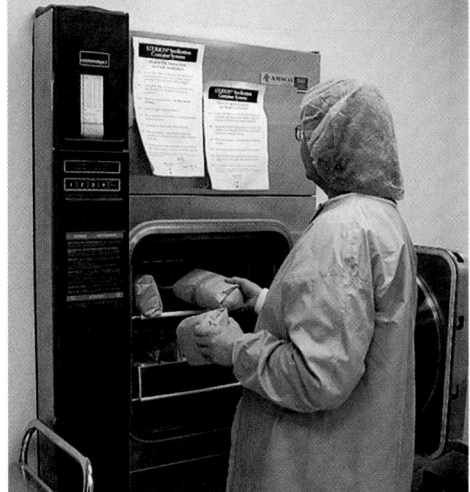

Fig. 15-11 An autoclave.

temperatures destroy plastic and rubber items. They are not autoclaved. Steam under pressure sterilizes objects in 30 to 45 minutes.

See *Focus on Long-Term Care and Home Care: Sterilization,* p. 222.

Other Aseptic Measures

Hand hygiene, cleaning, disinfection, and sterilization are important aseptic measures. So are the measures listed in Box 15-4, p. 222. They are useful in home, work, and everyday life.

FOCUS ON LONG-TERM CARE AND HOME CARE
Sterilization

Home Care
You can use boiling water to sterilize items in the home.
* Use a pot with a lid. The pot must be big enough to hold the items.
* Wash all items to be sterilized. Use soap and hot water.
* Fill the pot with cold water. Completely cover all items with water.
* Put the lid on the pot.
* Bring the water to a full boil. Steam will escape under the lid.
* Boil the items for 5 to 15 minutes. Follow agency policy.
* Turn off the heat.
* Let the pot cool.
* Remove the items to a clean towel. Use tongs to remove the items.
* Let the items air-dry.
* Put the items away as the family prefers or as the nurse instructs.

  Many people use dishwashers for baby bottles (Fig. 15-12). However, many dishwashers do not get hot enough to actually sterilize items.

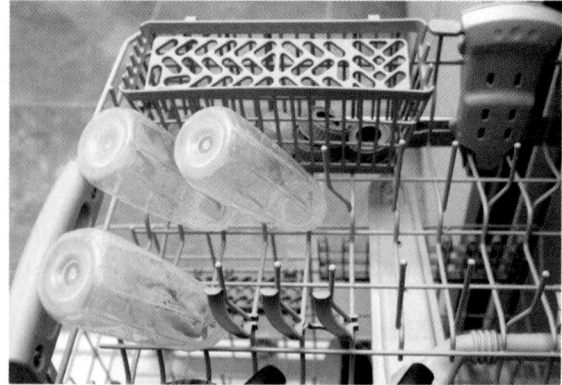

Fig. 15-12 A dishwasher is used to clean baby bottles.

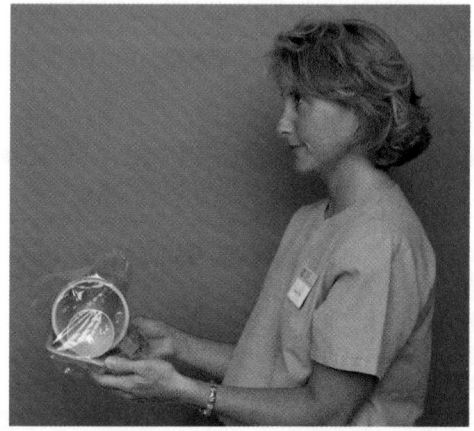

Fig. 15-13 Hold equipment away from your uniform.

BOX 15-4 ASEPTIC MEASURES

Controlling Reservoirs (Hosts–You or the Person)
* Provide for the person's hygiene needs (Chapter 20).
* Wash contaminated areas with soap and water. Feces, urine, and blood can contain microbes. So can body fluids, secretions, and excretions.
* Use leak-proof plastic bags for soiled tissues, linens, and other items.
* Keep tables, counters, wheelchair trays, and other surfaces clean and dry.
* Label bottles with the person's name and the date the bottle was opened.
* Keep bottles and fluid containers tightly capped or covered.
* Keep drainage containers below the drainage site (Chapters 22 and 33).
* Empty drainage containers and dispose of drainage following agency policy. Usually drainage containers are emptied every shift. Follow the nurse's directions if you need to empty them more often.

Controlling Portals of Exit
* Cover your nose and mouth when coughing or sneezing.
* Provide the person with tissues to use when coughing or sneezing.
* Wear PPE as needed (p. 227).

Controlling Transmission
* Provide all persons with their own personal care equipment. This includes wash basins, bedpans, urinals, commodes, and eating and drinking utensils.
* Do not take equipment from one person's room to use for another person. Even if un-used, do not take the item from one room to another.
* Hold equipment and linens away from your uniform (Fig. 15-13).
* Practice hand hygiene. See Box 15-3.
* Assist the person with hand washing:
  * Before and after eating
  * After elimination
  * After changing tampons, sanitary napkins, or other personal hygiene products
  * After contact with blood, body fluids, secretions, or excretions
* Prevent dust movement. Do not shake linens or equipment. Use a damp cloth for dusting.
* Clean from the cleanest area to the dirtiest. This prevents soiling a clean area.
* Clean away from your body. Do not dust, brush, or wipe toward yourself. Otherwise you transmit microbes to your skin, hair, and clothing.

BOX 15-4	**ASEPTIC MEASURES—cont'd**

Controlling Transmission—cont'd

- Flush urine and feces down the toilet. Avoid splatters and splashes.
- Pour contaminated liquids directly into sinks or toilets. Avoid splashing onto other areas.
- Do not sit on the person's bed or chair. You will pick up microbes. You will transfer them to the next surface that you sit on.
- Do not use items that are on the floor. The floor is contaminated.
- Clean tubs, showers, and shower chairs after each use. Follow the agency's disinfection procedures.
- Clean bedpans, urinals, and commodes after each use. Follow the agency's disinfection procedures.
- Report pests—ants, spiders, mice, and so on.

Controlling Portals of Entry

- Provide for good skin care (Chapter 20). This promotes intact skin.
- Provide for good oral hygiene (Chapter 20). This promotes intact mucous membranes.

Controlling Portals of Entry—cont'd

- Protect the skin from injury.
  - Do not let the person lie on tubes or other items.
  - Make sure linens are dry and wrinkle-free (Chapter 19).
  - Turn and re-position the person as directed by the nurse and care plan (Chapters 16 and 17).
- Assist with or clean the genital area after elimination. (See "Perineal Care" in Chapter 20.) Wipe and clean from the urethra (the cleanest area) to the rectum (the dirtiest area). This helps prevent urinary tract infections.
- Make sure drainage tubes are properly connected. This prevents microbes from entering the drainage system.

Protecting the Susceptible Host

- Follow the care plan to meet hygiene needs. This protects the skin and mucous membranes.
- Follow the care plan to meet nutrition and fluid needs (Chapter 24). This helps prevent infection.
- Assist with deep-breathing and coughing exercises as directed (Chapter 36). This helps prevent respiratory infections.

ISOLATION PRECAUTIONS

Blood, body fluids, secretions, and excretions can transmit pathogens. Sometimes barriers are needed to keep pathogens within a certain area. Usually the area is the person's room. This requires isolation procedures.

The *Guideline for Isolation Precautions: Preventing Transmission of Infectious Agents in Healthcare Settings 2007* is followed. The guideline was issued by the Centers for Disease Control and Prevention (CDC). Isolation precautions prevent the spread of *communicable diseases (contagious diseases). They are diseases caused by pathogens that spread easily.* See Table 15-1, p. 224 for common childhood communicable diseases.

Isolation precautions are based on *clean* and *dirty*. *Clean* areas or objects are free of pathogens. They are not contaminated. *Dirty* areas or objects are contaminated with pathogens. If a *clean* area or object has contact with something *dirty*, the clean area is now dirty. *Clean* and *dirty* also depend on how the pathogen is spread.

The CDC guideline has two tiers of precautions:

- Standard Precautions
- Transmission-Based Precautions

Standard Precautions

Standard Precautions are part of the CDC's isolation precautions (Box 15-5, p. 224). They reduce the risk of spreading pathogens. They also reduce the risk of spreading known and unknown infections. *Standard Precautions are used for all persons whenever care is given.* They prevent the spread of infection from:

- Blood.
- All body fluids, secretions, and excretions (except sweat) even if blood is not visible. Sweat is not known to spread infection.
- Non-intact skin (skin with open breaks).
- Mucous membranes.

TABLE 15-1	COMMON COMMUNICABLE CHILDHOOD DISEASES	
Disease	**Method of Transmission**	**Signs and Symptoms**
Chickenpox (varicella)	Direct contact and airborne contact with respiratory secretions; direct contact with skin lesions	Fever; rash; skin lesions
Diphtheria	Direct or indirect contact with respiratory secretions and skin lesions from the person or a carrier	Sore throat; fever; nasal discharge; enlarged lymph glands in the neck; cough; hoarseness; patches (lesions) on the tonsils, pharynx, larynx, nasal membranes, and skin
Measles (rubeola)	Direct or indirect contact with nasal secretions	Fever; cough; rash; inflammation of the mucous membranes of the nose; nasal discharge; bronchitis
Mumps	Direct contact with saliva droplets	Fever; headache; swollen salivary glands; earache
Whooping cough (pertussis)	Airborne or direct contact with droplets from the respiratory tract	Fever; sneezing; severe cough at night; coughs are short and rapid followed by a "whoop" or crowing sound with breathing in
Poliomyelitis	Airborne or direct contact with respiratory secretions; direct contact with feces	Fever; sore throat; headache; nausea and vomiting; loss of appetite; abdominal pain; neck and spinal stiffness; paralysis
German measles (rubella)	Airborne or direct contact with secretions from the nose and pharynx	Fever; headache; loss of appetite; nasal inflammation; sore throat; cough; rash
Scarlet fever	Airborne or direct contact with nasal and pharyngeal secretions	Fever; chills; headache; vomiting; abdominal pain; red and swollen tonsils and pharynx; rash

BOX 15-5	STANDARD PRECAUTIONS

Hand Hygiene
- Follow the rules for hand hygiene. See Box 15-3.
- Touch surfaces close to the person only when necessary. This prevents contamination of clean hands from environmental surfaces. It also prevents the transmission of pathogens from contaminated hands to other surfaces.
- Do not wear fake nails or nail extenders if you will have contact with persons at risk for infection or other adverse outcomes. (NOTE: Some agencies do not allow fake nails or nail extenders.)

Personal Protective Equipment (PPE)
- Wear PPE when contact with blood or body fluids is likely.
- Do not contaminate your clothing or skin when removing PPE.
- Remove and discard PPE before leaving the person's room or care setting.

Gloves
- Wear gloves when contact with the following is likely:
  - Blood
  - Potentially infectious materials (body fluids, secretions, and excretions are examples)
  - Mucous membranes
  - Non-intact skin
  - Skin that may be contaminated (for example, a person is incontinent of feces or urine)

Gloves—cont'd
- Wear gloves that fit and are appropriate for the task:
  - Wear disposable gloves to provide direct care to the person.
  - Wear disposable gloves or utility gloves for cleaning equipment or care settings.
- Remove gloves after contact with the person or the person's care setting. The care setting includes equipment used in the person's care.
- Remove gloves after contact with care equipment.
- Do not wear the same pair of gloves to care for more than one person. Remove gloves after contact with a person and before going to another person.
- Do not wash gloves for re-use with different persons.
- Change gloves during care if your hands will move from a contaminated body site to a clean body site.

Gowns
- Wear a gown that is appropriate to the task.
- Wear a gown to protect your skin and clothing when contact with blood, body fluids, secretions, or excretions is likely.
- Wear a gown for direct contact with a person if he or she has uncontained secretions or excretions.
- Remove the gown and perform hand hygiene before leaving the person's room or care setting.
- Do not re-use gowns, even for repeat contacts with the same person.

Modified from Siegel JD, Rhinehart E, Jackson M, Chiarello L, and the Healthcare Infection Control Practices Advisory Committee, *Guideline for isolation precautions: preventing transmission of infectious agents in healthcare settings 2007*, Atlanta, 2007, Centers for Disease Control and Prevention.

BOX 15-5 STANDARD PRECAUTIONS—cont'd

Mouth, Nose, and Eye Protection

- Wear PPE—masks, goggles, face shields—for procedures and tasks that are likely to cause splashes and sprays of blood, body fluids, secretions, or excretions.
- Wear PPE—mask, goggles, face shield—appropriate for the procedure or task.
- Wear gloves, a gown, and one of the following for procedures that are likely to cause sprays of respiratory secretions:
  - A face shield that fully covers the front and sides of the face
  - A mask with attached shield
  - A mask and goggles

Respiratory Hygiene/Cough Etiquette

- Instruct persons with respiratory symptoms to:
  - Cover the nose and mouth when coughing or sneezing.
  - Use tissues to contain respiratory secretions.
  - Dispose of tissues in the nearest waste container after use.
  - Perform hand hygiene after contact with respiratory secretions.
- Provide visitors with masks according to agency policy.

Care Equipment

- Wear appropriate PPE when handling care equipment that is visibly soiled with blood, body fluids, secretions, or excretions.
- Wear appropriate PPE when handling care equipment that may have been in contact with blood, body fluids, secretions, or excretions.
- Remove organic material before disinfection and sterilization procedures. Use cleaning agents according to agency policy.

Care of the Environment

- Follow agency policies and procedures for cleaning and maintaining surfaces. Environmental surfaces and care equipment are examples. Surfaces near the person may need more frequent cleaning and maintenance—door knobs, bed rails, overbed tables, toilet surfaces and areas, and so on.
- Clean and disinfect multi-use electronic equipment according to agency policy. This includes:
  - Items used by patients and residents
  - Items used to give care
  - Mobile devices that are moved in and out of patient or resident rooms

Care of the Environment—cont'd

- Follow these rules for children's toys. This includes toys in agency waiting areas:
  - Select toys that are easily cleaned and disinfected.
  - Do not allow the use of stuffed, furry toys if they will be shared.
  - Clean and disinfect large stationary toys (for example, climbing equipment) at least weekly and whenever visibly soiled.
  - Rinse toys with water after disinfection if they are likely to be mouthed by children. Or wash them in a dishwasher.
  - Clean and disinfect a toy immediately when it needs cleaning. Or store the toy in a labeled container away from toys that are clean and ready for use.

Textiles and Laundry

- Handle used textiles and fabrics (linens) with minimum agitation. This prevents contamination of air, surfaces, and other persons.

Worker Safety

- Protect yourself and others from exposure to bloodborne pathogens. This includes handling needles and other sharps. Follow federal and state standards and guidelines. See the Bloodborne Pathogen Standard (p. 235).
- Use a mouthpiece, resuscitation bag, or other ventilation device during resuscitation to prevent contact with the person's mouth and oral secretions. See Chapter 51.

Patient or Resident Placement

- A private room is preferred if the person is at risk for transmitting the infection to others.
- Follow the nurse's instructions if a private room is not available.

Transmission-Based Precautions

Some infections require Transmission-Based Precautions (Box 15-6, p. 226). (NOTE: In health care settings, Transmission-Based Precautions are commonly called "isolation precautions.") You must understand how certain infections are spread (see Fig. 15-2). This helps you understand the different types of Transmission-Based Precautions.

BOX 15-6   TRANSMISSION-BASED PRECAUTIONS

Contact Precautions

- Used for persons with known or suspected infections or conditions that increase the risk of contact transmission.
- Patient or resident placement:
  - A single room is preferred.
  - Do the following if a room is shared with another person who is not infected with the same agent:
    - Keep the privacy curtain between the beds closed.
    - Change PPE and practice hand hygiene between contact with persons in the same room. Do so regardless of whether one or both persons are on Contact Precautions.
- Gloves:
  - Don gloves upon entering the person's room or care setting.
  - Wear gloves whenever touching the person's intact skin.
  - Wear gloves whenever touching surfaces or items near the person.
- Gowns:
  - Wear a gown whenever clothing may have direct contact with the person.
  - Wear a gown whenever contact is likely with surfaces or equipment near the person.
  - Don the gown upon entering the person's room or care setting.
  - Remove the gown and practice hand hygiene before leaving the person's room or care setting.
  - Make sure your clothing and skin do not touch potentially contaminated surfaces after removing the gown.
- Patient or resident transport:
  - Limit transport and movement of the person outside of the room to medically-necessary purposes.
  - Cover the area of the person's body that is infected.
  - Remove and discard contaminated PPE and practice hand hygiene before transporting the person.
  - Don clean PPE to handle the person at the transport destination.
- Care equipment:
  - Follow Standard Precautions.
  - Use disposable equipment when possible. If possible, leave non-disposable equipment in the person's room.
  - Clean and disinfect non-disposable and multiple-use equipment before use on another person.

Droplet Precautions

- Used for persons known or suspected to be infected with pathogens transmitted by respiratory droplets. Such droplets come from a person who is coughing, sneezing, or talking.

Droplet Precautions—cont'd

- Patient or resident placement:
  - A single room is preferred.
  - Do the following if a room is shared with another person who is not infected with the same agent:
    - Keep the privacy curtain between the beds closed.
    - Change PPE and practice hand hygiene between contact with persons in the same room. Do so regardless of whether one or both persons are on Droplet Precautions.
- Personal protective equipment:
  - Don a mask upon entering the person's room or care setting.
- Patient or resident transport:
  - Limit transport and movement of the person outside of the room to medically necessary purposes.
  - Have the person wear a mask.
  - Instruct the person to follow Respiratory Hygiene/Cough Etiquette (see Box 15-5, "Standard Precautions").
  - No mask is required for health team members transporting the person.

Airborne Precautions

- Used for persons known or suspected to be infected with pathogens transmitted person-to-person by the airborne route. Tuberculosis (TB), measles, chicken pox, smallpox, and severe acute respiratory syndrome (SARS) are examples.
- The person is placed in an airborne infection isolation room (AIIR). If one is not available, the person is transferred to an agency with an AIIR.
- Staff susceptible to the infection are restricted from entering the room. This is if immune staff members are available.
- Personal protective equipment:
  - An approved respirator is worn on entering the room or home of a person with TB.
  - Respiratory protection is recommended for all staff when caring for persons with smallpox.
- Patient or resident transport:
  - Limit transport and movement of the person outside of the room to medically necessary purposes.
  - Have the person wear a surgical mask.
  - Instruct the person to follow Respiratory Hygiene/Cough Etiquette (see Box 15-5, "Standard Precautions").
  - Cover skin lesions infected with the microbe.
  - No mask or respirator is required for staff transporting the person.

Modified from Siegel JD, Rhinehart E, Jackson M, Chiarello L, and the Healthcare Infection Control Practices Advisory Committee, *Guideline for isolation precautions: preventing transmission of infectious agents in healthcare settings 2007*, Atlanta, 2007, Centers for Disease Control and Prevention.

Some agencies have airborne infection isolation rooms (AIIRs). An AIIR room is a private (single-person) room with a private bathroom. AIIR room practices include:

- All persons entering the room wear a tuberculosis (TB) respirator.
- The room door is kept closed except when someone enters or leaves the room.
- Treatments and procedures are done in the room.
- The person wears a mask during transport.

See *Focus on Communication: Transmission-Based Precautions.*

See *Delegation Guidelines: Transmission-Based Precautions.*

See *Promoting Safety and Comfort: Transmission-Based Precautions.*

See *Teamwork and Time Management: Transmission-Based Precautions.*

FOCUS ON COMMUNICATION
Transmission-Based Precautions

Some agencies require visitors to wear PPE when visiting a person needing isolation precautions. Visitors may question the need for PPE. They do not wear PPE around the person in his or her home or outside the agency. They do not understand the need. Some visitors ignore signs or requests to wear PPE. It is important to communicate with the person and visitors about PPE. You can politely say:

- "Your visitors will need to wear a gown and gloves while in your room."
- "Please wear this mask. It is our policy to protect you, your family member, and others."

Tell the nurse if the person or visitors have more questions. Also tell the nurse if someone refuses to follow isolation precautions.

You may see others on the health care team not wearing PPE when it is needed. Inform the person that PPE is needed. Offer to get the person PPE. For example, you can say:

- "A mask is needed when caring for Mrs. Stayton. I will get you one."
- "Here are gloves and a gown. They need to be worn in Mr. Parker's room."

Be polite. Tell the nurse if the person refuses.

DELEGATION GUIDELINES
Transmission-Based Precautions

You may assist in the care of persons who require isolation precautions. If so, review the type used with the nurse. You also need this information from the nurse and the care plan:

- What PPE to use
- What special safety measures are needed

PROMOTING SAFETY AND COMFORT
Transmission-Based Precautions

Safety

Preventing the spread of infection is important. Isolation precautions protect everyone—patients, residents, visitors, staff, and you. If you are careless, everyone's safety is at risk.

Comfort

Persons requiring isolation precautions usually must stay in their rooms. The person may feel lonely, especially if visitors are few. To help the person:

- Remember that the pathogen is undesirable, not the person.
- Treat the person with respect, kindness, and dignity.
- Provide newspapers, magazines, books, and other reading matter.
- Provide hobby materials if possible.
- Place a clock in the room.
- Suggest that the person call family and friends.
- Provide a current TV guide.
- Organize your work so you can stay to visit with the person.
- Say "hello" from the doorway often.

Items brought into the person's room become contaminated. Disinfect or discard the items according to agency policy.

TEAMWORK AND TIME MANAGEMENT
Transmission-Based Precautions

Donning (putting on) and removing PPE take time and effort. Once you don PPE, you must remove it before leaving the room. Therefore you need to plan your time and work so that you do not need to leave the room.

- Meet the needs of other patients or residents first.
- Ask a co-worker to answer signal lights for you. Ask politely and thank your co-worker for helping you.
- Gather needed care items to bring to the room.
- Make sure the person's needs are met before leaving the room.
- Complete a safety check of the room.
- Tell the person when you will return to the room.

Offer to help co-workers who care for persons needing isolation. Bring items to the room as needed. Also answer signal lights for your co-workers. Be sure to tell them about the care given and your observations.

Protective Measures

Agency policies may differ from those in this text. The rules in Box 15-7, p. 228 are a guide for giving safe care when using isolation precautions.

Isolation precautions involve wearing PPE—gloves, a gown, a mask, and goggles or a face shield.

Removing linens, trash, and equipment from the room may require double-bagging (p. 233). Follow agency procedures when collecting specimens and transporting persons.

See *Promoting Safety and Comfort: Protective Measures,* p. 228.

BOX 15-7 RULES FOR ISOLATION PRECAUTIONS

- Collect all needed items before entering the room.
- Do not contaminate equipment and supplies. Floors are contaminated. So is any object on the floor or that falls to the floor.
- Use mops wetted with a disinfectant solution to clean floors. Floor dust is contaminated.
- Prevent drafts. Some microbes are carried in the air by drafts.
- Use paper towels to handle contaminated items.
- Remove items from the room in leak-proof plastic bags.
- Double-bag items if the outer part of the bag is or can be contaminated (p. 233).
- Follow agency policy for removing and transporting disposable and re-usable items.
- Return re-usable dishes, drinking vessels, eating utensils, and trays to the food service (dietary) department. Discard disposable dishes, drinking vessels, eating utensils, and trays in the waste container in the person's room.
- Do not touch your hair, nose, mouth, eyes, or other body parts.
- Do not touch any clean area or object if your hands are contaminated.
- Wash your hands if they are visibly dirty or contaminated with blood, body fluids, secretions, or excretions.
- Place clean items on paper towels.
- Do not shake linens.
- Use paper towels to turn faucets on and off.
- Use a paper towel to open the door to the person's room. Discard it as you leave.
- Tell the nurse if you have any cuts, open skin areas, a sore throat, vomiting, or diarrhea.

PROMOTING SAFETY AND COMFORT
Protective Measures

Safety

The PPE needed for Standard Precautions depends on the tasks, procedures, and care measures you will do in the room. The PPE needed also depends on the type of Transmission-Based Precautions ordered for the person. Sometimes only gloves are needed. The nurse tells you when other PPE are needed.

According to the CDC's isolation guideline, gloves are always worn when gowns are worn. Sometimes other PPE are needed when gowns are worn. The isolation guideline shows PPE donned and removed in the following order:

- Donning PPE (Fig. 15-14, A):
  - Gown
  - Mask or respirator
  - Eyewear (goggles or face shield)
  - Gloves
- Removing PPE (removed at the doorway before leaving the person's room) (Fig. 15-14, B):
  - Gloves
  - Goggles or face shield
  - Gown
  - Mask or respirator

(Note: Some state competency tests require hand hygiene after removing each item of PPE. And some states use a different order for donning and removing PPE. Follow the procedures used in your state and agency.)

SEQUENCE FOR DONNING PERSONAL PROTECTIVE EQUIPMENT (PPE)	SECUENCIA PARA PONERSE EL EQUIPO DE PROTECCIÓN PERSONAL (PPE)

The type of PPE used will vary based on the level of precautions required; e.g., Standard and Contact, Droplet or Airborne Infection Isolation.

El tipo de PPE que se debe utilizar depende del nivel de precaución que sea necesario; por ejemplo, equipo Estándar y de Contacto o de Aislamiento de infecciones transportadas por gotas o por aire.

1. GOWN
- Fully cover torso from neck to knees, arms to end of wrists, and wrap around the back
- Fasten in back of neck and waist

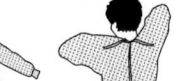

1. BATA
- *Cubra con la bata todo el torso desde el cuello hasta las rodillas, los brazos hasta la muñeca y dóblela alrededor de la espalda*
- *Átesela por detrás a la altura del cuello y la cintura*

2. MASK OR RESPIRATOR
- Secure ties or elastic bands at middle of head and neck
- Fit flexible band to nose bridge
- Fit snug to face and below chin
- Fit-check respirator

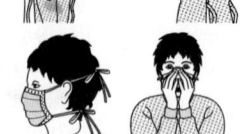

2. MÁSCARA O RESPIRADOR
- *Asegúrese los cordones o la banda elástica en la mitad de la cabeza y en el cuello*
- *Ajústese la banda flexible en el puente de la nariz*
- *Acomódesela en la cara y por debajo del mentón*
- *Verifique el ajuste del respirador*

A

3. GOGGLES OR FACE SHIELD
- Place over face and eyes and adjust to fit

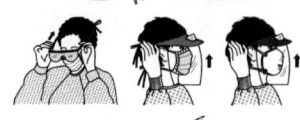

3. GAFAS PROTECTORAS O CARETAS
- *Colóquesela sobre la cara y los ojos y ajústela*

4. GLOVES
- Extend to cover wrist of isolation gown

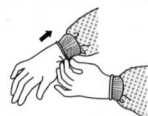

4. GUANTES
- *Extienda los guantes para que cubran la parte del puño en la bata de aislamiento*

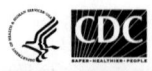

USE SAFE WORK PRACTICES TO PROTECT YOURSELF AND LIMIT THE SPREAD OF CONTAMINATION	UTILICE PRÁCTICAS DE TRABAJO SEGURAS PARA PROTEGERSE USTED MISMO Y LIMITAR LA PROPAGACIÓN DE LA CONTAMINACIÓN
■ Keep hands away from face ■ Limit surfaces touched ■ Change gloves when torn or heavily contaminated ■ Perform hand hygiene	■ *Mantenga las manos alejadas de la cara* ■ *Limite el contacto con superficies* ■ *Cambie los guantes si se rompen o están demasiado contaminados* ■ *Realice la higiene de las manos*

Fig. 15-14 A, Donning personal protective equipment.

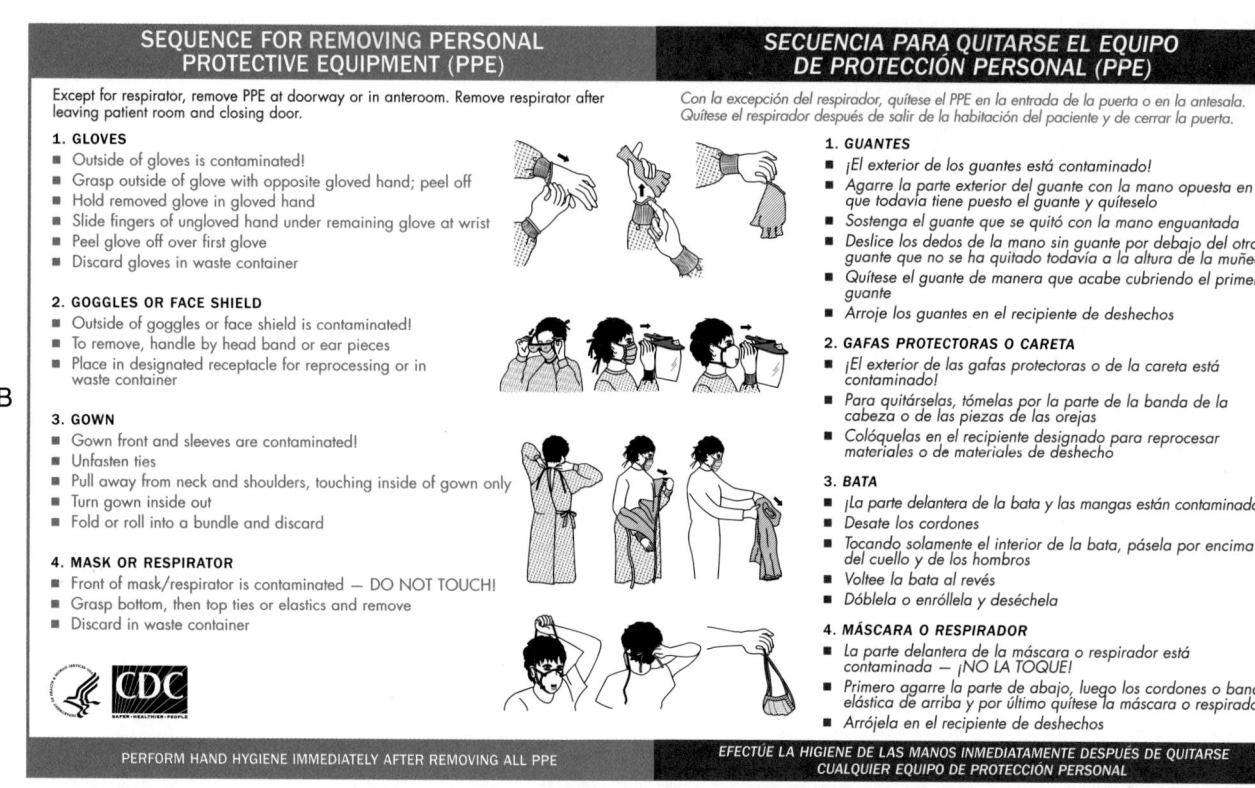

SEQUENCE FOR REMOVING PERSONAL PROTECTIVE EQUIPMENT (PPE)	SECUENCIA PARA QUITARSE EL EQUIPO DE PROTECCIÓN PERSONAL (PPE)

Except for respirator, remove PPE at doorway or in anteroom. Remove respirator after leaving patient room and closing door.

1. GLOVES
- Outside of gloves is contaminated!
- Grasp outside of glove with opposite gloved hand; peel off
- Hold removed glove in gloved hand
- Slide fingers of ungloved hand under remaining glove at wrist
- Peel glove off over first glove
- Discard gloves in waste container

2. GOGGLES OR FACE SHIELD
- Outside of goggles or face shield is contaminated!
- To remove, handle by head band or ear pieces
- Place in designated receptacle for reprocessing or in waste container

3. GOWN
- Gown front and sleeves are contaminated!
- Unfasten ties
- Pull away from neck and shoulders, touching inside of gown only
- Turn gown inside out
- Fold or roll into a bundle and discard

4. MASK OR RESPIRATOR
- Front of mask/respirator is contaminated — DO NOT TOUCH!
- Grasp bottom, then top ties or elastics and remove
- Discard in waste container

Con la excepción del respirador, quítese el PPE en la entrada de la puerta o en la antesala. Quítese el respirador después de salir de la habitación del paciente y de cerrar la puerta.

1. GUANTES
- ¡El exterior de los guantes está contaminado!
- Agarre la parte exterior del guante con la mano opuesta en la que todavía tiene puesto el guante y quíteselo
- Sostenga el guante que se quitó con la mano enguantada
- Deslice los dedos de la mano sin guante por debajo del otro guante que no se ha quitado todavía a la altura de la muñeca
- Quítese el guante de manera que acabe cubriendo el primer guante
- Arroje los guantes en el recipiente de deshechos

2. GAFAS PROTECTORAS O CARETA
- ¡El exterior de las gafas protectoras o de la careta está contaminado!
- Para quitárselas, tómelas por la parte de la banda de la cabeza o de las piezas de las orejas
- Colóquelas en el recipiente designado para reprocesar materiales o de materiales de deshecho

3. BATA
- ¡La parte delantera de la bata y las mangas están contaminadas!
- Desate los cordones
- Tocando solamente el interior de la bata, pásela por encima del cuello y de los hombros
- Voltee la bata al revés
- Dóblela o enróllela y deséchela

4. MÁSCARA O RESPIRADOR
- La parte delantera de la máscara o respirador está contaminada — ¡NO LA TOQUE!
- Primero agarre la parte de abajo, luego los cordones o banda elástica de arriba y por último quítese la máscara o respirador
- Arrójela en el recipiente de deshechos

PERFORM HAND HYGIENE IMMEDIATELY AFTER REMOVING ALL PPE	EFECTÚE LA HIGIENE DE LAS MANOS INMEDIATAMENTE DESPUÉS DE QUITARSE CUALQUIER EQUIPO DE PROTECCIÓN PERSONAL

Fig. 15-14, cont'd B, Removing personal protective equipment.

Gloves. The skin is a natural barrier. It prevents microbes from entering the body. Small skin breaks on the hands and fingers are common. Some are very small and hard to see. Disposable gloves act as a barrier. They protect you from pathogens in the person's blood, body fluids, secretions, and excretions. They also protect the person from microbes on your hands.

Wear gloves whenever contact with blood, body fluids, secretions, excretions, mucous membranes, or non-intact skin is likely. Contact may be direct. Or contact may be with items or surfaces contaminated with blood, body fluids, secretions, or excretions.

Wearing gloves is the most common protective measure used with Standard Precautions and Transmission-Based Precautions. Remember the following when using gloves:
- The outside of gloves is contaminated.
- Gloves are easier to put on when your hands are dry.
- Do not tear gloves when putting them on. Carelessness, long fingernails, and rings can tear gloves. Blood, body fluids, secretions, and excretions can enter the glove through the tear. This contaminates your hand.

- You need a new pair for every person.
- Remove and discard torn, cut, or punctured gloves at once. Practice hand hygiene. Then put on a new pair.
- Wear gloves once. Discard them after use.
- Put on clean gloves just before touching mucous membranes or non-intact skin.
- Put on new gloves whenever gloves become contaminated with blood, body fluids, secretions, or excretions. A task may require more than one pair of gloves.
- Change gloves whenever moving from a contaminated body site to a clean body site.
- Change gloves if interacting with the person involves touching portable computer keyboards or other mobile equipment that is transported from room to room.
- Put on gloves last when they are worn with other PPE.
- Make sure gloves cover your wrists. If you wear a gown, gloves cover the cuffs (Fig. 15-15, p. 230).
- Remove gloves so the inside part is on the outside. The inside is *clean.*
- Practice hand hygiene after removing gloves.
  See *Promoting Safety and Comfort: Gloves,* p. 230.

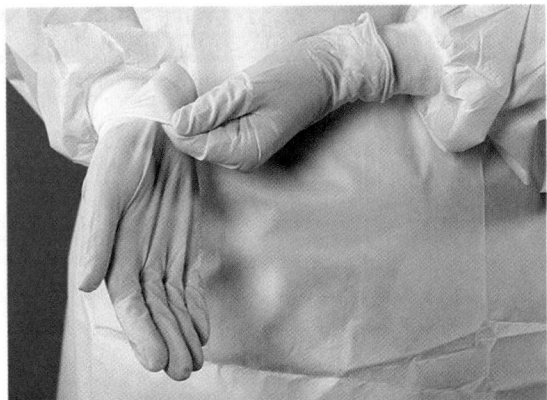

Fig. 15-15 The gloves cover the cuffs of the gown.

PROMOTING SAFETY AND COMFORT
Gloves

Safety

No special method is needed to put on non-sterile gloves. To remove gloves, see procedure: *Removing Gloves*.

Some gloves are made of latex (a rubber product). Latex allergies are common. They can cause skin rashes. Asthma and shock are more serious problems. Report skin rashes and breathing problems to the nurse at once.

You may have a latex allergy. Some patients and residents are allergic to latex. This is noted on the care plan and your assignment sheet. Latex-free gloves are worn for latex allergies.

Comfort

Many nurses and nursing assistants wear gloves for every patient and resident contact. Remember, gloves are needed whenever contact with blood, body fluids, secretions, excretions, mucous membranes, or non-intact skin is likely. Gloves are not needed when such contact is not likely. Back massages and brushing and combing hair are examples. To reduce exposure to latex, wear gloves only when needed.

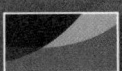 **REMOVING GLOVES**   VIDEO NNAAP® Skill

PROCEDURE

1 See *Promoting Safety and Comfort: Gloves*.
2 Make sure that glove touches only glove.
3 Grasp a glove at the palm (Fig. 15-16, A). Grasp it on the outside.
4 Pull the glove down over your hand so it is inside out (Fig. 15-16, B).
5 Hold the removed glove with your other gloved hand.
6 Reach inside the other glove. Use the first two fingers of the ungloved hand (Fig. 15-16, C).
7 Pull the glove down (inside out) over your hand and the other glove (Fig. 15-16, D).
8 Discard the gloves. Follow agency policy.
9 Practice hand hygiene.

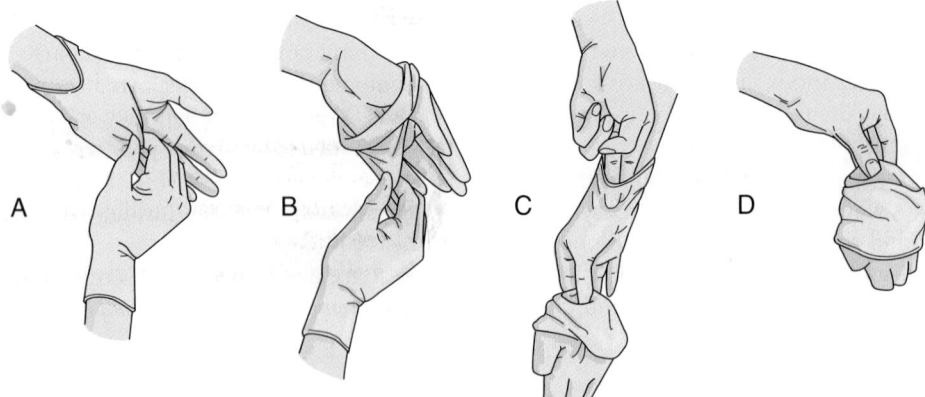

Fig. 15-16 Removing gloves. **A,** Grasp the glove at the palm. **B,** Pull the glove down over the hand. The glove is inside out. **C,** Insert the fingers of the ungloved hand inside the other glove. **D,** Pull the glove down and over the other hand and glove. The glove is inside out.

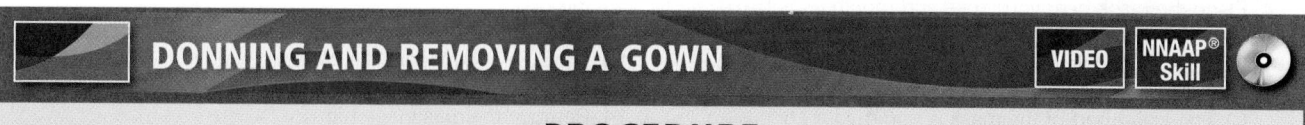

Gowns. Gowns prevent the spread of microbes. They protect your clothes and body from contact with blood, body fluids, secretions, and excretions. They also protect against splashes and sprays.

Gowns must completely cover you from your neck to your knees. The long sleeves have tight cuffs. The gown opens at the back. It is tied at the neck and waist. The gown front and sleeves are considered *contaminated*.

Gowns are used once. A wet gown is contaminated. Remove it and put on a dry one. Discard disposable gowns after use.

DONNING AND REMOVING A GOWN   VIDEO   NNAAP® Skill

PROCEDURE

1 Remove your watch and all jewelry.
2 Roll up uniform sleeves.
3 Practice hand hygiene.
4 Hold a clean gown out in front of you. Let it unfold. Do not shake the gown.
5 Put your hands and arms through the sleeves (see Fig. 15-14, A).
6 Make sure the gown covers you from your neck to your knees. It must cover your arms to the end of your wrists.
7 Tie the strings at the back of the neck (see Fig. 15-14, A).
8 Overlap the back of the gown. Make sure it covers your uniform. The gown should be snug, not loose.
9 Tie the waist strings. Tie them at the back or the side. Do not tie them in front.
10 Put on other PPE.
   a Mask or respirator (if needed).
   b Goggles or face shield (if needed).
   c Gloves. Make sure the gloves cover the gown cuffs.
11 Provide care.
12 Remove and discard the gloves.
13 Remove and discard the goggles or face shield if worn.
14 Remove the gown. Do not touch the outside of the gown.
   a Untie the neck and waist strings (see Fig. 15-14, B).
   b Pull the gown down from each shoulder toward the same hand (see Fig. 15-14, B).
   c Turn the gown inside out as it is removed. Hold it at the inside shoulder seams, and bring your hands together (Fig. 15-17).
15 Hold and roll up the gown away from you (see Fig. 15-14, B). Keep it inside out. Do not let the gown touch the floor.
16 Discard the gown.
17 Remove and discard the mask if worn.
18 Practice hand hygiene.

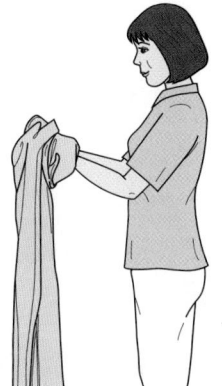

Fig. 15-17 The gown is turned inside out as it is removed.

Masks and Respiratory Protection. You wear masks for these reasons:

- For protection from contact with infectious materials from the person. Respiratory secretions and sprays of blood or body fluids are examples.
- During sterile procedures to protect the person from infectious agents carried in your mouth or nose.

Masks are disposable. A wet or moist mask is contaminated. Breathing can cause masks to become wet or moist. Apply a new mask when contamination occurs.

A mask fits snugly over your nose and mouth. Practice hand hygiene before putting on a mask. When removing a mask, touch only the ties or the elastic bands. The front of the mask is contaminated.

Tuberculosis respirators (Fig. 15-18, p. 232) are worn when caring for persons with TB. See Chapter 42 for more information about persons with TB.

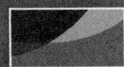

DONNING AND REMOVING A MASK

VIDEO

PROCEDURE

1 Practice hand hygiene.
2 Put on a gown if required.
3 Pick up a mask by its upper ties. Do not touch the part that will cover your face.
4 Place the mask over your nose and mouth (Fig. 15-19, A).
5 Place the upper strings above your ears. Tie them at the back in the middle of your head (Fig. 15-19, B).
6 Tie the lower strings at the back of your neck (Fig. 15-19, C). The lower part of the mask is under your chin.
7 Pinch the metal band around your nose. The top of the mask must be snug over your nose. If you wear eyeglasses, the mask must be snug under the bottom of the eyeglasses.
8 Make sure the mask is snug over your face and under your chin.

9 Put on goggles or a face shield if needed and if not part of the mask.
10 Put on gloves.
11 Provide care. Avoid coughing, sneezing, and unnecessary talking.
12 Change the mask if it becomes wet or contaminated.
13 Remove and discard the gloves. Remove the goggles or face shield and gown if worn.
14 Remove the mask (see Fig. 15-14, B).
  a Untie the lower strings of the mask.
  b Untie the top strings.
  c Hold the top strings. Remove the mask.
15 Discard the mask.
16 Practice hand hygiene.

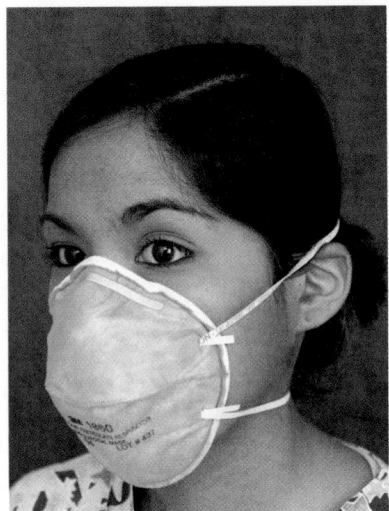

Fig. 15-18 Tuberculosis respirator.

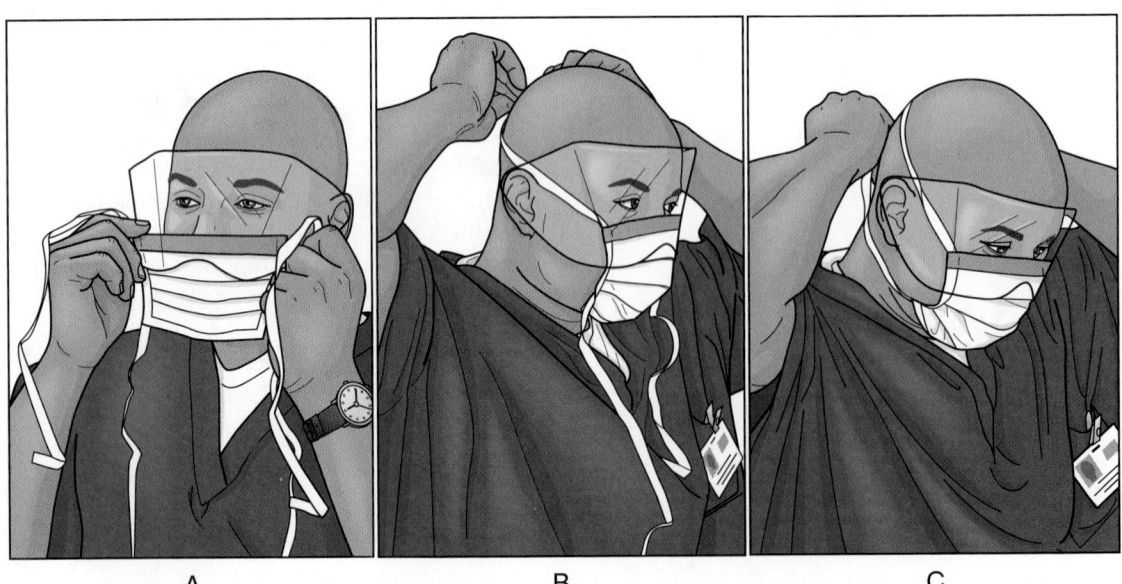

A   B   C

Fig. 15-19 Donning and removing a mask. NOTE: the mask has a face shield. **A,** The mask covers the nose and mouth. **B,** Upper strings are tied at the back of the head. **C,** Lower strings are tied at the back of the neck.

Goggles and Face Shields. Goggles and face shields protect your eyes, mouth, and nose from splashing or spraying of blood, body fluids, secretions, and excretions (see Fig. 15-19). Splashes and sprays can occur when giving care, cleaning items, or disposing of fluids.

The front (outside) of goggles or a face shield is contaminated. The ties, ear-pieces, or headband used to secure the device are "clean." Use them to remove the device after hand hygiene. They are safe to touch with bare hands.

Discard disposable goggles or face shields after use. Re-usable eyewear is cleaned before re-use. It is washed with soap and water. Then a disinfectant is used.

See *Promoting Safety and Comfort: Goggles and Face Shields.*

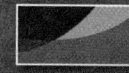 **Bagging Items.** Contaminated items are bagged to remove them from the person's room. Leak-proof plastic bags are used. They have the *BIOHAZARD* symbol (Fig. 15-20). *Biohazardous waste is items contaminated with blood, body fluids, secretions, or excretions.* (Bio *means* life. Hazardous *means* dangerous or harmful.)

Bag and transport linens following agency policy. Laundry bags with contaminated linen need a *BIOHAZARD* symbol. Melt-away bags are common. They dissolve in hot water. Once soiled linen is bagged, no one needs to handle it. Do not over-fill the bag. Tie the bag securely. Then place it in a laundry hamper lined with a biohazard plastic bag.

Trash is placed in a container labeled with the *BIOHAZARD* symbol. Follow agency policy for bagging and transporting trash, equipment, and supplies.

Usually one bag is needed. Double-bagging involves two bags. Double-bagging is needed if the outside of the bag is wet, soiled, or may be contaminated.

PROMOTING SAFETY AND COMFORT
Goggles and Face Shields

Safety

Eyeglasses and contact lenses do not provide eye protection. If you wear eyeglasses, use a face shield that fits over your glasses with minimal gaps.

Goggles do not provide splash or spray protection to other parts of your face.

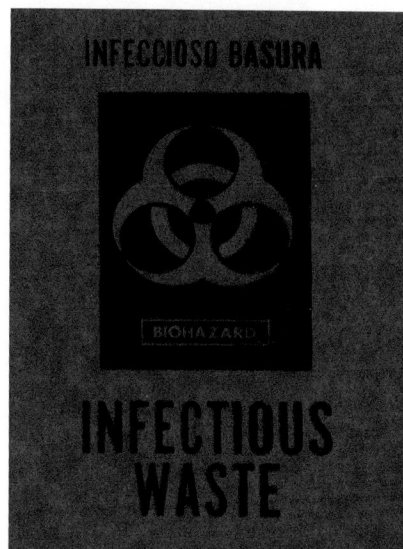

Fig. 15-20 *BIOHAZARD* symbol.

DOUBLE-BAGGING

PROCEDURE

1. Ask a co-worker to help you. He or she stands outside the doorway. You stand inside the doorway.
2. Place soiled linen, re-usable items, disposable supplies, and trash in the right containers. Containers are lined with leak-proof biohazard bags.
3. Seal the bags securely.
4. Ask your co-worker to make a wide cuff on the clean bag. It is held wide open. The cuff protects the hands from contamination (Fig. 15-21, A, p. 234).
5. Place the contaminated bag into the clean bag (Fig. 15-21, B, p. 234). Do not touch the outside of the clean bag.
6. Ask your co-worker to seal the bag. Have the bag labeled according to agency policy.
7. Repeat steps 4, 5, and 6 for other contaminated bags.
8. Ask your co-worker to take or send the bags to the appropriate department for disposal, disinfection, or sterilization.

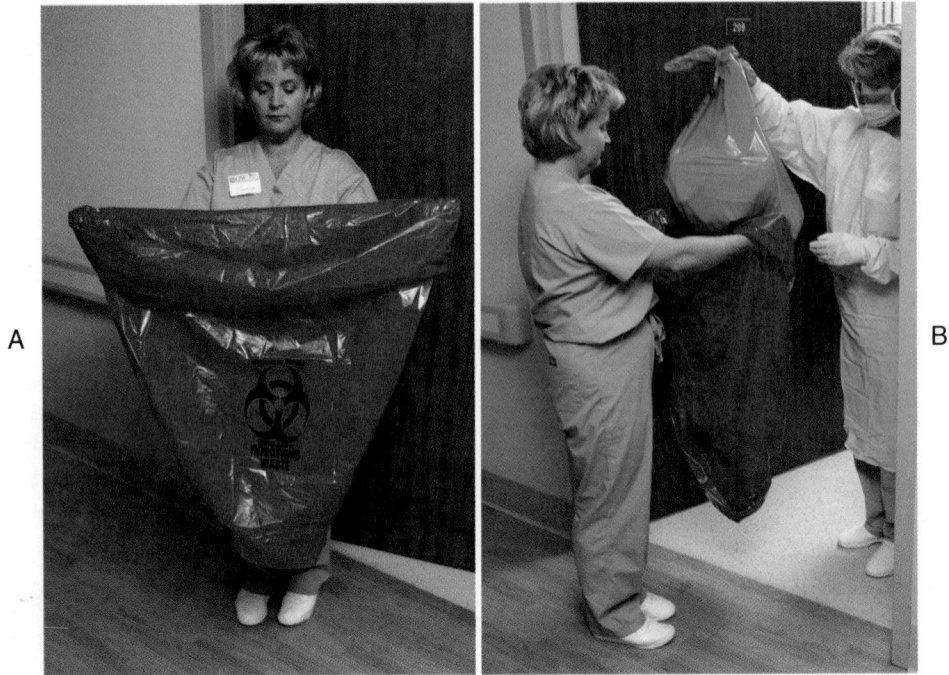

Fig. 15-21 Double-bagging. **A,** A cuff is made on a clean bag. **B,** One nursing assistant is in the room by the doorway. The other is outside the doorway. The "dirty" bag is placed inside the "clean" bag.

Collecting Specimens. Blood, body fluids, secretions, and excretions often require laboratory testing (Chapter 31). Specimens are transported to the laboratory in biohazard specimen bags. To collect a specimen:

- Label the specimen container and biohazard specimen bag. Apply warning labels according to agency policy.
- Wear gloves. Don other PPE as required.
- Put the specimen container and lid in the person's bathroom. Put them on a paper towel.
- Collect the specimen. Do not contaminate the outside of the container. Also avoid contamination when transferring the specimen from the collecting vessel to the specimen container.
- Put the lid on securely.
- Remove and discard PPE. Practice hand hygiene.
- Use a paper towel to pick up and take the container outside the room.
- Put the container in the biohazard bag.
- Discard the paper towels.
- Follow agency policy for storing the specimen.
- Practice hand hygiene.

Transporting Persons. Persons on Transmission-Based Precautions usually do not leave their rooms. Sometimes they go to other areas for treatments or tests.

Transporting procedures vary among agencies. Some require transport by bed. This prevents contaminating wheelchairs and stretchers. Others use wheelchairs and stretchers.

A safe transport means that other persons are protected from the infection. Follow agency procedures and these guidelines:

- Have the person wear a clean gown or pajamas and an isolation gown.
- Have the person wear a mask as required by the Transmission-Based Precautions used.
- Cover any draining wounds.
- Give the person tissues and a leak-proof bag. Used tissues are placed in the bag.
- Wear PPE as required.
- Place an extra layer of sheets and absorbent pads on the stretcher or wheelchair. This protects against draining body fluids.
- Do not let anyone else on the elevator. This reduces exposure to infection.
- Alert staff in the receiving area about the Transmission-Based Precautions. They wear gloves and PPE as needed.
- Disinfect the stretcher or wheelchair after use.

Meeting Basic Needs

The person has love, belonging, and self-esteem needs. Often they are unmet when Transmission-Based Precautions are used. Visitors and staff often avoid the person. They may need to put on PPE. This task takes extra effort before entering the room. Some are not sure what they can touch. They may fear getting the disease.

The person may feel lonely, unwanted, and rejected. Self-esteem suffers. The person knows the disease can be spread to others. He or she may feel dirty and undesirable. Without intending to, visitors and staff can make the person feel ashamed and guilty for having a contagious disease.

The nurse helps the person, visitors, and staff understand the need for Transmission-Based Precautions and how they affect the person. You can help meet love, belonging, and self-esteem needs. (See *Promoting Safety and Comfort: Transmission-Based Precautions*, p. 227.)

See *Focus on Communication: Meeting Basic Needs.*

See *Focus on Children and Older Persons: Meeting Basic Needs.*

FOCUS ON COMMUNICATION
Meeting Basic Needs

Some questions or statements can make the person feel dirty or ashamed. Be careful what you say. For example, do *not* say:

- "How did you get that?"
- "What were you doing?"
- "I'm afraid to touch you."
- "Don't breathe on me."

Always treat the person with respect, kindness, and dignity.

FOCUS ON CHILDREN AND OLDER PERSONS
Meeting Basic Needs

Children

Infants and children do not understand isolation. Goggles, face shields, masks, and gowns may scare them. Parents and staff look different. Gloves and gowns prevent skin-to-skin contact with parents. Because of likely contamination, toys and comfort items (blankets, stuffed animals) may be kept from the child. This adds to the child's distress.

The nurse prepares the child and family for isolation. Simple explanations are given to the child. If appropriate for his or her age, the child can have a mask and goggles or face shield to touch and play with.

Children need to see the faces of people entering the room. Let the child see your face before putting on a mask and goggles or a face shield. Say "hello" to the child, and state your name.

Older Persons

Persons with poor vision need to know who you are. Let them see your face before you put on a mask or goggles or a face shield. State your name and explain what you are going to do. Then put on PPE.

Persons with dementia do not understand the need for isolation precautions. Masks, gowns, goggles, and face shields may increase confusion and cause fear and agitation. These measures can help:

- Let the person see your face before putting on PPE.
- Tell the person who you are and what you are going to do.
- Use a calm, soothing voice.
- Do not hurry the person.
- Use touch to reassure the person.
- Follow the care plan and the nurse's instructions for other measures to help the person.
- Report signs of increased confusion or behavior changes.

BLOODBORNE PATHOGEN STANDARD

The human immunodeficiency virus (HIV) and the hepatitis B virus (HBV) are major health concerns (Chapters 40 and 43). The health team is at risk for exposure to these viruses. The Bloodborne Pathogen Standard is intended to protect them from exposure. It is a regulation of the Occupational Safety and Health Administration (OSHA). See Box 15-8, p. 236 for terms used in the standard.

HIV and HBV are found in the blood. They are bloodborne pathogens. They exit the body through blood. They are spread to others by blood. Other potentially infectious materials (OPIM) also spread the viruses (see Box 15-8, p. 236).

BOX 15-8	BLOODBORNE PATHOGEN STANDARD TERMS

blood Human blood, human blood components, and products made from human blood.

bloodborne pathogens Pathogens present in human blood and that can cause disease in humans. They include but are not limited to HBV and HIV.

contaminated The presence or reasonably anticipated presence of blood or OPIM on an item or surface.

contaminated laundry Laundry soiled with blood or OPIM or that may contain sharps.

contaminated sharps Any contaminated object that can penetrate the skin—needles, scalpels, broken glass, broken capillary tubes, exposed ends of dental wires, and so on.

decontamination The use of physical or chemical means to remove, inactivate, or destroy bloodborne pathogens on a surface or item. The infectious particles can no longer be transmitted. The surface or item is safe for handling, use, or disposal.

engineering controls Controls that isolate or remove the bloodborne pathogen hazard from the workplace (sharps disposal containers, self-sheathing needles).

exposure incident Eye, mouth, other mucous membrane, non-intact skin, or parenteral contact with blood or OPIM that results from an employee's duties.

hand washing facilities The adequate supply of running water, soap, single-use towels, or hot-air drying machines.

HBV Hepatitis B virus.

HIV Human immunodeficiency virus.

occupational exposure Reasonably anticipated skin, eye, mucous membrane, or parenteral contact with blood or OPIM that may result from an employee's duties.

other potentially infectious materials (OPIM):
- Human body fluids—semen, vaginal secretions, cerebrospinal fluid, synovial fluid, pleural fluid, pericardial fluid, peritoneal fluid, amniotic fluid, saliva in dental procedures, any body fluid that is visibly contaminated with blood, and all body fluids when it is difficult or impossible to differentiate between them

- Any tissue or organ (other than intact skin) from a human (living or dead)
- HIV-containing cell or tissue cultures, organ cultures, and HIV- or HBV-containing culture medium or other solutions; blood, organs, or other tissues from experimental animals infected with HIV or HBV

parenteral Piercing mucous membranes or the skin through needle-sticks, human bites, cuts, abrasions, and so on.

personal protective equipment (PPE) The clothing or equipment worn by staff for protection against a hazard.

regulated waste:
- Liquid or semi-liquid blood or OPIM
- Contaminated items that would release blood or OPIM in a liquid or semi-liquid state if compressed
- Items caked with dried blood or OPIM that can release these materials during handling
- Contaminated sharps
- Pathological and microbiological wastes containing blood or OPIM

source individual Any person (living or dead) whose blood or OPIM may be a source of occupational exposure to staff. Examples include but are not limited to:
- Hospital and clinic patients
- Clients in agencies for the developmentally disabled
- Trauma victims
- Clients of drug and alcohol treatment agencies
- Hospice and nursing center residents
- Human remains
- Persons who donate or sell blood or blood components

sterilize The use of a physical or chemical procedure to destroy all microbes, including spores.

work practice controls Controls that reduce the likelihood of exposure by changing the way the task is performed.

Exposure Control Plan

The agency has an exposure control plan. It identifies staff at risk for exposure to blood or OPIM. All caregivers and the laundry, central supply, and housekeeping staffs are at risk. The plan tells what to do for an exposure incident.

Staff at risk receive free training. It occurs upon employment and yearly. Training is also done for new or changed tasks involving exposure to bloodborne pathogens. Training includes:
- An explanation of the standard and where to get a copy
- The causes, signs, and symptoms of bloodborne diseases
- How bloodborne pathogens are spread
- An explanation of the exposure control plan and where to get a copy
- How to know which tasks might cause exposure
- The use and limits of safe work practices, engineering controls, and PPE

- Information about the hepatitis B vaccination
- Who to contact and what to do in an emergency
- Information on reporting an exposure incident, post-exposure evaluation, and follow-up
- Information on warning labels and color-coding

Preventive Measures

Preventive measures reduce the risk of exposure. Such measures follow.

Hepatitis B Vaccination. Hepatitis B is a liver disease caused by HBV. HBV is spread by blood and sexual contact.

The hepatitis B vaccine produces immunity against hepatitis B. *Immunity means that a person has protection against a certain disease.* He or she will not get the disease.

A *vaccination involves giving a vaccine to produce immunity against an infectious disease. A vaccine is a preparation containing dead or weakened microbes.* The hepatitis B vaccination involves 3 injections (shots). The second injection is given 1 month after the first. The third injection is given at least 4 months after the first one. The vaccination can be given before or after HBV exposure.

You can receive the hepatitis B vaccination within 10 working days of being hired. The agency pays for it. You can refuse the vaccination. If so, you must sign a statement refusing the vaccine. You can have the vaccination at a later date.

Engineering and Work Practice Controls. *Engineering controls* reduce employee exposure in the workplace. *Work practice controls* also reduce exposure risks. All tasks involving blood or OPIM are done in ways to limit splatters, splashes, and sprays. Producing droplets also is avoided. OSHA requires these work practice controls:

- Do not eat, drink, smoke, apply cosmetics or lip balm, or handle contact lenses in areas of exposure.
- Do not store food or drinks where blood or OPIM are kept.
- Practice hand hygiene after removing gloves.
- Wash hands as soon as possible after skin contact with blood or OPIM.
- Never re-cap, bend, or remove needles by hand. Instead, use mechanical means (forceps) or a one-handed method.
- Never shear or break needles.
- Discard needles and sharp instruments (such as razors) in containers that are closable, puncture-resistant, and leak-proof. Containers are color-coded in red and have the *BIOHAZARD* symbol. Containers must be upright and not allowed to over-fill.

Personal Protective Equipment (PPE). This includes gloves, goggles, face shields, masks, laboratory coats, gowns, shoe covers, and surgical caps. Blood or OPIM must not pass through them. They protect your clothes, undergarments, skin, eyes, mouth, and hair.

PPE is free to staff. Correct sizes are available. The agency makes sure that PPE is cleaned, laundered, repaired, replaced, or discarded. OSHA requires these measures for PPE:

- Remove PPE before leaving the work area.
- Remove PPE when a garment becomes contaminated.
- Place used PPE in marked areas or containers when being stored, washed, decontaminated, or discarded.
- Wear gloves when you expect contact with blood or OPIM.
- Wear gloves when handling or touching contaminated items or surfaces.
- Replace worn, punctured, or contaminated gloves.

- Never wash or decontaminate disposable gloves for re-use.
- Discard utility gloves that show signs of cracking, peeling, tearing, or puncturing. Utility gloves are decontaminated for re-use if the process will not ruin them.

Equipment. Contaminated equipment is cleaned and decontaminated. Decontaminate work surfaces with a proper disinfectant:

- Upon completing tasks
- At once when there is obvious contamination
- After any spill of blood or OPIM
- At the end of your work shift when surfaces became contaminated since the last cleaning

Use a brush and dustpan or tongs to clean up broken glass. Never pick up broken glass with your hands, not even with gloves. Discard broken glass into a puncture-resistant container.

Waste. Special measures are used to discard regulated waste:

- Liquid or semi-liquid blood or OPIM
- Items contaminated with blood or OPIM
- Items caked with blood or OPIM
- Contaminated sharps

Closable, puncture-resistant, and leak-proof containers are used. Containers are color-coded in red. They have the *BIOHAZARD* symbol.

See *Focus on Long-Term Care and Home Care: Waste,* p. 238.

Housekeeping. The agency must be kept clean and sanitary. A cleaning schedule is required. It includes decontamination methods and the tasks and procedures to be done.

Laundry. OSHA requires these measures for contaminated laundry:

- Handle it as little as possible.
- Wear gloves or other needed PPE.
- Bag contaminated laundry where it is used.
- Mark laundry bags or containers with the *BIOHAZARD* symbol for laundry sent off-site.
- Place wet, contaminated laundry in leak-proof containers before transport. The containers are color-coded in red or have the *BIOHAZARD* symbol.

Exposure Incidents

An *exposure incident* is any eye, mouth, other mucous membrane, non-intact skin, or parenteral contact with blood or OPIM. *Parenteral* means piercing the mucous membranes or the skin. Piercing occurs by needle-sticks, human bites, cuts, and abrasions.

Report exposure incidents at once. Medical evaluation, follow-up, and required tests are free. Your blood is tested for HIV and HBV. If you refuse testing, the blood sample is kept for at least 90 days. Testing is done later if you change your mind.

Home Care

Dressings, gloves, and other care items are used in home care. So are syringes, needles, and other sharps (such as razors). You do not use syringes or needles. However, you do use safety razors for shaving (Chapter 21) and lancets for blood glucose testing (Chapter 31). Proper disposal:

- Protects neighbors, children, pets, janitors, housekeepers, sanitation workers, and sewage treatment workers from injury and infection. HIV, AIDS, and hepatitis B and C are risks.
- Prevents needle sharing and the re-use of sharps.
- Protects the environment.
  According to the Environmental Protection Agency (EPA):
- Do not throw loose needles, syringes, or sharps into the garbage.
- Do not flush needles, syringes, or sharps down the toilet.
- Do not put needles, syringes, or sharps in recycling containers for bottles, plastics, and paper.
  Properly store used needles, syringes, and sharps. Put them in a commercial or household sharps container right after use. A household container can be a hard plastic bottle with a screw-on lid. Plastic bleach or detergent bottles with screw-on lids are examples. Secure the lid in place with heavy tape for added protection. The container must be puncture-resistant. Do not use soda cans, milk cartons, glass bottles, coffee cans, or other containers that are not puncture-resistant.

Many communities have disposal options. The nurse and care plan tell you what to use at the person's address. The EPA describes these disposal options:

- *Drop-boxes or supervised collection sites.* The filled sharps container is taken to a collection site. Hospitals, doctors' offices, clinics, pharmacies, health departments, and police and fire stations are examples.
- *Household hazardous waste collection sites.* The sharps container is taken to a hazardous waste collection site. The container is placed in a sharps collection bin.
- *Residential special waste pick-up services.* Used sharps are placed in a special recycling-type container. The container is placed outside the home for collection by special waste handlers. Programs have regular pick-up times or require a call for a pick-up.
- *Mail-back programs.* Used sharps are placed in a special container. The container is mailed to a collection site. U.S. Postal Service procedures are followed. This program works well for rural areas.
- *Syringe exchange programs.* Used needles and syringes are exchanged for new ones. The agency operating the program disposes of used ones.
- *Home needle destruction devices.* Such devices sever, melt, or burn the needle. The syringe and destroyed needle are placed in the garbage.
  Dressings, gloves, soiled bed protectors, and other care items also need proper disposal.
- Place them in plastic bags.
- Close the bags securely.
- Label each bag with a "Not for Recycling" label.
- Place the bags in a garbage can with a lid.
- Make sure animals cannot get into the garbage can. Trash scents can attract animals.

Confidentiality is important. You are told of the evaluation results. You also are told of any medical conditions that may need treatment. You receive a written opinion of the medical evaluation within 15 days after its completion.

The *source individual* is the person whose blood or body fluids are the source of an exposure incident. His or her blood is tested for HIV or HBV. The agency informs you about laws affecting the source's identity and test results.

SURGICAL ASEPSIS

Surgical asepsis (sterile technique) is the practice that keeps equipment and supplies free of all microbes. Sterile means the absence of all microbes, including spores. Surgical asepsis is required any time the skin or sterile tissues are entered.

Surgery and labor and delivery areas require surgical asepsis. So do many tests and nursing procedures. If a break occurs in sterile technique, microbes can enter the body. Infection is a risk.

Assisting With Sterile Procedures

You can assist nurses with sterile procedures. You may be allowed to perform certain sterile procedures. A sterile dressing change is an example.

See *Delegation Guidelines: Assisting With Sterile Procedures.*
See *Promoting Safety and Comfort: Assisting With Sterile Procedures.*

DELEGATION GUIDELINES
Assisting With Sterile Procedures

Before a sterile procedure, you need this information from the nurse:
- The name of the procedure and the reason for it
- What gloves to wear—sterile or non-sterile
- What you are expected to do
- When to report observations
- What you can and cannot touch
- What patient or resident concerns to report at once

Safety
Do not perform a sterile procedure unless:
* Your state allows you to perform the procedure.
* The procedure is in your job description.
* You received the necessary education and training.
* You review the procedure with the nurse.
* A nurse is available for questions and guidance.

Principles of Surgical Asepsis

All items in contact with the person are kept sterile. If an item is contaminated, infection is a risk. A sterile field is needed. A *sterile field* is *a work area free of* all *pathogens and non-pathogens (including spores)*. Box 15-9 lists the principles and practices of surgical asepsis. Follow them to maintain a sterile field.

BOX 15-9 PRINCIPLES AND PRACTICES FOR SURGICAL ASEPSIS

* A sterile item can touch only another sterile item:
  * If a sterile item touches a clean item, the sterile item is contaminated.
  * If a clean item touches a sterile item, the sterile item is contaminated.
  * A sterile package is contaminated if open, torn, punctured, wet, or moist.
  * A sterile package is contaminated when the expiration date has passed.
  * Place only sterile items on a sterile field.
  * Use sterile gloves or sterile forceps to handle other sterile items (Fig. 15-22).
  * Consider any item to be contaminated if not sure of its sterility.
  * Do not use contaminated items. They are discarded or re-sterilized.
* A sterile field or sterile items are always kept within your vision and above your waist:
  * If you cannot see an item, the item is contaminated.
  * If the item is below your waist, the item is contaminated.
  * Keep sterile-gloved hands above your waist and within your sight.
  * Do not leave a sterile field unattended.
  * Do not turn your back on a sterile field.
* Airborne microbes can contaminate sterile items or a sterile field:
  * Prevent drafts. Close the door, and avoid extra movements. Ask other staff in the room to avoid extra movements.
* Avoid coughing, sneezing, talking, or laughing over a sterile field. Turn your head away from the sterile field if you must talk.
* Wear a mask if you need to talk during the procedure.
* Do not perform or assist with sterile procedures if you have a respiratory infection.
* Do not reach over a sterile field.
* Fluid flows downward, in the direction of gravity:
  * Hold wet items down (see Fig. 15-22). If held up, fluid flows down into a contaminated area.
* The sterile field is kept dry, unless the area below it is sterile:
  * The sterile field is contaminated if it gets wet and the area below it is not sterile.
  * Avoid spilling and splashing when pouring sterile fluids into sterile containers.
* The edges of a sterile field are contaminated:
  * A 1-inch (2.5 centimeter [cm]) margin around the sterile field is considered contaminated (Fig. 15-23).
  * Place all sterile items inside the 1-inch (2.5 cm) margin of the sterile field.
  * Items outside the 1-inch (2.5 cm) margin are contaminated.
* Honesty is essential to sterile technique:
  * You know when you contaminate an item or sterile field. Be honest with yourself even if other staff are not present.
  * Remove the contaminated item, and correct the matter. If necessary, start over with sterile supplies.
  * Report the contamination to the nurse.

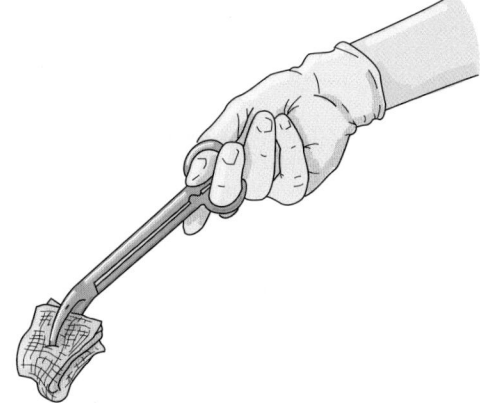

Fig. 15-22 Sterile forceps are used to handle sterile items.

Fig. 15-23 A 1-inch (2.5 cm) margin around the sterile field is considered contaminated. The shading and slash marks show that the 1-inch margin is contaminated.

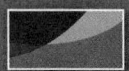 **Sterile Gloving**

Before donning sterile gloves, the sterile field is set up. After sterile gloves are on, you can handle sterile items within the sterile field. Do not touch anything outside the sterile field.

Sterile gloves are disposable. They come in many sizes so they fit snugly. The insides are powdered for ease in donning the gloves. The right and left gloves are marked on the package.

See *Promoting Safety and Comfort: Sterile Gloving.*

PROMOTING SAFETY AND COMFORT
Sterile Gloving

Safety

Always keep sterile gloved hands above your waist and within your vision. Touch only items within the sterile field. If you contaminate the gloves, remove them. Tell the nurse what happened. Practice hand hygiene, and put on a new pair. Replace gloves that are torn, cut, or punctured.

Comfort

If you or the nurse contaminates your gloves, they must be removed. This means leaving the bedside to get another pair. Care is delayed. The person's comfort is affected if the care is painful or involves an uncomfortable position. When collecting supplies, get an extra pair of gloves. The gloves are in the room if the first pair is contaminated. Care can continue with little delay.

STERILE GLOVING

PROCEDURE

1 Follow *Delegation Guidelines: Assisting With Sterile Procedures,* p. 238. See *Promoting Safety and Comfort:*
   a *Assisting With Sterile Procedures,* p. 239
   b *Sterile Gloving*
2 Practice hand hygiene.
3 Inspect the package of sterile gloves for sterility.
   a Check the expiration date.
   b See if the package is dry.
   c Check for tears, holes, punctures, and watermarks.
4 Arrange a work surface.
   a Make sure you have enough room.
   b Arrange the work surface at waist level and within your vision.
   c Clean and dry the work surface.
   d Do not reach over or turn your back on the work surface.
5 Open the package. Grasp the flaps. Gently peel them back.
6 Remove the inner package. Place it on your work surface.
7 Read the manufacturer's instructions on the inner package. It may be labeled with *left, right, up,* and *down.*
8 Arrange the inner package for left, right, up, and down. The left glove is on your left. The right glove is on your right. The cuffs are near you; the fingers point away from you.
9 Grasp the folded edges of the inner package. Use the thumb and index finger of each hand.
10 Fold back the inner package to expose the gloves (Fig. 15-24, A). Do not touch or otherwise contaminate the inside of the package or the gloves. The inside of the inner package is a sterile field.
11 Note that each glove has a cuff about 2 to 3 inches wide. The cuffs and insides of the gloves are *not sterile.*
12 Put on the right glove if you are right-handed. Put on the left glove if you are left-handed.
   a Pick up the glove with your other hand. Use your thumb and index and middle fingers (Fig. 15-24, B).
   b Touch only the cuff and inside of the glove.
   c Turn the hand to be gloved palm side up.
   d Lift the cuff up. Slide your fingers and hand into the glove (Fig. 15-24, C).
   e Pull the glove up over your hand. If some fingers get stuck, leave them that way until the other glove is on. *Do not use your ungloved hand to straighten the glove. Do not let the outside of the glove touch any non-sterile surface.*
   f Leave the cuff turned down.
13 Put on the other glove. Use your gloved hand.
   a Reach under the cuff of the second glove. Use the 4 fingers of your gloved hand (Fig. 15-24, D). Keep your gloved thumb close to your gloved palm.
   b Pull on the second glove (Fig. 15-24, E). Your gloved hand cannot touch the cuff or any surface. Hold the thumb of your first gloved hand away from the gloved palm.
14 Adjust each glove with the other hand. The gloves should be smooth and comfortable (Fig. 15-24, F).
15 Slide your fingers under the cuffs to pull them up (Fig. 15-24, G).
16 Touch only sterile items.
17 Remove and discard the gloves. See Figure 15-16.
18 Practice hand hygiene.

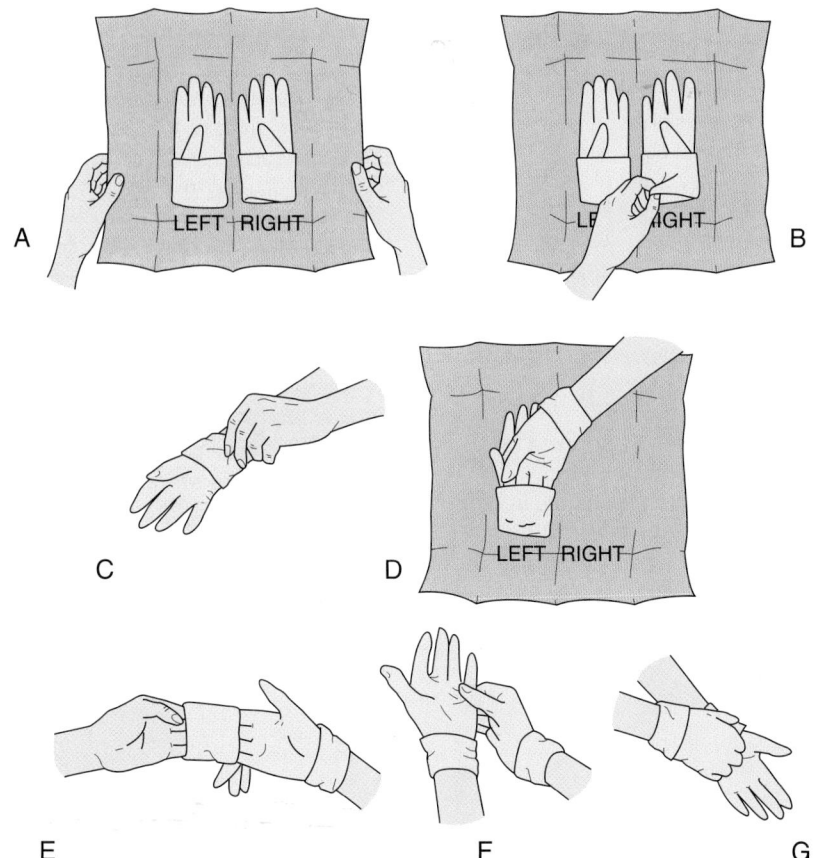

Fig. 15-24 Sterile gloving. **A,** Open the inner wrapper to expose the gloves. **B,** Pick up the glove at the cuff with your thumb and index and middle fingers. **C,** Slide your fingers and hand into the glove. **D,** Reach under the cuff of the other glove with your fingers. **E,** Pull on the second glove. **F,** Adjust each glove for comfort. **G,** Slide your fingers under the cuffs to pull them up.

FOCUS ON PRIDE

The Person, Family, and Yourself

Personal and Professional Responsibility

You have an important role in preventing the spread of infection. Your actions affect the person's risk for infection. You are responsible for following the guidelines in this chapter. Practice good hand hygiene before and after giving care. Follow Standard Precautions and Transmission-Based Precautions.

When assisting with or performing a procedure, remove items that become contaminated. If necessary, stop and get new supplies. Do not use a contaminated item. You may be alone. Be honest with yourself. Be responsible. Do the right thing, even if other staff are not present. Take pride in providing care that prevents the spread of infection.

Rights and Respect

Caring for persons who need Transmission-Based Precautions can be a challenge. Extra time and effort are needed to apply and remove PPE and clean equipment used in the room. You must plan carefully when gathering supplies before entering the room. If an item is forgotten, you must wait for help or remove and re-apply PPE. You may feel frustrated.

The person must not feel as if he or she is a burden. The person deserves the same kindness and respect you give others. You must:

- Watch your verbal and nonverbal communication (Chapter 8).
- Avoid complaining.
- Practice good teamwork and time management.
- Tell the nurse if you are feeling overwhelmed.

Independence and Social Interaction

Patients and residents are often unable to perform hygiene measures they would normally do independently. Hand hygiene is an example. Ask patients and residents if they would like to wash their hands often. Assist them to wash their hands before and after eating, after voiding or having a bowel movement, after coughing or sneezing, and any time their hands are dirty. Hand hygiene is not only important for you. It is also important for patients and residents. When independence is limited, help protect the person and others by promoting hand hygiene.

Continued

FOCUS ON **PRIDE**—cont'd

Delegation and Teamwork

Before making delegation decisions, the nurse must assess and plan (Chapter 7). The nurse considers the person's needs and risks. Some persons are more at risk for infection than others. Burn, transplant, and chemotherapy patients are examples. The nurse must make delegation decisions carefully. If delegated care of persons at increased risk for infection, you must:

- Practice medical asepsis at all times.
- Practice surgical asepsis when assisting with sterile procedures.
- Practice hand hygiene.
- Follow Standard Precautions and the Bloodborne Pathogen Standard at all times.
- Follow any Transmission-Based Precautions ordered for the person.
- Wear PPE as directed by the nurse.
- Follow the person's care plan.
- Report any sign or symptom of infection at once.
- Provide good oral hygiene and skin care (Chapter 20).
- Tell the nurse if you have any sign or symptom of infection.

Communication is an important part of delegation. Do not be offended or annoyed if the nurse reminds you to perform these actions. Measures to prevent infection are very important for these persons. The nurse must make sure the person's health and safety are protected.

Ethics and Laws

The following is a real case showing how failure to follow infection control procedures led to patient harm.

A patient, Mr. Helman, had hip surgery (August 1) following a car accident in which he suffered many injuries. His roommate, Mr. Hagerup, had a back injury that caused paralysis from the waist down. The men shared a room for about 2 weeks.

Eight days after Mr. Helman's hip surgery (August 9), Mr. Hagerup complained of a boil under his right arm. (A boil is a local skin infection. The infection causes a painful red bump. When opened, purulent drainage comes from the boil. Purulent drainage is thick and green, yellow, or brown in color.) The boil was treated with hot compresses. On August 10, there was purulent drainage from the boil. On the same day, a drainage specimen was sent to the laboratory. On August 13, the laboratory report showed the boil drainage contained a type of staphylococcus. Mr. Hagerup was moved at once to an isolation room.

Between August 10 and August 13, the nursing team cared for Mr. Helman and Mr. Hagerup. They "moved from one patient to the other, changed sheets, gave sponge baths, changed dressings, administered back rubs . . . [and] carried out the necessary hospital routine for the care of the two men. They did not observe sterile techniques . . . [to be used] where infection is suspected; they did not wash their hands or leave the room between administering to the patients."

On August 13, Mr. Helman's surgical wound opened and drained a large amount of purulent drainage. Laboratory tests showed that the drainage contained the same microbe found in Mr. Hagerup's wound. Mr. Helman's wound infection destroyed bone, tissue, and ligaments. He had another surgery on October 28. His hip was fused in "a nearly immovable position." (To fuse means to unite two or more bones together.) He was discharged from the hospital on March 14. He needed home care and doctor's care.

In a lawsuit against the hospital, the jury returned a verdict in favor of Mr. Helman. The hospital appealed the verdict. The court hearing the appeal upheld the verdict in favor of Mr. Helman.

(G. E. Helman et al. v Sacred Heart Hospital, Wash., 1963.)

The health team must prevent the spread of microbes and infection. Even one careless act can spread microbes. This affects the person's health and safety. Be very careful about your work. Take pride in providing care that protects the person from infection.

REVIEW QUESTIONS

Circle T if the statement is TRUE or F if it is FALSE.

1. T F Microbes are pathogens in their natural sites.
2. T F A pathogen can cause an infection.
3. T F An infection results when microbes invade and grow in the body.
4. T F An item is sterile if non-pathogens are present.
5. T F You hold your hands and forearms up during hand washing.
6. T F Un-used items in the person's room are used for another person.
7. T F A person received the hepatitis B vaccine. The person will develop the disease.
8. T F The 1-inch edge around a sterile field is considered contaminated.
9. T F The inside and cuffs of sterile gloves are considered contaminated.
10. T F You can flush household sharps down the toilet.
11. T F You can throw household sharps in the garbage.

Circle the BEST answer.

12. Most pathogens need the following to grow *except*
    a Water
    b Light
    c Oxygen
    d Nourishment

13. Signs and symptoms of infection include the following *except*
    a Fever, nausea, vomiting, rash, and/or sores
    b Pain or tenderness, redness, and/or swelling
    c Fatigue, loss of appetite, and/or a discharge
    d A wound and/or bleeding

14. Which is *not* a portal of exit?
    a Respiratory tract
    b Blood
    c Reproductive system
    d Intact skin

15. Which does *not* prevent healthcare-associated infections?
    a Hand hygiene before and after giving care
    b Sterilizing all care items
    c Surgical asepsis
    d Standard Precautions

16 Your hands are soiled with blood. What should you do?
   a Wash your hands with soap and water.
   b Practice hand hygiene.
   c Rinse your hands.
   d Tell the nurse.

17 During care, you move from a contaminated body site to a clean body site. Your hands are not visibly soiled. What should you do?
   a Change your gloves.
   b Practice hand hygiene.
   c Rinse your hands.
   d Put on sterile gloves.

18 You are going to use an alcohol-based hand rub. Which action is *not* correct?
   a Wash your hands before applying the hand rub.
   b Rub your hands together.
   c Cover all surfaces of your hands and fingers.
   d Rub your hands together until your hands are dry.

19 When cleaning equipment, do the following *except*
   a Rinse the item in cold water before cleaning
   b Wash the item with soap and hot water
   c Use a brush if necessary
   d Work from dirty to clean areas

20 Isolation precautions
   a Prevent infection
   b Destroy pathogens
   c Keep pathogens within a certain area
   d Destroy all microbes

21 Standard Precautions
   a Are used for all persons
   b Prevent the spread of pathogens through the air
   c Require gowns, masks, gloves, and goggles
   d Require a doctor's order

22 You wear utility gloves for contact with
   a Blood
   b Body fluids
   c Secretions and excretions
   d Cleaning solutions

23 A mask
   a Can be re-used
   b Is clean on the inside
   c Is contaminated when moist
   d Should fit loosely for breathing

24 These statements are about PPE. Which is *false*?
   a Wash disposable gloves for re-use.
   b Remove PPE before leaving the work area.
   c Discard cracked or torn utility gloves.
   d Wear gloves when touching contaminated items or surfaces.

25 Contaminated surfaces are cleaned at the following times *except*
   a After completing a task
   b When there is obvious contamination
   c After blood is spilled
   d After removing gloves

26 Goggles or a face shield is worn
   a When using Standard Precautions
   b When splashing body fluids is likely
   c If you have an eye infection
   d When assisting with sterile procedures

27 According to the Bloodborne Pathogen Standard, you should *not*
   a Wear gloves
   b Discard sharp items into a biohazard container
   c Store food and blood in different places
   d Eat and drink in care settings

28 You were exposed to a bloodborne pathogen. Which is *true*?
   a You do not have to report the exposure.
   b You pay for required tests.
   c You can refuse HIV and HBV testing.
   d The source individual can refuse testing.

29 These statements are about surgical asepsis. Which is *false*?
   a A sterile item can touch only another sterile item.
   b Wet items are held up.
   c If you cannot see an item, it is considered contaminated.
   d Sterile items are kept above your waist.

30 You have on sterile gloves. You can touch
   a Anything on the sterile field
   b Anything on your work surface
   c Anything below your waist
   d Any part of your uniform

Answers to these questions are on p. 833.

16 Body Mechanics

OBJECTIVES

- Define the key terms and key abbreviations listed in this chapter.
- Explain the purpose and rules of body mechanics.
- Explain how ergonomics can prevent work-related injuries.
- Identify the causes, signs, and symptoms of back injuries.
- Position persons in the basic bed positions and in a chair.
- Explain how to promote PRIDE in the person, the family, and yourself.

KEY TERMS

base of support The area on which an object rests

body alignment The way the head, trunk, arms, and legs are aligned with one another; posture

body mechanics Using the body in an efficient and careful way

dorsal recumbent position The back-lying or supine position

ergonomics The science of designing a job to fit the worker

Fowler's position A semi-sitting position; the head of the bed is raised between 45 and 60 degrees

lateral position The person lies on one side or the other; side-lying position

posture See "body alignment"

prone position Lying on the abdomen with the head turned to one side

semi-prone side position See "Sims' position"

side-lying position See "lateral position"

Sims' position A left side-lying position in which the upper leg (right leg) is sharply flexed so it is not on the lower leg (left leg) and the lower arm (left arm) is behind the person; semi-prone side position

supine position The back-lying or dorsal recumbent position

KEY ABBREVIATIONS

MSD Musculo-skeletal disorder	**OSHA** Occupational Safety and Health Administration

ody mechanics *means using the body in an efficient and careful way.* It involves good posture, balance, and using your strongest and largest muscles for work. Fatigue, muscle strain, and injury can result from the improper use and positioning of the body during activity or rest. Focus on the person's and your own body mechanics. Good body mechanics reduce the risk of injury.

See *Body Structure and Function Review: The Musculo-Skeletal System.*

BODY STRUCTURE AND FUNCTION REVIEW: THE MUSCULO-SKELETAL SYSTEM

The musculo-skeletal system:
- Provides the framework for the body.
- Lets the body move.
- Protects internal organs.
- Gives the body shape.

Bones

Bones are hard, rigid structures. They are made up of living cells.
- *Long bones* bear the body's weight. Leg bones are long bones. The human body has 206 bones.
- *Short bones* allow skill and ease in movement. Bones in the wrists, fingers, ankles, and toes are short bones.
- *Flat bones* protect the organs. They include the ribs, skull, pelvic bones, and shoulder blades.
- *Irregular bones* are the vertebrae in the spinal column. They allow various degrees of movement and flexibility.

Joints

A *joint* is the point at which two or more bones meet. Joints allow movement. There are three major types of joints (Fig. 16-1):
- *Ball-and-socket joint* allows movement in all directions. It is made up of the rounded end of one bone and the hollow end of another bone. The rounded end of one fits into the hollow end of the other. The joints of the hips and shoulders are ball-and-socket joints.
- *Hinge joint* allows movement in one direction. The elbow is a hinge joint.
- *Pivot joint* allows turning from side to side. A pivot joint connects the skull to the spine.
- Some joints are immovable. They connect the bones of the skull.

Muscles

The human body has more than 500 *muscles* (Fig 16-2, p. 246).
- *Voluntary muscles* can be consciously controlled. Muscles attached to bones *(skeletal muscles)* are voluntary. Arm muscles do not work unless you move your arm; likewise for leg muscles. Skeletal muscles are *striated.* That is, they look striped or streaked.

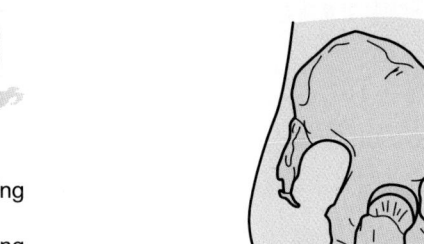
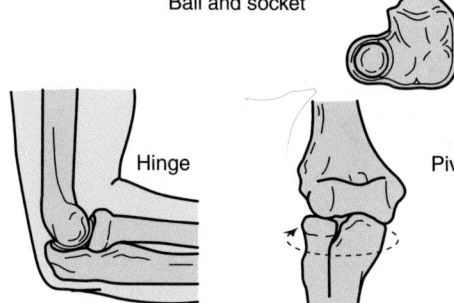

Ball and socket

Hinge   Pivot

Fig. 16-1 Types of joints.

Muscles—cont'd
- *Involuntary muscles* work automatically. You cannot control them. They control the action of the stomach, intestines, blood vessels, and other body organs.

Muscles have three functions:
- Movement of body parts
- Maintenance of posture or muscle tone
- Production of body heat

Some muscles constantly contract to maintain the body's posture. When muscles contract, they burn food for energy. Heat is produced. The more muscle activity, the greater the amount of heat produced.

Continued

BODY STRUCTURE AND FUNCTION REVIEW: THE MUSCULO-SKELETAL SYSTEM—cont'd

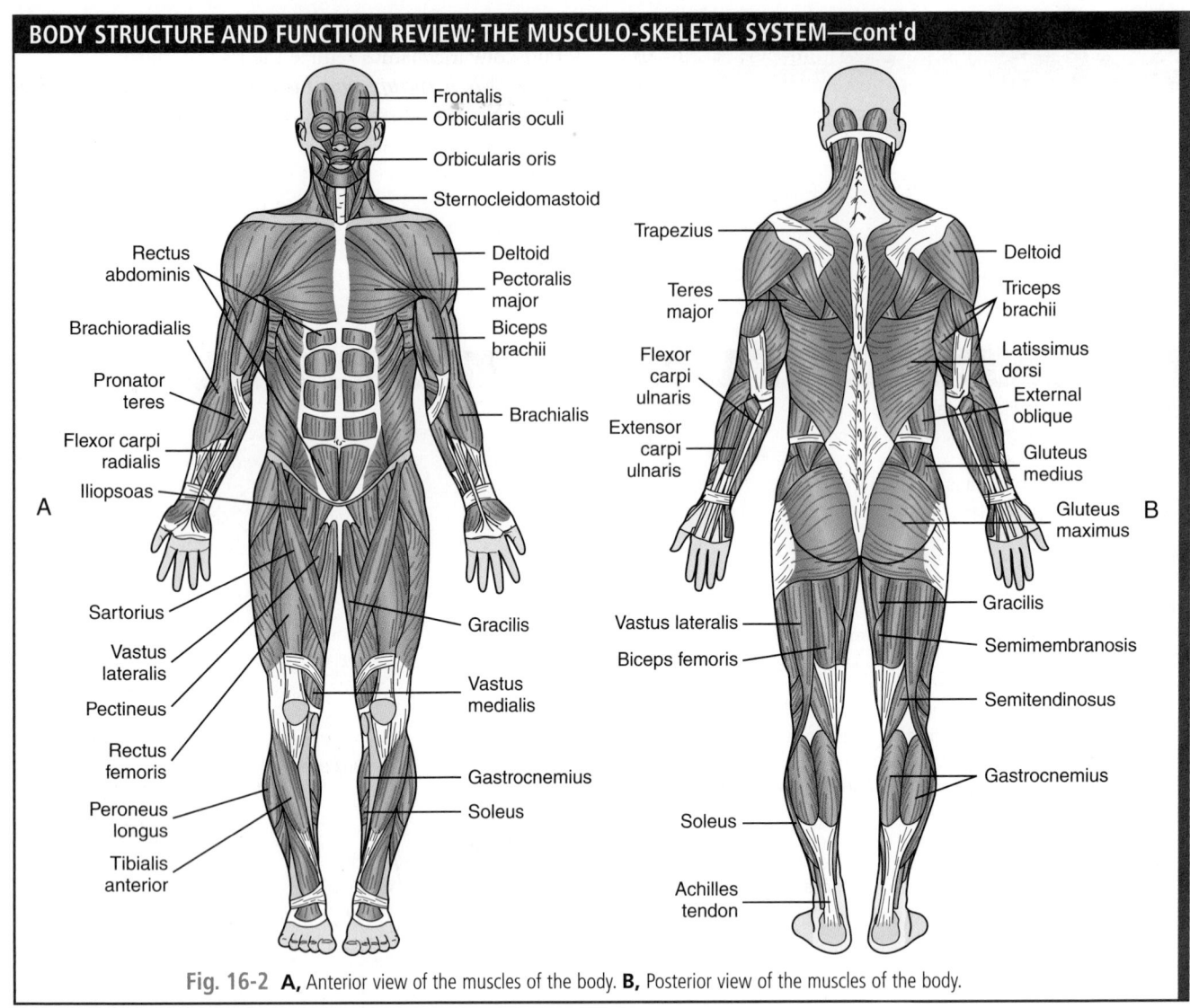

Fig. 16-2 **A,** Anterior view of the muscles of the body. **B,** Posterior view of the muscles of the body.

PRINCIPLES OF BODY MECHANICS

Body alignment (posture) is the way the head, trunk, arms, and legs are aligned with one another. Good alignment lets the body move and function with strength and efficiency. Standing, sitting, and lying down require good alignment.

Base of support is the area on which an object rests. A good base of support is needed for balance (Fig. 16-3). When standing, your feet are your base of support. Stand with your feet apart for a wider base of support and more balance.

Your strongest and largest muscles are in the shoulders, upper arms, hips, and thighs. Use these muscles to handle and move persons and heavy objects. Otherwise, you place strain and exertion on smaller and weaker muscles. This causes fatigue and injury. *Back injuries are a major risk.* For good body mechanics:

- Bend your knees and squat to lift a heavy object (Fig. 16-4). Do not bend from your waist. Bending from the waist places strain on small back muscles.
- Hold items close to your body and base of support (see Fig. 16-4). This involves upper arm and shoulder muscles. Holding objects away from your body places strain on small muscles in your lower arms.

All activities require good body mechanics. You must safely and efficiently handle and move persons and heavy objects. Follow the rules in Box 16-1.

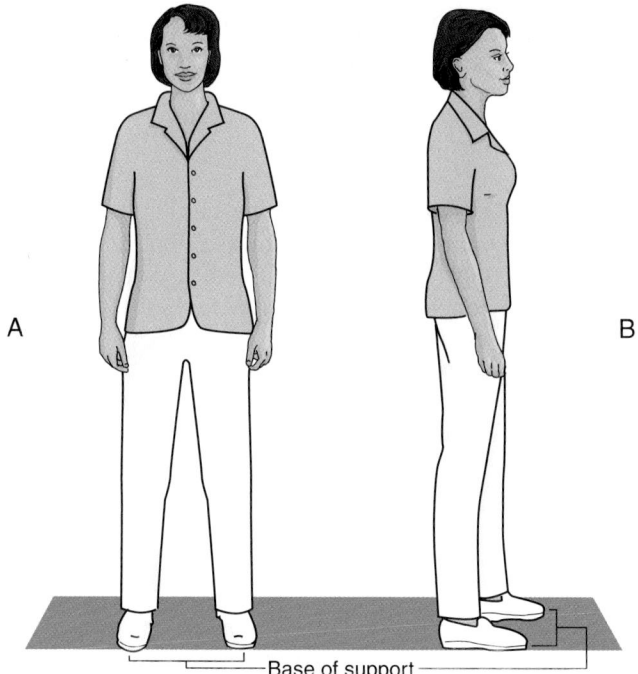

A

B

— Base of support —

Fig. 16-3 A, Anterior (front) view of an adult in good body alignment. The feet are apart for a wide base of support. **B,** Lateral (side) view of an adult with good posture and alignment.

ERGONOMICS

Ergonomics is the science of designing a job to fit the worker. (*Ergo* means work. *Nomos* means law.) It involves changing the task, work station, equipment, and tools to help reduce stress on the worker's body. The goal is to eliminate a serious and disabling work-related musculo-skeletal disorder (MSD). MSDs are caused or made worse by the work setting.

Work-Related MSDs

MSDs are injuries and disorders of the muscles, tendons, ligaments, joints, and cartilage. They can involve the nervous system. The arms and back are often affected. So are the hands, fingers, neck, wrists, legs, and shoulders. MSDs are painful and disabling. They can develop slowly over weeks, months, and years. Or they can occur from one event. Pain, numbness, tingling, stiff joints, difficulty moving, and muscle loss can occur. Sometimes there is paralysis.

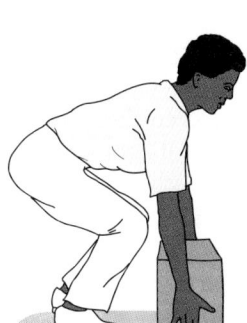
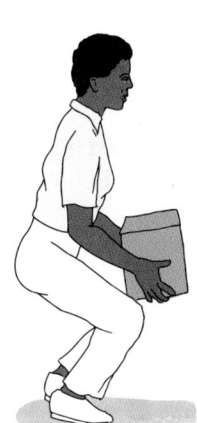
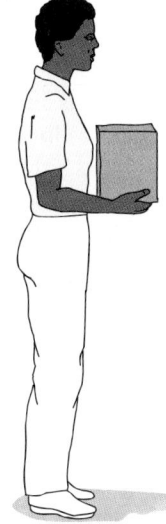

Fig. 16-4 Picking up a box using good body mechanics.

BOX 16-1	RULES FOR BODY MECHANICS

- Keep your body in good alignment with a wide base of support.
- Use an upright working posture. Bend your legs. Do not bend your back.
- Use the stronger and larger muscles in your shoulders, upper arms, thighs, and hips.
- Keep objects close to your body when you lift, move, or carry them (see Fig. 16-4).
- Avoid unnecessary bending and reaching. Raise the bed so it is close to your waist. Adjust the overbed table so it is at your waist level.
- Face your work area. This prevents unnecessary twisting.
- Push, slide, or pull heavy objects whenever you can rather than lifting them. Pushing is easier than pulling.
- Widen your base of support when pushing or pulling. Move your front leg forward when pushing. Move your rear leg back when pulling (Fig. 16-5, p. 248).

- Use both hands and arms to lift, move, or carry objects.
- Turn your whole body when changing the direction of your movement. Move and turn your feet in the direction of the turn instead of twisting your body.
- Work with smooth and even movements. Avoid sudden or jerky motions.
- Do not lean over a person to give care.
- *Get help from a co-worker to move heavy objects. Do not lift or move them by yourself.*
- Bend your hips and knees to lift heavy objects from the floor (see Fig. 16-4). Straighten your back as the object reaches thigh level. Your leg and thigh muscles work to raise the item off the floor and to waist level.
- Do not lift objects higher than chest level. Do not lift above your shoulders. Use a step stool or ladder to reach an object higher than chest level.

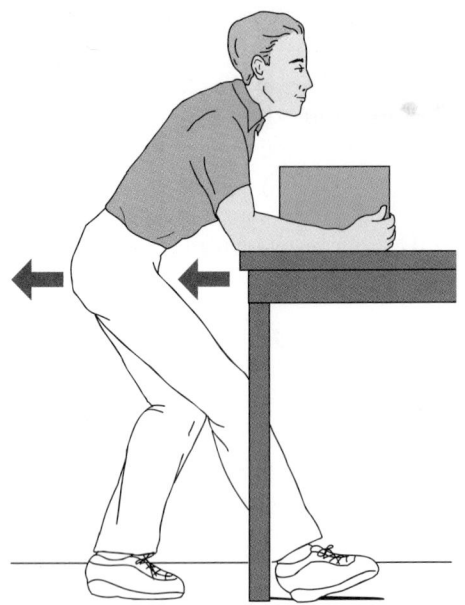

Fig. 16-5 Move your rear leg back when pulling an item.

MSDs are workplace health hazards. Early signs and symptoms include pain, limited joint movement, or soft tissue swelling. Time off work is often needed. According to the U.S. Department of Labor, nursing assistants are at great risk.

Always report a work-related injury as soon as possible. Early attention can help prevent the problem from becoming worse. Also injuries are often less serious and less costly to treat with early attention. In later stages, the problem can become more serious and harder and more costly to treat.

The following tasks are known to be high risk for MSDs:
- Transfers—to and from beds, chairs, wheelchairs, Geri-chairs, toilets, stretchers, and bathtubs
- Trying to stop a person from falling
- Picking up a person from the floor to the bed
- Lifting alone
- Lifting persons who are confused or uncooperative
- Lifting persons who cannot support their own weight
- Lifting heavy persons
- Weighing a person
- Moving a person up in bed
- Re-positioning a person in a bed or in a chair
- Changing an incontinence product
- Making beds
- Dressing and undressing a person
- Feeding a person in bed
- Giving a bed bath
- Applying anti-embolism stockings
- Prolonged holding of a body part for care measures—arm, leg, abdomen, skin fold

The Occupational Safety and Health Administration (OSHA) has identified MSD risk factors for the nursing team. An MSD is more likely if risk factors are combined. For example, a task involves both force and repeating actions.
- *Force*—the amount of physical effort needed to perform a task. Lifting or transferring heavy persons, preventing falls, and unexpected or sudden motions are examples.
- *Repeating action*—doing the same motion or series of motions continually or frequently. Re-positioning persons and transfers to and from beds, chairs, and commodes without adequate rest breaks are examples. So is frequently cranking manual beds.
- *Awkward postures*—assuming positions that place stress on the body. Examples are reaching above shoulder height, kneeling, squatting, leaning over a bed, bending, or twisting the torso while lifting.
- *Heavy lifting*—manually lifting people who cannot move themselves.

OSHA requires a safe work setting. The setting must be free of hazards that cause or are likely to cause death or serious physical harm to staff. The employer must make reasonable attempts to prevent or reduce the hazard. OSHA inspection teams enforce this law.

Back Injuries

Back injuries are major threats. Back injuries can occur from repeated activities or from one event. Signs and symptoms include:
- Pain when trying to assume a normal posture
- Decreased mobility
- Pain when standing or rising from a seated position

These and other factors can lead to back disorders:
- Reaching while lifting
- Poor posture when sitting or standing
- Staying in one position too long
- Poor body mechanics when lifting, pushing, pulling, or carrying objects
- Poor physical condition—not having the strength or endurance to perform tasks without strain
- Repeated lifting of awkward items, equipment, or persons
- Shifting weight when a person loses balance or strength while moving
- Twisting while lifting
- Bending while lifting
- Maintaining a bent posture such as leaning over a bed
- Reaching over raised bed rails
- Working in a confined, crowded, or cluttered area (rooms, bathrooms, hallways)
- Fatigue
- Poor footing such as on slippery floors
- Lifting with forceful movement

Follow the rules in Box 16-1. They help prevent back injuries. Also, be extra careful when performing tasks associated with back injuries.

See *Promoting Safety and Comfort: Back Injuries.*

Back Injuries

Safety

According to OSHA, these activities are associated with back injuries in nursing centers:

- Moving a person who totally depends on others for care.
- Moving a person who is combative.
- Transferring a person who is on the floor to the bed or a chair.
- Re-positioning a person in bed or in a chair.
- Transferring a person from bed to chair or from chair to bed.
- Transferring a person from one chair to another. This includes transfers to and from the wheelchair and toilet.
- Bending to bathe, dress, or feed a person.
- Bending to make a bed or change linens.
- Weighing a person.
- Changing an incontinence product.
- Trying to stop a person from falling.
  Use good body mechanics to protect yourself from injury.

Do not work alone. Avoid lifting whenever possible.

POSITIONING THE PERSON

The person must be properly positioned at all times. Regular position changes and good alignment promote comfort and well-being. Breathing is easier. Circulation is promoted. Pressure ulcers and contractures are prevented. A *contracture* is the lack of joint mobility caused by abnormal shortening of a muscle (Chapter 27).

For comfort, you move and turn when in bed or a chair. Many patients and residents do too. Some need reminding to adjust their positions. Others need help. Still others depend entirely on the nursing team for position changes.

Whether in bed or chair, the person is re-positioned at least every 2 hours. Some people are re-positioned more often. Follow the nurse's instructions and the care plan. To safely position a person:

- Use good body mechanics.
- Ask a co-worker to help you if needed.
- Explain the procedure to the person.
- Be gentle when moving the person.
- Provide for privacy.
- Use pillows as directed by the nurse for support and alignment.
- Provide for comfort after positioning. (See the inside of the front book cover.)
- Place the signal light within reach after positioning.
- Complete a safety check before leaving the room. (See the inside of the front book cover.)

  See *Focus on Communication: Positioning the Person.*
  See *Delegation Guidelines: Positioning the Person.*
  See *Promoting Safety and Comfort: Positioning the Person.*

Positioning the Person

Moving is painful for many persons. Some older persons have painful joints. Most persons have pain after surgery or an injury. Make sure that you do not cause pain when positioning the person. Tell the person what you are going to do before and during the procedure. Move the person slowly and gently. Give the person time to tell you if a movement is painful. Make sure the person is comfortable. You can say:

- "Am I hurting you?"
- "Please tell me if I'm moving you too fast."
- "Please tell me if you feel pain or discomfort."
- "Do you need a pillow adjusted?"
- "Are you comfortable?"
- "How can I help make you more comfortable?"

Positioning the Person

Many delegated tasks involve positioning and re-positioning. You need this information from the nurse and the care plan:

- Position or positioning limits ordered by the doctor
- How often to turn and re-position the person
- How many staff members need to help you
- What assist devices to use (Chapter 17)
- What skin care measures to perform (Chapter 20)
- What range-of-motion exercises to perform (Chapter 27)
- Where to place pillows
- What positioning devices are needed and how to use them (Chapter 27)
- What observations to report and record
- When to report observations
- What patient or resident concerns to report at once

Positioning the Person

Safety

Pressure ulcers (Chapter 34) are serious threats from lying or sitting too long in one place. Wet, soiled, and wrinkled linens are other causes. Whenever you re-position a person, make sure linens are clean, dry, and wrinkle-free. Change or straighten linens as needed.

Contractures can develop from staying in one position too long (Chapter 27). Re-positioning, exercise, and activity help prevent contractures.

Comfort

Pillows and positioning devices support body parts and keep the person in good alignment. This promotes comfort. Place pillows and positioning devices as directed by the nurse and the care plan.

Most older persons do not tolerate the prone position. They have limited range of motion in their necks. Usually the Sims' position is not comfortable for them. Check with the nurse before placing any older person in the prone position or Sims' position.

Fowler's Position

Fowler's position is a semi-sitting position. The head of the bed is raised between 45 and 60 degrees (Fig. 16-6). The knees may be slightly elevated. For good alignment:
- The spine is straight.
- The head is supported with a small pillow.
- The arms are supported with pillows.

The nurse may have you place small pillows under the lower back, thighs, and ankles. Persons with heart and respiratory disorders usually breathe easier in Fowler's position.

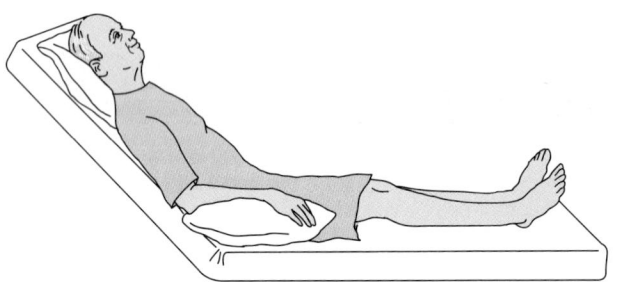

Fig. 16-6 Fowler's position.

Supine Position

The *supine position (dorsal recumbent position) is the back-lying position* (Fig. 16-7).

For good alignment:
- The bed is flat.
- The head and shoulders are supported on a pillow.
- Arms and hands are at the sides. You can support the arms with regular pillows. Or you can support the hands on small pillows with the palms down.

The nurse may have you place a folded or rolled towel under the lower back and a small pillow under the thighs. A pillow under the lower legs lifts the heels off of the bed. This prevents them from rubbing on the sheets.

Prone Position

In the *prone position, the person lies on the abdomen with the head turned to one side.* For good alignment:
- The bed is flat.
- Small pillows are placed under the head, abdomen, and lower legs (Fig. 16-8).
- Arms are flexed at the elbows with the hands near the head.

You also can position a person with the feet hanging over the end of the mattress (Fig. 16-9). A pillow is not needed under the feet.

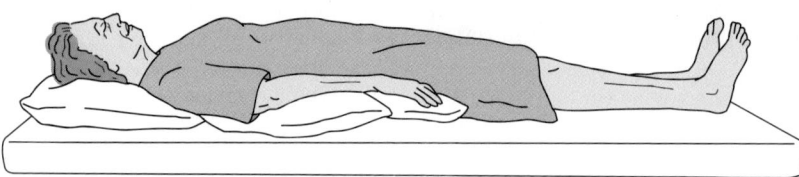

Fig. 16-7 Supine position.

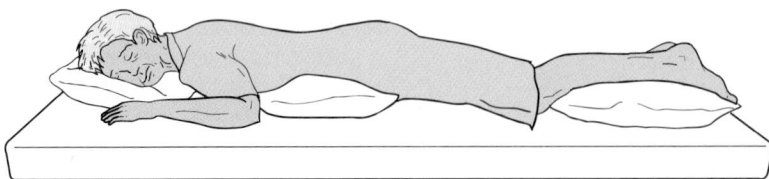

Fig. 16-8 Prone position.

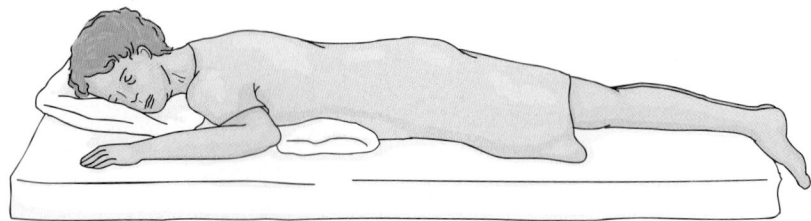

Fig. 16-9 Prone position with the feet hanging over the edge of the mattress.

Lateral Position

In the *lateral position (side-lying position), the person lies on one side or the other* (Fig. 16-10):

* The bed is flat.
* A pillow is under the head and neck.
* The upper leg is in front of the lower leg. (The nurse may ask you to position the upper leg behind the lower leg, not on top of it.)
* The ankle, upper leg, and thigh are supported with pillows.
* A small pillow is positioned against the person's back. The person rolls back against the pillow so that his or her back is at a 45-degree angle with the mattress.
* A small pillow is under the upper hand and arm.

Sims' Position

The *Sims' position (semi-prone side position) is a left side-lying position. The upper leg (right leg) is sharply flexed so it is not on the lower leg (left leg). The lower arm (left arm) is behind the person* (Fig. 16-11). For good alignment:

* The bed is flat.
* A pillow is under the person's head and shoulder.
* The upper leg (right leg) is supported with a pillow.
* A pillow is under the upper arm (right arm) and hand (right hand).

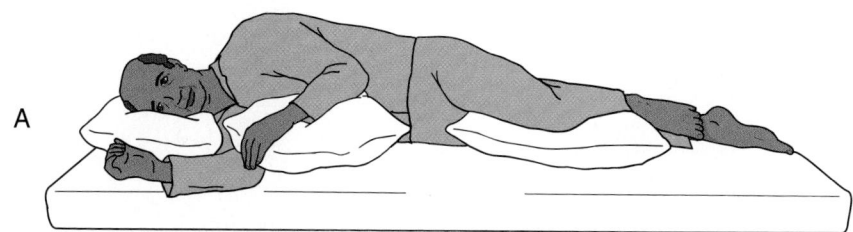

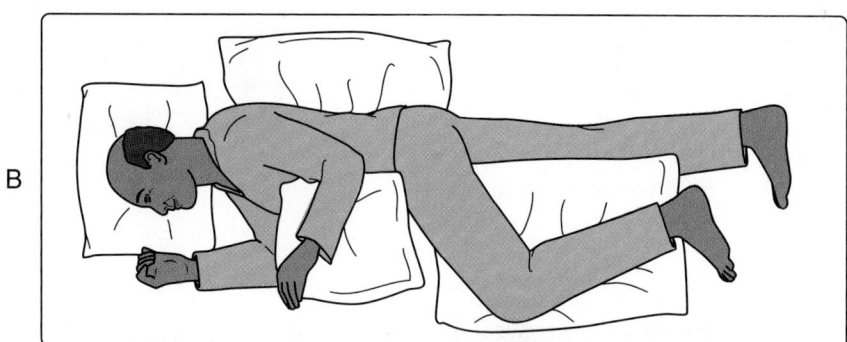

Fig. 16-10 Lateral position. **A,** Pillows are placed under the head and neck, under the upper hand and arm, and under the lower front leg. **B,** A pillow is placed against the person's back. The back is at a 45-degree angle to the mattress.

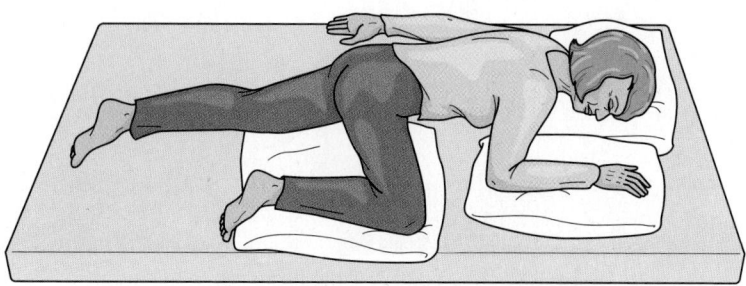

Fig. 16-11 Sims' position.

Chair Position

Persons who sit in chairs must hold their upper bodies and heads erect. If not, poor alignment results. For good alignment:

- The person's back and buttocks are against the back of the chair.
- Feet are flat on the floor or wheelchair footplates. Never leave feet unsupported.
- Backs of the knees and calves are slightly away from the edge of the seat (Fig. 16-12).

The nurse may have you put a small pillow between the person's lower back and the chair. This supports the lower back. *Remember, a pillow is not used behind the back if restraints are used* (Chapter 14).

Paralyzed arms are supported on pillows. Some persons have positioners (Fig. 16-13). Ask the nurse about their proper use. The nurse may have you position the wrists at a slight upward angle.

Some people require postural supports if they cannot keep their upper bodies erect (Fig. 16-14). Postural supports help keep them in good alignment. The health team selects the best product for the person's needs. The person's safety, dignity, and function are considered.

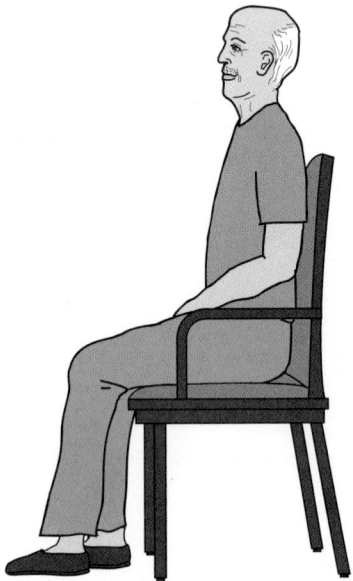

Fig. 16-12 The person is positioned in a chair. The person's feet are flat on the floor, the calves do not touch the chair. The back is straight and against the back of the chair.

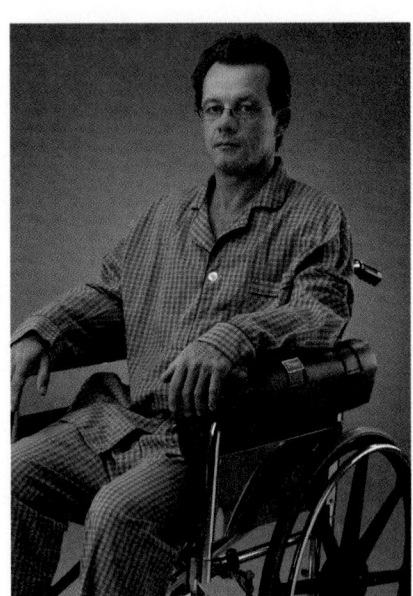

Fig. 16-13 Elevated armrest.

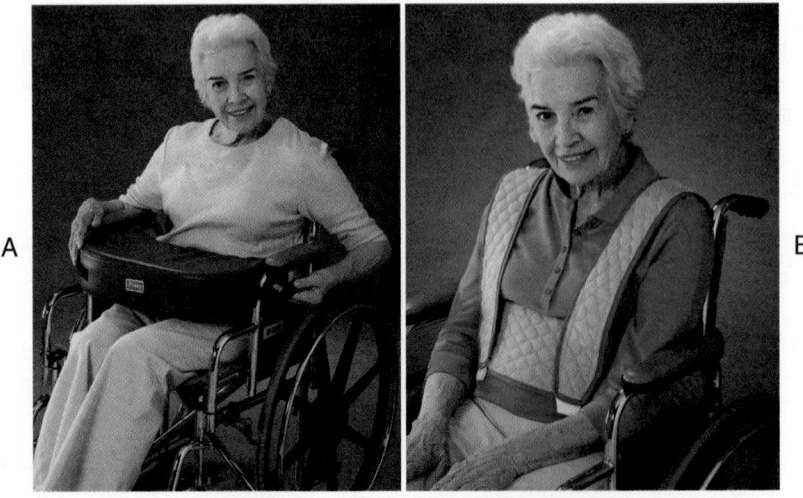

Fig. 16-14 Postural supports. **A,** Posey Hugger. **B,** Torso support.

FOCUS ON PRIDE

The Person, Family, and Yourself

Personal and Professional Responsibility

Moving persons causes strain on your body. Injuries can occur. Some factors increase your risk for injury. For example:

- Poor physical condition—not having the strength or endurance to perform tasks
- Fatigue
- Poor posture when sitting or standing
- Poor body mechanics when lifting, pushing, pulling, or carrying objects
- Repeated lifting of patients or residents or repeated lifting of awkward items or equipment
- Twisting or bending while lifting or maintaining a bent posture
- Reaching over raised bed rails
- Trying to lift or move an object or person alone

You must protect yourself from injury. Avoid the factors listed above. Also, follow the rules for body mechanics in Box 16-1. Use good judgment when you re-position and transfer patients and residents (Chapter 17). Ask for help when needed. Take responsibility for protecting yourself from harm.

Rights and Respect

OSHA requires that employers provide a safe work setting. You have the right to ask potential or current employers about safety plans to reduce your risk of injury. Ask about training or orientation programs related to body mechanics, safe handling of persons, and workplace hazards. Know and follow agency procedures for reporting problems.

Independence and Social Interaction

Remaining independent to the extent possible promotes dignity, self-esteem, and pride. Let the person choose bed or chair positioning as allowed by the nurse and the care plan. Let the person help as much as safely possible. Talk with the person while moving him or her. Ask about his or her preferences. Doing so promotes comfort, independence, and social interaction.

Delegation and Teamwork

Moving and positioning are safer when done by 2 or more workers. This is very important when caring for bariatric persons. You may need the help of 3, 4, or more co-workers to safely move such persons. Or special equipment may be needed. See Chapter 17. Follow the person's care plan.

Never try to move a person without enough help. You can harm yourself, your co-workers, and the person. Work as a team to protect yourself and others from injury.

Ethics and Laws

Proper body mechanics help prevent injuries that could affect health and ability to function. Failure to move and position the person correctly places the person at risk. For example:

- A person is left slumped in a chair for 3 hours. The person develops a pressure ulcer.
- A person is not re-positioned as instructed in the care plan. The person's contracture worsens.
- A person is moved without enough help. The move is rough. The person is injured.

You must provide care in a manner that maintains or improves each person's quality of life, health, and safety. It is the right thing to do.

REVIEW QUESTIONS

Circle the BEST answer.

1 Good body mechanics involve the following *except*
   a Good posture
   b Balance
   c Using the strongest and largest muscles
   d Having the job fit the worker

2 Good alignment means
   a The area on which an object rests
   b Having the head, trunk, arms, and legs aligned with one another
   c Using muscles, tendons, ligaments, and joints correctly
   d The back-lying or supine position

3 These actions are about body mechanics. Which action is *not* correct?
   a Hold objects away from your body when lifting, moving, or carrying them.
   b Face the direction you are working to prevent twisting.
   c Push, pull, or slide heavy objects.
   d Use both hands and arms to lift, move, or carry heavy objects.

4 Which action is easier?
   a Pushing   c Sliding
   b Pulling   d Lifting

5 The purpose of ergonomics is to
   a Reduce stress on the worker's body
   b Safely position a person
   c Promote quality of life
   d Use good body mechanics

6 Risk factors for MSDs include the following *except*
   a Repeating actions
   b Awkward postures
   c Bending your hips and knees
   d Force

7 Patients and residents are re-positioned at least every
   a 15 minutes   c 2 hours
   b 30 minutes   d 3 hours

8 The back-lying position is called
   a Fowler's position   c The prone position
   b The supine position   d Sims' position

9 Breathing is usually easier in
   a Fowler's position   c The lateral position
   b The supine position   d Sims' position

10 For Fowler's position
   a The bed is flat
   b The head of the bed is raised 45 to 60 degrees
   c The person's head is turned toward one side
   d The person's feet hang over the edge of the mattress

11 A pillow is placed against the person's back in
   a Fowler's position   c The lateral position
   b The prone position   d Sims' position

12 When in a chair, the person's feet
   a Must be flat on the floor
   b Are positioned on footplates
   c Dangle
   d Are positioned on pillows

Answers to these questions are on p. 833.

17 Safely Moving and Transferring the Person

OBJECTIVES

- Define the key terms and key abbreviations listed in this chapter.
- Identify comfort and safety measures for moving and transferring the person.
- Explain how to prevent work-related injuries when moving and transferring persons.
- Describe four levels of dependence.
- Identify the information needed from the nurse and care plan before moving and transferring persons.
- Perform the procedures described in this chapter.
- Explain how to promote PRIDE in the person, the family, and yourself.

KEY TERMS

friction The rubbing of one surface against another
logrolling Turning the person as a unit, in alignment, with one motion

shearing When skin sticks to a surface while muscles slide in the direction the body is moving
transfer Moving the person from one place to another

KEY ABBREVIATIONS

ID Identification

OSHA Occupational Safety and Health Administration

You will turn and re-position persons often. You move them in bed. You transfer them to and from beds, chairs, wheelchairs, stretchers, and toilets. *Transfer means moving the person from one place to another.* During these and other tasks, you must use your body correctly. This protects you and the person from injury.

See *Focus on Communication: Safely Moving and Transferring Persons.*
See *Promoting Safety and Comfort: Safely Moving and Transferring Persons.*
See *Teamwork and Time Management: Safely Moving and Transferring Persons.*

FOCUS ON COMMUNICATION
Safely Moving and Transferring Persons

Moving and transfers can be very painful following an injury or surgery. Many older persons have painful joints. Make sure the person is comfortable and that you are not causing pain. You can say:

- "Am I hurting you?"
- "Please tell me when you feel pain or discomfort."
- "Do you need a pillow adjusted?"
- "Are you comfortable?"
- "How can I help make you more comfortable?"

Before any move or transfer, you need to explain the procedure. Tell the person what you and your co-workers will do. Also explain what the person needs to do. Do so as you begin the procedure. Also, remind the person just before the move.

The procedures in this chapter explain how to move the person "on the count of 3." Staff move the person at the same time. The person is moved smoothly. One co-worker leads the others by counting. Decide who will count before the move. Be sure the person and staff know who is leading and what to do. You can say:

We are going to help you stand. I will count "1, 2, 3." When I say "3," we will pull up on your transfer belt. We will steady your feet with our feet. You need to push on the mattress and stand when I say "3."

Safety

Many older persons have osteoporosis or arthritis (Chapter 41). They have fragile bones and joints. To prevent injuries:

* Follow the rules of body mechanics (Chapter 16).
* Always have help when moving a person.
* Move the person carefully to prevent injury or pain.
* Keep the person in good alignment during the procedure.
* Position the person in good alignment after moving or transferring him or her.
* Make sure his or her face, nose, and mouth are not obstructed by a pillow or other device.

Comfort

To promote mental comfort when moving or transferring the person:

* Always explain what you are going to do and how the person can help.
* Always screen and cover the person to protect the right to privacy.
  To promote physical comfort:
* Keep the person in good alignment.
* Make sure the person's head does not hit the head-board when he or she is moved up in bed. If the person can be without a pillow, place it upright against the head-board.
* Use pillows to position the person as directed by the nurse and the care plan. If a pillow is allowed under the person's head, make sure it is under the head and shoulders.
* Use other positioning devices as directed by the nurse and the care plan.

TEAMWORK AND TIME MANAGEMENT
Safely Moving and Transferring Persons

Patients and residents are moved, turned, transferred, and re-positioned. These tasks and procedures are best done by at least 2 staff members.

Friendships are common among co-workers. And some working relationships are better than others. Do not just ask your friends or those with whom you work well to help you. Include all co-workers. Do not just help your friends or those with whom you work well. Assist anyone who asks for your help. This includes new staff and those from other units.

PREVENTING WORK-RELATED INJURIES

You must prevent work-related injuries when moving and transferring patients and residents. Follow the rules in Box 17-1. The Occupational Safety and Health Administration (OSHA) recommends:

* Minimizing manual lifting in all cases.
* Eliminating manual lifting when possible.

To safely move and transfer the person, the nurse and health team determine:

* *The person's dependence level.* Dependence levels relate to the ability to move without help. Some persons move without help. Others totally depend on the staff. Know the person's dependence level before you move or transfer a person. See Box 17-2, p. 257.
* *The amount of assistance needed.* This depends on the person's height, weight, cognitive function, and dependence level. Some persons only need help from 1 staff member. Others need help from at least 2 or 3 staff members.
* *What procedure to use.* The nurse and care plan tell you what procedure to use.
* *The equipment needed.* Assist equipment and devices are presented throughout this chapter. The nurse and care plan tell you what to use. Always follow the manufacturer's instructions. Ask for training to use the equipment and devices safely.

See *Focus on Children and Older Persons: Preventing Work-Related Injuries,* p. 258.
See *Teamwork and Time Management: Preventing Work-Related Injuries,* p. 258.
See *Delegation Guidelines: Preventing Work-Related Injuries,* p. 258.
See *Promoting Safety and Comfort: Preventing Work-Related Injuries,* p. 258.

Text continued on p. 258

BOX 17-1	PREVENTING WORK-RELATED INJURIES

General Guidelines

* Wear shoes with good traction. Avoid shoes with worn-down soles. Good traction helps to prevent slips or falls.
* Use assist equipment and devices whenever possible instead of lifting and moving the person manually. Follow the care plan.
* Get help from other staff. The nurse and care plan tell you how many staff members are needed for a task.
* Plan and prepare for the task. For example, know what equipment is needed, where to place chairs or wheelchairs, and what side of the bed to work on.

General Guidelines—cont'd

* Schedule harder tasks early in your shift.
* Balance lighter and harder tasks. Plan your work to complete a lighter task after a harder one.
* Lock bed wheels and wheelchair or stretcher wheels.
* Tell the person how he or she can help. Give clear, simple instructions. Give the person time to respond.
* Do not hold or grab the person under the underarms.
* Do not let the person hold or grasp you around your neck.

Modified from Cal/OSHA: A back injury prevention guide for health care providers, Sacramento, Calif., 1997 and referenced in Occupational Safety and Health Administration: *Ergonomics: guidelines for nursing homes,* 2009.

Continued

BOX 17-1   PREVENTING WORK-RELATED INJURIES—cont'd

Manual Lifting

- Use good body mechanics.
  - Stand with good posture. Keep your back straight.
  - Bend your legs, not your back.
  - Use your legs to do the work.
  - Face the person.
  - Do not twist or turn. Pick up your feet, and pivot your whole body in the direction of the move.
- Keep what you are moving close to you—the person, equipment, or supplies.
- Move the person toward you, not away from you.
- Use slides and lateral transfers instead of manual lifting.
- Use a wide, balanced base of support. Stand with one foot slightly ahead of the other.
- Lower the person slowly by bending your legs. Do not bend your back. Return to an erect position as soon as possible.
- Use smooth, even movements. Avoid jerking movements.
- Lift on the "count of 3" when lifting with others. Everyone lifts at the same time.

Lateral Transfers

- Position surfaces as close as possible to each other (bed and chair; bed and stretcher).
- Adjust surfaces so that they are at about waist height. The receiving surface should be slightly lower to take advantage of gravity. For example, to transfer the person from bed to a chair, the chair surface is lower than the bed.
- Make sure bed rails are down. Make sure stretcher side rails are down.
- Use drawsheets, turning pads, large incontinence pads, or other friction reducing devices. Such devices include sliding boards, slide sheets, and low-friction mattress covers.
- Get a good hand-hold. Roll up drawsheets, turning pads, and large incontinence pads. Or use assist devices with handles.
- Kneel on the bed or stretcher. This prevents extended reaches and bending your back.
- Have staff on both sides of the bed or other surface. Move the person on the "count of 3." Use a smooth, push-pull motion. Do not reach across the person.

Gait/Transfer Belts

- Keep the person as close to you as possible.
- Avoid bending, reaching, or twisting when:
  - Applying or removing a belt
  - Lowering the person to a chair, the bed, the toilet, or the floor
  - Helping the person walk
- Use a gentle rocking motion to assist the person to stand. The rocking motion gives strength and force as you pull the person to standing position.
- See Chapter 13.

Stand-Pivot Transfers

- Use assist devices as directed. Follow the care plan.
- Use a gait/transfer belt with handles.
- Keep your feet at least shoulder-width apart.
- Lower the bed so the person can place his or her feet on the floor.
- Plan the transfer so that the person moves his or her strong side first.
- Get the person close to the edge of the bed or the chair. Ask the person to lean forward as he or she stands.
- Block the person's weak leg with your legs or knees. If the position is awkward, do the following:
  - Use a transfer belt with handles.
  - Straddle your legs around the person's weak leg.
- Bend your legs. Do not bend your back.
- Pivot with your feet to turn.
- Use a gentle rocking motion to assist the person to stand. The rocking motion gives strength and force as you pull the person to standing position.

Lifting or Moving the Person in Bed

- Adjust the height of the bed, stretcher, or other surface so that it is at waist level.
- Lower the bed rail or the stretcher side rail.
- Work on the side where the person will be closest to you.
- Place equipment or other items close to you and at waist level.
- Use drawsheets, turning pads, large incontinence pads, or slide sheets.

Transporting the Person and Equipment

- Push, do not pull.
- Keep the load close to your body.
- Use an upright posture.
- Push with your whole body, not just your arms.
- Move down the center of the hallway. This helps avoid collisions.
- Watch out for door handles and high thresholds on floors. These can cause abrupt stops.

Transferring the Person From the Floor

- Use a mechanical lift if possible (p. 278). If not, place a sling, blanket, drawsheet, cot, or other assist device under the person as directed by the nurse.
- Position at least two staff members on each side of the person. More staff is needed if the person is large.
- Bend your knees, not your back. Do not twist.
- Roll the person onto his or her side to position the assist device. Do not reach across the person.
- Lower the hoist (if using a mechanical lift) to attach the sling. The hoist should be low enough to easily attach the sling.
- Do the following for a manual lift:
  - Kneel on one knee.
  - Grasp the blanket, drawsheet, cot, or other device.
  - Lift smoothly with your legs as you stand on the "count of 3." Do not bend your back.

Modified from Cal/OSHA: A back injury prevention guide for health care providers, Sacramento, Calif., 1997 and referenced in Occupational Safety and Health Administration: *Ergonomics: guidelines for nursing homes*, 2009.

BOX 17-2 LEVELS OF DEPENDENCE

Code 4: Total Dependence. The person cannot help with the transfer. The task or procedure is done by the staff.

- The person is lifted and transferred with a full-sling mechanical lift (Fig. 17-1). The lift is used for transfers between beds, chairs, and toilets. It is also used for transfers to and from bathtubs and weighing scales.

Code 3: Extensive Assistance. The person can bear some weight, can sit up with help, and may be able to pivot to transfer.

- The person is lifted and transferred with a mechanical lift. The lift is used for transfers between beds, chairs, and toilets. It is also used for transfers to and from bathtubs and weighing scales. The type of lift is noted on the person's care plan—full-sling mechanical lift or stand-assist lift (Fig. 17-2).

Code 2: Limited Assistance. The person is highly involved in the moving or transfer procedure. He or she needs some help moving the legs. The person can stand (bear weight). The person has upper body strength and can sit up. He or she can pivot transfer.

- Stand-assist devices may be needed. Some attach to the bed or chair (Fig. 17-3). Other stand-assist devices include walkers (Chapter 27) and gait/transfer belts with handles (Chapter 13).
- Sliding boards are useful for transfers to and from beds and chairs (Fig. 17-4).

Code 1: Supervision. The staff need to look after, encourage, or cue the person. To *cue* means to remind the person what to do.

- The devices for Code 2 may be needed.

Code 0: Independent. The person can walk without help. Sometimes the person may need limited assistance.

- Mechanical assistance is not normally required for transfers, lifting, or re-positioning.

Modified from Nelson AL: *Patient care ergonomics resource guide: safe patient handling and movement,* 2005, Patient Safety Center of Inquiry (Tampa, Florida), Veterans Health Administration and Department of Defense.

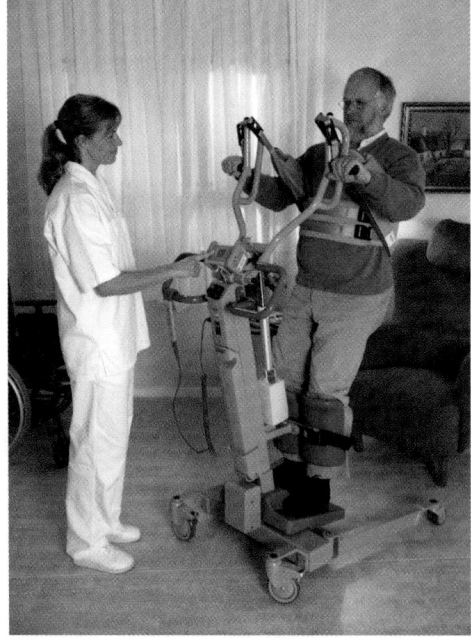

Fig. 17-2 Stand-assist lift.

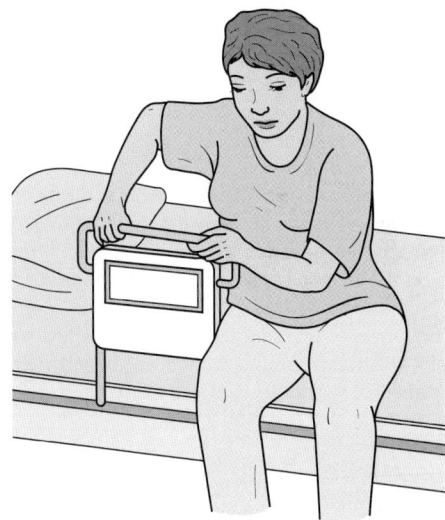

Fig. 17-3 Stand-assist bed attachment.

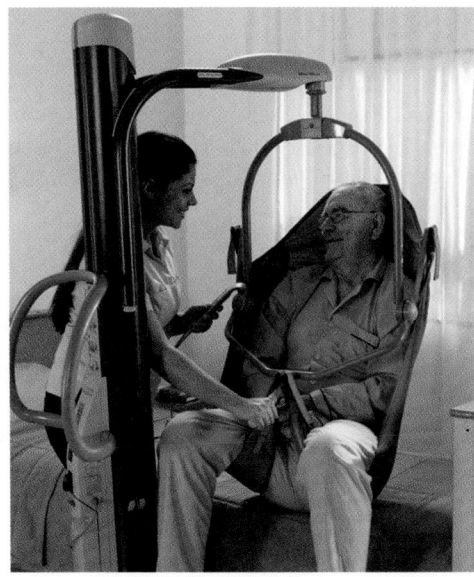

Fig. 17-1 Full-sling mechanical lift.

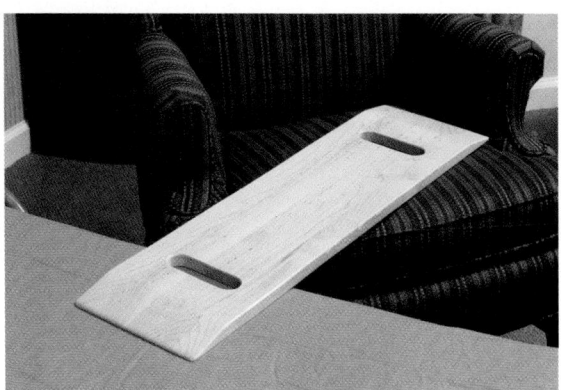

Fig. 17-4 Sliding board for transferring to and from surfaces.

FOCUS ON CHILDREN AND OLDER PERSONS
Preventing Work-Related Injuries

Older Persons

Persons with dementia may not understand what you are doing. They may resist your moving and transfer efforts. The person may shout at you, grab you, or try to hit you. Always have a co-worker help you. Do not force the person. The rules and guidelines in Box 17-1 apply. The person's care plan also has measures for safe care. For example:

- Proceed slowly.
- Use a calm, pleasant voice.
- Divert the person's attention. For example, let the person hold on to a washcloth or other soft object. This helps distract the person and keeps his or her hands busy.

Tell the nurse at once if you have problems moving or transferring the person.

TEAMWORK AND TIME MANAGEMENT
Preventing Work-Related Injuries

Some agencies have "lift teams." These teams perform most of the lifting, moving, and transfer procedures. They use assist equipment and do not manually lift or move patients and residents unless necessary.

The nurse advises the lift team of scheduled procedures. The team is called by beeper, pager, wireless phone, or other device for unscheduled transfers.

Do not assume that the lift team will lift, move, or transfer your assigned patients and residents. Follow agency policy for checking or adding to the lift team's schedule. Do not neglect or omit a procedure because the agency has a lift team. If the person is on the team's schedule, always check to make sure that the procedure was done. Sometimes the team can get delayed because of unscheduled or unexpected events. Always thank the team for the work that they do. Their work protects patients, residents, and you from injury.

DELEGATION GUIDELINES
Preventing Work-Related Injuries

Many tasks involve moving and transferring persons. Before doing so, you need this information from the nurse and the care plan:

- The person's height and weight.
- The person's dependence level (see Box 17-2).
- The person's physical abilities. For example, can the person sit up, stand up, or walk without help? Does the person have strength in his or her arms?
- If the person has a weak side. If yes, which side is weak?
- If the person has a medical condition that increases the risk of injury. Dizziness, confusion, hearing or vision problems, recent surgery, and fragile skin are examples.
- Any doctor's orders for moving or transferring the person.
- The person's ability to follow directions.
- If behavior problems are likely. Combative, agitated, uncooperative, and unpredictable behaviors are examples.
- The amount of assistance needed.
- How many staff members are needed to complete the task safely.
- What procedure to use.
- What equipment to use.

PROMOTING SAFETY AND COMFORT
Preventing Work-Related Injuries

Safety

Decide how to move the person before starting the procedure. If you need help from other staff, ask them to help before you begin. Also plan how to protect drainage tubes or containers connected to the person.

Beds are raised to move persons in bed (Chapter 19). This reduces bending and reaching. You must:

- Use the bed correctly.
- Protect the person from falling when the bed is raised.
- Follow the rules of body mechanics (Chapter 16).

MOVING PERSONS IN BED

Some persons can move and turn in bed. Others need help from at least 1 person. Those who are weak, unconscious, paralyzed, or in casts need help. Sometimes 2 or 3 people or a mechanical lift is needed.

- *Code 4: Total Dependence*—a mechanical lift or friction-reducing device and at least 2 staff members.
- *Code 3: Extensive Assistance*—a mechanical lift or friction-reducing device and at least 2 staff members.
- *The person weighs less than 200 pounds*—2 to 3 staff members and a friction-reducing device.
- *The person weighs more than 200 pounds*—at least 3 staff members and a friction-reducing device.

See *Delegation Guidelines: Moving Persons in Bed.*

DELEGATION GUIDELINES
Moving Persons in Bed

Many tasks involve moving the person in bed. Before moving a person, you need this information from the nurse and the care plan:
- What procedure to use.
- How many staff are needed to safely move the person.
- The person's position limits and restrictions.
- How far you can lower the head of the bed.
- Any limits in the person's ability to move or be re-positioned.
- What pillows you can remove before moving the person.
- What equipment is needed—trapeze, lift sheet, slide sheet, mechanical lift.
- If you need to apply an abdominal binder. For the person with bariatric needs, an abdominal binder may be used if the person's abdomen is in the way. See Chapter 33.
- How to position the person.
- If the person uses bed rails.
- What observations to report and record:
  - Who helped you with the procedure
  - How much help the person needed
  - How the person tolerated the procedure
  - How you positioned the person
  - Complaints of pain or discomfort
- When to report observations.
- What patient or resident concerns to report at once.

FOCUS ON CHILDREN AND OLDER PERSONS
Protecting the Skin

Older Persons
Older persons are at great risk for shearing. Their fragile skin is easily torn. Many have arthritis and osteoporosis (Chapter 41). They have fragile bones and joints. Protect them from pain and injury.

Ask a co-worker to help you move older persons. Use a friction-reducing device. Move older persons carefully and gently.

Persons with dementia may try to resist your efforts. Do not force the person. Proceed slowly. Use a calm voice. Divert the person's attention if necessary.

Protecting the Skin

Protect the person's skin during moving and transfer procedures. Friction and shearing injure the skin. Both cause infection and pressure ulcers (Chapter 34).
- *Friction is the rubbing of one surface against another.* When moved in bed, the person's skin rubs against the sheet.
- *Shearing is when the skin sticks to a surface while muscles slide in the direction the body is moving* (Fig. 17-5). It occurs when the person slides down in bed or is moved in bed.

To reduce friction and shearing when moving the person in bed:
- Roll the person.
- Use friction-reducing devices. Such devices include a lift sheet (turning sheet). A cotton drawsheet (Chapter 19) serves as a lift sheet (turning sheet). Turning pads, large incontinence products, and slide sheets (p. 263) are other friction-reducing devices.

See *Focus on Children and Older Persons: Protecting the Skin.*

Raising the Person's Head and Shoulders

Sometimes you raise the person's head and shoulders to give care. Simply turning or removing a pillow requires this procedure. You can raise the person's head and shoulders easily and safely by locking arms with the person. *Do not pull on the person's arm or shoulder.* Have help with older persons and with those who are heavy or hard to move. This protects the person and you from injury.

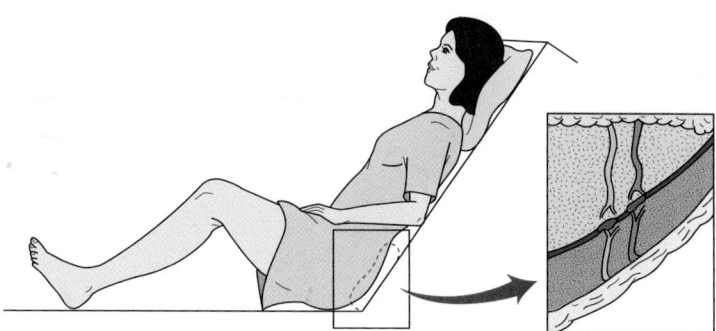

Fig. 17-5 Shearing. When the head of the bed is raised to a sitting position, skin on the buttocks stays in place. However, internal structures move forward as the person slides down in bed. This pinches the skin between the mattress and the hip bones.

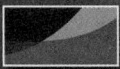

RAISING THE PERSON'S HEAD AND SHOULDERS

QUALITY OF LIFE

Remember to:
- Knock before entering the person's room.
- Address the person by name.
- Introduce yourself by name and title.

- Explain the procedure to the person before beginning and during the procedure.
- Protect the person's rights during the procedure.
- Handle the person gently during the procedure.

PRE-PROCEDURE

1. Follow *Delegation Guidelines:*
   a. *Preventing Work-Related Injuries,* p. 258
   b. *Moving Persons in Bed,* p. 259
   See *Promoting Safety and Comfort:*
   a. *Safely Moving and Transferring Persons,* p. 255
   b. *Preventing Work-Related Injuries,* p. 258
2. Ask a co-worker to assist if you need help.
3. Practice hand hygiene.

4. Identify the person. Check the ID (identification) bracelet against the assignment sheet. Also call the person by name.
5. Provide for privacy.
6. Lock the bed wheels.
7. Raise the bed for body mechanics. Bed rails are up if used.

PROCEDURE

8. Have your co-worker stand on the other side of the bed. Lower the bed rails if up.
9. Ask the person to put the near arm under your near arm and behind your shoulder. His or her hand rests on top of your shoulder. If you are standing on the right side, the person's right hand rests on your right shoulder (Fig. 17-6, A). The person does the same with your co-worker. The person's left hand rests on your co-worker's left shoulder (Fig. 17-7, A).
10. Put your arm nearest to the person under his or her arm. Your hand is on the person's shoulder. Your co-worker does the same.

11. Put your free arm under the person's neck and shoulders (Fig. 17-6, B). Your co-worker does the same (Fig. 17-7, B). Support the neck.
12. Help the person rise to a sitting or semi-sitting position on the "count of 3" (Figs. 17-6, C and 17-7, C).
13. Use the arm and hand that supported the person's neck and shoulders to give care (Fig. 17-6, D). Your co-worker supports the person (Fig. 17-7, D).
14. Help the person lie down. Provide support with your locked arm. Support the person's neck and shoulders with your other arm. Your co-worker does the same.

POST-PROCEDURE

15. Provide for comfort. (See the inside of the front book cover.)
16. Place the signal light within reach.
17. Lower the bed to its lowest position.
18. Raise or lower bed rails. Follow the care plan.

19. Unscreen the person.
20. Complete a safety check of the room. (See the inside of the front book cover.)
21. Practice hand hygiene.
22. Report and record your observations.

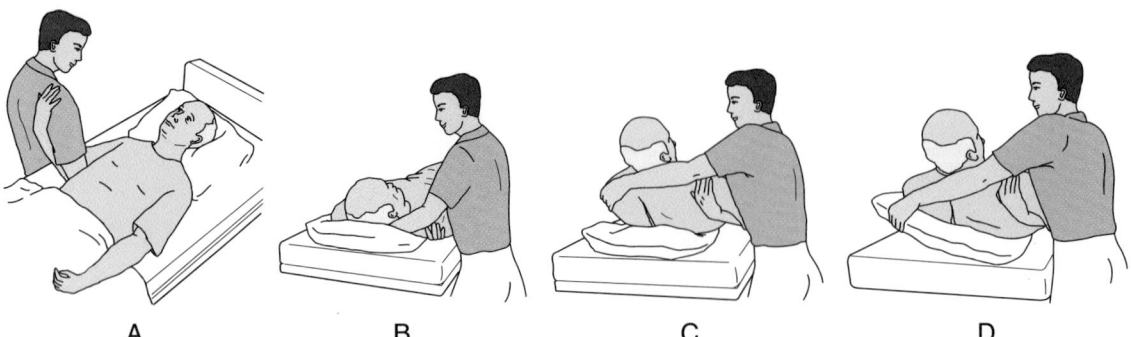

A   B   C   D

Fig. 17-6 Raising the person's head and shoulders by locking arms with the person. **A,** The person's near arm is under the nursing assistant's near arm and behind the shoulder. **B,** The nursing assistant's far arm is under the person's neck and shoulders. The near arm is under the person's near arm. **C,** The person is raised to a semi-sitting position by locking arms. **D,** The nursing assistant lifts the pillow while the person is in a semi-sitting position.

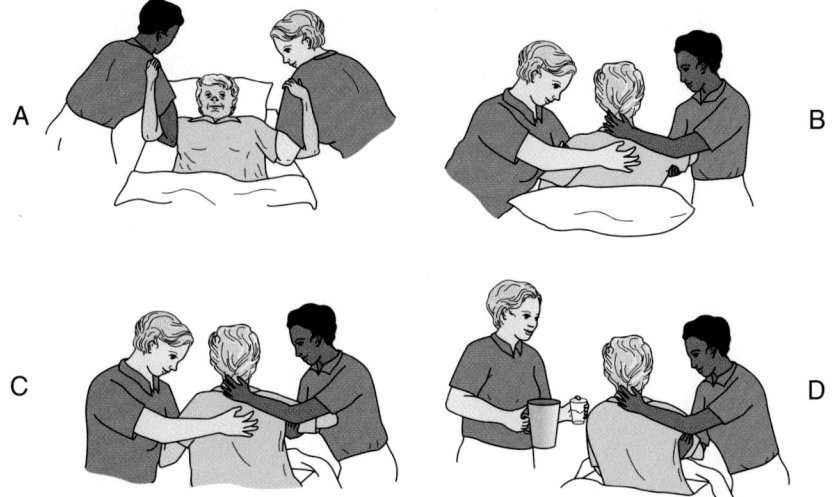

Fig. 17-7 Raising the person's head and shoulders with a co-worker. **A,** Two nursing assistants lock arms with the person. **B,** The nursing assistants each have an arm under the person's head and neck. **C,** The nursing assistants raise the person to a semi-sitting position. **D,** One nursing assistant supports the person in the semi-sitting position. The other gives care.

Moving the Person Up in Bed

When the head of the bed is raised, it is easy to slide down toward the middle and foot of the bed (Fig. 17-8). You move the person up in bed for good alignment and comfort.

You can sometimes move lightweight adults up in bed alone if they can assist using a trapeze. However, it is best done with help and an assist device—lift sheet, large incontinence product, slide sheet (p. 263). For heavy, weak, and very old persons, 2 or more staff members are needed. Always protect the person and yourself from injury.

See *Promoting Safety and Comfort: Moving the Person Up in Bed.*

> **PROMOTING SAFETY AND COMFORT**
> **Moving the Person Up in Bed**
>
> **Safety**
> *This procedure is best done with at least 2 staff members.* Use assist devices as directed by the nurse and care plan. Ask any questions before you begin the procedure.
> Perform this procedure alone *only if:*
> * The person is small in size.
> * The person can follow directions.
> * The person can assist with much of the moving.
> * The person uses a trapeze.
> * The person can push against the mattress with his or her feet.
> * The nurse says it is safe to do so.
> * You are comfortable doing so.

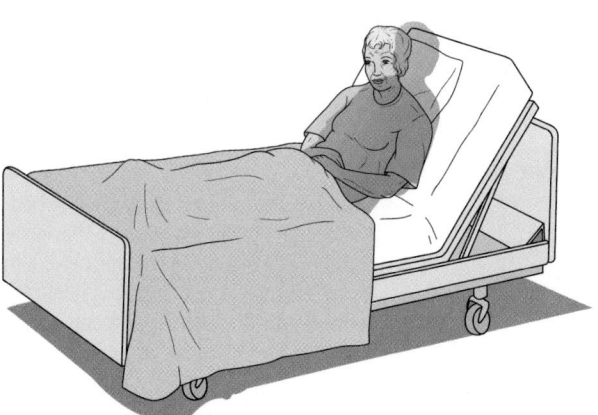

Fig. 17-8 The person is in poor alignment after sliding down in bed.

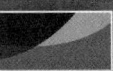

MOVING THE PERSON UP IN BED

VIDEO

QUALITY OF LIFE

Remember to:
- Knock before entering the person's room.
- Address the person by name.
- Introduce yourself by name and title.

- Explain the procedure to the person before beginning and during the procedure.
- Protect the person's rights during the procedure.
- Handle the person gently during the procedure.

PRE-PROCEDURE

1 Follow *Delegation Guidelines:*
  a *Preventing Work-Related Injuries,* p. 258
  b *Moving Persons in Bed,* p. 259
  See *Promoting Safety and Comfort:*
  a *Safely Moving and Transferring Persons,* p. 255
  b *Preventing Work-Related Injuries,* p. 258
  c *Moving the Person Up in Bed,* p. 261
2 Ask a co-worker to help you.

3 Practice hand hygiene.
4 Identify the person. Check the ID bracelet against the assignment sheet. Also call the person by name.
5 Provide for privacy.
6 Lock the bed wheels.
7 Raise the bed for body mechanics. Bed rails are up if used.

PROCEDURE

8 Lower the head of the bed to a level appropriate for the person. It is as flat as possible.
9 Stand on one side of the bed. Your co-worker stands on the other side.
10 Lower the bed rails if up.
11 Remove pillows as directed by the nurse. Place a pillow upright against the head-board if the person can be without it.
12 Stand with a wide base of support. Point the foot near the head of the bed toward the head of the bed. Face the head of the bed.
13 Bend your hips and knees. Keep your back straight.

14 Place one arm under the person's shoulder and one arm under the thighs. Your co-worker does the same. Grasp each other's forearms (Fig. 17-9).
15 Ask the person to grasp the trapeze.
16 Have the person flex both knees.
17 Explain that:
  a You will count "1, 2, 3."
  b The move will be on "3."
  c On "3," the person pushes against the bed with the feet if able. And the person pulls up with the trapeze.
18 Move the person to the head of the bed on the count of "3." Shift your weight from your rear leg to your front leg (see Fig. 17-9). Your co-worker does the same.
19 Repeat steps 12 through 18 if necessary.

POST-PROCEDURE

20 Put the pillow under the person's head and shoulders. Straighten linens.
21 Position the person in good alignment. Raise the head of the bed to a level appropriate for the person.
22 Provide for comfort. (See the inside of the front book cover.)
23 Place the signal light within reach.

24 Lower the bed to its lowest position.
25 Raise or lower bed rails. Follow the care plan.
26 Unscreen the person.
27 Complete a safety check of the room. (See the inside of the front book cover.)
28 Practice hand hygiene.
29 Report and record your observations.

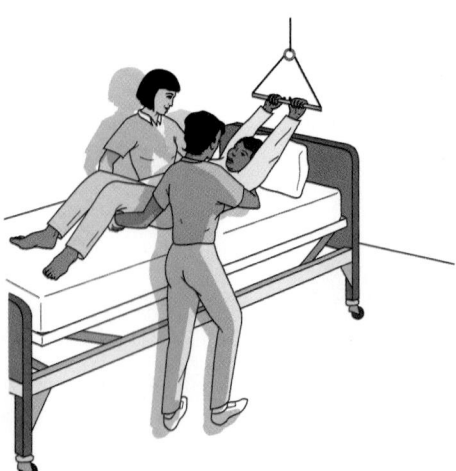

Fig. 17-9 A person is moved up in bed by two nursing assistants. Each has one arm under the person's shoulders and the other under the thighs. They have locked arms under the person. The person grasps the trapeze and flexes the knees. The nursing assistants shift their weight from the rear leg to the front leg as the person is moved up in bed.

Moving the Person Up in Bed With an Assist Device

You use assist devices to move some persons up in bed. Such assist devices include a drawsheet (lift sheet), flat sheet folded in half, turning pad (Fig. 17-10), slide sheet (Fig. 17-11), and large incontinence product. With these devices, the person is moved more evenly. And the devices reduce shearing and friction.

Place the device under the person from the head to above the knees or lower. At least 2 staff members are needed. This procedure is used for most patients and residents. It is used:

- Following the guidelines for "Moving Persons in Bed," p. 258
- For persons recovering from spinal cord surgery or spinal cord injuries
- For older persons
  See *Promoting Safety and Comfort: Moving the Person Up in Bed With an Assist Device.*

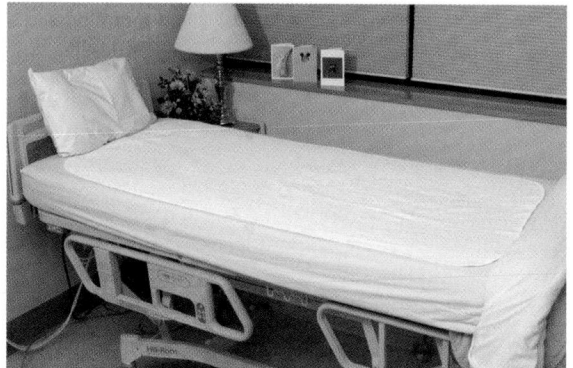

Fig. 17-10 Turning pad.

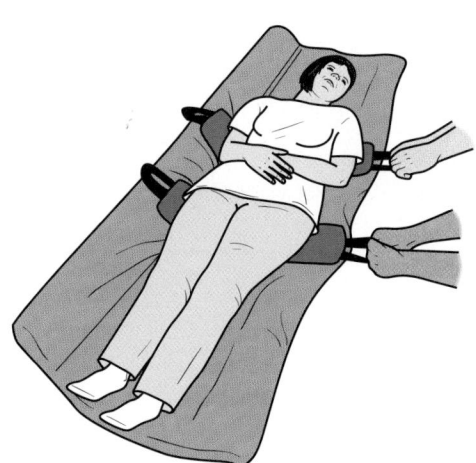

Fig. 17-11 Slide sheet.

PROMOTING SAFETY AND COMFORT

Moving the Person Up in Bed With an Assist Device

Safety

Not all incontinence products are used as assist devices. Disposable, single-use underpads are not strong enough to hold the person's weight during the move. Re-usable underpads are stronger. For safety, the underpad must:

- Be strong enough to support the person's weight.
- Extend from under the person's head to above the knees or lower.
- Be wide enough for you and other staff to get a firm grip for the lift.

Ask the nurse if the person's underpad is safe as an assist device.

To use a slide sheet, place it under the person. See procedure: *Making an Occupied Bed* in Chapter 19 for this step. After moving the person up in bed, remove the slide sheet. The person is in danger of sliding down in bed or off the bed if the slide sheet is not removed.

For persons with bariatric needs, the care plan may include:

- Performing the task with a friction-reducing device or bariatric lift and:
  - At least 2 staff members if the person can assist with the move.
  - At least 3 staff members if the person cannot assist with the move.
  - Positioning the bed in Trendelenburg's position. This position allows the use of gravity to pull the person up in bed. The position is used only if tolerated by the person.
- Leaving the friction-reducing device under the person. The device is covered with a drawsheet. Leaving the device under the person reduces the risk of injuries to the person and staff. The person is not turned from side-to-side to place and remove the friction-reducing device.

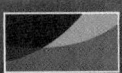

MOVING THE PERSON UP IN BED WITH AN ASSIST DEVICE

QUALITY OF LIFE

Remember to:
- Knock before entering the person's room.
- Address the person by name.
- Introduce yourself by name and title.

- Explain the procedure to the person before beginning and during the procedure.
- Protect the person's rights during the procedure.
- Handle the person gently during the procedure.

PRE-PROCEDURE

1 Follow *Delegation Guidelines:*
  a *Preventing Work-Related Injuries,* p. 258
  b *Moving Persons in Bed,* p. 259
  See *Promoting Safety and Comfort:*
  a *Safely Moving and Transferring Persons,* p. 255
  b *Preventing Work-Related Injuries,* p. 258
  c *Moving the Person Up in Bed,* p. 261
  d *Moving the Person Up in Bed With an Assist Device,* p. 263

2 Ask a co-worker to help you.
3 Practice hand hygiene.
4 Identify the person. Check the ID bracelet against the assignment sheet. Also call the person by name.
5 Provide for privacy.
6 Lock the bed wheels.
7 Raise the bed for body mechanics. Bed rails are up if used.

PROCEDURE

8 Lower the head of the bed to a level appropriate for the person. It is as flat as possible.
9 Stand on one side of the bed. Your co-worker stands on the other side.
10 Lower the bed rails if up.
11 Remove pillows as directed by the nurse. Place a pillow upright against the headboard if the person can be without it.
12 Stand with a broad base of support. Point the foot near the head of the bed toward the head of the bed. Face that direction.

13 Roll the sides of the assist device up close to the person. (NOTE: Omit this step if the device has handles.)
14 Grasp the rolled-up assist device firmly near the person's shoulders and hips (Fig. 17-12). Or grasp it by the handles. Support the head.
15 Bend your hips and knees.
16 Move the person up in bed on the count of "3." Shift your weight from your rear leg to your front leg.
17 Repeat steps 12 through 16 if necessary.
18 Unroll the assist device. (NOTE: Omit this step if the device has handles.)

POST-PROCEDURE

19 Put the pillow under the person's head and shoulders.
20 Position the person in good alignment. Raise the head of the bed to a level appropriate for the person.
21 Provide for comfort. (See the inside of the front book cover.)
22 Place the signal light within reach.
23 Lower the bed to its lowest position.

24 Raise or lower bed rails. Follow the care plan.
25 Unscreen the person.
26 Complete a safety check of the room. (See the inside of the front book cover.)
27 Practice hand hygiene.
28 Report and record your observations.

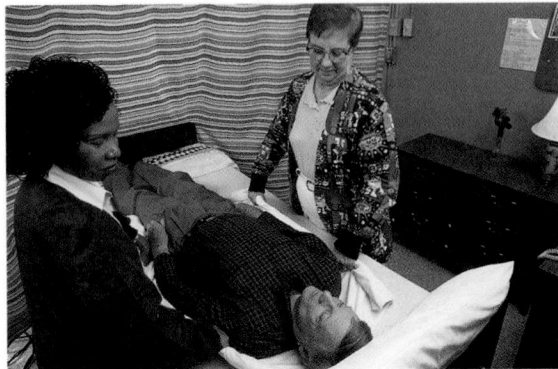

Fig. 17-12 A drawsheet is used to move the person up in bed. It extends from the person's head to above the knees. Rolled close to the person, the drawsheet is held near the shoulders and hips.

Moving the Person to the Side of the Bed

Re-positioning and care procedures require moving the person to the side of the bed. Move the person to the side of the bed before turning. Otherwise, after turning, the person lies on the side of the bed—not in the middle.

Sometimes you have to reach over the person. Giving a bed bath is an example. You reach less if the person is near you.

One method involves moving the person in segments (Fig. 17-13). Sometimes you can do this alone. With at least 1 co-worker, use a mechanical lift (p. 278) or an assist device:

- Following the guidelines for "Moving Persons in Bed," p. 258
- For older persons
- For persons with arthritis
- For persons recovering from spinal cord injuries or spinal cord surgery

Assist devices for this procedure include a drawsheet (lift sheet), flat sheet folded in half, turning pad, slide sheet, and large incontinence product. Using an assist device helps prevent pain and skin damage. It also helps prevent injury to the bones, joints, and spinal cord.

See *Promoting Safety and Comfort: Moving the Person to the Side of the Bed.*

PROMOTING SAFETY AND COMFORT
Moving the Person to the Side of the Bed

Safety

Use the method and equipment that are best for the person. Get this information from the nurse and the care plan for tasks that involve moving the person to the side of the bed. Such tasks include re-positioning, bedmaking, bathing, and range-of-motion exercises.

The wrong method could seriously injure a person. This is very important for persons who are very old, have arthritis, or have spinal cord involvement.

When using an assist device, you need at least 1 co-worker to help you. Depending on the person's size, 3 staff members may be needed. Then ask 2 co-workers to help you.

To use a slide sheet, place it under the person. After moving the person up in bed, remove the device.

To move the person in segments, move the person toward you not away from you. This helps protect you from injury.

Comfort

After moving the person to the side of the bed, move the pillow too. Position the pillow correctly. It should be under the person's head and shoulders.

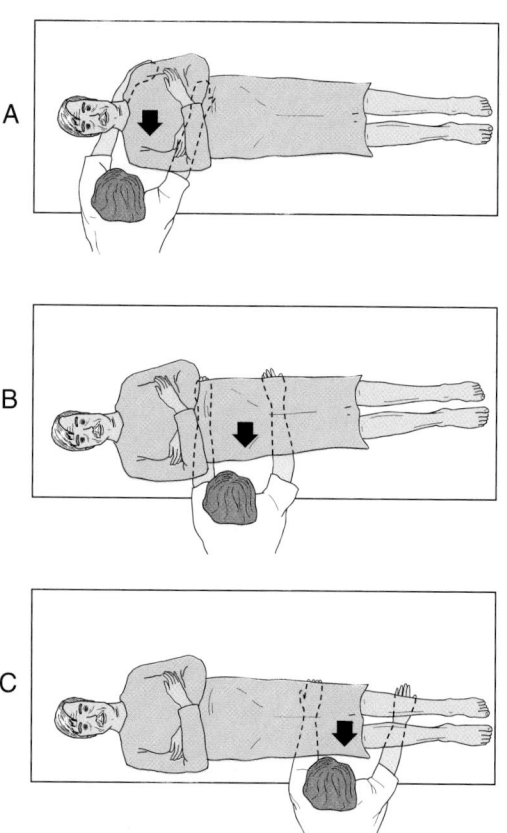

Fig. 17-13 Moving the person to the side of the bed in segments. **A,** The upper part of the body is moved. **B,** The lower part of the body is moved. **C,** The legs and feet are moved.

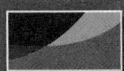

MOVING THE PERSON TO THE SIDE OF THE BED

QUALITY OF LIFE

Remember to:
- Knock before entering the person's room.
- Address the person by name.
- Introduce yourself by name and title.

- Explain the procedure to the person before beginning and during the procedure.
- Protect the person's rights during the procedure.
- Handle the person gently during the procedure.

PRE-PROCEDURE

1 Follow *Delegation Guidelines:*
   a *Preventing Work-Related Injuries,* p. 258
   b *Moving Persons in Bed,* p. 259
   See *Promoting Safety and Comfort:*
   a *Safely Moving and Transferring Persons,* p. 255
   b *Preventing Work-Related Injuries,* p. 258
   c *Moving the Person to the Side of the Bed,* p. 265
2 Ask 1 or 2 co-workers to help you if using an assist device.

3 Practice hand hygiene.
4 Identify the person. Check the ID bracelet against the assignment sheet. Also call the person by name.
5 Provide for privacy.
6 Lock the bed wheels.
7 Raise the bed for body mechanics. Bed rails are up if used.

PROCEDURE

8 Lower the head of the bed to a level appropriate for the person. It is as flat as possible.
9 Stand on the side of the bed to which you will move the person.
10 Lower the bed rail near you if bed rails are used. (Both bed rails are lowered for step 15.)
11 Remove pillows as directed by the nurse.
12 Stand with your feet about 12 inches apart. One foot is in front of the other. Flex your knees.
13 Cross the person's arms over the person's chest.
14 *Method 1—Moving the person in segments:*
   a Place your arm under the person's neck and shoulders. Grasp the far shoulder.
   b Place your other arm under the mid-back.
   c Move the upper part of the person's body toward you. Rock backward and shift your weight to your rear leg (see Fig. 17-13, A).
   d Place one arm under the person's waist and one under the thighs.

   e Rock backward to move the lower part of the person toward you (see Fig. 17-13, B).
   f Repeat the procedure for the legs and feet (see Fig. 17-13, C). Your arms should be under the person's thighs and calves.
15 *Method 2—Moving the person with a drawsheet:*
   a Roll up the drawsheet close to the person (see Fig. 17-12).
   b Grasp the rolled-up drawsheet near the person's shoulder's and hips. Your co-worker does the same. Support the person's head.
   c Rock backward on the count of "3" moving the person toward you. Your co-worker rocks backward slightly and then forward toward you while keeping the arms straight.
   d Unroll the drawsheet. Remove any wrinkles.

POST-PROCEDURE

16 Position the person in good alignment.
17 Provide for comfort. (See the inside of the front book cover.)
18 Place the signal light within reach.
19 Lower the bed to its lowest position.
20 Raise or lower bed rails. Follow the care plan.

21 Unscreen the person.
22 Complete a safety check of the room. (See the inside of the front book cover.)
23 Practice hand hygiene.
24 Report and record your observations.

TURNING PERSONS

Turning persons onto their sides helps prevent complications from bedrest (Chapter 27). Certain procedures and care measures also require the side-lying position. You turn the person toward you or away from you. The direction depends on the person's condition and the situation.

After turning the person, position him or her in good alignment. Use pillows to support the person in the side-lying position.

Some persons turn and re-position themselves in bed. Others need help. Some totally depend on the nursing staff for care. After turning, make sure the person's face, nose, and mouth are not obstructed by a pillow or other device.

Many older persons suffer from arthritis in their spines, hips, and knees. When turning these persons, logrolling is preferred (p. 269). Logrolling may be less painful for these persons.

See *Delegation Guidelines: Turning Persons.*
See *Promoting Safety and Comfort: Turning Persons.*

DELEGATION GUIDELINES
Turning Persons

Before turning and re-positioning a person, you need this information from the nurse and the care plan:
- The person's dependency level (see Box 17-2)
- How much help the person needs
- How many staff members are needed to safely complete the procedure
- The person's comfort level and what body parts are painful
- Which procedure to use
- What assist devices to use
- What supportive devices are needed for positioning (Chapter 27)
- Where to place pillows
- What observations to report and record:
  - Who helped you with the procedure
  - How much help the person needed
  - How the person tolerated the procedure
  - How you positioned the person
  - Complaints of pain or discomfort
- When to report observations
- What patient or resident concerns to report at once

PROMOTING SAFETY AND COMFORT
Turning Persons

Safety

Use good body mechanics when turning a person in bed (Chapter 16). Follow the rules in Box 17-1.

The person must be in good alignment. Otherwise, musculo-skeletal injuries, skin breakdown, or pressure ulcers could occur.

If using an assist device, ask a co-worker to help you.

Do not turn a person away from you with the far bed rail down. Raise the bed rail on the side near you. Then go to the other side of the bed. Lower that bed rail if up. Turn the person toward you.

Comfort

After turning, position the person in good alignment. Use pillows as directed to support the person in the side-lying position (Chapter 16).

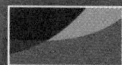 ### TURNING AND RE-POSITIONING THE PERSON

QUALITY OF LIFE

Remember to:
- Knock before entering the person's room.
- Address the person by name.
- Introduce yourself by name and title.

- Explain the procedure to the person before beginning and during the procedure.
- Protect the person's rights during the procedure.
- Handle the person gently during the procedure.

PRE-PROCEDURE

1 Follow *Delegation Guidelines:*
  a *Preventing Work-Related Injuries,* p. 258
  b *Moving Persons in Bed,* p. 259
  c *Turning Persons*
  See *Promoting Safety and Comfort:*
  a *Safely Moving and Transferring Persons,* p. 255
  b *Preventing Work-Related Injuries,* p. 258
  c *Moving the Person to the Side of the Bed,* p. 265
  d *Turning Persons*

2 Practice hand hygiene.
3 Identify the person. Check the ID bracelet against the assignment sheet. Also call the person by name.
4 Provide for privacy.
5 Lock the bed wheels.
6 Raise the bed for body mechanics. Bed rails are up.

Continued

TURNING AND RE-POSITIONING THE PERSON—cont'd

VIDEO | VIDEO CLIP | NNAAP® Skill

PROCEDURE

7 Lower the head of the bed to a level appropriate for the person. It is as flat as possible.
8 Stand on the side of the bed opposite to where you will turn the person.
9 Lower the near bed rail.
10 Move the person to the side near you. (See procedure: *Moving the Person to the Side of the Bed,* p. 266.)
11 Cross the person's arms over the person's chest. Cross the leg near you over the far leg.
12 *Turning the person away from you:*
   a Stand with a wide base of support. Flex the knees.
   b Place one hand on the person's shoulder. Place the other on the hip near you.
   c Roll the person gently away from you toward the raised bed rail (Fig. 17-14, A). Shift your weight from your rear leg to your front leg.

13 *Turning the person toward you:*
   a Raise the bed rail.
   b Go to the other side of the bed. Lower the bed rail.
   c Stand with a wide base of support. Flex your knees.
   d Place one hand on the person's far shoulder. Place the other on the far hip.
   e Roll the person toward you gently (Fig. 17-14, B).
14 Position the person. Follow the nurse's directions and the care plan. The following is common:
   a Place a pillow under the head and neck.
   b Adjust the shoulder. The person should not lie on an arm.
   c Place a small pillow under the upper hand and arm.
   d Position a pillow against the back.
   e Flex the upper knee. Position the upper leg in front of the lower leg.
   f Support the upper leg and thigh on pillows. Make sure the ankle is supported.

POST-PROCEDURE

15 Provide for comfort. (See the inside of the front book cover.)
16 Place the signal light within reach.
17 Lower the bed to its lowest position.
18 Raise or lower bed rails. Follow the care plan.

19 Unscreen the person.
20 Complete a safety check of the room. (See the inside of the front book cover.)
21 Practice hand hygiene.
22 Report and record your observations.

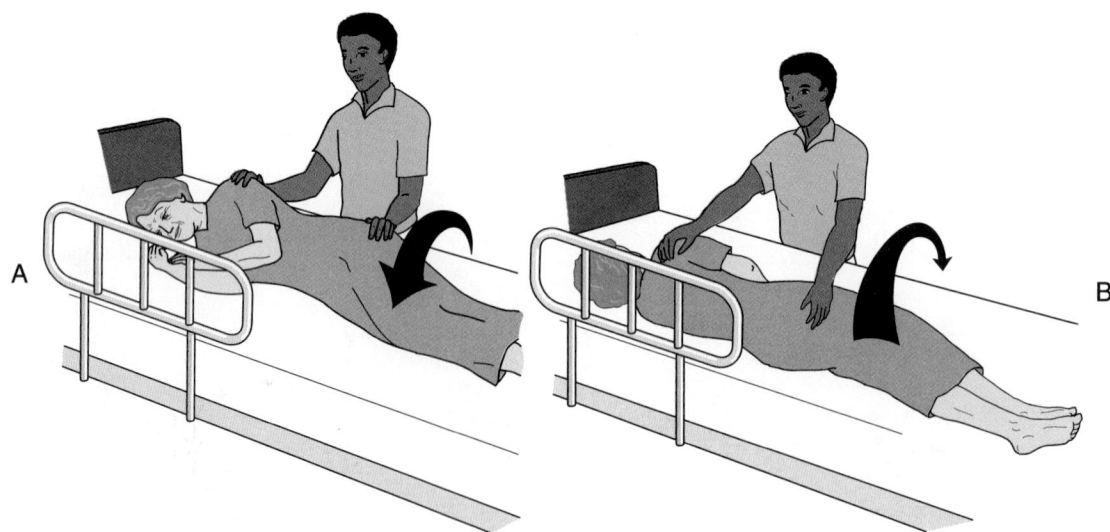

Fig. 17-14 Turning the person. **A,** Turning the person away from you, **B,** Turning the person toward you.
NOTE: Non-standard bed rails are used to show positioning and hand placement.

Logrolling

Logrolling is turning the person as a unit, in alignment, with one motion. The spine is kept straight. The procedure is used to turn:

- Older persons with arthritic spines or knees.
- Persons recovering from hip fractures.
- Persons with spinal cord injuries. The spine is kept straight at all times after spinal cord injury.
- Persons recovering from spinal surgery. The spine is kept straight at all times after spinal surgery.
  See *Promoting Safety and Comfort: Logrolling.*

PROMOTING SAFETY AND COMFORT
Logrolling

Safety

To logroll a person, 2 or 3 staff members are needed. If the person is tall or heavy, 3 are needed. Sometimes you use an assist device—drawsheet, turning pad, large incontinence product, slide sheet.

Comfort

After spinal cord injury or surgery, the spine and neck are kept straight. Therefore, *usually a pillow is not allowed under the head and neck.* Follow the nurse's directions and the care plan to position the person and use pillows.

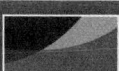

LOGROLLING THE PERSON

QUALITY OF LIFE

Remember to:
- Knock before entering the person's room.
- Address the person by name.
- Introduce yourself by name and title.

- Explain the procedure to the person before beginning and during the procedure.
- Protect the person's rights during the procedure.
- Handle the person gently during the procedure.

PRE-PROCEDURE

1 Follow *Delegation Guidelines:*
  a *Preventing Work-Related Injuries,* p. 258
  b *Moving Persons in Bed,* p. 259
  c *Turning Persons,* p. 267
  See *Promoting Safety and Comfort:*
  a *Safely Moving and Transferring Persons,* p. 255
  b *Preventing Work-Related Injuries,* p. 258
  c *Turning Persons,* p. 267
  d *Logrolling*

2 Ask a co-worker to help you.
3 Practice hand hygiene.
4 Identify the person. Check the ID bracelet against the assignment sheet. Also call the person by name.
5 Provide for privacy.
6 Lock the bed wheels.
7 Raise the bed for body mechanics. Bed rails are up if used.

PROCEDURE

8 Make sure the bed is flat.
9 Stand on the side opposite to which you will turn the person. Your co-worker stands on the other side.
10 Lower the bed rails if used.
11 Move the person as a unit to the side of the bed near you. Use the assist device. (If the person has a spinal cord injury, assist the nurse as directed.)
12 Place the person's arms across the chest. Place a pillow between the knees.
13 Raise the bed rail if used.
14 Go to the other side.
15 Stand near the shoulders and chest. Your co-worker stands near the hips and thighs.

16 Stand with a broad base of support. One foot is in front of the other.
17 Ask the person to hold his or her body rigid.
18 Roll the person toward you (Fig. 17-15, A, p. 270). Or use the assist device (Fig. 17-15, B, p. 270). Turn the person as a unit.
19 Position the person in good alignment. Use pillows as directed by the nurse and the care plan. The following is common (unless the spinal cord is involved):
  a One pillow against the back for support
  b One pillow under the head and neck if allowed
  c One pillow or a folded bath blanket between the legs
  d A small pillow under the upper arm and hand

POST-PROCEDURE

20 Provide for comfort. (See the inside of the front book cover.)
21 Place the signal light within reach.
22 Lower the bed to its lowest position.
23 Raise or lower bed rails. Follow the care plan.

24 Unscreen the person.
25 Complete a safety check of the room. (See the inside of the front book cover.)
26 Practice hand hygiene.
27 Report and record your observations.

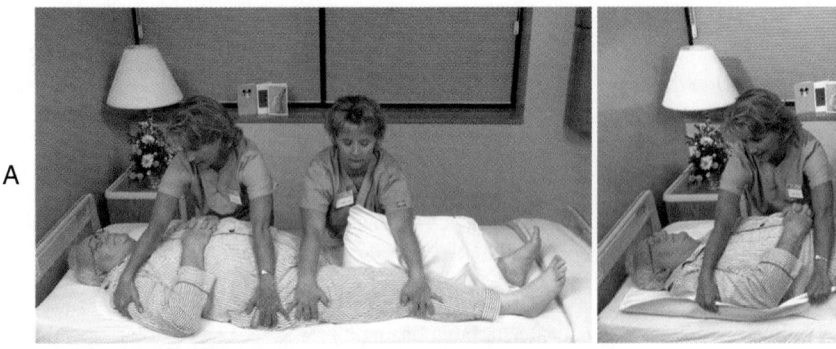

Fig. 17-15 Logrolling. **A,** A pillow is between the person's legs. The arms are crossed on the chest. The person is on the far side of the bed. **B,** The assist device is used to logroll the person.

SITTING ON THE SIDE OF THE BED (DANGLING)

Patients and residents sit on the side of the bed *(dangle)* for many reasons. Many older persons become dizzy or faint when getting out of bed too fast. They may need to sit on the side of the bed for 1 to 5 minutes before walking or transferring. Some persons increase activity in stages—bedrest, to sitting on the side of the bed, and then to sitting in a chair. Walking is the next step.

While dangling the legs, the person coughs and deep breathes. He or she moves the legs back and forth in circles. This stimulates circulation.

Two staff members may be needed. Persons with balance and coordination problems need support. If dizziness or fainting occurs, lay the person down.

See *Focus on Children and Older Persons: Dangling.*
See *Delegation Guidelines: Dangling.*
See *Promoting Safety and Comfort: Dangling.*

FOCUS ON CHILDREN AND OLDER PERSONS
Dangling

Older Persons
Many older persons have circulatory changes. They may become dizzy or faint when getting up too fast. Let them sit on the side of the bed for a few minutes before a transfer or walking.

DELEGATION GUIDELINES
Dangling

The nurse may ask you to help a person sit on the side of the bed. The procedure is part of other tasks—assisting the person to stand, transferring from bed to chair, partial bath, and others. Before the dangling procedure, you need this information from the nurse and the care plan:

- Areas of weakness. For example, if the arms are weak, the person cannot hold on to the side of the mattress for support. If the left side is weak, turn the person onto the stronger right side. The person uses the right arm to help move from the lying to sitting position.
- The person's dependence level (see Box 17-2).
- The amount of help the person needs.
- If you need a co-worker to help you.
- If the bed is raised or in its lowest position.
- How long the person needs to sit on the side of the bed.
- What exercises the person needs to perform while dangling:
  - Range-of-motion exercises (Chapter 27)
  - Deep-breathing and coughing exercises (Chapter 36)
- If the person will walk or transfer to a chair after dangling. If yes, the bed is in its lowest position.
- What observations to report and record (Fig. 17-16):
  - Pulse and respiratory rates (Chapter 26)
  - Pale or bluish skin color *(cyanosis)*
  - Complaints of dizziness, light-headedness, or difficulty breathing
  - Who helped you with the procedure
  - How well the activity was tolerated
  - The length of time the person dangled
  - The amount of help needed
  - Other observations and complaints
- When to report observations.
- What patient or resident concerns to report at once.

PROMOTING SAFETY AND COMFORT
Dangling

Safety

This procedure is *not* used for persons with a:
- Code 4: Total Dependence
- Code 3: Extensive Assistance

Sitting and balance problems often occur after illness, injury, surgery, and bedrest. Some persons who are disabled also have problems sitting and with balance. Support the person who is sitting on the side of the bed. Have a co-worker help you. This protects the person from falling and other injuries.

Comfort

Provide for the person's warmth during the dangling procedure. Help the person put on a robe. Or cover the person's shoulders and back with a bath blanket.

The person may want to perform hygiene measures while sitting on the side of the bed. Oral hygiene and washing the face and hands are examples. These measures are refreshing and stimulate circulation. Follow the nurse's directions and the care plan.

Date	Time	Nursing Margin	Other Depts Margin
9/9	0900	Assisted to sit on the side of the bed with assistance of one. Active leg exercises performed. Tolerated procedure without complaints of pain or discomfort. No c/o dizziness. BP-130/78 L arm sitting, P-74 regular rate and rhythm, R-20 unlabored. Color good. Assisted to lie down after 5 minutes. Positioned on L side. Bed in low position, signal light within reach. Adam Aims, CNA ————	

Fig. 17-16 Charting sample.

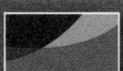

SITTING ON THE SIDE OF THE BED (DANGLING)

QUALITY OF LIFE

Remember to:
- Knock before entering the person's room.
- Address the person by name.
- Introduce yourself by name and title.
- Explain the procedure to the person before beginning and during the procedure.
- Protect the person's rights during the procedure.
- Handle the person gently during the procedure.

PRE-PROCEDURE

1 Follow *Delegation Guidelines:*
 a *Preventing Work-Related Injuries,* p. 258
 b *Dangling*
 See *Promoting Safety and Comfort:*
 a *Safely Moving and Transferring Persons,* p. 255
 b *Preventing Work-Related Injuries,* p. 258
 c *Dangling*
2 Ask a co-worker to help you if the person will dangle.
3 Practice hand hygiene.
4 Identify the person. Check the ID bracelet against the assignment sheet. Also call the person by name.
5 Provide for privacy.
6 Decide what side of the bed to use.
7 Move furniture to provide moving space.
8 Lock the bed wheels.
9 Raise the bed for body mechanics. Bed rails are up if used.

Continued

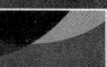

SITTING ON THE SIDE OF THE BED (DANGLING)—cont'd

PROCEDURE

10 Lower the bed rail if up.
11 Position the person in a side-lying position facing you. The person lies on the strong side.
12 Raise the head of the bed to a sitting position.
13 Stand by the person's hips. Face the foot of the bed.
14 Stand with your feet apart. The foot near the head of the bed is in front of the other foot.
15 Slide one arm under the person's neck and shoulders. Grasp the far shoulder. Place your other hand over the thighs near the knees (Fig. 17-17, A).
16 Pivot toward the foot of the bed while moving the person's legs and feet over the side of the bed. As the legs go over the edge of the mattress, the trunk is upright (Fig. 17-17, B).
17 Ask the person to hold on to the edge of the mattress. This supports the person in the sitting position. If possible, raise a half-length bed rail for the person to grasp. Raise the bed rail on the person's strong side. Have your co-worker support the person at all times.

18 Do not leave the person alone. Provide support at all times.
19 Check the person's condition:
   a Ask how the person feels. Ask if the person feels dizzy or light-headed.
   b Check the pulse and respirations.
   c Check for difficulty breathing.
   d Note if the skin is pale or bluish in color *(cyanosis)*.
20 Reverse the procedure to return the person to bed. (Or prepare to transfer the person to a chair or wheelchair. Lower the bed to its lowest position so the person's feet are flat on the floor. Support the person at all times.)
21 Lower the head of the bed after the person returns to bed. Help him or her move to the center of the bed.
22 Position the person in good alignment.

POST-PROCEDURE

23 Provide for comfort. (See the inside of the front book cover.)
24 Place the signal light within reach.
25 Lower the bed to its lowest position.
26 Raise or lower bed rails. Follow the care plan.
27 Return furniture to its proper place.

28 Unscreen the person.
29 Complete a safety check of the room. (See the inside of the front book cover.)
30 Practice hand hygiene.
31 Report and record your observations.

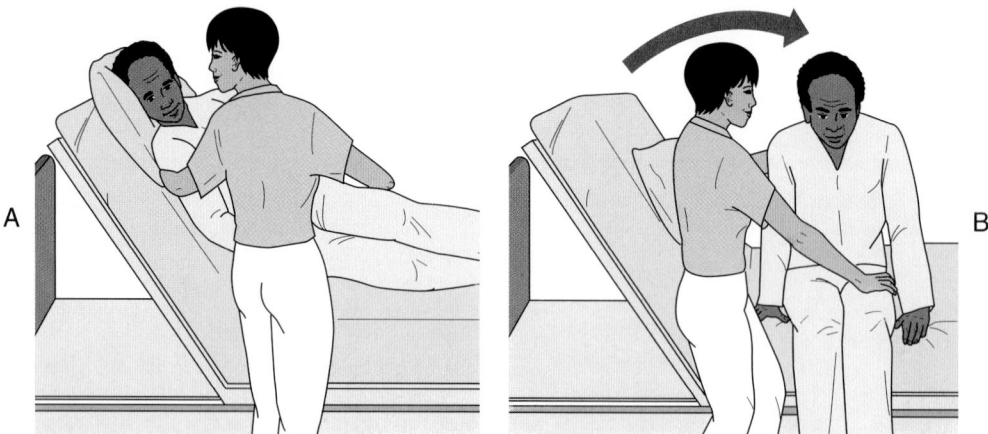

Fig. 17-17 Helping the person sit on the side of the bed. **A,** The person's shoulders and thighs are supported. **B,** The person sits upright as the legs and feet are pulled over the edge of the bed.

TRANSFERRING PERSONS

Patients and residents are moved to and from beds, chairs, wheelchairs, shower chairs, commodes, toilets, and stretchers. The amount of help needed and the method used vary with the person's dependency level (see Box 17-2). Some persons transfer by themselves or need little help. Some persons need help from at least 1, 2, or 3 people.

The rules of body mechanics apply to transfers (Chapter 16). So do the guidelines in Box 17-1. Arrange the room so there is enough space for a safe transfer. Correct placement of the chair, wheelchair, or other device also is needed for a safe transfer.

See *Delegation Guidelines: Transferring Persons.*
See *Promoting Safety and Comfort: Transferring Persons.*
See *Teamwork and Time Management: Transferring Persons.*

Transfer Belts

Transfer belts were discussed in Chapter 13. Also called gait belts, they are used to support patients and residents during transfers. They also are used for re-positioning in chairs and wheelchairs (p. 285).

Wider belts have padded handles. They are easier to grip and allow better control should the person fall.

DELEGATION GUIDELINES
Transferring Persons

Before a transfer procedure, you need this information from the nurse and the care plan:
* What procedure to use.
* The person's dependency level (see Box 17-2).
* The amount of help the person needs.
* What equipment to use—transfer belt, wheelchair, mechanical assist device, positioning devices, wheelchair cushion, and so on.
* The person's height and weight.
* The number of staff needed to complete the task safely.
* Areas of weakness. For example, if the arms are weak, the person cannot hold on to the mattress for support. If the left side is weak, he or she gets out of bed on the stronger right side. The person uses the right arm to help move from the lying to sitting position.
* What observations to report and record:
  * Pulse rate before and after the transfer (Chapter 26)
  * Complaints of light-headedness, pain, discomfort, difficulty breathing, weakness, or fatigue
  * The amount of help needed to transfer the person
  * Who helped you with the procedure
  * How the person helped with the transfer
  * How you positioned the person
* When to report observations.
* What patient or resident concerns to report at once.

PROMOTING SAFETY AND COMFORT
Transferring Persons

Safety

The person wears non-skid footwear for transfers. Such footwear protects the person from falls. Slipping and sliding are prevented. Tie shoelaces securely. Otherwise the person can trip and fall.

Check the length of the person's gown or robe if necessary. Long gowns and robes can cause falls. Also, avoid robes with long ties. The person can trip and fall.

Lock bed, wheelchair, and stretcher wheels and wheels on other devices. This prevents the bed and the device from moving during the transfer. Otherwise, the person can fall. You also are at risk for injury.

Comfort

After the transfer, position the person in good alignment. Place needed items within reach.

TEAMWORK AND TIME MANAGEMENT
Transferring Persons

Mechanical assist devices are used to transfer some persons. After using such a device, return it to the storage area. It needs to be there for other staff. Do not leave a device in a person's room or other area. Co-workers should not have to assume that an assist device is in use or take time looking for one.

Many mechanical assist devices are battery-operated. The battery must be charged for the device to work properly. Follow agency policy to charge or replace batteries.

You may need help from 1 or 2 co-workers for a safe transfer. Politely ask co-workers to help you. Tell them what time you need the help and for how long. This helps them plan their own work. Always thank your co-workers for helping you. Willingly help them when asked.

Bed to Chair or Wheelchair Transfers

Safety is important for chair, wheelchair, commode, and shower chair transfers. Help the person out of bed on his or her strong side. If the left side is weak and the right side strong, get the person out of bed on the right side. In transferring, the strong side moves first. It pulls the weaker side along. Transfers from the weak side are awkward and unsafe.

The following stand and pivot transfers are used if:
* The person's legs are strong enough to bear some or all of his or her weight.
* The person is cooperative and can follow directions.
* The person can assist with the transfer.

See *Promoting Safety and Comfort: Bed to Chair or Wheelchair Transfers, p. 274.*

Text continued on p. 277

PROMOTING SAFETY AND COMFORT
Bed to Chair or Wheelchair Transfers

Safety

The chair, wheelchair, or other device must support the person's weight. The number of staff needed for a transfer depends on the person's abilities, condition, and size. Sometimes you will use mechanical assist devices (p. 278).

The person must not put his or her arms around your neck. Otherwise the person can pull you forward or cause you to lose your balance. Neck, back, and other injuries from falls are possible.

If not using a mechanical assist device, using a gait/transfer belt is the preferred method for chair or wheelchair transfers. It is safer for the person and you. Putting your arms around the person and grasping the shoulder blades is the other method. It can cause the person discomfort. And it can be stressful for you. Use this method *only* if instructed to do so by the nurse and the care plan.

Safety—cont'd

Bed and wheelchair wheels are locked for a safe transfer. After the transfer, unlock the wheelchair wheels to position the wheelchair as the person prefers. After positioning the chair, lock the wheels or keep them unlocked according to the care plan. Locked wheels may be viewed as restraints if the person cannot unlock them to move the wheelchair (Chapter 14). However, falls and other injuries are risks if the person tries to stand when the wheelchair wheels are unlocked.

Comfort

Most wheelchairs and bedside chairs have vinyl seats and backs. Vinyl holds body heat. The person becomes warm and perspires more. If the nurse allows, cover the back and seat with a folded bath blanket. This increases the person's comfort in the chair. Some people have wheelchair cushions or positioning devices. Ask the nurse how to use and place the devices. Also follow the manufacturer's instructions.

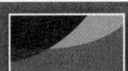 # TRANSFERRING THE PERSON TO A CHAIR OR WHEELCHAIR

QUALITY OF LIFE

Remember to:
- Knock before entering the person's room.
- Address the person by name.
- Introduce yourself by name and title.

- Explain the procedure to the person before beginning and during the procedure.
- Protect the person's rights during the procedure.
- Handle the person gently during the procedure.

PRE-PROCEDURE

1 Follow *Delegation Guidelines:*
   a *Preventing Work-Related Injuries,* p. 258
   b *Transferring Persons,* p. 273
   See *Promoting Safety and Comfort:*
   a *Transfer/Gait Belts* (Chapter 13)
   b *Safely Moving and Transferring Persons,* p. 255
   c *Preventing Work-Related Injuries,* p. 258
   d *Transferring Persons,* p. 273
   e *Bed to Chair or Wheelchair Transfers*
2 Collect:
   - Wheelchair or arm chair
   - Bath blanket

- Lap blanket
- Robe and non-skid footwear
- Paper or sheet
- Transfer belt (if needed)
- Seat cushion (if needed)
3 Practice hand hygiene.
4 Identify the person. Check the ID bracelet against the assignment sheet. Also call the person by name.
5 Provide for privacy.
6 Decide which side of the bed to use. Move furniture for a safe transfer.

PROCEDURE

7 Raise the wheelchair footplates. Remove or swing front rigging out of the way if possible. Position the chair or wheelchair near the bed on the person's strong side:
   a If at the head of the bed, it faces the foot of the bed.
   b If at the foot of the bed, it faces the head of the bed.
   c The armrest almost touches the bed.
8 Place a folded bath blanket or cushion on the seat (if needed).
9 Lock the wheelchair wheels.

10 Lower the bed to its lowest position. Lock the bed wheels.
11 Fan-fold top linens to the foot of the bed.
12 Place the paper or sheet under the person's feet. (This protects the person's linens from the footwear.) Put footwear on the person.
13 Help the person sit on the side of the bed (p. 271). His or her feet touch the floor.
14 Help the person put on a robe.

TRANSFERRING THE PERSON TO A CHAIR OR WHEELCHAIR—cont'd

PROCEDURE—cont'd

15 Apply the transfer belt if needed (Chapter 13). It is applied at the waist over clothing.

16 *Method 1: Using a transfer belt:*
- **a** Stand in front of the person.
- **b** Have the person hold on to the mattress.
- **c** Make sure the person's feet are flat on the floor.
- **d** Have the person lean forward.
- **e** Grasp the transfer belt at each side. Grasp the handles or grasp the belt from underneath. See Chapter 13.
- **f** Prevent the person from sliding or falling. Do one of the following:
  - **(1)** Brace your knees against the person's knees. Block his or her feet with your feet (Fig. 17-18, p. 276).
  - **(2)** Use the knee and foot of one leg to block the person's weak leg or foot. Place your other foot slightly behind you for balance.
  - **(3)** Straddle your legs around the person's weak leg.
- **g** Explain the following:
  - **(1)** You will count "1, 2, 3."
  - **(2)** The move will be on "3."
  - **(3)** On "3," the person pushes down on the mattress and stands.
- **h** Ask the person to push down on the mattress and to stand on the count of "3." Pull the person to a standing position as you straighten your knees (Fig. 17-19, p. 276).

17 *Method 2: No transfer belt:* (NOTE: Use this method only if directed by the nurse and the care plan.)
- **a** Follow steps 16, a–c.
- **b** Place your hands under the person's arms. Your hands are around the person's shoulder blades (Fig. 17-20, p. 276).
- **c** Have the person lean forward.

- **d** Prevent the person from sliding or falling. Do one of the following:
  - **(1)** Brace your knees against the person's knees. Block his or her feet with your feet.
  - **(2)** Use the knee and foot of one leg to block the person's weak leg or foot. Place your other foot slightly behind you for balance.
  - **(3)** Straddle your legs around the person's weak leg.
- **e** Explain the "count of 3." See step 16, g.
- **f** Ask the person to push down on the mattress and to stand on the count of "3." Pull the person up into a standing position as you straighten your knees.

18 Support the person in the standing position. Hold the transfer belt, or keep your hands around the person's shoulder blades. Continue to prevent the person from sliding or falling.

19 Turn the person so he or she can grasp the far arm of the chair or wheelchair. The legs will touch the edge of the seat (Fig. 17-21, p. 276).

20 Continue to turn the person until the other armrest is grasped.

21 Lower him or her into the chair or wheelchair as you bend your hips and knees. To assist, the person leans forward and bends the elbows and knees (Fig. 17-22, p. 276).

22 Make sure the hips are to the back of the seat. Position the person in good alignment.

23 Attach the wheelchair front rigging. Position the person's feet on the wheelchair footplates.

24 Cover the person's lap and legs with a lap blanket. Keep the blanket off the floor and the wheels.

25 Remove the transfer belt if used.

26 Position the chair as the person prefers. Lock the wheelchair wheels according to the care plan.

POST-PROCEDURE

27 Provide for comfort. (See the inside of the front book cover.)

28 Place the signal light and other needed items within reach.

29 Unscreen the person.

30 Complete a safety check of the room. (See the inside of the front book cover.)

31 Practice hand hygiene.

32 Report and record your observations.

33 See procedure: *Transferring the Person From a Chair or Wheelchair to Bed* (p. 277) to return the person to bed.

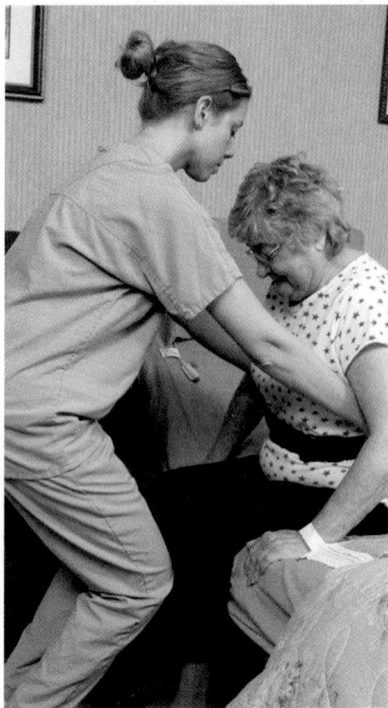

Fig. 17-18 The person's feet and knees are blocked by the nursing assistant's feet and knees. This prevents the person from sliding or falling.

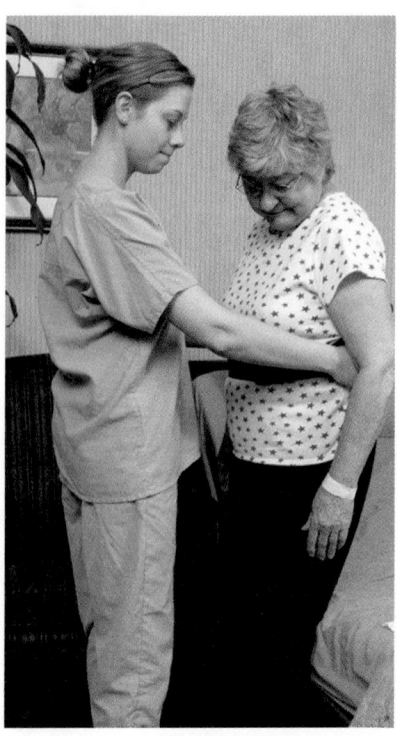

Fig. 17-19 The person is pulled up to a standing position and supported by holding the transfer belt and blocking the person's knees and feet.

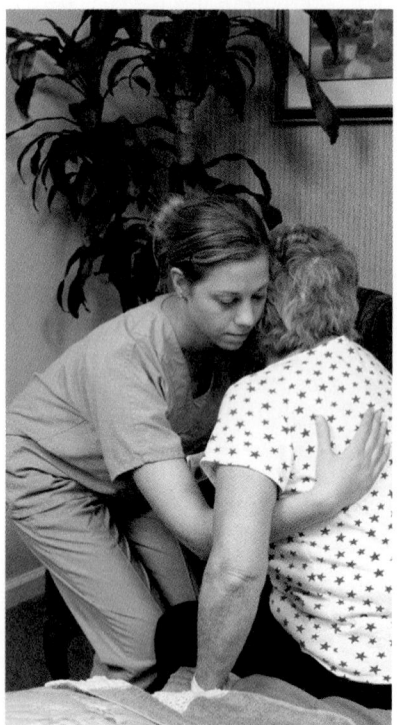

Fig. 17-20 The person is being prepared to stand. The hands are placed under the person's arms and around the shoulder blades.

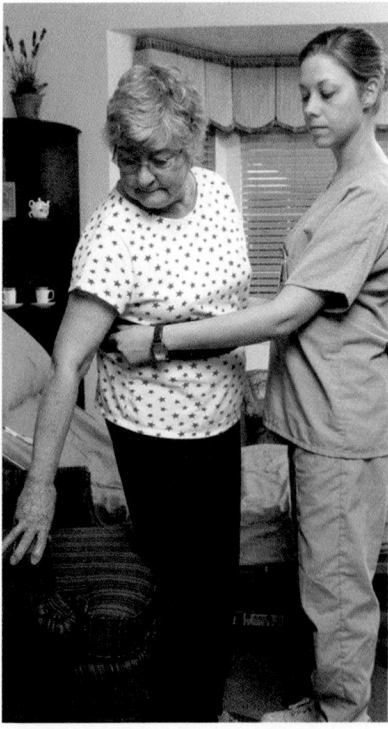

Fig. 17-21 The person is supported as he or she grasps the far arm of the chair. The legs are against the chair.

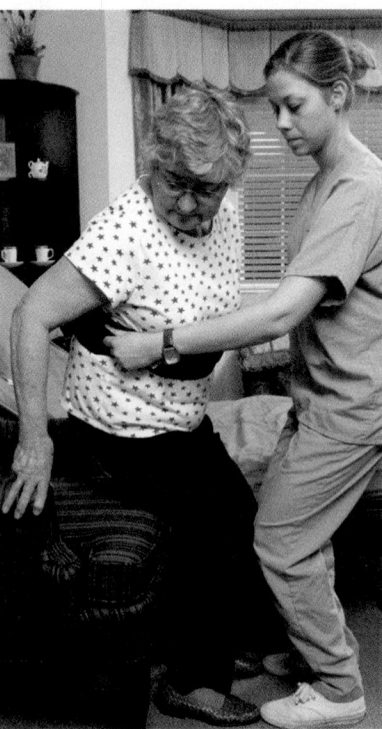

Fig. 17-22 The person holds the armrests, leans forward, and bends the elbows and knees while being lowered into the chair.

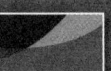

Chair or Wheelchair to Bed Transfers

Chair or wheelchair to bed transfers have the same rules as bed to chair transfers. If the person is weak on one side, transfer the person so that the strong side moves first. Or position the chair or wheelchair so the person's strong side is near the bed. The strong side moves first.

For example, Mrs. Lee's right side is weak. Her left side is strong. To transfer her from bed to chair, the chair was on the left side of the bed. This allowed her left side (strong side) to move first. Now you will transfer Mrs. Lee back to bed. If the chair is on the left side of the bed, her weak right side is near the bed. Moving the weak side first is not safe. Move the chair to the other side of the bed or turn the chair around. Mrs. Lee's stronger left side will be near the bed. The stronger side moves first for a safe transfer.

TRANSFERRING THE PERSON FROM A CHAIR OR WHEELCHAIR TO BED

QUALITY OF LIFE

Remember to:
- Knock before entering the person's room.
- Address the person by name.
- Introduce yourself by name and title.

- Explain the procedure to the person before beginning and during the procedure.
- Protect the person's rights during the procedure.
- Handle the person gently during the procedure.

PRE-PROCEDURE

1 Follow *Delegation Guidelines:*
  a *Preventing Work-Related Injuries,* p. 258
  b *Transferring Persons,* p. 273
  See *Promoting Safety and Comfort:*
  a *Transfer/Gait Belts* (Chapter 13)
  b *Safely Moving and Transferring Persons,* p. 255
  c *Preventing Work-Related Injuries,* p. 258

  d *Transferring Persons,* p. 273
  e *Bed to Chair or Wheelchair Transfers,* p. 274
2 Collect a transfer belt if needed.
3 Practice hand hygiene.
4 Identify the person. Check the ID bracelet against the assignment sheet. Also call the person by name.
5 Provide for privacy.

PROCEDURE

6 Move furniture for moving space.
7 Raise the head of the bed to a sitting position. The bed is in the lowest position.
8 Move the signal light so it is on the strong side when the person is in bed.
9 Position the chair or wheelchair so the person's strong side is next to the bed (Fig. 17-23, p. 278). Have a co-worker help you if necessary.
10 Lock the wheelchair and bed wheels.
11 Remove and fold the lap blanket.
12 Remove the person's feet from the footplates. Raise the footplates. Remove or swing the front rigging out of the way. (The person has on non-skid footwear.)
13 Apply the transfer belt (if needed).
14 Make sure the person's feet are flat on the floor.
15 Stand in front of the person.
16 Ask the person to hold on to the armrests. (If the nurse directs you to do so, place your arms under the person's arms. Your hands are around the shoulder blades.)
17 Have the person lean forward.
18 Grasp the transfer belt on each side if using it. Grasp underneath the belt.

19 Prevent the person from sliding or falling. Do one of the following:
  a Brace your knees against the person's knees. Block his or her feet with your feet.
  b Use the knee and foot of one leg to block the person's weak leg or foot. Place your other foot slightly behind you for balance.
  c Straddle your legs around the person's weak leg.
20 Explain the "count of 3." (See procedure: *Transferring the Person to a Chair or Wheelchair,* p. 274.)
21 Ask the person to push down on the armrests on the count of "3." Pull the person into a standing position as you straighten your knees.
22 Support the person in the standing position. Hold the transfer belt, or keep your hands around the person's shoulder blades. Continue to prevent the person from sliding or falling.
23 Turn the person so he or she can reach the edge of the mattress. The legs will touch the mattress.
24 Continue to turn the person until he or she can reach the mattress with both hands.
25 Lower him or her onto the bed as you bend your hips and knees. To assist, the person leans forward and bends the elbows and knees.
26 Remove the transfer belt.
27 Remove the robe and footwear.
28 Help the person lie down.

Continued

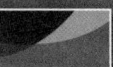

TRANSFERRING THE PERSON FROM A CHAIR OR WHEELCHAIR TO BED—cont'd

POST-PROCEDURE

29 Provide for comfort. (See the inside of the front book cover.)
30 Place the signal light and other needed items within reach.
31 Raise or lower bed rails. Follow the care plan.
32 Arrange furniture to meet the person's needs.

33 Unscreen the person.
34 Complete a safety check of the room. (See the inside of the front book cover.)
35 Practice hand hygiene.
36 Report and record your observations.

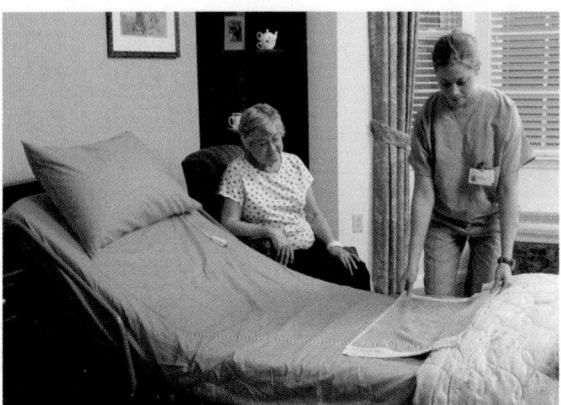

Fig. 17-23 The chair is positioned so the person's strong side is near the bed.

Mechanical Lifts

Persons who cannot help themselves are transferred with mechanical lifts (Fig. 17-24). So are persons too heavy for the staff to transfer. Use the devices for transfers to and from beds, chairs, stretchers, tubs, shower chairs, toilets, commodes, whirlpools, or vehicles.

There are manual, battery-operated, and electric lifts. Some lifts are mounted on the ceiling. Your agency may have bariatric lifts—floor-based or ceiling (Fig. 17-25).

Slings. The type of sling used depends on the person's size, condition, and other needs. Slings are padded, unpadded, or made of mesh.

- *Standard full sling*—for normal transfers.
- *Extended length sling*—for persons with extra large thighs.
- *Bathing sling*—to transfer the person directly from the bed or chair into a bathtub. The sling is left in place and attached to the lift during the bath.
- *Toileting sling*—the sling bottom is open. For infection control, each person has his or her own toileting sling.

- *Amputee sling*—for the person who has had both legs amputated (double amputee).
- *Bariatric sling*—for use with a bariatric lift. There are also bariatric bathing and toileting slings. The nurse may have you leave the sling under the person at all times. The person is not turned from side-to-side to place and remove the sling each time he or she is moved or transferred. This reduces the risk of injury to the person and staff.

Follow agency policy and the manufacturer's instructions for washing slings. Also follow agency policy for handling and washing contaminated slings. A sling is contaminated if it:

- Has any visible sign of blood, body fluids, secretions, or excretions.
- Is used on a person's bare skin.
- Is used to bathe a person.

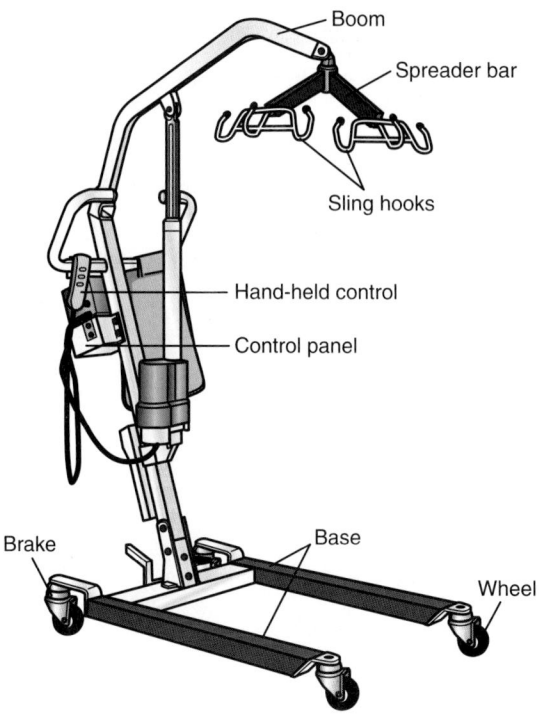

Fig. 17-24 Parts of a mechanical lift.

Boom
Spreader bar
Sling hooks
Hand-held control
Control panel
Brake
Base
Wheel

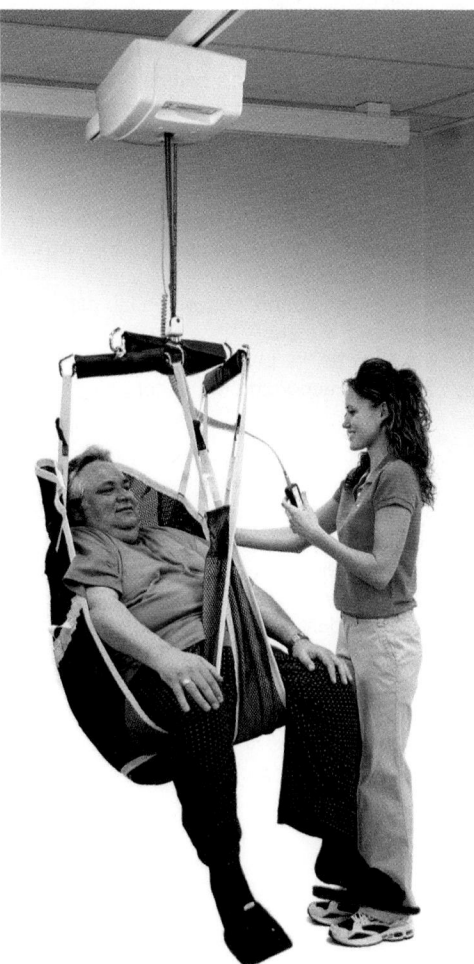

Fig. 17-25 Bariatric ceiling lift.

Using a Mechanical Lift. Before using a lift:
- You must be trained in its use.
- It must work.
- The sling, straps, hooks, and chains must be in good repair.
- The person's weight must not exceed the lift's capacity.
- At least 2 staff members are needed.

There are different types of mechanical lifts. Always follow the manufacturer's instructions. The procedure on p. 280 is used as a guide.

See *Delegation Guidelines: Using a Mechanical Lift.*
See *Promoting Safety and Comfort: Using a Mechanical Lift.*

DELEGATION GUIDELINES
Using a Mechanical Lift

Before using a mechanical lift, you need this information from the nurse and the care plan:
- The person's dependency level (see Box 17-2).
- What lift to use.
- If you need to apply an abdominal binder. For the person with bariatric needs, an abdominal binder may be used if the person's abdomen is in the way. See Chapter 33.
- What sling to use—full, extended length, bathing, toileting, amputee, bariatric.
- If a padded, unpadded, or mesh sling is needed.
- What size sling to use.
- How many co-workers are needed to perform the task safely.

PROMOTING SAFETY AND COMFORT
Using a Mechanical Lift

Safety

Always follow the manufacturer's instructions. Knowing how to use one lift does not mean that you know how to use others.

If you have questions, ask the nurse. If you have not used a certain lift before, ask for needed training. Ask the nurse to help you until you are comfortable using the lift.

Mechanical lifts must be in good working order. Tell the nurse when a lift needs repair or is not working properly.

Some mechanical lifts are powered by batteries. The batteries must be well-charged. Follow the manufacturer's instructions and agency policy.

For persons with bariatric needs:
- Make sure the receiving surface (bed, chair, wheelchair, stretcher, and so on) has expanded capacity for the person's weight.
- Use a chair or wheelchair with arms that you can remove or lower.

Comfort

The person is lifted up and off the bed or chair. Falling from the lift is a common fear. To promote the person's mental comfort, always explain the procedure before you begin. Also show the person how the lift works.

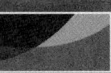 **TRANSFERRING THE PERSON USING A MECHANICAL LIFT** `VIDEO`

QUALITY OF LIFE

Remember to:
- Knock before entering the person's room.
- Address the person by name.
- Introduce yourself by name and title.

- Explain the procedure to the person before beginning and during the procedure.
- Protect the person's rights during the procedure.
- Handle the person gently during the procedure.

PRE-PROCEDURE

1 Follow *Delegation Guidelines:*
  a *Preventing Work-Related Injuries,* p. 258
  b *Transferring Persons,* p. 273
  c *Using a Mechanical Lift,* p. 279
  See *Promoting Safety and Comfort:*
  a *Safely Moving and Transferring Persons,* p. 255
  b *Preventing Work-Related Injuries,* p. 258
  c *Transferring Persons,* p. 273
  d *Using a Mechanical Lift,* p. 279
2 Ask a co-worker to help you.

3 Collect:
  a Mechanical lift and sling
  b Arm chair or wheelchair
  c Footwear
  d Bath blanket or cushion
  e Lap blanket
4 Practice hand hygiene.
5 Identify the person. Check the ID bracelet against the assignment sheet. Also call the person by name.
6 Provide for privacy.

PROCEDURE

7 Raise the bed for body mechanics. Bed rails are up if used.
8 Lower the head of the bed to a level appropriate for the person. It is as flat as possible.
9 Stand on one side of the bed. Your co-worker stands on the other side.
10 Lower the bed rails if up. Lock the bed wheels.
11 Center the sling under the person (Fig. 17-26, A). To position the sling, turn the person from side to side as if making an occupied bed (Chapter 19). Follow the manufacturer's instructions to position the sling.
12 Position the person in semi-Fowler's position.
13 Place the chair at the head of the bed. It is even with the head-board and about 1 foot away from the bed. Place a folded bath blanket or cushion in the chair.
14 Lower the bed to its lowest position.
15 Raise the lift so you can position it over the person.
16 Position the lift over the person (Fig. 17-26, B).
17 Lock the lift wheels in position.
18 Attach the sling to the sling hooks (Fig. 17-26, C).

19 Raise the head of the bed to a sitting position.
20 Cross the person's arms over the chest.
21 Raise the lift high enough until the person and sling are free of the bed (Fig. 17-26, D).
22 Have your co-worker support the person's legs as you move the lift and the person away from the bed (Fig. 17-26, E).
23 Position the lift so the person's back is toward the chair.
24 Position the chair so you can lower the person into it.
25 Lower the person into the chair. Guide the person into the chair (Fig. 17-26, F).
26 Lower the spreader bar to unhook the sling. Remove the sling from under the person unless otherwise indicated.
27 Put footwear on the person. Position the person's feet on the wheelchair footplates.
28 Cover the person's lap and legs with a lap blanket. Keep it off the floor and wheels.
29 Position the chair as the person prefers. Lock the wheelchair wheels according to the care plan.

POST-PROCEDURE

30 Provide for comfort. (See the inside of the front book cover.)
31 Place the signal light and other needed items within the person's reach.
32 Unscreen the person.

33 Complete a safety check of the room. (See the inside of the front book cover.)
34 Practice hand hygiene.
35 Report and record your observations.
36 Reverse the procedure to return the person to bed.

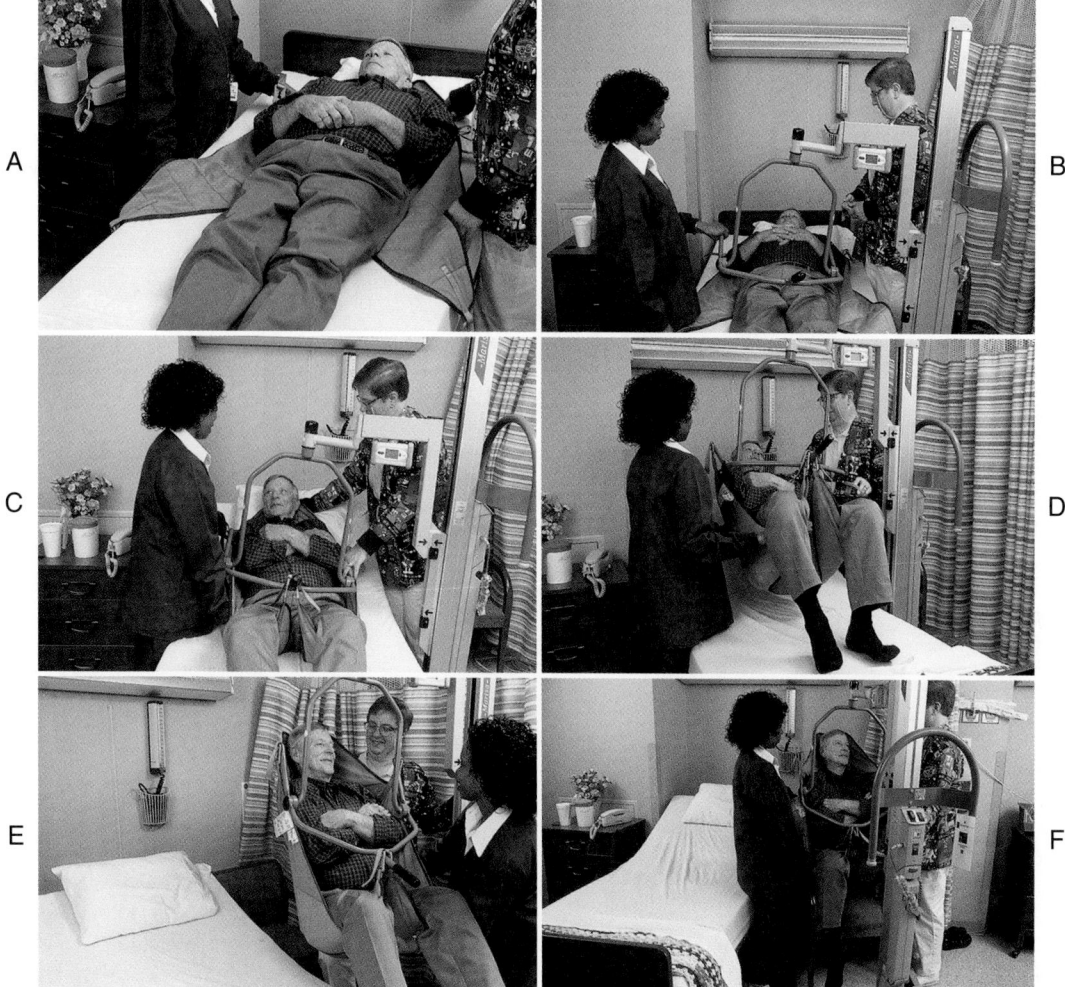

Fig. 17-26 Using a mechanical lift. **A,** The sling is positioned under the person. **B,** The lift is over the person. **C,** The sling is attached to the spreader bar. **D,** The lift is raised until the sling and person are off of the bed. **E,** The person's legs are supported as the person and lift are moved away from the bed. **F,** The person is guided into a chair.

Transferring the Person To and From the Toilet

Using the bathroom for elimination promotes dignity, self-esteem, and independence. It also is more private than using a bedpan, urinal, or bedside commode. However, getting to the toilet is hard for persons who use wheelchairs. Bathrooms are often small. There is little room for you or a wheelchair. Therefore transfers involving wheelchairs and toilets are often hard. Falls and work-related injuries are risks.

Sometimes mechanical lifts are used to transfer the person to and from a toilet. A sliding board (see Fig. 17-4) may be used if:

- The wheelchair armrests can be removed.
- The person has upper body strength.
- The person has good sitting balance.
- There is enough room to position the wheelchair next to the toilet.

The procedure on p. 282 can be used if the person can stand and pivot from the wheelchair to the toilet.

See *Promoting Safety and Comfort: Transferring the Person to and From the Toilet,* p. 282.

Safety

Make sure the person has a raised toilet seat. The toilet seat and wheelchair are at the same level.

A standard toilet has a weight limit of 350 pounds. For persons with bariatric needs:

- Do not have the person use a wall-mounted toilet. A steel, floor-mounted toilet is best.
- Obtain a bariatric commode (Chapter 22) if the person's room does not have a floor-mounted toilet.

Check the grab bars by the toilet. If they are loose, tell the nurse. Do not transfer the person to the toilet if the grab bars are not secure.

Follow Standard Precautions and the Bloodborne Pathogen Standard. Wear gloves if the person is incontinent of urine or feces.

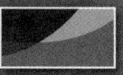

TRANSFERRING THE PERSON TO AND FROM THE TOILET

QUALITY OF LIFE

Remember to:
- Knock before entering the person's room.
- Address the person by name.
- Introduce yourself by name and title.

- Explain the procedure to the person before beginning and during the procedure.
- Protect the person's rights during the procedure.
- Handle the person gently during the procedure.

PRE-PROCEDURE

1 Follow *Delegation Guidelines:*
  a *Preventing Work-Related Injuries,* p. 258
  b *Transferring Persons,* p. 273
  See *Promoting Safety and Comfort:*
  a *Transfer/Gait Belts* (Chapter 13)
  b *Safely Moving and Transferring Persons,* p. 255

  c *Preventing Work-Related Injuries,* p. 258
  d *Transferring Persons,* p. 273
  e *Bed to Chair or Wheelchair Transfers,* p. 274
  f *Transferring the Person To and From the Toilet*
2 Practice hand hygiene.

PROCEDURE

3 Have the person wear non-skid footwear.
4 Position the wheelchair next to the toilet if there is enough room. If not, position the chair at a right angle (90-degree angle) to the toilet (Fig. 17-27). It is best if the person's strong side is near the toilet.
5 Lock the wheelchair wheels.
6 Raise the footplates. Remove or swing the front rigging out of the way.
7 Apply the transfer belt.
8 Help the person unfasten clothing.
9 Use the transfer belt to help the person stand and to turn to the toilet. (See procedure: *Transferring the Person to a Chair or Wheelchair,* p. 274.) The person uses the grab bars to turn to the toilet.
10 Support the person with the transfer belt while he or she lowers clothing. Or have the person hold on to the grab bars for support. Lower the person's pants and undergarments.
11 Use the transfer belt to lower the person onto the toilet seat. Make sure he or she is properly positioned on the toilet.
12 Remove the transfer belt.
13 Tell the person you will stay nearby. Remind the person to use the signal light or call for you when help is needed. Stay with the person if required by the care plan.

14 Close the bathroom door to provide for privacy.
15 Stay near the bathroom. Complete other tasks in the person's room. Check on the person every 5 minutes.
16 Knock on the bathroom door when the person calls for you.
17 Help with wiping, perineal care (Chapter 20), flushing, and hand washing as needed. Wear gloves and practice hand hygiene after removing and discarding the gloves.
18 Apply the transfer belt.
19 Use the transfer belt to help the person stand.
20 Help the person raise and secure clothing.
21 Use the transfer belt to transfer the person to the wheelchair. (See procedure: *Transferring the Person to a Chair or Wheelchair,* p. 274.)
22 Make sure the person's buttocks are to the back of the seat. Position the person in good alignment.
23 Position the person's feet on the footplates.
24 Remove the transfer belt.
25 Cover the person's lap and legs with a lap blanket. Keep the blanket off the floor and wheels.
26 Position the chair as the person prefers. Lock the wheelchair wheels according to the care plan.

POST-PROCEDURE

27 Provide for comfort. (See the inside of the front book cover.)
28 Place the signal light and other needed items within the person's reach.
29 Unscreen the person.

30 Complete a safety check of the room. (See the inside of the front book cover.)
31 Practice hand hygiene.
32 Report and record your observations.

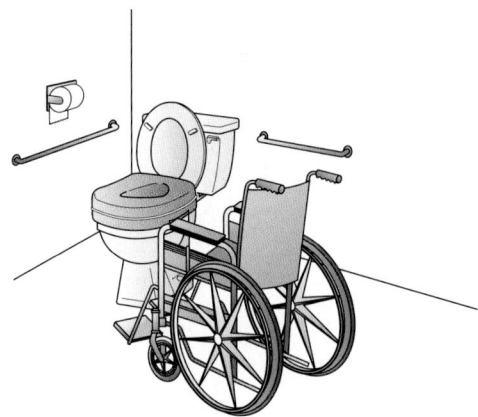

Fig. 17-27 The wheelchair is placed at a right angle (90-degree angle) to the toilet.

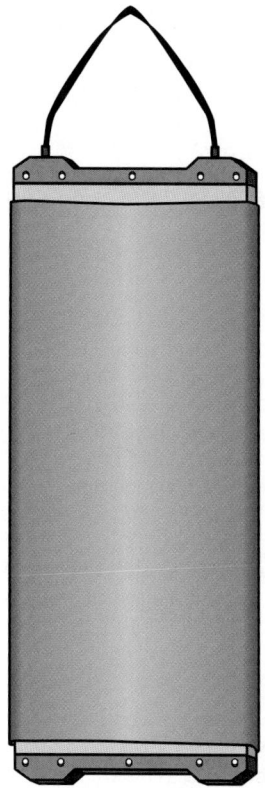

Fig. 17-28 Lateral transfer device with slide board.

Moving the Person to a Stretcher

Stretchers (gurneys) are used to transport persons to other areas. They are used for persons who:

- Cannot sit up
- Must stay in a lying position
- Are seriously ill

The stretcher is covered with a folded flat sheet or bath blanket. A pillow and extra blankets are on hand. If the nurse allows, raise the head of the stretcher to a Fowler's or semi-Fowler's position (Chapter 18). This increases the person's comfort.

A drawsheet, turning pad, large incontinence underpad, slide sheet, or lateral transfer device with slide board (Fig. 17-28) is used. At least 2 or 3 staff are needed for a safe transfer. OSHA recommends the following:

- If the person weighs less than 100 pounds—use a lateral sliding aid and 2 staff members
- If the person weighs 100 to 200 pounds—use a lateral sliding aid or a friction-reducing device and 2 staff members
- If the person weighs more than 200 pounds, use one of the following:
  - A lateral sliding aid and 3 staff members
  - A friction-reducing device or lateral transfer device and 2 staff members
  - A mechanical lateral transfer device with a built-in slide board

Safety straps are used when the person is on the stretcher. Side rails are kept up during the transport. The stretcher is moved feet first. This is so the staff member at the head of the stretcher can watch the person's breathing and color during the transport. Never leave a person on a stretcher alone.

See *Delegation Guidelines: Moving the Person to a Stretcher.*

See *Promoting Safety and Comfort: Moving the Person to a Stretcher.*

DELEGATION GUIDELINES

Moving the Person to a Stretcher

For persons with bariatric needs, the nurse and care plan may direct staff to:

- Use a bariatric stretcher. Check for the "EC" (expanded capacity) sticker and the weight limit.
- Raise or lower the stretcher so that it is ½ inch lower than the bed.
- Use a friction-reducing device or a mechanical lateral transfer device.
- Transfer the person from his or her stronger side.
- Apply an abdominal binder if the person's abdomen is in the way. See Chapter 33.

PROMOTING SAFETY AND COMFORT

Moving the Person to a Stretcher

Safety

Protect yourself and the person from injury:

- Position the stretcher and bed surfaces as close as possible to each other.
- Avoid extended reaches and bending your back. You may need to kneel on the bed or stretcher.
- Follow the rules for stretcher safety (Chapter 12).
- Make sure the bed and stretcher wheels are locked.
- Practice good body mechanics (Chapter 16) and follow the guidelines in Box 17-1.
- Keep the person in good alignment.
- Make sure you have enough help.
- Hold the person securely. You must not drop the person onto the floor.

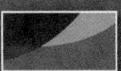 **MOVING THE PERSON TO A STRETCHER**

QUALITY OF LIFE

Remember to:
- Knock before entering the person's room.
- Address the person by name.
- Introduce yourself by name and title.

- Explain the procedure to the person before beginning and during the procedure.
- Protect the person's rights during the procedure.
- Handle the person gently during the procedure.

PRE-PROCEDURE

1 Follow *Delegation Guidelines:*
   a *Preventing Work-Related Injuries,* p. 258
   b *Transferring Persons,* p. 273
   c *Moving the Person to a Stretcher,* p. 283
   See *Promoting Safety and Comfort:*
   a *Safely Moving and Transferring Persons,* p. 255
   b *Preventing Work-Related Injuries,* p. 258
   c *Transferring Persons,* p. 273
   d *Moving the Person to a Stretcher,* p. 283
2 Ask 1 or 2 staff members to help you.

3 Collect:
   - Stretcher covered with a sheet or bath blanket
   - Bath blanket
   - Pillow(s) if needed
   - Slide sheet, lateral transfer device with slide board, drawsheet, or other assist device
4 Practice hand hygiene.
5 Identify the person. Check the ID bracelet against the assignment sheet. Also call the person by name.
6 Provide for privacy.
7 Raise the bed and stretcher for body mechanics.

PROCEDURE

8 Position yourself and co-workers:
   a One or two workers stand on the side of the bed where the stretcher will be.
   b One worker stands on the other side of the bed.
9 Lower the head of the bed. It is as flat as possible.
10 Lower the bed rails if used.
11 Cover the person with a bath blanket. Fan-fold top linens to the foot of the bed.
12 Position the assist device. Or loosen the drawsheet on each side.
13 Use the assist device to move the person to the side of the bed. This is the side where the stretcher will be.
14 Protect the person from falling. Hold the far arm and leg.

15 Have your co-workers position the stretcher next to the bed. They stand behind the stretcher (Fig. 17-29, A).
16 Lock the bed and stretcher wheels.
17 Grasp the assist device (Fig. 17-29, B).
18 Transfer the person to the stretcher on the count of "3." Center the person on the stretcher.
19 Place a pillow or pillows under the person's head and shoulders if allowed. Raise the head of the stretcher if allowed.
20 Cover the person. Provide for comfort.
21 Fasten the safety straps. Raise the side rails.
22 Unlock the stretcher wheels. Transport the person.

POST-PROCEDURE

23 Practice hand hygiene.
24 Report and record:
   - The time of the transport
   - Where the person was transported to

   - Who went with him or her
   - How the transfer was tolerated
25 Reverse the procedure to return the person to bed.

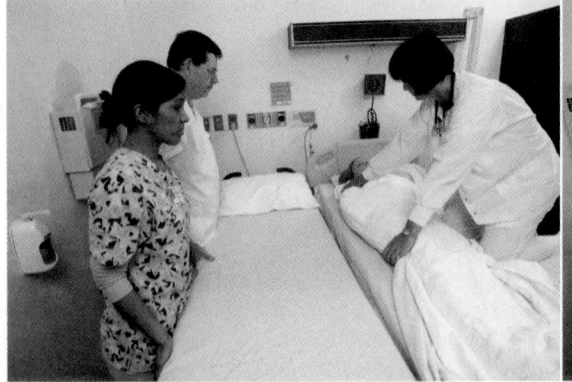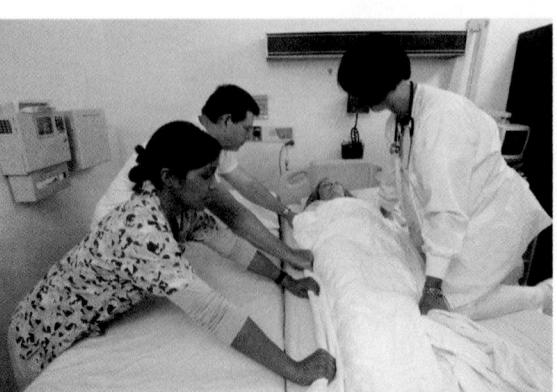

Fig. 17-29 Transferring the person to a stretcher. **A,** The stretcher is against the bed and is held in place. **B,** A drawsheet is used to transfer the person from the bed to a stretcher.

RE-POSITIONING IN A CHAIR OR WHEELCHAIR

The person can slide down into the chair. For good alignment and safety, the person's back and buttocks must be against the back of the chair.

Some persons can help with re-positioning. Others need help. If the person cannot help, use a mechanical lift to re-position the person. Follow the nurse's directions and the care plan for the best way to re-position a person in a chair or wheelchair. *Do not pull the person from behind the chair or wheelchair.*

If the person's chair reclines:

- Ask a co-worker to help you. (For persons with bariatric needs, at least 3 staff members are needed.)
- Lock the wheels.
- Recline the chair.
- Position a friction-reducing device (drawsheet or slide sheet) under the person.
- Use the device to move the person up. See procedure: *Moving the Person Up in Bed With an Assist Device*, p. 264.

Use this method if the person is alert and cooperative. The person must be able to follow directions. And the person must have the strength to help.

- Lock the wheelchair wheels.
- Remove or swing the front rigging out of the way.
- Position the person's feet flat on the floor.
- Apply a transfer belt.
- Position the person's arms on the armrests.
- Stand in front of the person. Block his or her knees and feet with your knees and feet.
- Grasp the transfer belt on each side while the person leans forward.
- Ask the person to push with his or her feet and arms on the count of "3."
- Move the person back into the chair on the count of "3" as the person pushes with his or her feet and arms (Fig. 17-30).

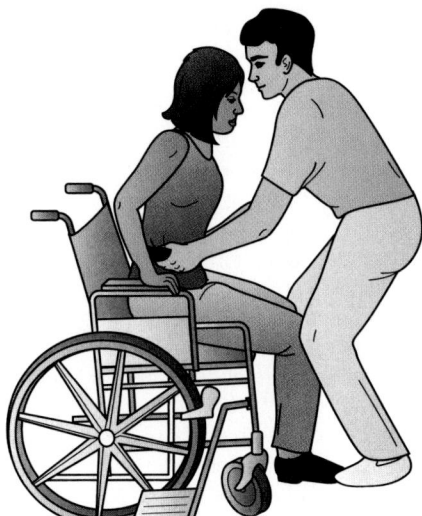

Fig. 17-30 Re-positioning the person in a wheelchair. A transfer belt is used to move the person to the back of the chair.

FOCUS ON **PRIDE**—cont'd

Ethics and Laws

The following is a real example of a lawsuit filed against a hospital. The person accused the nurse of injuring her during a transfer.

Admitted to the hospital for a respiratory problem, the patient had a history of shoulder injuries and surgeries. A nurse positioned the patient in a sitting position. The patient testified that she had immediate pain and heard a popping sound in her arm. The patient sued the hospital for a shoulder injury.

In her lawsuit, the patient claimed that:

- *A large sign warned the staff not to touch her arms. The sign was posted by her husband.*
- *The nurse was negligent for not reading the sign and the patient's chart.*

The hospital claimed that:

- *There was no sign.*
- *The nurse did not pull on the patient's arm.*
- *The patient caused her own injury.*

The jury found in favor of the hospital.

(T. Rosen v Verdugo Hills Hospital, Calif., 1999.)

In this case, the hospital did not have to pay damages (Chapter 4) to the patient. But the lawsuit cost time, money, effort, and stress for all involved.

Always be careful. Follow delegation guidelines, the care plan, and the nurse's instructions. Also, listen to the person. Ask the nurse if you are unsure about how to safely move a person. Do not put yourself in a position where you may be at fault.

REVIEW QUESTIONS

Circle the BEST answer.

1 A person's skin rubs against the sheet. This is called
a Shearing
b Friction
c Ergonomics
d Posture

2 Which occurs when a person slides down in bed?
a Shearing
b Friction
c Ergonomics
d Posture

3 Which protects the skin when moving the person in bed?
a Rolling the person
b Sliding the person up in bed
c Moving the mattress
d Using ergonomics

4 When you move or transfer a person, you must
a Allow personal choice
b Protect the person's privacy
c Use pillows for support
d Get help from a co-worker

5 You are delegated tasks that involve moving persons in bed. Which is *true*?
a The nurse tells you how to position the person.
b You decide which procedure to use.
c Bed rails are used at all times.
d Three workers are needed to complete the task safely.

6 As an assist device, a drawsheet is placed so that it
a Covers the person's body
b Is under the person from the head to above the knees
c Extends from the mid-back to mid-thigh level
d Covers the entire mattress

7 Before turning a person onto his or her side, you
a Move the person to the side of the bed
b Move the person to the middle of the bed
c Lock arms with the person
d Position pillows for comfort

8 The logrolling procedure
a Is used after spinal cord injuries or surgeries
b Requires a transfer belt
c Requires a mechanical lift
d Involves a stretcher and a drawsheet

9 A person is going to sit on the side of the bed. You need to know
a Which side is stronger
b If bed rails are used
c If a mechanical lift is needed
d If a transfer belt is needed

10 For chair and wheelchair transfers, the person must
a Wear non-skid footwear
b Have the bed rails up
c Use a mechanical lift
d Have a drawsheet or other assist device

11 Before transferring a person to or from a bed, you must
a Have the person wear non-skid footwear
b Lock the bed wheels
c Apply a transfer belt
d Position pillows for support

12 When transferring the person to bed, a chair, or the toilet
a The strong side moves first
b The weak side moves first
c Pillows are used for support
d The transfer belt is removed

13 To use a mechanical lift, you must do the following *except*
a Follow the manufacturer's instructions
b Make sure the lift works
c Compare the person's weight to the lift's weight limit
d Use a transfer belt

14 To safely transfer a person with a mechanical lift, at least
a 1 worker is needed
b 2 workers are needed
c 3 workers are needed
d 4 workers are needed

15 These statements are about transfers to and from a toilet. Which is *false*?
a The person wears non-skid footwear.
b Wheelchair wheels must be locked.
c The person uses the towel bars for support.
d A transfer belt is used.

16 These statements are about transfers to and from a stretcher? Which is *false*?
a The bed and stretcher wheels must be locked.
b The stretcher's side rails are raised when the person is on the stretcher.
c Once on the stretcher, the person can be left alone.
d At least 2 workers are needed for a safe transfer.

Answers to these questions are on p. 833.

The Person's Unit

OBJECTIVES

- Define the key terms and key abbreviations listed in this chapter.
- Identify the room temperatures required by OBRA and the CMS.
- Describe how to protect the person from drafts.
- List ways to prevent or reduce odors and noise.
- Explain how lighting affects comfort.
- Describe the basic bed positions.
- Identify the persons at risk for entrapment in the hospital bed system.
- Identify hospital bed system entrapment zones.
- Explain how to use the furniture and equipment in the person's unit.
- Describe how a bathroom is equipped for the person's use.
- Describe how to provide for safety, privacy, and comfort in the person's unit.
- Explain how to maintain the person's unit.
- Describe OBRA and CMS requirements for resident rooms.
- Explain how to promote PRIDE in the person, the family, and yourself.

KEY TERMS

Fowler's position A semi-sitting position; the head of the bed is raised between 45 and 60 degrees

full visual privacy Having the means to be completely free from public view while in bed

high-Fowler's position A semi-sitting position; the head of the bed is raised 60 to 90 degrees

reverse Trendelenburg's position The head of the bed is raised and the foot of the bed is lowered

semi-Fowler's position The head of the bed is raised 30 degrees; or the head of the bed is raised 30 degrees and the knee portion is raised 15 degrees

Trendelenburg's position The head of the bed is lowered and the foot of the bed is raised

KEY ABBREVIATIONS

CMS	Centers for Medicare & Medicaid Services
CNA	Certified nursing assistant
F	Fahrenheit
FDA	Food and Drug Administration
IV	Intravenous
OBRA	Omnibus Budget Reconciliation Act of 1987

The *person's unit* is the personal space, furniture, and equipment provided for the person by the agency (Fig. 18-1, p. 288). The person's unit is a private area. Many agencies have private rooms. A private room is for 1 person. Semi-private rooms are for 2 people. Some agencies have rooms that are shared by 4 people. Patient and resident rooms are designed to provide comfort, safety, and privacy.

See *Focus on Long-Term Care and Home Care: The Person's Unit.*

COMFORT

Age, illness, and activity affect comfort. So do temperature, ventilation, noise, odors, and lighting. These factors are controlled to meet the person's needs.

See *Focus on Communication: Comfort*, p. 288.

FOCUS ON LONG-TERM CARE AND HOME CARE
The Person's Unit

Long-Term Care

Some residents have private rooms. Others share a room with another person. The person's unit is private. It is treated like the person's home.

The Omnibus Budget Reconciliation Act of 1987 (OBRA) and the Centers for Medicare & Medicaid Services (CMS) have requirements for resident rooms. See Box 18-1, p. 288. OBRA requires that resident units be as personal and home-like as possible. Residents are allowed to bring and use some furniture and personal items from home. This promotes dignity and self-esteem.

As space allows, the person chooses where to place personal items. However, a resident cannot take or use another person's space. Doing so violates the other person's rights.

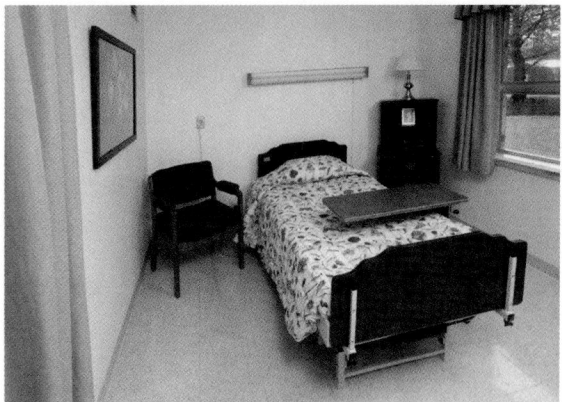

Fig. 18-1 Furniture and equipment in a resident's unit in a nursing center.

FOCUS ON COMMUNICATION

Comfort

What is comfortable for one person may not be comfortable for another. Ask about the person's comfort. You can say:
- "How is the temperature? Is it too hot or too cold?"
- "Is the noise level okay?"
- "Please let me know if you notice any bad odors."
- "How is the lighting? Is it too bright or too dark?"
- "Are you comfortable?"

Temperature and Ventilation

Heating and air conditioning systems maintain a comfortable temperature. Most healthy people are comfortable when the temperature is 68°F (Fahrenheit) to 74°F. This range may be too hot or too cold for others. Older persons and those who are ill may need higher temperatures for comfort.

Less active persons usually do not like cool areas. Nor do those needing help to move about. They need to dress warmly. They also need warm room temperatures. You may find the rooms rather warm.

Stale room air and lingering odors affect comfort and rest. Ventilation systems provide fresh air and move room air. Drafts occur as air moves. Infants, older persons, and those who are ill are sensitive to drafts. To protect them from drafts:
- Have them wear the correct clothing.
- Have them wear enough clothing.
- Offer lap robes to those in chairs and wheelchairs. Lap robes cover the legs.
- Provide enough blankets for warmth.
- Cover them with bath blankets when giving care.
- Move them from drafty areas.
  See *Focus on Children and Older Persons: Temperature and Ventilation.*

BOX 18-1 | **OBRA AND CMS REQUIREMENTS FOR RESIDENT ROOMS**

- Rooms are designed for 1 to 4 persons.
- Rooms have a direct access to an exit corridor.
- Rooms are designed or equipped for full visual privacy—ceiling-suspended privacy curtain that extends around the bed, movable screens, window coverings, doors.
- Rooms have at least 1 window to the outside.
- Each person has closet space with racks and shelves.
- Toilet facilities are in the room or nearby (includes bathing facilities).
- Rooms, bathrooms, and bathing areas have a functioning call system.
- The person has a bed of proper height and size.
- The person has a clean, comfortable mattress.
- Bed and bath linens (towels and washcloths) are clean and in good condition.
- Bed linens are appropriate to the weather and climate.
- The room has furniture for clothing, personal items, and a chair for visitors.
- Rooms are clean and orderly.
- Room temperature levels are between 71°F and 81°F.
- Ventilation, humidity, and odor levels are acceptable.
- Non-smoking areas are identified.
- Sound levels are comfortable.
- Lighting is adequate and comfortable with little glare.
- Rooms have clean, orderly drawers and shelves for personal items.
- The room is free of pests and rodents.
- Hand rails are in good repair.
- Floors are clean and dry.
- The person's setting is free of clutter.
- Personal supplies and items are labeled and stored appropriately.
- Items are within reach for use in bed or bathroom.
- There is space for wheelchair or walker use.
- The person has a raised toilet seat (if needed).

FOCUS ON CHILDREN AND OLDER PERSONS

Temperature and Ventilation

Older Persons

Poor circulation and loss of the skin's fatty tissue layer occur with aging. Therefore older persons are sensitive to cold (Chapter 11). They must wear enough clothing. Many wear sweaters in warm weather. Respect the person's wishes and choices.

Odors

Odors occur in health care settings and in home care. Food aromas and flower scents are pleasant. Bowel movements and urine have embarrassing odors. So do draining wounds and vomitus. Body, breath, and smoking odors may offend others.

Some people are very sensitive to odors. They may become nauseated. Good nursing care, ventilation, and housekeeping practices help prevent odors. To reduce odors:

- Empty, clean, and disinfect bedpans, urinals, commodes, and kidney basins promptly.
- Make sure toilets are flushed.
- Check incontinent persons often (Chapters 22 and 23).
- Clean persons who are wet or soiled from urine, feces, vomitus, or wound drainage.
- Change wet or soiled linens and clothing promptly.
- Keep laundry containers closed.
- Follow agency policy for wet or soiled linens and clothing.
- Dispose of incontinence and ostomy products promptly (Chapters 22 and 23).
- Provide good hygiene to prevent body and breath odors (Chapter 20).
- Use room deodorizers as needed and allowed by agency policy. Sometimes odors remain after removing the cause. Do not use sprays around persons with breathing problems. Ask the nurse if you are unsure.

Smoke odors present special problems. Residents, visitors, and staff smoke only in the areas allowed. If you smoke, follow the agency's policy. Practice hand washing after handling smoking materials and before giving care. Give careful attention to your uniforms, hair, and breath because of smoke odors.

Noise

According to the CMS, a "comfortable" sound level:

- Does not interfere with a person's hearing.
- Promotes privacy when privacy is desired.
- Allows the person to take part in social activities.

Common health care sounds may disturb some patients and residents. Examples include:

- The clanging of equipment
- The clatter of dishes and meal trays
- Loud voices, TVs, radios, music players, and so on
- Ringing phones
- Intercom systems and signal lights
- Equipment needing repair
- Squeaky wheels on stretchers, wheelchairs, carts, and other items needing oil
- Cleaning and housekeeping equipment

Loud talking and laughter in hallways and at the nurses' station are common. Patients and residents may think that the staff are talking and laughing about them.

People want to know the cause and meaning of new sounds. This relates to safety and security needs. Some

---

sounds seem dangerous, frightening, or irritating. Patients and residents may become upset, anxious, and uncomfortable. What is noise to one person may not be noise to another. For example, some people enjoy loud music. It disturbs others.

Health care agencies are designed to reduce noise. Window coverings, carpets, and acoustical tiles absorb noise. Plastic items make less noise than metal equipment (bedpans, urinals, wash basins). To decrease noise:

- Control your voice.
- Handle equipment carefully.
- Keep equipment in good working order.
- Answer phones, signal lights, and intercoms promptly.
  See *Focus on Children and Older Persons: Noise.*
  See *Focus on Communication: Noise.*

Lighting

According to the CMS, comfortable lighting:

- Lessens glares.
- Lets the person control the intensity, location, and direction of light.
- Lets visually impaired persons maintain or increase independent functioning.

Good lighting is needed for safety and comfort. Glares, shadows, and dull lighting can cause falls, headaches, and eyestrain. A bright room is cheerful. Dim light is better for relaxing and rest.

Adjust lighting to meet the person's changing needs. The overbed light provides soft, medium, or bright lighting. Ceiling lights provide soft to very bright light. Also adjust window coverings as needed.

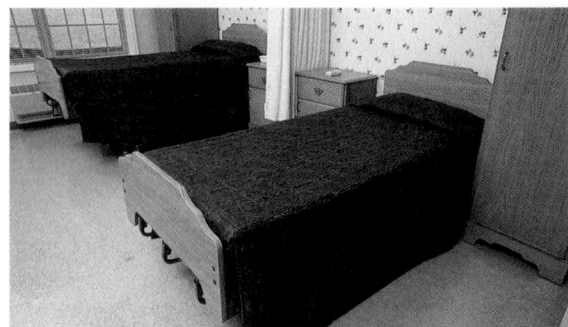

Fig. 18-2 The far bed is in the highest horizontal position. The near bed is in the lowest horizontal position.

Persons with poor vision need bright light. This is very important at meal time and when moving about in the room and agency. Bright lighting also helps the staff perform procedures.

Always keep light controls within the person's reach. This protects the right to personal choice.

See *Focus on Children and Older Persons: Lighting.*

ROOM FURNITURE AND EQUIPMENT

Rooms are furnished and equipped to meet basic needs—comfort, sleep, elimination, nutrition, hygiene, and activity. There is equipment to communicate with staff, family, and friends. The right to privacy is considered.

The Bed

Beds have electrical or manual controls. Beds are raised horizontally to give care. This reduces bending and reaching. The lowest horizontal position lets the person get out of bed with ease (Fig. 18-2). The head of the bed is flat or raised varying degrees.

Electric bed controls are on a side panel, bed rail, or the foot-board (Fig. 18-3, A). Some controls are hand-held devices (Fig. 18-3, B). Patients and residents are taught to use the controls safely. They are warned not to raise the bed to the high position or to adjust the bed to harmful positions. They are told of any position limits or restrictions.

The staff can lock most electric beds into any position. The person cannot adjust the bed to unsafe positions. Persons restricted to certain positions may need their beds locked. So may persons with confusion or dementia.

Manual beds have cranks at the foot of the bed (Fig. 18-4):
- Left crank—raises or lowers the head of the bed.
- Right crank—adjusts the knee portion.
- Center crank—raises or lowers the entire bed horizontally.

The cranks are pulled up for use. Keep them down at all other times. Cranks in the "up" position are safety hazards. Anyone walking past may bump into them.

See *Focus on Long-Term Care and Home Care: The Bed.*
See *Promoting Safety and Comfort: The Bed.*

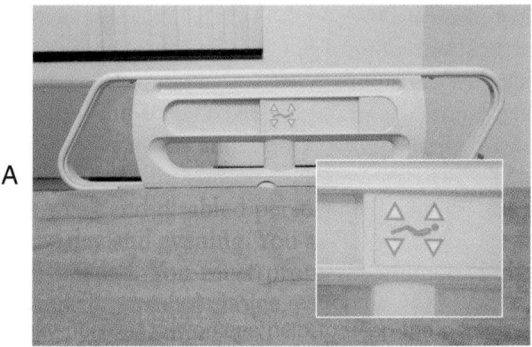
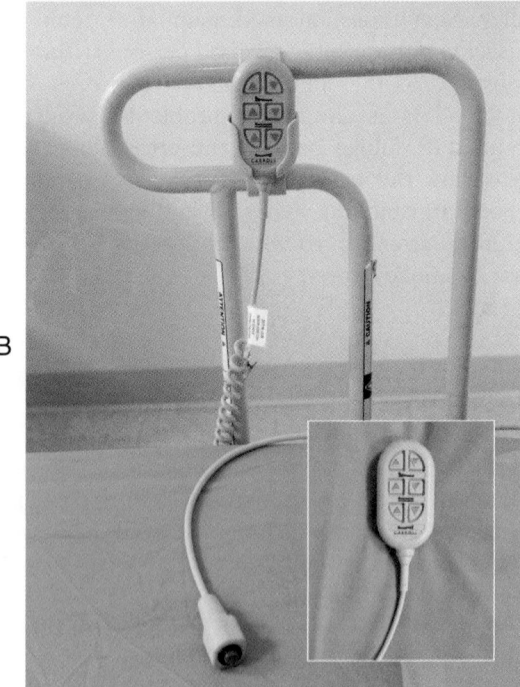

Fig. 18-3 Controls for an electric bed. **A,** Controls in the bed rail. **B,** Hand-held bed control (see inset) can be attached to the bed rail.

Bed Positions. The six basic bed positions are:

- *Flat*—This is the usual sleeping position. The position is used after spinal cord injury or surgery and for cervical traction.
- *Fowler's position*—*Fowler's position is a semi-sitting position. The head of the bed is raised between 45 and 60 degrees* (Fig. 18-5). See Chapter 16.
- *High-Fowler's position*—*High-Fowler's position is a semi-sitting position. The head of the bed is raised 60 to 90 degrees* (Fig. 18-6, p. 292).
- *Semi-Fowler's position*—In *semi-Fowler's position, the head of the bed is raised 30 degrees* (Fig. 18-7, p. 292). Some agencies define semi-Fowler's position as when *the head of the bed is raised 30 degrees and the knee portion is raised 15 degrees*. This position is comfortable and prevents sliding down in bed. However, raising the knee portion can interfere with circulation in the legs. For safe care, know the definition used by your agency. Also check with the nurse before using this position.
- *Trendelenburg's position*—In *Trendelenburg's position, the head of the bed is lowered and the foot of the bed is raised* (Fig. 18-8, p. 292). A doctor orders the position. Blocks are placed under the legs at the foot of the bed. Or the bed frame is tilted.
- *Reverse Trendelenburg's position*—In *reverse Trendelenburg's position, the head of the bed is raised and the foot of the bed is lowered* (Fig. 18-9, p. 292). A doctor orders this position. Blocks are placed under the legs at the head of the bed. Or the bed frame is tilted.

See *Focus on Long-Term Care and Home Care: Bed Positions*, p. 292.

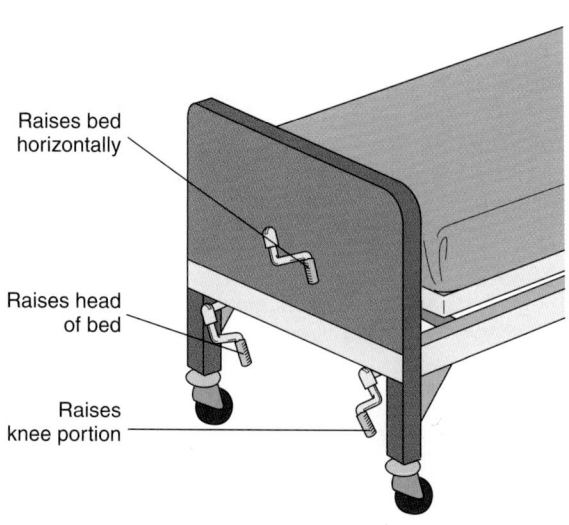

Raises bed horizontally

Raises head of bed

Raises knee portion

Fig. 18-4 Manually operated bed.

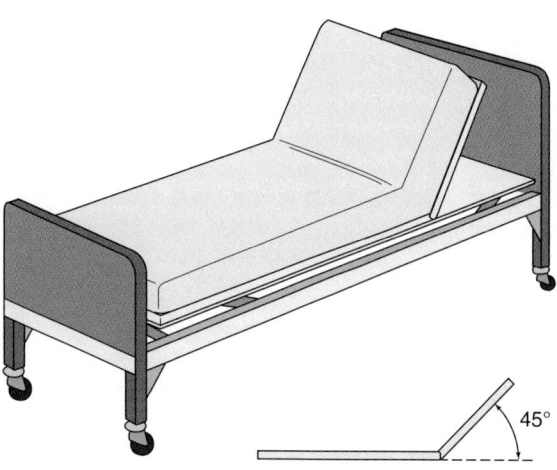

45°

Fig. 18-5 Fowler's position.

FOCUS ON LONG-TERM CARE AND HOME CARE
The Bed

Home Care

Some home care patients have hospital beds. Others use their regular beds. You cannot raise regular beds to give care. Therefore you will bend more when giving care. To avoid injuring yourself, use good body mechanics.

PROMOTING SAFETY AND COMFORT
The Bed

Safety

Beds have bed rails and wheels (Chapter 13). Bed wheels are locked at all times except when moving the bed. They must be locked when you:

- Give bedside care.
- Transfer the person to and from the bed. The person can be injured if the bed moves. So can you.

Use bed rails as the nurse and care plan direct. Otherwise the person could suffer injury or harm.

Comfort

Some persons spend a lot of time in bed. Adjust the bed to meet the person's needs. Tell the nurse if the person complains about the bed or mattress.

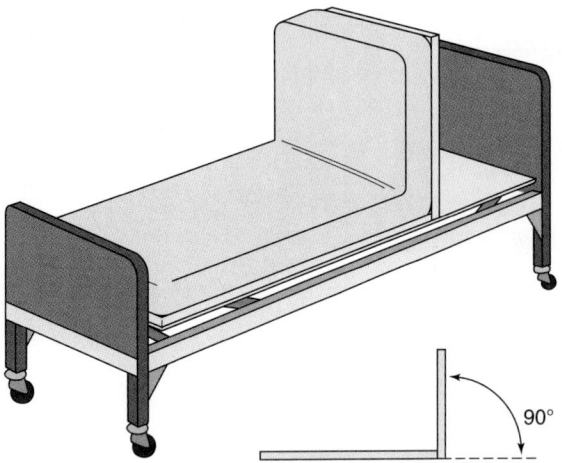

90°

Fig. 18-6 High-Fowler's position.

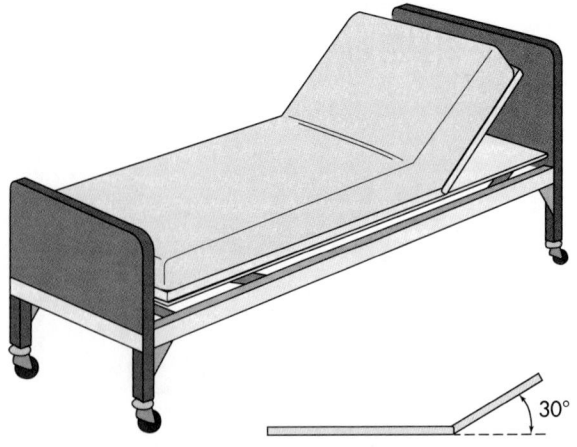

30°

Fig. 18-7 Semi-Fowler's position.

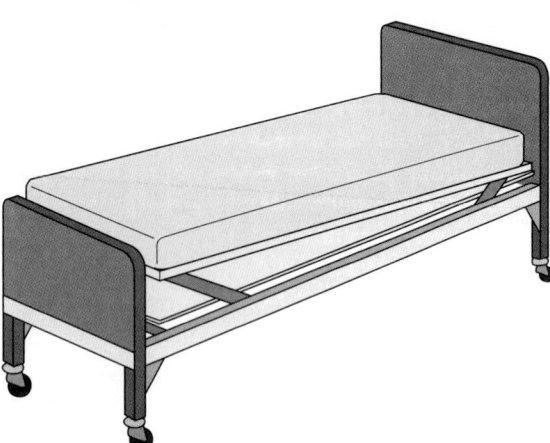

Fig. 18-8 Trendelenburg's position.

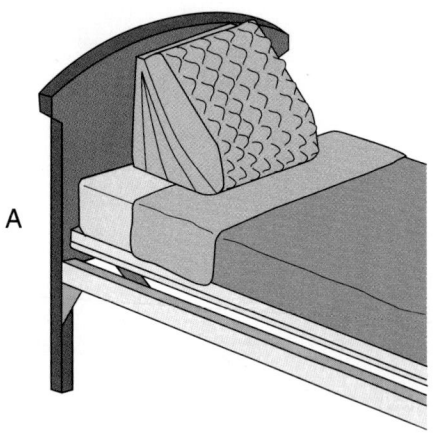

A

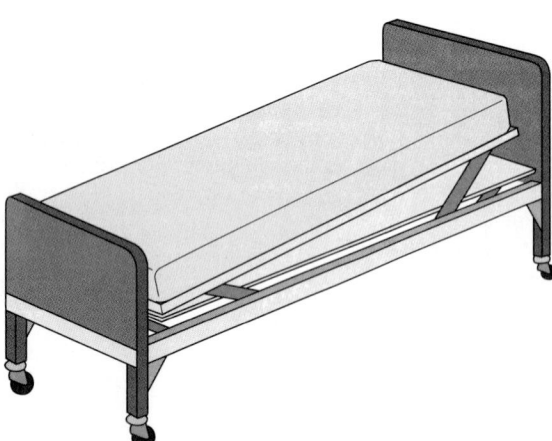

Fig. 18-9 Reverse Trendelenburg's position.

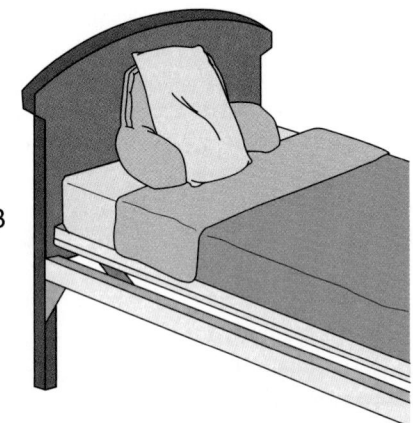

B

Fig. 18-10 Backrests for regular beds. **A,** Wedge pillow. **B,** Study pillow (dorm pillow) with armrests. A pillow provides added support.

FOCUS ON LONG-TERM CARE AND HOME CARE
Bed Positions

Home Care
Backrests are used with regular beds for Fowler's and semi-Fowler's positions (Fig. 18-10). Large, sturdy sofa pillows can be used. Check the head-board to make sure it is sturdy. It needs to provide support when the person leans against the backrest.

Zone 1: Within the rail

Zone 2: Between the top
of the compressed
mattress and the
bottom of the rail,
between the supports

Zone 3: Between the rail
and the mattress

Zone 4: Between the top
of the compressed
mattress and the
bottom of the rail,
at the end of the rail

Zone 5: Between the split
bed rails

Zone 6: Between the end of the
rail and the side edge of
the head-board or foot-board

Zone 7: Between the head or foot
board and the mattress end

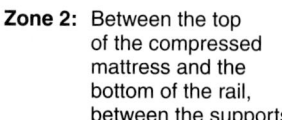

Fig. 18-11 Hospital bed system entrapment zones.

Bed Safety. Bed safety involves the *hospital bed system.* The Food and Drug Administration (FDA) defines the hospital bed system as the bed frame and its parts. The parts include the mattress, bed rails, head- and foot-boards, and bed attachments.

Entrapment within parts of the hospital bed system is a risk. That is, the person can get caught, trapped, or entangled in spaces created by bed rails, the mattress, the bed frame, the head-board, or the foot-board. Serious injuries and deaths have occurred from head, neck, and chest entrapment. Arm and leg entrapment also can occur. Persons at greatest risk:

- Are older.
- Are frail.
- Are confused or disoriented.
- Are restless.
- Have uncontrolled body movements.
- Have poor muscle control.
- Are small in size.
- Are restrained (Chapter 14).

Hospital bed systems have seven entrapment zones (Fig. 18-11 and Fig. 18-12, p. 294). You may feel that a person is at risk for entrapment. Report your concerns to the nurse at once. Also, always check the person for entrapment. If a person is caught, trapped, or entangled in the bed or any of its parts, try to release the person. Also call for the nurse at once.

See *Focus on Children and Older Persons: Bed Safety.*

FOCUS ON CHILDREN AND OLDER PERSONS
Bed Safety

Children

Entrapment can occur in cribs. To prevent entrapment, the mattress and crib must be the same size. When the mattress is smaller than the crib, gaps occur between:

- The crib rail and mattress
- The crib rail and head-board
- The crib rail and foot-board

Tell the nurse if you have concerns about a baby's crib.

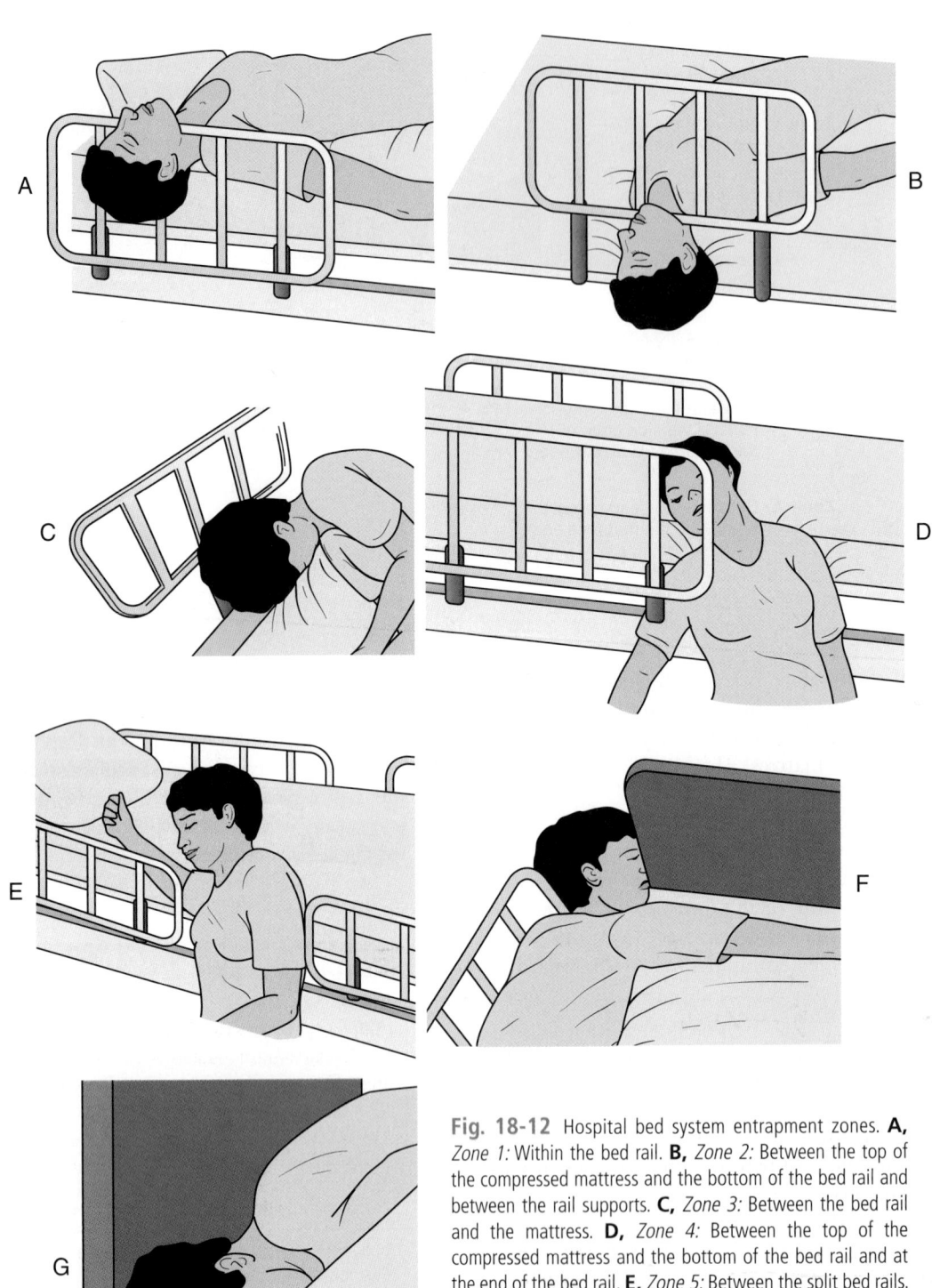

Fig. 18-12 Hospital bed system entrapment zones. **A,** *Zone 1:* Within the bed rail. **B,** *Zone 2:* Between the top of the compressed mattress and the bottom of the bed rail and between the rail supports. **C,** *Zone 3:* Between the bed rail and the mattress. **D,** *Zone 4:* Between the top of the compressed mattress and the bottom of the bed rail and at the end of the bed rail. **E,** *Zone 5:* Between the split bed rails. **F,** *Zone 6:* Between the end of the bed rail and the side edge of the head-board or foot-board. **G,** *Zone 7:* Between the head-board or foot-board and the end of the mattress.

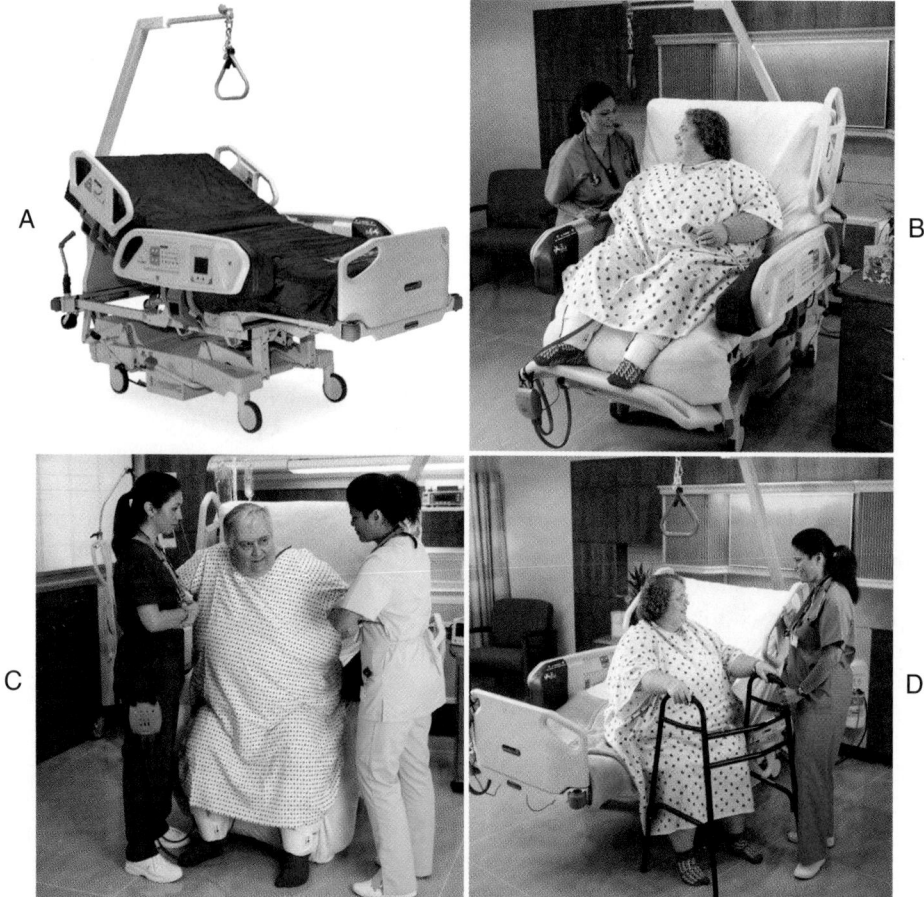

Fig. 18-13 A, Bariatric bed with a trapeze. **B,** Bariatric bed converted to a chair. **C,** The bariatric bed allows the person to get out of bed from the chair position. **D,** The person gets out of the bariatric bed from the side.

Bariatric Beds. Bariatric beds may have these and other features:

- A wide frame with a weight capacity from 500 to 1000 pounds (Fig. 18-13, A). Some frames can be adjusted for the person's height. For example, the bed length is shortened so the person's feet touch the foot-board. This prevents the person from sliding down in bed. Or the frame is lengthened for a taller person.
- A chair position. The bed converts into a chair without moving the person (Fig. 18-13, B). The foot-board becomes a footrest.
- Front and side egress positions. *Egress* means to *go out* or *leave*. By adjusting the foot-board out of the way, the person can move from a lying to sitting to standing position (Fig. 18-13, C). Or the person can get out of bed on the side (Fig. 18-13, D).
- Power transport to move the bed. The bed is used to transport the person. The person is not transferred to a stretcher.
- A pressure relief surface to prevent pressure ulcers. The surface can be used to turn the person for care measures.

- A trapeze for the person to re-position himself or herself.
- A built-in scale.

Bariatric beds vary depending on the model. Follow the manufacturer's instructions to use the bed safely.

See *Focus on Communication: Bariatric Beds.*

FOCUS ON COMMUNICATION

Bariatric Beds

Many obese persons have been disrespected for much of their lives. They have faced insult and judgment by others. This can cause low self-esteem and emotional problems. Obese persons may be sensitive to comments about their weight or size.

Always think before you speak. Consider if the comment may offend the person. For example, do not say: "The nurse is trying to get a bed big enough for you." Instead, you can say: "The nurse is getting a bed that will be more comfortable for you."

Be aware of your verbal and nonverbal communication. Your words and actions must always show dignity and respect.

The Overbed Table

The overbed table (see Fig. 18-1) is moved over the bed by sliding the base under the bed. The table is raised or lowered for the person in bed or in a chair. Turn the handle or push the lever to adjust the table height. The table is used for meals, writing, reading, and other activities. Some overbed tables have a storage area for beauty, hair care, shaving, or other personal items.

The nursing team uses the overbed table as a work area. Place only clean and sterile items on the table. Never place bedpans, urinals, or soiled linen on the overbed table. Clean the table after using it for a work surface. Also clean it before serving meal trays.

The Bedside Stand

The bedside stand is next to the bed. It is used to store personal items and personal care equipment. It has a top drawer and a lower cabinet with shelves or just drawers (Fig. 18-14). The top drawer is used for money, eyeglasses, books, and other items.

The top shelf or middle drawer is used for the wash basin. The wash basin holds personal items—soap and soap dish, powder, lotion, deodorant, towels, washcloth, bath blanket, and sleepwear. An emesis basin or kidney basin (shaped like a kidney) holds oral hygiene items. The kidney basin is stored in the top drawer, middle drawer, or on the top shelf. The bedpan and its cover, the urinal, and toilet paper are stored on the lower shelf or in the bottom drawer.

The stand top is often used for tissues and other personal items. A clock, photos, phone, flowers, cards, and gifts are examples. Some stands have a side or back rod for towels and washcloths.

Place only clean and sterile items on the bedside stand. Never place bedpans, urinals, or soiled linen on the top of the stand. Clean the bedside stand after using it for a work surface.

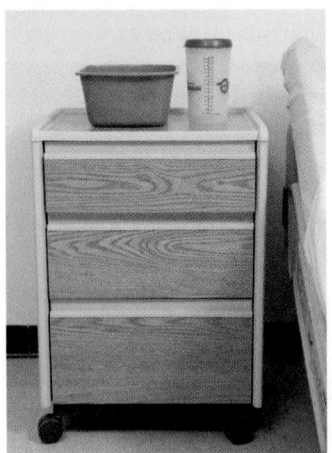

Fig. 18-14 The bedside stand.

Chairs

The person's unit has a chair for personal and visitor use (see Fig. 18-1 and Fig. 18-15). It must be comfortable and sturdy. It must not move or tip during transfers. The person should be able to get in and out of the chair with ease. It should not be too low or too soft. Nursing center residents may bring chairs from home.

Privacy Curtains

The person's unit has a privacy curtain that extends around the bed. The curtain is pulled around the bed to provide privacy for the person (Chapter 4). Rooms with more than one bed have a privacy curtain between the units. *Always pull the curtain completely around the bed before giving care.*

Privacy curtains prevent others from seeing the person. They do not block sounds or voices. Others in the room can hear sounds or talking behind the curtain.

See *Focus on Long-Term Care and Home Care: Privacy Curtains.*

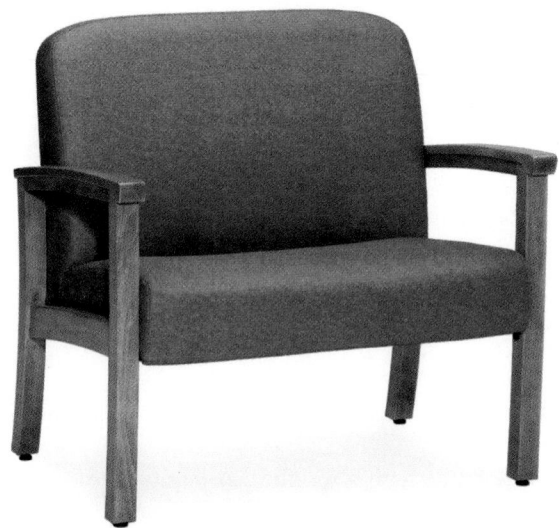

Fig. 18-15 The bariatric chair is wider and has expanded capacity.

FOCUS ON LONG-TERM CARE AND HOME CARE
Privacy Curtains

Long-Term Care

According to OBRA and the CMS, each person has the right to full visual privacy. *Full visual privacy is having the means to be completely free from public view while in bed.* The privacy curtain helps provide full visual privacy.

Home Care

Portable screens or room dividers help provide privacy in the home setting (Fig. 18-16). Decorator styles provide color and are pleasant to look at.

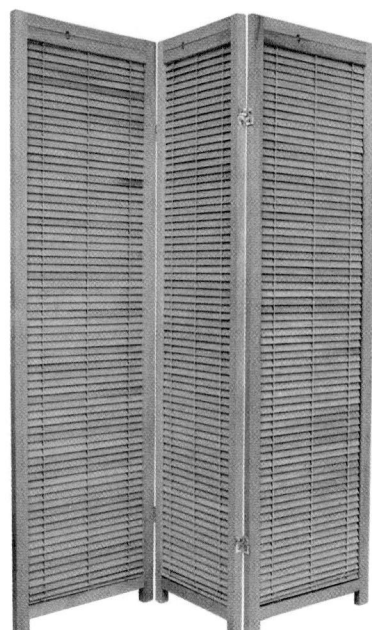

Fig. 18-16 A portable screen provides privacy in the home.

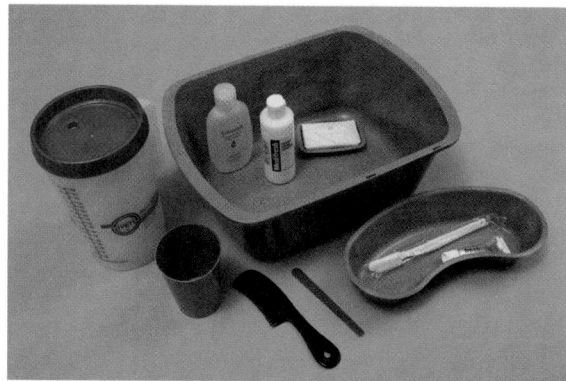

Fig. 18-17 Personal care items.

Personal Care Items

Personal care items are used for hygiene and elimination. A bedpan and urinal are provided. The agency also provides a wash basin, kidney basin, water pitcher and cup, and soap and a soap dish (Fig. 18-17). Some provide powder, lotion, toothbrush, toothpaste, mouthwash, tissues, and a comb.

Some persons provide their own oral hygiene equipment, hair care supplies, and deodorant. Some also prefer their own soap, lotion, and powder. Respect the person's choices in personal care products.

The Call System

Each patient and resident has a call system. When in their rooms, using the toilet, or in a bathing area, they must be able to contact the staff at the nurses' station. The call system lets the person signal for help. The signal light is at the end of a long cord (Fig. 18-18, p. 298). It attaches to the bed or chair. (See p. 299 for signal lights in bathrooms and shower or tub rooms.) Always keep the signal light within the person's reach—in the room, bathroom, and shower or tub room.

To get help, the person presses a button at the end of the signal light. The signal light at the bedside (bathroom, shower or tub room) is connected to a light above the room door. The signal light also connects to a computer, light panel, or intercom system at the nurses' station (Fig. 18-19, p. 298). These tell the staff that the person needs help. The staff member shuts off the light at the bedside when responding to the call for help.

An intercom system lets the staff talk with the person from the nurses' station. The person tells what is needed. Then the light is turned off at the station. Hard-of-hearing persons may have problems using an intercom. Be careful when using an intercom. Remember confidentiality. Persons nearby can hear what you and the person say.

Some signal lights are turned on by tapping with a hand or fist (Fig. 18-20, p. 298). They are useful for persons with limited hand mobility.

The person is taught how to use the call system when admitted to the agency. Some people cannot use signal lights. Examples are persons who are confused or in a coma. The care plan lists special communication measures. Check these persons often. Make sure their needs are met.

The phrase "signal light" is used in this book when referring to the call system. You must:

- Keep the signal light within the person's reach. Even if the person cannot use the signal light, keep it within reach for use by visitors and staff. They may need to signal for help.
- Place the signal light on the person's strong side.
- Remind the person to signal when help is needed.
- Answer signal lights promptly. The person signals when help is needed. For example, the person may have an urgent need to use the bathroom. Promptly helping the person to the bathroom prevents embarrassing problems. You also help prevent infection, skin breakdown, pressure ulcers, and falls.
- Answer bathroom and shower or tub room signal lights at once.

See *Focus on Communication: The Call System*, p. 299.

See *Focus on Long-Term Care and Home Care: The Call System*, p. 299.

See *Teamwork and Time Management: The Call System*, p. 299.

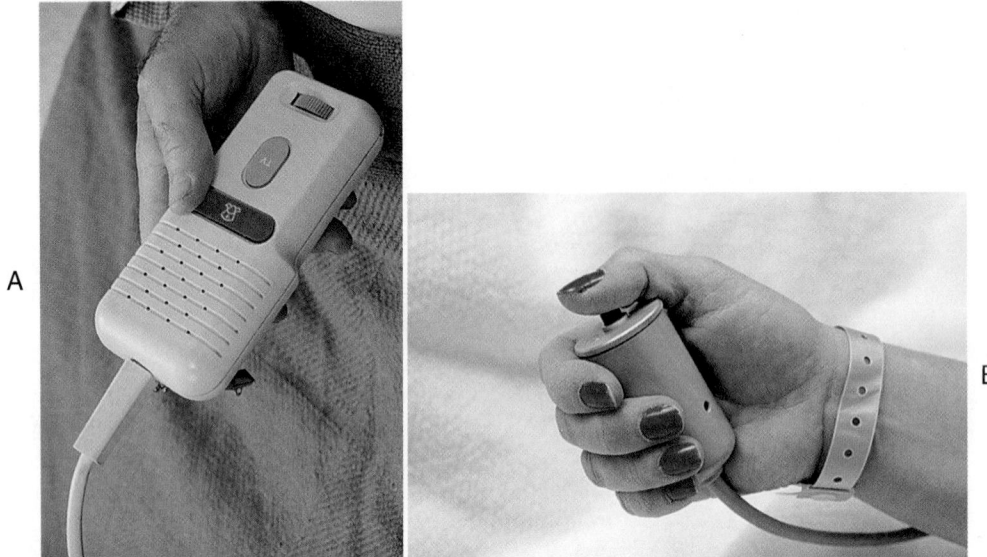

Fig. 18-18 The signal light button is pressed when help is needed. NOTE: There are different types of signal lights.

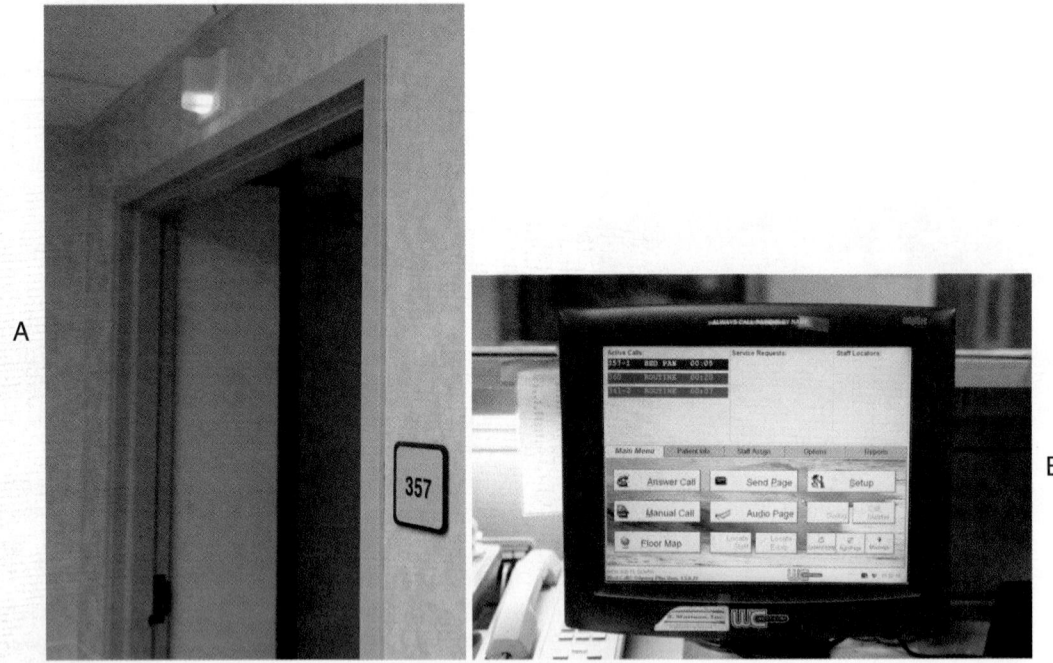

Fig. 18-19 A, Light above the room door. With this system, the color signals what type of help the person is asking for with the hand-held signal light—red for a nurse, green for pain, yellow for elimination needs. **B,** Computer monitor at the nurses' station.

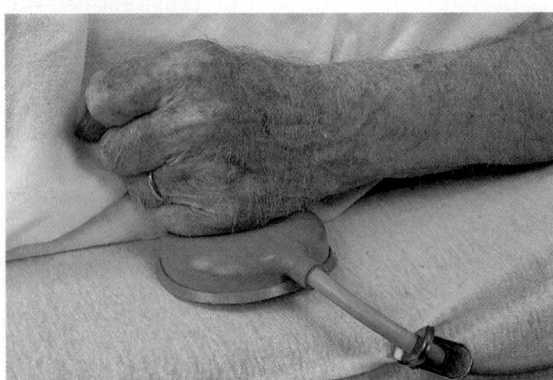

Fig. 18-20 Signal light for a person with limited hand mobility.

FOCUS ON COMMUNICATION
The Call System

You will answer signal lights for co-workers. You may not know their patients and residents and they may not know you. To promote quality of life and safe care, you can say:

- "My name is Kate Hines. I'm a nursing assistant. How can I help you?"
- "Mrs. Janz, I'll need to check your care plan before I bring you more salt. I'll be right back, but is there anything else I can do before I leave?"
- "Mr. Duncan, I'll be happy to take your meal tray. I'll tell your nursing assistant what you ate."
- "Mrs. Palmer, do you use the bathroom or the bedpan?"

Sometimes patients and residents signal for help often. Do not delay in meeting their needs. Never take signal lights away from them. This is not safe. Avoid statements that make a person feel as if he or she is a burden. For example, do not say:

- "I just helped you to the bathroom. Can't you wait?"
- "I was just in your room. What do you want now?"

Do not discourage the person from asking for help. The person may try to do something alone. This could cause injury. Tell the nurse. Your co-workers can help you meet the person's needs.

FOCUS ON LONG-TERM CARE AND HOME CARE
The Call System

Home Care

Some home care patients stay in bed or in a certain part of the home. They need a way to call for help. Tap bells, dinner bells, baby monitors, and other devices are useful (Fig. 18-21). Or you can give the person a small can with a few coins inside. Children's toys with bells, horns, and whistles may be useful.

TEAMWORK AND TIME MANAGEMENT
The Call System

Patients and residents use their signal lights when they need help. A person may put on a signal light when you are with another person. The same may happen to another nursing team member. If nursing team members answer signal lights for each other, lights are answered promptly. Patients and residents receive quality care. Everyone is responsible for answering signal lights even if not assigned to the person.

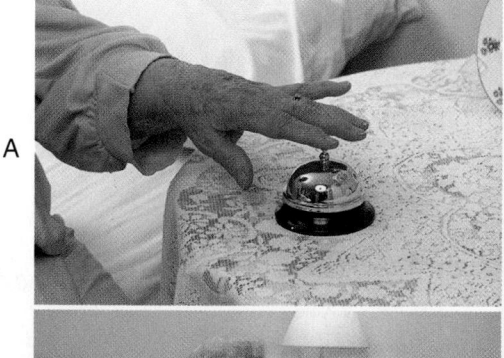
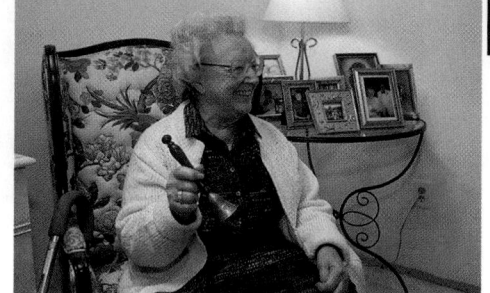
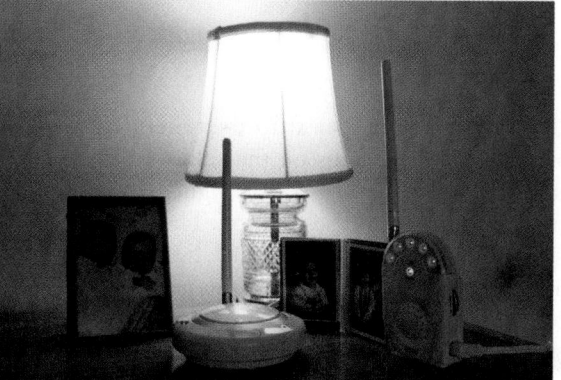

Fig. 18-21 **A,** Tap bell. **B,** Dinner bell. **C,** Baby monitor.

The Bathroom

Patient and resident rooms have toilet facilities. A toilet, sink, call system, and mirror are standard equipment (Fig. 18-22, p. 300). Some bathrooms have showers.

Grab bars are by the toilet for safety. The person uses them for support when lowering to or raising from the toilet. Some bathrooms have higher toilets or raised toilet seats. They make wheelchair transfers easier. They also are helpful for persons with joint problems.

Towel racks, toilet paper, soap, paper towel dispenser, and a wastebasket are in the bathroom. They are placed within easy reach of the person.

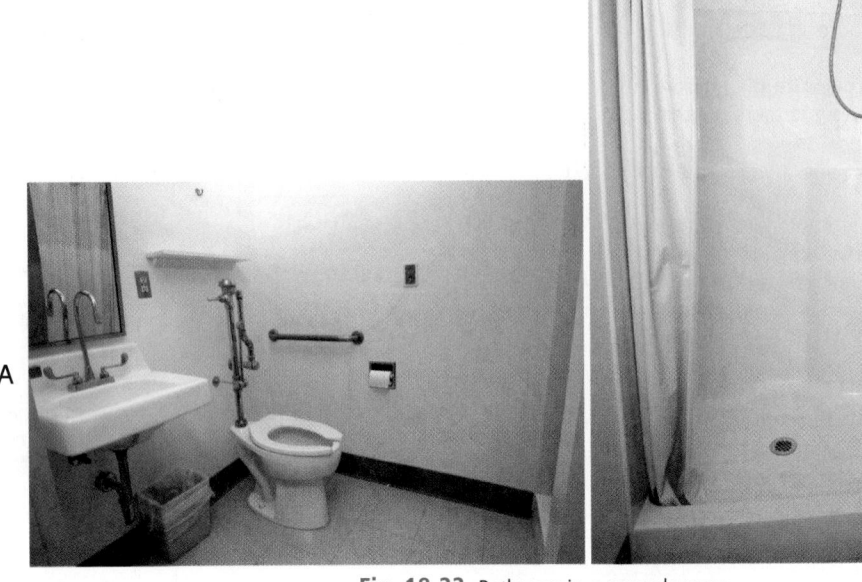

Fig. 18-22 Bathroom in a person's room.

Usually the signal light is next to the toilet. Pressing a button or pulling a cord turns on the signal light. When the bathroom signal light is used, the light flashes above the room door and at the nurses' station. The sound at the nurses' station is different from signal lights in rooms. These differences alert the staff that the person is in the bathroom. Someone must respond at once when a person needs help in a bathroom.

Closet and Drawer Space

Closet and drawer space are provided for clothing. OBRA and the CMS require that nursing centers provide each person with closet space. The closet space must have shelves and a clothes rack (Fig. 18-23). The person must have free access to the closet and its contents.

Items in closets and drawers are the person's private property. You must have the person's permission to open or search closets or drawers.

Sometimes people hoard items—drugs, napkins, straws, food, sugar, salt, pepper, and so on. Hoarding can cause safety or health risks. The staff can inspect a person's closet or drawers if hoarding is suspected. The person is informed of the inspection. He or she is present when it takes place.

See *Promoting Safety and Comfort: Closet and Drawer Space*.

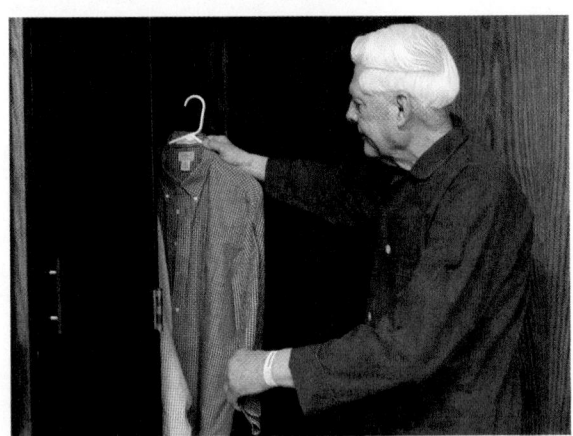

Fig. 18-23 The resident can reach items in his closet.

PROMOTING SAFETY AND COMFORT
Closet and Drawer Space

Safety

The nurse may ask you to inspect a person's closet, drawers, or personal items. If so, the person must be present. Also have a co-worker with you. Your co-worker is a witness to what you are doing. This protects you if the person claims that something was stolen or damaged.

Other Equipment

Many agencies furnish rooms with other equipment. A TV, radio, and clock provide comfort and relaxation. Many rooms have phones, a computer, and Internet access.

Blood pressure equipment is often mounted on walls. There also are wall outlets for oxygen and suction (Fig. 18-24). Oxygen tanks and portable suction equipment are common in nursing centers and home care settings. For intravenous (IV) infusions, an IV pole (IV standard) is used to hang IV bags or feeding bags.

GENERAL RULES

Everyone involved in the person's care must keep the unit clean, neat, safe, and comfortable. To maintain the person's unit, follow the rules in Box 18-2.

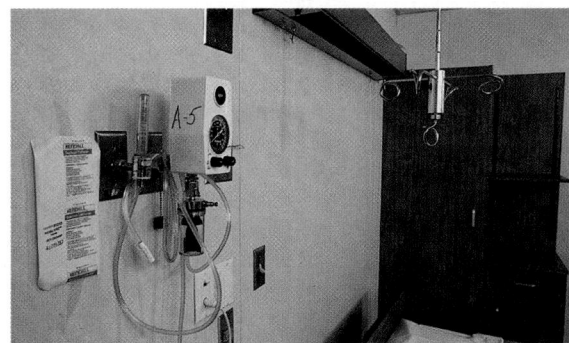

Fig. 18-24 This room has a hanging IV rod and oxygen and suction outlets.

BOX 18-2 MAINTAINING THE PERSON'S UNIT

- Keep the signal light within the person's reach at all times.
- Meet the needs of persons who cannot use the call system.
- Make sure the person can reach the overbed table and the bedside stand.
- Arrange personal items as the person prefers. Make sure they are easily reached.
- Make sure the person can reach the phone, TV, bed, and light controls.
- Provide the person with enough tissues and toilet paper.
- Adjust lighting, temperature, and ventilation for the person's comfort.
- Handle equipment carefully to prevent noise.
- Explain the causes of strange noises.
- Empty wastebaskets in the person's room and bathroom. Empty them every shift or at least once a day. Empty them more often if they become full.
- Respect the person's belongings. An item may not have importance or value to you. Yet it has great meaning for the person. Even a scrap of paper can have great meaning to the person.
- Do not throw away any items belonging to the person.
- Do not move furniture or the person's belongings. Persons with poor vision rely on memory or feel for the location of items.
- Straighten bed linens and towels as often as needed.
- Complete a safety check before leaving the room. (See the inside of the front book cover.)

Continued

FOCUS ON P R I D E

The Person, Family, and Yourself

Personal and Professional Responsibility

Loud talking and laughter in hallways and at the nurses' station are common. Patients, residents, and visitors overhear this noise. They may think the staff are not working. Or they may think the staff are talking about or laughing at them. Some may find this irritating or upsetting. Some may become anxious, uncomfortable, or angry.

Reducing noise requires cooperation from all staff. It is not your responsibility alone. But you can help. Do your part to reduce noise. Politely remind others to speak softly if needed. Take pride in providing patients and residents with a quiet and comfortable setting.

Rights and Respect

Nursing center residents have left their homes. Each had furniture, appliances, a private bathroom, and personal items. Now the person lives in a strange place. He or she may have a roommate. Leaving one's home is a hard part of growing old with poor health.

Nursing center residents have the right to make their units as home-like as possible. Some bring personal items from home. Photos, TVs, radios, books, religious items, and plants are examples. A chair, footstool, lamp, and small table are often allowed.

Allow personal choice when arranging items. When helping the person choose the best places for items, make sure the person's choices:
- Are safe.
- Will not cause falls or other accidents.
- Do not interfere with the rights of others.

The center is the person's home. A home-like setting is important for quality of life.

Independence and Social Interaction

People want to be independent. They do not want to rely on others for simple, everyday things. Often accidents and injuries occur when the person tries to get needed items. The person has to reach too far and falls. Or he or she tries to get up without help.

The location of items in the person's unit can help prevent injuries. To promote independence and safety:
- Keep needed personal items within reach.
- Place assistive devices nearby. Walkers and canes are examples.
- Place the signal light within the person's reach. Answer signal lights and tend to the person's needs promptly.

FOCUS ON PRIDE—cont'd

Delegation and Teamwork

Some nursing units check on the person at regular intervals. For example, every hour nursing staff ask about the person's needs, positioning, comfort, and the placement of personal items. The person's needs are addressed, and the person is reminded that a staff member will return in one hour. Nursing staff sign a form each time. The person may still use the signal light for urgent needs. Non-urgent needs are met when staff return at the scheduled time. The process is explained to the person upon admission.

Some nursing units rotate assigned times among team members. For example, a nurse is assigned the even hours and a nursing assistant is assigned the odd hours. The team works together to meet the person's needs. If your unit uses this practice:

- Be prompt. Check on the person at the correct time.
- Be honest. Do not sign the form if you did not check on the person. Also, do not sign the form early.
- Have a good attitude. Do not complain. The agency has reasons for using this practice. The agency may be trying to improve care, decrease signal light use, or help nurses with time management.

Ethics and Laws

This chapter focused on the objects and surroundings in the person's unit and how those affect the person's comfort and well-being. You are also a part of that setting. You must help the person feel safe, secure, and comfortable. The following is an example of a nursing assistant who failed to do so.

A certified nursing assistant (CNA) worked at a nursing home in Arizona. In February 2002, she was counseled to improve on her poor attendance and for having negative outbursts. In August 2002, it was noted that she gave poor care:

- *Residents were not turned and/or briefs were not changed every 2 hours according to facility policy.*
- *She continued to have negative outbursts.*

Later, reports were made that she had failed to provide care and meet a resident's needs. It was reported to the Arizona State Board of Nursing that she abused a resident for failure to provide care and not meeting his needs.

- *The resident was described as alert, paralyzed, on a ventilator for chronic respiratory failure, and totally dependent for all needs.*
- *The CNA was in his room many times during the night. She did not provide the care he requested.*
- *The CNA placed his signal light out of reach. He used his head to use the signal light for assistance.*

In November 2003, the CNA was terminated from employment for resident abuse. The CNA was hired by another agency in December 2003. She worked there until March 2004. On March 17 she was counseled for:

- *Telling a resident that if she did not speak English she should go back to her country*
- *Being rough, rude, and verbally abusive to residents*
- *Refusing to work on a nursing unit "because all patients 'stink'"*
- *Being critical and judgmental with new staff*
- *Leaving residents soaking wet at the end of her shift*
- *Telling a resident to "pee in your britches" rather than helping him to the bathroom*

Her employment was terminated on March 19, 2004.

In January 2004, the Arizona State Board of Nursing sent the CNA a questionnaire. It was returned to the Board as undeliverable. The CNA failed to notify the Board of an address change within the 30 days required by law.

The Board revoked the CNA's certificate for unprofessional conduct. She violated the following aspects of the state's Nurse Practice Act:

- *Conduct or practice that is or might be harmful or dangerous to the health of a patient or the public*
- *Failing to follow an employer's policies and procedures designed to safeguard the client*
- *Failing to respect client rights and dignity*
- *Neglecting or abusing a client physically, verbally, or financially*
- *Practicing in any other manner that gives the Board reasonable cause to believe that the health of a client or the public may be harmed*
- *Failing to notify the board in writing within 30 days of any address change*

(Arizona State Board of Nursing, May 18, 2006. NOTE: Names withheld by request of the Arizona State Board of Nursing.)

Your words and actions are heard and seen by others. Bad conduct reduces quality of care and reflects poorly on you. You can lose your job and the ability to work as a nursing assistant. Always provide care in a way that promotes the person's comfort, safety, and quality of life.

REVIEW QUESTIONS

Circle the BEST answer.

1 Which temperature range is required by OBRA and the CMS?
   a 61°F to 68°F
   b 68°F to 74°F
   c 71°F to 81°F
   d 76°F to 81°F

2 Which does *not* protect a person from drafts?
   a Wearing enough clothing
   b Being covered with enough blankets
   c Being moved from a drafty area
   d Sitting by a fan

3 Which does *not* prevent or reduce odors?
   a Placing flowers in the room
   b Emptying bedpans promptly
   c Using room deodorizers
   d Practicing good hygiene

4 To prevent odors, you need to do the following *except*
   a Check incontinent persons often
   b Dispose of ostomy products at the end of your shift
   c Keep laundry containers closed
   d Clean persons who are wet or soiled

5 Which does *not* control noise?
   a Using plastic items
   b Handling dishes with care
   c Speaking softly
   d Talking with others in the hallway

6 Beds are raised horizontally to
   a Prevent bending and reaching when giving care
   b Let the person get in and out of bed with ease
   c Raise the head of the bed
   d Lock the bed in position

7 The head of the bed is raised 30 degrees. This is called
   a Fowler's position
   b Semi-Fowler's position
   c Trendelenburg's position
   d Reverse Trendelenburg's position

8 These statements are about hospital bed system entrapment. Which is *false*?
   a Serious injuries and death can occur.
   b Older, frail, and confused persons are at risk.
   c The head, neck, and chest are areas of entrapment.
   d Bed rails present the only risk for entrapment.

9 The overbed table is *not* used
   a For eating
   b As a working surface
   c For the urinal
   d To store shaving items

10 The bedpan is stored in the
   a Closet
   b Bedside stand
   c Overbed table
   d Bathroom

11 Signal lights are answered
   a When you have time
   b At the end of your shift
   c Promptly
   d When you are near the person's room

12 To maintain the person's unit, you can do the following *except*
   a Save items that do not look important
   b Provide enough tissues and toilet paper
   c Place personal items as you choose
   d Straighten bed linens as needed

Circle T if the statement is TRUE or F if it is FALSE.

13 T F The person's unit is considered private.
14 T F Persons with dementia may have extreme reactions to strange sounds.
15 T F The privacy curtain prevents others from hearing conversations.
16 T F Soft, dim lighting is relaxing.
17 T F The signal light must always be within the person's reach.
18 T F The overbed table and bedside stand should be within the person's reach.
19 T F You should explain the cause of strange noises.
20 T F The person must be able to reach items in the closet.
21 T F You can adjust the person's room temperature for your comfort.
22 T F You can look through a person's closet and drawers.

Answers to these questions are on p. 833.

19 Bedmaking

OBJECTIVES

- Define the key terms listed in this chapter.
- Describe open, closed, occupied, and surgical beds.
- Explain when to change linens.
- Explain how to use drawsheets.
- Handle linens following the rules of medical asepsis.
- Perform the procedures described in this chapter.
- Explain how to promote PRIDE in the person, the family, and yourself.

KEY TERMS

cotton drawsheet A drawsheet made of cotton; it helps keep the mattress and bottom linens clean
drawsheet A small sheet placed over the middle of the bottom sheet
waterproof drawsheet A drawsheet made of plastic, rubber, or absorbent material used to protect the mattress and bottom linens from dampness and soiling

Beds are made every day. Clean, dry, and wrinkle-free linens:
- Promote comfort.
- Prevent skin breakdown.
- Prevent pressure ulcers.

Beds are usually made in the morning after baths. Or they are made while the person is in the shower, up in the chair, or out of the room. Beds are made and rooms straightened before visitors arrive.

To keep beds neat and clean:
- Change linens when they are wet, soiled, or damp.
- Straighten linens whenever loose or wrinkled.
- Straighten loose or wrinkled linens at bedtime.
- Check for and remove food and crumbs after meals and snacks.
- Check linens for dentures, eyeglasses, hearing aids, sharp objects, and other items.
- Follow Standard Precautions and the Bloodborne Pathogen Standard. Contact with blood, body fluids, secretions, or excretions is likely.

TYPES OF BEDS

Beds are made in these ways:
- A *closed bed* is not in use. Top linens are not folded back (Fig. 19-1). Or the bed is ready for a new patient or resident. In nursing centers, closed beds are made for residents who are up during the day.
- An *open bed* is in use. Top linens are fan-folded back so the person can get into bed. A closed bed becomes an open bed by fan-folding back the top linens (Fig. 19-2).
- An *occupied bed* is made with the person in it (Fig. 19-3).

- A *surgical bed* is made to transfer a person from a stretcher to bed (Fig. 19-4). This bed also is made for persons who arrive by ambulance.

LINENS

When handling linens and making beds, practice medical asepsis. Your uniform is considered "dirty." Always hold linens away from your body and uniform (Fig. 19-5). Never shake linens. Shaking them spreads microbes. Place clean linens on a clean surface. Never put clean or dirty linens on the floor.

Collect enough linens. If the person has two pillows, get two pillowcases. The person may need extra blankets for warmth. Do not bring unneeded linens to a person's room. Once in the person's room, extra linen is considered contaminated. Do not use it for another person.

Collect linens in the order you will use them:
- Mattress pad (if needed)
- Bottom sheet (flat or fitted)
- Waterproof drawsheet or waterproof pad (if needed)
- Cotton drawsheet (if needed)
- Top sheet
- Blanket
- Bedspread
- Pillowcase(s)
- Bath towel(s)
- Hand towel
- Washcloth
- Gown or pajamas
- Bath blanket

Use one arm to hold the linens. Use your other hand to pick them up. The first item to use is at the bottom of your stack. (You picked up the mattress pad first. It is at the

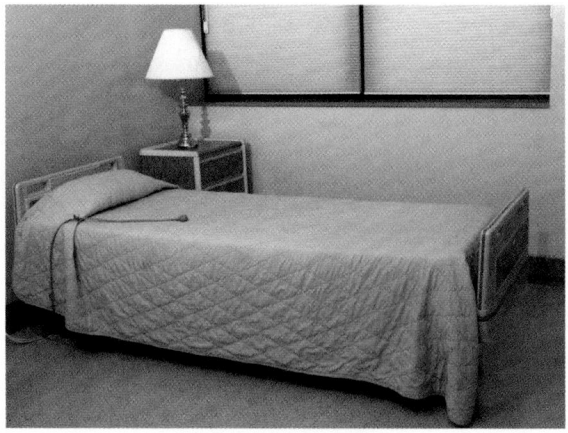

Fig. 19-1 Closed bed.

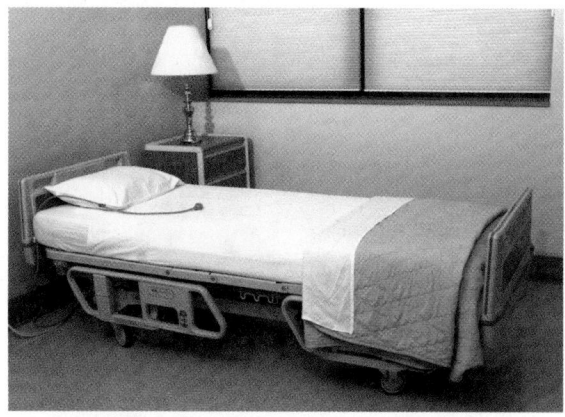

Fig. 19-2 Open bed. Top linens are fan-folded to the foot of the bed.

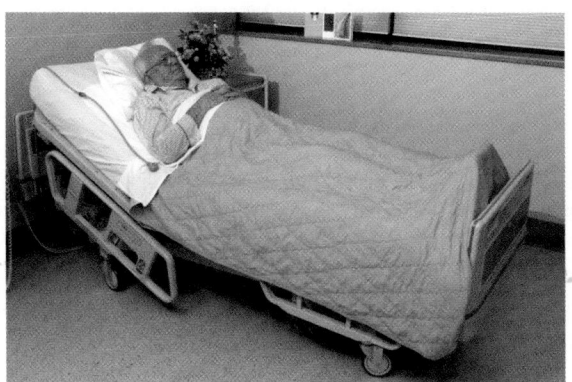

Fig. 19-3 Occupied bed.

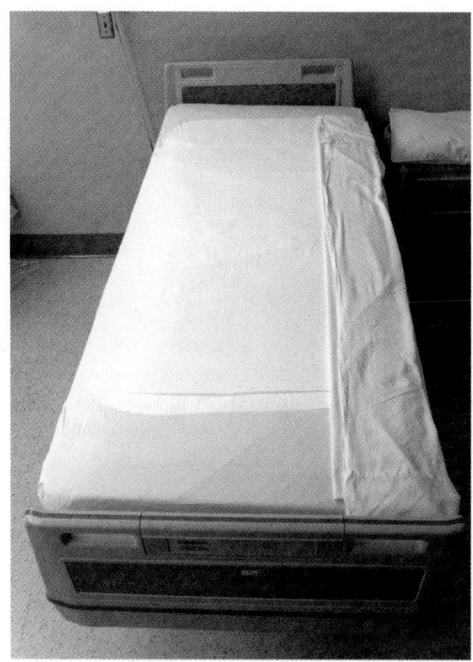

Fig. 19-4 Surgical bed.

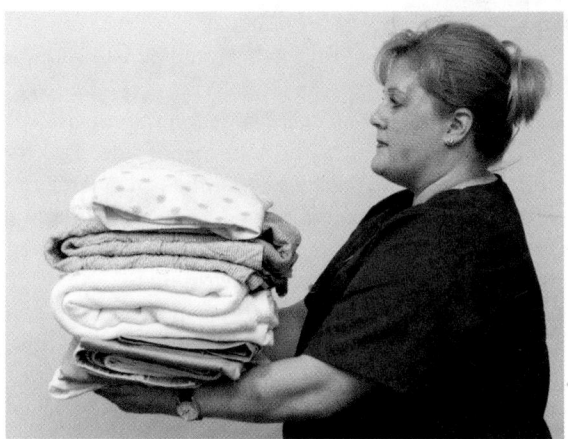

Fig. 19-5 Hold linens away from your body and uniform.

bottom. The bath blanket is on top.) You need the mattress pad first. To get it on top, place your arm over the bath blanket. Then turn the stack over onto the arm on the bath blanket (Fig. 19-6, p. 306). The arm that held the linens is now free. Place the clean linen on a clean surface.

Remove dirty linen one piece at a time. Roll each piece away from you. The side that touched the person is inside the roll and away from you (Fig. 19-7, p. 306).

In hospitals, top and bottom sheets, the cotton drawsheet, and pillowcases are changed daily. The mattress pad, plastic drawsheet, blanket, and bedspread are re-used for the same person. They are not re-used if soiled, wet, or wrinkled. Change wet, damp, or soiled linens right away. Wear gloves and follow Standard Precautions and the Bloodborne Pathogen Standard.

See *Focus on Long-Term Care and Home Care: Linens,* p. 306.

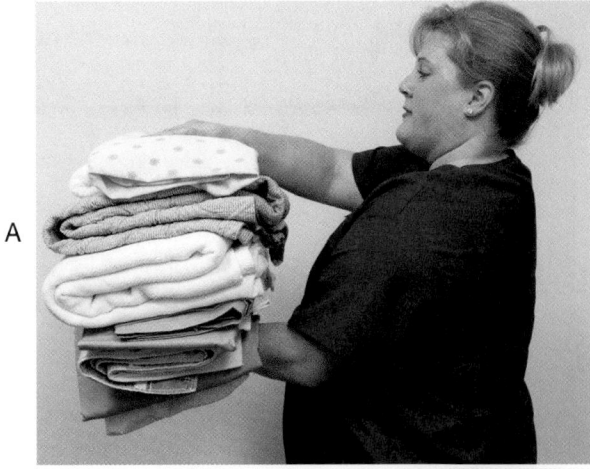

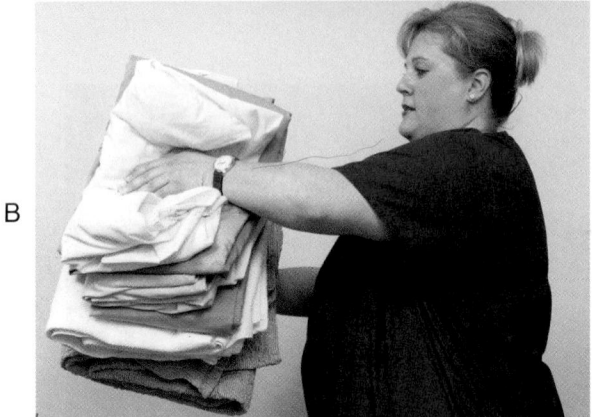

Fig. 19-6 Collecting linens. Linens are held away from the body and uniform. **A,** The arm is placed over the top of the stack of linens. **B,** The stack of linens is turned onto the arm. The linens are held away from the body.

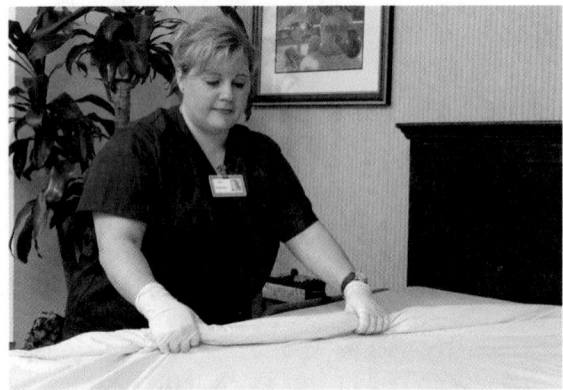

Fig. 19-7 Roll dirty linen away from you.

FOCUS ON LONG-TERM CARE AND HOME CARE
Linens

Long-Term Care
In nursing centers, linens are not changed every day. The center is the person's home. People do not change linens every day at home. A complete linen change is usually done on the person's bath day. This may be once or twice a week. Pillowcases, top and bottom sheets, and drawsheets (if used) are changed twice a week. Linens are always changed if wet, damp, soiled, or very wrinkled.

Some residents bring bedspreads, pillows, sheets, blankets, quilts, or afghans from home. Use them to make the bed. These items are the person's property. Make sure the items are labeled with the person's name. This prevents loss or confusion with another person's property.

Some centers have colored or printed linens. If so, let the person choose what color to use. Also let him or her decide how many pillows or blankets to use. If possible, the person chooses the time when you make the bed. The resident has the right to personal choice.

Home Care
Linen changes in the home are usually done weekly. Follow the person's routine. Change linens more often if the person asks you to do so. Always change linens that are wet, damp, soiled, or very wrinkled. Contact the nurse if the person refuses to have linens changed.

Drawsheets

A *drawsheet is a small sheet placed over the middle of the bottom sheet.*
- A *cotton drawsheet is made of cotton. It helps keep the mattress and bottom linens clean.*
- A *waterproof drawsheet is a drawsheet made of plastic, rubber, or absorbent material. It protects the mattress and bottom linens from dampness and soiling.* Some are rubber or plastic on one side—the waterproof side. The waterproof side is placed down, away from the person. The other side is cotton. It is placed up, toward the person. Other waterproof drawsheets are disposable. They are discarded when wet, soiled, or wrinkled.

The cotton drawsheet protects the person from contact with plastic or rubber and absorbs moisture. However, discomfort and skin breakdown may occur. Plastic and rubber retain heat. Waterproof drawsheets are hard to keep tight and wrinkle-free. Many agencies use incontinence products (Chapter 22) to keep the person and linens dry. Others use waterproof pads or disposable bed protectors (Fig. 19-8).

Cotton drawsheets are often used without waterproof drawsheets. Plastic-covered mattresses cause some persons to perspire heavily. This causes discomfort. A cotton drawsheet reduces heat retention and absorbs moisture. Cotton drawsheets are often used as assist devices to move and transfer persons in bed (Chapter 17). If used as an assist device, do not tuck it in at the sides.

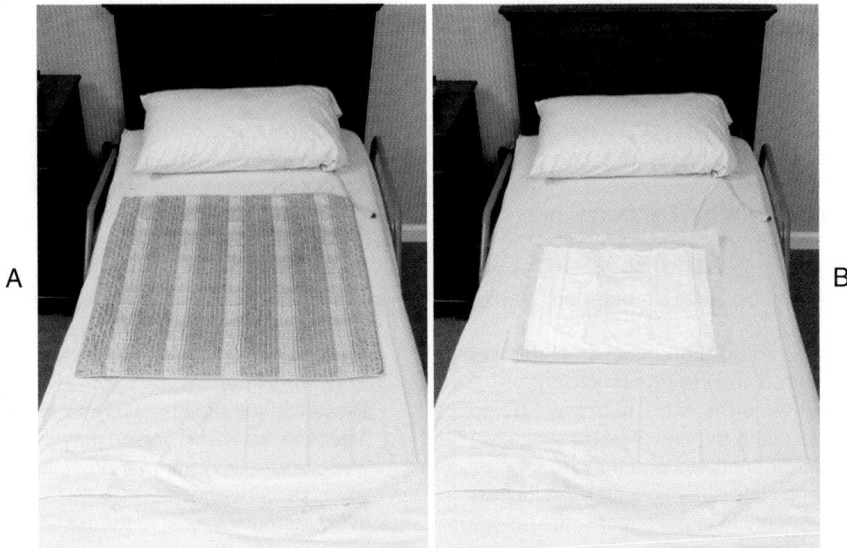

Fig. 19-8 A, Waterproof pad. **B,** Disposable bed protector.

The procedures that follow include waterproof and cotton drawsheets. This is so you learn how to use them. Ask the nurse about the type used in your agency.

See *Focus on Long-Term Care and Home Care: Drawsheets.*

MAKING BEDS

Safety and medical asepsis are important for bedmaking. Follow the rules in Box 19-1.

See *Focus on Children and Older Persons: Making Beds,* p. 308.

See *Focus on Long-Term Care and Home Care: Making Beds,* p. 308.

See *Delegation Guidelines: Making Beds,* p. 308.

See *Promoting Safety and Comfort: Making Beds,* p. 309.

See *Teamwork and Time Management: Making Beds,* p. 309.

FOCUS ON LONG-TERM CARE AND HOME CARE
Drawsheeets

Home Care

A flat sheet folded in half can serve as a cotton drawsheet. A twin-size sheet is easier to use for this purpose. The nurse tells you what to use.

Medical supply stores sell waterproof drawsheets and waterproof pads. The nurse discusses the need for these items with the person and family.

Some people use plastic mattress protectors. They protect mattresses but do not protect bottom linens (cotton drawsheet, bottom sheet, and mattress pad). Some people place plastic under the drawsheet. The nurse tells you what is safe for the person.

Do not use plastic trash bags or dry-cleaning bags. They are not strong enough to protect the linens and mattress. They slide easily and move out of place. Suffocation is a risk if the bag covers the person's nose and mouth.

BOX 19-1 RULES FOR BEDMAKING

- Use good body mechanics at all times (Chapter 16).
- Follow the rules in Chapter 17 to safely move and transfer the person.
- Follow the rules of medical asepsis.
- Follow Standard Precautions and the Bloodborne Pathogen Standard.
- Practice hand hygiene before handling clean linen.
- Practice hand hygiene after handling dirty linen.
- Bring enough linen to the person's room. Do not bring extra linens.
- Bring only the linens that you will need. You cannot use extra linen for another person.
- Place clean linen on a clean surface. Use the bedside chair, overbed table, or bedside stand. Place a barrier (towel, paper towels) between the clean surface and the linens if required by agency policy.
- Do not use extra linen in the person's room for another resident. Extra linen is considered contaminated. Put it with the dirty laundry.
- Do not use torn or frayed linen.
- Never shake linens. Shaking spreads microbes.
- Hold linens away from your body and uniform. Do not let dirty or clean linen touch your uniform.
- Never put dirty linens on the floor or on clean linens. Follow agency policy for dirty linen.
- Keep bottom linens tucked in and wrinkle-free.
- Cover a waterproof drawsheet with a cotton drawsheet. Plastic or rubber must not touch the person's body.
- Straighten and tighten loose sheets, blankets, and bedspreads as needed.
- Make as much of one side of the bed as possible before going to the other side. This saves time and energy.
- Change wet, damp, and soiled linens right away.

FOCUS ON CHILDREN AND OLDER PERSONS
Making Beds

Children

Cribs and crib linens present safety hazards. Mattresses, linens, and bumper pads pose many dangers. They can strangle and suffocate the baby. Follow the safety measures in Chapters 12 and 18. Also note the following. Report any hazard to the nurse.

- New cribs must meet December 2010 safety standards. Used or antique cribs with drop sides do not meet current safety standards.
- The crib mattress must be firm. A soft mattress can cover the baby's nose and mouth. This prevents breathing.
- The mattress must fit tight into the crib. There must be no gaps between the mattress and the crib. The baby can get trapped in gaps between the mattress and the crib.
- The space between the crib slats is no more than $2\frac{3}{8}$ inches. This is the width of a soda can. In larger spaces, the baby's head can get caught between the slats. The baby can suffocate.
- The mattress is at least 26 inches lower than the top of the crib sides. This prevents the baby from falling out of the crib. The mattress is lowered to the lowest position when the baby starts to stand in the crib.
- The end-panels must not have cut-outs. The baby's head can get trapped in cut-outs.
- Corner posts must be at least 16 inches above the end-panels. This prevents the baby's sleepwear or other garments from getting caught on the corner posts.
- Bumper pads are not used. If used, bumper pads:
  - Must cover the entire inside of the crib.
  - Must fit snugly against the slats. If not, the baby's head can get caught between the bumper pads and the slats.
  - Tie or snap in place. At least 6 ties or straps are needed. They are secured:
    - At the top and bottom edges of each corner (4 ties or snaps)
    - In the middle at each long side (2 ties or snaps)
  - Are placed so the ties or straps are away from the baby.
  - Must not have long ties or straps—no longer than 8 inches. Extra length is cut off. The baby can get entangled in long ties or straps.
  - Are removed from the crib when the baby starts to stand.
- Plastic trash bags, dry-cleaning bags, or plastic packaging materials are not used to protect the mattress. The plastic can cling to the baby's face, nose, and mouth. This prevents breathing and causes suffocation.
- The mattress is covered with a crib sheet. The crib sheet fits snugly.
- Only crib sheets are used in cribs. Sheets for twin, regular, queen, king, and other beds are not used.
- Sheets are not used if they are frayed, worn, or have loose threads or stitching.
- Pillows, blankets, comforters, quilts, sheepskin, sleep positioners, and pillow-like stuffed toys, and other soft products are not placed in the crib.
- Keep drop-side rails up and locked at all times. See Chapters 12 and 13.

FOCUS ON LONG-TERM CARE AND HOME CARE
Making Beds

Home Care

Many home care patients do not have hospital beds. You will use twin-, regular-, queen-, and king-sized beds. Water beds, sofa sleepers, cots, and recliners are common. Make the bed as the person wishes. Follow the rules in Box 19-1. If the person's wishes are not safe, contact the nurse.

Your assignment may include doing laundry. Wash linen when soiling is fresh to help prevent staining. Urine, feces, vomit, and blood can stain linens. Follow these guidelines:

- Wear gloves. Linens may contain blood, body fluids, secretions, or excretions.
- Rinse the item in cold water to remove the substance.
- Treat the stain. The person may use a stain-removing agent. Read and follow the manufacturer's instructions. Or follow the nurse's directions.
- Wash and dry linens as the person prefers.

DELEGATION GUIDELINES
Making Beds

Before making a bed, you need this information from the nurse and the care plan:

- What type of bed to make—closed, open, occupied, or surgical.
- If you need to use a cotton drawsheet.
- If you need to use a waterproof drawsheet, waterproof pad, or incontinence product.
- Position restrictions or limits in the person's movement or activity.
- If the person uses bed rails.
- The person's treatment, therapy, and activity schedule. For example, Mr. Smith needs a treatment in bed. Change linens after the treatment. Make Mrs. Chapman's bed while she is in physical therapy.
- How to position the person and the positioning devices needed.
- If the bed needs to be locked into a certain position (Chapter 18).
- When to report observations.
- What patient or resident concerns to report at once.

PROMOTING SAFETY AND COMFORT
Making Beds

Safety
You need to raise the bed for body mechanics. The bed also must be flat. If the bed is locked, unlock it. Then adjust the bed. Return the bed to the correct position when you are done. Then lock the bed.

Wear gloves to remove linen from the person's bed. Also follow other aspects of Standard Precautions and the Bloodborne Pathogen Standard. Linens may contain blood, body fluids, secretions, or excretions.

After making a bed, lower the bed to the correct level for the person. Follow the care plan. For an occupied bed, raise or lower bed rails according to the care plan.

Comfort
For an occupied bed, cover the person with a bath blanket before removing the top sheet. Do not leave the person uncovered when making the bed. The bath blanket provides for warmth and privacy.

Adjust the person's pillow as needed during the procedure. After the procedure, position the person as directed by the nurse and the care plan. Always make sure linens are straight and wrinkle-free.

TEAMWORK AND TIME MANAGEMENT
Making Beds

To save time and energy, make beds with a co-worker. Make one side of the bed while your co-worker makes the other.

Making beds with a co-worker is faster, easier, and safer for patients, residents, you, and your co-worker. Always thank your co-worker for helping you. Also help your co-worker make beds when asked to do so.

The Closed Bed
Closed beds are made for:
- Residents and home care patients who are up for most or all of the day. Top linens are folded back at bedtime. Clean linens are used as needed.
- New patients and residents. The bed is made after the bed frame and mattress are cleaned and disinfected. Clean linens are needed for the entire bed.

Text continued on p. 313

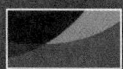 **MAKING A CLOSED BED**

QUALITY OF LIFE

Remember to:
- Knock before entering the person's room.
- Address the person by name.
- Introduce yourself by name and title.

- Explain the procedure to the person before beginning and during the procedure.
- Protect the person's rights during the procedure.
- Handle the person gently during the procedure.

PRE-PROCEDURE

1 Follow *Delegation Guidelines: Making Beds.* See *Promoting Safety and Comfort: Making Beds.*
2 Practice hand hygiene.
3 Collect clean linen:
- Mattress pad (if needed)
- Bottom sheet (flat sheet or fitted sheet)
- Waterproof drawsheet or waterproof pad (if needed)
- Cotton drawsheet (if needed)
- Top sheet
- Blanket
- Bedspread
- A pillowcase for each pillow

- Bath towel(s)
- Hand towel
- Washcloth
- Gown or pajamas
- Bath blanket
- Gloves
- Laundry bag
- Paper towels (if you need a barrier for clean linens)
4 Place linen on a clean surface. Use the paper towels as a barrier between the clean surface and clean linen if required by agency policy.
5 Raise the bed for body mechanics. Bed rails are down.

PROCEDURE

6 Put on the gloves.
7 Remove linen. Roll each piece away from you. Place each piece in a laundry bag. (NOTE: Discard incontinence products or disposable bed protectors in the trash. Do not put them in the laundry bag.)

8 Clean the bed frame and mattress (if this is your job).
9 Remove and discard gloves. Practice hand hygiene.
10 Move the mattress to the head of the bed.
11 Put the mattress pad on the mattress. It is even with the top of the mattress.

Continued

MAKING A CLOSED BED—cont'd

PROCEDURE—cont'd

12 Place the bottom sheet on the mattress pad (Fig. 19-9). Unfold it length-wise. Place the center crease in the middle of the bed. If using a flat sheet:

  a Position the lower edge even with the bottom of the mattress.

  b Place the large hem at the top and the small hem at the bottom.

  c Face hem-stitching downward, away from the person.

13 Open the sheet. Fan-fold it to the other side of the bed (Fig. 19-10, A and B).

14 Tuck the corners of a fitted sheet over the mattress at the top and then the foot of the bed. For a flat sheet, tuck the top of the sheet under the mattress. The sheet is tight and smooth.

15 Make a mitered corner at the top if using a flat sheet (Fig. 19-11).

16 Place the waterproof drawsheet on the bed. It is in the middle of the mattress. Or put the waterproof pad on the bed.

17 Open the waterproof drawsheet. Fan-fold it to the other side of the bed.

18 Place a cotton drawsheet over the waterproof drawsheet. It covers the entire waterproof drawsheet (Fig. 19-12).

19 Open the cotton drawsheet. Fan-fold it to the other side of the bed.

20 Tuck both drawsheets under the mattress. Or tuck each in separately.

21 Go to the other side of the bed.

22 Miter the top corner of the flat bottom sheet.

23 Pull the bottom sheet tight so there are no wrinkles. Tuck in the sheet.

24 Pull the drawsheets tight so there are no wrinkles. Tuck both in together or separately (Fig. 19-13, p. 312).

25 Go to the other side of the bed.

26 Put the top sheet on the bed.

  a Unfold it length-wise. Place the center crease in the middle.

  b Place the large hem even with the top of the mattress.

  c Open the sheet. Fan-fold it to the other side.

  d Face hem-stitching outward, away from the person.

  e Do not tuck the bottom in yet.

  f Never tuck top linens in on the sides.

27 Place the blanket on the bed:

  a Unfold it so the center crease is in the middle.

  b Put the upper hem about 6 to 8 inches from the top of the mattress.

  c Open the blanket. Fan-fold it to the other side.

  d If steps 33 and 34 are not done, turn the top sheet down over the blanket. Hem-stitching is down, away from the person.

28 Place the bedspread on the bed:

  a Unfold it so the center crease is in the middle.

  b Place the upper hem even with the top of the mattress.

  c Open and fan-fold the bedspread to the other side.

  d Make sure the bedspread facing the door is even. It covers all top linens.

29 Tuck in top linens together at the foot of the bed so they are smooth and tight. Make a mitered corner.

30 Go to the other side.

31 Straighten all top linen. Work from the head of the bed to the foot.

32 Tuck in top linens together at the foot of the bed. Make a mitered corner.

33 Turn the top hem of the bedspread under the blanket to make a cuff (Fig. 19-14, p. 312).

34 Turn the top sheet down over the bedspread. Hem-stitching is down. (Steps 33 and 34 are not done in some agencies. The bedspread covers the pillow. If so, tuck the bedspread under the pillow.)

35 Put the pillowcase on the pillow as in Figure 19-15, p. 312 or Figure 19-16, p. 312. Fold extra material under the pillow at the seam end of the pillowcase.

36 Place the pillow on the bed. The open end of the pillowcase is away from the door. The seam is toward the head of the bed.

POST-PROCEDURE

37 Provide for comfort. (See the inside of the front book cover.) NOTE: Omit this step if the bed is prepared for a new patient or resident.

38 Attach the signal light to the bed. Or place it within the person's reach.

39 Lower the bed to its lowest position. Lock the bed wheels.

40 Put the towels, washcloth, gown or pajamas, and bath blanket in the bedside stand.

41 Complete a safety check of the room. (See the inside of the front book cover.)

42 Follow agency policy for dirty linen.

43 Practice hand hygiene.

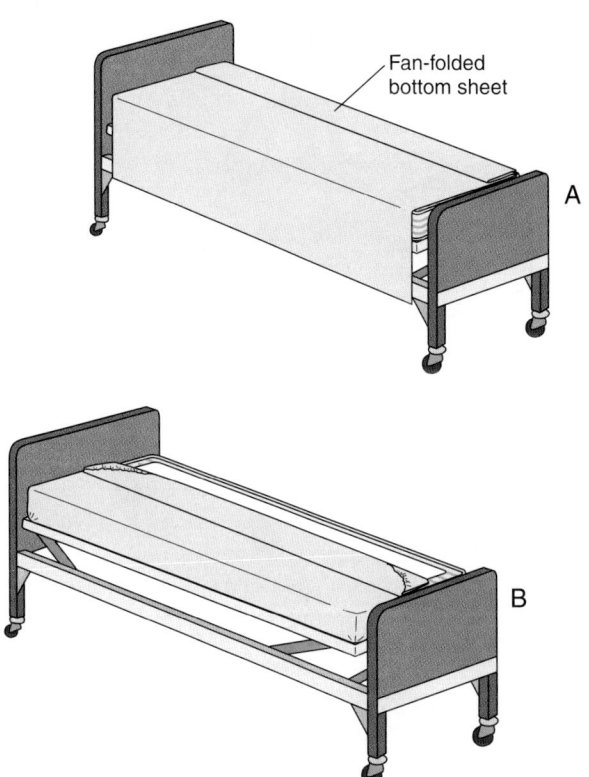

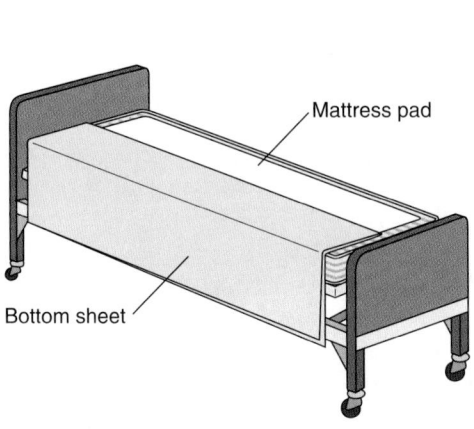

Fig. 19-9 A flat bottom sheet is on the bed with the center crease in the middle. The lower hem of the sheet is even with the bottom of the mattress.

Fig. 19-10 **A,** The flat bottom sheet is fan-folded to the other side of the bed. **B,** A fitted sheet is on the bed with the center crease in the middle.

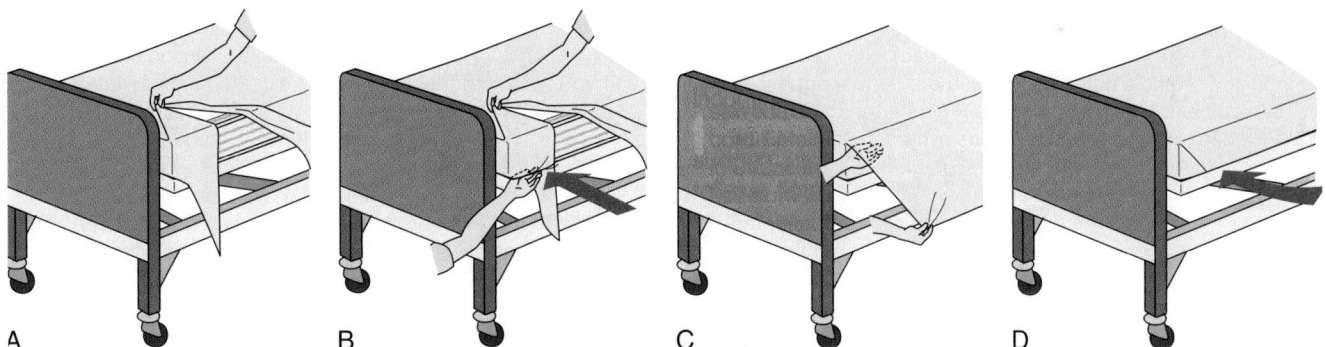

Fig. 19-11 Making a mitered corner. **A,** The flat bottom sheet is tucked under the mattress at the head of the bed. The side of the sheet is raised onto the mattress. **B,** The remaining portion of the sheet is tucked under the mattress. **C,** The raised portion of the sheet is brought off the mattress. **D,** The entire side of the sheet is tucked under the mattress.

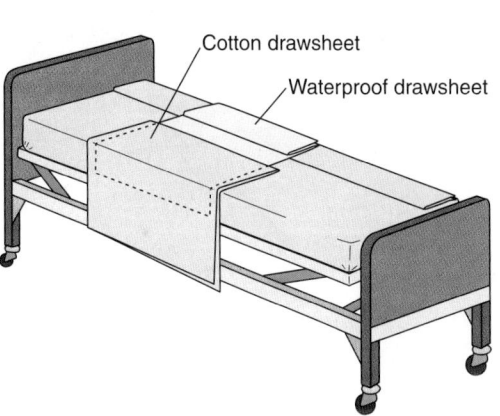

Fig. 19-12 A cotton drawsheet is over the waterproof drawsheet. The cotton drawsheet completely covers the waterproof drawsheet.

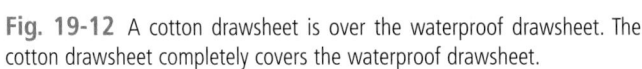

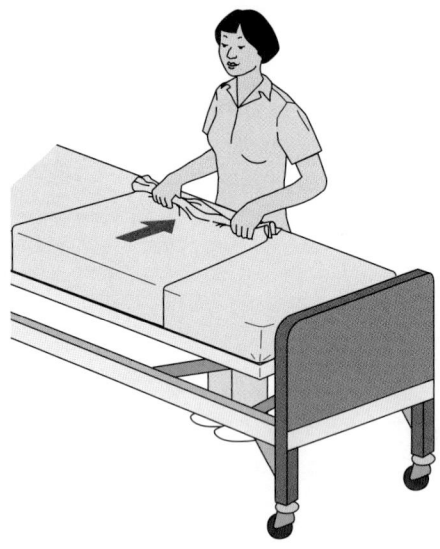

Fig. 19-13 The drawsheet is pulled tight to remove wrinkles.

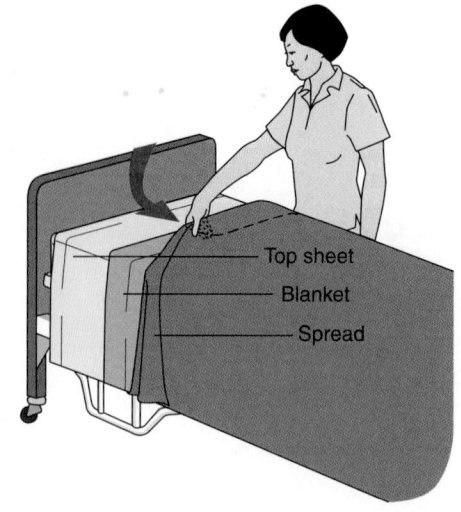

Top sheet
Blanket
Spread

Fig. 19-14 The top hem of the bedspread is turned under the top hem of the blanket to make a cuff.

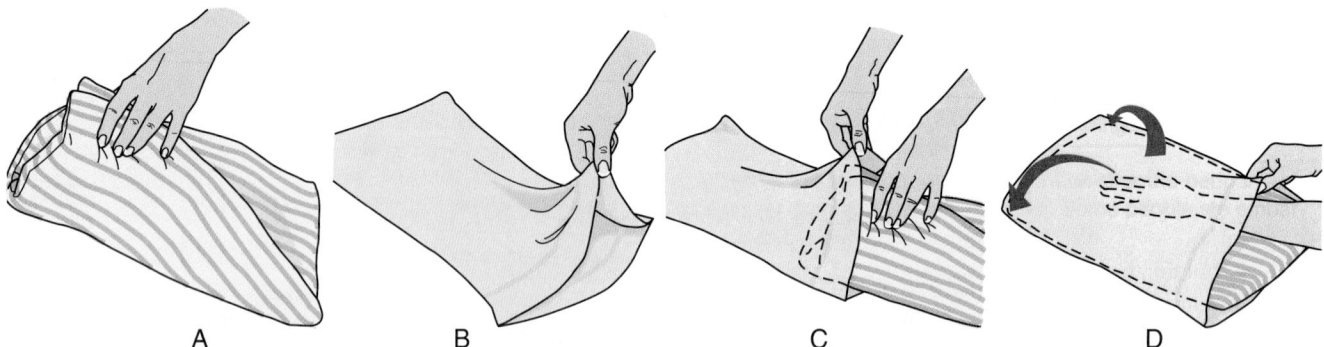

A   B   C   D

Fig. 19-15 Putting a pillowcase on a pillow. **A,** Grasp the corners of the pillow at the seam end and form a "V" with the pillow. **B,** Open the pillowcase with your free hand. **C,** Guide the "V" end of the pillow into the pillowcase. **D,** Let the "V" end of the pillow fall into the corners of the pillowcase.

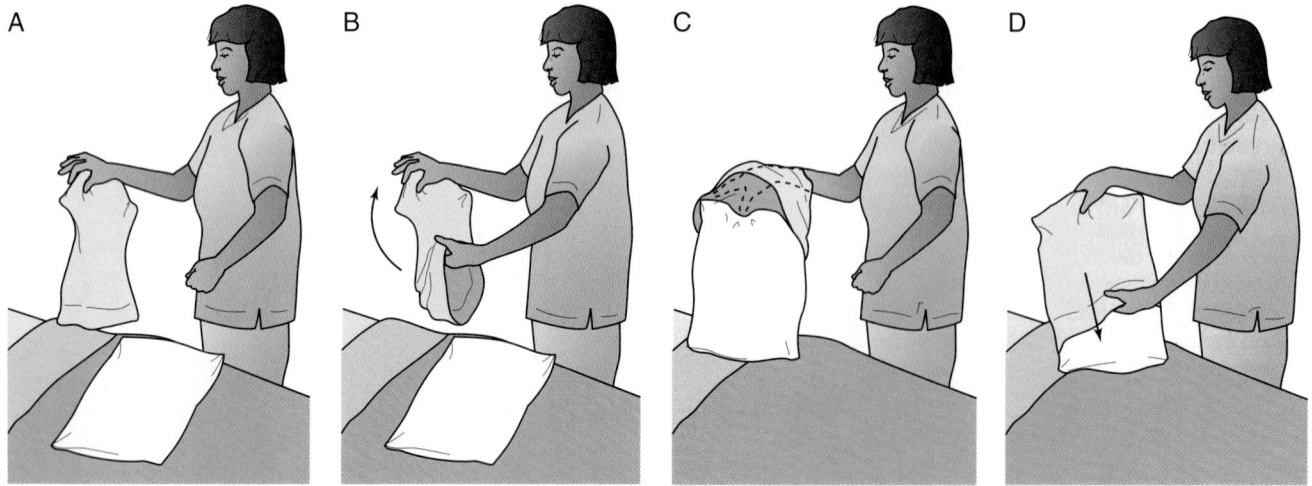

A   B   C   D

Fig. 19-16 Putting a pillowcase on a pillow. **A,** Grasp the closed end of the pillowcase. **B,** Using your other hand, gather up the pillowcase. The pillowcase should cover your hand holding the closed end. **C,** Grasp the pillow with the hand covered by the pillowcase. **D,** Pull the pillowcase down over the pillow with your other hand.

The Open Bed

A closed bed becomes an open bed by fan-folding back the top linen. The person can get into bed with ease. Make this bed for:

- Newly admitted persons arriving by wheelchair
- Persons who are getting ready for bed
- Persons who are out of bed for a short time

The Occupied Bed

You make an occupied bed when the person stays in bed. Keep the person in good alignment. Follow restrictions or limits in the person's movement or position.

Explain each procedure step to the person before it is done. This is important even if the person cannot respond to you or is in a coma.

See *Focus on Communication: The Occupied Bed.*

See *Promoting Safety and Comfort: The Occupied Bed.*

Text continued on p. 316

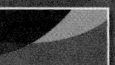 ## MAKING AN OPEN BED

QUALITY OF LIFE

Remember to:
- Knock before entering the person's room.
- Address the person by name.
- Introduce yourself by name and title.

- Explain the procedure to the person before beginning and during the procedure.
- Protect the person's rights during the procedure.
- Handle the person gently during the procedure.

PROCEDURE

1 Follow *Delegation Guidelines: Making Beds,* p. 308. See *Promoting Safety and Comfort: Making Beds,* p. 309.
2 Practice hand hygiene.
3 Collect linen for a closed bed.

4 Make a closed bed. See procedure: *Making a Closed Bed,* p. 309.
5 Fan-fold top linens to the foot of the bed (see Fig. 19-2).

POST-PROCEDURE

6 Attach the signal light to the bed.
7 Lower the bed to its lowest position.
8 Put the towels, washcloth, gown or pajamas, and bath blanket in the bedside stand.
9 Provide for comfort. (See the inside of the front book cover.)

10 Place the signal light within the person's reach.
11 Complete a safety check of the room. (See the inside of the front book cover.)
12 Follow agency policy for dirty linen.
13 Practice hand hygiene.

FOCUS ON COMMUNICATION
The Occupied Bed

After making an occupied bed, make sure the person is comfortable. You can ask:
- "Are you comfortable?"
- "How can I make you more comfortable?"
- "Are you warm enough?"
- "Do you feel any creases or wrinkles?"
- "Can I adjust your pillow?"

After making the bed, thank the person for cooperating.

PROMOTING SAFETY AND COMFORT
The Occupied Bed

Safety

The person lies on one side of the bed and then the other. Protect the person from falling out of bed. If bed rails are used, the far bed rail is up. If the person does not use bed rails, have a co-worker help you. You work on one side of the bed. Your co-worker works on the other.

Comfort

To make an occupied bed, the person lies on his or her side. You tuck dirty bottom linens under the person. Then you put clean linens on the bed. These, too, are tucked under the person. The tucked linens create a "bump" in the middle of the bed. To make the other side, the person rolls over the "bump" to the other side of the bed. To promote comfort, make the "bump" as low as possible. Do this by fan-folding dirty and clean bottom linens neatly and flatly.

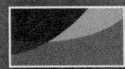

MAKING AN OCCUPIED BED

QUALITY OF LIFE

Remember to:
- Knock before entering the person's room.
- Address the person by name.
- Introduce yourself by name and title.

- Explain the procedure to the person before beginning and during the procedure.
- Protect the person's rights during the procedure.
- Handle the person gently during the procedure.

PROCEDURE

1 Follow *Delegation Guidelines: Making Beds,* p. 308. See *Promoting Safety and Comfort:*
   a *Making Beds,* p. 309
   b *The Occupied Bed,* p. 313
2 Practice hand hygiene.
3 Collect the following:
   - Gloves
   - Laundry bag
   - Clean linen (see procedure: *Making a Closed Bed,* p. 309)
   - Paper towels (if you need a barrier for clean linens)

4 Place linen on a clean surface. Place the paper towels between the clean surface and clean linen if a barrier is required by agency policy.
5 Identify the person. Check the ID (identification) bracelet against the assignment sheet. Also call the person by name.
6 Provide for privacy.
7 Remove the signal light.
8 Raise the bed for body mechanics. Bed rails are up if used. Bed wheels are locked.
9 Lower the head of the bed. It is as flat as possible.

PROCEDURE

10 Practice hand hygiene. Put on gloves.
11 Loosen top linens at the foot of the bed.
12 Lower the bed rail near you if up.
13 Remove the bedspread (Fig. 19-17). Then remove the blanket in the same way. Place each over the chair.
14 Cover the person with a bath blanket. Use the one in the bedside stand.
   a Unfold the bath blanket over the top sheet.
   b Ask the person to hold on to the bath blanket. If he or she cannot, tuck the top part under the person's shoulders.
   c Grasp the top sheet under the bath blanket at the shoulders. Bring the sheet down toward the foot of the bed. Remove the sheet from under the blanket (Fig. 19-18, p. 316).
15 Position the person on the side of the bed away from you. Adjust the pillow for comfort.
16 Loosen bottom linens from the head to the foot of the bed.
17 Fan-fold bottom linens one at a time toward the person. Start with the cotton drawsheet (Fig. 19-19, p. 316). If re-using the mattress pad, do not fan-fold it.
18 Place a clean mattress pad on the bed. Unfold it length-wise. The center crease is in the middle. Fan-fold the top part toward the person. If re-using the mattress pad, straighten and smooth any wrinkles.
19 Place the bottom sheet on the mattress pad. Hem-stitching is away from the person. Unfold the sheet so the crease is in the middle. If using a flat sheet, the small hem is even with the bottom of the mattress. Fan-fold the top part toward the person.
20 Tuck the corners of a fitted sheet over the mattress. If using a flat sheet, make a mitered corner at the head of the bed. Tuck the sheet under the mattress from the head to the foot.

21 Pull the waterproof drawsheet (if re-used) toward you over the bottom sheet. Tuck excess material under the mattress. Do the following for a clean waterproof drawsheet (Fig. 19-20, p. 316).
   a Place the waterproof drawsheet on the bed. It is in the middle of the mattress.
   b Fan-fold the top part toward the person.
   c Tuck in excess fabric.
22 Place the cotton drawsheet over the waterproof drawsheet. It covers the entire waterproof drawsheet. Fan-fold the top part toward the person. Tuck in excess fabric.
23 Explain to the person that he or she will roll over a "bump." Assure the person that he or she will not fall.
24 Help the person turn to the other side. Adjust the pillow for comfort.
25 Raise the bed rail. Go to the other side, and lower the bed rail.
26 Loosen bottom linens. Remove one piece at a time. Place each piece in the laundry bag. (NOTE: Discard disposable bed protectors and incontinence products in the trash. Do not put them in the laundry bag.)
27 Remove and discard the gloves. Practice hand hygiene.
28 Straighten and smooth the mattress pad.
29 Pull the clean bottom sheet toward you. Tuck the corners of a fitted sheet over the mattress. If using a flat sheet, make a mitered corner at the top. Tuck the sheet under the mattress from the head to the foot of the bed.
30 Pull the drawsheets tightly toward you. Tuck both under together or separately.
31 Position the person supine in the center of the bed. Adjust the pillow for comfort.
32 Put the top sheet on the bed. Unfold it length-wise. The crease is in the middle. The large hem is even with the top of the mattress. Hem-stitching is on the outside.

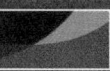 **MAKING AN OCCUPIED BED—cont'd**

PROCEDURE—cont'd

33 Ask the person to hold the top sheet so you can remove the bath blanket. Or tuck the top sheet under the person's shoulders. Remove and discard the bath blanket.

34 Place the blanket on the bed. Unfold it so the crease is in the middle and it covers the person. The upper hem is 6 to 8 inches from the top of the mattress.

35 Place the bedspread on the bed. Unfold it so the center crease is in the middle and it covers the person. The top hem is even with the mattress top.

36 Turn the top hem of the bedspread under the blanket to make a cuff.

37 Bring the top sheet down over the bedspread to form a cuff.

38 Go to the foot of the bed.

39 Make a toe pleat. Make a 2-inch pleat across the foot of the bed. The pleat is about 6 to 8 inches from the foot of the bed.

40 Lift the mattress corner with one arm. Tuck all top linens under the mattress. Make a mitered corner.

41 Raise the bed rail. Go to the other side, and lower the bed rail.

42 Straighten and smooth top linens.

43 Tuck all top linens under the mattress. Make a mitered corner.

44 Change the pillowcase(s).

POST-PROCEDURE

45 Provide for comfort. (See the inside of the front book cover.)

46 Place the signal light within reach.

47 Lower the bed to its lowest position. The bed wheels are locked.

48 Raise or lower bed rails. Follow the care plan.

49 Put the clean towels, washcloth, gown or pajamas, and bath blanket in the bedside stand.

50 Unscreen the person.

51 Complete a safety check of the room. (See the inside of the front book cover.)

52 Follow agency policy for dirty linen.

53 Practice hand hygiene.

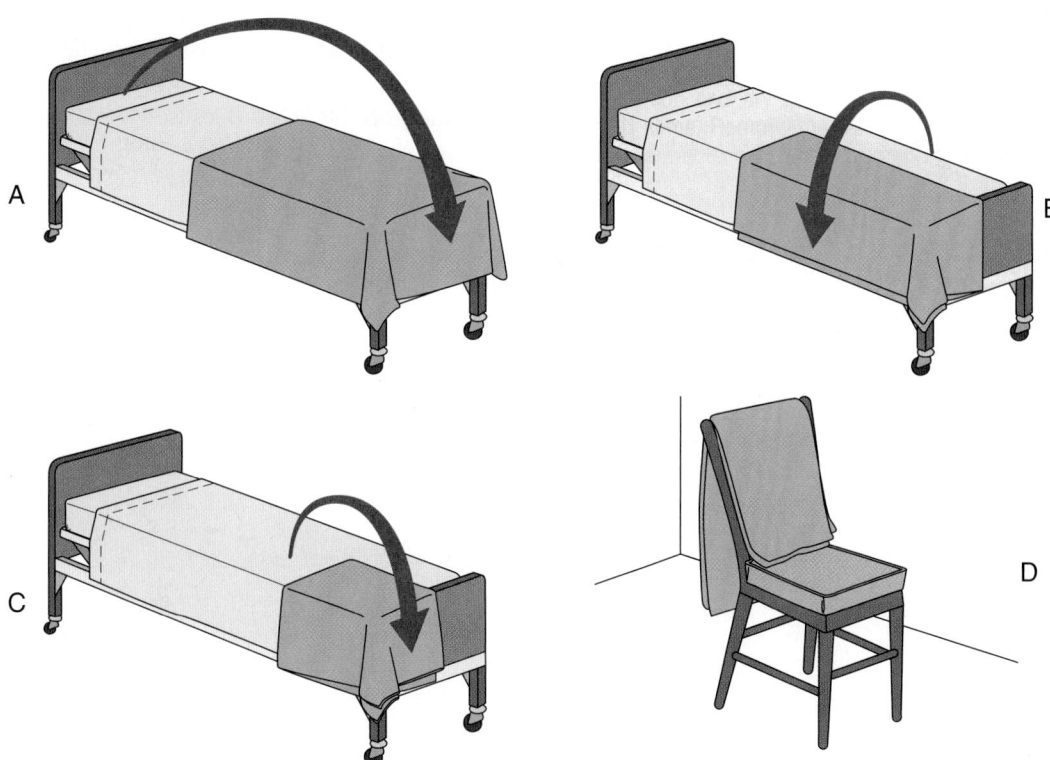

Fig. 19-17 Folding linen for re-use. **A,** Fold the top edge of the bedspread down to the bottom edge. **B,** Fold the bedspread from the far side of the bed to the near side. **C,** Fold the top edge of the bedspread down to the bottom edge again. **D,** Place the folded bedspread over the back of the chair.

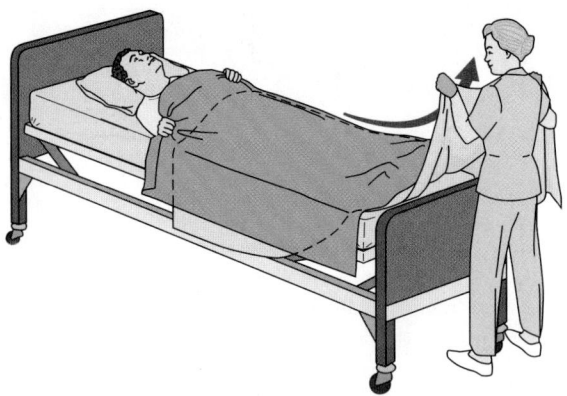

Fig. 19-18 The person holds on to the bath blanket. The top sheet is removed from under the bath blanket. (NOTE: Bed rails are used according to the care plan.)

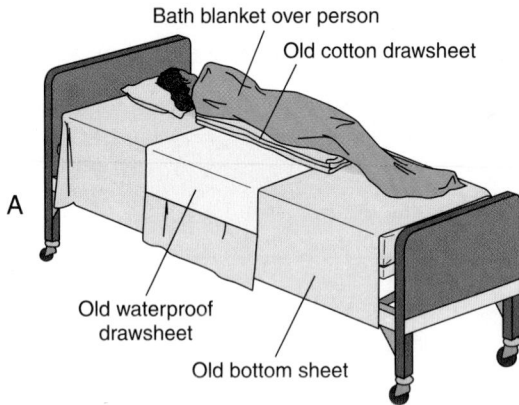

Bath blanket over person
Old cotton drawsheet

A

Old waterproof drawsheet

Old bottom sheet

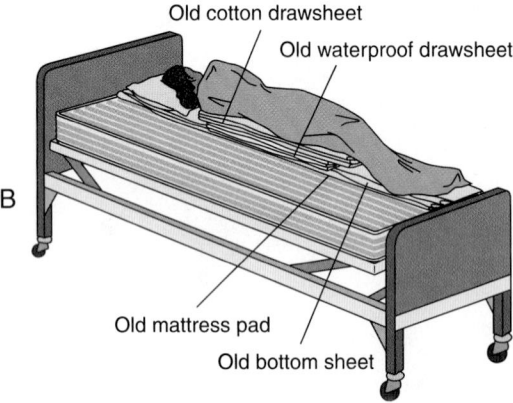

Old cotton drawsheet
Old waterproof drawsheet

B

Old mattress pad
Old bottom sheet

Fig. 19-19 A, The cotton drawsheet is fan-folded and tucked under the person. **B,** All bottom linens are tucked under the person. (NOTE: Bed rails are used according to the care plan.)

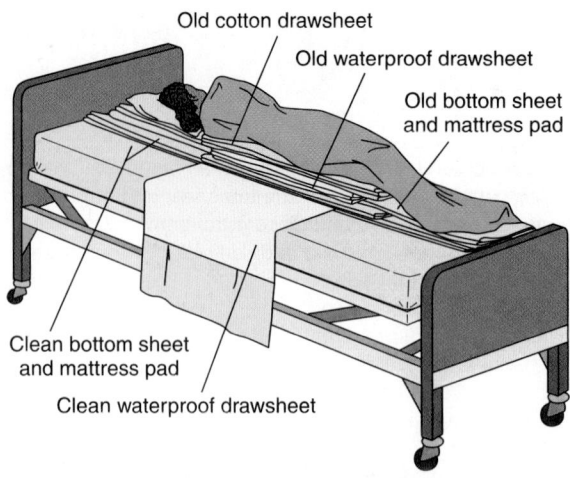

Old cotton drawsheet
Old waterproof drawsheet
Old bottom sheet and mattress pad

Clean bottom sheet and mattress pad
Clean waterproof drawsheet

Fig. 19-20 A clean bottom sheet and waterproof drawsheet are on the bed with both fan-folded and tucked under the person. (NOTE: Bed rails are used according to the care plan.)

The Surgical Bed

The surgical bed also is called a *recovery bed* or *post-operative bed*. It is a form of the open bed. Top linens are folded to transfer the person from a stretcher to the bed. These beds are made for persons:

- Returning to their rooms from surgery. A complete linen change is needed.
- Who arrive at the agency by ambulance. A complete linen change is needed if the person is a new patient or resident or is returning to the agency from the hospital.
- Who go by stretcher to treatment or therapy areas. A complete linen change is not needed.
- Using portable tubs. Because the person has a bath, a complete linen change is needed.

See *Promoting Safety and Comfort: The Surgical Bed.*

PROMOTING SAFETY AND COMFORT

The Surgical Bed

Safety

To safely transfer a person from a stretcher to a surgical bed, see procedure: *Moving the Person to a Stretcher* (Chapter 17). Also follow the rules for stretcher safety (Chapter 12). After the transfer, lower the bed to its lowest position. Make sure the bed wheels are locked. Raise or lower bed rails according to the care plan.

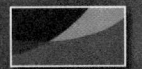

MAKING A SURGICAL BED

VIDEO

PROCEDURE

1 Follow *Delegation Guidelines: Making Beds,* p. 308. See *Promoting Safety and Comfort:*
   a *Making Beds,* p. 309
   b *The Surgical Bed*
2 Practice hand hygiene.
3 Collect the following:
   • Clean linen (see procedure: *Making a Closed Bed,* p. 309)
   • Gloves
   • Laundry bag
   • Equipment requested by the nurse
   • Paper towels (if you need a barrier for clean linens)
4 Place linen on a clean surface. Place the paper towels between the clean surface and clean linen if a barrier is required by agency policy.
5 Remove the signal light.
6 Raise the bed for body mechanics.
7 Remove all linen from the bed. Wear gloves. Practice hand hygiene after removing and discarding them.
8 Make a closed bed (see procedure: *Making a Closed Bed,* p. 309). Do not tuck top linens under the mattress.

9 Fold all top linens at the foot of the bed back onto the bed. The fold is even with the edge of the mattress (Fig. 19-21, A).
10 Know on which side of the bed the stretcher will be placed. Fan-fold linen length-wise to the other side of the bed (Fig. 19-21, B).
11 Put the pillowcase(s) on the pillow(s).
12 Place the pillow(s) on a clean surface.
13 Leave the bed in its highest position.
14 Leave both bed rails down.
15 Put the clean towels, washcloth, gown or pajamas, and bath blanket in the bedside stand.
16 Move furniture away from the bed. Allow room for the stretcher and the staff.
17 Do not attach the signal light to the bed.
18 Complete a safety check of the room. (See the inside of the front book cover.)
19 Follow agency policy for soiled linen.
20 Practice hand hygiene.

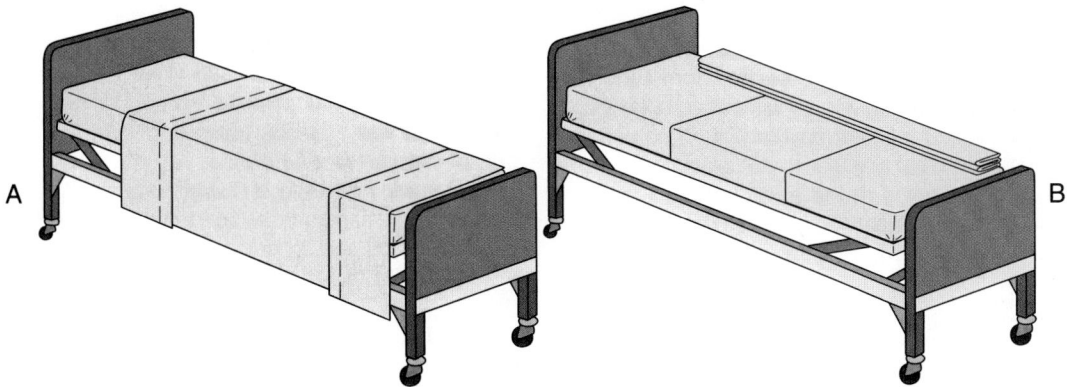

Fig. 19-21 Surgical bed. **A,** The bottom of the top linens is folded back onto the bed. The fold is even with the bottom edge of the mattress. **B,** Top linens are fan-folded length-wise to the opposite side of the bed.

FOCUS ON PRIDE

The Person, Family, and Yourself

Personal and Professional Responsibility

The bed is the largest item in the person's unit. The person, family, and visitors notice if the bed is unmade, messy, or dirty. They question the quality of care.

You are responsible for providing a neat and orderly setting. The bed must be clean and well made. If the person stays in bed, straighten and tighten sheets and other linen as needed. These actions promote comfort and quality of life.

Rights and Respect

Nursing center residents have the right to make their settings as home-like as possible. Residents often bring bedspreads, blankets, quilts, and so on from home. The items have meaning and value. For example, Mr. Baker wants his afghan on his bed at night. His wife made it years ago. Mr. Baker moved in to the nursing center after his wife died. The sight and smell of the afghan remind him of his wife and home.

Protect personal items from loss and damage. Handle the person's belongings with care and respect.

Independence and Social Interaction

Allow personal choice when possible. What is best for you, may not be best for the person. For example, you planned to make Mrs. Beck's bed and straighten her room after breakfast. However, her family comes to visit at that time. Mrs. Beck wants her bed made before or during breakfast.

Ask about the person's preferences. Consider them when planning your day and managing your time. The more choices allowed, the greater the person's sense of control and independence.

Delegation and Teamwork

Agencies have different ways of handling dirty linen. Some have containers in each room. Others have carts in the hallways. The carts are emptied each shift or as needed. Some agencies have a room where dirty linen is placed. Others have chutes.

When handling dirty linen:
- Wear gloves.
- Follow agency policy for dirty linen.
- Do not over-fill the bag or container. The person who empties the bag or cart may be injured.
- Work as a team. Some units assign a person to empty linen containers. Linen must not overflow from carts. If you see a full cart, empty it. Do so without complaining. The person assigned the task may be busy. If no one is assigned the task, work together to complete it.
- Clean up after yourself. If you fill a cart, empty it. If you place an item in a cart that will cause an odor, empty it.
- Place dirty linen in the correct location. Do not place dirty linen in a room or cart where it does not belong. If chutes are used, use the correct chute. Other chutes in the same area may be for trash.

Ethics and Laws

Patients and residents must always be treated with dignity, care, and kindness. The following is a real event in which a nurse ignored these values.

On August 2, 1990, a patient had back surgery. She was on complete bedrest until August 4 when the doctor changed the order. The new order was "increase activity up as tolerated with assist." According to the facts reported in the court case, the following occurred between the patient and a nurse:

- *On August 5 the patient was awakened when the nurse bumped into her bed. The nurse told the patient that she had to get up and have her bed made. The patient explained that she had an uncomfortable night, could not sleep, and wanted to rest. Despite pleas to stay in bed, the nurse told the patient that she [the nurse] had to make the bed.*
- *The nurse then pulled the patient by her arm. The patient pleaded with the nurse to leave her alone because she wanted to sleep. The patient also told the nurse that it hurt to have her arm pulled that way.*
- *The nurse let go of the patient's arm. The patient laid down in bed.*
- *The nurse then pulled the patient's feet off of the bed. In extreme pain, the patient "started to yell, to plead with the nurse not to do what she was doing and told her that it hurt."*
- *The nurse insisted that the patient had to get up. The nurse insisted that she had to make the bed. The nurse forced the patient into a standing position. The patient, in pain, told the nurse that she was going to "throw up or faint."*
- *The nurse shoved the patient "into a straight back chair using her hands to press down hard on the [patient's] shoulders."*
- *In extreme pain, the patient pleaded with the nurse and said that she was going to faint.*
- *The nurse then forced the patient's head between her knees down to her lap. The patient felt extreme pain in the middle of her back.*
- *The nurse then raised the patient's back. In extreme pain, the patient could not get up when she tried to do so. The patient continued to plead with the nurse to put her back to bed.*
- *The nurse again told the patient that she had to make the bed. The nurse "ripped the sheet off the bed and used it to tie [the patient] in the chair with a knot towards the back."*
- *The patient "tried to reach forward to push the nurse's call button . . . [The nurse] kicked and pushed the table out at the same time, away and out of the [patient's] grasp." The patient said that she wanted to call a nurse.*
- *The nurse left the room for 10 minutes. "She came back and made the bed with a laboratory technician." After making the bed, they put the patient back in bed. The patient was crying.*

The Appellate Court of Illinois reviewing the case said the "negligence here was . . . grossly apparent. . . ." The case was sent back to the trial court for a full trial.

(R. Prairie v University of Chicago Hospitals, 1998.)

Treating a person in such a way is unethical and is abuse. If you see a person being mistreated, take action. Get help. Protect the person.

REVIEW QUESTIONS

Circle T if the statement is TRUE or F if it is FALSE.

1 T F In nursing centers, complete linen changes are required for closed beds and surgical beds.

2 T F In home care, complete linen changes are done daily.

3 T F Twin-size sheets can be used in baby cribs.

4 T F You can place pillows and blankets in a baby's crib.

5 T F Hem-stitching of the bottom sheet is placed away from the person.

6 T F To remove crumbs from the bed, you shake linens in the air.

7 T F The upper hem of the bedspread is even with the top of the mattress.

8 T F Top linens are fan-folded to the foot of the bed for an open bed.

9 T F A cotton drawsheet is used only with a waterproof drawsheet.

10 T F Residents can bring bed coverings from home.

Circle the BEST answer.

11 You will transfer a person from a stretcher to the bed. Which bed should you make?
   a A closed bed
   b An open bed
   c An occupied bed
   d A surgical bed

12 When handling linens
   a Put dirty linens on the floor
   b Hold linens away from your body and uniform
   c Shake linens to unfold them
   d Take extra linen to another person's room

13 A resident is out of the bed most of the day. Which bed should you make?
   a A closed bed
   b An open bed
   c An occupied bed
   d A surgical bed

14 A complete linen change is done when
   a The bottom linens are wet or soiled
   b The bed is made for a new person
   c The person will transfer from a stretcher to a bed
   d Linens are loose or wrinkled

15 You are using a waterproof drawsheet. Which is *true*?
   a A cotton drawsheet must completely cover the waterproof drawsheet.
   b Waterproof pads are needed.
   c The person's consent is needed.
   d The plastic or rubber is in contact with the person's skin.

16 To make an occupied bed, you do the following *except*
   a Cover the person with a bath blanket
   b Screen the person
   c Raise the far bed rail
   d Fan-fold top linens to the foot of the bed

17 A surgical bed is kept
   a In Fowler's position
   b In the lowest position
   c In the highest position
   d In the supine position

Answers to these questions are on p. 833.

20 Personal Hygiene

OBJECTIVES

- Define the key terms and key abbreviations listed in this chapter.
- Explain why personal hygiene is important.
- Describe the care given before and after breakfast, after lunch, and in the evening.
- Describe the rules for bathing.
- Identify safety measures for tub baths and showers.

- Explain the purposes of a back massage.
- Explain the purposes of perineal care.
- Identify the observations to report and record when assisting with hygiene.
- Perform the procedures described in this chapter.
- Explain how to promote PRIDE in the person, the family, and yourself.

KEY TERMS

AM care See "early morning care"
aspiration Breathing fluid, food, vomitus, or an object into the lungs
denture An artificial tooth or a set of artificial teeth
diaphoresis Profuse (excessive) sweating
early morning care Routine care given before breakfast; AM care
evening care Care given in the evening at bedtime; PM care
morning care Care given after breakfast; hygiene measures are more thorough at this time

oral hygiene Mouth care
pericare See "perineal care"
perineal care Cleaning the genital and anal areas; pericare
plaque A thin film that sticks to the teeth; it contains saliva, microbes, and other substances
PM care See "evening care"
tartar Hardened plaque

KEY ABBREVIATIONS

C Centigrade
F Fahrenheit

ID Identification

Hygiene promotes comfort, safety, and health. The skin is the body's first line of defense against disease. Intact skin prevents microbes from entering the body and causing an infection. Likewise, mucous membranes of the mouth, genital area, and anus must be clean and intact. Besides cleansing, good hygiene prevents body and breath odors. It is relaxing and increases circulation.

Culture and personal choice affect hygiene. (See *Caring About Culture: Personal Hygiene*, p. 322.) Some people take showers. Others take tub baths. Some bathe at bedtime. Others bathe in the morning. Bathing frequency also varies. Some bathe 1 or 2 times a day—before work and after work or exercise. Some people do not have water for bathing. Others cannot afford soap, deodorant, shampoo, toothpaste, or other hygiene products.

Many factors affect hygiene needs—perspiration (sweating), elimination, vomiting, drainage from wounds or body openings, bedrest, and activity. Illness and aging changes can affect self-care abilities. Some people need help with hygiene. The nurse uses the nursing process to meet the person's hygiene needs. Follow the nurse's directions and the care plan.

See *Body Structure and Function Review: Teeth, Gums, and Skin.*

See *Focus on Communication: Personal Hygiene*, p. 322.

See *Focus on Children and Older Persons: Personal Hygiene*, p. 322.

BODY STRUCTURE AND FUNCTION REVIEW: TEETH, GUMS, AND SKIN

The Teeth and Gums
The *teeth* cut, chop, and grind food into small bits for digestion and swallowing. A tooth has three main parts: the *crown, neck,* and *root* (Fig. 20-1). The crown is the outer part. It is covered by enamel. The neck is surrounded by *gums (gingivae)*. The root fits into the bone of the lower or upper jaw.

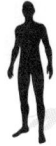

The Skin
The skin is the largest system. It is the body's natural covering. There are two layers (Fig. 20-2).
- The *epidermis* is the outer layer. It has living cells and dead cells. Dead cells constantly flake off and are replaced by living cells. Living cells also die and flake off. Living cells of the epidermis contain *pigment*. The epidermis has no blood vessels and few nerve endings.
- The *dermis* is the inner layer. It is made up of connective tissue. Blood vessels, nerves, sweat glands, oil glands, and hair roots are found in the dermis.

Sweat glands help regulate body temperature. Sweat is secreted through the skin's pores. The body is cooled as sweat

The Skin—cont'd
evaporates. Oil glands secrete an oily substance into the space near the hair shaft. Oil travels to the skin surface. The oil helps keep the hair and skin soft and shiny.

The skin has many functions:
- Provides the body's protective covering.
- Prevents microbes and other substances from entering the body.
- Prevents excess amounts of water from leaving the body.
- Protects organs from injury.
- Contains sensory structures. Nerve endings in the skin sense both pleasant and unpleasant stimulation. They sense cold, pain, touch, and pressure to protect the body from injury.
- Helps regulate body temperature. Blood vessels dilate (widen) when temperature outside the body is high. More blood is brought to the body surface for cooling during evaporation. When blood vessels constrict (narrow), the body retains heat. This is because less blood reaches the skin.
- Stores fats and water.

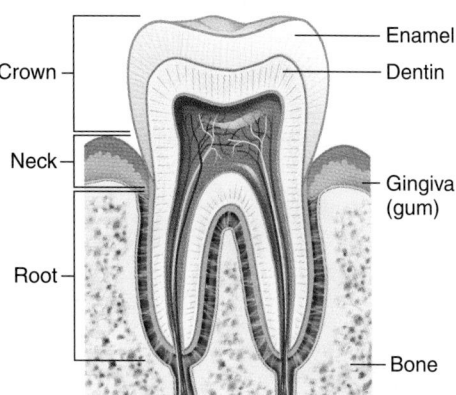

Fig. 20-1 Parts of the tooth.

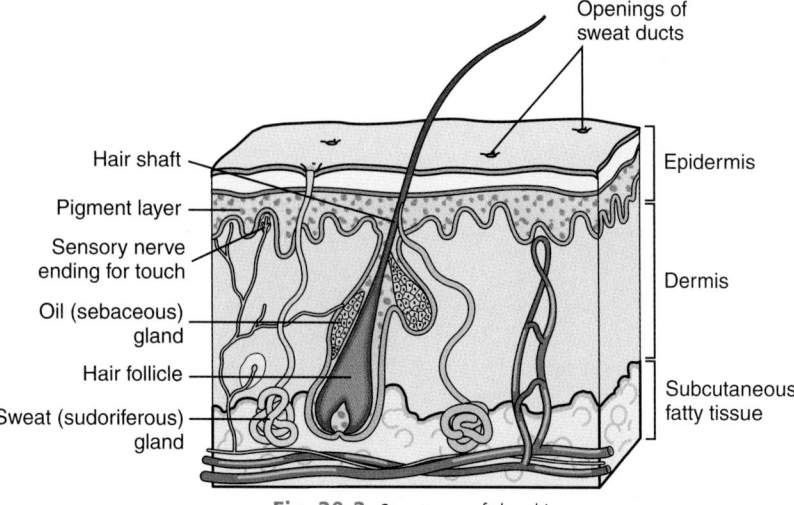

Fig. 20-2 Structures of the skin.

✿ CARING ABOUT CULTURE
Personal Hygiene

Personal hygiene is very important to *East Indian Hindus*. Their religion requires at least one bath a day. Some believe bathing after a meal is harmful. Another belief is that a cold bath prevents a blood disease. Some believe that eye injuries can occur if a bath is too hot. Hot water can be added to cold water. However, cold water is not added to hot water. After bathing, the body is carefully dried with a towel.

From Giger JN, Davidhizar RE: *Transcultural nursing: assessment and intervention*, ed 5, St Louis, 2008, Mosby.

FOCUS ON COMMUNICATION
Personal Hygiene

During hygiene procedures, make sure that the person is warm enough. You can ask:
- "Is the water warm enough?" "Is it too hot?" "Is it too cold?"
- "Are you warm enough?"
- "Do you need another bath blanket?"
- "Is the water starting to cool?"
- "Is the room warm enough?"

FOCUS ON CHILDREN AND OLDER PERSONS
Personal Hygiene

Older Persons

Some older persons resist your efforts to assist with hygiene. Illness, disability, dementia, and personal choice are common reasons. Follow the care plan to meet the person's needs. Also see Chapter 46.

Bending and reaching are hard for some older and disabled persons. Some have weak hand grips. They cannot hold soap or a washcloth. Adaptive devices for hygiene promote independence (Fig. 20-3). Always let the person do as much for himself or herself as safely possible.

DAILY CARE

Most people have hygiene routines and habits. For example, teeth are brushed and the face and hands washed after sleep. These and other hygiene measures are often done before and after meals and at bedtime.

Infants and young children need help with hygiene. So do some weak and disabled persons. Routine care is given during the day and evening. You assist with hygiene whenever it is needed. You must protect the person's right to privacy and to personal choice.

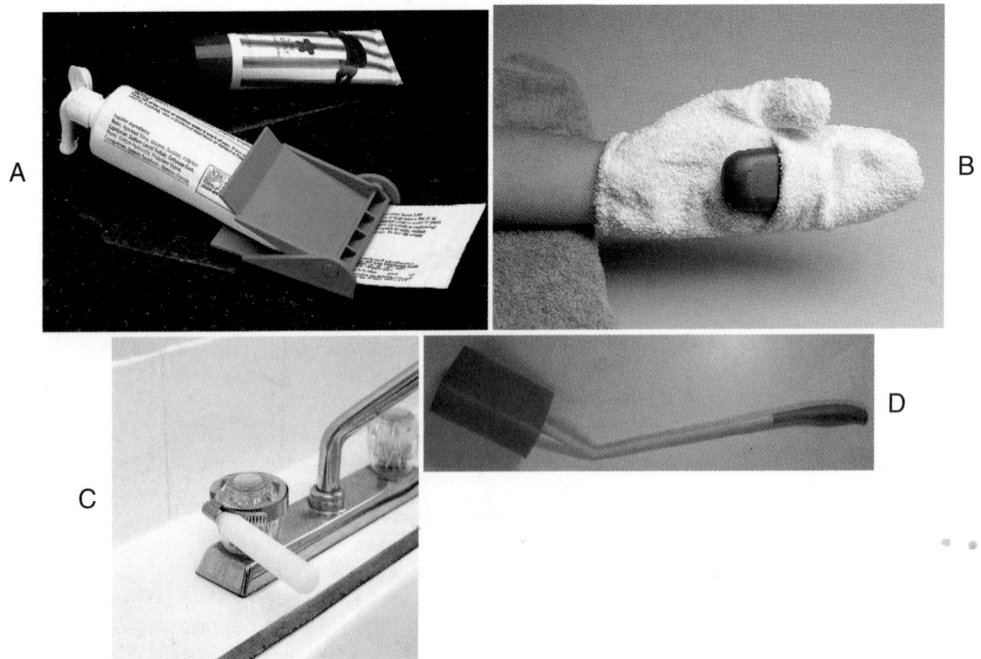

Fig. 20-3 Adaptive devices for hygiene. **A,** Tube squeezer for toothpaste. **B,** The wash mitt holds a bar of soap. **C,** A tap turner makes round knobs easy to turn. **D,** A long-handled sponge is used for hard to reach body parts.

Before Breakfast

Routine care given before breakfast is called early morning care or AM care. Night shift or day shift staff members give AM care. They get patients and residents ready for breakfast or morning tests. AM care includes:

- Assisting with elimination
- Cleaning incontinent persons
- Changing wet or soiled linens and garments
- Assisting with hygiene—face and hand washing and oral hygiene
- Assisting with dressing and hair care
- Positioning persons for breakfast—dining room, bed-side chair, or in bed
- Making beds and straightening units

After Breakfast

Morning care is given after breakfast. Hygiene measures are more thorough at this time. They usually involve:

- Assisting with elimination
- Cleaning incontinent persons
- Changing wet or soiled linens and garments
- Assisting with hygiene—face and hand washing, oral hygiene, bathing, back massage, and perineal care
- Assisting with grooming—hair care, shaving, dressing, and undressing
- Assisting with activity—range-of-motion exercises and ambulation
- Making beds and straightening units

Afternoon Care

Routine hygiene is done after lunch and before the evening meal. It is done before the person takes a nap, has visitors, or attends activity programs. Afternoon care involves:

- Assisting with elimination before and after naps
- Cleaning incontinent persons before and after naps
- Changing wet or soiled linen before and after naps
- Changing wet or soiled garments before and after naps
- Assisting with hygiene and grooming—face and hand washing, oral hygiene, and hair care
- Assisting with activity—range-of-motion exercises and ambulation
- Straightening beds and units

Evening Care

Care given in the evening at bedtime is called evening care or PM care. Evening care is relaxing and promotes comfort. Measures performed before sleep include:

- Assisting with elimination
- Cleaning incontinent persons
- Changing wet or soiled linens and garments
- Assisting with hygiene—face and hand washing, oral hygiene, and back massages
- Helping persons change into sleepwear
- Straightening beds and units

ORAL HYGIENE

Oral hygiene (mouth care) does the following:

- Keeps the mouth and teeth clean
- Prevents mouth odors and infections
- Increases comfort
- Makes food taste better
- Reduces the risk for *cavities (dental caries)* and *periodontal disease*

Periodontal disease *(gum disease, pyorrhea)* is an inflammation of tissues around the teeth. Plaque and tartar build up from poor oral hygiene. *Plaque is a thin film that sticks to teeth. It contains saliva, microbes, and other substances.* Plaque causes tooth decay *(cavities). Hardened plaque is called tartar.* Tartar builds up at the gum line near the neck of the tooth. Tartar buildup causes periodontal disease. The gums are red and swollen and bleed easily. As the disease progresses, bone is destroyed and teeth loosen. Tooth loss is common.

Illness, disease, and some drugs often cause:

- A bad taste in the mouth.
- A whitish coating in the mouth and on the tongue.
- Redness and swelling in the mouth and on the tongue.
- Dry mouth. Dry mouth also is common from oxygen, smoking, decreased fluid intake, and anxiety.

The nurse assesses the person's need for mouth care. So may the speech/language pathologist and the dietitian.

See *Focus on Children and Older Persons: Oral Hygiene.*

FOCUS ON CHILDREN AND OLDER PERSONS
Oral Hygiene

Children

Infants need mouth care to remove food and bacteria. This helps prevent *baby bottle tooth decay (early childhood tooth decay)*. More common in the upper front teeth, it can occur in all teeth (Fig. 20-4, p. 324). To prevent baby bottle tooth decay, the American Dental Association recommends the following:

- Wipe the baby's gums with a clean, damp gauze pad or washcloth after each feeding.
- Brush the teeth when they begin to erupt. Use a child's soft toothbrush. Brush gently.
- Fill baby bottles only with formula, milk, or breastmilk. Do not fill bottles with sugar water, juice, or soft drinks. Bacteria in the mouth use sugars in such drinks for nourishment.
- Do not put the baby to bed with a bottle. Bottles should be finished before bedtime or naptime.
- Provide a clean pacifier.
  - Do not dip a pacifier in sugar or honey.
  - Do not put a pacifier in your mouth to clean it.
- Use toothpaste when the child can spit. This is usually around 2 years of age. He or she should not swallow toothpaste. Use a pea-sized amount of toothpaste.
- Brush the child's teeth until he or she is 6 years old. Children learn to brush their teeth around 3 years of age. They may not be thorough. Older children can do a thorough job. Remind them when to brush.

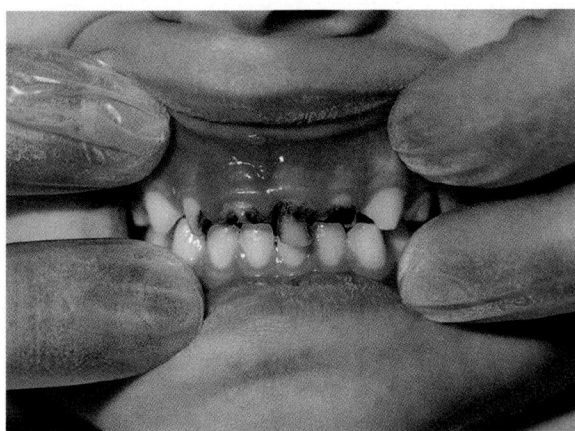

Fig. 20-4 Baby bottle tooth decay.

Flossing

Dental floss is a soft thread used to clean between the teeth. Flossing removes plaque and tartar. These substances cause periodontal disease (p. 323). Flossing also removes food from between the teeth. Usually done after brushing, it can be done at other times. Some people floss after meals. If done once a day, bedtime is the best time to floss. You need to floss for persons who cannot do so themselves.

See *Focus on Children and Older Persons: Flossing.*

Equipment

A toothbrush, toothpaste, dental floss, and mouthwash are needed. A toothbrush with soft bristles is best.

Sponge swabs are used for persons with sore, tender mouths. They also are used for unconscious persons. Use sponge swabs with care. Check the foam pad to make sure it is tight on the stick. The person could choke on the foam pad if it comes off the stick.

You also need a kidney basin, water cup, straw, tissues, towels, and gloves. Many persons bring oral hygiene equipment from home.

See *Delegation Guidelines: Oral Hygiene.*
See *Promoting Safety and Comfort: Oral Hygiene.*

Brushing and Flossing Teeth

Many people perform oral hygiene themselves. Others need help gathering and setting up equipment for oral hygiene. You perform oral hygiene for persons who:
- Are very weak.
- Cannot move or use their arms.
- Are too confused to brush their teeth.

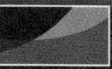

ASSISTING THE PERSON TO BRUSH AND FLOSS THE TEETH

QUALITY OF LIFE

Remember to:
- Knock before entering the person's room.
- Address the person by name.
- Introduce yourself by name and title.

- Explain the procedure to the person before beginning and during the procedure.
- Protect the person's rights during the procedure.
- Handle the person gently during the procedure.

PRE-PROCEDURE

1. Follow *Delegation Guidelines: Oral Hygiene*. See *Promoting Safety and Comfort: Oral Hygiene*.
2. Practice hand hygiene.
3. Collect the following:
   - Toothbrush with soft bristles
   - Toothpaste
   - Mouthwash (or solution noted on the care plan)
   - Dental floss (if used)
   - Water cup with cool water
   - Straw
   - Kidney basin
   - Hand towel
   - Paper towels
   - Gloves
4. Place the paper towels on the overbed table. Arrange items on top of them.
5. Identify the person. Check the ID (identification) bracelet against the assignment sheet. Also call the person by name.
6. Provide for privacy.
7. Lower the bed rail near you if up.

PROCEDURE

8. Position the person so he or she can brush with ease.
9. Place the towel over the person's chest. This protects garments and linens from spills.
10. Adjust the overbed table in front of the person.
11. Let the person perform oral hygiene. This includes brushing the teeth and tongue, rinsing the mouth, flossing, and using mouthwash or other solution.
12. Remove the towel when the person is done.
13. Move the overbed table to the side of the bed.

POST-PROCEDURE

14. Provide for comfort. (See the inside of the front book cover.)
15. Place the signal light within reach.
16. Raise or lower bed rails. Follow the care plan.
17. Rinse the toothbrush. Clean, rinse, and dry equipment. Return the toothbrush and equipment to their proper place. Wear gloves.
18. Wipe off the overbed table with the paper towels. Discard the paper towels.
19. Unscreen the person.
20. Complete a safety check of the room. (See the inside of the front book cover.)
21. Follow agency policy for dirty linen.
22. Remove and discard the gloves. Practice hand hygiene.
23. Report and record your observations.

BRUSHING AND FLOSSING THE PERSON'S TEETH

QUALITY OF LIFE

Remember to:
- Knock before entering the person's room.
- Address the person by name.
- Introduce yourself by name and title.

- Explain the procedure to the person before beginning and during the procedure.
- Protect the person's rights during the procedure.
- Handle the person gently during the procedure.

PRE-PROCEDURE

1. Follow *Delegation Guidelines: Oral Hygiene*. See *Promoting Safety and Comfort: Oral Hygiene*.
2. Practice hand hygiene.
3. Collect the following:
   - Toothbrush with soft bristles
   - Toothpaste
   - Mouthwash (or solution noted on the care plan)
   - Dental floss (if used)
   - Water cup with cool water
   - Straw
   - Kidney basin
   - Hand towel
   - Paper towels
   - Gloves
4. Place the paper towels on the overbed table. Arrange items on top of them.
5. Identify the person. Check the ID bracelet against the assignment sheet. Also call the person by name.
6. Provide for privacy.
7. Raise the bed for body mechanics. Bed rails are up if used.

Continued

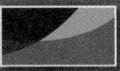

BRUSHING AND FLOSSING THE PERSON'S TEETH—cont'd

PROCEDURE

8 Lower the bed rail near you if up.

9 Assist the person to a sitting position or to a side-lying position near you. (NOTE: Some state competency tests require that the person is at a 75 to 90 degree angle.)

10 Place the towel across the person's chest.

11 Adjust the overbed table so you can reach it with ease.

12 Practice hand hygiene. Put on the gloves.

13 Hold the toothbrush over the kidney basin. Pour some water over the brush.

14 Apply toothpaste to the toothbrush.

15 Brush the teeth gently (Fig. 20-5).

16 Brush the tongue gently.

17 Let the person rinse the mouth with water. Hold the kidney basin under the person's chin (Fig. 20-6). Repeat this step as needed.

18 Floss the person's teeth (optional):

  a Break off an 18-inch piece of dental floss from the dispenser.

  b Hold the floss between the middle fingers of each hand (Fig. 20-7, A).

  c Stretch the floss with your thumbs.

  d Start at the upper back tooth on the right side. Work around to the left side.

  e Move the floss gently up and down between the teeth (Fig. 20-7, B). Move the floss up and down against the side of the tooth. Work from the top of the crown to the gum line.

  f Move to a new section of floss after every second tooth.

  g Floss the lower teeth. Use up and down motions as for the upper teeth. Start on the right side. Work around to the left side.

19 Let the person use mouthwash or other solution. Hold the kidney basin under the chin.

20 Wipe the person's mouth. Remove the towel.

21 Remove and discard the gloves. Practice hand hygiene.

POST-PROCEDURE

22 Provide for comfort. (See the inside of the front book cover.)

23 Place the signal light within reach.

24 Lower the bed to its lowest position.

25 Raise or lower bed rails. Follow the care plan.

26 Rinse the toothbrush. Clean, rinse, and dry equipment. Return the toothbrush and equipment to their proper place. Wear gloves.

27 Wipe off the overbed table with the paper towels. Discard the paper towels.

28 Unscreen the person.

29 Complete a safety check of the room. (See the inside of the front book cover.)

30 Follow agency policy for dirty linen.

31 Remove and discard the gloves. Practice hand hygiene.

32 Report and record your observations.

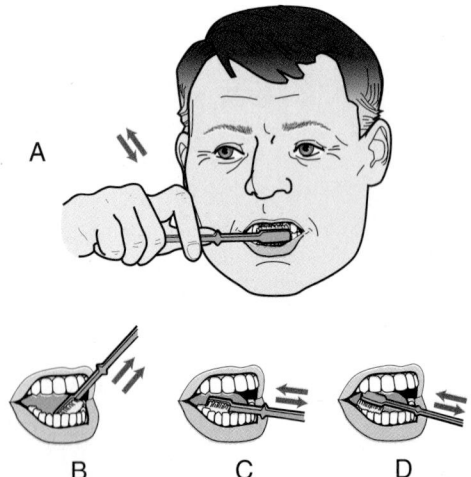

Fig. 20-5 Brushing teeth. **A,** The brush is held at a 45-degree angle to the gums. Teeth are brushed with short strokes. **B,** The brush is at a 45-degree angle against the inside of the front teeth. Teeth are brushed from the gum to the crown of the tooth with short strokes. **C,** The brush is held horizontally against the inner surfaces of the teeth. The teeth are brushed back and forth. **D,** The brush is positioned on the biting surfaces of the teeth. The teeth are brushed back and forth.

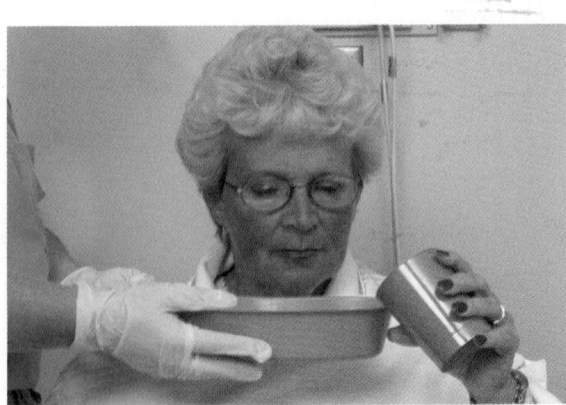

Fig. 20-6 The kidney basin is held under the person's chin.

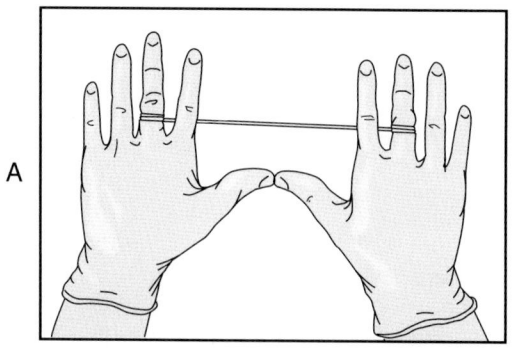
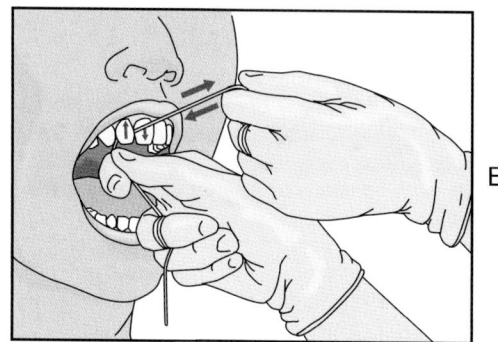

Fig. 20-7 Flossing. **A,** Floss is wrapped around the middle fingers. **B,** Floss is moved in up-and-down motions between the teeth. Floss is moved up and down from the crown to the gum line.

Mouth Care for the Unconscious Person

Unconscious persons cannot eat or drink. Some breathe with their mouths open. Many receive oxygen. These factors cause mouth dryness. They also cause crusting on the tongue and mucous membranes. Oral hygiene keeps the mouth clean and moist. It also helps prevent infection.

The care plan tells you what cleaning agent to use. Use sponge swabs to apply the cleaning agent. Apply a lubricant (check the care plan) to the lips after cleaning. It prevents cracking of the lips.

Unconscious persons usually cannot swallow. Protect them from choking and aspiration. *Aspiration is breathing fluid, food, vomitus, or an object into the lungs.* It can cause pneumonia and death. To prevent aspiration:

- Position the person on one side with the head turned well to the side (Fig. 20-8). In this position, excess fluid runs out of the mouth.
- Use only a small amount of fluid to clean the mouth.
- Do not insert dentures. Dentures are not worn when the person is unconscious.

Keep the person's mouth open with a padded tongue blade (Fig. 20-9). Do not use your fingers. The person can bite down on them. The bite breaks the skin and creates a portal of entry for microbes. Infection is a risk.

Mouth care is given at least every 2 hours. Follow the nurse's directions and the care plan.

See *Focus on Communication: Mouth Care for the Unconscious Person*, p. 328.

See *Promoting Safety and Comfort: Mouth Care for the Unconscious Person*, p. 328.

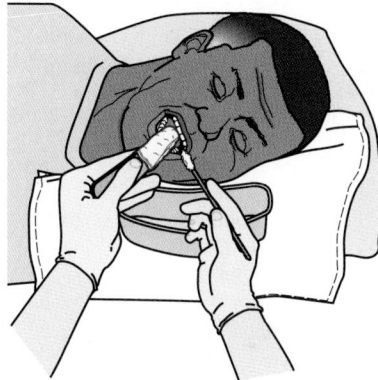

Fig. 20-8 The unconscious person's head is turned well to the side to prevent aspiration. A padded tongue blade is used to keep the mouth open while cleaning the mouth with swabs.

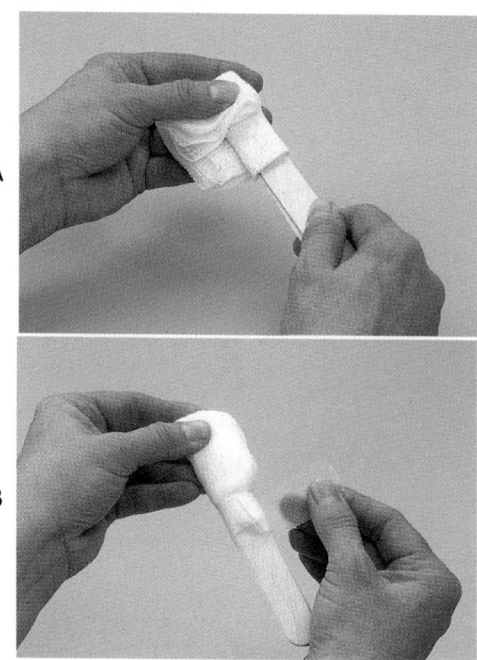

Fig. 20-9 Making a padded tongue blade. **A,** Place two wooden tongue blades together. Wrap gauze around the top half. **B,** Tape the gauze in place.

FOCUS ON COMMUNICATION
Mouth Care for the Unconscious Person

Unconscious persons cannot speak or respond to you. However, some can hear. Always assume that unconscious persons can hear. Explain what you are doing step-by-step. Also, tell the person when you are done, when you are leaving the room, and when you will return.

PROMOTING SAFETY AND COMFORT
Mouth Care for the Unconscious Person

Safety

Use sponge swabs with care. Make sure the sponge pad is tight on the stick. The person could aspirate or choke on the sponge if it comes off the stick.

Comfort

Unconscious persons are re-positioned at least every 2 hours. To promote comfort, combine mouth care with skin care, re-positioning, and other comfort measures.

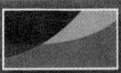 # PROVIDING MOUTH CARE FOR THE UNCONSCIOUS PERSON

QUALITY OF LIFE

Remember to:
- Knock before entering the person's room.
- Address the person by name.
- Introduce yourself by name and title.

- Explain the procedure to the person before beginning and during the procedure.
- Protect the person's rights during the procedure.
- Handle the person gently during the procedure.

PRE-PROCEDURE

1 Follow *Delegation Guidelines: Oral Hygiene*, p. 324. See *Promoting Safety and Comfort:*
  a *Oral Hygiene*, p. 324
  b *Mouth Care for the Unconscious Person*
2 Practice hand hygiene.
3 Collect the following:
   - Cleaning agent (check the care plan)
   - Sponge swabs
   - Padded tongue blade
   - Water cup with cool water
   - Hand towel
   - Kidney basin
   - Lip lubricant
   - Paper towels
   - Gloves
4 Place the towels on the overbed table. Arrange items on top of them.
5 Identify the person. Check the ID bracelet against the assignment sheet. Also call the person by name.
6 Provide for privacy.
7 Raise the bed for body mechanics. Bed rails are up if used.

PROCEDURE

8 Lower the bed rail near you if up.
9 Practice hand hygiene. Put on the gloves.
10 Position the person in a side-lying position near you. Turn his or her head well to the side.
11 Place the towel under the person's face.
12 Place the kidney basin under the chin.
13 Separate the upper and lower teeth. Use the padded tongue blade. Be gentle. Never use force. If you have problems, ask the nurse for help.
14 Clean the mouth using sponge swabs moistened with the cleaning agent (see Fig. 20-8).
   a Clean the chewing and inner surfaces of the teeth.
   b Clean the gums and outer surfaces of the teeth.
   c Swab the roof of the mouth, inside of the cheeks, and the lips.
   d Swab the tongue.
   e Moisten a clean swab with water. Swab the mouth to rinse.
   f Place used swabs in the kidney basin.
15 Remove the kidney basin and supplies.
16 Wipe the person's mouth. Remove the towel.
17 Apply lubricant to the lips.
18 Remove and discard the gloves. Practice hand hygiene.

POST-PROCEDURE

19 Provide for comfort. (See the inside of the front book cover.)
20 Place the signal light within reach.
21 Lower the bed to its lowest position.
22 Raise or lower bed rails. Follow the care plan.
23 Clean, rinse, dry, and return equipment to its proper place. Discard disposable items. (Wear gloves.)
24 Wipe off the overbed table with paper towels. Discard the paper towels.
25 Unscreen the person.
26 Complete a safety check of the room. (See the inside of the front book cover.)
27 Tell the person that you are leaving the room. Tell him or her when you will return.
28 Follow agency policy for dirty linen.
29 Remove and discard the gloves. Practice hand hygiene.
30 Report and record your observations.

Denture Care

A *denture is an artificial tooth or a set of artificial teeth* (Fig. 20-10). They are often called "false teeth." Dentures replace missing teeth. People lose teeth because of gum disease, tooth decay, or injury. Full and partial dentures are common:

- *Full denture.* The person has no upper or no lower natural teeth. Dentures replace the upper or lower teeth.
- *Partial denture.* The person has some natural teeth. The partial denture replaces the missing teeth.

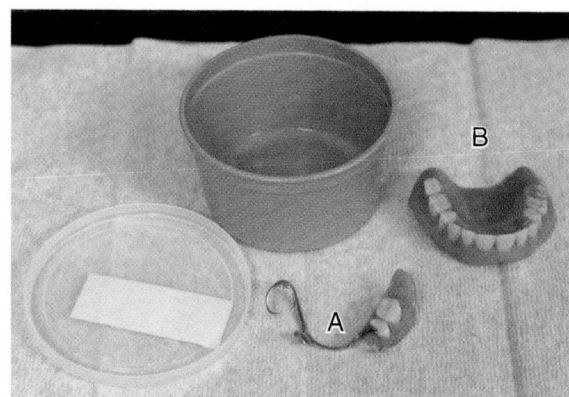

Fig. 20-10 Dentures. **A,** Partial denture. **B,** Full denture.

Mouth care is given and dentures cleaned as often as natural teeth. Dentures are slippery when wet. They easily break or chip if dropped onto a hard surface (floors, sinks, counters). Hold them firmly when removing or inserting them. During cleaning, firmly hold them over a basin of water lined with a towel. This prevents them from falling onto a hard surface.

Persons with dentures need a denture cleaner, denture cup, and denture brush or toothbrush. Use only denture cleaning products. Otherwise, you could damage dentures.

To use a cleaning agent, follow the manufacturer's instructions. They tell how to use the cleaning agent and what water temperature to use. Hot water causes dentures to lose their shape (warp). If not worn after cleaning, store dentures in a container with cool or warm water or a denture soaking solution. Otherwise they can dry out and warp.

Dentures are usually removed at bedtime. Some people do not wear their dentures. Others wear dentures for eating and remove them after meals. Remind them not to wrap dentures in tissues or napkins. Otherwise, they are easily discarded.

Many people clean their own dentures. Some need help collecting items used to clean dentures. They may need help getting to the bathroom. You clean dentures for those who cannot do so.

See *Promoting Safety and Comfort: Denture Care.*

PROMOTING SAFETY AND COMFORT
Denture Care

Safety

Dentures are the person's property. They are costly. Handle them very carefully. Label the denture cup with the person's name and room and bed number. Report lost or damaged dentures to the nurse at once. Losing or damaging dentures is negligent conduct.

Never carry dentures in your hands. Always use a denture cup or kidney basin. You could easily drop the dentures as you move from the bedside to the bathroom. Or you could drop them when moving from the bathroom to the bedside.

Comfort

Many people do not like being seen without their dentures. Privacy is important. Allow privacy when the person cleans dentures. If you clean dentures, return them to the person as quickly as possible.

Persons with dentures may have some natural teeth. They need to brush and floss the natural teeth. See procedure: *Assisting the Person to Brush and Floss the Teeth*, p. 325. Or see procedure: *Brushing and Flossing the Person's Teeth*, p. 325.

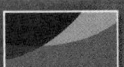 **PROVIDING DENTURE CARE**

QUALITY OF LIFE

Remember to:
- Knock before entering the person's room.
- Address the person by name.
- Introduce yourself by name and title.

- Explain the procedure to the person before beginning and during the procedure.
- Protect the person's rights during the procedure.
- Handle the person gently during the procedure.

PRE-PROCEDURE

1 Follow *Delegation Guidelines: Oral Hygiene*, p. 324. See *Promoting Safety and Comfort:*
   a *Oral Hygiene*, p. 324
   b *Denture Care*, p. 329
2 Practice hand hygiene.
3 Collect the following:
   - Denture brush or toothbrush (for cleaning dentures)
   - Denture cup labeled with the person's name and room and bed number
   - Denture cleaning agent
   - Soft-bristled toothbrush or sponge swabs (for oral hygiene)
   - Toothpaste
   - Water cup with cool water

   - Straw
   - Mouthwash (or other noted solution)
   - Kidney basin
   - Two hand towels
   - Gauze squares
   - Paper towels
   - Gloves
4 Place the paper towels on the overbed table. Arrange items on top of them.
5 Identify the person. Check the ID bracelet against the assignment sheet. Also call the person by name.
6 Provide for privacy.
7 Raise the bed for body mechanics.

PROCEDURE

8 Lower the bed rail near you if used.
9 Practice hand hygiene. Put on the gloves.
10 Place a towel over the person's chest.
11 Ask the person to remove the dentures. Carefully place them in the kidney basin.
12 Remove the dentures if the person cannot do so. Use gauze squares for a good grip on the slippery dentures.
   a Grasp the denture with your thumb and index finger (Fig. 20-11). Move it up and down slightly to break the seal. Gently remove the denture. Place it in the kidney basin.
   b Grasp and remove the lower denture with your thumb and index finger. Turn it slightly, and lift it out of the person's mouth. Place it in the kidney basin.
13 Follow the care plan for raising bed rails.
14 Take the kidney basin, denture cup, denture brush, and denture cleaning agent to the sink.
15 Line the bottom of the sink with a towel. Fill the sink halfway with water.
16 Rinse each denture under cool or warm running water. Follow agency policy for water temperature.
17 Return dentures to the kidney basin or denture cup.
18 Apply the denture cleaning agent to the brush.
19 Brush the dentures as in Figure 20-12. Brush the inner, outer, and chewing surfaces.
20 Rinse the dentures under running water. Use warm or cool water as directed by the cleaning agent manufacturer.

21 Rinse the denture cup and lid. Place dentures in the denture cup. Cover the dentures with cool or warm water. Follow agency policy for water temperature.
22 Clean the kidney basin.
23 Take the denture cup and kidney basin to the overbed table.
24 Lower the bed rail if up.
25 Position the person for oral hygiene.
26 Clean the person's gums and tongue. Use toothpaste and the toothbrush (or sponge swabs).
27 Have the person use mouthwash (or noted solution). Hold the kidney basin under the chin.
28 Ask the person to insert the dentures. Insert them if the person cannot.
   a Hold the upper denture firmly with your thumb and index finger. Raise the upper lip with the other hand. Insert the denture. Gently press on the denture with your index fingers to make sure it is in place.
   b Hold the lower denture with your thumb and index finger. Pull the lower lip down slightly. Insert the denture. Gently press down on it to make sure it is in place.
29 Place the denture cup in the top drawer of the bedside stand if the dentures are not worn. The dentures must be in water or in a denture soaking solution.
30 Wipe the person's mouth. Remove the towel.
31 Remove and discard the gloves. Practice hand hygiene.

PROVIDING DENTURE CARE—cont'd

| VIDEO | VIDEO CLIP | NNAAP® Skill |

POST-PROCEDURE

32 Assist with hand washing.
33 Provide for comfort. (See the inside of the front book cover.)
34 Place the signal light within reach.
35 Lower the bed to its lowest position.
36 Raise or lower bed rails. Follow the care plan.
37 Remove the towel from the sink. Drain the sink.
38 Rinse the brushes. Clean, rinse, and dry equipment. Return the brushes and equipment to their proper place. Discard disposable items. Wear gloves for this step.

39 Wipe off the overbed table with the paper towels. Discard the paper towels.
40 Unscreen the person.
41 Complete a safety check of the room. (See the inside of the front book cover.)
42 Follow agency policy for dirty linen.
43 Remove and discard the gloves. Practice hand hygiene.
44 Report and record your observations.

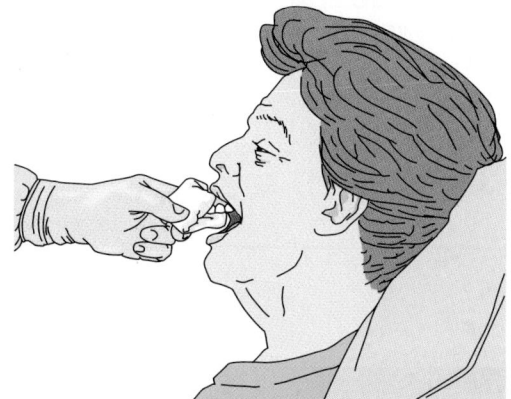

Fig. 20-11 Remove the upper denture by grasping it with the thumb and index finger of one hand. Use a piece of gauze to grasp the slippery denture.

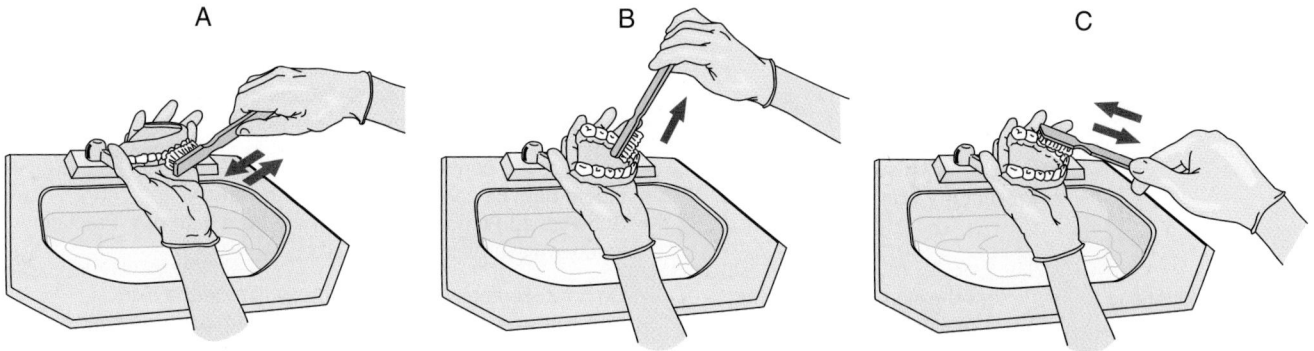

A B C

Fig. 20-12 Cleaning dentures. **A,** Brush the outer surfaces of the denture with back-and-forth motions. (Note that the denture is held over the sink. The sink is filled half-way with water and is lined with a towel.) **B,** Position the brush vertically to clean the inner surfaces of the denture. Use upward strokes. **C,** Brush the chewing surfaces with back-and-forth motions.

BATHING

Bathing cleans the skin. It also cleans the mucous membranes of the genital and anal areas. Microbes, dead skin, perspiration, and excess oils are removed. A bath is refreshing and relaxing. Circulation is stimulated and body parts exercised. Observations are made, and you have time to talk to the person.

Complete or partial baths, tub baths, or showers are given. The method depends on the person's condition, self-care abilities, and personal choice. In hospitals, bathing is common after breakfast. In nursing centers, bathing usually occurs after breakfast or the evening meal. The person's choice of bath time is respected whenever possible.

Bathing frequency is a personal matter. Some people bathe daily. Others bathe once or twice a week. Personal choice, weather, activity, and illness affect bathing frequency. Ill persons may have fevers and perspire heavily. They need frequent bathing. Other illnesses and dry skin may limit bathing to every 2 or 3 days.

The rules for bed baths, showers, and tub baths are listed in Box 20-1. Table 20-1 describes common skin care products.

See *Focus on Communication: Personal Hygiene*, p. 322.
See *Focus on Children and Older Persons: Bathing.*
See *Delegation Guidelines: Bathing.*
See *Promoting Safety and Comfort: Bathing*, p. 334.

Text continued on p. 334

BOX 20-1 **RULES FOR BATHING**

- Follow the care plan for bathing method and skin care products.
- Allow personal choice whenever possible.
- Follow Standard Precautions and the Bloodborne Pathogen Standard.
- Collect needed items before starting the procedure.
- Provide for privacy. Screen the person. Close doors and window coverings—drapes, shades, blinds, shutters, and so on.
- Assist the person with elimination. Bathing stimulates the need to urinate. Comfort and relaxation increase if urination needs are met.
- Cover the person for warmth and privacy.
- Reduce drafts. Close doors and windows.
- Protect the person from falling.
- Use good body mechanics at all times.

- Follow the rules to safely move and transfer the person (Chapter 17).
- Know what water temperature to use. See *Delegation Guidelines: Bathing.*
- Keep bar soap in the soap dish between latherings. This prevents soapy water. It also reduces the chances of slipping and falls in showers and tubs.
- Wash from the cleanest areas to the dirtiest areas.
- Encourage the person to help as much as is safely possible.
- Rinse the skin thoroughly. You must remove all soap.
- Pat the skin dry to avoid irritating or breaking the skin. Do not rub the skin.
- Dry under the breasts, between skin folds, in the perineal area, and between the toes.
- Bathe skin when urine or feces are present. This prevents skin breakdown and odors.

TABLE 20-1 **SKIN CARE PRODUCTS**

Type	Purpose	Care Considerations
Soaps	• Clean the skin • Remove dirt, dead skin, skin oil, some microbes, and perspiration	• Tend to dry and irritate the skin. Dry skin is easily injured and causes itching and discomfort. • Skin must be thoroughly rinsed to remove all soap. • Not needed for every bath. Plain water can clean the skin. • Plain water is often used for older persons due to dry skin. • People with dry skin may use soaps containing bath oils. • Not used if a person has very dry skin.
Bath oils	• Keep the skin soft • Prevent dry skin	• Some soaps contain bath oil. • Liquid bath oil can be added to bath water. • Showers and tubs become slippery from bath oils. Practice safety measures to prevent falls.
Creams and lotions	• Protect the skin from the drying effect of air and evaporation	• Do not feel greasy but leave an oily film on the skin. • Lotion is applied to bony areas after bathing to prevent skin breakdown (back, elbows, knees, and heels). • Lotion is used for back massages. • Most are scented.
Powders	• Absorb moisture • Prevent friction when two skin surfaces rub together	• Usually applied under the breasts, under the arms, and in the groin area, and sometimes between the toes. • Applied after drying the skin in a thin, even layer. • Excessive amounts cause caking and crusts that can irritate the skin.
Deodorants	• Mask and control body odors	• Applied to the underarms. • Not applied to irritated skin. • Do not replace bathing.
Antiperspirants	• Reduce the amount of perspiration	• Applied to the underarms. • Not applied to irritated skin. • Do not replace bathing.

FOCUS ON CHILDREN AND OLDER PERSONS
Bathing

Children

The nurse collects information about the child's bathing practices on admission. The care plan reflects the child's normal practices and needs during illness.

Many older children enjoy showers. The nurse tells you how much help and supervision the child needs. Remember, independence and privacy are important to older children.

See "Bathing an Infant" in Chapter 49.

Older Persons

Dry skin occurs with aging. Soap also dries the skin. Dry skin is easily damaged. Therefore, older persons usually need a complete bath or shower twice a week. Partial baths are taken the other days. Some bathe daily but not with soap. Thorough rinsing is needed when using soap. Lotions and oils help keep the skin soft.

Bathing procedures can threaten persons with dementia. They do not understand what is happening or why. And they may fear harm or danger. Confusion can increase. Therefore, they may resist care and become agitated and combative. They may shout at you and cry out for help. You must be calm, patient, and soothing.

The nurse assesses the person's behaviors and routines. The person may be calmer and less confused or agitated during a certain time of the day. Bathing is scheduled for the person's calm times. The nurse decides if a bed bath, tub bath, shower, or towel bath (p. 338) is best for the person.

The rules in Box 20-1 apply when bathing these persons. The care plan also includes measures to help the person through the bath. Such measures may include:

- Use terms such as "cleaned up" or "washed" rather than "shower" or "bath."

Older Persons—cont'd

- Complete pre-procedure activities. For example, ready supplies and linens. Make sure you have everything that you need.
- Provide for warmth. Increase the room temperature before starting the bath or shower. Have extra towels and a robe nearby.
- Play soft music to help the person relax.
- Provide for safety.
  - Use a hand-held shower nozzle.
  - Have the person use a shower chair or shower bench.
  - Do not use bath oil. It can make the tub or shower slippery. And it may cause a urinary tract infection.
  - Do not leave the person alone in the tub or shower.
- Draw bath water ahead of time. Test the water temperature. Add warm or cold water as needed.
- Tell the person what you are doing step-by-step. Use clear, simple statements.
- Let the person help as much as possible. For example, give the person a washcloth. Ask him or her to wash the arms. If the person does not know what to do, still let the person hold the washcloth if it is safe to do so.
- Put a towel over the person's shoulder or lap (tub bath or shower). This helps the person feel less exposed.
- Do not rush the person.
- Use a calm, pleasant voice.
- Distract the person if needed.
- Calm the person.
- Handle the person gently.
- Try giving a partial bath if a shower or tub bath agitates the person.
- Try the bath later if the person continues to resist care.

DELEGATION GUIDELINES
Bathing

To assist with bathing, you need this information from the nurse and the care plan:

- What bath to give—complete bed bath, partial bath, tub bath, shower, towel bath, or bag bath.
- How much help the person needs.
- The person's activity or position limits.
- What water temperature to use. Bath water cools rapidly. Heat is lost to the bath basin, overbed table, washcloth, and your hands. Therefore water temperature for complete bed baths and partial bed baths is usually between 110°F and 115°F (Fahrenheit) (43.3°C and 46.1°C [centigrade]) for adults. Older persons have fragile skin. They need lower water temperatures.
- What skin care products to use and what the person prefers.

- What observations to report and record:
  - The color of the skin, lips, nail beds, and sclera (whites of the eyes)
  - If the skin appears pale, grayish, yellow (*jaundice*—Chapter 43), bluish (*cyanotic*)
  - The location and description of rashes
  - Skin texture—smooth, rough, scaly, flaky, dry, moist
  - *Diaphoresis*—profuse (excessive) sweating
  - Bruises or open skin areas
  - Pale or reddened areas, particularly over bony parts
  - Drainage or bleeding from wounds or body openings
  - Swelling of the feet and legs
  - Corns or calluses on the feet
  - Skin temperature (cold, cool, warm, hot)
  - Complaints of pain or discomfort
- When to report observations.
- What patient or resident concerns to report at once.

Safety

Hot water can burn delicate and fragile skin. Measure water temperature according to agency policy. If unsure if the water is too hot, ask the nurse to check it.

Protect the person from falls and other injuries. Practice the safety measures presented in Chapters 12 and 13. Also protect the person from drafts.

Use caution when applying powder. Do not use powders near persons with respiratory disorders. Inhaling powder can irritate the airway and lungs. Before using powder, check with the nurse and care plan. To safely apply powder:

* Turn away from the person.
* Sprinkle a small amount of powder onto your hand or a cloth. Do not shake or sprinkle powder onto the person.
* Apply the powder in a thin layer.
* Make sure powder does not get on the floor. Powder is slippery and can cause falls.

You make beds after baths. After making the bed, lower the bed to its lowest position. For an occupied bed, raise or lower bed rails according to the care plan. Make sure the bed wheels are locked.

Protect the person and yourself from infection. When giving baths and making beds, contact with blood, body fluids, secretions, and excretions is likely. Follow Standard Precautions and the Bloodborne Pathogen Standard.

Comfort

Before bathing, let the person meet elimination needs (Chapters 22 and 23). Bathing stimulates the need to urinate. The person has greater comfort if his or her bladder is empty. Also, bathing is not interrupted.

Comfort—cont'd

Oral hygiene is a common part of bathing routines. Some persons do so before the bathing procedure; others do so after. Allow personal choice and follow the person's care plan.

Provide for warmth. Cover the person with a bath blanket. Make sure the water is warm enough for the person. Cool water causes chilling.

If the person prefers, remove the person's gown or pajamas after washing the eyes, face, ears, and neck. Removing sleepwear at this time helps the person feel less exposed and provides more mental comfort with the bath.

If the person is able, let him or her wash the genital area. This promotes privacy and helps prevent embarrassment. You need to:

1. Provide clean water. See step 14 in procedure: *Giving Female Perineal Care*, p. 348.
2. Adjust the overbed table so he or she can reach the wash basin, soap, and towels with ease.
3. Make sure the person understands what to do.
4. Place the signal light within reach. Ask the person to signal when finished.
5. Lower the bed to its lowest level.
6. Remove and discard the gloves. Practice hand hygiene.
7. Leave the room.
8. Answer the signal light promptly. Knock before entering the room.
9. Raise the bed for body mechanics.
10. Practice hand hygiene. Put on gloves.
11. Make sure the person has cleaned thoroughly.
12. Finish the bathing procedure.

Persons With Bariatric Needs

Persons with bariatric needs often have problems providing their own hygiene. They may not be able to reach body parts. Skin folds are common. Good hygiene and skin care are needed for comfort and to prevent pressure ulcers.

The rules for bathing in Box 20-1 apply. Always follow the person's care plan. The care plan will include:

* How often to bathe the person.
* The bathing method—bed bath, shower, whirlpool.
* How many staff members are needed.
* What equipment is needed. For example, the person may need a bariatric shower chair.
* What cleansing agent to use. Harsh soaps are avoided. They can dry and injure the skin.
* How often to clean under skin folds. The person may perspire heavily. Moisture can collect between skin folds providing a place for microbes to live and grow.
* How to dry under skin folds. The nurse may have you use a hand-held hair dryer on the "cool" setting.
* What product to place under skin folds. The nurse may have you place gauze or a cotton-fabric under the folds. The material reduces friction and absorbs moisture.
* What skin care products to use—powder, lotion, and so on.

See *Teamwork and Time Management: Persons With Bariatric Needs*.

Bathing bariatric persons requires teamwork and planning. Even if the person can assist, you will often need help from co-workers. You may need help to hold skin folds while you clean, dry, and apply skin care products. Or you need to turn or transfer the person. Ask your co-workers for help in advance. Plan a time that is best for you, your co-workers, and the person.

Also allow extra time to complete hygiene measures. Plan your work to avoid seeming rushed. The person must not feel as if he or she is a burden. If unsure how much time to allow, ask other staff who have cared for the person. They can give advice on how much time and help are needed.

The Complete Bed Bath

For a complete bed bath, you wash the person's entire body in bed. You give such baths to persons who cannot bathe themselves. Bed baths are usually needed by persons who are:

- Unconscious
- Paralyzed
- In casts or traction
- Weak from illness or surgery

A bed bath is new to some people. Some are embarrassed to have their bodies seen. Some fear exposure. Explain how you give the bath. Also explain how you cover the body for privacy.

Text continued on p. 338

GIVING A COMPLETE BED BATH

QUALITY OF LIFE

Remember to:

- Knock before entering the person's room.
- Address the person by name.
- Introduce yourself by name and title.
- Explain the procedure to the person before beginning and during the procedure.
- Protect the person's rights during the procedure.
- Handle the person gently during the procedure.

PRE-PROCEDURE

1 Follow *Delegation Guidelines: Bathing*, p. 333. See *Promoting Safety and Comfort: Bathing*.
2 Practice hand hygiene.
3 Identify the person. Check the ID bracelet against the assignment sheet. Also call the person by name.
4 Collect clean linen. See procedure: *Making a Closed Bed* in Chapter 19. Place linen on a clean surface.
5 Collect the following:
   - Wash basin
   - Soap
   - Bath thermometer
   - Orangewood stick or nail file
   - Washcloth
   - Two bath towels and two hand towels
   - Bath blanket
   - Clothing or sleepwear
   - Lotion
   - Powder
   - Deodorant or antiperspirant
   - Brush and comb
   - Other grooming items as requested
   - Paper towels
   - Gloves
6 Cover the overbed table with paper towels. Arrange items on the overbed table. Adjust the height as needed.
7 Provide for privacy.
8 Raise the bed for body mechanics. Bed rails are up if used.

PROCEDURE

9 Remove the signal light.
10 Practice hand hygiene. Put on gloves.
11 Remove the sleepwear. Do not expose the person. Follow agency policy for dirty sleepwear.
12 Cover the person with a bath blanket. Remove top linens (see procedure: *Making an Occupied Bed* in Chapter 19).
13 Lower the head of the bed. It is as flat as possible. The person has at least one pillow.
14 Fill the wash basin ⅔ (two-thirds) full with water. Follow the care plan for water temperature. Water temperature is usually 110°F to 115°F (43.3°C to 46.1°C) for adults. Measure water temperature. Use the bath thermometer. Or test the water by dipping your elbow or inner wrist into the basin.
15 Lower the bed rail near you if up.
16 Ask the person to check the water temperature. Adjust the water temperature if it is too hot or too cold. Raise the bed rail before leaving the bedside. Lower it when you return.

17 Place the basin on the overbed table.
18 Place a hand towel over the person's chest.
19 Make a mitt with the washcloth (Fig. 20-13, p. 337). Use a mitt for the entire bath.
20 Wash around the person's eyes with water. Do not use soap.
   a Clean the far eye. Gently wipe from the inner to the outer aspect of the eye with a corner of the mitt (Fig. 20-14, p. 337).
   b Clean around the eye near you. Use a clean part of the washcloth for each stroke.
21 Ask the person if you should use soap to wash the face.
22 Wash the face, ears, and neck. Rinse and pat dry with the towel on the chest.
23 Help the person move to the side of the bed near you.

Continued

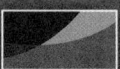

GIVING A COMPLETE BED BATH—cont'd

PROCEDURE—cont'd

24 Expose the far arm. Place a bath towel length-wise under the arm. Apply soap to the washcloth.

25 Support the arm with your palm under the person's elbow. His or her forearm rests on your forearm.

26 Wash the arm, shoulder, and underarm. Use long, firm strokes (Fig. 20-15). Rinse and pat dry.

27 Place the basin on the towel. Put the person's hand into the water (Fig. 20-16). Wash it well. Clean under the fingernails with an orangewood stick or nail file.

28 Have the person exercise the hand and fingers.

29 Remove the basin. Dry the hand well. Cover the arm with the bath blanket.

30 Repeat steps 24 to 29 for the near arm.

31 Place a bath towel over the chest cross-wise. Hold the towel in place. Pull the bath blanket from under the towel to the waist. Apply soap to the washcloth.

32 Lift the towel slightly, and wash the chest (Fig. 20-17). Do not expose the person. Rinse and pat dry, especially under the breasts.

33 Move the towel length-wise over the chest and abdomen. Do not expose the person. Pull the bath blanket down to the pubic area. Apply soap to the washcloth.

34 Lift the towel slightly, and wash the abdomen (Fig. 20-18, p. 338). Rinse and pat dry.

35 Pull the bath blanket up to the shoulders, covering both arms. Remove the towel.

36 Change soapy or cool water. Measure bath water temperature as in step 14. If bed rails are used, raise the bed rail near you before leaving the bedside. Lower it when you return.

37 Uncover the far leg. Do not expose the genital area. Place a towel length-wise under the foot and leg. Apply soap to the washcloth.

38 Bend the knee, and support the leg with your arm. Wash it with long, firm strokes. Rinse and pat dry.

39 Place the basin on the towel near the foot.

40 Lift the leg slightly. Slide the basin under the foot.

41 Place the foot in the basin (Fig. 20-19, p. 338). Use an orangewood stick or nail file to clean under toenails if necessary. If the person cannot bend the knees:
   a Wash the foot. Carefully separate the toes. Rinse and pat dry.
   b Clean under the toenails with an orangewood stick or nail file if necessary.

42 Remove the basin. Dry the leg and foot. Apply lotion to the foot if directed by the nurse and care plan. Cover the leg with the bath blanket. Remove the towel.

43 Repeat steps 37 to 42 for the near leg.

44 Change the water. Measure water temperature as in step 14. Raise the bed rail near you before leaving the bedside. Lower it when you return.

45 Turn the person onto the side away from you. The person is covered with the bath blanket.

46 Uncover the back and buttocks. Do not expose the person. Place a towel length-wise on the bed along the back. Apply soap to the washcloth.

47 Wash the back. Work from the back of the neck to the lower end of the buttocks. Use long, firm, continuous strokes (Fig. 20-20, p. 338). Rinse and dry well.

48 Turn the person onto his or her back.

49 Change the water for perineal care (p. 346). See step 14 in procedure: *Giving Female Perineal Care* (p. 348) for water temperature. (Some state competency tests also require changing gloves and hand hygiene at this time.) Raise the bed rail near you before leaving the bedside. Lower it when you return.

50 Provide perineal care if the person cannot do so (p. 346). (Practice hand hygiene and wear gloves for perineal care.)

51 Remove and discard the gloves. Practice hand hygiene.

52 Give a back massage (p. 344).

53 Apply deodorant or antiperspirant. Apply lotion and powder as requested. See *Promoting Safety and Comfort: Bathing*, p. 334.

54 Put clean garments on the person.

55 Comb and brush the hair (Chapter 21).

56 Make the bed.

POST-PROCEDURE

57 Provide for comfort. (See the inside of the front book cover.)

58 Place the signal light within reach.

59 Lower the bed to its lowest position.

60 Raise or lower bed rails. Follow the care plan.

61 Put on clean gloves.

62 Empty, clean, rinse, and dry the wash basin. Return it and other supplies to their proper place.

63 Wipe off the overbed table with paper towels. Discard the paper towels.

64 Unscreen the person.

65 Complete a safety check of the room. (See the inside of the front book cover.)

66 Follow agency policy for dirty linen.

67 Remove and discard the gloves. Practice hand hygiene.

68 Report and record your observations.

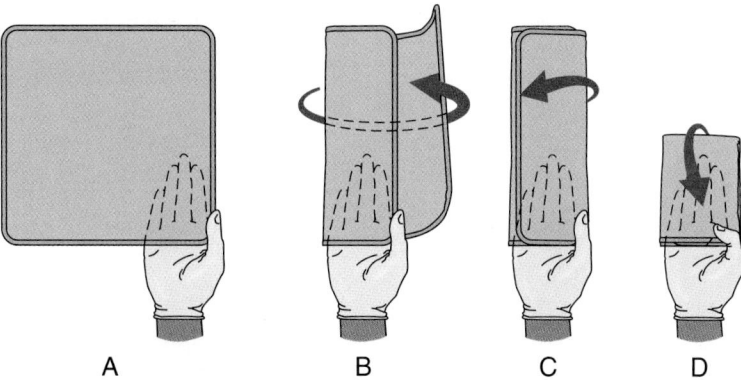

Fig. 20-13 Making a mitted washcloth. **A,** Grasp the near side of the washcloth with your thumb. **B,** Bring the washcloth around and behind your hand. **C,** Fold the side of the washcloth over your palm as you grasp it with your thumb. **D,** Fold the top of the washcloth down and tuck it under next to your palm.

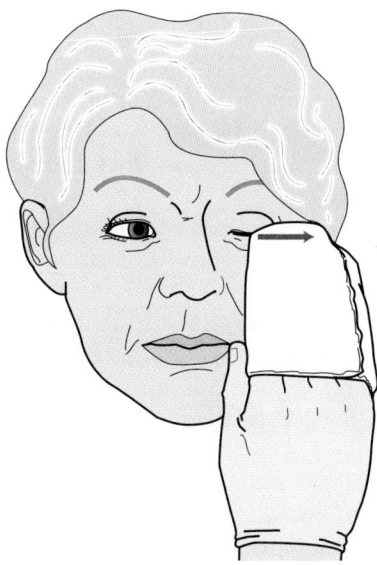

Fig. 20-14 Wash the person's eyes with a mitted washcloth. Wipe from the inner to the outer aspect of the eye.

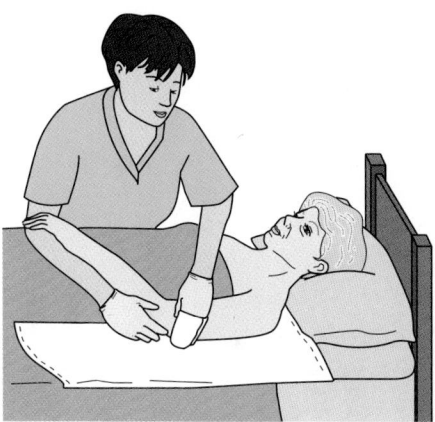

Fig. 20-15 The person's arm is washed with firm, long strokes using a mitted washcloth.

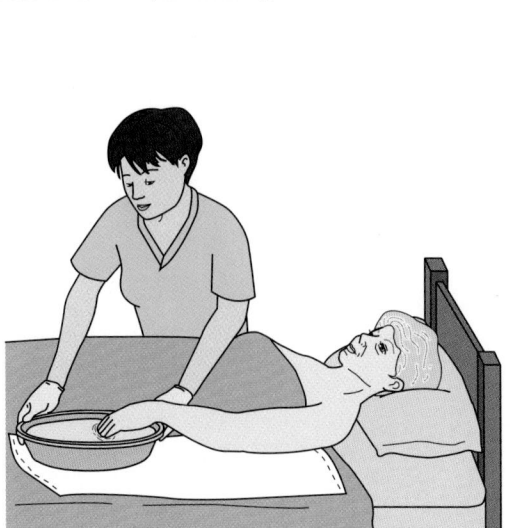

Fig. 20-16 The person's hand is washed by placing the wash basin on the bed.

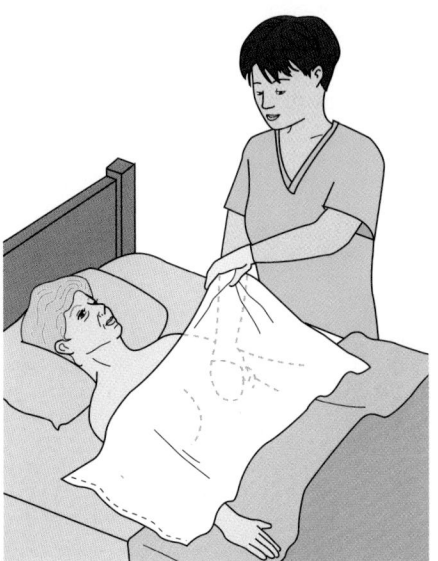

Fig. 20-17 The person's breasts are not exposed during the bath. A bath towel is placed horizontally over the chest area. The towel is lifted slightly to reach under to wash the breasts and chest.

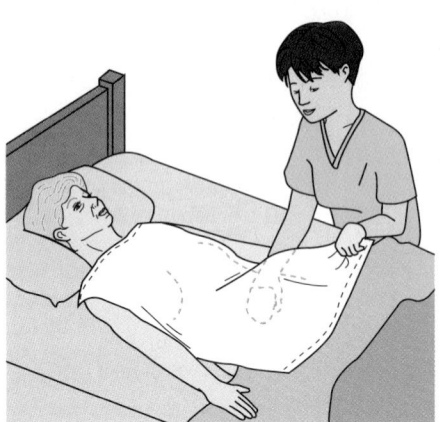

Fig. 20-18 The bath towel is turned so that it is vertical to cover the breasts and abdomen. The towel is lifted slightly to bathe the abdomen. The bath blanket covers the pubic area.

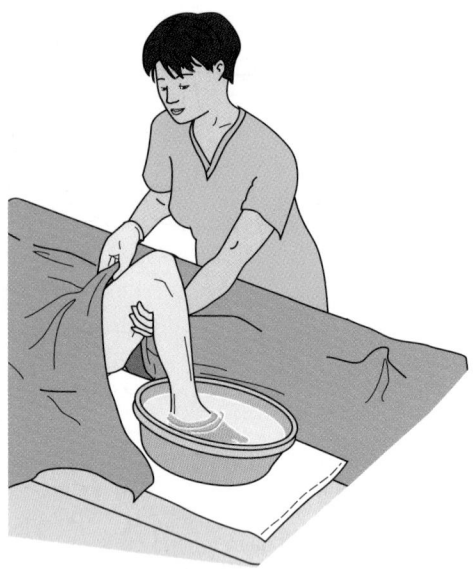

Fig. 20-19 The foot is washed by placing it in the wash basin on the bed.

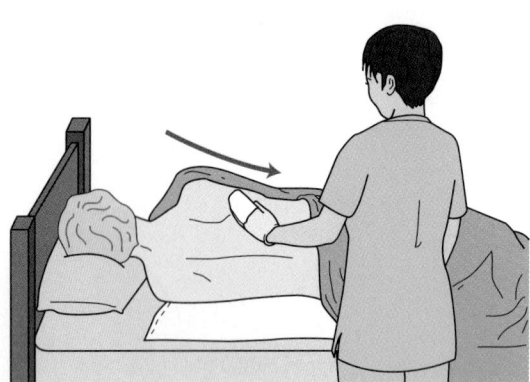

Fig. 20-20 The back is washed with long, firm, continuous strokes. Note that the person is in a side-lying position. A towel is placed length-wise on the bed to protect the linens from water.

Towel Baths

For a towel bath, an over-sized towel is used. It covers the body from the neck to the feet. The towel is completely wet with a solution—water and cleaning, skin-softening, and drying agents. The drying agent promotes fast drying of the person's body. The nurse and care plan tell you when to use a towel bath. To give a towel bath, follow agency policy.

See *Focus on Children and Older Persons: Towel Baths.*

Bag Baths

Bag baths are commercially prepared or prepared at the agency. A plastic bag has 8 to 10 washcloths. They are moistened with a cleaning agent that does not need rinsing. To give a bag bath:

- Warm the washcloths in a microwave oven. Follow the manufacturer's instructions for what microwave setting to use.
- Use a new washcloth for each body part.
- Let the skin air-dry. You do not need towels.
- Discard the washcloths following agency policy. Do not flush them down the toilet.

The Partial Bath

The *partial bath* involves bathing the face, hands, axillae (underarms), back, buttocks, and perineal area. Odors or discomfort occur if these areas are not clean. Some persons bathe themselves in bed or at the sink. You assist as needed. Most need help washing the back. You give partial baths to persons who cannot bathe themselves.

The rules for bathing apply (see Box 20-1). So do the complete bed bath considerations.

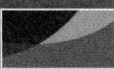 ## ASSISTING WITH THE PARTIAL BATH

QUALITY OF LIFE

Remember to:
- Knock before entering the person's room.
- Address the person by name.
- Introduce yourself by name and title.

- Explain the procedure to the person before beginning and during the procedure.
- Protect the person's rights during the procedure.
- Handle the person gently during the procedure.

PRE-PROCEDURE

1 Follow *Delegation Guidelines: Bathing,* p. 333. See *Promoting Safety and Comfort: Bathing,* p. 334.

2 Follow steps 2 through 7 in procedure: *Giving a Complete Bed Bath,* p. 335.

PROCEDURE

3 Make sure the bed is in the lowest position.
4 Practice hand hygiene. Put on gloves.
5 Cover the person with a bath blanket. Remove top linens.
6 Fill the wash basin ⅔ (two-thirds) full with water. Water temperature is usually 110°F to 115°F (43.3°C to 46.1°C) or as directed by the nurse. Measure water temperature with the bath thermometer. Or test bath water by dipping your elbow or inner wrist into the basin.
7 Ask the person to check the water temperature. Adjust the water temperature if it is too hot or too cold.
8 Place the basin on the overbed table.
9 Position the person in Fowler's position. Or assist him or her to sit at the bedside.
10 Adjust the overbed table so the person can reach the basin and supplies.
11 Help the person undress. Provide for privacy and warmth with the bath blanket.
12 Ask the person to wash easy to reach body parts (Fig. 20-21). Explain that you will wash the back and areas the person cannot reach.
13 Place the signal light within reach. Ask him or her to signal when help is needed or bathing is complete.

14 Remove and discard the gloves. Practice hand hygiene. Then leave the room.
15 Return when the signal light is on. Knock before entering. Practice hand hygiene.
16 Change the bath water. Measure bath water temperature as in step 6.
17 Raise the bed for body mechanics. The far bed rail is up if used.
18 Ask what was washed. Put on gloves. Wash and dry areas the person could not reach. The face, hands, underarms, back, buttocks, and perineal area are washed for the partial bath.
19 Remove and discard the gloves. Practice hand hygiene.
20 Give a back massage (p. 344).
21 Apply lotion, powder, and deodorant or antiperspirant as requested.
22 Help the person put on clean garments.
23 Assist with hair care and other grooming needs.
24 Assist the person to a chair. (Lower the bed if the person transfers to a chair.) Or turn the person onto the side away from you.
25 Make the bed. (Raise the bed for body mechanics.)

POST-PROCEDURE

26 Provide for comfort. (See the inside of the front book cover.)
27 Place the signal light within reach.
28 Lower the bed to its lowest position.
29 Raise or lower bed rails. Follow the care plan.
30 Put on clean gloves.
31 Empty, clean, rinse, and dry the bath basin. Return the basin and supplies to their proper place.

32 Wipe off the overbed table with the paper towels. Discard the paper towels.
33 Unscreen the person.
34 Complete a safety check of the room. (See the inside of the front book cover.)
35 Follow agency policy for dirty linen.
36 Remove and discard the gloves. Practice hand hygiene.
37 Report and record your observations.

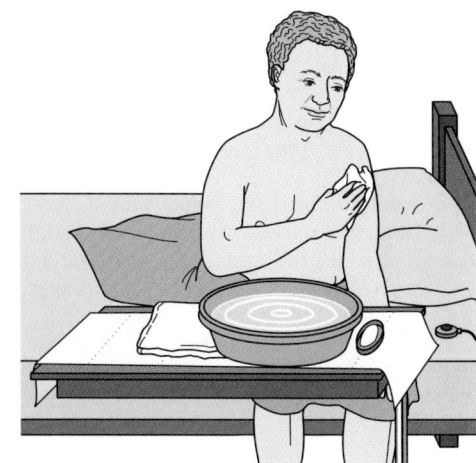

Fig. 20-21 The person is bathing himself while sitting on the side of the bed. Necessary equipment is within his reach.

Tub Baths and Showers

Some people like tub baths. Others like showers. Falls, burns, and chilling from water are risks. Safety is important (Box 20-2). The measures in Box 20-1 also apply. If other measures are needed, follow the nurse's directions and the care plan.

Some bathrooms have showers. If not, reserve the shower or tub room for the person.

Tub Baths. Tub baths are relaxing. A tub bath can make a person feel faint, weak, or tired. These are great risks for person who were on bedrest. A tub bath lasts no longer than 20 minutes.

To get in and out of the tub, the person may use:
- A shower bench (Fig. 20-22).
- A tub with a side entry door (Fig. 20-23).
- Wheelchair or stretcher lift. The person is transferred to the tub room by wheelchair or stretcher. Then the device and person are lifted into the tub (Fig. 20-24).
- Mechanical lift (Chapter 17).

Whirlpool tubs have a cleansing action. You wash the upper body. Carefully wash under the breasts and between skin folds. Also wash the perineal area. Pat dry the person with towels after the bath.

BOX 20-2	SAFETY MEASURES FOR TUB BATHS AND SHOWERS

- Know what water temperature to use. See *Delegation Guidelines: Tub Baths and Showers,* p. 342.
- Clean and disinfect the tub or shower before and after use.
- Dry the tub or shower room floor.
- Check hand rails, grab bars, hydraulic lifts, and other safety aids. They must be in working order.
- Place a bath mat in the tub or on the shower floor. This is not needed if there are non-skid strips or a non-skid surface.
- Cover the person for warmth and privacy. This includes during transport to and from the shower or tub room.
- Place needed items within the person's reach.
- Place the signal light within the person's reach.
- Show the person how to use the signal light in the shower or tub room.
- Have the person use the grab bars when getting in and out of the tub. The person must not use towel bars for support.
- Turn cold water on first, then hot water. Turn hot water off first, then cold water.
- Adjust water temperature and pressure to prevent chilling or burns. Do this before the person gets into the shower. If a shower chair is used, position it first.
- Direct water away from the person while adjusting water temperature and pressure.
- Fill the tub before the person gets into it. If using a tub with a side entry door, follow the manufacturer's instructions.
- Measure the water temperature. For showers and tub baths, use the digital display. Or you can use a bath thermometer for a tub bath.
- Keep the water spray directed toward the person during the shower. This helps keep him or her warm. (NOTE: Do not direct the water spray toward the person's face. This can frighten the person.)
- Keep bar soap in the soap dish between latherings. This reduces the risk of slipping and falls in showers and tubs. It also prevents soapy tub water.
- Avoid using bath oils. They make tub and shower surfaces slippery.
- Do not leave weak or unsteady persons unattended.
- Stay within hearing distance if the person can be left alone. Wait outside the shower curtain or door. You must be nearby if the person calls for you or has an accident.
- Drain the tub before the person gets out of the tub. Turn off the shower before the person gets out of the shower. Cover him or her to provide privacy and prevent chilling.

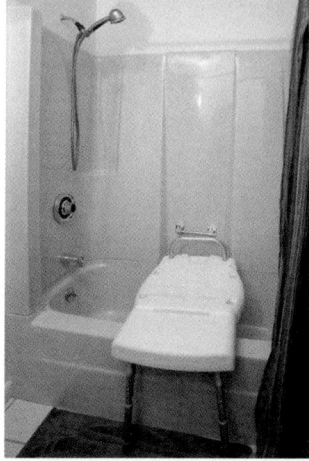

Fig. 20-22 A shower bench is positioned for the person's use in getting into and out of the tub.

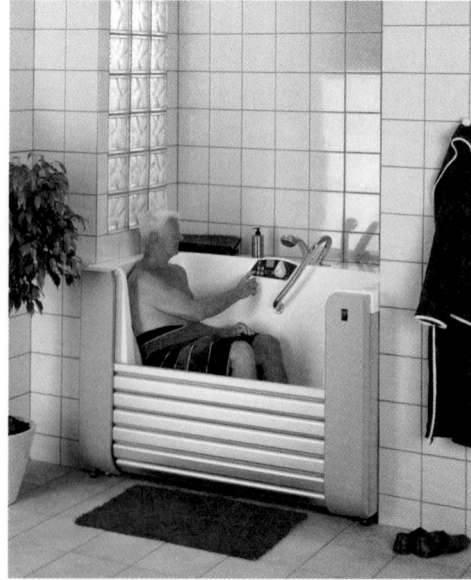

Fig. 20-23 Tub with a side entry door.

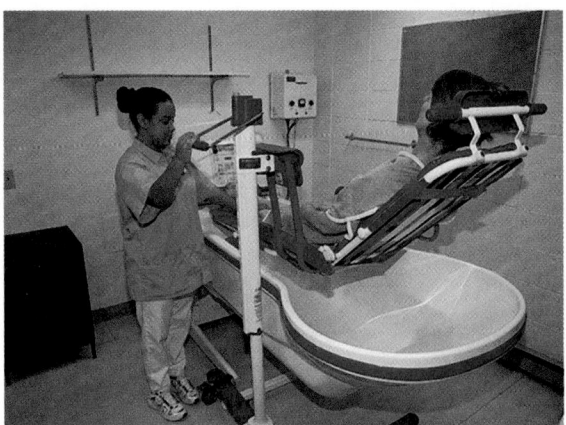

Fig. 20-24 The stretcher and person are lowered into the tub.

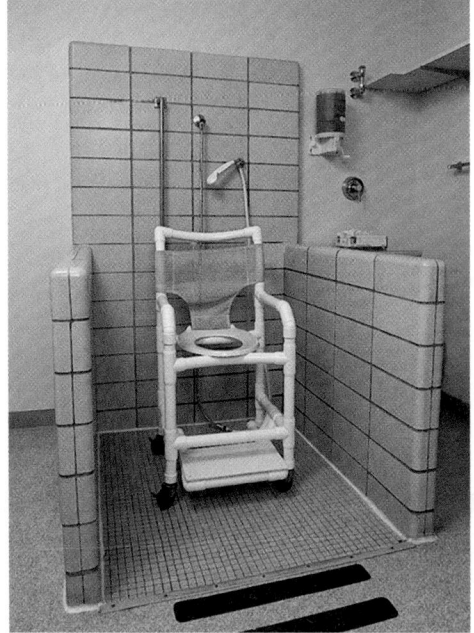

Fig. 20-25 A shower chair in a shower stall.

Showers. Some people can stand and use a regular shower. They use the grab bars for support. Like tubs, showers have non-skid surfaces. If not, a bath mat is used. Never let weak or unsteady persons stand in the shower. They need to use:

- *Shower chairs.* Water drains through an opening (Fig. 20-25). You use the chair to transport the person to and from the shower. Lock the wheels during the shower to prevent the chair from moving.
- *Shower stalls or cabinets.* The person walks into the device or is wheeled in on a wheelchair (Fig. 20-26). Use the hand-held nozzle.
- *Shower trolleys (portable tubs).* The person has a shower lying down (Fig. 20-27, p. 342). You lower the sides to transfer the person from the bed to the trolley. Raise the side rails after the transfer. Then transport the person to the tub or shower room. Use the hand-held nozzle to give the shower in the usual manner.

Some shower rooms have two or more stations. Provide for privacy. The person has the right not to have his or her body seen by others. Properly screen and cover the person. Also close doors and the shower curtain.

See *Focus on Long-Term Care and Home Care: Tub Baths and Showers*, p. 342.
See *Delegation Guidelines: Tub Baths and Showers*, p. 342.
See *Promoting Safety and Comfort: Tub Baths and Showers*, p. 342.
See *Teamwork and Time Management: Tub Baths and Showers*, p. 342.

Text continued on p. 344

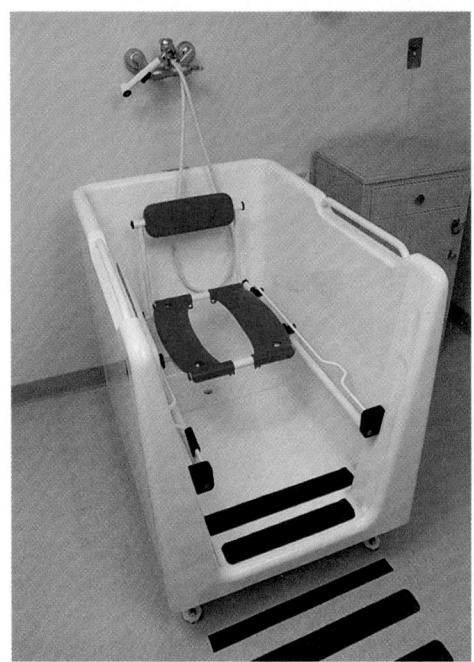

Fig. 20-26 A shower cabinet.

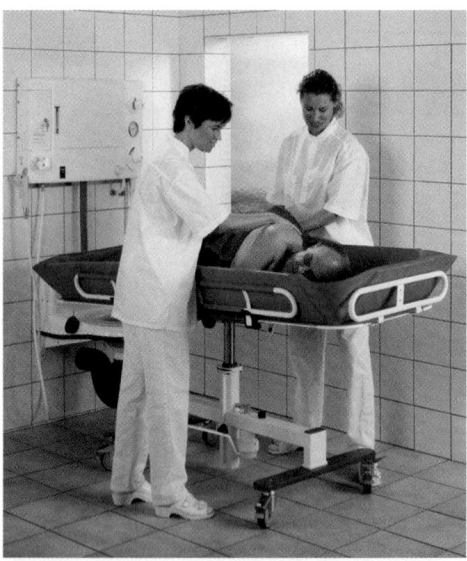

Fig. 20-27 Shower trolley. The sides are lowered for transfers into and out of the trolley.

FOCUS ON LONG-TERM CARE AND HOME CARE
Tub Baths and Showers

Home Care

Many homes have shower stalls or bathtub-shower units. To step into the tub or shower, the person needs to use grab bars. Help the person get in and out of the shower as needed.

The person can buy or rent a shower chair. Or a sturdy chair can be used. A sturdy lawn chair is an example. The nurse helps the person and family find a safe chair for shower use.

The bathtub unit may not have a shower. A hand-held shower nozzle can be installed.

DELEGATION GUIDELINES
Tub Baths and Showers

Before assisting with a tub bath or shower, you need this information from the nurse and the care plan:
- If the person takes a tub bath or shower
- What water temperature to use (usually 105°F; 40.5°C)
- What equipment is needed—shower chair, shower cabinet, shower trolley, and so on
- How much help the person needs
- If the person can bathe himself or herself
- What observations to report and record:
  - Dizziness
  - Light-headedness
  - See *Delegation Guidelines: Bathing*, p. 333
- When to report observations
- What patient or resident concerns to report at once

PROMOTING SAFETY AND COMFORT
Tub Baths and Showers

Safety

Some persons are very weak. At least 2 persons are needed to safely assist them with tub baths and showers. If the person is heavy, 3 or more staff members may be needed.

The person may use a tub with a side entry door, a shower chair, a shower trolley, or other device. Always follow the manufacturer's instructions.

Protect the person from falls, chilling, and burns. Follow the safety measures in Chapters 12 and 13. Remember to measure water temperature.

Clean and disinfect the tub or shower before and after use. This prevents the spread of microbes and infection.

Comfort

Warmth and privacy promote comfort during tub baths and showers. You need to:
- Make sure the tub or shower room is warm.
- Provide for privacy. Close the room door, screen the person, and close window coverings.
- Make sure water temperature is warm enough for the person.
- Have the person remove his or her clothing or robe and footwear just before getting into the tub or shower. Do not let the person remain exposed longer than necessary.
- Leave the room if the person can be alone.

TEAMWORK AND TIME MANAGEMENT
Tub Baths and Showers

The agency may not have tub and shower equipment for each person. You need to reserve the room and equipment for the person. Your co-workers do the same for their patients and residents.

Consider the needs of others. For example, you reserve the shower room from 0945 to 1030. Do your very best to follow the schedule. Make sure the shower room is clean and ready for the next person. Or you and a co-worker schedule something for the same time. Plan a new schedule with your co-worker.

All bed linens are changed on the person's bath or shower day. Ask co-workers to make the person's bed while you assist with the tub bath or shower. Also ask them to straighten the person's unit. The person returns to a clean bed and unit. Return the favor when your co-workers are assisting with tub baths, showers, or other care measures.

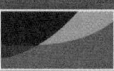 **ASSISTING WITH A TUB BATH OR SHOWER**

QUALITY OF LIFE

Remember to:
- Knock before entering the person's room.
- Address the person by name.
- Introduce yourself by name and title.

- Explain the procedure to the person before beginning and during the procedure.
- Protect the person's rights during the procedure.
- Handle the person gently during the procedure.

PRE-PROCEDURE

1 Follow *Delegation Guidelines:*
   a *Bathing,* p. 333
   b *Tub Baths and Showers*
   See *Promoting Safety and Comfort:*
   a *Bathing,* p. 334
   b *Tub Baths and Showers*
2 Reserve the bathtub or shower.
3 Practice hand hygiene.
4 Identify the person. Check the ID bracelet against the assignment sheet. Also call the person by name.

5 Collect the following:
   - Washcloth and two bath towels
   - Soap
   - Bath thermometer (for a tub bath)
   - Clothing or sleepwear
   - Grooming items as requested
   - Robe and non-skid footwear
   - Rubber bath mat if needed
   - Disposable bath mat
   - Gloves
   - Wheelchair, shower chair, transfer bench, and so on as needed

PROCEDURE

6 Place items in the tub or shower room. Use the space provided or a chair.
7 Clean and disinfect the tub or shower.
8 Place a rubber bath mat in the tub or on the shower floor. Do not block the drain.
9 Place the disposable bath mat on the floor in the front of the tub or shower.
10 Put the OCCUPIED sign on the door.
11 Return to the person's room. Provide for privacy. Practice hand hygiene.
12 Help the person sit on the side of the bed.
13 Help the person put on a robe and non-skid footwear. Or the person can leave on clothing.
14 Assist or transport the person to the tub room or shower.
15 Have the person sit on a chair if he or she walked to the tub or shower room.
16 Provide for privacy.
17 For a tub bath:
   a Fill the tub half-way with warm water (usually 105°F; 40.5°C). Follow the care plan for water temperature.
   b Measure water temperature. Use the bath thermometer or check the digital display.
   c Ask the person to check the water temperature. Adjust the water temperature if it is too hot or too cold.
18 For a shower:
   a Turn on the shower.
   b Adjust water temperature and pressure. Check the digital display.
   c Ask the person to check the water temperature. Adjust the water temperature if it is too hot or too cold.

19 Help the person undress and remove footwear.
20 Help the person into the tub or shower. Position the shower chair, and lock the wheels.
21 Assist with washing as necessary. Wear gloves.
22 Ask the person to use the signal light when done or when help is needed. Remind the person that a tub bath lasts no longer than 20 minutes.
23 Place a towel across the chair.
24 Leave the room if the person can bathe alone. If not, stay in the room or nearby. Remove and discard the gloves and practice hand hygiene if you will leave the room.
25 Check the person at least every 5 minutes.
26 Return when he or she signals for you. Knock before entering. Practice hand hygiene.
27 Turn off the shower, or drain the tub. Cover the person while the tub drains.
28 Help the person out of the shower or tub and onto the chair.
29 Help the person dry off. Pat gently. Dry under the breasts, between skin folds, in the perineal area, and between the toes.
30 Assist with lotion and other grooming items as needed.
31 Help the person dress and put on footwear.
32 Help the person return to the room. Provide for privacy.
33 Assist the person to a chair or into bed.
34 Provide a back massage if the person returns to bed.
35 Assist with hair care and other grooming needs.

Continued

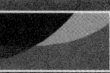

ASSISTING WITH A TUB BATH OR SHOWER—cont'd

VIDEO   VIDEO CLIP

POST-PROCEDURE

36 Provide for comfort. (See the inside of the front book cover.)
37 Place the signal light within reach.
38 Raise or lower bed rails. Follow the care plan.
39 Unscreen the person.
40 Complete a safety check of the room. (See the inside of the front book cover.)
41 Clean and disinfect the tub or shower. Remove soiled linen. Wear gloves.
42 Discard disposable items. Put the UNOCCUPIED sign on the door. Return supplies to their proper place.
43 Follow agency policy for dirty linen.
44 Remove and discard the gloves. Practice hand hygiene.
45 Report and record your observations.

THE BACK MASSAGE

The back massage (back rub) relaxes muscles and stimulates circulation. You give back massages after baths and showers and with evening care. You also give them at other times. Examples include after re-positioning or helping the person to relax.

Back massages last 3 to 5 minutes. Observe the skin before the massage. Look for breaks in the skin, bruises, reddened areas, and other signs of skin breakdown.

Lotion reduces friction during the massage. Warm the lotion before it is applied. Do one of the following:
- Rub some lotion between your hands.
- Place the bottle in the bath water.
- Hold the bottle under warm water.

Use firm strokes. Also keep your hands in contact with the person's skin. After the massage, apply some lotion to the elbows, knees, and heels. This keeps the skin soft. These bony areas are at risk for skin breakdown.

See *Delegation Guidelines: The Back Massage.*
See *Promoting Safety and Comfort: The Back Massage.*

DELEGATION GUIDELINES
The Back Massage

Before giving a back massage, you need this information from the nurse and the care plan:
- If the person can have a back massage (see *Promoting Safety and Comfort: The Back Massage*)
- How to position the person
- If the person has position limits
- When the person is to have a back massage
- If the person needs frequent back massages for comfort and to relax
- What observations to report and record:
  - Breaks in the skin
  - Bruising
  - Reddened areas
  - Signs of skin breakdown
- When to report observations
- What patient or resident concerns to report at once

PROMOTING SAFETY AND COMFORT
The Back Massage

Safety
Back massages are dangerous for persons with certain heart diseases, back injuries, back and other surgeries, skin diseases, and lung disorders. Check with the nurse and the care plan before giving back massages to persons with these conditions.

Do not massage reddened bony areas. Reddened areas signal skin breakdown and pressure ulcers. Massage can lead to more tissue damage.

Wear gloves if the person's skin is not intact. Always follow Standard Precautions and the Bloodborne Pathogen Standard.

Comfort
The prone position is best for a massage. The side-lying position is often used. Older and disabled persons usually find the side-lying position more comfortable.

The back massage involves stroking down the back and over the buttocks. Some persons may not want the buttocks exposed and touched for a massage. Explain the procedure to the person. Obtain the person's consent to expose and touch the buttocks. If the person does not give consent, modify the procedure as in step 14 of the procedure: *Giving a Back Massage.*

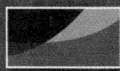 **GIVING A BACK MASSAGE**

QUALITY OF LIFE

Remember to:
- Knock before entering the person's room.
- Address the person by name.
- Introduce yourself by name and title.

- Explain the procedure to the person before beginning and during the procedure.
- Protect the person's rights during the procedure.
- Handle the person gently during the procedure.

PRE-PROCEDURE

1 Follow *Delegation Guidelines: The Back Massage*. See *Promoting Safety and Comfort: The Back Massage*.
2 Practice hand hygiene.
3 Identify the person. Check the ID bracelet against the assignment sheet. Also call the person by name.

4 Collect the following:
  - Bath blanket
  - Bath towel
  - Lotion
5 Provide for privacy.
6 Raise the bed for body mechanics. Bed rails are up if used.

PROCEDURE

7 Lower the bed rail near you if up.
8 Position the person in the prone or side-lying position. The back is toward you.
9 Expose the back, shoulders, upper arms, and buttocks. Cover the rest of the body with the bath blanket. Expose the buttocks only if the person gives consent.
10 Lay the towel on the bed along the back. Do this if the person is in a side-lying position.
11 Warm the lotion.
12 Explain that the lotion may feel cool and wet.
13 Apply lotion to the lower back area.
14 Stroke up from the buttocks to the shoulders. Then stroke down over the upper arms. Stroke up the upper arms, across the shoulders, and down the back to the buttocks (Fig. 20-28, p. 346). Use firm strokes. Keep your hands in contact with the person's skin. If the person does not want the buttocks exposed, stroke down the back to the waist and up the back to the shoulders.

15 Repeat step 14 for at least 3 minutes.
16 Knead the back (Fig. 20-29, p. 346):
  a Grasp the skin between your thumb and fingers.
  b Knead half of the back. Start at the buttocks and move up to the shoulder. Then knead down from the shoulder to the buttocks.
  c Repeat on the other half of the back.
17 Apply lotion to bony areas. Use circular motions with the tips of your index and middle fingers. (Do not massage reddened bony areas.)
18 Use fast movements to stimulate. Use slow movements to relax the person.
19 Stroke with long, firm movements to end the massage. Tell the person you are finishing.
20 Straighten and secure clothing or sleepwear.
21 Cover the person. Remove the towel and bath blanket.

POST-PROCEDURE

22 Provide for comfort. (See the inside of the front book cover.)
23 Place the signal light within reach.
24 Lower the bed to its lowest position.
25 Raise or lower bed rails. Follow the care plan.
26 Return lotion to its proper place.

27 Unscreen the person.
28 Complete a safety check of the room. (See the inside of the front book cover.)
29 Follow agency policy for dirty linen.
30 Practice hand hygiene.
31 Report and record your observations.

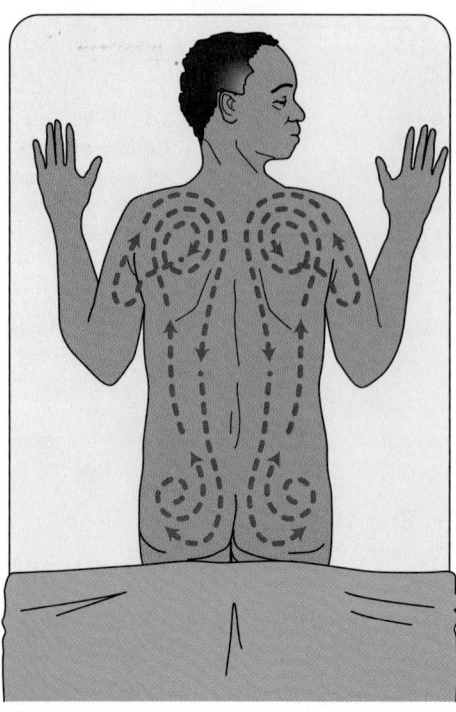

Fig. 20-28 The person lies in the prone position for a back massage. Stroke upward from the buttocks to the shoulders, down over the upper arms, back up the upper arms, across the shoulders, and down the back to the buttocks.

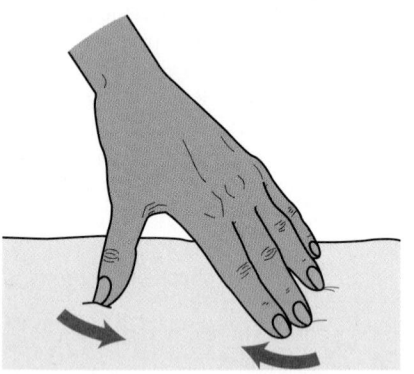 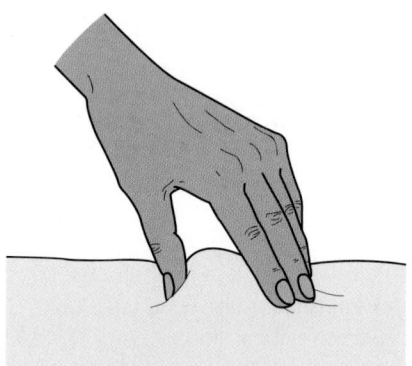

Fig. 20-29 Kneading is done by picking up tissue between the thumb and fingers.

PERINEAL CARE

Perineal care (pericare) involves cleaning the genital and anal areas. These areas provide a warm, moist, and dark place for microbes to grow. Cleaning prevents infection and odors, and it promotes comfort.

Perineal care is done daily during the bath. It also is done whenever the area is soiled with urine or feces. Perineal care is very important for persons who:

- Have urinary catheters (Chapter 22).
- Have had rectal or genital surgery.
- Are menstruating (Chapter 9).
- Are incontinent of urine or feces.

- Are uncircumcised (Fig. 20-30). Being *circumcised* means that the fold of skin (foreskin) covering the glans of the penis was surgically removed. Being *uncircumcised* means that the person has foreskin covering the head of the penis.

The person does perineal care if able. Otherwise, it is given by the nursing staff. This procedure embarrasses many people and staff, especially when it involves the other sex.

Perineal and *perineum* are not common terms. Most people understand *privates*, *private parts*, *crotch*, *genitals*, or

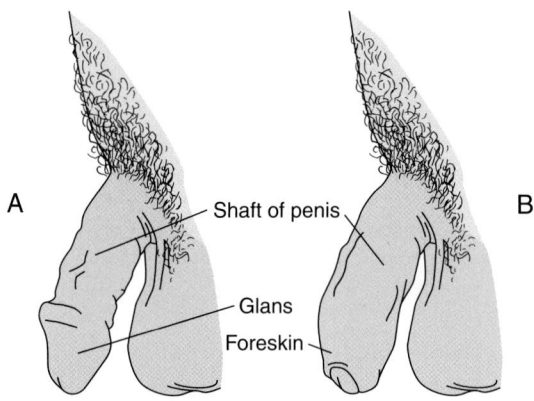

Fig. 20-30 **A,** Circumcised male. **B,** Uncircumcised male.

FOCUS ON COMMUNICATION
Perineal Care

Talking to the person about perineal care may be difficult. You may be embarrassed. However, you must explain the procedure to the person.

When a person performs his or her own perineal care, you can say:

- "Mrs. Bell, I'll give you some privacy while you finish your bath. Can you reach everything you need? Please call me if you need help. Here is your signal light."
- "Mr. Baker, I'll give you time to finish your bath. Please wash your genital and rectal areas. Signal for me when you're done or need help."

If you provide perineal care for the person, you can say:

- "Mrs. Allan, next I'll clean between your legs. I'll keep you covered with the bath blanket. I'll tell you before I touch you. Please tell me if you feel any pain or discomfort."
- "Mr. Scott, I'll clean your private parts now. Please let me know if you feel any pain or discomfort."

DELEGATION GUIDELINES
Perineal Care

Before giving perineal care, you need this information from the nurse and the care plan:

- When to give perineal care.
- What terms the person understands—perineum, privates, private parts, crotch, genitals, area between the legs, and so on.
- How much help the person needs.
- What water temperature to use—usually 105°F to 109°F (40.5°C to 42.7°C). Water in a basin cools rapidly.
- What cleaning agent to use.
- Any position restrictions or limits.
- What observations to report and record:
  - Odors
  - Redness, swelling, discharge, bleeding, or irritation
  - Complaints of pain, burning, or other discomfort
  - Signs of urinary or fecal incontinence
- When to report observations.
- What patient or resident concerns to report at once.

PROMOTING SAFETY AND COMFORT
Perineal Care

Safety

Hot water can burn delicate perineal tissues. To prevent burns, measure water temperature according to agency policy. If the water seems too hot, ask the nurse to check it.

Protect yourself and the person from infection. Contact with blood, body fluids, secretions, or excretions is likely during perineal care. Follow Standard Precautions and the Bloodborne Pathogen Standard.

Persons who are incontinent need perineal care. Protect the person and dry garments and linens from the wet or soiled items. Remove the wet or soiled incontinence products, garments, and linen. Then apply clean, dry ones.

Comfort

To avoid embarrassment, it is best if the person does perineal care. If you provide this care, explain how you protect privacy. Act in a professional manner at all times.

Perineal care involves touching the genital and anal areas. The person may prefer that someone of the same sex provide this care. Or the person may fear sexual assault. Always obtain the person's consent before providing perineal care. For mental comfort, the person may want a family member or another staff member present to witness the procedure. Ask if he or she wants someone present and that person's name.

the *area between the legs.* Use terms the person understands. The term must be in good taste professionally.

Standard Precautions, medical asepsis, and the Bloodborne Pathogen Standard are followed. Work from the cleanest area to the dirtiest. This is commonly called cleaning from "front to back." The urethral area (the front) is the cleanest. The anal area (the back) is the dirtiest. Therefore clean from the urethra to the anal area. This prevents the transmission of bacteria from the anal area to the vagina and urinary system.

The perineal area is delicate and easily injured. Use warm water, not hot. Use washcloths, towelettes, cotton balls, or swabs according to agency policy. Rinse thoroughly. Pat dry after rinsing. This reduces moisture and promotes comfort.

See *Focus on Communication: Perineal Care.*
See *Delegation Guidelines: Perineal Care.*
See *Promoting Safety and Comfort: Perineal Care.*

Text continued on p. 351

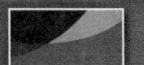 **GIVING FEMALE PERINEAL CARE**   VIDEO | VIDEO CLIP | NNAAP® Skill

QUALITY OF LIFE

Remember to:
- Knock before entering the person's room.
- Address the person by name.
- Introduce yourself by name and title.

- Explain the procedure to the person before beginning and during the procedure.
- Protect the person's rights during the procedure.
- Handle the person gently during the procedure.

PRE-PROCEDURE

1 Follow *Delegation Guidelines: Perineal Care,* p. 347. See *Promoting Safety and Comfort: Perineal Care,* p. 347.
2 Practice hand hygiene.
3 Collect the following:
   - Soap or other cleaning agent as directed
   - At least 4 washcloths
   - Bath towel
   - Bath blanket
   - Bath thermometer
   - Wash basin

   - Waterproof pad
   - Gloves
   - Paper towels
4 Cover the overbed table with paper towels. Arrange items on top of them.
5 Identify the person. Check the ID bracelet against the assignment sheet. Also call the person by name.
6 Provide for privacy.
7 Raise the bed for body mechanics. Bed rails are up if used.

PROCEDURE

8 Lower the bed rail near you if up.
9 Practice hand hygiene. Put on gloves.
10 Cover the person with a bath blanket. Move top linens to the foot of the bed.
11 Position the person on the back.
12 Drape the person as in Figure 20-31.
13 Raise the bed rail if used.
14 Fill the wash basin. Water temperature is usually 105°F to 109°F (40.5°C to 42.7°C). Follow the care plan for water temperature. Measure water temperature according to agency policy.
15 Ask the person to check the water temperature. Adjust the water temperature if it is too hot or too cold. Raise the bed rail before leaving the bedside. Lower it when you return.
16 Place the basin on the overbed table.
17 Lower the bed rail if up.
18 Help the person flex her knees and spread her legs. Or help her spread her legs as much as possible with the knees straight.
19 Place a waterproof pad under her buttocks. Remove any wet or soiled incontinence products.
20 Fold the corner of the bath blanket between her legs onto her abdomen.
21 Wet the washcloths.
22 Squeeze out excess water from a washcloth. Make a mitted washcloth. Apply soap.
23 Separate the labia. Clean downward from front to back with one stroke (Fig. 20-32).

24 Repeat steps 22 and 23 until the area is clean. Use a clean part of the washcloth for each stroke. Use more than one washcloth if needed.
25 Rinse the perineum with a clean washcloth. Separate the labia. Stroke downward from front to back. Repeat as necessary. Use a clean part of the washcloth for each stroke. Use more than one washcloth if needed.
26 Pat the area dry with the towel. Dry from front to back.
27 Fold the blanket back between her legs.
28 Help the person lower her legs and turn onto her side away from you.
29 Apply soap to a mitted washcloth.
30 Clean the rectal area. Clean from the vagina to the anus with one stroke (Fig. 20-33).
31 Repeat steps 29 and 30 until the area is clean. Use a clean part of the washcloth for each stroke. Use more than one washcloth if needed.
32 Rinse the rectal area with a washcloth. Stroke from the vagina to the anus. Repeat as necessary. Use a clean part of the washcloth for each stroke. Use more than one washcloth if needed.
33 Pat the area dry with the towel. Dry from front to back.
34 Remove the waterproof pad.
35 Remove and discard the gloves. Practice hand hygiene. Put on clean gloves.
36 Provide clean and dry linens and incontinence products as needed.

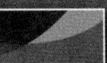

GIVING FEMALE PERINEAL CARE—cont'd

POST-PROCEDURE

37 Cover the person. Remove the bath blanket.

38 Provide for comfort. (See the inside of the front book cover.)

39 Place the signal light within reach.

40 Lower the bed to its lowest position.

41 Raise or lower bed rails. Follow the care plan.

42 Empty, clean, rinse, and dry the wash basin.

43 Return the basin and supplies to their proper place.

44 Wipe off the overbed table with the paper towels. Discard the paper towels.

45 Unscreen the person.

46 Complete a safety check of the room. (See the inside of the front book cover.)

47 Follow agency policy for dirty linen.

48 Remove and discard the gloves. Practice hand hygiene.

49 Report and record your observations.

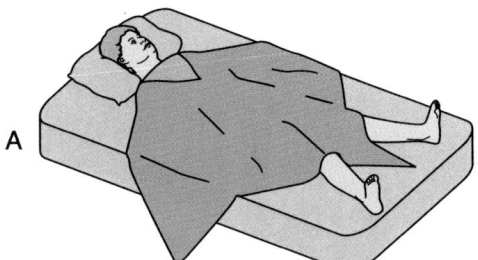 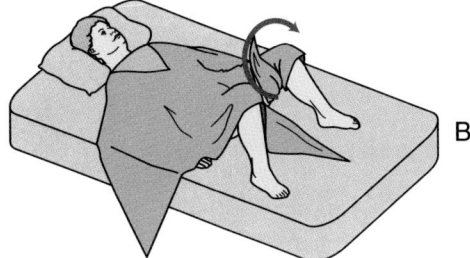

Fig. 20-31 Draping for perineal care. **A,** Position the bath blanket like a diamond: one corner is at the neck, there is a corner at each side, and one corner is between the person's legs. **B,** Wrap the blanket around the leg by bringing the corner around under the leg and over the top. Tuck the corner under the hip.

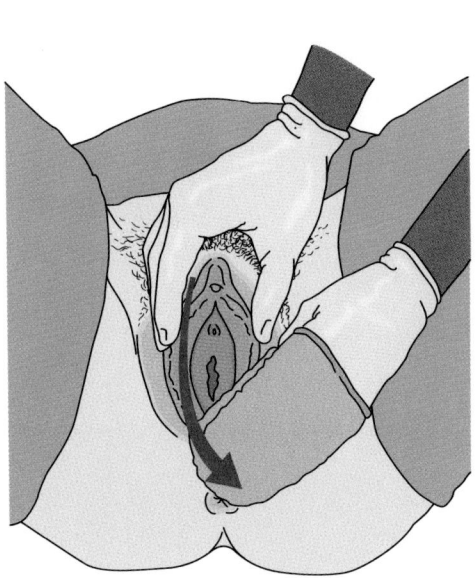 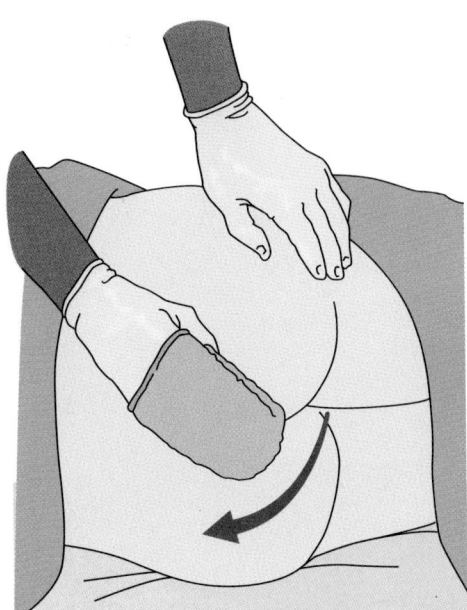

Fig. 20-32 Separate the labia with one hand. Use a mitted washcloth to cleanse between the labia with downward strokes.

Fig. 20-33 The rectal area is cleaned by wiping from the vagina to the anus. The side-lying position allows the anal area to be cleaned more thoroughly.

GIVING MALE PERINEAL CARE

VIDEO | VIDEO CLIP

QUALITY OF LIFE

Remember to:
- Knock before entering the person's room.
- Address the person by name.
- Introduce yourself by name and title.

- Explain the procedure to the person before beginning and during the procedure.
- Protect the person's rights during the procedure.
- Handle the person gently during the procedure.

PROCEDURE

1. Follow steps 1 through 17 in procedure: *Giving Female Perineal Care,* p. 348. Drape the person as in Figure 20-31.
2. Place a waterproof pad under his buttocks. Remove any wet or soiled incontinence products.
3. Retract the foreskin if the person is uncircumcised (Fig. 20-34).
4. Grasp the penis.
5. Clean the tip. Use a circular motion. Start at the meatus of the urethra, and work outward (Fig. 20-35). Repeat as needed. Use a clean part of the washcloth each time.
6. Rinse the area with another washcloth.
7. Return the foreskin to its natural position immediately after rinsing.
8. Clean the shaft of the penis. Use firm downward strokes. Rinse the area.

9. Help the person flex his knees and spread his legs. Or help him spread his legs as much as possible with his knees straight.
10. Clean the scrotum. Rinse well. Observe for redness and irritation of the skin folds.
11. Pat dry the penis and the scrotum. Use the towel.
12. Fold the bath blanket back between his legs.
13. Help him lower his legs and turn onto his side away from you.
14. Clean the rectal area (see procedure: *Giving Female Perineal Care,* p. 348). (NOTE: For males, clean from the scrotum to the anus.) Rinse and dry well.
15. Remove the waterproof pad.
16. Remove and discard the gloves. Practice hand hygiene. Put on clean gloves.
17. Provide clean and dry linens and incontinence products.

POST-PROCEDURE

18. Follow steps 37 through 49 in procedure: *Giving Female Perineal Care,* p. 349.

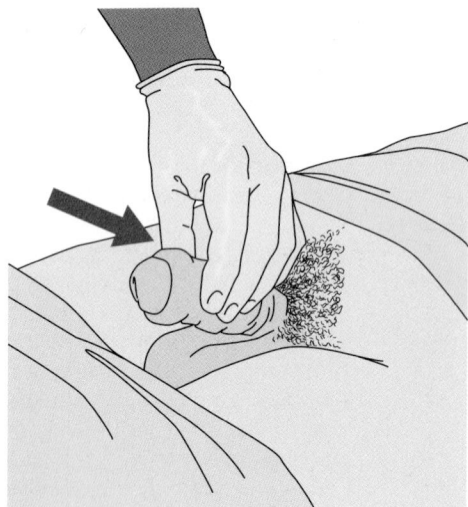

Fig. 20-34 The foreskin of the uncircumcised male is pulled back for perineal care. It is returned to the normal position immediately after cleaning and rinsing.

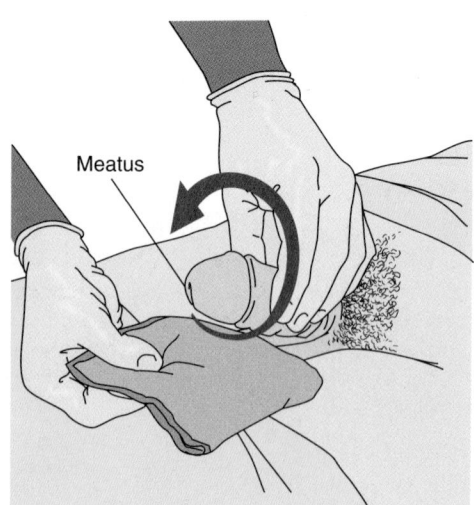

Meatus

Fig. 20-35 The penis is cleaned with circular motions starting at the meatus.

REPORTING AND RECORDING

You make many observations while assisting with hygiene. Report the following at once:

- Bleeding
- Signs of skin breakdown
- Discharge from the vagina or urinary tract
- Unusual odors
- Changes from prior observations

Also report and record the care given. (See "Flow Sheets" in Chapter 6.) If care is not recorded, it is assumed that care was not given. This can cause serious legal problems.

FOCUS ON PRIDE

The Person, Family, and Yourself

Personal and Professional Responsibility

Patients and residents depend on you to meet their hygiene needs. You are responsible for providing care in a way that maintains or improves the person's quality of life, health, and safety. To do so:

- Follow the guidelines and procedures presented in this chapter.
- Focus on the *Quality of Life* section at the beginning of each procedure.
- View the person as an individual with unique needs. Ask about the person's needs and preferences.

Take pride in providing care that benefits the person's overall well-being.

Rights and Respect

Privacy promotes dignity and respect. To protect the right to privacy:

- Do not expose the person.
- Ask visitors to leave the room before you give care.
- Close doors, privacy curtains, and window coverings before giving care.
- Cover the person when going to and from tubs or shower rooms.
- Expose only the body part involved in the procedure.

Independence and Social Interaction

Personal choice helps the person remain independent. Hygiene is a very personal matter. Allow personal choice in such matters as bath time, products used, and what to wear. Encourage the person to do as much self-care as safely possible. Doing so promotes independence and improves self-esteem.

Delegation and Teamwork

Some agencies have commercial warmers for bag baths that show which bags are warm. When you remove a pack, replace it with another pack. Then the warmer is full for other staff. If you see the warmer is getting low, fill it. Otherwise, staff find an empty warmer when going to get a pack. They must wait for a pack to heat up. Or the warmer is almost empty, and the other person has to fill it. Avoid having the attitude that "someone else can do it." This shows poor teamwork and work ethics. Take pride in being a helpful and courteous member of the team.

Ethics and Laws

You will perform some tasks often. Bathing and other personal hygiene measures are examples. Over time, some staff become less careful with routine tasks. They may forget about dangers. Or they think that nothing bad will happen. This is very unsafe.

Accidents happen. Mistakes are made. The following examples show how harm can occur during routine bathing.

A patient (Mr. Genza) was paralyzed on his right side because of a stroke. He could not walk or talk. He could stand with difficulty. He died at age 51 from burns suffered during a shower.

A wrongful death suit was filed for what was claimed to be negligent care. According to the facts reported in the court case, the following occurred:

- *An attendant took the patient to the shower. He was taken in a wheelchair.*
- *The attendant undressed the patient. The patient was placed on a chair and under running water in the shower.*
- *The attendant claimed that he tested the water.*
- *The shower room was supervised by an RN. The RN testified that an attendant was required to be present at all times while a paralyzed patient was receiving a shower.*
- *The attendant stated that he washed the patient's back and head. Then he went to attend to another patient 5 or 6 feet from the shower. A tub was between the attendant and Mr. Genza.*
- *When the attendant asked if he wanted to get out of the shower, Mr. Genza indicated that he did not.*
- *Two minutes later, the attendant was getting another patient out of the tub. The attendant heard Mr. Genza shout and saw that the shower handle was moved from its original setting.*
- *Two days later, Mr. Genza died from burns.*
- *On the day of the accident, the hot water gauge read 171°F. It tested at 158°F to 159°F.*
- *An expert witness stated that 110°F is hot enough for shower room use.*
- *In the Court's opinion, the home was grossly negligent for:*
  - *Failing to provide the supervision needed by a helpless person*
  - *Providing water facilities that were dangerous and a threat to the lives of anyone using them*

(M. Lewinski v State of Illinois, 1967.)

In another case, a daughter filed a complaint for the wrongful death of her mother. According to the complaint, on August 29, 1993, a nurse's aide ran water in a whirlpool bath for the nursing home resident. The nurse's aide tested the water with her bare arm and hand. She found the water satisfactory. The resident also tested the water by putting her foot in the water, which showed that the water was okay. Using a lift chair, the resident was transferred into the tub.

After the bath, the nurse's aide asked two co-workers to help her get the resident out of the tub. After getting her out, a co-worker noted a small spot on the resident's left hip. The resident had no burns on her body before the bath. However, redness of her extremities was noted over the next 30 minutes. Blisters began and continued to form.

The resident had second and third degree burns from her mid-back down over the buttocks, the perineal area, and lower extremities. (Author note: a first degree burn means the epidermis is damaged. A second degree burn involves the epidermis and part of the dermis. A third degree burn involves the epidermis and the entire dermis.) The resident was transferred to the hospital. She died on September 1, 1993.

Continued

FOCUS ON PRIDE—cont'd

The daughter sued the county, the nursing home and hospital, the nursing home administrator, hospital board members, and the nurse's aide. The trial court dismissed the case on a legal technicality. However, the Appellate Court reversed the dismissal by the trial court and returned the case to court for trial.

(D. Burton v Choctaw County, Mississippi, Choctaw Hospital d/b/a Choctaw County Nursing Home; and others, 1997.)

You must always be careful. Harm can result from routine care measures. Follow the safety measures in this chapter at all times.

REVIEW QUESTIONS

Circle T if the statement is TRUE or F if it is FALSE.

1 T F Hygiene is needed for comfort, safety, and health.
2 T F After lunch, Mrs. Bell asks for a back massage. You can give the back massage.
3 T F A toothbrush with hard bristles is good for oral hygiene.
4 T F A baby's teeth are flossed when two baby teeth touch.
5 T F Unconscious persons are supine for mouth care.
6 T F You use your fingers to keep an unconscious person's mouth open for oral hygiene.
7 T F You clean dentures over a towel on a counter.
8 T F A person has a partial denture. Natural teeth are brushed.
9 T F Bath oils cleanse and soften the skin.
10 T F Powders absorb moisture and prevent friction.
11 T F Deodorants reduce the amount of perspiration.
12 T F To wash the eye, wash from the outer to the inner aspect.
13 T F A tub bath lasts 30 minutes.
14 T F You can give permission for showers but not tub baths.
15 T F Weak persons are left alone in the shower if they are sitting.
16 T F A back massage relaxes muscles and stimulates circulation.
17 T F Perineal care helps prevent infection.
18 T F Foreskin is returned to its normal position immediately after cleaning.

Circle the BEST answer.

19 Oral hygiene does the following *except*
   a Prevent mouth odors   c Increase comfort
   b Prevent infection   d Coat and dry the mouth
20 A person flosses once a day. When is the best time to floss?
   a In the morning   c After meals
   b Before meals   d At bedtime
21 Which is *not* reported to the nurse?
   a Bleeding, swelling, or redness of the gums
   b Irritations, sores, or white patches in the mouth or on the tongue
   c Lips that are dry, cracked, swollen, or blistered
   d Food between the teeth
22 Which is *not* a purpose of bathing?
   a Increasing circulation
   b Promoting drying of the skin
   c Exercising body parts
   d Refreshing and relaxing the person
23 To apply powder you should
   a Turn toward the person
   b Sprinkle a small amount onto your hand
   c Apply a thick layer of powder
   d Shake the powder onto the person
24 Soaps do the following *except*
   a Remove dirt and dead skin
   b Soften the skin
   c Remove skin oil
   d Dry the skin
25 Which action is *wrong* when bathing a person?
   a Covering the person for warmth and privacy
   b Rinsing the skin thoroughly to remove all soap
   c Washing from the dirtiest to the cleanest area
   d Patting the skin dry
26 Water for a complete bed bath is at least
   a 100°F   c 110°F
   b 105°F   d 120°F
27 You are assisting with a shower. You should do the following *except*
   a Measure water temperature
   b Direct the water spray at the person's face
   c Keep bar soap in the soap dish
   d Turn the shower off before the person gets out of the shower
28 You are going to give a back massage. Which is *false*?
   a It should last 3 to 5 minutes.
   b Lotion is warmed before being applied.
   c Your hands are always in contact with the skin.
   d The side-lying position is best.
29 Water temperature for perineal care is at least
   a 100°F   c 110°F
   b 105°F   d 120°F
30 These statements are about perineal care. Which is *false*?
   a The perineal area is easily injured.
   b The person does perineal care if he or she is able.
   c You clean from "back to front."
   d You follow Standard Precautions.

Answers to these questions are on p. 833.

Grooming 21

KEY TERMS

alopecia Hair loss
anticoagulant A drug that prevents or slows down (*anti*) blood clotting (*coagulate*)
dandruff Excessive amounts of dry, white flakes from the scalp
hirsutism Excessive body hair
lice See "pediculosis"
mite A very small spider-like organism

pediculosis Infestation with wingless insects; lice
pediculosis capitis Infestation of the scalp (*capitis*) with lice; head lice
pediculosis corporis Infestation of the body (*corporis*) with lice
pediculosis pubis Infestation of the pubic (*pubis*) hair with lice

KEY ABBREVIATIONS

C	Centigrade	**ID**	Identification
F	Fahrenheit	**IV**	Intravenous

Hair care, shaving, and nail and foot care are important to many people. Like hygiene, these grooming measures prevent infection and promote comfort. They also affect love, belonging, and self-esteem needs.

People differ in their grooming measures. Some want only clean hair. Others want a certain hairstyle. Some want only clean hands. Others want clean, manicured, and polished nails. Many men shave and groom their beards.

Likewise, many women shave their legs and underarms. Some women have facial hair. They may shave or use other hair removal methods.

As with hygiene, the person should tend to grooming measures to the extent possible. This promotes independence and quality of life. The person may use adaptive devices for grooming (Fig. 21-1, p. 354).

See *Teamwork and Time Management: Grooming*, p. 354.

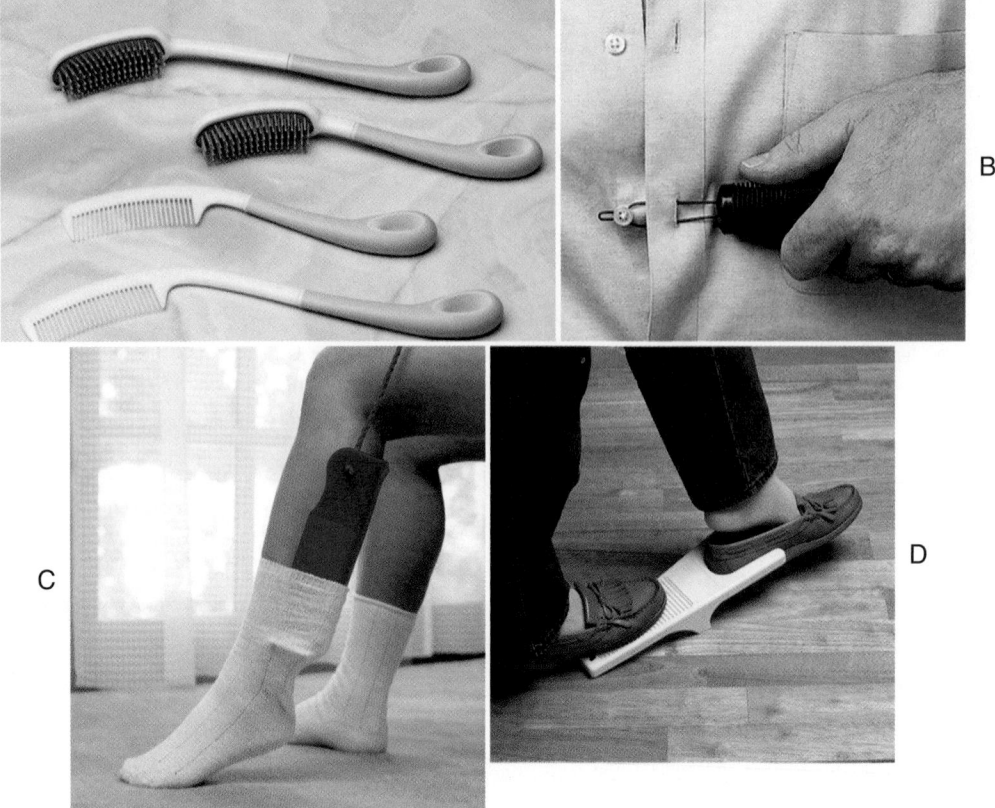

Fig. 21-1 Grooming aids. **A,** Long-handled combs and brushes are used for hair care. **B,** A button hook is used to button and zip clothing. **C,** A sock assist is used to pull on socks and stockings. **D,** A shoe remover is used to take off shoes.

TEAMWORK AND TIME MANAGEMENT

Grooming

Some grooming equipment is shared among patients and residents. Shampoo trays, electric shavers, and whirlpool foot baths are examples. Let other team members know when you need an item. Schedule the item following agency policy. After the procedure, promptly clean and return the item to its proper place. Do not make your co-workers look for or clean an item.

HAIR CARE

The look and feel of hair affect mental well-being. Some people cannot perform hair care. You assist with hair care whenever needed.

The nursing process reflects the person's culture, personal choice, skin and scalp condition, health history, and self-care ability.

See *Focus on Long-Term Care and Home Care: Hair Care.*

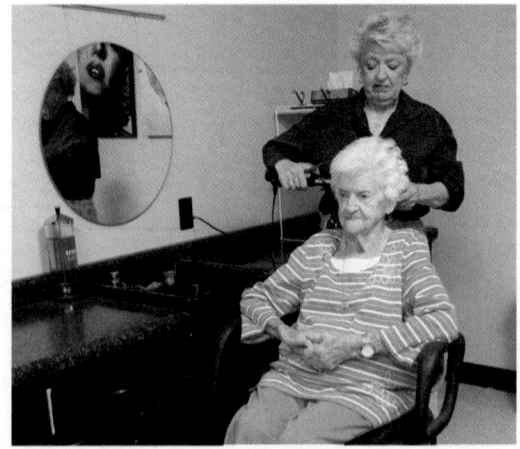

Fig. 21-2 Beauty shop in a nursing center.

FOCUS ON LONG-TERM CARE AND HOME CARE

Hair Care

Long-Term Care

Many nursing centers have beauty and barber shops (Fig. 21-2). Residents can have their hair shampooed, cut, and styled. Men also can have their mustaches and beards groomed.

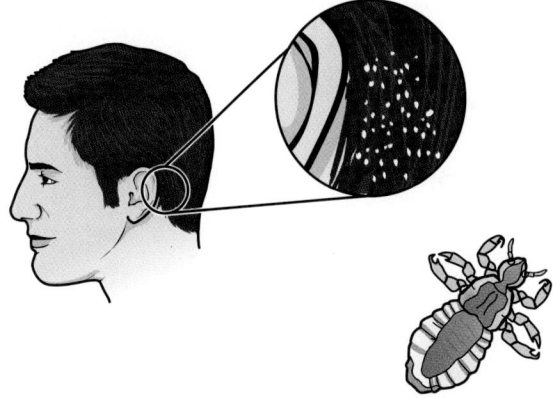

Fig. 21-3 Head lice.

Skin and Scalp Conditions

Skin and scalp conditions include hair loss, excessive body hair, dandruff, lice, and scabies.

See *Focus on Communication: Skin and Scalp Conditions.*

Alopecia, Hirsutism, and Dandruff. *Alopecia means hair loss.* Hair loss may be complete or partial. Male pattern baldness occurs with aging. It results from heredity. Hair also thins in some women with aging. Cancer treatments (radiation therapy to the head and chemotherapy) often cause alopecia in persons of all ages. Skin disease is another cause. Stress, poor nutrition, pregnancy, some drugs, and hormone changes are other causes. Except for hair loss from aging, hair usually grows back.

Hirsutism is excessive body hair. It can occur in men, women, and children. It results from heredity and abnormal amounts of male hormones.

Dandruff is the excessive amount of dry, white flakes from the scalp. Itching is common. Sometimes eyebrows and ear canals are involved. Medicated shampoos correct the problem.

Lice. *Pediculosis (lice) is the infestation with wingless insects.* See Figure 21-3. *Infestation* means being in or on a host. Lice attach their eggs (*nits*) to hair shafts. Nits are oval and yellow to white in color. They hatch in about one week.

After hatching, lice feed on blood to live. They bite the scalp or skin. Adult lice are about the size of a sesame seed. They are tan to grayish-white in color. Lice bites cause severe itching in the affected body area.

- *Pediculosis capitis is the infestation of the scalp* (capitis) *with lice.* It is commonly called "head lice."
- *Pediculosis pubis is the infestation of the pubic* (pubis) *hair with lice.* This form of lice is also called "crabs."
- *Pediculosis corporis is the infestation of the body* (corporis) *with lice.*

Lice easily spread to others through clothing, head coverings, furniture, beds, towels, bed linen, and sexual contact. They also are spread by sharing combs and brushes. Lice are treated with medicated shampoos, lotions, and creams specific for lice. Thorough bathing is needed. So is washing clothing and linens in hot water.

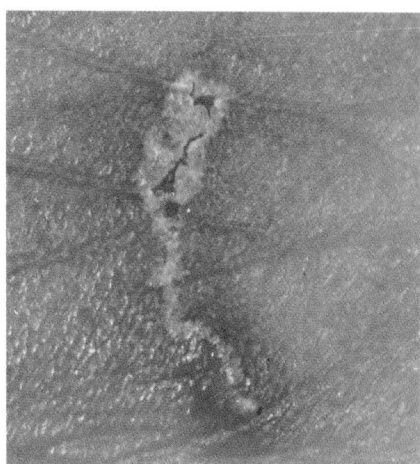

Fig. 21-4 Scabies.

Report signs and symptoms of lice to the nurse at once:
- Complaints of a tickling feeling or something moving in the hair
- Itching
- Irritability
- Sores on the head or body caused by scratching
- Rash

Scabies. Scabies is a skin disorder caused by a female mite (Fig. 21-4). A *mite is a very small spider-like organism* (Fig. 21-5, p. 356). The female mite burrows into the skin and lays eggs. When the eggs hatch, the females produce more eggs. The person becomes infested with mites.

The person has a rash and intense itching. Common sites are between the fingers, around the wrists, in the underarm area, on the thighs, and in the genital area. Other sites include the breasts, waist, and buttocks.

Scabies is highly contagious. It is transmitted to others by close contact. Persons living in crowded living settings are at risk. So are persons with weakened immune systems. Special creams are ordered to kill the mites. The person's room is cleaned. Clothing and linens are washed in hot water.

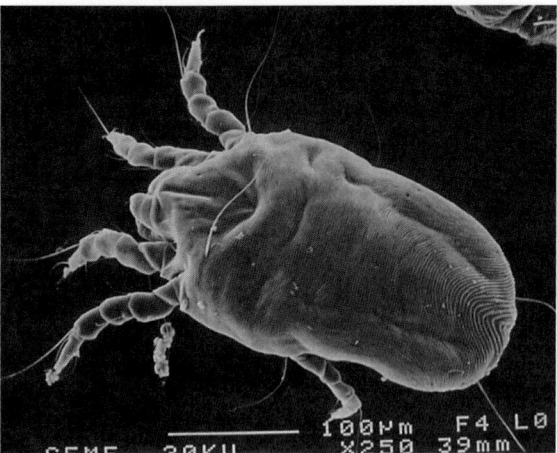

Fig. 21-5 Dust mite.

Brushing and Combing Hair

Brushing and combing hair are part of early morning care, morning care, and afternoon care. And they are done whenever needed. Some people also brush and comb hair at bedtime. Make sure you provide hair care before visitors arrive.

Encourage patients and residents to do their own hair care. Assist as needed. Provide hair care for those who cannot do so. The person chooses how to brush, comb, and style hair.

Brushing increases blood flow to the scalp. And it brings scalp oils along the hair shaft. Scalp oils help keep hair soft and shiny. Brushing and combing prevent tangled and matted hair. To brush and comb hair, start at the scalp. Then brush or comb to the hair ends.

Long hair easily mats and tangles. Daily brushing and combing prevent the problem. So does braiding. You need the person's consent to braid hair. *Never cut matted or tangled hair.* Tell the nurse if the person has matted or tangled hair. The nurse may have you comb or brush through the matting and tangling from the hair ends to the scalp.

Special measures are needed for curly, coarse, and dry hair. Use a wide-tooth comb for curly hair. Start at the neckline. Working upward, lift and fluff hair outward. Continue to the forehead. Wet hair or apply conditioner or petroleum jelly as directed. This makes combing easier.

The person may have certain hair care practices and products. They are part of the care plan. Also, let the person guide you when giving hair care.

See *Caring about Culture: Brushing and Combing Hair.*
See *Focus on Children and Older Persons: Brushing and Combing Hair.*
See *Delegation Guidelines: Brushing and Combing Hair.*
See *Promoting Safety and Comfort: Brushing and Combing Hair.*

BRUSHING AND COMBING THE PERSON'S HAIR

QUALITY OF LIFE

Remember to:
- Knock before entering the person's room.
- Address the person by name.
- Introduce yourself by name and title.

- Explain the procedure to the person before beginning and during the procedure.
- Protect the person's rights during the procedure.
- Handle the person gently during the procedure.

PRE-PROCEDURE

1 Follow *Delegation Guidelines: Brushing and Combing Hair.* See *Promoting Safety and Comfort: Brushing and Combing Hair.*
2 Practice hand hygiene.
3 Identify the person. Check the ID (identification) bracelet against the assignment sheet. Also call the person by name.

4 Ask the person how to style hair.
5 Collect the following:
- Comb and brush
- Bath towel
- Other hair care items as requested
6 Arrange items on the bedside stand.
7 Provide for privacy.

PROCEDURE

8 Lower the bed rail if up.
9 Help the person to the chair. The person puts on a robe and non-skid footwear when up. (If the person is in bed, raise the bed for body mechanics. Bed rails are up if used. Lower the bed rail near you. Assist the person to a semi-Fowler's position if allowed.)
10 Place a towel across the person's back and shoulders or across the pillow.
11 Ask the person to remove eyeglasses. Put them in the eyeglass case. Put the case inside the bedside stand.
12 *Brush and comb hair that is* not *matted or tangled:*
   a Use the comb to part the hair.
      (1) Part hair down the middle into 2 sides (Fig. 21-6, A).
      (2) Divide 1 side into 2 smaller sections (Fig. 21-6, B).

b Brush 1 of the small sections of hair. Start at the scalp, and brush toward the hair ends (Fig. 21-7). Do the same for the other small section of hair.
c Repeat steps 12, a(2) and 12, b for the other side.
13 *Brush and comb matted and tangled hair:*
   a Take a small section of hair near the ends.
   b Comb or brush through to the hair ends.
   c Add small sections of hair as you work up to the scalp.
   d Comb or brush through each longer section to the hair ends.
   e Brush or comb from the scalp to the hair ends.
14 Style the hair as the person prefers.
15 Remove the towel.
16 Let the person put on the eyeglasses.

POST-PROCEDURE

17 Provide for comfort. (See the inside of the front book cover.)
18 Place the signal light within reach.
19 Lower the bed to its lowest position.
20 Raise or lower bed rails. Follow the care plan.
21 Clean and return hair care items to their proper place.

22 Unscreen the person.
23 Complete a safety check of the room. (See the inside of the front book cover.)
24 Follow agency policy for dirty linen.
25 Practice hand hygiene.

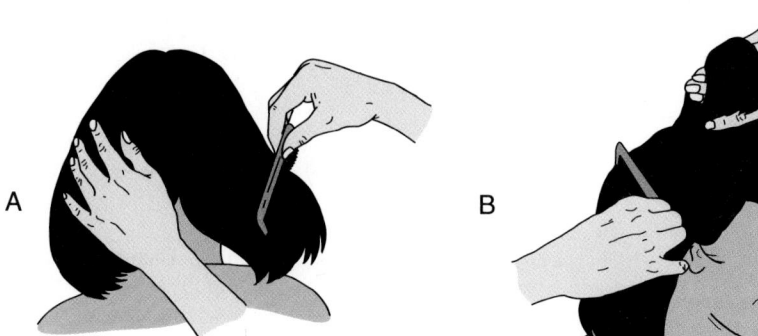

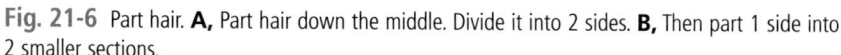

Fig. 21-6 Part hair. **A,** Part hair down the middle. Divide it into 2 sides. **B,** Then part 1 side into 2 smaller sections.

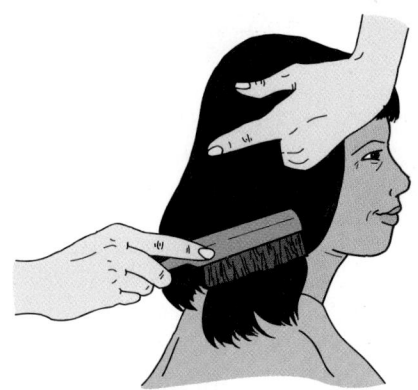

Fig. 21-7 Brush hair by starting at the scalp. Brush down to the hair ends.

SHAMPOOING

Most people shampoo at least once a week. Some shampoo 2 or 3 times a week. Others shampoo every day. Many factors affect frequency. They include the condition of the hair and scalp, hairstyle, and personal choice.

Some persons use certain shampoos and conditioners. Others used medicated products ordered by the doctor.

The person may need help shampooing. Shampoo hair when the nurse tells you to do so. The nurse tells you what method to use. The shampoo method depends on the person's condition, safety factors, and personal choice.

- *Shampoo during the shower or tub bath.* The person shampoos in the shower. You use a hand-held nozzle for those using shower chairs or taking tub baths. You direct a spray of water at the hair.
- *Shampoo at the sink.* The person sits facing away from the sink. A folded towel is placed over the sink edge to protect the neck. The person's head is tilted back over the edge of the sink. You use a water pitcher or hand-held nozzle to wet and rinse the hair.
- *Shampoo on a stretcher.* The stretcher is in front of the sink. A towel is placed under the neck. The head is tilted over the edge of the sink (Fig. 21-8). You use a water pitcher or hand-held nozzle to wet and rinse the hair.
- *Shampoo in bed.* The person's head and shoulders are moved to the edge of the bed if possible. You place a shampoo tray under the head to protect the linens and mattress from water. The tray drains into a basin placed on a chair by the bed (Fig. 21-9). You use a water pitcher to wet and rinse the hair. This method is used for persons who need complete bed baths. It also is used for persons who cannot use a chair, wheelchair, or stretcher.

Some agencies have commercially prepared shampoo caps. Each cap contains a cleaning agent that does not need rinsing. Some caps also contain conditioner. To use a shampoo cap:

- Warm the package in a microwave oven or commercial warmer. Follow the manufacturer's instructions for microwave settings and warming times.
- Check the cap's temperature. The cap should be warm. Do not use a cap that is too hot.
- Apply the cap to the person's head.
- Massage the cap gently. Follow the manufacturer's instructions for how long to massage. One to three minutes is common. Longer hair may require more time.
- Remove the cap. You do not need to rinse the hair. Dry the hair with a towel if needed.
- Comb the hair.

Dry and style hair as quickly as possible after the shampoo. Women may want hair curled or rolled up before drying. Check with the nurse before doing so.

See *Focus on Children and Older Persons: Shampooing.*
See *Focus on Long-Term Care and Home Care: Shampooing.*
See *Delegation Guidelines: Shampooing.*
See *Promoting Safety and Comfort: Shampooing.*

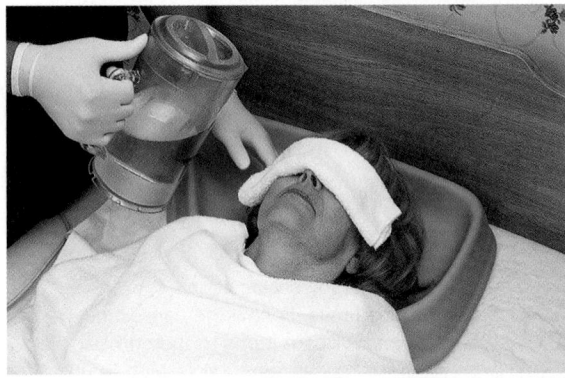

Fig. 21-9 A shampoo tray is used to shampoo a person in bed. The tray is directed to the side of the bed so water drains into a collecting basin.

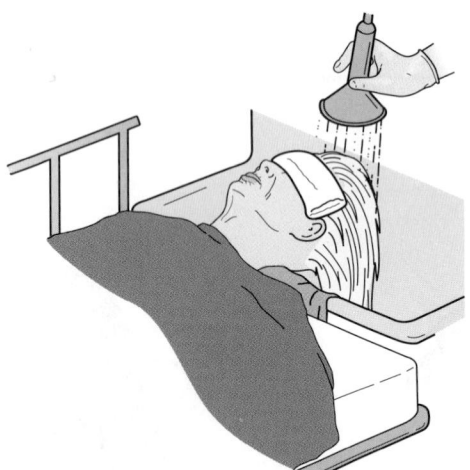

Fig. 21-8 Shampooing while the person is on a stretcher. The stretcher is in front of the sink.

FOCUS ON CHILDREN AND OLDER PERSONS
Shampooing

Children
Oil gland secretion increases with puberty. Therefore adolescents tend to have oily hair. They may need to shampoo often.

Older Persons
Oil gland secretion decreases with aging. Therefore, older persons have dry hair. They may shampoo less often than younger adults do.

FOCUS ON LONG-TERM CARE AND HOME CARE
Shampooing

Long-Term Care
Shampooing is usually done weekly on the person's bath or shower day. If a person's hair is done by a hairdresser or barber, do not shampoo the hair. The person wears a shower cap during the tub bath or shower.

Home Care
You can make a shampoo trough from a plastic shower curtain or tablecloth. Or use a sturdy plastic drop cloth for painting. Do not use plastic trash bags or dry-cleaning bags. They slip and slide easily and are not sturdy.

Place the plastic under the person's head. Make a raised edge around the plastic to prevent water from spilling over the sides. Tape the plastic in place if necessary. Direct the ends of the plastic into a basin. Water flows into the basin.

DELEGATION GUIDELINES
Shampooing

To shampoo a person, you need this information from the nurse and the care plan:
- When to shampoo the person's hair
- What method to use
- What shampoo and conditioner to use
- The person's position restrictions or limits
- What water temperature to use—usually 105°F (Fahrenheit) (40.5°C [centigrade])
- If hair is curled or rolled up before drying
- What observations to report and record:
  - Scalp sores
  - Flaking
  - Itching
  - The presence of nits or lice
  - Patches of hair loss
  - Hair falling out in patches
  - Very dry or very oily hair
  - Matted or tangled hair
  - How the person tolerated the procedure
- When to report observations
- What patient or resident concerns to report at once

PROMOTING SAFETY AND COMFORT
Shampooing

Safety
Keep shampoo away from and out of the eyes. Have the person hold a washcloth over the eyes. When rinsing, cup your hand at the person's forehead. This keeps soapy water from running down the person's forehead and into the eyes.

Return medicated products to the nurse. Never leave them at the bedside unless the nurse tells you to do so.

Wear gloves if the person has scalp sores. Follow Standard Precautions and the Bloodborne Pathogen Standard.

For a shampoo on a stretcher, follow the rules for stretcher use (Chapter 12). To safely transfer the person to and from the stretcher, see procedure: *Moving the Person to a Stretcher* (Chapter 17). Lock the stretcher wheels and use the safety straps and side rails. The far side rail is raised during the procedure.

Some people can shampoo themselves during a tub bath or shower. Place an extra towel, shampoo, and hair conditioner within the person's reach. Assist as needed.

Comfort
When shampooing during the tub bath or shower, the person tips his or her head back to keep shampoo and water out of the eyes. Support the back of the person's head with one hand. Shampoo with your other hand. Some persons cannot tip their heads back. They lean forward and hold a folded washcloth over the eyes. Support the forehead with one hand as you shampoo with the other. Make sure that the person can breathe easily.

Many people have limited range of motion in their necks. They are not shampooed at the sink or on a stretcher.

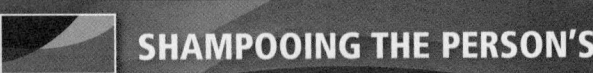 **SHAMPOOING THE PERSON'S HAIR**

QUALITY OF LIFE

Remember to:
- Knock before entering the person's room.
- Address the person by name.
- Introduce yourself by name and title.

- Explain the procedure to the person before beginning and during the procedure.
- Protect the person's rights during the procedure.
- Handle the person gently during the procedure.

PRE-PROCEDURE

1 Follow *Delegation Guidelines: Shampooing*, p. 359. See *Promoting Safety and Comfort: Shampooing*, p. 359.
2 Practice hand hygiene.
3 Collect the following:
   - Two bath towels
   - Washcloth
   - Shampoo
   - Hair conditioner (if requested)
   - Bath thermometer
   - Pitcher or hand-held nozzle (if needed)
   - Shampoo tray (if needed)
   - Basin or pan (if needed)

   - Waterproof pad (if needed)
   - Gloves (if needed)
   - Comb and brush
   - Hair dryer
4 Arrange items nearby.
5 Identify the person. Check the ID bracelet against the assignment sheet. Also call the person by name.
6 Provide for privacy.
7 Raise the bed for body mechanics for a shampoo in bed. Bed rails are up if used.
8 Practice hand hygiene.

PROCEDURE

9 Lower the bed rail near you if up.
10 Cover the person's chest with a bath towel.
11 Brush and comb the hair to remove snarls and tangles.
12 Position the person for the method you will use. To shampoo the person in bed:
   a Lower the head of the bed and remove the pillow.
   b Place the waterproof pad and shampoo tray under the head and shoulders.
   c Support the head and neck with a folded towel if necessary.
13 Raise the bed rail if used.
14 Obtain water. Water temperature is usually 105°F (40.5°C). Test water temperature according to agency policy. Also ask the person to check the water. Adjust the water temperature as needed. Raise the bed rail before leaving the bedside.
15 Lower the bed rail near you if up.
16 Put on gloves (if needed).
17 Ask the person to hold a washcloth over the eyes. It should not cover the nose and mouth. (NOTE: A damp washcloth is easier to hold. It will not slip. However, some state competency tests require a dry washcloth.)

18 Use the pitcher or nozzle to wet the hair.
19 Apply a small amount of shampoo.
20 Work up a lather with both hands. Start at the hairline. Work toward the back of the head.
21 Massage the scalp with your fingertips. Do not scratch the scalp with your fingernails.
22 Rinse the hair until the water runs clear.
23 Repeat steps 19 through 22.
24 Apply conditioner. Follow directions on the container.
25 Squeeze water from the person's hair.
26 Cover the hair with a bath towel.
27 Remove the shampoo tray, basin, and waterproof pad.
28 Dry the person's face with the towel. Use the towel on the person's chest.
29 Help the person raise the head if appropriate. For the person in bed, raise the head of the bed.
30 Rub the hair and scalp with the towel. Rub gently. Use the second towel if the first one is wet.
31 Comb the hair to remove snarls and tangles.
32 Dry and style hair as quickly as possible.
33 Remove and discard the gloves (if used). Practice hand hygiene.

POST-PROCEDURE

34 Provide for comfort. (See the inside of the front book cover.)
35 Place the signal light within reach.
36 Lower the bed to its lowest position.
37 Raise or lower bed rails. Follow the care plan.
38 Unscreen the person.
39 Complete a safety check of the room. (See the inside of the front book cover.)

40 Clean, rinse, dry, and return equipment to its proper place. Remember to clean the brush and comb. Discard disposable items.
41 Follow agency policy for dirty linen.
42 Practice hand hygiene.
43 Report and record your observations.

■ SHAVING

Many men shave for comfort and mental well-being. Many women shave their legs and underarms. Some women shave facial hair. Or they may use other hair removal methods—waxing, hair removal products, plucking, threading. See Box 21-1 for shaving rules.

Safety razors or electric shavers are used (Fig. 21-10). Patients and residents may have their own electric shavers. If the agency's shaver is used, clean it after every use. Follow the manufacturer's instructions for brushing out whiskers. Also follow agency policy for cleaning electric shavers.

Safety razors (blade razors) involve razor blades. They can cause nicks and cuts. Older persons with wrinkled skin are at risk for nicks and cuts. Therefore safety razors are not used on persons who have healing problems or for those taking anticoagulant drugs. An *anticoagulant is a drug that prevents or slows down* (anti) *blood clotting* (coagulate). Bleeding occurs easily and is hard to stop. A nick or cut can cause serious bleeding. Electric shavers are used.

Soften the beard before shaving. To do so, apply a moist, warm washcloth or towel for a few minutes. Then pat dry the face and apply talcum powder if using an electric shaver. For a safety razor, lather the face with soap and water or shaving cream.

See *Focus on Children and Older Persons: Shaving.*
See *Delegation Guidelines: Shaving.*
See *Promoting Safety and Comfort: Shaving,* p. 362.

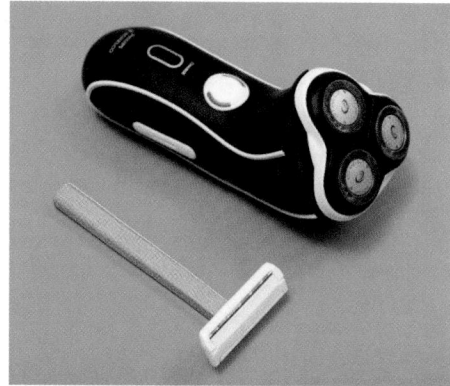

Fig. 21-10 Electric shaver and safety razor.

FOCUS ON CHILDREN AND OLDER PERSONS
Shaving

Older Persons

Safety razors are not used to shave persons with dementia. They may not understand what you are doing. They may resist care and move suddenly. Serious nicks and cuts can occur. Use electric shavers for these persons.

DELEGATION GUIDELINES
Shaving

To shave a person, you need this information from the nurse and the care plan:
- What shaver to use—electric or safety
- If the person takes anticoagulant drugs
- When to shave the person
- What facial hair to shave
- The location of tender or sensitive areas on the person's face
- What observations to report and record:
  - Nicks (report at once)
  - Cuts (report at once)
  - Bleeding (report at once)
  - Irritation
- When to report observations
- What patient or resident concerns to report at once

BOX 21-1   RULES FOR SHAVING

- Use electric shavers for persons taking anticoagulant drugs. Never use safety razors.
- Protect bed linens. Place a towel under the part being shaved. Or place a towel across the person's chest and shoulders to protect clothing.
- Soften the skin before shaving. Apply a warm, moist washcloth or towel to the face for a few minutes.
- Encourage the person to do as much as safely possible.
- Hold the skin taut as needed.
- Shave in the correct direction:
  - Shaving the face with a safety razor—shave in the direction of hair growth.
  - Shaving the underarms with a safety razor—shave in the direction of hair growth.
  - Shaving the legs with a safety razor—shave up from the ankles. This is against hair growth.
  - Using an electric shaver—shave against the direction of hair growth. If using a rotary-type shaver, move the shaver in small circles over the face. (NOTE: Some state competency tests require shaving in the direction of hair growth. Follow the rules in your state and agency. Also follow the manufacturer's instructions.)
- Do not cut, nick, or irritate the skin.
- Rinse the body part thoroughly.
- Apply direct pressure to nicks or cuts (Chapter 51).
- Report nicks, cuts, or irritation to the nurse at once.

PROMOTING SAFETY AND COMFORT

Shaving

Safety

Safety razors are very sharp. Protect the person and yourself from nicks or cuts. Prevent contact with blood. For an electrical shaver, follow safety measures for electrical equipment (Chapter 12).

Rinse the safety razor often during the procedure. Rinsing removes whiskers and lather. Then wipe the razor. To protect yourself from cuts:

- Place several thicknesses of tissues or paper towels on the overbed table. Do not hold them in your hand.
- Wipe the razor on the tissues or paper towels.

Follow Standard Precautions and the Bloodborne Pathogen Standard. Discard used razor blades and disposable shavers in the sharps container. Do not recap the razor.

Comfort

In some men, the neck area below the jaw is tender and sensitive. Some electric shavers become very warm or hot while in use. Such heat can irritate the skin. Shave tender areas first while the shaver is cool. Then move to the other areas of the face.

Some people apply lotion or after-shave to the skin after shaving. Lotion softens the skin. After-shave closes skin pores. To soften the skin, heat is applied before shaving. It also opens pores.

SHAVING THE PERSON'S FACE WITH A SAFETY RAZOR 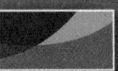 VIDEO

QUALITY OF LIFE

Remember to:
- Knock before entering the person's room.
- Address the person by name.
- Introduce yourself by name and title.

- Explain the procedure to the person before beginning and during the procedure.
- Protect the person's rights during the procedure.
- Handle the person gently during the procedure.

PRE-PROCEDURE

1. Follow *Delegation Guidelines: Shaving*, p. 361. See *Promoting Safety and Comfort: Shaving*.
2. Practice hand hygiene.
3. Collect the following:
   - Wash basin
   - Bath towel
   - Hand towel
   - Washcloth
   - Safety razor
   - Mirror
   - Shaving cream, soap, or lotion
   - Shaving brush
   - After-shave or lotion
   - Tissues or paper towels
   - Paper towels
   - Gloves
4. Arrange paper towels and supplies on the overbed table.
5. Identify the person. Check the ID bracelet against the assignment sheet. Also call the person by name.
6. Provide for privacy.
7. Raise the bed for body mechanics. Bed rails are up if used.

PROCEDURE

8. Fill the wash basin with warm water.
9. Place the basin on the overbed table.
10. Lower the bed rail near you if up.
11. Practice hand hygiene. Put on gloves.
12. Assist the person to semi-Fowler's position if allowed or to the supine position.
13. Adjust lighting to clearly see the person's face.
14. Place the bath towel over the person's chest and shoulders.
15. Adjust the overbed table for easy reach.
16. Tighten the razor blade to the shaver if necessary.
17. Wash the person's face. Do not dry.
18. Wet the washcloth or towel. Wring it out.
19. Apply the washcloth or towel to the face for a few minutes.

20. Apply shaving cream with your hands. Or use a shaving brush to apply lather.
21. Hold the skin taut with one hand.
22. Shave in the direction of hair growth. Use shorter strokes around the chin and lips (Fig. 21-11).
23. Rinse the razor often. Wipe it with tissues or paper towels.
24. Apply direct pressure to any bleeding areas (Chapter 51).
25. Wash off any remaining shaving cream or soap. Pat dry with a towel.
26. Apply after-shave or lotion if requested. (If there are nicks or cuts, do not apply after-shave or lotion.)
27. Remove and discard the towel and gloves. Practice hand hygiene.

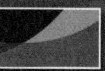

SHAVING THE PERSON'S FACE WITH A SAFETY RAZOR—cont'd | VIDEO |

POST-PROCEDURE

28 Provide for comfort. (See the inside of the front book cover.)
29 Place the signal light within reach.
30 Lower the bed to its lowest position.
31 Raise or lower bed rails. Follow the care plan.
32 Clean, rinse, dry, and return equipment and supplies to their proper place. Discard a razor blade or a disposable razor into the sharps container. Discard other disposable items. Wear gloves.

33 Wipe off the overbed table with paper towels. Discard the paper towels.
34 Unscreen the person.
35 Complete a safety check of the room. (See the inside of the front book cover.)
36 Follow agency policy for dirty linen.
37 Remove and discard the gloves. Practice hand hygiene.
38 Report nicks, cuts, irritation, or bleeding to the nurse at once. Also report and record other observations.

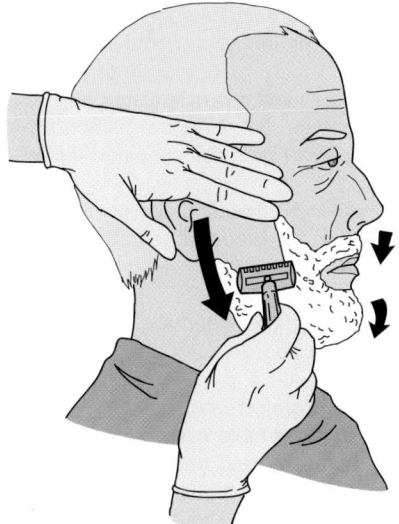

Fig. 21-11 Shave the face in the direction of hair growth. Use longer strokes on the larger areas of the face. Use short strokes around the chin and lips.

Caring for Mustaches and Beards

Mustaches and beards need daily care. Food can collect in the whiskers. So can mouth and nose drainage. Daily washing and combing are needed. Ask the person how to groom his mustache or beard. *Never trim a mustache or beard without the person's consent.*

Shaving Legs and Underarms

Many women shave their legs and underarms. This practice varies among cultures. Some women shave only the lower legs. Others shave to mid-thigh or the entire leg.

To shave the legs and underarms:
• Follow the rules in Box 21-1.
• Collect shaving items with bath items.
• Shave after bathing. The skin is soft at this time.
• Use soap and water, shaving cream, or lotion for the lather. Follow the care plan.
• Use the kidney basin to rinse the razor. Do not use the bath water.

NAIL AND FOOT CARE

Nail and foot care prevents infection, injury, and odors. Hangnails, ingrown nails (nails that grow in at the side), and nails torn away from the skin cause skin breaks. These breaks are portals of entry for microbes. Long or broken nails can scratch skin or snag clothing.

The feet are easily infected and injured. Dirty feet, socks, or stockings harbor microbes and cause odors. Shoes and socks provide a warm, moist environment for microbes to grow. Injuries occur from stubbing toes, stepping on sharp objects, or being stepped on. Shoes that fit poorly cause blisters.

Poor circulation prolongs healing. Diabetes and vascular diseases are common causes of poor circulation. Infections or foot injuries are very serious for older persons and persons with circulatory disorders. Gangrene and amputation are serious complications (Chapter 41). Trimming and clipping toenails can easily cause injuries.

Nails are easier to trim and clean right after soaking or bathing. Use nail clippers to cut fingernails. *Never use scissors.* Use extreme caution to prevent damage to nearby tissues.

Some agencies do not let nursing assistants cut or trim toenails. Follow agency policy.

See *Focus on Long-Term Care and Home Care: Nail and Foot Care*, p. 364.
See *Delegation Guidelines: Nail and Foot Care*, p. 364.
See *Promoting Safety and Comfort: Nail and Foot Care*, p. 364.
See *Teamwork and Time Management: Nail and Foot Care*, p. 364.

FOCUS ON LONG-TERM CARE AND HOME CARE
Nail and Foot Care

Home Care

The feet soak during a tub bath. Or the person can sit on the side of the tub and soak the feet. Make sure the person can step into and out of the tub. Or have the person use a shower bench for getting in and out of the tub (Chapter 20). Otherwise, soak the feet in a basin or a whirlpool foot bath.

If comfortable for the person, he or she can soak the fingers in the sink. Or use a bowl if you do not have a small basin.

DELEGATION GUIDELINES
Nail and Foot Care

To give nail and foot care, you need this information from the nurse and the care plan:
- What water temperature to use
- How long to soak fingernails (usually 5 to 10 minutes)
- How long to soak feet (usually 15 to 20 minutes)
- What observations to report and record:
  - Dry, reddened, irritated, or callused areas
  - Breaks in the skin
  - Corns (Chapter 33) on top of and between the toes
  - Blisters
  - Very thick nails
  - Loose nails
- When to report observations
- What patient or resident concerns to report at once

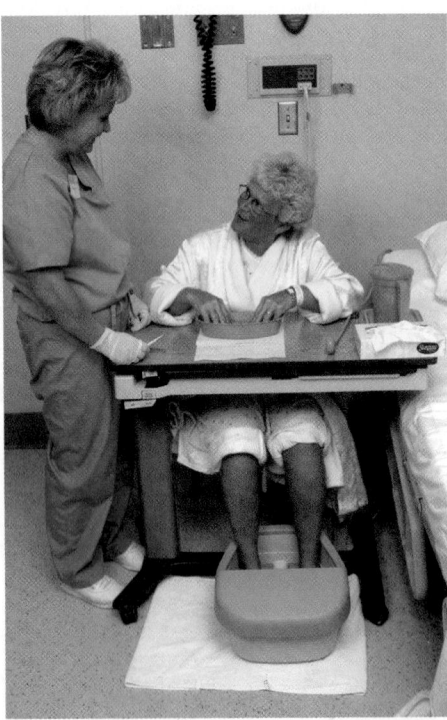

Fig. 21-12 Nail and foot care. The feet soak in a whirlpool foot bath. The fingers soak in a kidney basin.

PROMOTING SAFETY AND COMFORT
Nail and Foot Care

Safety

Remember, some states and agencies do not let nursing assistants cut and trim toenails. The RN or podiatrist (foot [pod] doctor) cuts toenails and provides foot care for the following persons. *You do not cut or trim the toenails for persons who:*
- Have diabetes.
- Have poor circulation to the legs and feet.
- Take drugs that affect blood clotting.
- Have very thick nails or ingrown toenails.

Check between the toes for cracks and sores. These areas are often overlooked. If not treated, a serious infection could occur.

The feet are easily burned. Persons with decreased sensation or circulatory problems may not feel hot temperatures.

After soaking, apply lotion or petroleum jelly to the feet. This can cause slippery feet. Help the person put on non-skid footwear before you transfer the person or let the person walk.

Breaks in the skin and bleeding can occur. Follow Standard Precautions and the Bloodborne Pathogen Standard.

Comfort

Sometimes you just trim the fingernails. Sometimes you just give foot care. When you do both, the person sits at the overbed table (Fig. 21-12). Provide for warmth and comfort.

Promote your own comfort when giving nail and foot care. Sit in front of the overbed table when cleaning and trimming fingernails. For foot care, rest the person's lower leg and foot on your lap. Or position the feet on the floor and kneel on the floor. Lay a towel across your lap or a bath mat on the floor to protect your uniform. Use good body mechanics. However you position yourself, you must support the person's foot and ankle when giving foot care.

TEAMWORK AND TIME MANAGEMENT
Nail and Foot Care

Use your time well when giving nail and foot care. The fingernails soak for 5 to 10 minutes. The feet soak for 15 to 20 minutes. You can make the person's bed or straighten the person's unit while the fingernails and feet soak. Or you could assist with brushing and combing hair. Check your assignment sheet for other ways to meet the person's needs.

GIVING NAIL AND FOOT CARE

QUALITY OF LIFE

Remember to:
- Knock before entering the person's room.
- Address the person by name.
- Introduce yourself by name and title.

- Explain the procedure to the person before beginning and during the procedure.
- Protect the person's rights during the procedure.
- Handle the person gently during the procedure.

PRE-PROCEDURE

1 Follow *Delegation Guidelines: Nail and Foot Care.* See *Promoting Safety and Comfort: Nail and Foot Care.*
2 Practice hand hygiene.
3 Collect the following:
- Wash basin or whirlpool foot bath
- Soap
- Bath thermometer
- Bath towel
- Hand towel
- Washcloth
- Kidney basin
- Nail clippers
- Orangewood stick

- Emery board or nail file
- Lotion for the hands
- Lotion or petroleum jelly for the feet
- Paper towels
- Bath mat
- Gloves

4 Arrange paper towels and other items on the overbed table.
5 Identify the person. Check the ID bracelet against the assignment sheet. Also call the person by name.
6 Provide for privacy.
7 Assist the person to the bedside chair. Remove footwear and socks or stockings. Place the signal light within reach.

PROCEDURE

8 Place the bath mat under the feet.
9 Fill the wash basin or whirlpool foot bath ⅔ (two-thirds) full with water. The nurse tells you what water temperature to use. (Measure water temperature with a bath thermometer. Or test it by dipping your elbow or inner wrist into the basin. Follow agency policy.) Also ask the person to check the water temperature. Adjust the water temperature as needed.
10 Place the basin or foot bath on the bath mat.
11 Put on gloves.
12 Help the person put his or her bare feet into the basin or foot bath. Make sure both feet are completely covered by water.
13 Adjust the overbed table in front of the person.
14 Fill the kidney basin ⅔ (two-thirds) full with water. See step 9 for water temperature.
15 Place the kidney basin on the overbed table.
16 Place the person's fingers into the basin. Position the arms for comfort (see Fig. 21-12).
17 Let the fingers soak for 5 to 10 minutes. Let the feet soak for 15 to 20 minutes. Re-warm water as needed.
18 Remove the kidney basin.
19 Clean under the fingernails with the orangewood stick. Use a towel to wipe the orangewood stick after each nail.
20 Dry the hands and between the fingers thoroughly.

21 Clip fingernails straight across with the nail clippers (Fig. 21-13, p. 366).
22 Shape nails with an emery board or nail file. Nails are smooth with no rough edges. Check each nail for smoothness. File as needed.
23 Push cuticles back with the orangewood stick or a washcloth (Fig. 21-14, p. 366).
24 Apply lotion to the hands. Warm lotion before applying it.
25 Move the overbed table to the side.
26 Lift a foot out of the water. Support the foot and ankle with one hand. With your other hand, wash the foot and between the toes with soap and a washcloth. Return the foot to the water for rinsing. Make sure you rinse between the toes.
27 Repeat step 26 for the other foot.
28 Remove the feet from the basin or foot bath. Dry thoroughly, especially between the toes. Support the foot and ankle as needed.
29 Apply lotion or petroleum jelly to the tops, soles, and heels of the feet. Do not apply between the toes. Warm lotion or petroleum jelly before applying it. Remove excess lotion or petroleum jelly with a towel. Support the foot and ankle as needed.
30 Remove and discard the gloves. Practice hand hygiene.
31 Help the person put on non-skid footwear.

POST-PROCEDURE

32 Provide for comfort. (See the inside of the front book cover.)
33 Place the signal light within reach.
34 Raise or lower bed rails. Follow the care plan.
35 Clean, rinse, dry, and return equipment and supplies to their proper place. Discard disposable items. Wear gloves for this step.

36 Unscreen the person.
37 Complete a safety check of the room. (See the inside of the front book cover.)
38 Follow agency policy for dirty linen.
39 Remove and discard the gloves. Practice hand hygiene.
40 Report and record your observations.

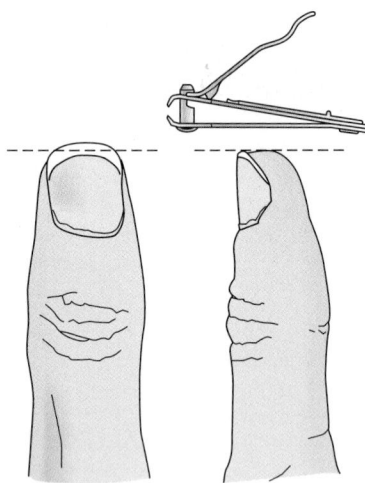

Fig. 21-13 Clip fingernails straight across. Use a nail clipper.

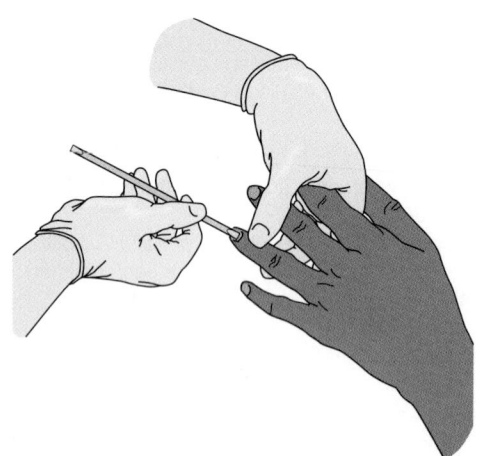

Fig. 21-14 Push the cuticle back with an orangewood stick.

CHANGING CLOTHING AND HOSPITAL GOWNS

Patients and residents change into clean sleepwear or gowns after bathing. Some people wear street clothes during the day. They undress and put on sleepwear at bedtime. Garments are changed whenever wet or soiled.

You may need to assist with changing garments. Follow these rules:

- Provide for privacy. Do not expose the person.
- Encourage the person to do as much as possible.
- Let the person choose what to wear. Make sure the person chooses the right undergarments.
- Make sure garments and footwear are the correct size. Many agencies have gowns and footwear for persons with bariatric needs.
- Remove clothing from the strong or "good" side first. This is often called the *unaffected side*.
- Put clothing on the weak side first. This is often called the *affected side*.

- Support the arm or leg when removing or putting on a garment.
- Move and handle the body gently. Do not force a joint beyond its range of motion or to the point of pain. See Chapter 27.

◼ Dressing and Undressing

Clothing changes are usually necessary on admission and discharge. Some people enter and leave the agency in a gown or pajamas. Most wear street clothes. The rules on this page are followed for dressing and undressing.

See *Focus on Communication: Dressing and Undressing.*

See *Focus on Children and Older Persons: Dressing and Undressing.*

See *Focus on Long-Term Care and Home Care: Dressing and Undressing.*

See *Delegation Guidelines: Dressing and Undressing.*

Text continued on p. 371

FOCUS ON COMMUNICATION

Dressing and Undressing

Make sure you allow for personal choice and independence when assisting with dressing and undressing. You can ask:

- "What would you like to wear today?"
- "There's a concert today in the lounge. Do you want to wear something special?"
- "Can I help you with those buttons?"
- "Would you like me to help you with that zipper?"

FOCUS ON CHILDREN AND OLDER PERSONS

Dressing and Undressing

Older Persons

Persons with dementia may not want to change clothes. Or they may not know how. For example, a person tries to put slacks on over his or her head. Or a person wears the wrong clothes for the season or weather. The Alzheimer's Disease Education and Referral Center (ADEAR) suggests the following:

- Try to assist with dressing at the same time each day. The person learns to expect dressing as a part of his or her daily routine.
- Let the person dress himself or herself to the extent possible. Allow extra time for this task. Do not rush the person.
- Let the person choose what to wear from 2 or 3 outfits. If the person has a favorite outfit, the family may buy several of the same outfit. This makes dressing easier if the person insists on wearing the same outfit.
- Choose comfortable clothes that are easy to get on and off. Garments with elastic waistbands and Velcro closures are examples. The person does not have to handle zippers, buttons, hooks, snaps, or other closures.
- Stack clothes in the order that they are put on. The person sees one item at a time. For example, underpants or undershorts are put on first. The item is on top of the stack.
- Give clear, simple, step-by-step directions.

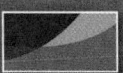 ## UNDRESSING THE PERSON

QUALITY OF LIFE

Remember to:
- Knock before entering the person's room.
- Address the person by name.
- Introduce yourself by name and title.

- Explain the procedure to the person before beginning and during the procedure.
- Protect the person's rights during the procedure.
- Handle the person gently during the procedure.

PRE-PROCEDURE

1 Follow *Delegation Guidelines: Dressing and Undressing*.
2 Practice hand hygiene.
3 Collect a bath blanket and clothing requested by the person.
4 Identify the person. Check the ID bracelet against the assignment sheet. Also call the person by name.
5 Provide for privacy.

6 Raise the bed for body mechanics. Bed rails are up if used.
7 Lower the bed rail on the person's weak side.
8 Position him or her supine.
9 Cover the person with a bath blanket. Fan-fold linens to the foot of the bed.

PROCEDURE

10 Remove garments that open in the back.
  a Raise the head and shoulders. Or turn him or her onto the side away from you.
  b Undo buttons, zippers, ties, or snaps.
  c Bring the sides of the garment to the sides of the person (Fig. 21-15, p. 368). If in a side-lying position, tuck the far side under the person. Fold the near side onto the chest (Fig. 21-16, p. 368).
  d Position the person supine.
  e Slide the garment off the shoulder on the strong side. Remove it from the arm (Fig. 21-17, p. 369).
  f Remove the garment from the weak side.
11 Remove garments that open in the front:
  a Undo buttons, zippers, ties, or snaps.
  b Slide the garment off the shoulder and arm on the strong side.
  c Assist the person to sit up or raise the head and shoulders. Bring the garment over to the weak side (Fig. 21-18, p. 369).
  d Lower the head and shoulders. Remove the garment from the weak side.

  e If you cannot raise the head and shoulders:
    (1) Turn the person toward you. Tuck the removed part under the person.
    (2) Turn him or her onto the side away from you.
    (3) Pull the side of the garment out from under the person. Make sure he or she will not lie on it when supine.
    (4) Return the person to the supine position.
    (5) Remove the garment from the weak side.
12 Remove pullover garments:
  a Undo any buttons, zippers, ties, or snaps.
  b Remove the garment from the strong side.
  c Raise the head and shoulders. Or turn the person onto the side away from you. Bring the garment up to the person's neck (Fig. 21-19, p. 369).
  d Bring the garment over the person's head.
  e Remove the garment from the weak side.
  f Position him or her in the supine position.

Continued

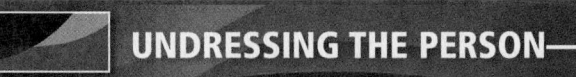 **UNDRESSING THE PERSON—cont'd**

PROCEDURE—cont'd

13 Remove pants or slacks:
   a Remove footwear and socks.
   b Position the person supine.
   c Undo buttons, zippers, ties, snaps, or buckles.
   d Remove the belt.
   e Ask the person to lift the buttocks off the bed. Slide the pants down over the hips and buttocks (Fig. 21-20). Have the person lower the hips and buttocks.

   f If the person cannot raise the hips off the bed:
     (1) Turn the person toward you.
     (2) Slide the pants off the hip and buttock on the strong side (Fig. 21-21).
     (3) Turn the person away from you.
     (4) Slide the pants off the hip and buttock on the weak side (Fig. 21-22).
   g Slide the pants down the legs and over the feet.
14 Dress the person. See procedure: *Dressing the Person*, p. 370.

POST-PROCEDURE

15 Provide for comfort. (See the inside of the front book cover.)
16 Place the signal light within reach.
17 Lower the bed to its lowest position.
18 Raise or lower bed rails. Follow the care plan.
19 Unscreen the person.

20 Complete a safety check of the room. (See the inside of the front book cover.)
21 Follow agency policy for soiled clothing.
22 Practice hand hygiene.
23 Report and record your observations.

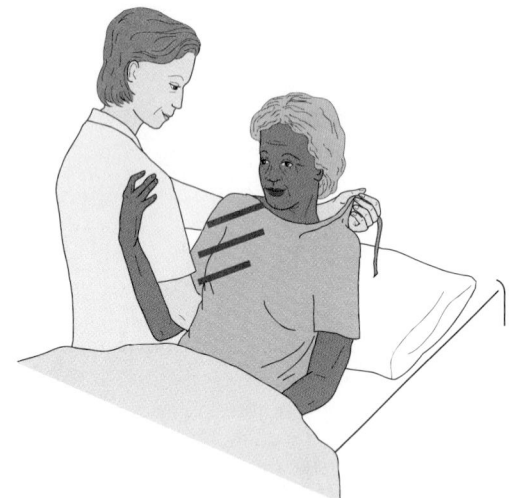

Fig. 21-15 The sides of the garment are brought from the back to the sides of the person. (Note that the "weak" side is *indicated by slash marks.*)

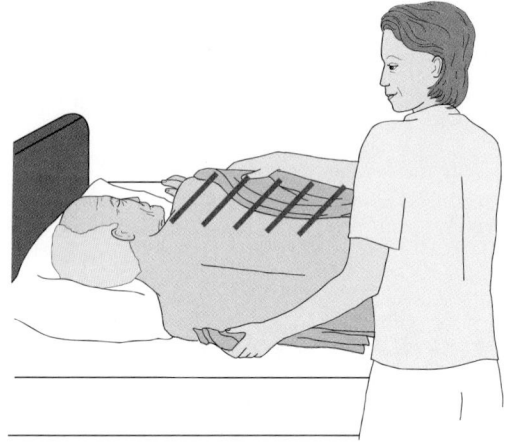

Fig. 21-16 A garment that opens in the back is removed from the person in the side-lying position. The far side of the garment is tucked under the person. The near side is folded onto the person's chest. (Note that the "weak" side is *indicated by slash marks.*)

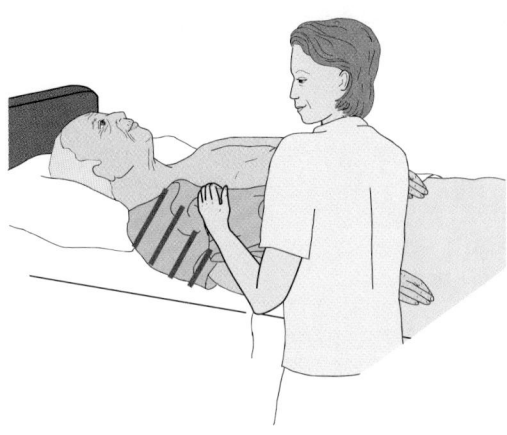

Fig. 21-17 The garment is removed from the strong side first. (Note that the "weak" side is *indicated by slash marks.*)

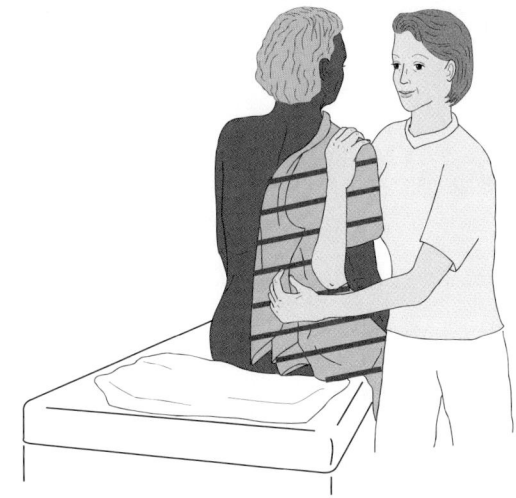

Fig. 21-18 A front-opening garment is removed with the person's head and shoulders raised. The garment is removed from the strong side first. Then it is brought around the back to the weak side. (Note that the "weak" side is *indicated by slash marks.*)

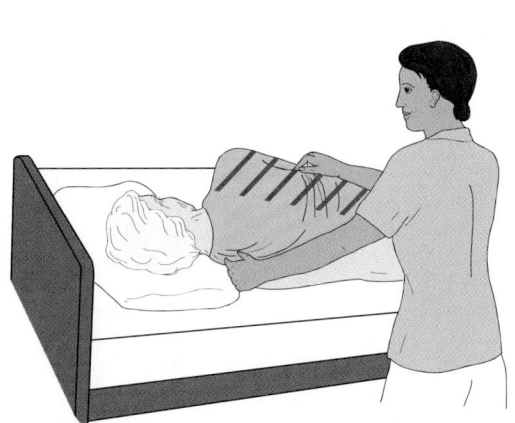

Fig. 21-19 A pullover garment is removed from the strong side first. Then the garment is brought up to the person's neck so that it can be removed from the weak side. (Note that the "weak" side is *indicated by slash marks.*)

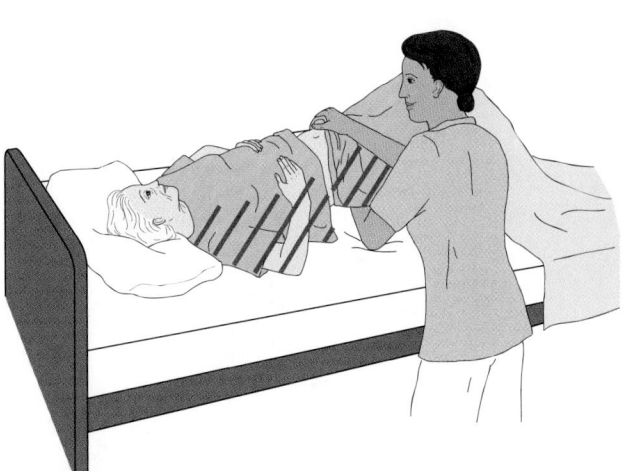

Fig. 21-20 The person lifts the hips and buttocks for removing the pants. The pants are slid down over the hips and buttocks. (Note that the "weak" side is *indicated by slash marks.*)

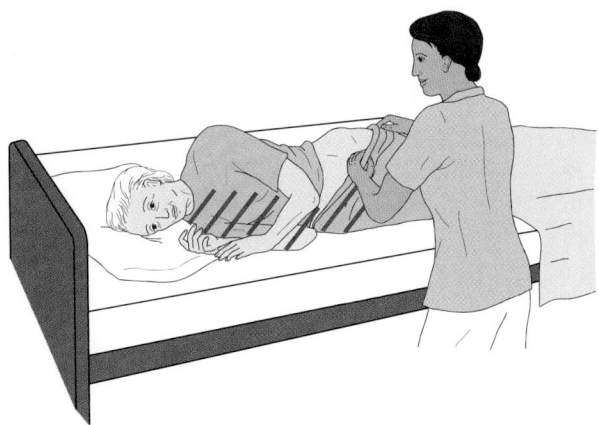

Fig. 21-21 Pants are removed in the side-lying position. They are removed from the strong side first. They are slid over the hip and buttock. (Note that the "weak" side is *indicated by slash marks.*)

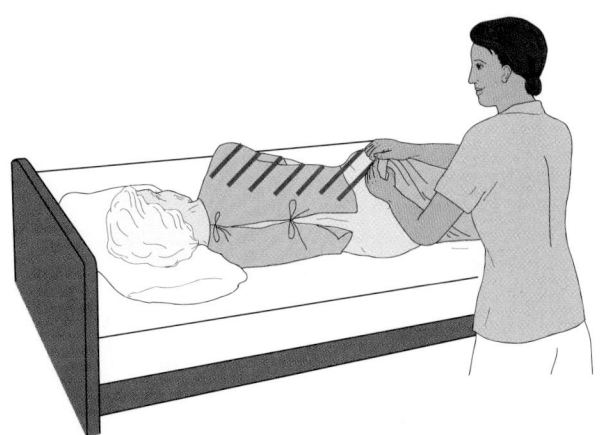

Fig. 21-22 The person is turned onto the strong side. The pants are removed from the weak side. (Note that the "weak" side is *indicated by slash marks.*)

QUALITY OF LIFE

Remember to:
- Knock before entering the person's room.
- Address the person by name.
- Introduce yourself by name and title.

- Explain the procedure to the person before beginning and during the procedure.
- Protect the person's rights during the procedure.
- Handle the person gently during the procedure.

PRE-PROCEDURE

1 Follow *Delegation Guidelines: Dressing and Undressing*, p. 367.
2 Practice hand hygiene.
3 Ask the person what he or she would like to wear.
4 Get a bath blanket and clothing requested by the person.
5 Identify the person. Check the ID bracelet against the assignment sheet. Also call the person by name.
6 Provide for privacy.

7 Raise the bed for body mechanics. Bed rails are up if used.
8 Lower the bed rail (if up) on the person's strong side.
9 Position the person supine.
10 Cover the person with a bath blanket. Fan-fold linens to the foot of the bed.
11 Undress the person. (See procedure: *Undressing the Person*, p. 367.)

PROCEDURE

12 Put on garments that open in the back:
  a Slide the garment onto the arm and shoulder of the weak side.
  b Slide the garment onto the arm and shoulder of the strong side.
  c Raise the person's head and shoulders.
  d Bring the sides to the back.
  e If you cannot raise the person's head and shoulders:
    (1) Turn the person toward you.
    (2) Bring one side of the garment to the person's back (Fig. 21-23, A).
    (3) Turn the person away from you.
    (4) Bring the other side to the person's back (Fig. 21-23, B).
  f Fasten buttons, zippers, snaps, or other closures.
  g Position the person supine.
13 Put on garments that open in the front:
  a Slide the garment onto the arm and shoulder on the weak side.
  b Raise the head and shoulders. Bring the side of the garment around to the back. Lower the person down. Slide the garment onto the arm and shoulder of the strong arm.
  c If the person cannot raise the head and shoulders:
    (1) Turn the person away from you.
    (2) Tuck the garment under him or her.
    (3) Turn the person toward you.
    (4) Pull the garment out from under him or her.
    (5) Turn the person back to the supine position.
    (6) Slide the garment over the arm and shoulder of the strong arm.
  d Fasten buttons, zippers, ties, snaps, or other closures.
14 Put on pullover garments:
  a Position the person supine.
  b Slide the arm and shoulder of the garment onto the weak side.

  c Raise the person's head and shoulders.
  d Bring the neck of the garment over the head.
  e Bring the garment down.
  f Slide the arm and shoulder of the garment onto the strong side.
  g If the person cannot assume a semi-sitting position:
    (1) Turn the person away from you.
    (2) Tuck the garment under the person.
    (3) Turn the person toward you.
    (4) Pull the garment out from under him or her.
    (5) Position the person supine.
    (6) Slide the arm and shoulder of the garment onto the strong side.
  h Fasten buttons, zippers, ties, snaps, or other closures.
15 Put on pants or slacks:
  a Slide the pants over the feet and up the legs.
  b Ask the person to raise the hips and buttocks off the bed.
  c Bring the pants up over the buttocks and hips.
  d Ask the person to lower the hips and buttocks.
  e If the person cannot raise the hips and buttocks:
    (1) Turn the person onto the strong side.
    (2) Pull the pants over the buttock and hip on the weak side.
    (3) Turn the person onto the weak side.
    (4) Pull the pants over the buttock and hip on the strong side.
    (5) Position the person supine.
  f Fasten buttons, zippers, ties, snaps, a belt buckle, or other closures.
16 Put socks and non-skid footwear on the person. Make sure socks are up all the way and smooth.
17 Help the person get out of bed. If the person will stay in bed, cover the person. Remove the bath blanket.

POST-PROCEDURE

18 Provide for comfort. (See the inside of the front book cover.)
19 Place the signal light within reach.
20 Lower the bed to its lowest position.
21 Raise or lower bed rails. Follow the care plan.
22 Unscreen the person.

23 Complete a safety check of the room. (See the inside of the front book cover.)
24 Follow agency policy for soiled clothing.
25 Practice hand hygiene.
26 Report and record your observations.

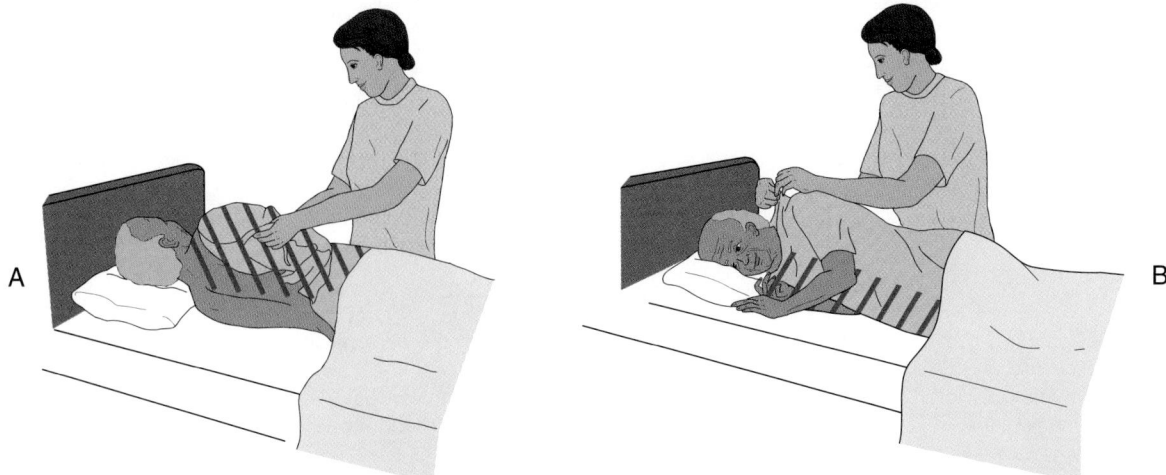

Fig. 21-23 Dressing a person. **A,** The side-lying position can be used to put on garments that open in the back. Turn the person toward you after the garment is put on the arms. The side of the garment is brought to the person's back. **B,** Then turn the person away from you. The other side of the garment is brought to the back and fastened. (Note that the "weak" side is *indicated by slash marks.*)

Changing Hospital Gowns

Many hospital patients wear gowns. So do some nursing center residents. Gowns are usually worn for IV (intravenous) therapy (Chapter 25). Some agencies have special gowns for IV therapy. They open along the sleeve and close with ties, snaps, or Velcro. Sometimes standard gowns are used.

If there is injury or paralysis, remove the gown from the strong arm first. Support the weak arm while removing the gown. Put the clean gown on the weak arm first and then on the strong arm.

See *Delegation Guidelines: Changing Hospital Gowns.*
See *Promoting Safety and Comfort: Changing Hospital Gowns.*

DELEGATION GUIDELINES
Changing Hospital Gowns

Before changing a gown, you need this information from the nurse and the care plan:
- Which arm has the IV
- If the person has an IV pump (see *Promoting Safety and Comfort: Changing Hospital Gowns*)

PROMOTING SAFETY AND COMFORT
Changing Hospital Gowns

Safety

IV pumps control how fast fluid enters a vein. This is called the *flow rate.* If the person has an IV pump and a standard gown, do not use the procedure on p. 372. The arm with the IV is not put through the sleeve.

Changing the gown can cause the IV flow rate to change. Always ask the nurse to check the flow rate after you change a gown.

Do not disconnect or remove any part of the IV set-up.

Comfort

Some hospital gowns are secured with ties at the upper back. The back and buttocks are exposed when the person stands. Cover the person for warmth and privacy. A robe or second gown may be used. Other gowns overlap in the back and tie at the side. These gowns provide more privacy. Because they tie at the side, uncomfortable bows and knots at the back are avoided.

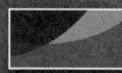

CHANGING THE GOWN OF THE PERSON WITH AN IV

QUALITY OF LIFE

Remember to:
- Knock before entering the person's room.
- Address the person by name.
- Introduce yourself by name and title.

- Explain the procedure to the person before beginning and during the procedure.
- Protect the person's rights during the procedure.
- Handle the person gently during the procedure.

PRE-PROCEDURE

1 Follow *Delegation Guidelines: Changing Hospital Gowns,* p. 371. See *Promoting Safety and Comfort: Changing Hospital Gowns,* p. 371.
2 Practice hand hygiene.
3 Get a clean gown and a bath blanket.

4 Identify the person. Check the ID bracelet against the assignment sheet. Also, call the person by name.
5 Provide for privacy.
6 Raise the bed for body mechanics. Bed rails are up if used.

PROCEDURE

7 Lower the bed rail near you (if up).
8 Cover the person with a bath blanket. Fan-fold linens to the foot of the bed.
9 Untie the gown. Free parts that the person is lying on.
10 Remove the gown from the arm with *no IV.*
11 Gather up the sleeve of the arm *with the IV.* Slide it over the IV site and tubing. Remove the arm and hand from the sleeve (Fig. 21-24, A).
12 Keep the sleeve gathered. Slide your arm along the tubing to the bag (Fig. 21-24, B).
13 Remove the bag from the pole. Slide the bag and tubing through the sleeve (Fig. 21-24, C). Do not pull on the tubing. Keep the bag above the person.

14 Hang the IV bag on the pole.
15 Gather the sleeve of the clean gown that will go on the arm with the IV infusion.
16 Remove the bag from the pole. Slip the sleeve over the bag at the shoulder part of the gown (Fig. 21-24, D). Hang the bag.
17 Slide the gathered sleeve over the tubing, hand, arm, and IV site. Then slide it onto the shoulder.
18 Put the other side of the gown on the person. Fasten the gown.
19 Cover the person. Remove the bath blanket.

POST-PROCEDURE

20 Provide for comfort. (See the inside of the front book cover.)
21 Place the signal light within reach.
22 Lower the bed to its lowest position.
23 Raise or lower bed rails. Follow the care plan.
24 Unscreen the person.

25 Complete a safety check of the room. (See the inside of the front book cover.)
26 Follow agency policy for dirty linen.
27 Practice hand hygiene.
28 Ask the nurse to check the flow rate.
29 Report and record your observations.

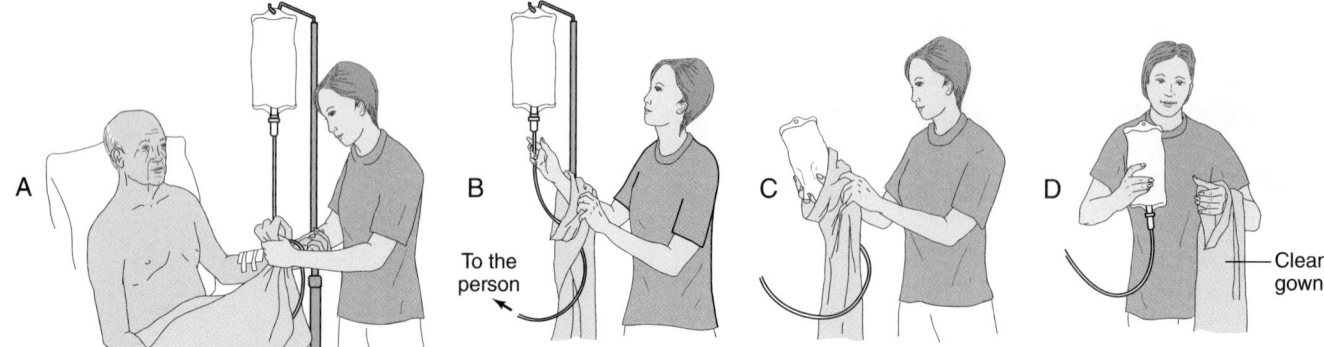

Fig. 21-24 Changing a gown. **A,** The gown is removed from the arm with no IV. The sleeve on the arm with the IV is gathered up, slipped over the IV site and tubing, and removed from the arm and hand. **B,** The gathered sleeve is slipped along the IV tubing to the bag. **C,** The IV bag is removed from the pole and passed through the sleeve. **D,** The gathered sleeve of the clean gown is slipped over the IV bag at the shoulder part of the gown.

FOCUS ON PRIDE

The Person, Family, and Yourself

Personal and Professional Responsibility

Grooming promotes comfort. Self-esteem and body image improve when the person likes how he or she looks. Clean hair, nails, and garments all help mental well-being. So does a clean-shaven face or a well-groomed beard or mustache.

Your attitude is reflected in the way you give care. To show that you value the person's self-esteem and comfort:

- Be pleasant. Talk with the person.
- Ask about the person's preferences. Allow personal choice.
- Avoid seeming rushed. Let the person know that you have time for him or her.
- Avoid thinking that care measures are tasks to be completed. You are caring for a *person*. Show that you care about the person's needs and feelings.
- Do a good job. Be thorough and careful.
- Clean up after yourself. Leave the person's setting neat and orderly.

Also, care for your own appearance. Patients, residents, and family members notice when others are not well groomed. If you are not groomed well, they may question the quality of care you provide. Have a professional appearance.

Rights and Respect

People have different grooming preferences. Ask what the person prefers. For example, ask what he or she would like to wear. Or ask how to style the person's hair. Follow the person's grooming routines whenever possible.

You may not like the person's hairstyle or clothing choices. Or you may not agree with the person's choice of personal care products. Do not judge the person by your own standards or impose your choices on the person. Do not make the person feel badly about his or her choices. Respect the person's right to choose. Assist with grooming in a way that improves the person's self-esteem.

Independence and Social Interaction

Sometimes family members want to help with grooming. For example, they want to style the person's hair. Or they want to apply lotion to the person's hands and feet.

With the person's permission, allow family members to assist with grooming measures as much as safely possible. This promotes social interaction. It also involves the family in the person's care.

Delegation and Teamwork

Grooming takes time. You, the person, the nurse, and other team members work together to plan and organize care. For example, Mr. Horn had a stroke and is hospitalized. He needs help with grooming. He eats breakfast at 0800, has speech therapy at 0930, has physical therapy at 1030, and his wife visits during lunchtime. Mr. Horn prefers to comb his hair, shave, and change his clothes after breakfast but before his wife visits. He also likes to rest after physical therapy. You plan to assist Mr. Horn with grooming after breakfast and before speech therapy.

Grooming is important. You must not neglect grooming because of a busy schedule. Plan ahead to meet the person's needs at a time best for the person and the team.

Ethics and Laws

Patients and residents have the right to be free from mistreatment and restraint (Chapter 2). The following is a case where a nurse did not follow these ethical principles:

A nurse told a patient that she was going to cut his hair and trim his beard. The patient repeatedly stated that he did not want a haircut or his beard trimmed. The patient protested and resisted the nurse's actions. She continued her actions while two other staff members restrained the patient.

The patient reported the incident to his social worker. An internal investigation was conducted.

The nurse lost her job. The United States Court of Appeals agreed that the nurse's termination was warranted because of:

- *The nature and seriousness of the offense*
- *The restraint of the patient after he repeatedly objected*

(L. Taylor v Department of Veterans Affairs, 2006.)

Never force a care measure on a person. If a person resists or refuses care, stop. Do not proceed. Politely ask the person for the reason. Tell the nurse. You, the nurse, and the person can discuss a solution.

Special care measures are needed for persons with confusion or dementia who resist care. See Chapter 46. Patience, kindness, and problem solving are needed. A co-worker or family member may need to give care. Or care may need to be given at a different time. Provide care in a way that protects the person's rights and shows dignity and respect.

REVIEW QUESTIONS

Circle the BEST answer.

1 A person has alopecia. This is
   a Excessive body hair
   b Dry, white flakes from the scalp
   c An infestation with lice
   d Hair loss

2 Which prevents hair from matting and tangling?
   a Bedrest
   b Daily brushing and combing
   c Daily shampooing
   d Cutting hair

3 A person's hair is *not* matted or tangled. When brushing hair, start at
   a The forehead and brush backward
   b The hair ends
   c The scalp
   d The back of the neck and brush forward

4 Brushing keeps the hair
   a Soft and shiny
   b Clean
   c Free of lice
   d Long

5 A person requests a shampoo. You should
   a Shampoo the hair during the person's shower
   b Shampoo hair at the sink
   c Shampoo the person in bed
   d Follow the care plan

6 When shaving a person's face, do the following *except*
   a Practice Standard Precautions
   b Follow the Bloodborne Pathogen Standard
   c Shave in the direction of hair growth
   d Shave when the skin is dry

7 A person is nicked during shaving. Your first action is to
   a Wash your hands
   b Apply direct pressure
   c Tell the nurse
   d Apply a bandage

8 Fingernails are cut with
   a An emery board
   b Scissors
   c A nail file
   d Nail clippers

9 Fingernails are trimmed
   a Before soaking
   b After soaking
   c Before trimming toenails
   d After trimming toenails

Circle T if the statement is TRUE or F if it is FALSE.

10 T F Mr. Polk has a mustache and beard. To promote comfort, you can shave his beard and mustache.

11 T F Clothing is removed from the strong side first.

12 T F The person chooses what to wear.

13 T F A person has poor circulation in the legs and feet. You can cut and trim the person's toenails.

14 T F You can cut matted hair.

Answers to these questions are on p. 833.

Urinary Elimination 22

OBJECTIVES

- Define the key terms and key abbreviations listed in this chapter.
- Describe normal urine.
- Describe the rules for normal urinary elimination.
- Identify the observations to report to the nurse.
- Describe urinary incontinence and the care required.
- Describe straight, indwelling, and condom catheters.

- Explain why catheters are used.
- Explain how to care for persons with catheters.
- Describe the bladder training methods.
- Perform the procedures described in this chapter.
- Explain how to promote PRIDE in the person, the family, and yourself.

KEY TERMS

catheter A tube used to drain or inject fluid through a body opening

catheterization The process of inserting a catheter

dysuria Painful or difficult *(dys)* urination *(uria)*

Foley catheter See "indwelling catheter"

functional incontinence The person has bladder control but cannot use the toilet in time

hematuria Blood *(hemat)* in the urine *(uria)*

indwelling catheter A catheter left in the bladder so urine drains constantly into a drainage bag; retention or Foley catheter

micturition See "urination"

mixed incontinence The combination of stress incontinence and urge incontinence

nocturia Frequent urination *(uria)* at night *(noct)*

oliguria Scant amount *(olig)* of urine *(uria)*; less than 500 mL in 24 hours

overflow incontinence Small amounts of urine leak from a full bladder

polyuria Abnormally large amounts *(poly)* of urine *(uria)*

reflex incontinence Urine is lost at predictable intervals when the bladder is full

retention catheter See "indwelling catheter"

straight catheter A catheter that drains the bladder and then is removed

stress incontinence When urine leaks during exercise and certain movements that cause pressure on the bladder

transient incontinence Temporary or occasional incontinence that is reversed when the cause is treated

urge incontinence The loss of urine in response to a sudden, urgent need to void; the person cannot get to a toilet in time

urinary frequency Voiding at frequent intervals

urinary incontinence The involuntary loss or leakage of urine

urinary retention The inability to void

urinary urgency The need to void at once

urination The process of emptying urine from the bladder; micturition or voiding

voiding See "urination"

KEY ABBREVIATIONS

C	Centigrade	IV	Intravenous
CMS	Centers for Medicare & Medicaid Services	mL	Milliliter
F	Fahrenheit	UTI	Urinary tract infection
ID	Identification		

BODY STRUCTURE AND FUNCTION REVIEW: THE URINARY SYSTEM

The two *kidneys* (Fig. 22-1) lie in the upper abdomen against the muscles of the back on each side of the spine. Blood passes through the two kidneys. *Urine* is formed in the kidneys.

Urine consists of wastes and excess fluids filtered out of the blood. Urine flows through the two *ureters* to the *urinary bladder*. Urine is stored in the bladder. The *urethra* connects the bladder to the outside of the body. Urine passes from the body through the urethra.

See Chapter 9 for more information.

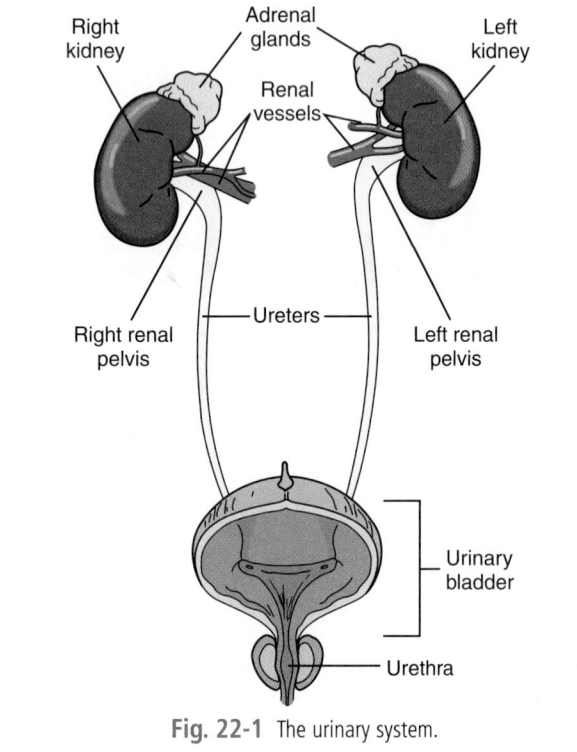

Right kidney
Adrenal glands
Left kidney
Renal vessels
Right renal pelvis
Ureters
Left renal pelvis
Urinary bladder
Urethra

Fig. 22-1 The urinary system.

BOX 22-1 RULES FOR NORMAL URINATION

- Practice medical asepsis.
- Follow Standard Precautions and the Bloodborne Pathogen Standard.
- Provide fluids as the nurse and care plan direct.
- Follow the person's voiding routines and habits. Check with the nurse and the care plan.
- Help the person to the bathroom when the request is made. Or provide the commode, bedpan, or urinal. The need to void may be urgent.
- Help the person assume a normal position for voiding if possible. Women sit or squat. Men stand.
- Warm the bedpan or urinal.
- Cover the person for warmth and privacy.
- Provide for privacy. Pull the curtain around the bed, close room and bathroom doors, and close window coverings. Leave the room if the person can be alone.
- Tell the person that running water, flushing the toilet, or playing music can mask voiding sounds. Voiding with others close by embarrasses some people.
- Stay nearby if the person is weak or unsteady.
- Place the signal light and toilet tissue within reach.
- Allow enough time. Do not rush the person.
- Promote relaxation. Some people like to read.
- Run water in a sink if the person cannot start the stream. Or place the person's fingers in warm water.
- Provide perineal care as needed (Chapter 20).
- Assist with hand washing after voiding. Provide a wash basin, soap, washcloth, and towel.
- Assist the person to the bathroom or offer the bedpan, urinal, or commode at regular times. Some people are embarrassed or are too weak to ask for help.

Eliminating waste is a physical need. The respiratory, digestive, integumentary, and urinary systems remove body wastes. The digestive system rids the body of solid wastes. The lungs remove carbon dioxide. Sweat contains water and other substances. Blood contains waste products from body cells burning food for energy. The urinary system removes waste products from the blood. It also maintains the body's water balance.

See *Body Structure and Function Review: The Urinary System.*

NORMAL URINATION

The healthy adult produces about 1500 mL (milliliters) or 3 pints of urine a day. Many factors affect urine production. They include age, disease, the amount and kinds of fluid ingested, dietary salt, body temperature, perspiration (sweating), and some drugs. Some substances increase urine production—coffee, tea, alcohol, and some drugs. A diet high in salt causes the body to retain water. So do some drugs. When water is retained, less urine is produced.

Urination, micturition, and *voiding mean the process of emptying urine from the bladder.* The amount of fluid intake, habits, and available toilet facilities affect frequency. So do activity, work, and illness. People usually void at bedtime, after sleep, and before meals. Some people void every 2 to 3 hours. The need to void at night disturbs sleep.

Some persons need help getting to the bathroom. Others use bedpans, urinals, or commodes. Follow the rules in Box 22-1 and the person's care plan.

See *Focus on Communication: Normal Urination.*
See *Focus on Children and Older Persons: Normal Urination.*
See *Teamwork and Time Management: Normal Urination.*

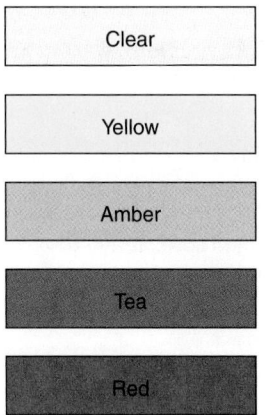

Fig. 22-2 Color chart for urine.

Observations

Normal urine is pale yellow, straw-colored, or amber (Fig. 22-2). It is clear with no particles. A faint odor is normal. Observe urine for color, clarity, odor, amount, particles, and blood.

Some foods affect urine color. Red food dyes, beets, blackberries, and rhubarb cause red-colored urine. Carrots and sweet potatoes cause bright yellow urine. Certain drugs change urine color. Asparagus causes a urine odor.

Ask the nurse to observe urine that looks or smells abnormal. Report complaints of urgency, burning on urination, or painful or difficult urination. Also report the problems in Table 22-1. The nurse uses the information for the nursing process.

TABLE 22-1	URINARY ELIMINATION PROBLEMS	
Problem	**Definition**	**Causes**
Dysuria	*Painful or difficult* (dys) *urination* (uria)	Urinary tract infection (UTI), trauma, urinary tract obstruction
Hematuria	*Blood* (hemat) *in the urine* (uria)	Kidney disease, UTI, trauma
Nocturia	*Frequent urination* (uria) *at night* (noct)	Excess fluid intake, kidney disease, prostate disease
Oliguria	*Scant amount* (olig) *of urine* (uria); *less than 500 mL in 24 hours*	Poor fluid intake, shock, burns, kidney disease, heart failure
Polyuria	*Abnormally large amounts* (poly) *of urine* (uria)	Drugs, excess fluid intake, diabetes, hormone imbalance
Urinary frequency	*Voiding at frequent intervals*	Excess fluid intake, UTI, pressure on the bladder, drugs
Urinary incontinence	*The involuntary loss or leakage of urine*	Trauma, disease, UTI, reproductive or urinary tract surgeries, aging, fecal impaction, constipation, not getting to the bathroom in time
Urinary retention	*The inability to void*	Prostate enlargement, nerve damage, UTI, drugs, surgery, kidney stones, constipation, trauma
Urinary urgency	*The need to void at once*	UTI, fear of incontinence, full bladder, stress

Bedpans

Bedpans are used by persons who cannot be out of bed. Women use bedpans for voiding and bowel movements. Men use them for bowel movements.

The *standard bedpan* is shown in Figure 22-3. The wide rim is placed under the buttocks. A *fracture pan* has a thin rim. It is only about ½-inch deep at one end (see Fig. 22-3). The smaller end is placed under the buttocks (Fig. 22-4). Fracture pans are used:

- By persons with casts
- By persons in traction
- By persons with limited back motion
- After spinal cord injury or surgery
- After a hip fracture
- After hip replacement surgery

Like a fracture pan, the small end of a bariatric bedpan is placed under the buttocks (Fig. 22-5). Some have a weight capacity of 1200 pounds.

See *Delegation Guidelines: Bedpans.*
See *Promoting Safety and Comfort: Bedpans.*

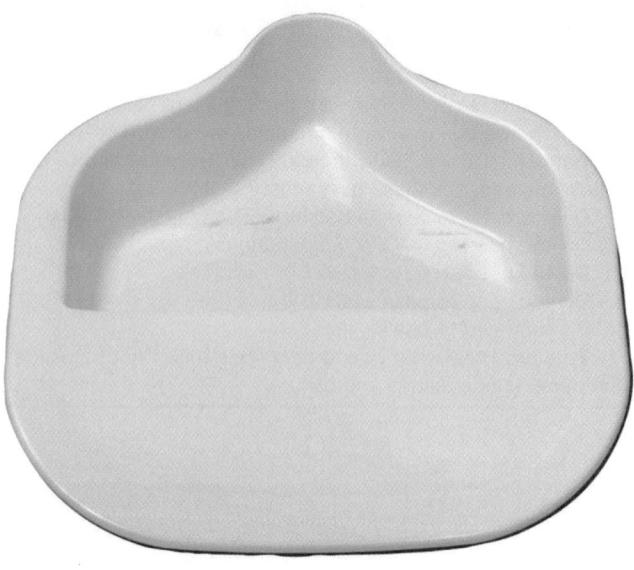

Fig. 22-5 Bariatric bedpan.

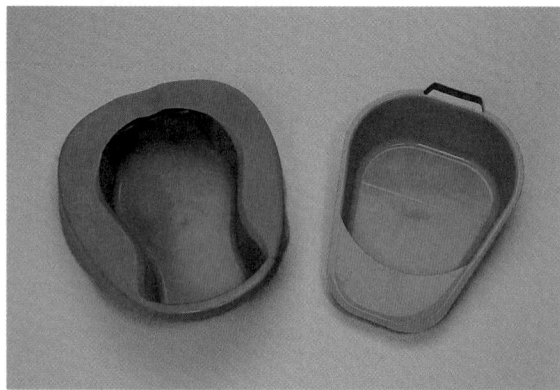

Fig. 22-3 Standard bedpan *(left)* and the fracture pan *(right).*

DELEGATION GUIDELINES

Bedpans

To assist with a bedpan, you need this information from the nurse and the care plan:

- What bedpan to use—standard bedpan, fracture pan, bariatric bedpan
- Position or activity limits
- If you can leave the room or if you need to stay with the person
- If the nurse needs to observe the results before disposing of the contents
- What observations to report and record:
  - Urine color, clarity, and odor
  - Amount
  - Presence of particles
  - Blood in the urine
  - Cloudy urine
  - Complaints of urgency, burning, dysuria, or other problems (see Table 22-1, p. 377)
  - For bowel movements, see Chapter 23
- When to report observations
- What patient or resident concerns to report at once

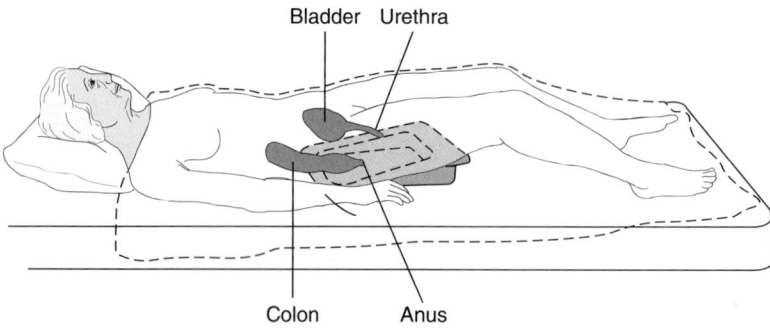

Bladder   Urethra

Colon   Anus

Fig. 22-4 A person positioned on a fracture pan. The small end is under the buttocks.

PROMOTING SAFETY AND COMFORT
Bedpans

Safety

Urine and bowel movements may contain blood and microbes. Microbes can live and grow in dirty bedpans. Follow Standard Precautions and the Bloodborne Pathogen Standard when handling bedpans and their contents. Thoroughly clean and disinfect bedpans after use.

Remember to raise the bed as needed for good body mechanics. Lower the bed before leaving the room. Raise or lower the bed rails according to the care plan.

Comfort

Some older persons have fragile bones from osteoporosis or painful joints from arthritis (Chapter 41). For them, fracture pans provide more comfort than standard bedpans.

Most bedpans are made of plastic. Some are made of metal. Metal bedpans are often cold. Warm them with warm water and then dry them before use.

The person must not sit on a bedpan for a long time. Bedpans are uncomfortable. And they can lead to pressure ulcers from prolonged pressure (Chapter 34).

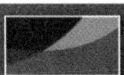 **GIVING THE BEDPAN**

QUALITY OF LIFE

Remember to:
- Knock before entering the person's room.
- Address the person by name.
- Introduce yourself by name and title.

- Explain the procedure to the person before beginning and during the procedure.
- Protect the person's rights during the procedure.
- Handle the person gently during the procedure.

PRE-PROCEDURE

1 Follow *Delegation Guidelines: Bedpans.* See *Promoting Safety and Comfort: Bedpans.*
2 Provide for privacy.
3 Practice hand hygiene.
4 Put on gloves.

5 Collect the following:
- Bedpan
- Bedpan cover
- Toilet tissue
- Waterproof pad (if required by the agency)
6 Arrange equipment on the chair or bed.

PROCEDURE

7 Lower the bed rail near you if up.
8 Lower the head of the bed. Position the person supine. Or raise the head of the bed slightly for the person's comfort.
9 Fold the top linens and gown out of the way. Keep the lower body covered.
10 Ask the person to flex the knees and raise the buttocks by pushing against the mattress with his or her feet.
11 Slide your hand under the lower back. Help raise the buttocks. If using a waterproof pad, place it under the person's buttocks.
12 Slide the bedpan under the person (Fig. 22-6, p. 380).
13 If the person cannot assist in getting on the bedpan:
  a Place the waterproof pad under the person's buttocks if using one.
  b Turn the person onto the side away from you.
  c Place the bedpan firmly against the buttocks (Fig. 22-7, A, p. 381).
  d Push the bedpan down and toward the person (Fig. 22-7, B, p. 381).
  e Hold the bedpan securely. Turn the person onto his or her back.
  f Make sure the bedpan is centered under the person.
14 Cover the person.

15 Raise the head of the bed so the person is in a sitting position (Fowler's position) if the person uses a standard bedpan. (NOTE: Some state competency tests require that you remove gloves and wash your hands before raising the head of the bed.)
16 Make sure the person is correctly positioned on the bedpan (Fig. 22-8, p. 381).
17 Raise the bed rail if used.
18 Place the toilet tissue and signal light within reach. (NOTE: Some state competency tests require that you ask the person to use hand wipes to clean the hands after wiping with toilet tissue.)
19 Ask the person to signal when done or when help is needed.
20 Remove and discard the gloves. Practice hand hygiene.
21 Leave the room and close the door.
22 Return when the person signals. Or check on the person every 5 minutes. Knock before entering.
23 Practice hand hygiene. Put on gloves.
24 Raise the bed for body mechanics. Lower the bed rail (if used) and lower the head of the bed.
25 Ask the person to raise the buttocks. Remove the bedpan. Or hold the bedpan and turn him or her onto the side away from you.

Continued

GIVING THE BEDPAN—cont'd

VIDEO | VIDEO CLIP | NNAAP® Skill

PROCEDURE—cont'd

26 Clean the genital area if the person cannot do so. Clean from front (urethra) to back (anus) with toilet tissue. Use fresh tissue for each wipe. Provide perineal care if needed. Remove and discard the waterproof pad if using one.

27 Cover the bedpan. Take it to the bathroom. Raise the bed rail (if used) before leaving the bedside.

28 Note the color, amount, and character of urine or feces.

29 Empty the bedpan contents into the toilet and flush.

30 Rinse the bedpan. Pour the rinse into the toilet and flush.

31 Clean the bedpan with a disinfectant.

32 Remove and discard soiled gloves. Practice hand hygiene and put on clean gloves.

33 Return the bedpan and clean cover to the bedside stand.

34 Help the person with hand washing. (Wear gloves for this step.)

35 Remove and discard the gloves. Practice hand hygiene.

POST-PROCEDURE

36 Provide for comfort. (See the inside of the front book cover.)

37 Place the signal light within reach.

38 Lower the bed to its lowest position.

39 Raise or lower bed rails. Follow the care plan.

40 Unscreen the person.

41 Complete a safety check of the room. (See the inside of the front book cover.)

42 Follow agency policy for soiled linen.

43 Practice hand hygiene.

44 Report and record your observations.

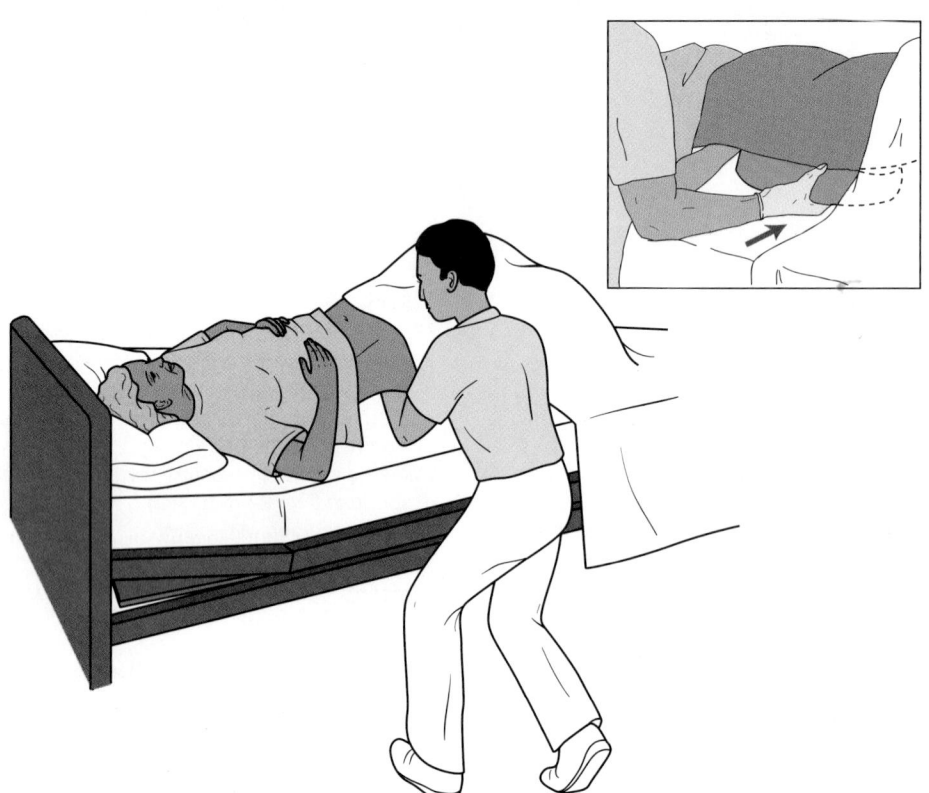

Fig. 22-6 The person raises the buttocks off the bed with help. The bedpan is slid under the person.

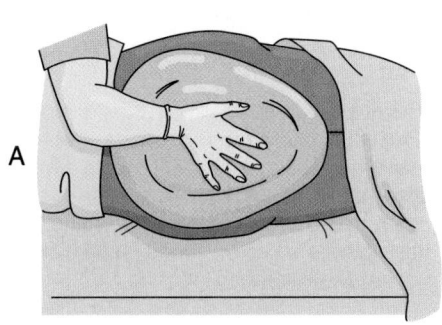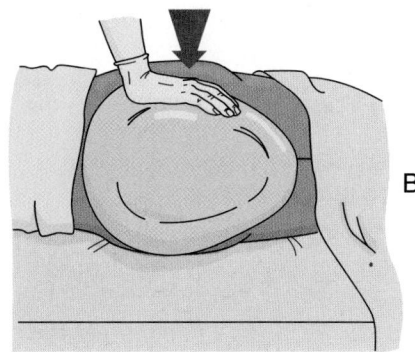

Fig. 22-7 Giving a bedpan. **A,** Position the person on one side. Place the bedpan firmly against the buttocks. **B,** Push downward on the bedpan and toward the person.

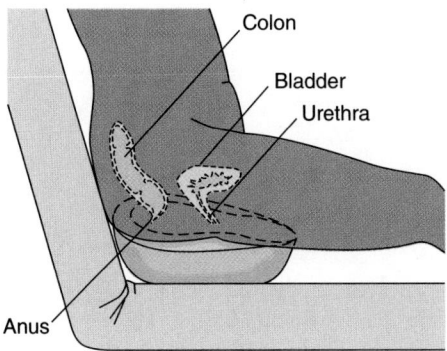

Fig. 22-8 The person is positioned on the bedpan so the urethra and anus are directly over the opening.

Urinals

Men use urinals to void (Fig. 22-9). Plastic urinals have caps and hook-type handles. The urinal hooks to the bed rail within the man's reach. He stands to use the urinal if possible. Or he sits on the side of the bed or lies in bed to use it. Some men need support when standing. You may have to place and hold the urinal for some men.

After voiding, the urinal cap is closed. This prevents urine spills. Remind men to hang urinals on bed rails and to signal after using them. Remind them not to place urinals on overbed tables and bedside stands. Overbed tables are used for eating and as a work surface. Bedside stands are used for personal items and supplies. These surfaces must not be contaminated with urine.

Some beds may not have bed rails. Follow agency policy for where to place urinals.

See *Focus on Communication: Urinals.*
See *Delegation Guidelines: Urinals,* p. 382.
See *Promoting Safety and Comfort: Urinals,* p. 382.

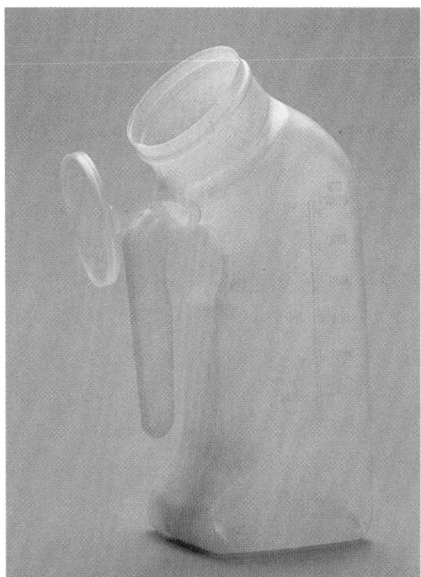

Fig. 22-9 Male urinal.

FOCUS ON COMMUNICATION

Urinals

Some men cannot use a urinal on their own. You may need to assist them. You may need to stay with the person. For the person's comfort, explain why you must help him. You can say:

- "Mr. Turner, I'll help you use your urinal. I need to stay with you to make sure you don't fall."
- "Mr. Gomez, I'll help you place and remove your urinal so it doesn't spill."

DELEGATION GUIDELINES
Urinals

To assist with urinals, you need this information from the nurse and the care plan:

- How the urinal is used—standing, sitting, or lying in bed
- If help is needed to place or hold the urinal
- If the man needs support to stand (if yes, how many staff are needed)
- If you can leave the room or if you need to stay with the person
- If the nurse needs to observe the urine before its disposal
- What observations to report and record (see *Delegation Guidelines: Bedpans*, p. 378)
- When to report observations
- What patient or resident concerns to report at once

PROMOTING SAFETY AND COMFORT
Urinals

Safety

Urine may contain microbes and blood. Follow Standard Precautions and the Bloodborne Pathogen Standard when handling urinals and their contents. Empty them promptly to prevent odors and the spread of microbes. A filled urinal spills easily, causing safety hazards. Also, it is an unpleasant sight and a source of odor. Urinals are cleaned and disinfected like bedpans.

Comfort

You may have to place the urinal for some men. This means placing the penis in the urinal. This may embarrass both the person and you. Act in a professional manner at all times.

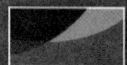 **GIVING THE URINAL**   VIDEO

QUALITY OF LIFE

Remember to:
- Knock before entering the person's room.
- Address the person by name.
- Introduce yourself by name and title.

- Explain the procedure to the person before beginning and during the procedure.
- Protect the person's rights during the procedure.
- Handle the person gently during the procedure.

PRE-PROCEDURE

1 Follow *Delegation Guidelines: Urinals.* See *Promoting Safety and Comfort: Urinals.*
2 Provide for privacy.
3 Determine if the man will stand, sit, or lie in bed.
4 Practice hand hygiene.
5 Put on gloves.
6 Collect the following:
   - Urinal
   - Non-skid footwear if the man will stand to void

PROCEDURE

7 Give him the urinal if he is in bed. Remind him to tilt the bottom down to prevent spills.
8 If he is going to stand:
   a Help him sit on the side of the bed.
   b Put non-skid footwear on him.
   c Help him stand. Provide support if he is unsteady.
   d Give him the urinal.
9 Position the urinal if necessary. Place his penis in the urinal if he cannot do so.
10 Place the signal light within reach. Ask him to signal when done or when he needs help.
11 Provide for privacy.
12 Remove and discard the gloves. Practice hand hygiene.
13 Leave the room and close the door.
14 Return when he signals for you. Or check on him every 5 minutes. Knock before entering.
15 Practice hand hygiene. Put on gloves.
16 Close the cap on the urinal. Take it to the bathroom.
17 Note the color, amount, and clarity of urine.
18 Empty the urinal into the toilet and flush.
19 Rinse the urinal with cold water. Pour rinse into the toilet and flush.
20 Clean the urinal with a disinfectant.
21 Return the urinal to its proper place.
22 Remove and discard soiled gloves. Practice hand hygiene and put on clean gloves.
23 Assist with hand washing.
24 Remove and discard the gloves. Practice hand hygiene.

POST-PROCEDURE

25 Provide for comfort. (See the inside of the front book cover.)
26 Place the signal light within reach.
27 Raise or lower bed rails. Follow the care plan.
28 Unscreen him.
29 Complete a safety check of the room. (See the inside of the front book cover.)
30 Follow agency policy for soiled linen.
31 Practice hand hygiene.
32 Report and record your observations.

Commodes

A commode is a chair or wheelchair with an opening for a container (Fig. 22-10). Persons unable to walk to the bathroom often use commodes. The commode allows a normal position for elimination. The commode arms and back provide support and help prevent falls.

Some commodes are wheeled into bathrooms and placed over toilets. They are useful for persons who need support when sitting. The container is removed if the commode is used with the toilet. Wheels are locked after the commode is positioned over the toilet.

See *Delegation Guidelines: Commodes.*
See *Promoting Safety and Comfort: Commodes.*

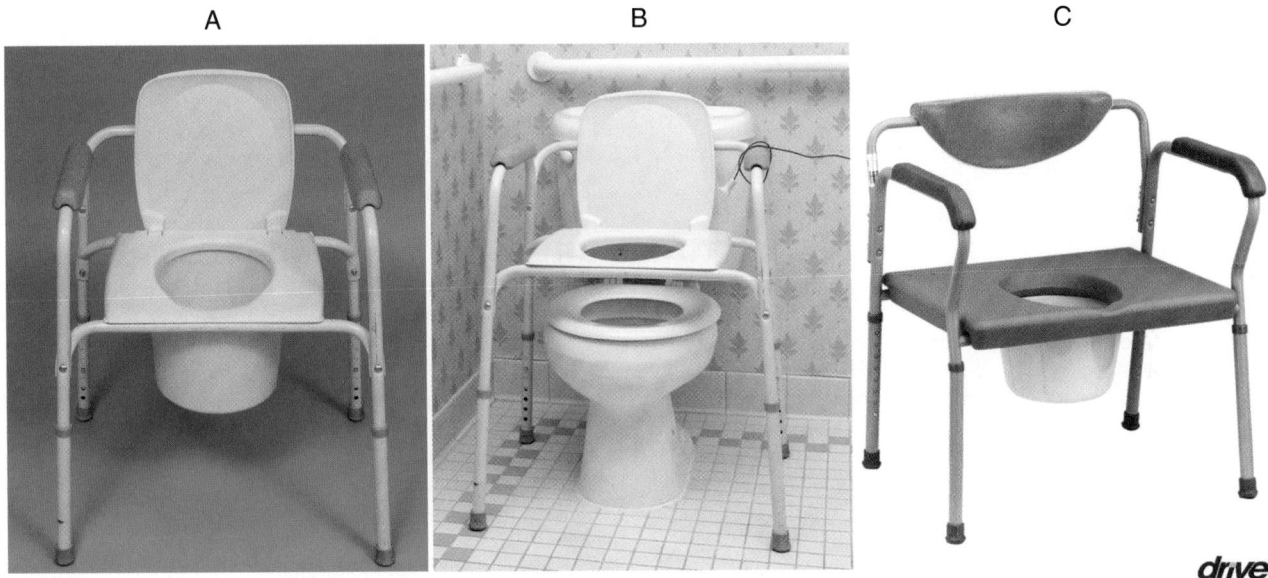

Fig. 22-10 **A,** The commode has a toilet seat with a container. The container slides out from under the seat for emptying. **B,** The container is removed. The commode chair is placed over the toilet. **C,** Bariatric commode.

DELEGATION GUIDELINES
Commodes

You need this information from the nurse and care plan when assisting with commodes:
- If the commode is used at the bedside or over the toilet
- How much help the person needs
- If you can leave the room or if you need to stay with the person
- If the nurse needs to observe urine or bowel movements
- What observations to report and record (see *Delegation Guidelines: Bedpans*, p. 378)
- When to report observations
- What patient or resident concerns to report at once

PROMOTING SAFETY AND COMFORT
Commodes

Safety

For commode use, transfer the person from the bed, chair, or wheelchair to the commode. Practice safe transfer procedures (Chapter 17). Use the transfer belt and lock the wheels. Remember to remove the transfer belt after the transfer. See "Transfer/Gait Belts" in Chapter 13.

Urine and feces may contain blood and microbes. Follow Standard Precautions and the Bloodborne Pathogen Standard. Thoroughly clean and disinfect the commode container after use. Clean and disinfect the seat and other commode parts if necessary.

Comfort

After the person transfers to the commode, cover his or her lap and legs with a bath blanket. This promotes warmth and privacy.

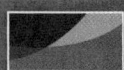 **HELPING THE PERSON TO THE COMMODE** | VIDEO |

QUALITY OF LIFE

Remember to:
- Knock before entering the person's room.
- Address the person by name.
- Introduce yourself by name and title.

- Explain the procedure to the person before beginning and during the procedure.
- Protect the person's rights during the procedure.
- Handle the person gently during the procedure.

PRE-PROCEDURE

1 Follow *Delegation Guidelines: Commodes*, p. 383. See *Promoting Safety and Comfort: Commodes*, p. 383.
2 Provide for privacy.
3 Practice hand hygiene.
4 Put on gloves.

5 Collect the following:
- Commode
- Toilet tissue
- Bath blanket
- Transfer belt
- Robe and non-skid footwear

PROCEDURE

6 Bring the commode next to the bed. Raise the lid and remove the container cover.
7 Help the person sit on the side of the bed. Lower the bed rail if used.
8 Help him or her put on a robe and non-skid footwear.
9 Apply the transfer belt.
10 Assist the person to the commode. Use the transfer belt.
11 Remove the transfer belt. Cover the person with a bath blanket for warmth.
12 Place the toilet tissue and signal light within reach.
13 Ask him or her to signal when done or when help is needed. (Stay with the person if necessary. Be respectful. Provide as much privacy as possible.)
14 Remove and discard the gloves. Practice hand hygiene.
15 Leave the room. Close the door.
16 Return when the person signals. Or check on the person every 5 minutes. Knock before entering.
17 Practice hand hygiene. Put on the gloves.
18 Help the person clean the genital area as needed. Remove and discard the gloves. Practice hand hygiene.

19 Apply the transfer belt. Help the person back to bed using the transfer belt. Remove the transfer belt, robe, and footwear. Raise the bed rail if used.
20 Put on clean gloves. Remove and cover the commode container. Clean the commode.
21 Take the container to the bathroom.
22 Observe urine and feces for color, amount, and character.
23 Empty the container contents into the toilet and flush.
24 Rinse the container. Pour the rinse into the toilet and flush.
25 Clean and disinfect the container.
26 Return the container to the commode. Close the lid on the commode.
27 Return other supplies to their proper place.
28 Remove and discard the soiled gloves. Practice hand hygiene and put on clean gloves.
29 Assist with hand washing.
30 Remove and discard the gloves. Practice hand hygiene.

POST-PROCEDURE

31 Provide for comfort. (See the inside of the front book cover.)
32 Place the signal light within reach.
33 Raise or lower bed rails. Follow the care plan.
34 Unscreen the person.

35 Complete a safety check of the room. (See the inside of the front book cover.)
36 Follow agency policy for dirty linen.
37 Practice hand hygiene.
38 Report and record your observations.

URINARY INCONTINENCE

Urinary incontinence is the involuntary loss or leakage of urine. While it occurs in some older persons, it is not a normal part of aging. However, older persons are at risk for incontinence because of changes in the urinary tract, medical and surgical conditions, and drug therapy.

Types of Incontinence

Incontinence may be temporary or permanent. The basic types of incontinence are:
- *Stress incontinence. Urine leaks during exercise and certain movements that cause pressure on the bladder.* Urine loss is small (less than 50 mL). Often called *dribbling,* it occurs with laughing, sneezing, coughing, lifting, or other activities. Obesity and late pregnancy also are causes. The problem is common in women and may begin during menopause. Pelvic muscles weaken from pregnancies and with aging.

- *Urge incontinence. Urine is lost in response to a sudden, urgent need to void. The person cannot get to a toilet in time.* Urinary frequency, urinary urgency, and night-time voidings are common. Causes include UTIs, Alzheimer's disease, nervous system disorders, bladder cancer, and an enlarged prostate.
- *Overflow incontinence. Small amounts of urine leak from a full bladder.* The person feels like the bladder is not empty. The person only dribbles or has a weak urine stream. Diabetes, enlarged prostate, and some drugs are causes. So are spinal cord injuries.
- *Functional incontinence. The person has bladder control but cannot use the toilet in time.* Immobility, restraints, unanswered signal lights, no signal light within reach, and not knowing where to find the bathroom are causes. So is difficulty removing clothing. Confusion and disorientation are other causes.
- *Reflex incontinence. Urine is lost at predictable intervals when the bladder is full.* The person does not feel the need to void. Nervous system disorders and injuries are common causes.
- *Mixed incontinence. The person has a combination of stress incontinence and urge incontinence.* Many older women have this type.
- *Transient incontinence. This refers to temporary or occasional incontinence that is reversed when the cause is treated. (Transient means for a short time.)* Common causes are delirium (Chapter 46), UTI, some drugs, increased urine production, restricted mobility, and fecal impaction (Chapter 23).

Sometimes incontinence results from intestinal, rectal, and reproductive system surgeries. Incontinence may result from a physical illness or drugs. Some causes can be reversed. Others cannot. If incontinence is a new problem, tell the nurse at once.

Managing Incontinence

The Centers for Medicare & Medicaid Services (CMS) require appropriate treatment and services for persons who are incontinent. The goals are to:

- Prevent UTIs.
- Restore as much normal bladder function as possible.

Incontinence is embarrassing. Garments get wet, and odors develop. The person is uncomfortable. Skin irritation, infection, and pressure ulcers are risks. Falling is a risk when trying to get to the bathroom quickly. Pride, dignity, and self-esteem are affected. Social isolation, loss of independence, and depression are common. Quality of life suffers.

The person's care plan may include some of the measures listed in Box 22-2. *Good skin care and dry garments and linens are essential.* Promoting normal urinary elimination prevents incontinence in some people (see Box 22-1). Others need bladder training (p. 403). Sometimes catheters are needed (p. 392).

Incontinence is linked to abuse, mistreatment, and neglect. Frequent care is needed. The person may wet again right after skin care and changing wet garments and linens. Remember, incontinence is beyond the person's control. It is not something the person chooses to do. Be patient. The

---

BOX 22-2 **NURSING MEASURES FOR PERSONS WITH URINARY INCONTINENCE**

- Record the person's voidings—times and amount. This includes incontinent times and successful use of the toilet, commode, bedpan, or urinal.
- Answer signal lights promptly. The need to void may be urgent.
- Promote normal urinary elimination (see Box 22-1).
- Promote normal bowel elimination (Chapter 23).
- Assist with elimination after sleep, before and after meals, and at bedtime.
- Follow the person's bladder training program (p. 403).
- Make sure the person has a clear pathway to the bathroom.
- Have the person wear easy-to-remove clothing. Incontinence can occur while trying to deal with buttons, zippers, other closures, and undergarments.
- Encourage the person to do pelvic muscle exercises as instructed by the nurse.
- Check the person often to make sure he or she is clean and dry.
- Help prevent UTIs:
  - Promote fluid intake as the nurse directs.
  - Have the person wear cotton underwear.
  - Keep the perineal area clean and dry.
- Decrease fluid intake at bedtime.

- Provide good skin care.
- Apply a barrier cream or moisturizer (cream, lotion, paste) as directed by the nurse. The cream prevents irritation and skin damage.
- Provide dry garments and linens.
- Observe for signs of skin breakdown (Chapters 33 and 34).
- Use incontinence products as the nurse directs. Follow the manufacturer's instructions.
- Do not leave urinals in place to catch urine in men who are incontinent.
- Keep the perineal area clean and dry (Chapter 20). Remember to:
  - Use soap and water or a no-rinse incontinence cleanser (perineal rinse). Follow the care plan. If using soap and water, use a safe and comfortable water temperature.
  - Follow Standard Precautions and the Bloodborne Pathogen Standard.
  - Protect the person and dry garments and linen from the wet incontinence product.
  - Expose only the perineal area.
  - Dry the perineal area and buttocks.
  - Remove wet incontinence products, garments, and linen. Apply clean, dry ones.

FOCUS ON CHILDREN AND OLDER PERSONS
Managing Incontinence

Children

Urinary incontinence is common in children. Day-time wetting is more common in girls. Night-time wetting is more common in boys. After age 5, wetting at night is often called *bedwetting* or *sleepwetting*. More common in boys, the cause is unknown. Possible factors include:

- Slower physical development
- Long sleeping periods
- More urine is produced at night
- Not being able to recognize a full bladder
- Anxiety
- Family history of bedwetting

Waiting for incontinence to disappear naturally is one treatment. This usually happens after age 5. The bladder grows in size and can hold more urine. The child learns to respond to the body's signal that it is time to void. Sometimes incontinence is caused by stress and anxiety. As the child grows older, stressful and anxiety-producing events may pass.

Other treatments include diet changes, moisture alarms, drugs, and bladder training.

Older Persons

Urinary incontinence is common in older persons. They are at risk for nervous, endocrine, and reproductive system disorders. Dementia, tumors, and poor mobility are risks.

Complications from incontinence pose serious problems for older persons. These include falls, pressure ulcers, and UTIs. Long hospital or long-term care stays are often necessary. The resulting health care costs are high.

Persons with dementia may develop incontinence. They may void in the wrong places. Trash cans, planters, heating vents,

Older Persons—cont'd

and closets are examples. Some persons remove incontinence products and throw them on the floor or in the toilet. Others resist staff efforts to keep them clean and dry.

You must provide safe care for these persons. The care plan lists needed measures. The care plan may include these measures recommended by the Alzheimer's Disease Education and Referral Center (ADEAR):

- Follow the person's bathroom routine as closely as possible. For example, take the person to the bathroom every 2 to 3 hours during the day. Do not wait for the person to ask.
- Observe for signs that the person may need to void. Restlessness and pulling at clothes are examples. Respond quickly.
- Stay calm when the person is incontinent. Re-assure the person if he or she becomes upset.
- Tell the nurse when the person is incontinent. Report the time, what the person was doing, and other observations. A pattern may emerge to the person's incontinence. If so, measures are planned to prevent the problem.
- Prevent episodes of incontinence during sleep. Limit the type and amount of fluids in the evening. Follow the care plan.
- Plan ahead if the person will leave the agency. Have the person wear clothing that is easy to remove. Pack an extra set of clothing. Know where to find restrooms.

You may need a co-worker's help to keep the person clean and dry. If you have questions, ask the nurse for help.

Remember, everyone has the right to safe care. They also have the right to be treated with dignity and privacy.

FOCUS ON LONG-TERM CARE AND HOME CARE
Managing Incontinence

Home Care

Incontinence is stressful for the family. They often have problems coping with the person's incontinence. It is a common reason for long-term care.

person's needs are great. If you are becoming short-tempered and impatient, talk to the nurse at once. The person has the right to be free from abuse, mistreatment, and neglect. Kindness, empathy, understanding, and patience are needed.

See *Focus on Children and Older Persons: Managing Incontinence.*

See *Focus on Long-Term Care and Home Care: Managing Incontinence.*

Applying Incontinence Products. Incontinence products help keep the person dry. Most products are disposable—used once. They usually have two layers and a waterproof back. Fluid passes through the first layer. It is absorbed by the lower layer. Many products are also available in bariatric sizes.

Common incontinence products include:

- *Complete incontinence brief* (Fig. 22-11, A). The product is secured at the sides with Velcro or tape tabs.
- *Pad and undergarment* (Fig. 22-11, B). Styles for men and for women, the undergarment looks like regular underwear. A pad (pant liner) is inserted into the built-in pouch.
- *Pull-on underwear* (Fig. 22-11, C). The product is designed to look like regular underwear. Some products come in styles for men and for women.
- *Belted undergarment* (Fig. 22-11, D). The belt is reusable. A pad is attached to the belt.

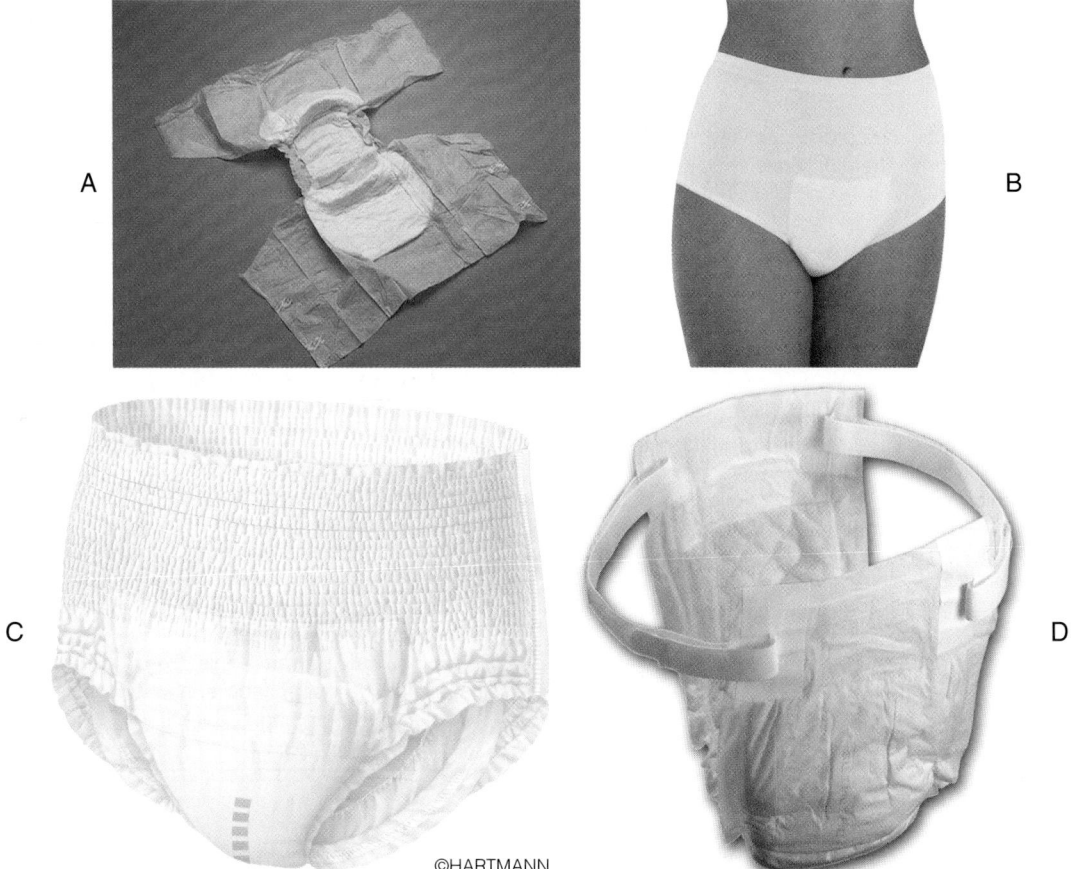

Fig. 22-11 Disposable garment protectors. **A,** Complete incontinence brief. **B,** Pad and undergarment. **C,** Pull-on underwear. **D,** Belted undergarment.

The nurse helps the person select products to meet his or her needs. To use them, follow the manufacturer's instructions and agency procedures.

See *Focus on Communication: Applying Incontinence Products.*

See *Delegation Guidelines: Applying Incontinence Products.*

See *Promoting Safety and Comfort: Applying Incontinence Products,* p. 388.

Text continued on p. 392

FOCUS ON COMMUNICATION

Applying Incontinence Products

Incontinence products are often called "adult diapers." The word "diaper" may offend the person or lower his or her self-esteem. Instead, you can say: "brief," "pad," or "underwear." Some persons prefer to say the brand name of the product they use. Use a term that promotes dignity and self-esteem.

DELEGATION GUIDELINES

Applying Incontinence Products

To apply an incontinence product, you need this information from the nurse and the care plan:

- What product to use.
- What size to use.
- If you need to apply a barrier cream. If yes, what cream to use.
- What observations to report and record:
  - Complaints of pain, burning, irritation, or the need to void
  - Signs and symptoms of skin breakdown: redness, irritation, blisters; and complaints of pain, burning, tingling, or itching
  - An estimate of the amount of urine: small, moderate, large
  - Urine color
  - Blood in the urine
  - Leakage
  - A poor product fit
- When to report observations.
- What patient or resident concerns to report at once.

PROMOTING SAFETY AND COMFORT
Applying Incontinence Products

Safety

To safely apply an incontinence product, always follow the manufacturer's instructions. The guidelines in Box 22-3 will help prevent:

* Leakage
* Skin irritation and blisters
* Tearing

Provide for safety if the person will stand for the procedure:

* Make sure the bed is in the lowest position.
* Lock the bed wheels.
* Have the person wear non-skid footwear.
* Make sure the person has something to hold on to for balance and stability.

Urine may contain microbes and blood. Follow Standard Precautions and the Bloodborne Pathogen Standard.

Comfort

For the person's comfort, always use the correct size. If the product is too large, urine can leak. If too small, the product will cause discomfort from being too tight.

BOX 22-3　GUIDELINES FOR APPLYING INCONTINENCE PRODUCTS

* Follow the manufacturer's instructions.
* Use the correct size. The nurse measures the person's hips and thighs. The largest measurement is used for the correct size.
* Note the front and back of the product.
* Center the product in the perineal area.
* Position the man's penis downward.
* Check for proper placement. The product should be in the creases between the thighs and the perineal area (groin area). It should fit the shape of the body.
* Note the amount of urine (small, moderate, large). Also note how often you change the product. The person may need an extended wear product for large amounts of urine or if he or she has diarrhea (Chapter 23).
* Do not let the plastic backing touch the person's skin.
* Provide perineal care after each incontinent episode.
* Do not use the product as a turning or lift sheet.
* Attach the tape tabs correctly. The product will tear if you try to unfasten the tape or change the tape's position.
  * Attach the lower tape first. Stretch the tape and attach it at a slightly upward angle. Do so for both sides.
  * Attach the upper tape after the lower tape is fastened. Stretch the tape and attach it in a horizontal manner. Do so for both sides.

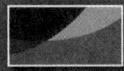 **APPLYING INCONTINENCE PRODUCTS**

QUALITY OF LIFE

Remember to:
* Knock before entering the person's room.
* Address the person by name.
* Introduce yourself by name and title.

* Explain the procedure to the person before beginning and during the procedure.
* Protect the person's rights during the procedure.
* Handle the person gently during the procedure.

PRE-PROCEDURE

1 Follow *Delegation Guidelines: Applying Incontinence Products*, p. 387. See *Promoting Safety and Comfort: Applying Incontinence Products.*
2 Practice hand hygiene.
3 Collect the following:
   * Incontinence product as directed by the nurse
   * Barrier cream as directed by the nurse
   * Cleanser
   * Items for perineal care (Chapter 20)
   * Waterproof pad
   * Paper towels
   * Trash bag
   * Gloves
   * Non-skid footwear if the person will stand

4 Cover the overbed table with paper towels. Arrange items on top of them.
5 Identify the person. Check the ID (identification) bracelet against the assignment sheet. Also call the person by name.
6 Provide for privacy.
7 Fill the wash basin. Water temperature is about 105°F (Fahrenheit) (40.5°C [centigrade]). Measure water temperature according to agency policy. Ask the person to check the water temperature. Adjust water temperature as needed.
8 Raise the bed for body mechanics. Bed rails are up if used. (Omit this step if the person will stand.)

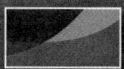 **APPLYING INCONTINENCE PRODUCTS—cont'd**

PROCEDURE

9 Lower the head of the bed. The bed is as flat as possible.
10 Lower the bed rail near you if up.
11 Practice hand hygiene. Put on the gloves.
12 Cover the person with a bath blanket. Lower top linens to the foot of the bed.
13 *To apply an incontinence brief with the person in bed:*
  a Place a waterproof pad under the buttocks. Ask the person to raise the buttocks off the bed. Or turn the person from side to side.
  b Loosen the tabs on each side of the product.
  c Turn the person onto the side away from you.
  d Remove the product from front to back. Observe the urine as you roll the product up (Fig. 22-12, A, p. 390).
  e Place the product in the trash bag. Set the bag aside.
  f Perform perineal care (Chapter 20).
  g Open the new brief. Fold it in half length-wise along the center (Fig. 22-12, B, p. 390).
  h Insert the product between the legs from front to back (Fig. 22-12, C, p. 390).
  i Unfold and spread the back panel (Fig. 22-12, D, p. 390).
  j Center the product in the perineal area.
  k Turn the person onto his or her back.
  l Unfold and spread the front panel. Provide a "cup" shape in the perineal area. For a man, position the penis downward.
  m Make sure the product is positioned high in the groin folds. This allows the product to fit the shape of the body.
  n Secure the product (Fig. 22-12, E, p. 390):
    (1) Pull the lower tape tab forward on the side near you. Attach it at a slightly upward angle. Do the same for the other side.
    (2) Pull the upper tape tab forward on the side near you. Attach it in a horizontal manner. Do the same for the other side.
  o Smooth out all wrinkles and folds.

14 *To apply a pad and undergarment with the person in bed:*
  a Place a waterproof pad under the buttocks. Ask the person to raise the buttocks off the bed. Or turn the person from side to side.
  b Turn the person onto the side away from you.
  c Pull the undergarment down. The waistband is over the knee (Fig. 22-13, A, p. 391).
  d Remove the pad from front to back. Observe the urine as you roll the product up (Fig. 22-13, B, p. 391).
  e Place the product in the trash bag. Set the bag aside.
  f Perform perineal care (Chapter 20).
  g Fold the new pad in half length-wise along the center (Fig. 22-13, C, p. 391).
  h Insert the pad between the legs from front to back (Fig. 22-13, D, p. 391).
  i Unfold and spread the back panel. See Figure 22-13, E, p. 391.
  j Center the pad in the perineal area.
  k Pull the undergarment up at the back (Fig. 22-13, F, p. 391).
  l Turn the person onto his or her back.
  m Unfold and spread the front panel (Fig. 22-13, G, p. 391). For a man, position the penis downward.
  n Pull the garment up in front (Fig. 22-13, H, p. 391).
  o Check and adjust the pad and undergarment for a good fit.
15 *To apply pull-on underwear with the person standing:*
  a Help the person put on non-skid footwear.
  b Help the person stand.
  c Tear the side seams to remove the used underwear (Fig. 22-14, A, p. 392).
  d Remove the product from front to back (Fig. 22-14, B, p. 392). Observe the urine as you roll the product up.
  e Place the product in the trash bag. Set the bag aside.
  f Perform perineal care (Chapter 20).
  g Have the person sit on the side of the bed.
  h Slide the underwear over the feet to past the knees (Fig. 22-14, C, p. 392).
  i Help the person stand.
  j Pull the underwear up (Fig. 22-14, D, p. 392).
  k Check for a good fit.
16 Remove and discard the gloves. Practice hand hygiene.

POST-PROCEDURE

17 Provide for comfort. (See the inside of the front book cover.)
18 Place the signal light within reach.
19 Lower the bed to its lowest position.
20 Raise or lower bed rails. Follow the care plan.
21 Unscreen the person.
22 Practice hand hygiene. Put on clean gloves.
23 Estimate the amount of urine in the old product: small, moderate, large. Open the product to observe for urine color and blood.
24 Clean, rinse, dry, and return the wash basin and other equipment. Return items to their proper place.
25 Remove and discard the gloves. Practice hand hygiene.
26 Complete a safety check of the room. (See the inside of the front book cover.)
27 Report and record your observations.

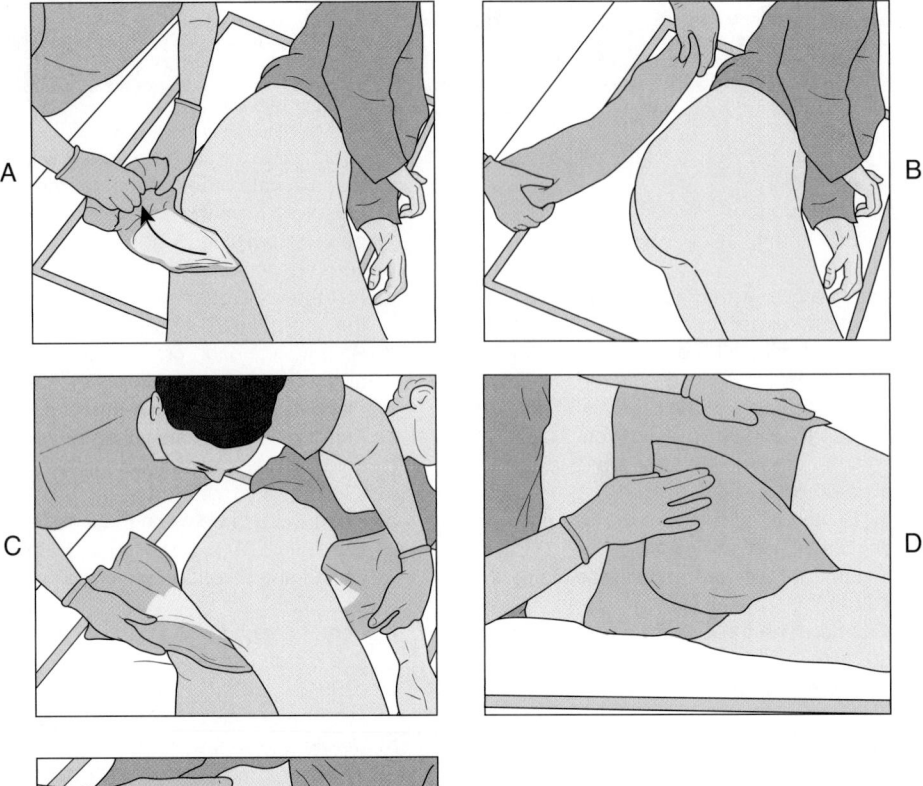

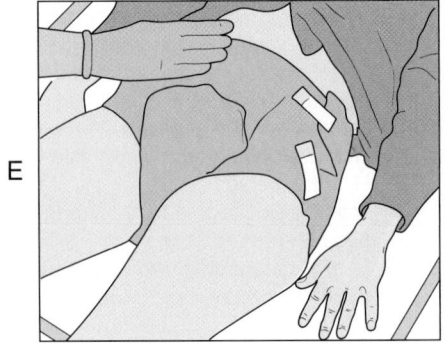

Fig. 22-12 Applying a complete incontinence brief. **A,** The product is removed from front to back. **B,** The new product is opened length-wise. **C,** The product is inserted length-wise between the legs from front to back. **D,** The back panel is spread open. **E,** The lower tape tab is attached at a slightly upward angle. The upper tape tab is attached in a horizontal manner.

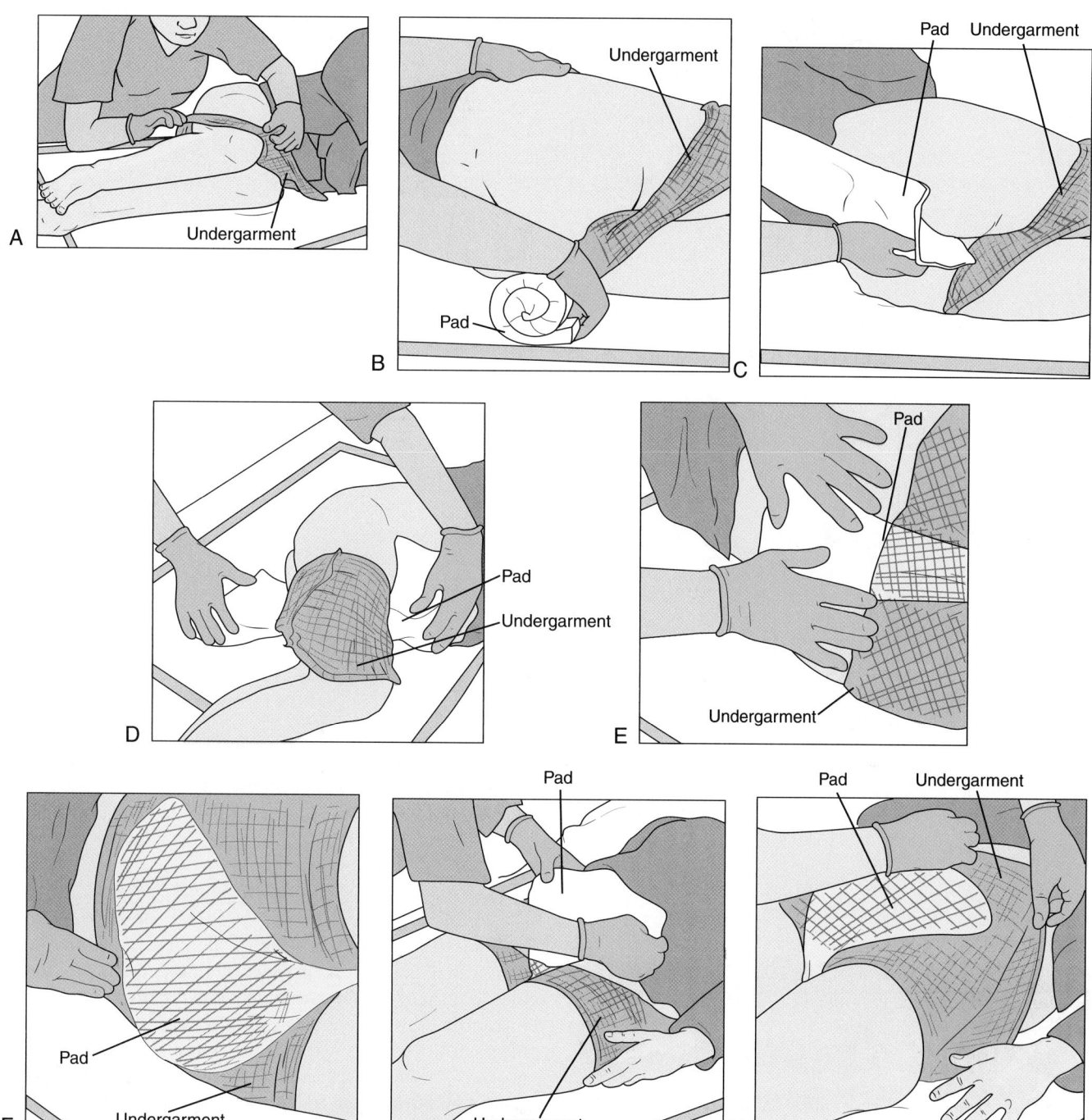

Fig. 22-13 Applying a pad and undergarment. **A,** The undergarment is pulled down. The waistband is over the knee. **B,** The pad is rolled up as it is removed from front to back. **C,** The new pad is folded in half length-wise along the center. **D,** The pad is inserted between the legs from front to back. **E,** The back panel is unfolded and spread out. **F,** The undergarment is pulled up at the back. **G,** The front panel is unfolded and spread open. **H,** The garment is pulled up in front.

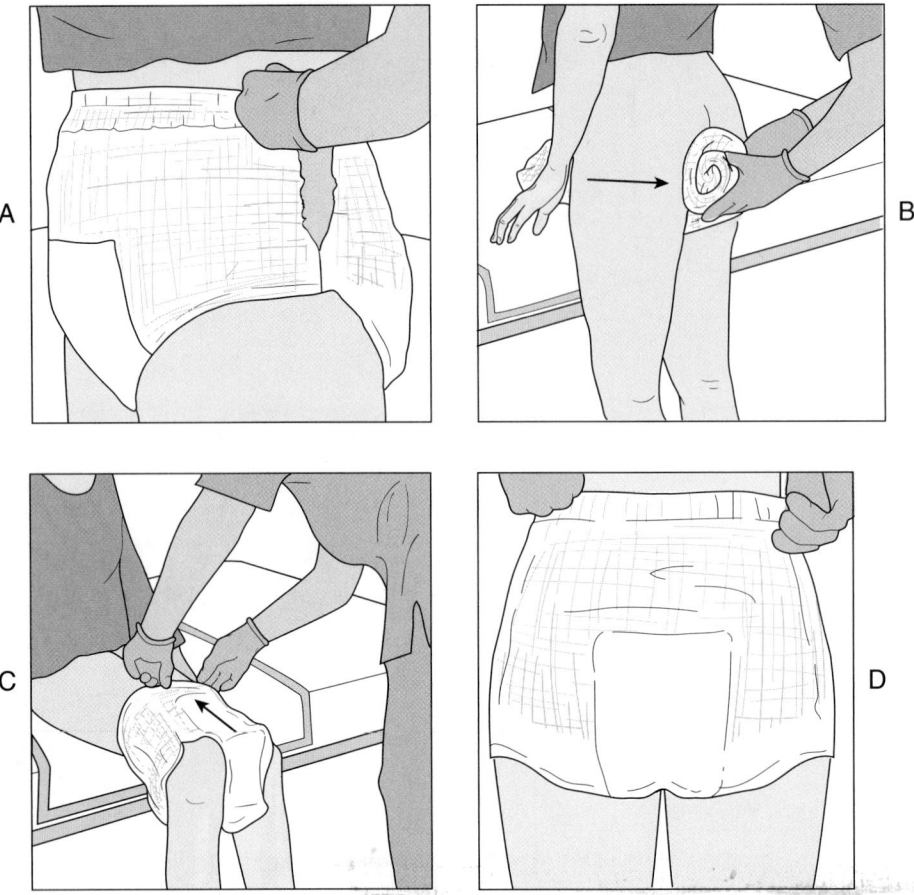

Fig. 22-14 Applying pull-on underwear. **A,** The side seams are torn to remove the used underwear. **B,** The product is removed from front to back. **C,** The underwear is slid over the feet to past the knees. **D,** The underwear is pulled up.

CATHETERS

A *catheter is a tube used to drain or inject fluid through a body opening.* Inserted through the urethra into the bladder, a urinary catheter drains urine.

- A *straight catheter drains the bladder and then is removed.*
- An *indwelling catheter (retention or Foley catheter) is left in the bladder. Urine drains constantly into a drainage bag.* A balloon near the tip is inflated with sterile water after the catheter is inserted. The balloon prevents the catheter from slipping out of the bladder (Fig. 22-15). Tubing connects the catheter to the drainage bag.

Catheterization is the process of inserting a catheter. It is done by a doctor or nurse. With the proper education and supervision, some states and agencies let nursing assistants insert and remove catheters.

Catheters often are used before, during, and after surgery. They keep the bladder empty. This reduces the risk of bladder injury during surgery. Also, the amount of urine can be monitored. After surgery, a full bladder causes pressure on nearby organs. Such pressure can lead to pain or discomfort.

Some people are too weak or disabled to use the bedpan, urinal, commode, or toilet. Dying persons are examples. For them, catheters can promote comfort and prevent incontinence. Catheters can protect wounds and pressure ulcers from contact with urine. They also allow hourly urinary output measurements. However, they are a last resort for incontinence. Catheters do not treat the cause of incontinence.

Catheters also are used to:
- Collect sterile urine specimens.
- Measure the amount of urine left in the bladder after the person voids. This is called *residual urine.*

You will care for persons with indwelling catheters. The risk of UTI is high. Follow the rules in Box 22-4 to promote safety and comfort.

See *Focus on Communication: Catheters*, p. 394.
See *Delegation Guidelines: Catheters*, p. 394.
See *Promoting Safety and Comfort: Catheters*, p. 394.

Text continued on p. 396

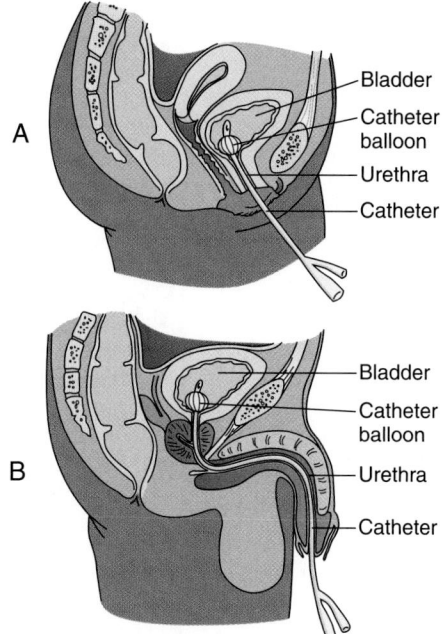

Fig. 22-15 Indwelling catheter. **A,** Indwelling catheter is in the female bladder. The inflated balloon at the tip prevents the catheter from slipping out through the urethra. **B,** Indwelling catheter with the balloon inflated is in the male bladder.

BOX 22-4 **CARING FOR PERSONS WITH INDWELLING CATHETERS**

- Follow the rules of medical asepsis.
- Follow Standard Precautions and the Bloodborne Pathogen Standard.
- Allow urine to flow freely through the catheter or tubing. Tubing should not have kinks. The person should not lie on the tubing.
- Keep the catheter connected to the drainage tubing. Follow the measures on p. 396 if the catheter and drainage tube are disconnected.
- Keep the drainage tube below the bladder. This prevents urine from flowing backward into the bladder.
- Move the bag to the other side of the bed when the person is turned and re-positioned on his or her other side.
- Attach the drainage bag to the bed frame, back of the chair, or lower part of an IV (intravenous) pole. *Never attach the drainage bag to the bed rail.* Otherwise it is higher than the bladder when the bed rail is raised.
- Do not let the drainage bag rest on the floor. This can contaminate the system.
- Coil the drainage tubing on the bed. Secure it to the bottom linen (Fig. 22-16, p. 394). Follow agency policy. Use a clip, bed sheet clamp, tape, safety pin with rubber band, or other device as directed by the nurse. Tubing must not loop below the drainage bag.
- Secure the catheter to the inner thigh (see Fig. 22-16, p. 394). Or secure it to the man's abdomen. This prevents excess catheter movement and friction at the insertion site. Secure the catheter with a tube holder, tape, or other device as the nurse directs.
- Check for leaks. Check the site where the catheter connects to the drainage bag. Report any leaks to the nurse at once.
- Provide catheter care according to the care plan—daily, twice a day, after bowel movements, or when vaginal discharge is present. (See procedure: *Giving Catheter Care,* p. 395). Some agencies consider perineal care to be sufficient. Follow the care plan.
- Provide perineal care daily or twice a day, after bowel movements, and when there is vaginal drainage. Follow the care plan.
- Empty the drainage bag at the end of the shift or as the nurse directs. Measure and record the amount of urine (see procedure: *Emptying a Urinary Drainage Bag,* p. 399). Report an increase or decrease in the amount of urine.
- Use a separate measuring container for each person. This prevents the spread of microbes from one person to another.
- Do not let the drain on the drainage bag touch any surface.
- Encourage fluid intake as directed by the nurse and the care plan.
- Report complaints to the nurse at once—pain, burning, the need to void, or irritation. Also report the color, clarity, and odor of urine and the presence of particles or blood.
- Observe for signs and symptoms of a UTI. Report the following at once:
  - Fever.
  - Chills.
  - Flank pain or tenderness. The flank area is in the back between the ribs and the hip.
  - Change in the urine—blood, foul smell, particles, cloudiness, oliguria.
  - Change in mental or functional status—confusion, decreased appetite, falls, decreased activity, tiredness, and so on.
  - Urine leakage around the catheter.

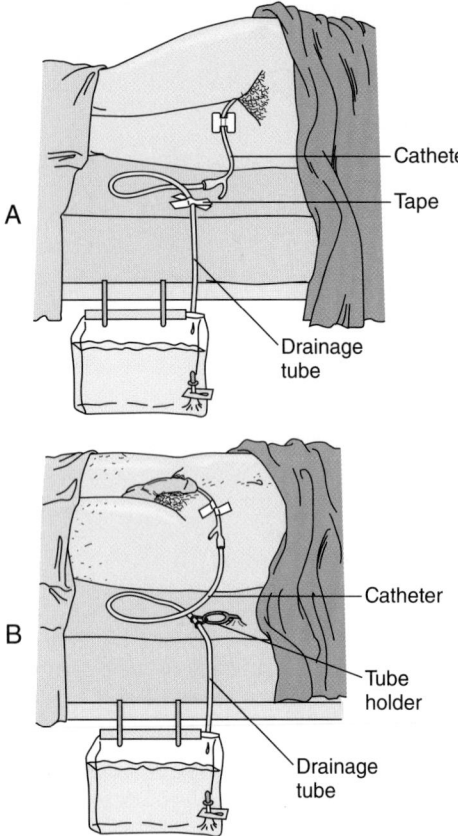

Fig. 22-16 Securing catheters. **A,** The catheter is secured to the inner thigh with a tube holder. The drainage tube is coiled on the bed and secured to bottom linens with tape. **B,** The catheter is secured to the man's abdomen with tape. Drainage tubing is secured to bottom linens with a clamp.

FOCUS ON COMMUNICATION
Catheters

Surveys are done to determine if the person is receiving appropriate treatment and services. The surveyor may ask you questions about:
- Your understanding of the person's bladder management program
- Your training related to handling catheters, catheter tubing, drainage bags, catheter care, UTIs, catheter-related injuries, dislodgement, and skin breakdown
- What observations to report, when to report them, and to whom you should report observations

Answer questions the best you can. If you do not know an answer, tell the surveyor who you would ask or where you would find the answer.

DELEGATION GUIDELINES
Catheters

The nurse may delegate catheter care to you. If so, you need this information from the nurse and the care plan:
- When to give catheter care—daily, twice a day, after bowel movements, or when vaginal discharge is present
- What water temperature to use for perineal care
- Where to secure the catheter—thigh or abdomen
- How to secure the catheter—tube holder, tape, or other device
- How to secure drainage tubing—clip, bed sheet clamp, tape, safety pin with rubber band, or other device
- What observations to report and record:
  - Complaints of pain, burning, irritation, or the need to void (report at once)
  - Crusting, abnormal drainage, or secretions
  - The color, clarity, and odor of urine
  - Particles in the urine
  - Blood in the urine
  - Cloudy urine
  - Urine leaking at the insertion site
  - Drainage system leaks
- When to report observations
- What patient or resident concerns to report at once

PROMOTING SAFETY AND COMFORT
Catheters

Safety
Urine may contain microbes and blood. Follow Standard Precautions and the Bloodborne Pathogen Standard.

Be very careful if using a safety pin and rubber band to secure the drainage tubing to the bottom linens:
- Check the safety pin and rubber band:
  - The safety pin must work properly. It must not be stretched out of shape.
  - The rubber band must be intact. It should not be frayed or over-stretched.
- Do not insert the pin through the catheter.
- Point the pin away from the person.

Comfort
The catheter must not pull at the insertion site. This causes discomfort and irritation. Hold the catheter securely during catheter care. Then properly secure the catheter. Make sure the tubing is not under the person. Besides obstructing urine flow, lying on the tubing is uncomfortable. It can also cause skin breakdown. To promote comfort, see Box 22-4.

GIVING CATHETER CARE

QUALITY OF LIFE

Remember to:
- Knock before entering the person's room.
- Address the person by name.
- Introduce yourself by name and title.

- Explain the procedure to the person before beginning and during the procedure.
- Protect the person's rights during the procedure.
- Handle the person gently during the procedure.

PRE-PROCEDURE

1 Follow *Delegation Guidelines:*
   a *Perineal Care* (Chapter 20)
   b *Catheters*
   See *Promoting Safety and Comfort:*
   a *Perineal Care* (Chapter 20)
   b *Catheters*
2 Practice hand hygiene.
3 Collect the following:
   - Items for perineal care (Chapter 20)
   - Gloves
   - Bath blanket

4 Cover the overbed table with paper towels. Arrange items on top of them.
5 Identify the person. Check the ID bracelet against the assignment sheet. Also call the person by name.
6 Provide for privacy.
7 Fill the wash basin. Water temperature is about 105°F (40.5°C). Measure water temperature according to agency policy. Ask the person to check the water temperature. Adjust water temperature as needed.
8 Raise the bed for body mechanics. Bed rails are up if used.

PROCEDURE

9 Lower the bed rail near you if up.
10 Practice hand hygiene. Put on the gloves.
11 Cover the person with a bath blanket. Fan-fold top linens to the foot of the bed.
12 Drape the person for perineal care (Chapter 20).
13 Fold back the bath blanket to expose the genital area.
14 Place the waterproof pad under the buttocks. Ask the person to flex the knees and raise the buttocks off the bed.
15 Separate the labia (female). In an uncircumcised male, retract the foreskin (Chapter 20). Check for crusts, abnormal drainage, or secretions.
16 Give perineal care (Chapter 20). Keep the foreskin of the uncircumcised male retracted until step 22.
17 Apply soap to a clean, wet washcloth.
18 Hold the catheter at the meatus. Do so for steps 19, 20, and 21.
19 Clean the catheter from the meatus down the catheter at least 4 inches (Fig. 22-17, p. 396). Clean downward, away from the meatus with 1 stroke. Do not tug or pull on the catheter. Repeat as needed with a clean area of the washcloth. Use a clean washcloth if needed.

20 Rinse the catheter with a clean washcloth. Rinse from the meatus down the catheter at least 4 inches. Rinse downward, away from the meatus with 1 stroke. Do not tug or pull on the catheter. Repeat as needed with a clean area of the washcloth. Use a clean washcloth if needed.
21 Dry the catheter with a towel. Dry from the meatus down the catheter at least 4 inches. Do not tug or pull on the catheter.
22 Return the foreskin to its natural position.
23 Pat dry the perineal area. Dry from front to back.
24 Secure the catheter. Coil and secure tubing (see Fig. 22-16).
25 Remove the waterproof pad.
26 Cover the person. Remove the bath blanket.
27 Remove and discard the gloves. Practice hand hygiene.

POST-PROCEDURE

28 Provide for comfort. (See the inside of the front book cover.)
29 Place the signal light within reach.
30 Lower the bed to its lowest position.
31 Raise or lower bed rails. Follow the care plan.
32 Clean, rinse, dry, and return equipment to its proper place. Discard disposable items. (Wear gloves for this step.)

33 Unscreen the person.
34 Complete a safety check of the room. (See the inside of the front book cover.)
35 Follow agency policy for soiled linen.
36 Remove and discard the gloves. Practice hand hygiene.
37 Report and record your observations (Fig. 22-18, p. 396).

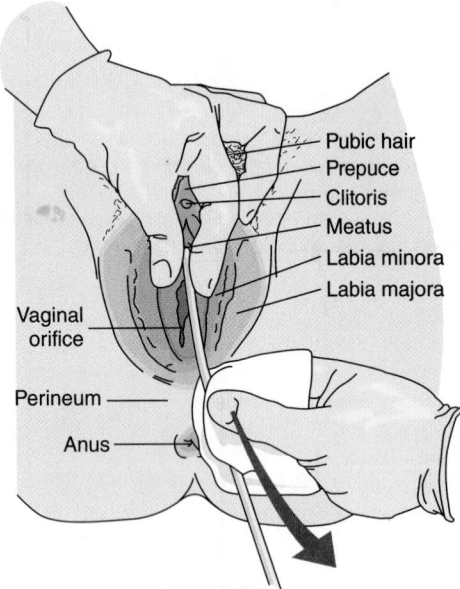

Fig. 22-17 The catheter is cleaned starting at the meatus. At least 4 inches of the catheter are cleaned.

Date	Time	Nursing Margin	Other Depts Margin
12/21	0900	Catheter care given. No drainage from around the catheter. Resident denies discomfort. Clear amber urine flowing freely. Catheter secured to abdomen with tape. Drainage tubing attached to bed with clip. Resident positioned on L side. Bed in low position. Signal light within reach. Adam Aims, CNA	

Fig. 22-18 Charting sample.

Drainage Systems

A closed drainage system is used for indwelling catheters. Nothing can enter the system from the catheter to the drainage bag. The urinary system is sterile. Infection can occur if microbes enter the drainage system. The microbes travel up the tubing or catheter into the bladder and kidneys. A UTI can threaten health and life.

The drainage system has drainage tubing and a drainage bag (see Fig. 22-16). Tubing attaches at one end to the catheter. At the other end, it attaches to the drainage bag.

The bag hangs from the bed frame, chair, or wheelchair. It must not touch the floor. The bag is always kept lower than the person's bladder (see Fig. 22-16). Some people wear leg bags when up. The leg bag attaches to the thigh or calf (p. 401).

Microbes can grow in urine. If the drainage bag is higher than the bladder, urine can flow back into the bladder. A UTI can occur. *Therefore do not hang the drainage bag on a bed rail.* Otherwise, when the bed rail is raised, the bag is higher than bladder level. When the person walks, the bag is held lower than the bladder.

Sometimes drainage systems become disconnected. If that happens, tell the nurse at once. Do not touch the ends of the catheter or tubing. Do the following:

- Practice hand hygiene. Put on gloves.
- Wipe the end of the tube with an antiseptic wipe.
- Wipe the end of the catheter with another antiseptic wipe.
- Do not put the ends down. Do not touch the ends after you clean them.
- Connect the tubing to the catheter.
- Discard the wipes into a biohazard bag.
- Remove the gloves. Practice hand hygiene.

Leg bags are changed to drainage bags when the person is in bed. This drainage bag stays lower than bladder level. You need to open the closed drainage system. You must prevent microbes from entering the system.

Drainage bags are emptied and urine is measured:

- At the end of every shift
- When changing from a leg bag to a drainage bag
- When changing from a drainage bag to a leg bag
- When the bag is becoming full
  See *Delegation Guidelines: Drainage Systems.*
  See *Promoting Safety and Comfort: Drainage Systems.*

Text continued on p. 400

DELEGATION GUIDELINES
Drainage Systems

Delegated tasks may involve urinary drainage systems. If so, you need this information from the nurse and the care plan:

- When to empty the drainage bag
- If the person uses a leg bag
- When to switch a drainage bag and leg bag
- If you should clean or discard the drainage bag
- What observations to report and record:
  - The amount of urine measured
  - The color, clarity, and odor of urine
  - Particles in the urine
  - Blood in the urine
  - Cloudy urine
  - Complaints of pain, burning, irritation, or the need to urinate
  - Drainage system leaks
- When to report observations
- What patient or resident concerns to report at once

Safety

Urine may contain microbes and blood. Follow Standard Precautions and the Bloodborne Pathogen Standard.

For the procedure: *Changing a Leg Bag to a Drainage Bag,* you will open sterile packages. You must keep sterile items free from contamination. Review "Surgical Asepsis" in Chapter 15.

A leg bag attaches to the thigh or calf (p. 401). Leg bags hold less than 1000 mL of urine. Most standard drainage bags hold at least 2000 mL of urine. Therefore leg bags fill faster than standard drainage bags. Check leg bags often. Empty the leg bag if it is becoming half full. Measure, report, and record the amount of urine in the bag.

Comfort

Urine in a drainage bag embarrasses some people. Visitors can see the urine when they are with the person. To promote mental comfort, have visitors sit on the side away from the drainage bag. Sometimes you can empty the bag before visitors arrive. Make sure you measure, report, and record the amount of urine.

Some agencies have drainage bag holders. The drainage bag is placed inside the holder. Urine cannot be seen.

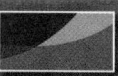

CHANGING A LEG BAG TO A DRAINAGE BAG

QUALITY OF LIFE

Remember to:
- Knock before entering the person's room.
- Address the person by name.
- Introduce yourself by name and title.

- Explain the procedure to the person before beginning and during the procedure.
- Protect the person's rights during the procedure.
- Handle the person gently during the procedure.

PRE-PROCEDURE

1 Follow *Delegation Guidelines: Drainage Systems.* See *Promoting Safety and Comfort: Drainage Systems.*
2 Practice hand hygiene.
3 Collect the following:
- Gloves
- Drainage bag and tubing
- Antiseptic wipes
- Waterproof pad
- Sterile cap and plug

- Catheter clamp
- Paper towels
- Bedpan
- Bath blanket

4 Arrange paper towels and equipment on the overbed table.
5 Identify the person. Check the ID bracelet against the assignment sheet. Also call the person by name.
6 Provide for privacy.

PROCEDURE

7 Have the person sit on the side of the bed.
8 Practice hand hygiene. Put on the gloves.
9 Expose the catheter and leg bag.
10 Clamp the catheter (Fig. 22-19, p. 398). This prevents urine from draining from the catheter into the drainage tubing.
11 Let urine drain from below the clamp into the drainage tubing. This empties the lower end of the catheter.
12 Help the person lie down.
13 Raise the bed rails if used. Raise the bed for body mechanics.
14 Lower the bed rail near you if up.
15 Cover the person with a bath blanket. Fan-fold top linens to the foot of the bed. Expose the catheter and leg bag.
16 Place the waterproof pad under the person's leg.
17 Open the antiseptic wipes. Set them on the paper towels.
18 Open the package with the sterile cap and plug. Set the package on the paper towels. Do not let anything touch the sterile cap or plug (Fig. 22-20, p. 398).
19 Open the package with the drainage bag and tubing.
20 Attach the drainage bag to the bed frame.
21 Disconnect the catheter from the drainage tubing. Do not let anything touch the ends.

22 Insert the sterile plug into the catheter end (Fig. 22-21, p. 398). Touch only the end of the plug. Do not touch the part that goes inside the catheter. (If you contaminate the end of the catheter, wipe the end with an antiseptic wipe. Do so before inserting the sterile plug.)
23 Place the sterile cap on the end of the leg bag drainage tube (see Fig. 22-21). (If you contaminate the tubing end, wipe the end with an antiseptic wipe. Do so before you put on the sterile cap.)
24 Remove the cap from the new drainage tubing.
25 Remove the sterile plug from the catheter.
26 Insert the end of the drainage tubing into the catheter.
27 Remove the clamp from the catheter.
28 Loop the drainage tubing on the bed. Secure the tubing to the bottom linens.
29 Remove the leg bag. Place it in the bedpan.
30 Remove and discard the waterproof pad.
31 Cover the person. Remove the bath blanket.
32 Take the bedpan to the bathroom.
33 Remove and discard the gloves. Practice hand hygiene.

Continued

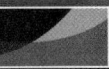

CHANGING A LEG BAG TO A DRAINAGE BAG—cont'd

POST-PROCEDURE

34 Provide for comfort. (See the inside of the front book cover.)

35 Place the signal light within reach.

36 Lower the bed to its lowest position.

37 Raise or lower bed rails. Follow the care plan.

38 Unscreen the person.

39 Put on clean gloves. Discard disposable items.

40 Empty the drainage bag. See procedure: *Emptying a Urinary Drainage Bag*.

41 Discard the drainage tubing and bag following agency policy. Or clean the bag following agency policy.

42 Clean and disinfect the bedpan. Place it in a clean cover.

43 Return the bedpan and other supplies to their proper place.

44 Remove and discard the gloves. Practice hand hygiene.

45 Complete a safety check of the room. (See the inside of the front book cover.)

46 Follow agency policy for soiled linen.

47 Practice hand hygiene.

48 Report and record your observations.

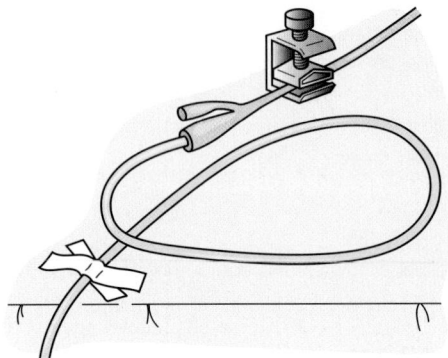

Fig. 22-19 The clamped catheter prevents urine from draining out of the bladder. The clamp is applied directly to the catheter—not to the drainage tube.

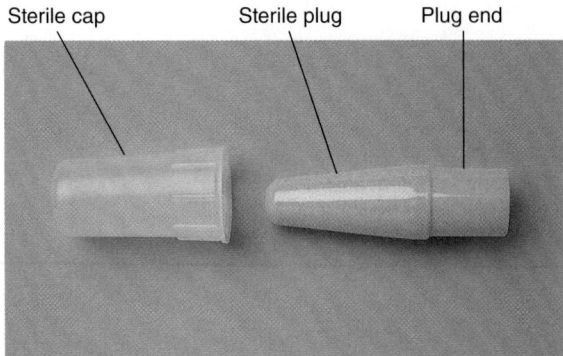

Fig. 22-20 Sterile cap and catheter plug. The inside of the cap is sterile. Touch only the end of the plug.

Sterile cap   Sterile plug   Plug end

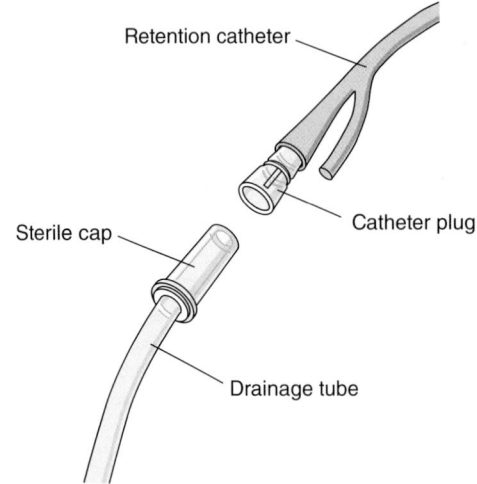

Retention catheter

Catheter plug

Sterile cap

Drainage tube

Fig. 22-21 Sterile plug is inserted into the end of the catheter. The sterile cap is on the end of the drainage tube.

EMPTYING A URINARY DRAINAGE BAG

VIDEO

QUALITY OF LIFE

Remember to:
- Knock before entering the person's room.
- Address the person by name.
- Introduce yourself by name and title.

- Explain the procedure to the person before beginning and during the procedure.
- Protect the person's rights during the procedure.
- Handle the person gently during the procedure.

PRE-PROCEDURE

1 Follow *Delegation Guidelines: Drainage Systems*, p. 396. See *Promoting Safety and Comfort: Drainage Systems*, p. 397.
2 Collect the following:
   - Graduate (measuring container)
   - Gloves
   - Paper towels
   - Antiseptic wipes

3 Practice hand hygiene.
4 Identify the person. Check the ID bracelet against the assignment sheet. Call the person by name.
5 Provide for privacy.

PROCEDURE

6 Put on the gloves.
7 Place a paper towel on the floor. Place the graduate on top of it.
8 Position the graduate under the collection bag.
9 Open the clamp on the drain.
10 Let all urine drain into the graduate. Do not let the drain touch the graduate (Fig. 22-22).
11 Clean the end of the drain with an antiseptic wipe.
12 Close and position the clamp (Fig. 22-23).
13 Measure urine.

14 Remove and discard the paper towel.
15 Empty the contents of the graduate into the toilet and flush.
16 Rinse the graduate. Empty the rinse into the toilet and flush.
17 Clean and disinfect the graduate.
18 Return the graduate to its proper place.
19 Remove and discard the gloves. Practice hand hygiene.
20 Record the time and amount of urine on the intake and output (I&O) record (Chapter 24).

POST-PROCEDURE

21 Provide for comfort. (See the inside of the front book cover.)
22 Place the signal light within reach.
23 Unscreen the person.

24 Complete a safety check of the room. (See the inside of the front book cover.)
25 Report and record the amount of urine and other observations.

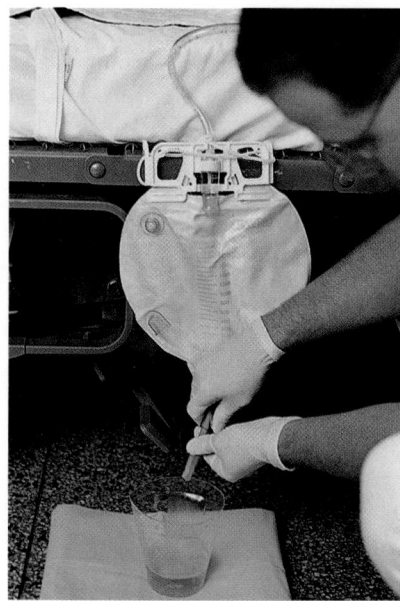

Fig. 22-22 The clamp on the drainage bag is opened. The drain is directed into the graduate. The drain must not touch the inside of the graduate.

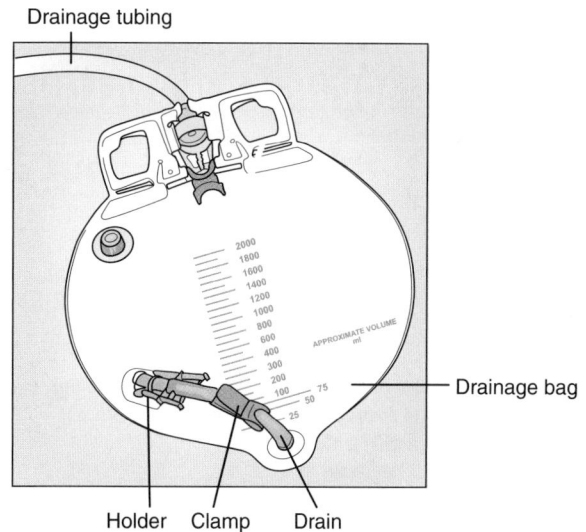

Fig. 22-23 The clamp is closed and positioned in the holder on the drainage bag.

Removing Indwelling Catheters

An indwelling catheter has two lumens (passage-ways). Sterile water is injected through one lumen to inflate the balloon (Fig. 22-24). The water is injected with a syringe. Urine drains from the bladder through the other lumen.

To remove the catheter, the balloon is deflated. You need a syringe large enough to hold all of the water in the balloon. Balloon size is marked at the end of the catheter.

A doctor's order is needed to remove a catheter. The person may need bladder training first (p. 403). Dysuria and urinary frequency are common after removing catheters.

See *Focus on Communication: Removing Indwelling Catheters.*

See *Delegation Guidelines: Removing Indwelling Catheters.*

See *Promoting Safety and Comfort: Removing Indwelling Catheters.*

FOCUS ON COMMUNICATION
Removing Indwelling Catheters

When removing an indwelling catheter, explain the procedure to the person before you begin and during the procedure. Also, tell the person about any discomfort that may be felt and when to expect discomfort. Instruct the person to tell you at once if he or she feels pain or needs you to stop the procedure. For example, you can say:

Mrs. Tanner, I'm going to remove your catheter. I will explain the procedure step-by-step. You may feel a little pressure or discomfort when the tube is removed. I will tell you before I remove it. Please tell me right away if you feel pain or if you need me to stop.

Instructing the person to breathe out (exhale) when removing the catheter may distract the person and promote relaxation. Explaining each step in a calm and professional manner also helps to reduce anxiety and provide comfort. Avoid seeming bossy or hurried. Politely tell the person what you will do and what he or she needs to do.

DELEGATION GUIDELINES
Removing Indwelling Catheters

Before removing a catheter, make sure that:
- Your state allows you to perform the procedure.
- The procedure is in your job description.
- You know how to use the agency's supplies and equipment.
- You review the procedure with the nurse.
- A nurse is available to answer questions and to supervise you.

If the above conditions are met, you need this information from the nurse:
- When to remove the catheter
- Balloon size
- Syringe size needed
- What observations to report and record:
  - The amount of urine in the drainage bag
  - Color, clarity, and odor of urine
  - Particles in the urine
  - Blood in the urine
  - How the person tolerated the procedure
  - Complaints of pain, burning, irritation, or the need to urinate
  - Any other observations
- When to report observations
- What patient or resident concerns to report at once

PROMOTING SAFETY AND COMFORT
Removing Indwelling Catheters

Safety

Before removing the catheter, you must remove all water from the balloon. If the balloon size is 5 mL, you must withdraw 5 mL of water into the syringe. Otherwise, injury to the urethra is likely as the catheter is removed. Do not remove the catheter if water remains in the balloon. Call for the nurse at once.

Urine may contain microbes and blood. Follow Standard Precautions and the Bloodborne Pathogen Standard.

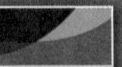

REMOVING AN INDWELLING CATHETER

QUALITY OF LIFE

Remember to:
- Knock before entering the person's room.
- Address the person by name.
- Introduce yourself by name and title.
- Explain the procedure to the person before beginning and during the procedure.
- Protect the person's rights during the procedure.
- Handle the person gently during the procedure.

PRE-PROCEDURE

1 Follow *Delegation Guidelines: Removing Indwelling Catheters.* See *Promoting Safety and Comfort: Removing Indwelling Catheters.*
2 Practice hand hygiene.
3 Collect the following:
   - Disposable towel
   - Syringe in the size as directed by the nurse
   - Disposable bag
   - Gloves
   - Bath blanket
4 Identify the person. Check the ID bracelet against the assignment sheet. Also call the person by name.
5 Provide for privacy.
6 Raise the bed for body mechanics. Bed rails are up if used.

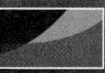

REMOVING AN INDWELLING CATHETER—cont'd

PROCEDURE

7 Lower the bed rail near you if up.

8 Practice hand hygiene. Put on the gloves.

9 Position and drape the person as for perineal care (Chapter 20).

10 Cover the person with a bath blanket.

11 Remove the tape or tube holder securing the catheter to the person.

12 Position the towel:
  a Female—between her legs
  b Male—over his thighs

13 Attach the syringe to the balloon port on the catheter (see Fig. 22-24).

14 Pull back on the syringe slowly. Withdraw all water from the balloon. Call for the nurse if you cannot remove all of the water.

15 Pull the catheter straight out. Remove the catheter gently. Do not remove the catheter if there is water in the balloon.

16 Discard the catheter into the bag.

17 Dry the perineal area with the towel. Discard the towel in the bag.

18 Remove and discard the gloves. Practice hand hygiene.

19 Cover the person. Remove the bath blanket.

POST-PROCEDURE

20 Provide for comfort. (See the inside of the front book cover.)

21 Place the signal light within reach.

22 Lower the bed to its lowest position.

23 Raise or lower bed rails. Follow the care plan.

24 Unscreen the person.

25 Put on clean gloves. Discard disposable items.

26 Empty the drainage bag. See procedure: *Emptying a Urinary Drainage Bag*, p. 399. Note the amount of urine.

27 Discard the drainage tubing and bag following agency policy.

28 Remove and discard the gloves. Practice hand hygiene.

29 Complete a safety check of the room. (See the inside of the front book cover.)

30 Practice hand hygiene.

31 Report and record your observations.

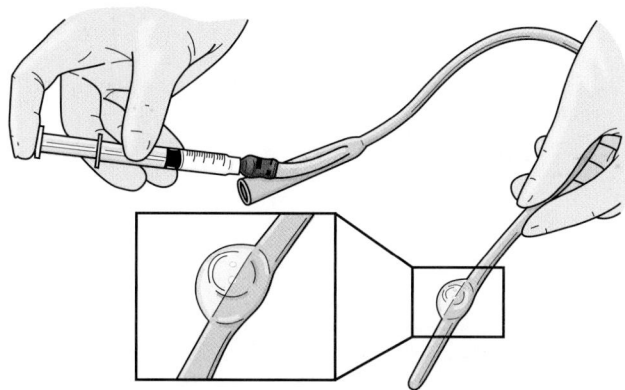

Fig. 22-24 The balloon of an indwelling catheter is inflated with water. A syringe is used to inject the water. A syringe also is used to remove the water.

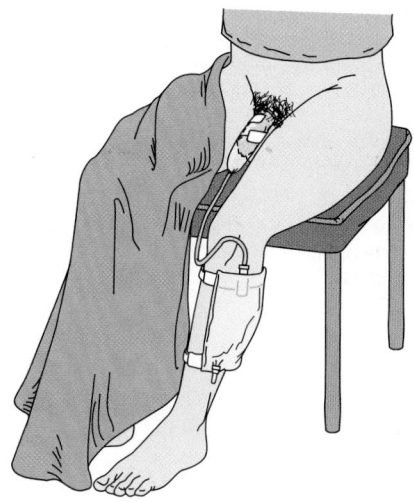

Fig. 22-25 Condom catheter attached to a leg bag.

Condom Catheters

Condom catheters are often used for incontinent men. They also are called *external catheters, Texas catheters,* and *urinary sheaths.* A condom catheter is a soft sheath that slides over the penis. Tubing connects the condom catheter and the drainage bag. Many men prefer leg bags (Fig. 22-25).

Condom catheters are changed daily after perineal care. To apply a condom catheter, follow the manufacturer's instructions. Thoroughly wash the penis with soap and water. Then dry it before applying the catheter.

Some condom catheters are self-adhering. Adhesive inside the catheter adheres to the penis. Other catheters are secured in place with elastic tape. Use the elastic tape packaged with the catheter. Elastic tape expands when the penis changes size. This allows blood flow to the penis. *Only use elastic tape. Never use adhesive or other tape to secure catheters. They do not expand. Blood flow to the penis is cut off, injuring the penis.*

See *Delegation Guidelines: Condom Catheters,* p. 402.

See *Promoting Safety and Comfort: Condom Catheters,* p. 402.

DELEGATION GUIDELINES
Condom Catheters

To remove or apply a condom catheter, you need this information from the nurse and the care plan:
- What size to use—small, medium, or large
- When to remove the catheter and apply a new one
- If a leg bag or standard drainage system is used
- What water temperature to use for perineal care
- What observations to report and record:
  - Reddened or open areas on the penis
  - Swelling of the penis
  - Color, clarity, and odor of urine
  - Particles in the urine
  - Blood in the urine
  - Cloudy urine
- When to report observations
- What patient or resident concerns to report at once

PROMOTING SAFETY AND COMFORT
Condom Catheters

Safety

Do not apply a condom catheter if the penis is red, irritated, or shows signs of skin breakdown. Report your observations to the nurse at once.

If you do not know how to use the condom catheters used at your agency, ask the nurse to show you the correct application. Then ask the nurse to observe you applying the catheter.

Blood must flow to the penis. If tape is needed, use the elastic tape packaged with the catheter. Apply it in a spiral.

Urine may contain microbes and blood. Follow Standard Precautions and the Bloodborne Pathogen Standard.

Comfort

To apply a condom catheter, you need to touch and handle the penis. This can embarrass the man. Some men become sexually aroused. Always act in a professional manner. If necessary, allow the man privacy. Provide for his safety and place the urinal within reach. Tell him when you will return, and then leave the room. Or ask him to use the signal light when he is ready for you to finish the procedure. Knock before entering the room again.

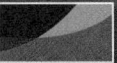 **APPLYING A CONDOM CATHETER** | VIDEO |

QUALITY OF LIFE

Remember to:
- Knock before entering the person's room.
- Address the person by name.
- Introduce yourself by name and title.

- Explain the procedure to the person before beginning and during the procedure.
- Protect the person's rights during the procedure.
- Handle the person gently during the procedure.

PRE-PROCEDURE

1 Follow *Delegation Guidelines:*
  a *Perineal Care* (Chapter 20)
  b *Condom Catheters*
  See *Promoting Safety and Comfort:*
  a *Perineal Care* (Chapter 20)
  b *Condom Catheters*
2 Practice hand hygiene.
3 Collect the following:
- Condom catheter
- Elastic tape
- Drainage bag or leg bag
- Cap for the drainage bag
- Basin of warm water
- Soap
- Towel and washcloths

- Bath blanket
- Gloves
- Waterproof pad
- Paper towels
4 Cover the overbed table with paper towels. Arrange items on top of them.
5 Identify the person. Check the ID bracelet against the assignment sheet. Also call the person by name.
6 Provide for privacy.
7 Fill the wash basin. Water temperature is about 105°F (40.5°C). Measure water temperature according to agency policy. Ask the person to check the water temperature. Adjust water temperature as needed.
8 Raise the bed for body mechanics. Bed rails are up if used.

APPLYING A CONDOM CATHETER—cont'd

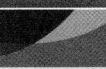

VIDEO

PROCEDURE

9 Lower the bed rail near you if up.
10 Practice hand hygiene. Put on the gloves.
11 Cover the person with a bath blanket. Lower top linens to the knees.
12 Ask the person to raise his buttocks off the bed. Or turn him onto his side away from you.
13 Slide the waterproof pad under his buttocks.
14 Have the person lower his buttocks. Or turn him onto his back.
15 Secure the drainage bag to the bed frame. Or have a leg bag ready. Close the drain.
16 Expose the genital area.
17 Remove the condom catheter.
  a Remove the tape. Roll the sheath off the penis.
  b Disconnect the drainage tubing from the condom. Cap the drainage tube.
  c Discard the tape and condom.
18 Provide perineal care (Chapter 20). Observe the penis for reddened areas, skin breakdown, and irritation.
19 Remove and discard the gloves. Practice hand hygiene. Put on clean gloves.

20 Remove the protective backing from the condom. This exposes the adhesive strip.
21 Hold the penis firmly. Roll the condom onto the penis. Leave a 1-inch space between the penis and the end of the catheter (Fig. 22-26).
22 Secure the condom.
  a For a self-adhering condom: press the condom to the penis.
  b For a condom secured with elastic tape: apply elastic tape in a spiral. See Figure 22-26. Do not apply tape completely around the penis.
23 Make sure the penis tip does not touch the condom. Make sure the condom is not twisted.
24 Connect the condom to the drainage tubing. Coil and secure excess tubing on the bed. Or attach a leg bag.
25 Remove the waterproof pad and gloves. Discard them. Practice hand hygiene.
26 Cover the person. Remove the bath blanket.

POST-PROCEDURE

27 Provide for comfort. (See the inside of the front book cover.)
28 Place the signal light within reach.
29 Lower the bed to its lowest position.
30 Raise or lower bed rails. Follow the care plan.
31 Unscreen the person.
32 Practice hand hygiene. Put on clean gloves.
33 Measure and record the amount of urine in the bag. Clean or discard the collection bag.

34 Clean, rinse, dry, and return the wash basin and other equipment. Return items to their proper place.
35 Remove and discard the gloves. Practice hand hygiene.
36 Complete a safety check of the room. (See the inside of the front book cover.)
37 Report and record your observations.

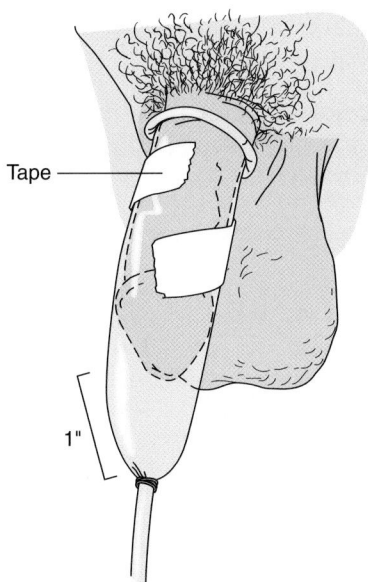

Tape

1"

Fig. 22-26 A condom catheter applied to the penis. A 1-inch space is between the penis and the end of the catheter. Elastic tape is applied in a spiral fashion to secure the condom catheter to the penis.

BLADDER TRAINING

Bladder training helps some persons with urinary incontinence. Some persons need bladder training after indwelling catheter removal. Control of urination is the goal. Bladder control promotes comfort and quality of life. It also increases self-esteem. You assist with bladder training as directed by the nurse and the care plan. Successful bladder retraining may take many weeks.

The rules for normal elimination are followed. The normal position for urination is assumed if possible. Privacy is important. The person's care plan may include one of the following:

- *Bladder retraining (bladder rehabilitation).* This requires that the person:
  - Resist or ignore the strong desire to urinate.
  - Postpone or delay voiding.
  - Urinate following a schedule rather than the urge to void.

  The time between voidings may be increased as bladder retraining progresses.

- *Prompted voiding.* The person voids at scheduled times. The person is taught to:
  - Recognize when the bladder is full.
  - Recognize the need to void.
  - Ask for help.
  - Respond when prompted to void.

- *Habit training/scheduled voiding.* Voiding is scheduled at regular times to match the person's voiding habits. This is usually every 3 to 4 hours while awake. The person does not delay or resist voiding. Timed-voiding is based on the person's usual voiding pattern.

- *Catheter clamping.* The catheter is clamped to prevent urine flow from the bladder (see Fig. 22-19). It is usually clamped for 1 hour at first. Over time, it is clamped for 3 to 4 hours. Urine drains when the catheter is unclamped. When the catheter is removed, voiding is encouraged every 3 to 4 hours or as directed by the nurse and the care plan.

FOCUS ON PRIDE

The Person, Family, and Yourself

Personal and Professional Responsibility

Some states allow nursing assistants to insert a catheter into the bladder. If your state and agency allow you to insert urinary catheters:

- The procedure must be in your job description.
- You must have the necessary education and training.
- You must know how to use the agency's supplies and equipment.
- A nurse must be available to answer questions and supervise you.

Rights and Respect

People usually void in private. Illness, disease, and aging can affect this very private act. Respect the person's right to privacy. Allow as much privacy as safely possible. Pull privacy curtains and close doors and window coverings. If you must stay in the room, allow as much privacy as possible. Stand just outside the bathroom door in case the person needs you. Or stand on the other side of the privacy curtain if safe to do so. The nurse helps you with ways to protect the person's privacy. Follow the nurse's directions and the care plan.

Empty urinals, bedpans, and commodes promptly. Urine-filled devices in the person's room do not respect the person's right to a neat and clean setting. It also may cause embarrassment. Do your best to promote comfort, dignity, and respect when assisting with elimination needs.

Independence and Social Interaction

Some persons can place bedpans and urinals themselves. Some can get on and off bedside commodes themselves. Others need some help but can be left alone to void. Allow persons to do as much as safely possible.

To safely promote independence, keep devices within reach for persons who use them without help. For persons who need some help, check on them often. Do not leave a person sitting on a bedpan or commode for a long time. Discomfort, odors, and skin breakdown are likely. Also, the person may think you forgot about him or her. The person may try to get off of the bedpan or commode alone. He or she may be harmed. Make sure the signal light is within reach. Respond promptly when a person calls for help.

Delegation and Teamwork

Reporting and recording what you have done and observed are parts of delegation. When assisting with elimination, accurate reporting and recording are important. The nurse needs correct information about urine appearance, odor, and amount. Changes in urination may lead to changes in the person's care. Report urinary problems and abnormal urine to the nurse. If you are unsure what to report or record, ask the nurse.

Ethics and Laws

Negligence occurs when a person does not act in a reasonable and careful manner and the person or the person's property is harmed (Chapter 4). Although the error is not intentional, the negligent person is responsible. The following is a real example of negligent care:

A patient was admitted to the hospital with a diagnosis of mild pneumonia. He was to be in the hospital for 24 to 48 hours. While in the hospital, he was left on a bedpan for 4 hours. Pressure ulcers resulted. He died of pneumonia after 41 days in the hospital.

His family sued the hospital. The jury awarded the family $800,000.

(Estate of D. Roberts v William Beaumont Hospital, Mich., 2002.)

The following practices can help you avoid this mistake:

- Be careful and focused when performing all procedures. Avoid distractions.
- Remind the person to press the signal light if you do not return promptly.
- Report and record promptly. When you report, the nurse knows what you did. When you record, there is a record of the care provided.
- Use reminders. This is very important when you are busy. For example, set a timer on your watch or write yourself a note.

Take pride in developing good habits that promote safety and quality care.

REVIEW QUESTIONS

Circle the BEST answer.

1 Which is *false?*
   a Urine is normally clear and yellow or amber in color.
   b Urine normally has an ammonia odor.
   c Micturition usually occurs before going to bed and after sleep.
   d A person normally voids 1500 mL a day.

2 Which is *not* a rule for normal elimination?
   a Help the person assume a normal position for voiding.
   b Provide for privacy.
   c Help the person to the bathroom or commode. Or provide the bedpan or urinal as soon as requested.
   d Stay with the person who uses the bedpan.

3 The person using a standard bedpan is in
   a Fowler's position
   b The supine position
   c The prone position
   d The side-lying position

4 After using the urinal, the man should
   a Put it on the bedside stand
   b Use the signal light
   c Put it on the overbed table
   d Empty it

5 After a person uses a commode, you should
   a Clean and disinfect the container, seat, and commode parts
   b Return the commode to the supply area
   c Get a new container
   d Get a new commode

6 Urinary incontinence
   a Is always permanent
   b Requires good skin care
   c Is treated with a catheter
   d Requires bladder training

7 Which is *not* a cause of functional incontinence?
   a Unanswered signal light
   b No signal light within reach
   c Problems removing clothing
   d UTI

8 When applying an incontinence product, you should
   a Let the plastic backing touch the person's skin
   b Remove the old product from back to front
   c Apply the new product from front to back
   d Use the product to turn and position the person after it is applied

9 A person has an indwelling catheter. Which is *not* correct?
   a Keep the drainage bag above the level of the bladder.
   b Keep drainage tubing free of kinks.
   c Coil the drainage tubing on the bed.
   d Secure the catheter according to agency policy.

10 A person has an indwelling catheter. Which is *not* correct?
   a Tape any leaks at the connection site.
   b Follow Standard Precautions and the Bloodborne Pathogen Standard.
   c Empty the drainage bag at the end of your shift.
   d Report complaints of pain, burning, the need to void, or irritation at once.

11 A person has an indwelling catheter. You are going to turn the person from the left side to the right side. What should you do with the drainage bag?
   a Move it to the right side.
   b Keep it on the left side.
   c Hang it from an IV pole.
   d Remove the catheter and the drainage bag.

12 When giving catheter care, you clean the catheter
   a From the meatus down the catheter at least 4 inches
   b From the meatus down the entire catheter
   c From the drainage tube connection up the catheter to the meatus
   d From the drainage tube connection up the catheter about 4 inches

13 You are going to remove an indwelling catheter. You
   a Attach a needle to the syringe
   b Check the balloon size
   c Tug on the catheter to see if it will come out
   d Use an antiseptic swab to clean the meatus

14 You are going to remove an indwelling catheter. It has a 5 mL balloon. You withdraw 3 mL. What should you do?
   a Call for the nurse.
   b Inject the fluid.
   c Pull the catheter out gently.
   d Cut the catheter.

15 For a condom catheter, you apply elastic tape
   a Completely around the penis
   b To the inner thigh
   c To the abdomen
   d In a spiral fashion

16 The goal of bladder training is to
   a Remove the catheter
   b Clamp the catheter
   c Allow the person to walk to the bathroom
   d Gain control of urination

17 A person is taught to ignore the urge to void. This type of bladder training is called
   a Bladder retraining
   b Prompted voiding
   c Habit training
   d Scheduled voiding

Answers to these questions are on p. 833.

23 Bowel Elimination

OBJECTIVES

- Define the key terms and key abbreviations listed in this chapter.
- Describe normal defecation.
- List the observations to make about defecation.
- Identify the factors that affect bowel elimination.
- Describe the common bowel elimination problems.
- Explain how to promote comfort and safety during defecation.
- Describe bowel training.
- Explain why enemas are given.
- Describe the common enema solutions.
- Describe the rules for giving enemas.
- Describe how to care for a person with an ostomy.
- Perform the procedures described in this chapter.
- Explain how to promote PRIDE in the person, the family, and yourself.

KEY TERMS

colostomy A surgically created opening *(stomy)* between the colon *(colo)* and abdominal wall

constipation The passage of a hard, dry stool

defecation The process of excreting feces from the rectum through the anus; a bowel movement

dehydration The excessive loss of water from tissues

diarrhea The frequent passage of liquid stools

enema The introduction of fluid into the rectum and lower colon

fecal impaction The prolonged retention and buildup of feces in the rectum

fecal incontinence The inability to control the passage of feces and gas through the anus

feces The semi-solid mass of waste products in the colon that is expelled through the anus

flatulence The excessive formation of gas or air in the stomach and intestines

flatus Gas or air passed through the anus

ileostomy A surgically created opening *(stomy)* between the ileum (small intestine *[ileo]*) and the abdominal wall

ostomy A surgically created opening for the elimination of body wastes; see "colostomy" and "ileostomy"

peristalsis The alternating contraction and relaxation of intestinal muscles

stoma A surgically created opening seen through the abdominal wall; see "colostomy" and "ileostomy"

stool Excreted feces

suppository A cone-shaped, solid drug that is inserted into a body opening; it melts at body temperature

KEY ABBREVIATIONS

BM	Bowel movement	**ID**	Identification
C	Centigrade	**IV**	Intravenous
CMS	Centers for Medicare & Medicaid Services	**mL**	Milliliter
F	Fahrenheit	**oz**	Ounce
GI	Gastro-intestinal	**SSE**	Soapsuds enema

Bowel elimination is a basic physical need. It is the excretion of wastes from the gastro-intestinal (GI) system (Chapter 9). Many factors affect bowel elimination. They include privacy, habits, age, diet, exercise and activity, fluids, and drugs. Problems easily occur. Promoting normal bowel elimination is important. You assist patients and residents in meeting elimination needs.

See *Body Structure and Function Review: The Gastro-Intestinal Tract.*

NORMAL BOWEL ELIMINATION

Some people have a bowel movement (BM) every day. Others have one every 2 to 3 days. Some people have 2 or 3 BMs a day. Many people have a BM after breakfast. Others do so in the evening.

Stools are normally brown. Bleeding in the stomach and small intestine causes black or tarry stools. Bleeding in the lower colon and rectum causes red-colored stools. So do beets, tomato juice or soup, red Jell-O, and foods with red food coloring. A diet high in green vegetables can cause

BODY STRUCTURE AND FUNCTION REVIEW: THE GASTRO-INTESTINAL TRACT

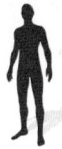

The GI tract is part of the digestive system (Chapter 9). Bowel elimination is the excretion of wastes through the GI tract. Food and fluids are normally taken in through the mouth. They are partially digested in the stomach. The partially digested food and fluids are called *chyme*.

Chyme passes from the stomach into the small intestine. Further digestion and absorption of nutrients occur as the chyme passes through the small bowel. Then chyme enters the large intestine (large bowel or colon) where fluid is absorbed. Chyme becomes less fluid and more solid in consistency. *Feces refer to the semi-solid mass of waste products in the colon that are expelled through the anus.*

Feces move through the intestines by peristalsis. *Peristalsis is the alternating contraction and relaxation of intestinal muscles.* The feces move through the large intestine to the rectum. Feces are stored in the rectum until excreted from the body (Fig. 23-1). *Defecation (bowel movement) is the process of excreting feces from the rectum through the anus. Stool refers to excreted feces.*

See Chapter 9 for more information.

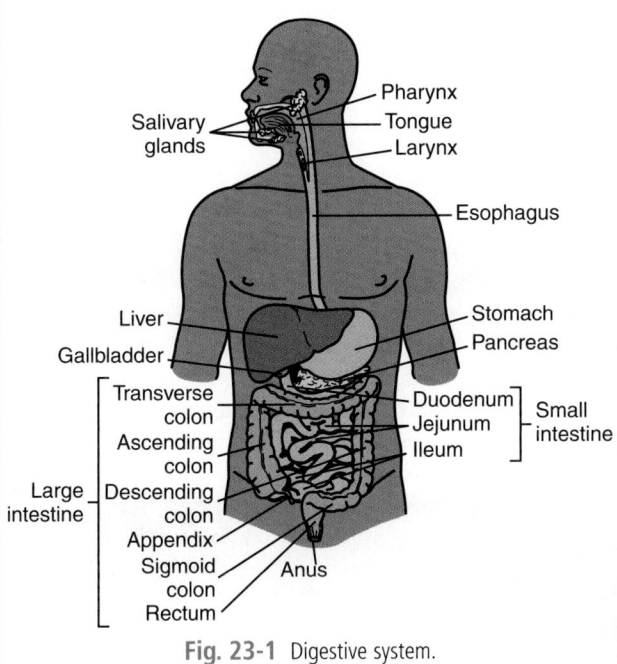

Fig. 23-1 Digestive system.

Labels: Pharynx, Tongue, Larynx, Esophagus, Salivary glands, Stomach, Pancreas, Liver, Gallbladder, Transverse colon, Ascending colon, Descending colon, Appendix, Sigmoid colon, Rectum, Large intestine, Duodenum, Jejunum, Ileum, Small intestine, Anus

Observations

Your observations are used for the nursing process. Carefully observe stools before disposing of them. Ask the nurse to observe abnormal stools. Observe and report the following to the nurse. If allowed to chart, also record the following:
- Color
- Amount
- Consistency
- Presence of blood or mucus
- Odor
- Shape
- Frequency of BMs
- Complaints of pain or discomfort
  See *Focus on Communication: Observations.*

green stools. Diseases and infection can cause clay-colored or white, pale, orange-colored, or green-colored stools and stools with mucus.

Stools are normally soft, formed, moist, and shaped like the rectum. They have a normal odor caused by bacterial action in the intestines. Certain foods and drugs also cause odors.

See *Focus on Children and Older Persons: Normal Bowel Elimination.*

BOWEL ELIMINATION RECORD

Bowel Movement Codes

Amount:	Consistency:	Frequency:
X = None **S** = Small **M** = Medium **L** = Large	**W** = Watery **S** = Soft **F** = Formed **H** = Hard	**X** = Times (#) (number of BMs of same amount and consistency)

Charting Instructions

Use the Bowel Movement Codes to chart the amount followed by the consistency of each BM and the frequency if needed. For multiple BMs of different amounts or consistencies, chart each BM separately.

Charting Example

Month: January

Shift	1	2	3	4
AM	X	X	X	SS
PM	X	SS	MWx2	X
Night	MF	X	MW, SS	X

Name: Marie Parker
Month: March

Shift	1	2	3	4	5	6	7	8	9	10	11	12	13	14	15	16	17	18	19	20	21	22	23	24	25	26	27	28	29	30	31
AM	MF	X																													
PM	X	SS x2																													
Night	X	X																													

Fig. 23-2 Bowel elimination record.

FACTORS AFFECTING BOWEL ELIMINATION

These factors affect stool frequency, consistency, color, and odor. They are part of the nursing process to meet the person's elimination needs. Normal, regular elimination is the goal.

- *Privacy.* A BM is a private act. Odors and sounds are embarrassing. Lack of privacy can prevent a BM despite the urge. Some people ignore the urge when people are present.
- *Habits.* Many people have a BM after breakfast. Some drink a hot beverage, read, or take a walk. These activities are relaxing. A BM is easier when a person is relaxed, not tense.
- *Diet—high-fiber foods.* High-fiber foods leave a residue for needed bulk. Fruits, vegetables, and whole-grain cereals and breads are high in fiber. Many people do not eat enough fruits and vegetables. Some cannot chew these foods. They may not have teeth. Or dentures fit poorly. Some people think that they cannot digest fruits and vegetables. So they refuse to eat them. Sometimes bran is added to cereal, prunes, or prune juice. These foods provide fiber and prevent constipation.
- *Diet—other foods.* Milk and milk products can cause constipation in some people. They cause diarrhea in others. Chocolate and other foods cause similar reactions. Spicy foods can irritate the intestines. Frequent stools or diarrhea can result. Gas-forming foods stimulate peristalsis, which aids a BM. Such foods include onions, beans, cabbage, cauliflower, radishes, and cucumbers.
- *Fluids.* Feces contain water. Stool consistency depends on the amount of water absorbed in the colon. The amount of fluid intake, urine output, and vomiting are factors. Feces harden and dry when large amounts of water are absorbed or when fluid intake is poor. Hard, dry feces move slowly through the colon. Constipation can occur. Drinking 6 to 8 glasses of water daily promotes normal bowel elimination. Warm fluids—coffee, tea, hot cider, warm water—increase peristalsis.
- *Activity.* Exercise and activity maintain muscle tone and stimulate peristalsis. Irregular elimination and constipation often occur from inactivity and bedrest. Inactivity may result from disease, surgery, injury, and aging.
- *Drugs.* Drugs can prevent constipation or control diarrhea. Other drugs have diarrhea or constipation as side effects. Drugs for pain relief often cause constipation. Antibiotics (used to fight or prevent infections) often cause diarrhea. Diarrhea occurs when the antibiotics kill normal flora in the colon. Normal flora is needed to form feces.
- *Disability.* Some people cannot control BMs. They have a BM whenever feces enter the rectum. A bowel training program is needed (p. 413).
- *Aging.* Age affects bowel elimination.
  See *Focus on Children and Older Persons: Factors Affecting Bowel Elimination.*

BOX 23-1	SAFETY AND COMFORT DURING BOWEL ELIMINATION

- Follow Standard Precautions and the Bloodborne Pathogen Standard.
- Provide for privacy:
  - Ask visitors to leave the room.
  - Close doors, privacy curtains, and window coverings.
- Help the person to the toilet or commode. Or provide the bedpan as soon as requested.
- Wheel the person into the bathroom on the commode if possible. Place the commode over the toilet. This provides privacy. Remember to lock the commode wheels.
- Make sure the bedpan is warm.
- Position the person in a normal sitting or squatting position.
- Cover the person for warmth and privacy.
- Allow enough time for a BM.
- Place the signal light and toilet tissue within reach.
- Leave the room if the person can be alone. Check on the person every 5 minutes.
- Stay nearby if the person is weak or unsteady.
- Provide perineal care.
- Dispose of stools promptly. This reduces odors and prevents the spread of microbes.
- Assist the person with hand washing after elimination.
- Follow the care plan if the person has fecal incontinence. The care plan tells you when to assist with elimination.

Safety and Comfort

The care plan has measures to meet the person's elimination needs. It may involve diet, fluids, and exercise. Follow the measures in Box 23-1 to promote safety and comfort.

See *Focus on Communication: Safety and Comfort.*

See *Teamwork and Time Management: Safety and Comfort.*

COMMON PROBLEMS

Common problems include constipation, fecal impaction, diarrhea, fecal incontinence, and flatulence.

Constipation

Constipation is the passage of a hard, dry stool. The person usually strains to have a BM. Stools are large or marble-size. Large stools cause pain as they pass through the anus. Constipation occurs when feces move slowly through the bowel. This allows more time for water absorption. Common causes of constipation include:

- A low-fiber diet
- Ignoring the urge to have a BM
- Decreased fluid intake
- Inactivity
- Drugs
- Aging
- Certain diseases

Dietary changes, fluids, and activity prevent or relieve constipation. The doctor may order one or more of the following:

- Stool softeners. These are drugs that soften feces. A BM is easier when feces are soft.
- Laxatives. Laxative comes from the Latin word that means *to loosen*. A *laxative* is a drug that promotes bowel elimination. It does so by increasing the bulk of feces, softening feces, and lubricating the intestinal wall.
- Suppositories (p. 414).
- Enemas (p. 415).

Fecal Impaction

A *fecal impaction is the prolonged retention and buildup of feces in the rectum.* Feces are hard or putty-like. Fecal impaction results if constipation is not relieved. The person cannot have a BM. More water is absorbed from the already hard feces. Liquid feces pass around the hardened fecal mass in the rectum. The liquid feces seep from the anus.

The person tries many times to have a BM. Abdominal discomfort, abdominal distention (swelling), nausea, cramping, and rectal pain are common. Older persons may have poor appetite or confusion. Some persons have a fever. Report these signs and symptoms to the nurse.

The nurse does a digital (finger) exam to check for an impaction. A lubricated, gloved finger is inserted into the rectum to feel for a hard mass (Fig. 23-3). The mass is felt in the lower rectum. Sometimes it is higher in the colon and out of reach. The digital exam often causes the urge to have a BM. The doctor may order drugs, suppositories, or enemas to remove the impaction.

Sometimes *digital removal of an impaction* is done. A lubricated, gloved finger is hooked around a piece of feces. Then the finger and feces are removed. The stool is dropped into the bedpan. The process is repeated as needed. The procedure can be uncomfortable and embarrassing.

Checking for and removing impactions are very dangerous. The vagus nerve can be stimulated. This nerve affects the heart. Stimulation of the vagus nerve slows the heart rate. The heart rate can slow to unsafe levels in some persons.

See *Focus on Long-Term Care and Home Care: Fecal Impaction.*
See *Delegation Guidelines: Fecal Impaction.*
See *Promoting Safety and Comfort: Fecal Impaction.*

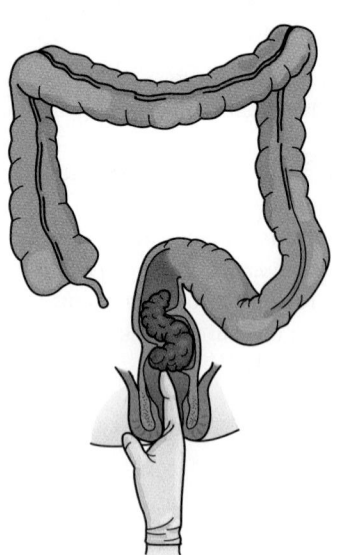

Fig. 23-3 A gloved index finger is used to check for a fecal impaction.

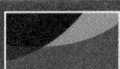 **CHECKING FOR A FECAL IMPACTION**

QUALITY OF LIFE

Remember to:
- Knock before entering the person's room.
- Address the person by name.
- Introduce yourself by name and title.

- Explain the procedure to the person before beginning and during the procedure.
- Protect the person's rights during the procedure.
- Handle the person gently during the procedure.

PRE-PROCEDURE

1 Follow *Delegation Guidelines: Fecal Impaction.* See *Promoting Safety and Comfort: Fecal Impaction.*
2 Practice hand hygiene.
3 Collect the following:
- Bedpan and cover
- Bath blanket
- Toilet tissue
- Gloves
- Lubricant
- Waterproof pad
- Basin of warm water
- Soap
- Washcloth
- Bath towel
4 Practice hand hygiene.
5 Identify the person. Check the ID (identification) bracelet against the assignment sheet. Also call the person by name.
6 Provide for privacy.
7 Raise the bed for body mechanics. Bed rails are up if used.

PROCEDURE

8 Lower the bed rail near you if up.
9 Cover the person with a bath blanket. Fan-fold top linens to the foot of the bed.
10 Position the person in Sims' position or in a left side-lying position.
11 Put on the gloves.
12 Place the waterproof pad under the buttocks.
13 Expose the anal area.
14 Lubricate your gloved index finger.
15 Ask the person to take a deep breath through his or her mouth.
16 Insert the gloved finger while the person is taking a deep breath.
17 Check for a fecal mass.
18 Remove your finger.
19 Remove and discard the gloves. Practice hand hygiene. Put on clean gloves.
20 Help the person onto the bedpan. Raise the head of the bed and raise the bed rail if used. Or assist the person to the bathroom or commode. The person wears a robe and non-skid footwear when up. The bed is in the lowest position.

21 Place the signal light and toilet tissue within reach. Remind the person not to flush the toilet.
22 Discard disposable items.
23 Remove and discard the gloves. Practice hand hygiene.
24 Leave the room if the person can be left alone.
25 Return when the person signals. Or check on the person every 5 minutes. Knock before entering.
26 Practice hand hygiene, and put on gloves. Lower the bed rail if up.
27 Observe stools for amount, color, consistency, shape, and odor.
28 Provide perineal care as needed.
29 Remove the waterproof pad.
30 Empty, rinse, clean, and disinfect equipment. If the person had a BM, flush the toilet after the nurse observes it.
31 Return equipment to its proper place.
32 Remove and discard the gloves. Practice hand hygiene after removing and discarding the gloves.
33 Assist with hand washing. Wear gloves for this step. Practice hand hygiene after removing and discarding the gloves.
34 Cover the person. Remove the bath blanket.

POST-PROCEDURE

35 Provide for comfort. (See the inside of the front book cover.)
36 Place the signal light within reach.
37 Lower the bed to its lowest position.
38 Raise or lower bed rails. Follow the care plan.
39 Unscreen the person.

40 Complete a safety check of the room. (See the inside of the front book cover.)
41 Follow agency policy for dirty linen and used supplies.
42 Practice hand hygiene.
43 Report and record your observations.

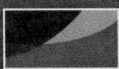 **REMOVING A FECAL IMPACTION**

QUALITY OF LIFE

Remember to:
- Knock before entering the person's room.
- Address the person by name.
- Introduce yourself by name and title.

- Explain the procedure to the person before beginning and during the procedure.
- Protect the person's rights during the procedure.
- Handle the person gently during the procedure.

PROCEDURE

1 Follow steps 1 through 10 in procedure: *Checking for a Fecal Impaction*, p. 411.
2 Check the person's pulse (Chapter 26). Note the rate and rhythm.
3 Practice hand hygiene. Put on the gloves.
4 Place the waterproof pad under the buttocks.
5 Expose the anal area.
6 Lubricate your gloved index finger.
7 Ask the person to take a deep breath through the mouth.
8 Insert your lubricated, gloved index finger.
9 Hook your index finger around a small piece of feces.
10 Remove your finger and the feces.

11 Drop the stool into the bedpan.
12 Clean your finger with toilet tissue. Place the toilet tissue in the bedpan.
13 Repeat steps 7 through 12 until you no longer feel feces.
14 *Check the person's pulse at intervals. Use your clean gloved hand. Note the rate and rhythm. Stop the procedure if the pulse rate has slowed or if the rhythm is irregular.*
15 Wipe the anal area with toilet tissue.
16 Follow steps 19 through 43 in procedure: *Checking for a Fecal Impaction*, p. 411.

Diarrhea

Diarrhea is the frequent passage of liquid stools. Feces move through the intestines rapidly. This reduces the time for fluid absorption. The need for a BM is urgent. Some people cannot get to a bathroom in time. Abdominal cramping, nausea, and vomiting may occur.

Causes of diarrhea include infections, some drugs, irritating foods, and microbes in food and water. Diet and drugs are ordered to reduce peristalsis. You need to:
- Assist with elimination needs promptly.
- Dispose of stools promptly. This prevents odors and the spread of microbes.
- Give good skin care. Liquid stools irritate the skin. So does frequent wiping with toilet tissue. Skin breakdown and pressure ulcers are risks.

Fluid lost through diarrhea must be replaced. Otherwise dehydration occurs. *Dehydration is the excessive loss of water from tissues.* The person has pale or flushed skin, dry skin, and a coated tongue. The urine is dark and scant in amount (oliguria). Thirst, weakness, dizziness, and confusion also occur. Falling blood pressure and increased pulse and respirations are serious signs. Death can occur. The nursing process is used to meet the person's fluid needs. The doctor may order IV (intravenous) fluids in severe cases (Chapter 25).

FOCUS ON CHILDREN AND OLDER PERSONS
Diarrhea

Children
Infants and young children have large amounts of body water. Dehydration is a risk. Death can be rapid. Report any liquid or watery stool at once. Ask the nurse to observe the stool. Note the number of wet diapers. Infants wet less when dehydrated.

Older Persons
Older persons are at risk for dehydration. The amount of body water decreases with aging. Many diseases common in older persons affect body fluids. So do many drugs. Report signs of diarrhea at once. Ask the nurse to observe the stool. Death is a risk when dehydration is not recognized and treated.

Microbes can cause diarrhea. Preventing the spread of infection is important. Always follow Standard Precautions and the Bloodborne Pathogen Standard when in contact with stools.

See *Focus on Children and Older Persons: Diarrhea.*
See *Promoting Safety and Comfort: Diarrhea.*

Safety

Clostridium difficile (C. difficile) is a microbe that causes diarrhea and intestinal infections. It can cause death. Persons at risk include those who are older, ill, or need the prolonged use of antibiotics. Signs and symptoms include:

- Watery diarrhea with a foul odor
- Fever
- Loss of appetite
- Nausea
- Abdominal pain or tenderness

The microbe is found in feces. A person becomes infected by touching items or surfaces contaminated with feces and then touching his or her mouth or mucous membranes. You can spread the microbe if your contaminated hands or gloves:

- Touch a person.
- Contaminate surfaces.

You must practice good hand hygiene. Alcohol-based hand rubs are not effective against *C. difficile*. You must wash your hands with soap and water. Also follow Standard Precautions.

Fecal Incontinence

Fecal incontinence is the inability to control the passage of feces and gas through the anus. Causes include:

- Intestinal diseases.
- Nervous system diseases and injuries.
- Fecal impaction.
- Diarrhea.
- Some drugs.
- Chronic illness.
- Aging.
- Mental health problems or dementia (Chapters 45 and 46). The person may not recognize the need for or act of having a BM.
- Not answering signal lights when help is needed with elimination.
- Not getting to the bathroom in time. The person may have mobility problems or he or she may walk slowly. Or the bathroom may be too far away.
- Not finding the bathroom when in a new setting.

Fecal incontinence affects the person emotionally. Frustration, embarrassment, anger, and humiliation are common. The person may need:

- Bowel training
- Help with elimination after meals and every 2 to 3 hours
- Incontinence products to keep garments and linens clean
- Good skin care

See *Focus on Children and Older Persons: Fecal Incontinence.*

Children

Infants and toddlers normally have fecal incontinence until toilet trained.

Older Persons

Persons with dementia may smear stools on themselves, furniture, and walls. Some are not aware of having BMs. Some resist care. Follow the person's care plan. The measures for urinary incontinence (Chapter 22) may be part of the care plan. Be patient. Ask for help from co-workers. Talk to the nurse if you have problems keeping the person clean.

Flatulence

Gas and air are normally in the stomach and intestines. They are expelled through the mouth (burping, belching, eructating) and anus. *Gas or air passed through the anus is called flatus. Flatulence is the excessive formation of gas or air in the stomach and intestines.* Causes include:

- Swallowing air while eating and drinking. This includes chewing gum, eating fast, drinking through a straw, and drinking carbonated beverages. Tense or anxious people may swallow large amounts of air when drinking.
- Bacterial action in the intestines.
- Gas-forming foods (onions, beans, cabbage, cauliflower, radishes, and cucumbers).
- Constipation.
- Bowel and abdominal surgeries.
- Drugs that decrease peristalsis.

If flatus is not expelled, the intestines distend. That is, they swell or enlarge from the pressure of gases. Abdominal cramping or pain, shortness of breath, and a swollen abdomen occur. "Bloating" is a common complaint. Exercise, walking, moving in bed, and the left side-lying position often produce flatus. Doctors may order enemas and drugs to relieve flatulence.

BOWEL TRAINING

Bowel training has two goals:

- To gain control of bowel movements.
- To develop a regular pattern of elimination. Fecal impaction, constipation, and fecal incontinence are prevented.

Meals, especially breakfast, stimulate the urge for a BM. The person's usual time of day for a BM is noted on the care plan. So is toilet, commode, or bedpan use. Offer help with elimination at the times noted. Factors that promote elimination are part of the care plan and bowel training program. These include a high-fiber diet, increased fluids, warm fluids, activity, and privacy. The nurse tells you about a person's bowel training program.

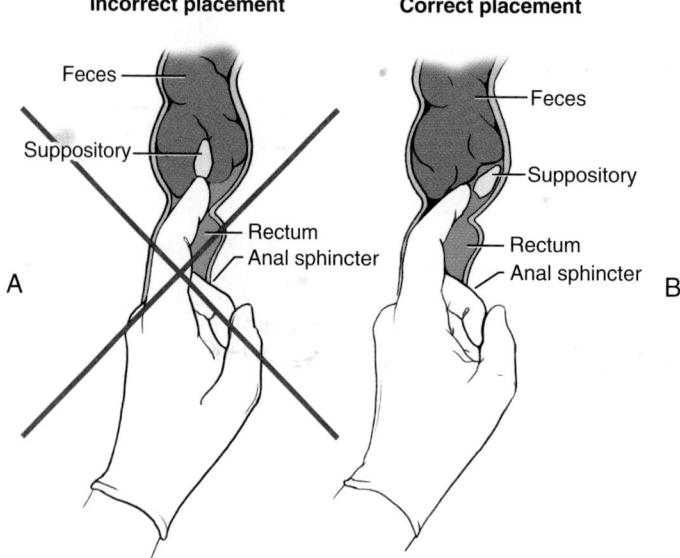

Fig. 23-4 A, The rectal suppository is not inserted into feces. **B,** The suppository is inserted into the rectum along the rectal wall.

SUPPOSITORIES

A *suppository is a cone-shaped, solid drug that is inserted into a body opening. It melts at body temperature.* A rectal suppository is inserted into the rectum (Fig. 23-4). A BM occurs about 30 minutes later.

The doctor may order a suppository to stimulate a BM for:

*   Constipation
*   Fecal impaction
*   Bowel training

See *Delegation Guidelines: Suppositories.*
See *Promoting Safety and Comfort: Suppositories.*

ENEMAS

An *enema is the introduction of fluid into the rectum and lower colon.* Doctors order enemas:

- To remove feces
- To relieve constipation, fecal impaction, or flatulence
- To clean the bowel of feces before certain surgeries and diagnostic procedures

Safety and comfort measures for bowel elimination are practiced when giving an enema (see Box 23-1). So are the rules in Box 23-2.

The doctor orders the enema solution. The solution depends on the enema's purpose—for cleansing, constipation, fecal impaction, or flatulence.

- *Tap water enema*—is obtained from a faucet.
- *Saline enema*—a solution of salt and water. For adults, add 1 to 2 teaspoons of table salt to 500 to 1000 mL (milliliters) of tap water.
- *Soapsuds enema (SSE)*—is for adults. Add 3 to 5 mL of castile soap to 500 to 1000 mL of tap water.
- *Small-volume enema*—the adult size contains about 120 mL (4 ounces [oz]) of solution. The child size contains about 60 mL (2 oz). The commercially prepared enema is ready to use.
- *Oil-retention enema*—has mineral, olive, or cottonseed oil. The adult size contains about 120 mL (4 oz) of solution. Children receive 60 mL (2 oz). The commercially prepared enema is ready to use.

Other enema solutions may be ordered. Consult with the nurse and use the agency's procedure manual to safely prepare and give enemas. You do not give enemas that contain drugs. Nurses give them.

See *Delegation Guidelines: Enemas.*
See *Promoting Safety and Comfort: Enemas*, p. 416.

| BOX 23-2 | SAFETY AND COMFORT MEASURES FOR GIVING ENEMAS |

- Have the person void first. This increases the person's comfort during the enema procedure.
- Measure solution temperature with a bath thermometer. See *Delegation Guidelines: Enemas.*
- Give the amount of solution ordered.
- Position the person as the nurse directs. The Sims' position or the left side-lying position is preferred.
- Ask the nurse and check the procedure manual for how far to insert the enema tubing. It is usually inserted 2 to 4 inches in adults.
- Lubricate the enema tip before inserting it.
- Stop tube insertion if you feel resistance, the person complains of pain, or bleeding occurs.
- Ask the nurse how high to raise the enema bag. For adults, it is usually held 12 inches above the anus.
- Give the solution slowly. Usually it takes 10 to 15 minutes to give 750 to 1000 mL.
- Hold the enema tube in place while giving the solution.
- Ask the nurse how long the person should retain the solution. The length of time depends on the amount and type of solution.
- Make sure the bathroom will be vacant when the person needs to have a BM. Make sure that another person will not use the bathroom. If the person uses the bedpan or commode, have the device ready.
- Ask the nurse to observe the enema results.

DELEGATION GUIDELINES
Enemas

Some states and agencies let nursing assistants give enemas. Others do not. Before giving an enema, make sure that:

- Your state allows you to perform the procedure.
- The procedure is in your job description.
- You have the necessary education and training.
- You review the procedure with a nurse.
- A nurse is available to answer questions and to supervise you.

If the above conditions are met, you need this information from the nurse:

- What type of enema to give—cleansing, small-volume, or oil-retention
- What size enema tube to use
- What lubricant to use
- When to give the enema
- How many times to repeat the enema
- The amount of solution ordered by the doctor—usually 500 to 1000 mL for a cleansing enema (for adults)
- How much castile soap to use for an SSE
- How much salt to use for a saline enema
- What the solution temperature should be—usually body temperature (98.6°F [Fahrenheit] or 37°C [centigrade]); sometimes warmer temperatures (105°F [40.5°C]) are used for adults
- How to position the person—Sims' or the left side-lying position
- How far to insert the enema tubing—usually 2 to 4 inches for adults
- How high to hold the solution container—usually 12 inches above the anus
- How fast to give the solution—750 to 1000 mL are usually given over 10 to 15 minutes
- How long the person should try to retain the solution
- What to report and record:
  - The amount of solution given
  - If you noted bleeding or resistance when inserting the tube
  - How long the person retained the enema solution
  - Color, amount, consistency, shape, and odor of stools
  - Complaints of cramping, pain, or discomfort
  - Complaints of nausea or weakness
  - How the person tolerated the procedure
- When to report observations
- What patient or resident concerns to report at once

Safety

Enemas are usually safe procedures. Many people give themselves enemas at home. However, enemas are dangerous for older persons and those with certain heart and kidney diseases.

Contact with stools is likely when giving enemas. Stools contain microbes and may contain blood. Follow Standard Precautions and the Bloodborne Pathogen Standard.

Comfort

Before starting the procedure, make sure that the bathroom is ready for the person's use. If the person will use the commode or bedpan, make sure the device is ready. Always keep a bedpan nearby in case the person starts to expel the enema solution and stools. Mental comfort is promoted when the person knows that the bathroom, commode, or bedpan is ready for use.

The person needs to retain the solution as long as possible. Make sure the person is comfortable in the Sims' or left side-lying position. When comfortable, it is easier for the person to tolerate the procedure.

To prevent cramping:
- Use the correct water temperature. Cool water causes cramping.
- Give the solution slowly.

The Cleansing Enema

Cleansing enemas clean the bowel of feces and flatus. They relieve constipation and fecal impaction. They are needed before certain surgeries and diagnostic procedures. Cleansing enemas take effect in 10 to 20 minutes.

The doctor orders a tap water, saline, or soapsuds enema. The doctor may order *enemas until clear*. This means that enemas are given until the return solution is clear and free of stools. Ask the nurse how many enemas to give. Agency policy may allow repeating enemas 2 or 3 times.

Tap-water enemas can be dangerous. The colon may absorb some of the water into the bloodstream. This creates a fluid imbalance. *Only 1 tap-water enema is given. Do not repeat the enema.* Repeated enemas increase the risk of excessive fluid absorption.

The *saline enema* solution is similar to body fluid. However, some of the salt solution may be absorbed. This too can cause a fluid imbalance. When excess salt is in the body, the body retains water.

Soapsuds enemas irritate the bowel's mucous lining. Repeated enemas can damage the bowel. So can using more than 3 to 5 mL of castile soap or stronger soaps.

See *Focus on Children and Older Persons: The Cleansing Enema.*

Children

Saline enemas are used for cleansing enemas in children. Check with the nurse for the amount of solution to give. These are guidelines:
- Infant—120 to 240 mL
- 2 to 4 years—240 to 360 mL
- 4 to 10 years—360 to 480 mL
- 11 years and older—480 to 720 mL

The nurse tells you how far to insert the enema tube. These are guidelines:
- Infants—1 inch
- 2 to 4 years—2 inches
- 4 to 10 years—2 to 3 inches
- 11 years and older—2 to 4 inches

Infants cannot tell you they hurt. If cramping occurs, the child will draw up the knees. The child's cry is higher-pitched than normal.

In children, cleansing enemas take effect in about 2 to 5 minutes.

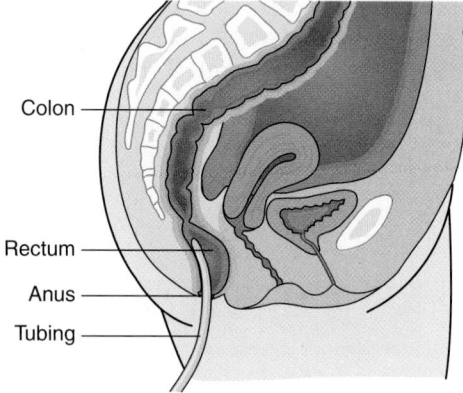

Fig. 23-5 Enema tubing inserted into the adult rectum.

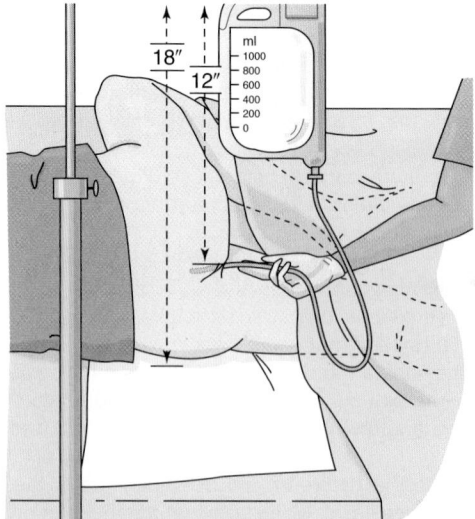

Fig. 23-6 Giving an enema. The person is in Sims' position. The enema bag hangs from an IV pole. The bag is 12 inches above the anus and 18 inches above the mattress.

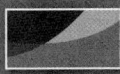 **GIVING A CLEANSING ENEMA** `VIDEO`

QUALITY OF LIFE

Remember to:
- Knock before entering the person's room.
- Address the person by name.
- Introduce yourself by name and title.

- Explain the procedure to the person before beginning and during the procedure.
- Protect the person's rights during the procedure.
- Handle the person gently during the procedure.

PRE-PROCEDURE

1 Follow *Delegation Guidelines: Enemas*, p. 415. See *Promoting Safety and Comfort: Enemas.*
2 Practice hand hygiene.
3 Collect the following before going to the person's room:
- Disposable enema kit as directed by the nurse (enema bag, tube, clamp, and waterproof pad)
- Bath thermometer
- Waterproof pad (if not in the enema kit)
- Water soluble lubricant
- 3 to 5 mL (1 teaspoon) castile soap or 1 to 2 teaspoons of salt
- IV pole
- Gloves
4 Arrange items in the person's room and bathroom.
5 Practice hand hygiene.

6 Identify the person. Check the ID bracelet against the assignment sheet. Also call the person by name.
7 Put on gloves.
8 Collect the following:
- Commode or bedpan and cover
- Toilet tissue
- Bath blanket
- Robe and non-skid footwear
- Paper towels
9 Remove and discard the gloves. Practice hand hygiene. Put on clean gloves.
10 Provide for privacy.
11 Raise the bed for body mechanics. Bed rails are up if used.

PROCEDURE

12 Lower the bed rail near you if up.
13 Cover the person with a bath blanket. Fan-fold top linens to the foot of the bed.
14 Position the IV pole so the enema bag is 12 inches above the anus. Or it is at the height directed by the nurse.
15 Raise the bed rail if used.
16 Prepare the enema:
- a Close the clamp on the tube.
- b Adjust water flow until it is lukewarm.
- c Fill the enema bag for the amount ordered.
- d Measure water temperature with the bath thermometer. The nurse tells you what temperature to use.
- e Prepare the solution as directed by the nurse:
  - (1) Tap water: add nothing.
  - (2) Saline enema: add salt as directed.
  - (3) SSE: add castile soap as directed.
- f Stir the solution with the bath thermometer. Scoop off any suds (SSE).
- g Seal the bag.
- h Hang the bag on the IV pole.
17 Lower the bed rail near you if up.
18 Position the person in Sims' position or in a left side-lying position.
19 Place a waterproof pad under the buttocks.
20 Expose the anal area.
21 Place the bedpan behind the person.
22 Position the enema tube in the bedpan. Remove the cap from the tubing.
23 Open the clamp. Let solution flow through the tube to remove air. Clamp the tube.
24 Lubricate the tube 2 to 4 inches from the tip.
25 Separate the buttocks to see the anus.
26 Ask the person to take a deep breath through the mouth.

27 Insert the tube gently 2 to 4 inches into the adult's rectum (Fig. 23-5). Do this when the person is exhaling. Stop if the person complains of pain, you feel resistance, or bleeding occurs.
28 Check the amount of solution in the bag.
29 Unclamp the tube. Give the solution slowly (Fig. 23-6).
30 Ask the person to take slow deep breaths. This helps the person relax.
31 Clamp the tube if the person needs to have a BM, has cramping, or starts to expel solution. Also, clamp the tube if the person is sweating or complains of nausea or weakness. Unclamp when symptoms subside.
32 Give the amount of solution ordered. Stop if the person cannot tolerate the procedure.
33 Clamp the tube before it is empty. This prevents air from entering the bowel.
34 Hold toilet tissue around the tube and against the anus. Remove the tube.
35 Discard toilet tissue into the bedpan.
36 Wrap the tubing tip with paper towels. Place it inside the enema bag.
37 Assist the person to the bathroom or commode. The person wears a robe and non-skid footwear when up. The bed is in the lowest position. Or help the person onto the bedpan. Raise the head of the bed. Raise or lower bed rails according to the care plan.
38 Place the signal light and toilet tissue within reach. Remind the person not to flush the toilet.
39 Discard disposable items.
40 Remove and discard the gloves. Practice hand hygiene.
41 Leave the room if the person can be left alone.
42 Return when the person signals. Or check on the person every 5 minutes. Knock before entering the room or bathroom.

Continued

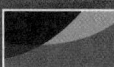

GIVING A CLEANSING ENEMA—cont'd   VIDEO

PROCEDURE—cont'd

43 Practice hand hygiene and put on gloves. Lower the bed rail if up.
44 Observe enema results for amount, color, consistency, shape, and odor. Call the nurse to observe the results.
45 Provide perineal care as needed.
46 Remove the waterproof pad.
47 Empty, rinse, clean, and disinfect equipment. Flush the toilet after the nurse observes the results.
48 Return equipment to its proper place.
49 Remove and discard the gloves. Practice hand hygiene.
50 Assist with hand washing. Wear gloves for this step. Practice hand hygiene after removing and discarding the gloves.
51 Cover the person. Remove the bath blanket.

POST-PROCEDURE

52 Provide for comfort. (See the inside of the front book cover.)
53 Place the signal light within reach.
54 Lower the bed to its lowest position.
55 Raise or lower bed rails. Follow the care plan.
56 Unscreen the person.
57 Complete a safety check of the room. (See the inside of the front book cover.)
58 Follow agency policy for dirty linen and used supplies.
59 Practice hand hygiene.
60 Report and record your observations.

The Small-Volume Enema

Small-volume enemas irritate and distend the rectum. This causes a BM. They are often ordered for constipation or when the bowel does not need complete cleansing.

These enemas are ready to give. The solution is usually given at room temperature. To give the enema, squeeze and roll up the plastic container from the bottom. Do not release pressure on the bottle. Otherwise, solution is drawn from the rectum back into the bottle.

Urge the person to retain the solution until he or she needs to have a BM. This usually takes about 5 to 10 minutes. Staying in the Sims' or left side-lying position helps retain the enema.

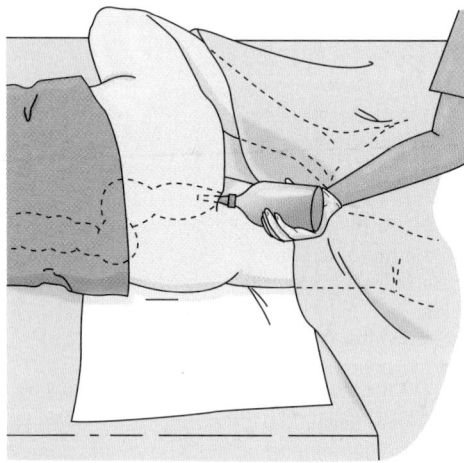

Fig. 23-7 The small-volume enema tip is inserted 2 inches into the rectum.

GIVING A SMALL-VOLUME ENEMA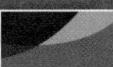

VIDEO

QUALITY OF LIFE

Remember to:
- Knock before entering the person's room.
- Address the person by name.
- Introduce yourself by name and title.

- Explain the procedure to the person before beginning and during the procedure.
- Protect the person's rights during the procedure.
- Handle the person gently during the procedure.

PRE-PROCEDURE

1. Follow *Delegation Guidelines: Enemas,* p. 415. See *Promoting Safety and Comfort: Enemas,* p. 416.
2. Practice hand hygiene.
3. Collect the following before going to the person's room:
   - Small-volume enema
   - Waterproof pad
   - Gloves
4. Arrange items in the person's room.
5. Practice hand hygiene.
6. Identify the person. Check the ID bracelet against the assignment sheet. Also call the person by name.
7. Put on gloves.
8. Collect the following:
   - Commode or bedpan
   - Toilet tissue
   - Robe and non-skid footwear
   - Bath blanket
9. Remove and discard the gloves. Practice hand hygiene. Put on clean gloves.
10. Provide for privacy.
11. Raise the bed for body mechanics. Bed rails are up if used.

PROCEDURE

12. Lower the bed rail near you if up.
13. Cover the person with a bath blanket. Fan-fold top linens to the foot of the bed.
14. Position the person in Sims' or a left side-lying position.
15. Place the waterproof pad under the buttocks.
16. Expose the anal area.
17. Position the bedpan near the person.
18. Remove the cap from the enema tip.
19. Separate the buttocks to see the anus.
20. Ask the person to take a deep breath through the mouth.
21. Insert the enema tip 2 inches into the adult's rectum (Fig. 23-7). Do this when the person is exhaling. Insert the tip gently. Stop if the person complains of pain, you feel resistance, or bleeding occurs.
22. Squeeze and roll up the container gently. Release pressure on the bottle after you remove the tip from the rectum.
23. Put the container into the box, tip first. Discard the container and box.
24. Assist the person to the bathroom or commode when he or she has the urge to have a BM. The person wears a robe and non-skid footwear when up. The bed is in the lowest position. Or help the person onto the bedpan, and raise the head of the bed. Raise or lower bed rails according to the care plan.
25. Place the signal light and toilet tissue within reach. Remind the person not to flush the toilet.
26. Discard disposable items.
27. Remove and discard the gloves. Practice hand hygiene.
28. Leave the room if the person can be left alone.
29. Return when the person signals. Or check on the person every 5 minutes. Knock before entering the room or bathroom.
30. Practice hand hygiene. Put on gloves.
31. Lower the bed rail if up.
32. Observe enema results for amount, color, consistency, shape, and odor. Call the nurse to observe the results.
33. Provide perineal care as needed.
34. Remove the waterproof pad.
35. Empty, rinse, clean, and disinfect equipment. Flush the toilet after the nurse observes the results.
36. Return equipment to its proper place.
37. Remove and discard the gloves. Practice hand hygiene.
38. Assist with hand washing. Wear gloves for this step. Practice hand hygiene after removing and discarding the gloves.
39. Cover the person. Remove the bath blanket.

POST-PROCEDURE

40. Provide for comfort. (See the inside of the front book cover.)
41. Place the signal light within reach.
42. Lower the bed to its lowest position.
43. Raise or lower bed rails. Follow the care plan.
44. Unscreen the person.
45. Complete a safety check of the room. (See the inside of the front book cover.)
46. Follow agency policy for dirty linen and used supplies.
47. Practice hand hygiene.
48. Report and record your observations.

The Oil-Retention Enema

Oil-retention enemas relieve constipation and fecal impactions. The oil is retained for 30 to 60 minutes or longer (1 to 3 hours). Retaining oil softens feces and lubricates the rectum. This lets feces pass with ease. Most oil-retention enemas are commercially prepared.

See *Promoting Safety and Comfort: The Oil-Retention Enema.*

PROMOTING SAFETY AND COMFORT
The Oil-Retention Enema

Safety

The oil-retention enema is retained for at least 30 to 60 minutes. Leave the room after giving the enema. Check on the person often. After checking on the person, tell him and her when you will return. Remind the person to signal for you if he or she needs help. Report any problems to the nurse at once.

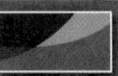 ## GIVING AN OIL-RETENTION ENEMA

QUALITY OF LIFE

Remember to:
- Knock before entering the person's room.
- Address the person by name.
- Introduce yourself by name and title.

- Explain the procedure to the person before beginning and during the procedure.
- Protect the person's rights during the procedure.
- Handle the person gently during the procedure.

PRE-PROCEDURE

1 Follow *Delegation Guidelines: Enemas*, p. 415. See *Promoting Safety and Comfort:*
   a *Enemas*, p. 416
   b *The Oil-Retention Enema*
2 Practice hand hygiene.
3 Collect the following:
- Oil-retention enema
- Waterproof pads

- Gloves
- Bath blanket
4 Arrange items in the person's room.
5 Practice hand hygiene.
6 Identify the person. Check the ID bracelet against the assignment sheet. Also call the person by name.
7 Provide for privacy.
8 Raise the bed for body mechanics. Bed rails are up if used.

PROCEDURE

9 Put on gloves.
10 Follow steps 12 through 23 in procedure: *Giving a Small-Volume Enema*, p. 419.
11 Cover the person. Leave him or her in the Sims' or left side-lying position.

12 Encourage him or her to retain the enema for the time ordered.
13 Place more waterproof pads on the bed if needed.
14 Remove and discard the gloves. Practice hand hygiene.

POST-PROCEDURE

15 Provide for comfort. (See the inside of the front book cover.)
16 Place the signal light within reach.
17 Lower the bed to its lowest position.
18 Raise or lower bed rails. Follow the care plan.
19 Unscreen the person.

20 Complete a safety check of the room. (See the inside of the front book cover.)
21 Follow agency policy for dirty linen and used supplies.
22 Practice hand hygiene.
23 Report and record your observations.
24 Check the person often.

THE PERSON WITH AN OSTOMY

Sometimes part of the intestines is removed surgically. Cancer, bowel disease, and trauma (stab or bullet wounds) are common reasons. An ostomy is sometimes necessary. An *ostomy is a surgically created opening for the elimination of body wastes. The opening seen through the abdominal wall is called a stoma.* The person wears a pouch over the stoma to collect stools and flatus.

Colostomy

A *colostomy is a surgically created opening* (stomy) *between the colon* (colo) *and abdominal wall.* Part of the colon is brought out onto the abdominal wall, and a stoma is made. Feces and flatus pass through the stoma instead of the anus.

Colostomies are temporary or permanent. If permanent, the diseased part of the colon is removed. A temporary colostomy gives the diseased or injured bowel time to heal. After healing, surgery is done to reconnect the bowel.

The colostomy site depends on the site of disease or injury (Fig. 23-8). Stool consistency—liquid to formed—depends on the colostomy site. The more colon remaining to absorb water, the more solid and formed the stool. If the colostomy is near the start of the colon, stools are liquid. If near the end of the colon, stools are formed.

Stools irritate the skin. Skin care prevents skin breakdown around the stoma. The skin is washed and dried. Then a skin barrier is applied around the stoma. It prevents stools from having contact with the skin. The skin barrier is part of the pouch or a separate device.

Ileostomy

An *ileostomy is a surgically created opening* (stomy) *between the ileum* (small intestine [ileo]) *and the abdominal wall.* Part of the ileum is brought out onto the abdominal wall, and a stoma is made. The entire colon is removed (Fig. 23-9, p. 422).

Liquid stools drain constantly from an ileostomy. Water is not absorbed because the colon was removed. Feces in the small intestine contain digestive juices that are very irritating to the skin. The ileostomy pouch must fit well. Stools must not touch the skin. Good skin care is required.

Ostomy Pouches

The pouch has an adhesive backing that is applied to the skin. Some pouches are secured to ostomy belts (Fig. 23-10, p. 422).

Pouches have a drain at the bottom that close with a clip, clamp, or wire closure. The drain is opened to empty the pouch. The pouch is emptied when stools are present. It is opened when it balloons or bulges with flatus. The drain is wiped with toilet tissue before it is closed.

The pouch is changed every 3 to 7 days and when it leaks. Frequent pouch changes can damage the skin.

Odors are prevented by:
- Performing good hygiene.
- Emptying the pouch.
- Avoiding gas-forming foods.
- Putting deodorants into the pouch. The nurse tells you what to use.

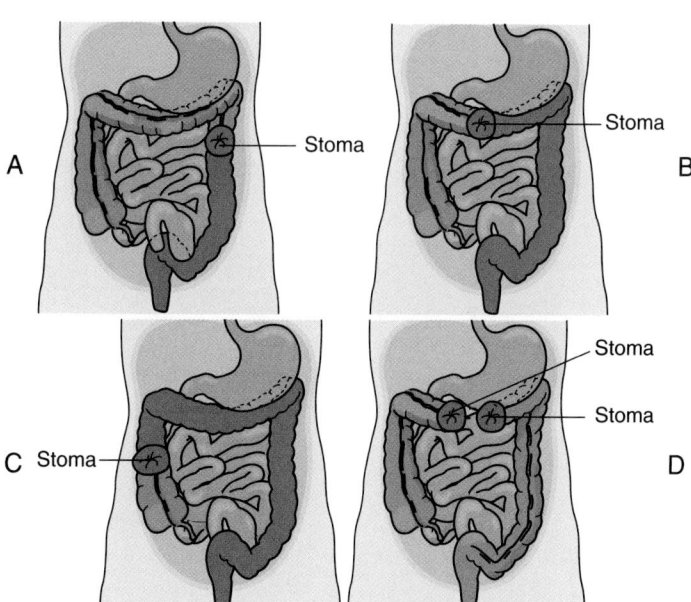

Fig. 23-8 Colostomy sites. *Shading* shows the part of the bowel surgically removed. **A,** Sigmoid or descending colostomy. **B,** Transverse colostomy. **C,** Ascending colostomy. **D,** Double-barrel colostomy has two stomas. One allows for the excretion of feces. The other is for the introduction of drugs to help the bowel heal. This type of colostomy is usually temporary.

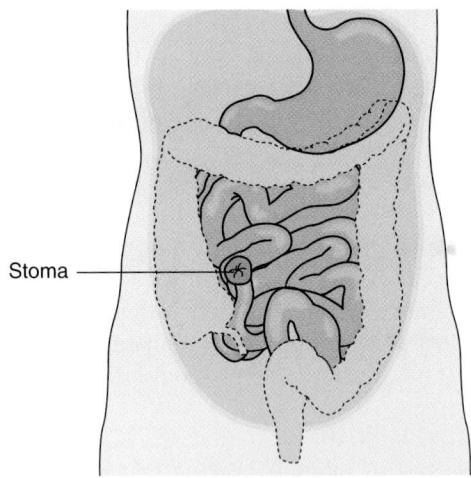

Fig. 23-9 An ileostomy. The entire large intestine is surgically removed.

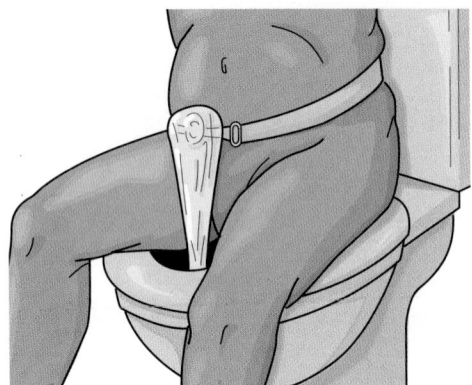

Fig. 23-10 The ostomy pouch is secured to an ostomy belt. The pouch is emptied by directing it into the toilet and opening the end.

The person wears normal clothes. However, tight garments can prevent feces from entering the pouch. Also, bulging from stools and flatus can be seen with tight clothes.

Peristalsis increases after eating and drinking. Therefore, stomas are usually quiet after sleep. That is, expelling feces is less likely at this time. If the person showers or bathes with the pouch off, it is best done before breakfast. Showers and baths are delayed for 1 to 2 hours after applying a new pouch. This gives adhesive time to seal to the skin.

Do not flush pouches down the toilet. Follow agency policy to dispose of them.

See *Focus on Children and Older Persons: Ostomy Pouches.*
See *Delegation Guidelines: Ostomy Pouches.*
See *Promoting Safety and Comfort: Ostomy Pouches.*

QUALITY OF LIFE

Remember to:
- Knock before entering the person's room.
- Address the person by name.
- Introduce yourself by name and title.
- Explain the procedure to the person before beginning and during the procedure.
- Protect the person's rights during the procedure.
- Handle the person gently during the procedure.

PRE-PROCEDURE

1 Follow *Delegation Guidelines: Ostomy Pouches.* See *Promoting Safety and Comfort: Ostomy Pouches.*
2 Practice hand hygiene.
3 Collect the following before going to the person's room:
- Clean pouch with skin barrier
- Pouch clamp, clip, or wire closure
- Clean ostomy belt (if used)
- Gauze pads or washcloths
- Adhesive remover wipes
- Skin paste (optional)
- Pouch deodorant
- Disposable bag
- Gloves
- Paper towels
4 Place the paper towels on the overbed table. Arrange supplies on top of the paper towels.

5 Practice hand hygiene.
6 Identify the person. Check the ID bracelet against the assignment sheet. Also call the person by name.
7 Put on gloves.
8 Collect the following:
- Bedpan with cover
- Waterproof pad
- Bath blanket
- Wash basin with warm water
9 Remove and discard the gloves. Practice hand hygiene. Put on clean gloves.
10 Provide for privacy.
11 Raise the bed for body mechanics. Bed rails are up if used.

PROCEDURE

12 Lower the bed rail near you if up.
13 Cover the person with a bath blanket. Fan-fold linens to the foot of the bed.
14 Place the waterproof pad under the buttocks.
15 Disconnect the pouch from the belt if one is worn. Remove the belt.
16 Remove and place the pouch and skin barrier in the bedpan. Gently push the skin down and lift up on the barrier. Use the adhesive remover wipes if necessary.
17 Wipe the stoma and around it with a gauze pad. This removes excess stool and mucus. Discard the gauze pad into the disposable bag.
18 Wet the gauze pads or the washcloth.
19 Wash the stoma and the skin around it with a gauze pad or washcloth. Wash gently. Do not scrub or rub the skin.
20 Pat dry with a gauze pad or the towel.
21 Observe the stoma and the skin around the stoma. Report bleeding, skin irritation, or skin breakdown.
22 Remove the backing from the new pouch.
23 Apply a thin layer of paste around the pouch opening. Let it dry following the manufacturer's instructions.

24 Pull the skin around the stoma taut. The skin must be wrinkle-free.
25 Center the pouch over the stoma. The drain is downward.
26 Press around the pouch and skin barrier so it seals to the skin. Apply gentle pressure with your fingers. Start at the bottom and work up around the sides to the top.
27 Maintain the pressure for 1 to 2 minutes. Follow the manufacturer's instructions.
28 Tug downward on the pouch gently. Make sure the pouch is secure.
29 Add deodorant to the pouch.
30 Close the pouch at the bottom. Use a clamp, clip, or wire closure.
31 Attach the ostomy belt if used. The belt should not be too tight. You should be able to slide 2 fingers under the belt.
32 Remove the waterproof pad.
33 Discard disposable supplies into the disposable bag.
34 Remove and discard the gloves. Practice hand hygiene.
35 Cover the person. Remove the bath blanket.

POST-PROCEDURE

36 Provide for comfort. (See the inside of the front book cover.)
37 Place the signal light within reach.
38 Lower the bed to its lowest position.
39 Raise or lower bed rails. Follow the care plan.
40 Unscreen the person.
41 Practice hand hygiene. Put on gloves.
42 Take the bedpan and disposable bag into the bathroom.
43 Empty the pouch and bedpan into the toilet. Observe the color, amount, consistency, and odor of stools. Flush the toilet.

44 Discard the pouch into the disposable bag. Discard the disposable bag.
45 Empty, rinse, clean, and disinfect equipment. Return equipment to its proper place.
46 Remove and discard the gloves. Practice hand hygiene.
47 Complete a safety check of the room. (See the inside of the front book cover.)
48 Follow agency policy for dirty linens.
49 Practice hand hygiene.
50 Report and record your observations.

The Person, Family, and Yourself

Personal and Professional Responsibility

You are responsible for knowing the legal limits of your role. Some states and agencies allow nursing assistants to insert some types of suppositories. If your state and agency allow this, you must know your limits. Because you are allowed to insert *some* types, does not mean you are allowed to insert *all* types.

For example, you may only be allowed to insert suppositories in persons who receive them regularly for constipation. You are not allowed to give a suppository for fever or vomiting. Know what you are and are not allowed to do. Never perform a task beyond the legal limits of your role.

Rights and Respect

Bowel elimination is typically done in private. Illness, disease, surgery, and aging can affect this private act. Some persons may feel embarrassed to have a BM in a strange environment. You can help the person feel more comfortable by respecting his or her privacy. To promote comfort and privacy:

- Ask others to leave the room.
- Close doors, curtains, and window coverings.
- Turn on water or music to mask sounds.
- Cover the person.
- Allow the person enough time. Place the signal light nearby and instruct the person to call if help is needed.
- Knock before entering the room. Tell the person who you are. Ask the person if you may enter before opening the door completely.
- Use a spray for odors that is provided by the agency.

Independence and Social Interaction

Persons with ostomies manage their own care if able. Some have had ostomies for a long time. They may have special routines or care measures. Do not react to things that seem odd to you. When you assist them, ask what they prefer. Listen to their requests. Follow their choices in ostomy care. To promote independence, allow personal choice and control as much as safely possible.

Delegation and Teamwork

The nurse may delegate a task to you that you have not done before. For example, a nurse asks you to give an enema or empty a colostomy bag. Never attempt a task that you are not comfortable doing. Make sure your state and agency allow you to perform the procedure. If those conditions are met, politely tell the nurse. You can say: "I'm sorry, but I have never done that task before. I do not feel comfortable doing it on my own. Would you please show me how it is done?" Take pride in making the right choice to tell the nurse about your delegation concern.

Ethics and Laws

Leaving a person sitting or lying in his or her urine or feces is neglect. It is a form of physical abuse. State laws, the Omnibus Budget Reconciliation Act of 1987 (OBRA), and the CMS require the reporting and investigating of abuse. If found guilty of abuse, neglect, or mistreatment of a patient or resident, you will lose your job. The offense is noted on your registry. You cannot work in a nursing center or on a skilled care nursing unit in a hospital. Protect yourself from being accused of neglect. Check on your patients or residents often. Do not allow them to be left sitting or lying in urine or feces.

Circle the BEST answer.

1 Which is *false*?
   a A person must have a BM every day.
   b Stools are normally brown, soft, and formed.
   c Diarrhea occurs when feces move rapidly through the bowels.
   d Constipation results when feces move slowly through the colon.

2 The prolonged retention and buildup of feces in the rectum is called
   a Constipation   c Diarrhea
   b Fecal impaction   d Fecal incontinence

3 Which does *not* promote comfort and safety for bowel elimination?
   a Asking visitors to leave the room
   b Helping the person to a sitting position
   c Offering the bedpan after meals
   d Telling the person that you will return very soon

4 Bowel training is aimed at
   a Bowel control and regular elimination
   b Ostomy control
   c Preventing fecal impaction, constipation, and fecal incontinence
   d Preventing bleeding

5 Your state and agency allow you to insert rectal suppositories. You insert a suppository
   a Into the feces   c Along the rectal wall
   b Into the stoma   d With an enema tube

6 Which is *not* used for a cleansing enema?
   a Castile soap   c Oil
   b Salt   d Tap water

7 Which is used for cleansing enemas in children?
   a Soapsuds   c Oil
   b Saline   d Tap water

8 These statements are about enemas. Which is *false*?
   a The solution should be cool.
   b The Sims' position is used.
   c The enema bag is held 12 inches above the anus.
   d The solution is given slowly.

9 In adults, the enema tube is inserted
   a 2 to 4 inches   c 6 to 8 inches
   b 4 to 6 inches   d 8 to 10 inches

10 The oil-retention enema is retained for at least
   a 10 to 15 minutes   c 30 to 60 minutes
   b 15 to 30 minutes   d 60 to 90 minutes

11 These statements are about ostomies. Which is *false*?
   a Good skin care around the stoma is needed.
   b Deodorants can control odors.
   c The person wears a pouch.
   d Stools are liquid.

12 An ostomy pouch is usually emptied
   a Every 4 to 6 hours
   b Every shift
   c Every 3 to 7 days
   d When stools are present

Answers to these questions are on p. 833.

Nutrition and Fluids

OBJECTIVES

- Define the key terms and key abbreviations listed in this chapter.
- Explain the purpose and use of the MyPlate symbol.
- Describe the functions and sources of nutrients.
- Explain how to read and use food labels.
- Describe the factors that affect eating and nutrition.
- Describe the OBRA requirements for serving food.
- Describe the special diets and between-meal snacks.
- Identify the signs, symptoms, and precautions for aspiration.
- Describe fluid requirements and the causes of dehydration.
- Explain how to assist with special fluid orders.

- Explain the purpose of intake and output records.
- Identify what to count as fluid intake.
- Explain how to assist with food and fluid needs.
- Explain how to assist with calorie counts.
- Explain how to provide drinking water.
- Explain how to prevent foodborne illnesses.
- Perform the procedures described in this chapter.
- Explain how to promote PRIDE in the person, the family, and yourself.

KEY TERMS

anorexia The loss of appetite
aspiration Breathing fluid, food, vomitus, or an object into the lungs
calorie The fuel or energy value of food
cholesterol A soft, waxy substance found in the bloodstream and all body cells
Daily Value (DV) How a serving fits into the daily diet; expressed in a percent (%) based on a daily diet of 2000 calories
dehydration A decrease in the amount of water in body tissues

dysphagia Difficulty *(dys)* swallowing *(phagia)*
edema The swelling of body tissues with water
graduate A measuring container for fluid
intake The amount of fluid taken in
nutrient A substance that is ingested, digested, absorbed, and used by the body
nutrition The processes involved in the ingestion, digestion, absorption, and use of foods and fluids by the body
output The amount of fluid lost

KEY ABBREVIATIONS

CMS	Centers for Medicare & Medicaid Services	**mg**	Milligram
DV	Daily Value	**mL**	Milliliter
F	Fahrenheit	**NPO**	*Non per os;* nothing by mouth
GI	Gastro-intestinal	**OBRA**	Omnibus Budget Reconciliation Act of 1987
ID	Identification	**oz**	Ounce
I&O	Intake and output	**USDA**	United States Department of Agriculture

Food and water are necessary for life. The person's diet affects physical and mental well-being. A poor diet and poor eating habits:
- Increase the risk for infection.
- Increase the risk of acute and chronic diseases.
- Cause chronic illnesses to become worse.
- Cause healing problems.

- Affect physical and mental function, increasing the risk for accidents and injuries.

Eating and drinking provide pleasure. They often are part of social times with family and friends. A friendly, social setting for meals is important. Otherwise, the person may eat poorly.

Many factors affect dietary practices. They include culture, finances, and personal choice. (See *Caring About Culture: Mealtime Practices.*) Dietary practices also include selecting, preparing, and serving food. The health team includes these factors in planning the person's nutrition needs.

See *Body Structure and Function Review: The Digestive System.*

See *Focus on Long-Term Care and Home Care: Nutrition and Fluids.*

⊛ CARING ABOUT CULTURE

Mealtime Practices

Many cultural groups have their main meal at mid-day. The *Austrians* do so. They eat light meals in the evening. Persons from *Brazil* also eat their main meal at noon. They have a light meal in the evening. A main meal at lunch also is common in *Finland*, *Germany*, and *Greece*. In *Iran*, the most important meal is eaten at mid-day.

Modified from D'Avanzo CE: *Pocket guide to cultural health assessment*, ed 4, St Louis, 2008, Mosby.

BODY STRUCTURE AND FUNCTION REVIEW: THE DIGESTIVE SYSTEM

The digestive system (*gastro-intestinal [GI] system*) breaks down food so it can be absorbed for use by the cells. This process is called *digestion*. The system also removes solid wastes from the body.

The digestive system involves the *alimentary canal (GI tract)* and the accessory organs of digestion (Fig. 24-1). The GI tract extends from the mouth to the anus.

Digestion begins in the *mouth (oral cavity)*. It receives food and prepares it for digestion. Using chewing motions, the *teeth* cut, chop, and grind food into small particles for digestion and swallowing. The *tongue* aids in chewing and swallowing. *Taste buds* on the tongue contain nerve endings. Taste buds allow for sensing sweet, sour, bitter, and salty tastes. *Salivary glands* in the mouth secrete saliva. Saliva moistens food particles to ease swallowing and begin digestion. During swallowing, the tongue pushes food into the pharynx.

The *pharynx* (throat) is a muscular tube. Swallowing continues as the pharynx contracts. Contraction of the pharynx pushes food into the esophagus. The *esophagus* is a muscular tube about 10 inches long. It extends from the pharynx to the stomach. Involuntary muscle contractions called *peristalsis* move food down the esophagus through the GI tract.

The *stomach* is a muscular, pouch-like sac. Strong stomach muscles stir and churn food to break it up into even smaller particles. A mucous membrane lines the stomach. It contains glands that secrete *gastric juices*. Food is mixed and churned with the gastric juices to form a semi-liquid substance called *chyme*. Through peristalsis, the chyme is pushed from the stomach into the small intestine.

The *small intestine* is about 20 feet long with 3 parts. The first part is the *duodenum*. There, more digestive juices are added to the chyme. One is called *bile*. Bile is a greenish liquid made in the *liver*. Bile is stored in the *gallbladder*. Juices from the *pancreas* and small intestine are added to the chyme. Digestive juices chemically break down food for absorption.

Peristalsis moves the chyme through the other parts of the small intestine: *jejunum* and *ileum*. Tiny projections called *villi* line the small intestine. Villi absorb the digested food into the capillaries. Most food absorption takes place in the jejunum and the ileum.

Some chyme is not digested. Undigested chyme passes from the small intestine into the *large intestine (large bowel or colon)*. More fluid is absorbed. The solid waste that remains is eliminated through the anus. See Chapters 9 and 23.

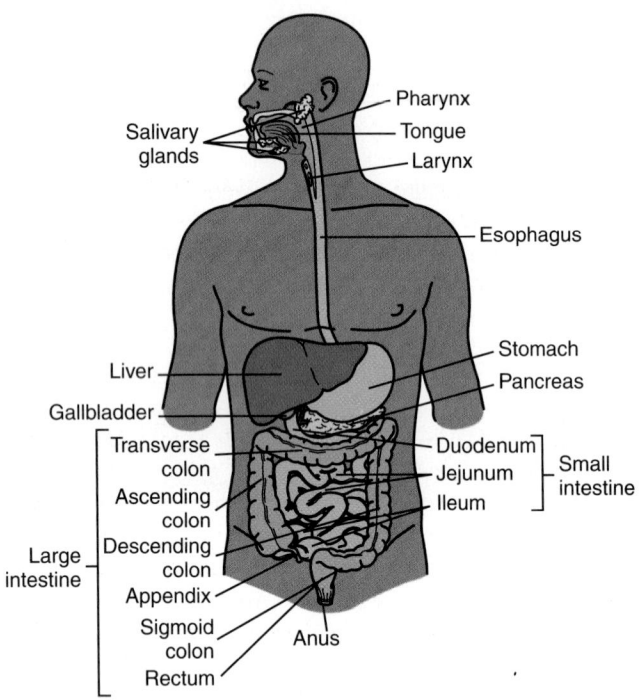

Salivary glands
Pharynx
Tongue
Larynx
Esophagus
Liver
Stomach
Pancreas
Gallbladder
Transverse colon
Ascending colon
Descending colon
Appendix
Sigmoid colon
Rectum
Large intestine
Duodenum
Jejunum
Ileum
Small intestine
Anus

Fig. 24-1 The digestive system.

BASIC NUTRITION

Nutrition is the processes involved in the ingestion, digestion, absorption, and use of foods and fluids by the body. Good nutrition is needed for growth, healing, and body functions. A well-balanced diet and correct calorie intake are needed. A high-fat, high-calorie diet causes weight gain and obesity. A low-calorie diet results in weight loss.

Foods and fluids contain nutrients. A *nutrient is a substance that is ingested, digested, absorbed, and used by the body.* Nutrients are grouped into fats, proteins, carbohydrates, vitamins, minerals, and water (p. 431).

Fats, proteins, and carbohydrates give the body fuel for energy. The amount of energy provided by a nutrient is measured in calories. A *calorie is the fuel or energy value of food:*

- 1 gram of fat—9 calories
- 1 gram of protein—4 calories
- 1 gram of carbohydrate—4 calories

Dietary Guidelines

The *Dietary Guidelines for Americans, 2010* (Appendix C) is for persons 2 years of age and older. It is also for persons at risk for chronic disease. Certain diseases are linked to poor diet and lack of physical activity. They include cardiovascular disease, hypertension (high blood pressure), diabetes, obesity, osteoporosis, and some cancers. The Dietary Guidelines help people:

- Attain and maintain a healthy weight.
- Reduce the risk of chronic disease.
- Promote over-all health.
  The Dietary Guidelines focus on:
- Consuming fewer calories
- Making informed food choices
- Being physically active

MyPlate

The MyPlate symbol (Fig. 24-2, p. 428) encourages healthy eating from 5 food groups. MyPlate, issued by the United States Department of Agriculture (USDA), helps you make wise food choices by:

- Balancing calories
  - Eating less
  - Avoiding over-sized portions
- Increasing certain foods
  - Making half of your plate fruits and vegetables
  - Making at least half of your grains whole grains
  - Drinking fat-free or low-fat (1%) milk
- Reducing certain foods
  - Choosing low-sodium foods
  - Drinking water instead of sugary drinks

The amount needed from each food group depends on age, sex, and physical activity (Table 24-1, p. 428). Activity should be moderate or vigorous (Box 24-1, p. 429). The USDA recommends that adults do at least one of the following:

- 2 hours and 30 minutes each week of moderate physical activity
- 1 hour and 15 minutes each week of vigorous physical activity

Physical activity at least 3 days a week is best. Each activity should be for at least 10 minutes at a time. Adults should also do strengthening activities at least 2 days a week. Push-ups, sit-ups, and weight-lifting are examples.

See *Focus on Children and Older Persons: MyPlate*, p. 429.

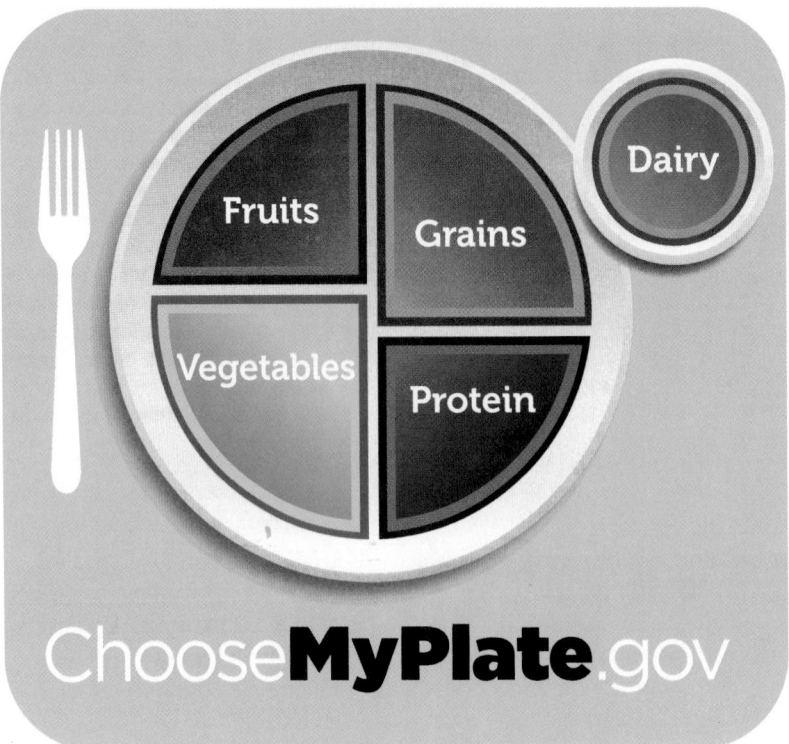

Fig. 24-2 The MyPlate Symbol.

TABLE 24-1	MYPLATE SERVING SIZES	
Group	**Daily Servings**	**Serving Sizes**
Grains	• Adult women: 5 to 6 ounces (oz); at least 3 oz from whole grains • Adult men: 6 to 8 oz; at least 3 to 4 oz from whole grains	1 oz = 1 slice of bread 1 oz = 1 cup of breakfast cereal 1 oz = ½ cup of cooked rice, cereal, or pasta
Vegetables	• Adult women: 2 to 2½ cups • Adult men: 2½ to 3 cups	1 cup = 1 cup of raw or cooked vegetables or vegetable juice 1 cup = 2 cups of raw leafy greens
Fruits	• Adult women: 1½ to 2 cups • Adult men: 2 cups	1 cup = 1 cup fruit 1 cup = 1 cup fruit juice 1 cup = ½ cup dried fruit
Dairy	• Adult women: 3 cups • Adult men: 3 cups	1 cup = 1 cup milk or yogurt 1 cup = 1½ oz natural cheese 1 cup = 2 oz processed cheese
Protein foods	• Adult women: 5 to 5½ oz • Adult men: 5½ to 6½ oz	1 oz = 1 oz of lean meat, poultry, or fish 1 oz = 1 egg 1 oz = 1 tablespoon peanut butter 1 oz = ¼ cup cooked dry beans 1 oz = ½ oz of nuts or seeds

Modified from MyPlate, U.S. Department of Agriculture, June 2011.

BOX 24-1	MODERATE AND VIGOROUS PHYSICAL ACTIVITIES

Moderate Physical Activities
- Walking briskly (about 3½ miles per hour)
- Bicycling (less than 10 miles per hour)
- Gardening (raking, trimming bushes)
- Dancing
- Golf (walking and carrying clubs)
- Water aerobics
- Canoeing
- Tennis (doubles)

Vigorous Physical Activities
- Running and jogging (5 miles per hour)
- Walking very fast (4½ miles per hour)
- Bicycling (more than 10 miles per hour)
- Heavy yard work (chopping wood)
- Swimming (freestyle laps)
- Aerobics
- Basketball (competitive)
- Tennis (singles)

From What Is Physical Activity? U.S. Department of Agriculture, June 4, 2011.

Children

The U.S. Department of Agriculture (USDA) offers these tips to help children eat vegetables and fruits. Some measures depend on the child's age.
- Serve vegetables and fruits with meals and as snacks.
- Let children choose vegetables, fruits, and what goes in salads.
- Let children help shop for vegetables and fruits. Let them choose new ones to try.
- Let children clean, peel, or cut up vegetables and fruits.
- Do not mix vegetables. Serve them separately. For example, do not combine peas and carrots.
- Decorate plates and serving dishes with fruit slices.
- Top cereal with berries.
- Make a "smiley face" with fruit. You can use banana slices for the eyes, raisins for the nose, and an orange slice for the mouth.
- Offer dried fruits and raisins in place of candy and chewy fruit snacks.
- Make fruit kabobs. Use pineapple chunks, bananas, grapes, and berries.
- Offer 100% fruit juices instead of soda or other drinks with sugar.

For physical activity, the USDA recommends the following for children 6 to 17 years of age:
- 60 minutes or more each day of moderate to vigorous physical activity.
- Vigorous activity at least 3 days a week.
- Muscle-strengthening activities daily. Climbing and jumping are examples.

Grains Group. Foods made from wheat, rice, oats, corn-meal, barley, or other cereal grain are grain products. Bread, pasta, oatmeal, breakfast cereals, tortillas, and grits are examples. The two types of grains are:
- *Whole grains* have the entire grain kernel. Whole-wheat flour, bulgur (cracked wheat), oatmeal, whole cornmeal, and brown rice are examples.
- *Refined grains* were processed to remove the grain kernel. These grains have a fine texture. White flour, white bread, and white rice are examples. They have less dietary fiber than whole grains.

Grains, especially whole grains, have these health benefits:
- Reduce the risk of heart disease.
- May prevent constipation.
- May help with weight management.
- May prevent certain birth defects.
- Contain these nutrients—dietary fiber, several B vitamins (thiamin, riboflavin, niacin, folate), and minerals (iron, magnesium, and selenium).

Vegetable Group. Vegetables can be eaten raw or cooked. They may be fresh, frozen, canned, dried, or juice. You can eat them whole, cut-up, or mashed. The 5 vegetable sub-groups are:
- *Dark green vegetables*—bok choy, broccoli, collard greens, dark green leafy lettuce, kale, mesclun, mustard greens, romaine lettuce, spinach, turnips, watercress
- *Red and orange vegetables*—acorn, butternut, and hubbard squashes; carrots; pumpkin; red peppers; sweet potatoes; tomatoes; tomato juice
- *Beans and peas*—black beans, black-eyed peas, garbanzo beans (chickpeas), kidney beans, lentils, navy beans, pinto beans, soybeans, split peas, and white beans
- *Starchy vegetables*—corn, green bananas, green peas, green lima beans, plantains, potatoes, taro, water chestnuts
- *Other vegetables*—artichokes, asparagus, bean sprouts, beets, Brussels sprouts, cabbage, cauliflower, celery, cucumbers, eggplant, green beans, green peppers, iceberg (head) lettuce, mushrooms, okra, onions, parsnips, turnips, wax beans, zucchini

Vegetables have these health benefits:
- May reduce the risk for stroke, heart disease, high blood pressure, cardiovascular diseases, and type 2 diabetes.
- May protect against certain cancers. Cancers of the mouth, stomach, and colon-rectum are examples.
- May reduce the risk of developing kidney stones.
- May reduce the risk of bone loss.
- May help lower calorie intake. Most vegetables are low in fat and calories.
- Contain no cholesterol. (*Cholesterol is a soft, waxy substance. It is found in the bloodstream and all body cells. Dietary sources are from animal foods—egg yolks, meat, poultry, shellfish, milk, and milk products.*)
- May prevent certain birth defects.
- Contain these nutrients—potassium, dietary fiber, folate (folic acid), vitamins A and C.

Fruit Group. Any fruit or 100% fruit juice counts as part of the fruit group. Fruits may be fresh, frozen, canned, or dried. They may be eaten whole, cut-up, or pureed. Avoid fruits canned in syrup. Syrup contains added sugar. Choose fruits canned in 100% fruit juice or water.

Fruits have these health benefits:
- May reduce the risk for stroke, heart disease, high blood pressure, cardiovascular diseases, obesity, and type 2 diabetes.
- May protect against certain cancers. Cancers of the mouth, stomach, and colon-rectum are examples.
- May reduce the risk of developing kidney stones.
- May reduce the risk of bone loss.
- May help prevent constipation.
- May help lower calorie intake. Most fruits are low in fat and calories.
- Contain no cholesterol.
- Are low in sodium.
- May prevent certain birth defects.
- Contain these nutrients—potassium, dietary fiber, vitamin C, and folate (folic acid).

Dairy Group. All fluid milk products are part of the dairy group. So are many foods made from milk. Low-fat or fat-free choices are best. The milk group includes all fluid milk, yogurt, and cheese. (Cream, cream cheese, and butter are not in this group.)

Milk has these health benefits:
- Helps build and maintain bone mass throughout life. This may reduce the risk of osteoporosis.
- May reduce the risk of cardiovascular disease, type 2 diabetes, and high blood pressure.
- Contains these nutrients—calcium, potassium, and vitamin D.

Protein Foods Group. This group includes all foods made from meat, poultry, seafood, eggs, processed soy products, nuts, and seeds. Beans and peas are included in this group as well as the vegetable group.

When selecting foods from this group, remember:
- To choose lean or low-fat meat and poultry. Higher fat choices include regular ground beef (75% to 80% lean) and chicken with skin.
- Using fat for cooking increases the calories. Fried chicken and eggs fried in butter are examples.
- Salmon, trout, and herring are rich in substances that may reduce the risk of heart disease.
- Liver and other organ meats are high in cholesterol.
- Egg yolks are high in cholesterol. Egg whites are cholesterol-free.
- Processed meats have added sodium (salt). They include ham, sausage, frankfurters, and luncheon and deli meats.

Many proteins are high in fat and cholesterol. Heart disease is a major risk. However, this group provides nutrients needed for health and body maintenance:
- Protein
- B vitamins (niacin, thiamin, riboflavin, and B_6) and vitamin E
- Iron, zinc, and magnesium

Oils. Oils are fats that are liquid at room temperature. Vegetable oils for cooking are examples. They include canola oil, corn oil, and olive oil. Oils come from plants and fish. Because they have nutrients, the USDA includes oils in food patterns. However, *oils are not a food group*.

Adult women are allowed 5 to 6 teaspoons of oils daily. Adult men are allowed 6 to 7 teaspoons daily. Some foods are high in oil—nuts, olives, some fish, and avocados.

When making oil choices, remember:
- Oils are high in calories.
- The best oil choices come from fish, nuts, and vegetable oils.
- Some foods are mainly oil. Mayonnaise, certain salad dressings, and soft margarine (tub or squeeze) are examples.
- Oils from plant sources do not contain cholesterol.
- *Solid fats* are solid at room temperature. Common solid fats include butter, milk fat, beef fat (tallow, suet), chicken fat, pork fat (lard), stick margarine, and shortening.
- Oils and solid fats have about 120 calories in each tablespoon.
- Enough oil is usually consumed daily from nuts, fish, cooking oil, and salad dressings.

Nutrients

No food or food group has every essential nutrient. A well-balanced diet ensures an adequate intake of essential nutrients.

- *Protein*—is the most important nutrient. It is needed for tissue growth and repair. Sources include meat, fish, poultry, eggs, milk and milk products, cereals, beans, peas, and nuts.
- *Carbohydrates*—provide energy and fiber for bowel elimination. They are found in fruits, vegetables, breads, cereals, and sugar. Carbohydrates break down into sugars during digestion. The sugars are absorbed into the bloodstream. Fiber is not digested. It provides the bulky part of chyme for elimination.
- *Fats*—provide energy. They provide flavor and help the body use certain vitamins. Sources include meats, lard, butter, shortening, oils, milk, cheese, egg yolks, and nuts. Unneeded dietary fat is stored as body fat (*adipose tissue*).
- *Vitamins*—are needed for certain body functions. The body stores vitamins A, D, E, and K. Vitamin C and the B complex vitamins are not stored. They must be ingested daily. The lack of a certain vitamin results in signs and symptoms of an illness. See Table 24-2.
- *Minerals*—are used for many body processes. Bone and tooth formation, nerve and muscle function, and fluid balance are examples. Foods containing calcium help prevent musculo-skeletal changes. See Table 24-3, p. 432.
- *Water*—is needed for all body processes (p. 439).

TABLE 24-2	FUNCTIONS AND SOURCES OF COMMON VITAMINS	
Vitamin	**Major Functions**	**Sources**
Vitamin A	Growth; vision; healthy hair, skin, and mucous membranes; resistance to infection	Liver, spinach, green leafy and yellow vegetables, yellow fruits, fish liver oils, egg yolks, butter, cream, whole milk
Vitamin B$_1$ (thiamin)	Muscle tone, nerve function, digestion, appetite, normal elimination, carbohydrate use	Pork, fish, poultry, eggs, liver, breads, pastas, cereals, oatmeal, potatoes, peas, beans, soybeans, peanuts
Vitamin B$_2$ (riboflavin)	Growth, healthy eyes, protein and carbohydrate metabolism, healthy skin and mucous membranes	Milk and milk products, liver, green leafy vegetables, eggs, breads, cereals
Vitamin B$_3$ (niacin)	Protein, fat, and carbohydrate metabolism; nervous system function; appetite; digestive system function	Meat, pork, liver, fish, peanuts, breads and cereals, green vegetables, dairy products
Vitamin B$_{12}$	Forming red blood cells, protein metabolism, nervous system function	Liver, meats, poultry, fish, eggs, milk, cheese
Folate (folic acid)	Forming red blood cells, intestinal function, protein metabolism	Liver, meats, fish, poultry, green leafy vegetables, whole grains
Vitamin C (ascorbic acid)	Forming substances that hold tissues together; healthy blood vessels, skin, gums, bones, and teeth; wound healing; preventing bleeding; resistance to infection	Citrus fruits, tomatoes, potatoes, cabbage, strawberries, green vegetables, melons
Vitamin D	Absorbing and metabolizing calcium and phosphorus, healthy bones	Fish liver oils, milk, butter, liver, exposure to sun light
Vitamin E	Normal reproduction, forming red blood cells, muscle function	Vegetable oils, milk, eggs, meats, cereals, green leafy vegetables
Vitamin K	Blood clotting	Liver, green leafy vegetables, egg yolks, cheese

TABLE 24-3	FUNCTIONS AND SOURCES OF COMMON MINERALS	
Mineral	**Major Functions**	**Sources**
Calcium	Forming teeth and bones, blood clotting, muscle contraction, heart function, nerve function	Milk and milk products, green leafy vegetables, whole grains, egg yolks, dried peas and beans, nuts
Phosphorus	Forming bones and teeth; use of proteins, fats, and carbohydrates; nerve and muscle function	Meat, fish, poultry, milk and milk products, nuts, egg yolks, dried peas and beans
Iron	Allows red blood cells to carry oxygen	Liver, meat, eggs, green leafy vegetables, breads and cereals, dried peas and beans, nuts
Iodine	Thyroid gland function, growth, metabolism	Iodized salt, seafood, shellfish
Sodium	Fluid balance, nerve and muscle function	Almost all foods
Potassium	Nerve function, muscle contraction, heart function	Fruits, vegetables, cereals, meats, dried peas and beans

Food Labels

Food labels are used to make informed food choices for a healthy diet. Figure 24-3 shows how to use a food label. Food labels contain information about:

- Serving size and the number of servings in each package.
- Calories and calories from fat. The number of servings eaten determines the number of calories of that food. For example: 1 cup of macaroni and cheese contains 250 calories with 110 of them from fat. If you eat 2 cups, you consume 500 calories—220 from fat.
- Nutrients—total fat (saturated fat and *trans* fat), cholesterol, sodium, carbohydrate (dietary fibers and sugar), protein, vitamins A and C, calcium, and iron.

How a serving fits into the daily diet is called the Daily Value (DV). The DV is a percent (%). The percent is based on 2000 calories daily. The % DV helps you decide if a food is high or low in a nutrient. According to the Food and Drug Administration (FDA), a 5% DV is low. A DV of 20% or more is high. In Figure 24-3, a serving of macaroni and cheese is low in dietary fiber, vitamins A and C, and iron. It is high in sodium and calcium.

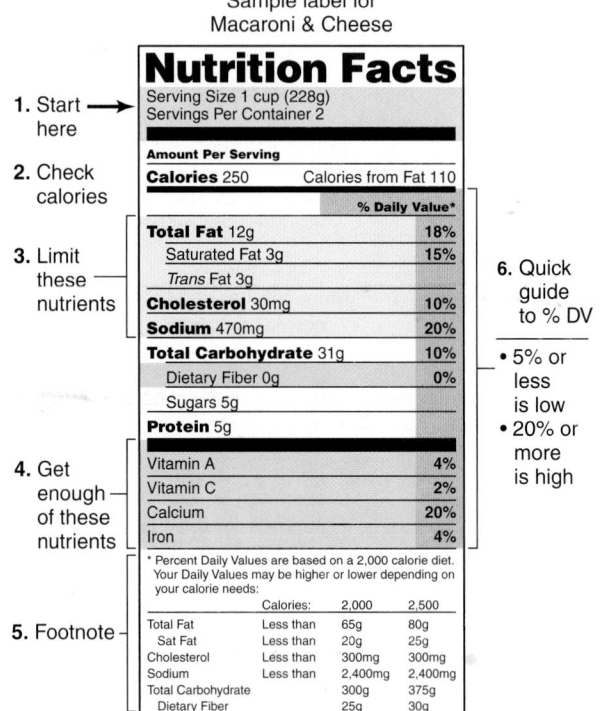

Fig. 24-3 Nutrition Facts Label.

MEETING NUTRITIONAL NEEDS

A team approach is needed to meet a person's nutritional needs. The person, nursing team, doctor, dietitian, speech-language pathologist, and occupational therapist are involved. So is the family if necessary. The person's likes, dislikes, and life-long habits are part of the nutritional care plan.

See *Focus on Long-Term Care and Home Care: Meeting Nutritional Needs*, p. 434.

See *Focus on Children and Older Persons: Meeting Nutritional Needs*, p. 435.

Factors Affecting Eating and Nutrition

Many factors affect eating and nutrition:

- *Culture*. Culture influences dietary practices, food choices, and food preparation. Frying, baking, smoking, or roasting food and eating raw food are cultural practices. So is using sauces, herbs, and spices. See *Caring About Culture: Food Practices*, p. 435.
- *Religion*. Selecting, preparing, and eating food often involve religious practices (Box 24-2, p. 435). A person may follow all, some, or none of the dietary practices of his or her faith. You must respect the person's religious practices.
- *Finances*. People with limited incomes often buy the cheaper carbohydrate foods. Their diets often lack protein and certain vitamins and minerals.
- *Appetite*. Appetite relates to the desire for food. When hungry, a person seeks food. He or she eats until the appetite is satisfied. Aromas and thoughts of food can stimulate the appetite. However, *loss of appetite (anorexia)* can occur. Causes include illness, drugs, anxiety, pain, and depression. Unpleasant sights, thoughts, and smells are other causes.

- *Personal choice*. Food likes and dislikes are personal. They begin in childhood with foods served in the home. As children grow older, they try new foods at school and social events. Food choices depend on how food looks, how it is prepared, its smell, and ingredients. Usually food likes expand with age and social experiences.
- *Body reactions*. People usually avoid foods that cause allergic reactions. They also avoid foods that cause nausea, vomiting, diarrhea, indigestion, gas, or headaches.
- *Illness*. Appetite usually decreases during illness and recovery from injuries. However, nutritional needs increase. The body must fight infection, heal tissue, and replace lost blood cells. Nutrients lost through vomiting and diarrhea need replacement.
- *Drugs*. Drugs can cause loss of appetite, confusion, nausea, constipation, impaired taste, or changes in GI function. They can cause inflammation of the mouth, throat, esophagus, and stomach.
- *Chewing problems*. Mouth, teeth, and gum problems can affect chewing. Examples include oral pain, dry or sore mouth, gum disease (Chapter 20), and dentures that fit poorly. Broken, decayed, or missing teeth also affect chewing, especially the meat group.
- *Swallowing problems*. Many health problems can affect swallowing. They include stroke; pain; confusion; dry mouth; and diseases of the mouth, throat, and esophagus. See "The Dysphagia Diet" on p. 438.
- *Disability*. Disease or injury can affect the hands, wrists, and arms. Assistive devices let the person eat independently. The speech-language pathologist and occupational therapist teach the person how to use them. Make sure each person has needed devices.
- *Impaired cognitive function*. Impaired cognitive function may affect the person's ability to use eating utensils. And it may affect eating, chewing, and swallowing. Follow the care plan to assist the person.

Text continued on p. 436

FOCUS ON LONG-TERM CARE AND HOME CARE
Meeting Nutritional Needs

Long-Term Care

The Omnibus Budget Reconciliation Act of 1987 (OBRA) has requirements for food served in nursing centers:

* Each person's nutritional and dietary needs are met.
* The person's diet is well-balanced. It is nourishing and tastes good. Food is well-seasoned. It is not too salty or too sweet.
* Food is appetizing. It has an appealing aroma and is attractive.
* Hot food is served hot. Cold food is served cold. Food servers keep food at the correct temperature.
* Food is served promptly. If not, hot food cools and cold food warms.
* Food is prepared to meet each person's needs. Some people need food cut, ground, or chopped. Others have special diets ordered by the doctor.
* Other foods are offered to residents who refuse the food served. The substituted food must have a similar nutritional value to the first foods served.
* Each person receives at least 3 meals a day. A bedtime snack is offered.
* The center provides needed adaptive equipment and utensils (Fig. 24-4).

Home Care

You may be assigned to shop for groceries, plan meals, and cook. You need to understand the MyPlate symbol, basic nutrition, and food labels. You also need to know the person's food likes and dislikes and eating habits. For example, some people have the same breakfast every day. Some people have their large meal in the evening, others at noon.

The nurse and dietitian advise you about what to prepare. Remember to:

* Review the foods allowed on the person's diet (p. 436).
* Use a good cookbook to plan and prepare meals.
* Plan menus for a full week.
* Check recipe ingredients. If not on hand, place needed items on your shopping list.
* Try to save money. Check newspapers for sales. Also check them and the Internet for coupons.
* Give all receipts to the person or family member.
* Store food properly. Refrigerate dairy products and most fresh fruits and vegetables right away. Do the same for the meat, fish, or poultry that you will use that day. Freeze the rest and frozen foods. Dried, packaged, canned, and bottled foods keep well in cabinets.
* See p. 450 for preventing "Foodborne Illnesses."

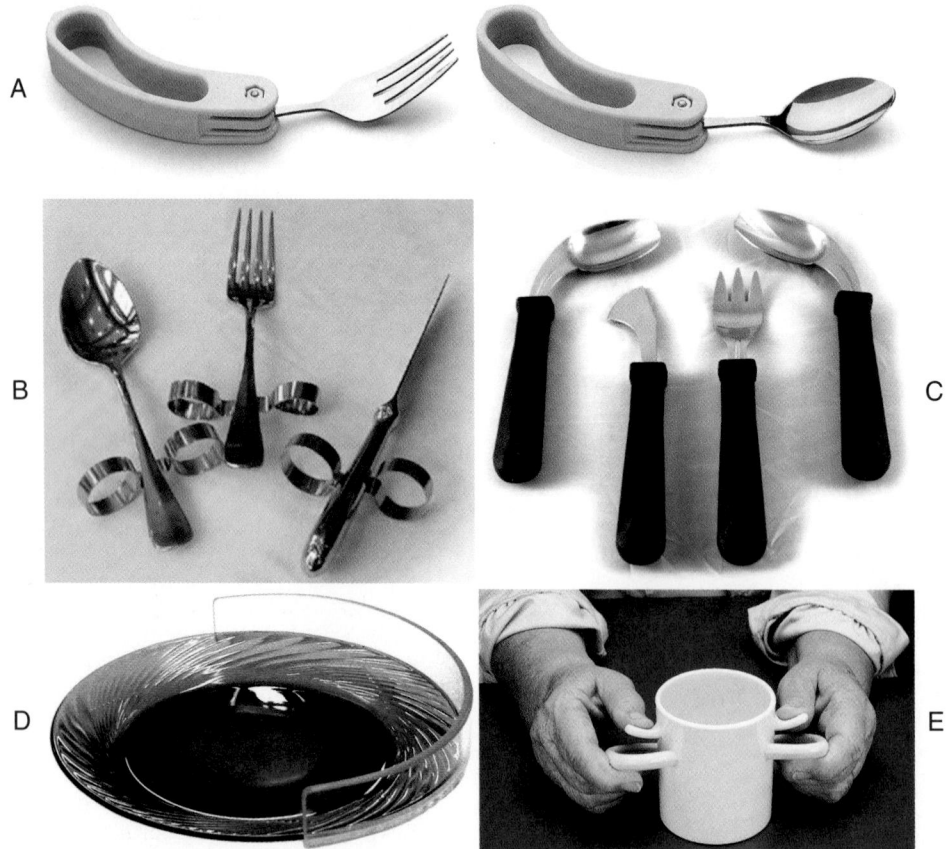

Fig. 24-4 Eating utensils for persons with special needs. **A,** The fork and spoon are angled. Fingers are inserted through the opening or wrapped around the handle. **B,** The utensils can be adjusted for the person's grip strength. **C,** Eating utensils have tapered and angled handles. The knife cuts with slicing and rocking motions. **D,** The plate guard helps keep food on the plate. **E,** The thumb grips on the cup help prevent spilling.

FOCUS ON CHILDREN AND OLDER PERSONS
Meeting Nutritional Needs

Children
The MyPlate symbol applies to children 2 years of age and older. The nurse tells you about the child's needs.

Older Persons
With aging, changes occur in the GI system:
* Taste and smell dull.
* Appetite decreases.
* Secretion of digestive juices decreases. Therefore fried and fatty foods are hard to digest. They may cause indigestion.

Some people have to avoid high-fiber foods needed for bowel elimination. High-fiber foods are hard to chew and can irritate the intestines. Such foods include apricots, celery, and fruits and vegetables with skins and seeds.

Foods providing soft bulk are often ordered for persons with chewing problems or constipation. These foods include whole-grain cereals and cooked fruits and vegetables.

Older persons need fewer calories than younger people do. Energy and activity levels are lower. Foods that contain calcium help prevent musculo-skeletal changes. Protein is needed for tissue growth and repair. The diets of some older persons may lack protein. High protein foods are costly.

✿ CARING ABOUT CULTURE
Food Practices

Food practices vary among cultural groups. Rice, corn, and beans are protein sources in *Mexico*. In the *Philippines,* rice is a main food. And fish, vegetables, and native fruits are preferred. A diet high in sugar and animal fat is common in *Poland*. In *China*, a meal of rice with meat, fish, and vegetables is common. High sodium content is from the use of soy sauce and dried and preserved foods.

Eating beef is common in the *United States*. In *India*, Hindus do not eat beef.

Modified from D'Avanzo CE: *Pocket guide to cultural health assessment*, ed 4, St Louis, 2008, Mosby.

BOX 24-2 | RELIGION AND DIETARY PRACTICES

Church of Jesus Christ of Latter Day Saints (Mormon)
* Alcohol, beverages containing caffeine (coffee, tea, colas), and chocolate are avoided.
* Fruits, vegetables, grains, and nuts take the place of meats.
* Meats, sugar, cheeses, and spices are avoided.
* Fasting is practiced.

Greek Orthodox
* Fasting is required during the Great Lent and before other holy days.
* Meat, fish, and dairy products are not eaten during a fast.

Hinduism
* Pork, fowl, ducks, snails, and crabs are avoided.
* No beef is eaten. The cow is a sacred animal to Hindus.
* Products from cows—milk, yogurt, and butter—are allowed.
* Days of fast include Hindu holidays, Sundays, birthdays, and marriage and death anniversaries.

Islam
* All pork and pork products are forbidden.
* Tea and coffee are discouraged.
* Alcohol is not allowed.
* Fasting is practiced on Mondays and Thursdays, for six days during the Shawwal (the tenth month of the Islamic calendar), and during the entire month of Ramadan (the ninth month of the Islamic calendar). Fasting means no food or drink from sunrise to sunset.

Judaism (Jewish Faith)
* Foods must be kosher. (*Kosher* means fit, proper, or correct.) Food must be prepared according to Jewish law.
* Meat of kosher animals can be eaten—cows, goats, and lambs.
* Chickens, ducks, and geese are kosher fowl.
* Kosher fish have scales and fins—tuna, sardines, carp, salmon, herring, whitefish, and so on. Lobster, shrimp, and clams are not allowed.
* Milk, milk products, and eggs from kosher animals and fowl are allowed.
* Meat and milk cannot be cooked together.
* Meat and milk products cannot be eaten at the same meal. They cannot be served on the same plate.
* Meat and milk products are not prepared or served with the same utensils and dishes. Two sets of utensils and dishes are needed. They are washed and stored separately.
* Fermented grain products are not consumed during Passover—cookies, noodles, alcohol, and so on.

Roman Catholic
* Fasting from meat is required on Ash Wednesday, Good Friday, and all Fridays during Lent.
* Not eating food is required for 1 hour before receiving Holy Communion. Water and drugs are allowed.

Seventh-Day Adventist
* Coffee, tea, and alcohol are avoided.
* Beverages with caffeine (colas) are avoided.
* Some groups have restrictions about meat, fish, and fowl.
* A vegetarian diet is encouraged.

SPECIAL DIETS

Doctors may order special diets for a nutritional deficiency or a disease (Table 24-4). They also order them for weight control (gain or loss) or to eliminate or decrease certain substances in the diet.

The health team considers the need for dietary changes, personal choices, religion, culture, and eating problems. They also consider food allergies and sensitivities. The nurse and dietitian teach the person and family about the diet.

Regular diet, general diet, and *house diet* mean no dietary limits or restrictions. Persons with diseases of the heart, kidneys, gallbladder, liver, stomach, or intestines often need special diets. High-protein diets are needed to heal wounds and pressure ulcers. Some persons have bran added to their food. It provides fiber for bowel elimination. Allergies, excess weight, and other disorders also require special diets.

The sodium-controlled diet is often ordered. So is a diabetes meal plan, p. 438. Persons with swallowing problems may need a dysphagia diet, p. 438.

TABLE 24-4 SPECIAL DIETS		
Diet	**Use**	**Foods Allowed**
Clear-liquid—foods liquid at body temperature and which leave small amounts of residue; non-irritating and non-gas forming	Post-operatively, acute illness, infection, nausea and vomiting, and to prepare for GI exams	Water, tea, and coffee (without milk or cream); carbonated drinks; gelatin; clear fruit juices (apple, grape, cranberry); fat-free clear broth; hard candy, sugar, and Popsicles
Full-liquid—foods liquid at room temperature or melt at body temperature	Advance from clear-liquid diet post-operatively; for stomach irritation, fever, nausea, and vomiting; for persons unable to chew, swallow, or digest solid foods	Foods on the clear-liquid diet; custard; eggnog; strained soups; strained fruit and vegetable juices; milk and milk shakes; strained, cooked cereals; plain ice cream and sherbet; pudding; yogurt
Mechanical soft—semi-solid foods that are easily digested	Advance from full-liquid diet, chewing problems, GI disorders, and infections	All liquids; eggs (not fried); broiled, baked, or roasted meat, fish, or poultry that is chopped or shredded; mild cheeses (American, Swiss, cheddar, cream, cottage); strained fruit juices; refined bread (no crust) and crackers; cooked cereal; cooked or pureed vegetables; cooked or canned fruit without skin or seeds; pudding; plain cakes and soft cookies without fruit or nuts
Fiber- and residue-restricted—food that leaves a small amount of residue in the colon	Diseases of the colon and diarrhea	Coffee, tea, milk, carbonated drinks, strained fruit juices; refined bread and crackers; creamed and refined cereal; rice; cottage and cream cheese; eggs (not fried); plain puddings and cakes; gelatin; custard; sherbet and ice cream; strained vegetable juices; canned or cooked fruit without skin or seeds; potatoes (not fried); strained cooked vegetables; plain pasta; *no raw fruits or vegetables*
High-fiber—foods that increase the amount of residue and fiber in the colon to stimulate peristalsis	Constipation and GI disorders	All fruits and vegetables; whole-wheat bread; whole-grain cereals; fried foods; whole-grain rice; milk, cream, butter, and cheese; meats
Bland—foods that are mechanically and chemically non-irritating and low in roughage; foods served at moderate temperatures; no strong spices or condiments	Ulcers, gallbladder disorders, and some intestinal disorders; after abdominal surgery	Lean meats; white bread; creamed and refined cereals; cream or cottage cheese; gelatin; plain puddings, cakes, and cookies; eggs (not fried); butter and cream; canned fruits and vegetables without skin and seeds; strained fruit juices; potatoes (not fried); pastas and rice; strained or soft cooked carrots, peas, beets, spinach, squash, and asparagus tips; creamed soups from allowed vegetables; no fried or spicy foods

TABLE 24-4	SPECIAL DIETS—cont'd	
Diet	**Use**	**Foods Allowed**
High-calorie—calorie intake is increased to about 3000 to 4000 daily; includes 3 full meals and between-meal snacks	Weight gain and some thyroid imbalances	Dietary increases in all foods; large portions of regular diet with 3 between-meal snacks
Calorie-controlled—provides adequate nutrients while controlling calories to promote weight loss and reduce body fat	Weight reduction	Foods low in fats and carbohydrates and lean meats; avoid butter, cream, rice, gravies, salad oils, noodles, cakes, pastries, carbonated and alcoholic drinks, candy, potato chips, and similar foods
High-iron—foods that are high in iron	Anemia, following blood loss, for women during the reproductive years	Liver and other organ meats, lean meats, egg yolks, shellfish, dried fruits, dried beans, green leafy vegetables, lima beans, peanut butter, enriched breads and cereals
Fat-controlled (low cholesterol)—foods low in fat and prepared without adding fat	Heart disease, gallbladder disease, disorders of fat digestion, liver disease, diseases of the pancreas	Skim milk (fat free) or buttermilk; cottage cheese (no other cheeses allowed); gelatin; sherbet; fruit; lean meat, poultry, and fish (baked, broiled, or roasted); fat-free broth; soups made with skim milk (fat free); margarine; rice, pasta, breads, and cereals; vegetables; potatoes
High-protein—aids and promotes tissue healing	For burns, high fever, infection, and some liver diseases	Meat, milk, eggs, cheese, fish, poultry; breads and cereals; green leafy vegetables
Sodium-controlled—a certain amount of sodium is allowed	Heart disease, fluid retention, liver disease, and some kidney diseases	Fruits and vegetables and unsalted butter are allowed; adding salt at the table is not allowed; highly salted foods and foods high in sodium are not allowed; the use of salt during cooking may be restricted
Diabetes meal plan—the same amount of carbohydrates, protein, and fat are eaten at the same time each day	Diabetes	Determined by nutritional and energy requirements

The Sodium-Controlled Diet

The average amount of sodium in the daily diet is 3000 to 5000 mg (milligrams). The body needs no more than 2300 mg a day. Healthy people excrete excess sodium in the urine.

The USDA recommends that sodium intake be reduced to 1500 mg daily for:
- Persons aged 51 and older
- African-Americans of any age (including children)
- Persons who have hypertension, diabetes, or chronic kidney disease (including children)

Heart, liver, and kidney diseases and certain drugs cause the body to retain extra sodium. Sodium causes the body to retain water. If there is too much sodium, the body retains more water. Tissues swell with water. There is excess fluid in the blood vessels. The heart has to work harder. That is, the workload of the heart increases. With heart disease, the extra workload can cause serious problems or death.

Sodium control decreases the amount of sodium in the body. The body retains less water. Less water in the tissues and blood vessels reduces the heart's workload.

The doctor orders the amount of sodium allowed. Sodium-controlled diets involve:
- Omitting high-sodium foods (Box 24-3, p. 438)
- Not adding salt to food at the table
- Limiting the amount of salt used in cooking
- Diet planning

BOX 24-3   HIGH-SODIUM FOODS

Grains
- Baked goods—biscuits, muffins, cakes, cookies, pies, pastries, sweet rolls, donuts, and so on
- Breads and rolls
- Cereals—cold, instant hot
- Noodle mixes
- Pancakes
- Salted snack foods—pretzels, corn chips, popcorn, crackers, chips, and so on
- Stuffing mixes
- Waffles

Vegetables
- Canned vegetables
- Olives
- Pickles and other pickled vegetables
- Relish
- Sauerkraut
- Tomato sauce or paste
- Vegetable juices—tomato, V8, Bloody Mary mixes
- Vegetables with sauces, creams, or seasonings

Fruits
- None—fruits are not high in sodium

Dairy Group
- Buttermilk
- Cheese
- Commercial dips made with sour cream

Protein Foods
- Bacon and Canadian bacon
- Canned meats and fish—chicken, tuna, salmon, anchovies, sardines
- Caviar
- Chipped, dried, and corned beef and other meats
- Deli meats—turkey, ham, bologna, salami, pastrami, and so on

Protein Foods—cont'd
- Dried fish
- Ham
- Herring
- Hot dogs (frankfurters)
- Liverwurst
- Lox and smoked salmon
- Mackerel
- Pepperoni
- Salt pork
- Sausages
- Scrapple
- Shellfish—shrimp, crab, clams, oysters, scallops, lobster

Other
- Asian foods—Chinese, Japanese, East Indian, Thai, Vietnamese
- Baking soda and baking powder
- Catsup (ketchup)
- Mayonnaise
- Salad dressings
- Cocoa mixes
- Commercially prepared dinners—frozen, canned, boxed, and so on
- Mexican foods
- Mustard
- Pasta dishes—lasagna, manicotti, ravioli
- Peanut butter
- Pizzas
- Pot pies
- Salted nuts or seeds
- Sauces—soy, teriyaki, Worcestershire, steak, barbecue, pasta, chili, cocktail
- Seasoning salts—garlic, onion, celery, meat tenderizers, monosodium glutamate (MSG), and so on
- Soups—canned, packaged, instant, dried, bouillon

Diabetes Meal Plan

Diabetes is a chronic illness in which the body cannot produce or use insulin properly (Chapter 43). The pancreas produces and secretes insulin. Insulin lets the body use sugar. Without enough insulin, sugar builds up in the bloodstream. It is not used by cells for energy. Diabetes is usually treated with insulin or other drugs, diet, and exercise.

A meal plan for healthy eating is developed. Consistency is key. It involves:
- The person's food preferences (likes, eating habits, meal times, culture, and life-style). It may involve limiting the amount of food or changing how it is prepared.
- Calories needed. The same amount of carbohydrates, protein, and fat are eaten each day.
- Eating meals and snacks at regular times. The person eats at regular times to maintain a certain blood sugar level.

Serve meals and snacks on time. Always check what was eaten. Report what the person did and did not eat. If all food was not eaten, a between-meal snack is needed (p. 448). The nurse tells you what to provide. It makes up for what was not eaten at the meal. The amount of insulin given also depends on daily food intake. Report changes in the person's eating habits.

The Dysphagia Diet

Dysphagia means *difficulty* (dys) *swallowing* (phagia). Food thickness is changed to meet the person's needs (Box 24-4). The doctor, speech-language pathologist, occupational therapist, dietitian, and nurse choose the right food thickness.

A *slow swallow* means the person has difficulty getting enough food and fluids for good nutrition and fluid balance. An *unsafe swallow* means that food enters the airway (aspiration). *Aspiration is breathing fluid, food, vomitus, or an object into the lungs* (Chapter 25).

BOX 24-4 DYSPHAGIA DIET

Consistency	Description
Thickened liquid	No lumps. Pureed with milk, gravy, or broth to thickness of baby food. Thickener is added to some foods and fluids as needed. Does not mound on a plate. May be called *creamy* or a *sauce*. Stir before serving if the food settles.
Medium thick (nectar-like)	The thickness of nectar or V8 juice (does not hold its shape). Stir right before serving.
Extra thick (honey-like)	Thick like honey. Mounds a bit on a spoon. Can drink from a cup. Stir before serving.
Yogurt-like	Thick like *yogurt* or *pudding*. Holds its shape. Served with a spoon.
Puree	No lumps; mounds on a plate. May be thick like mashed potatoes.

BOX 24-5 SIGNS AND SYMPTOMS OF DYSPHAGIA

- The person avoids food that needs chewing.
- The person avoids food with certain textures and temperatures.
- The person tires during a meal.
- Food spills out of the person's mouth while eating.
- Food "pockets" or is "squirreled" in the person's cheeks. This means that food remains or is hidden in the mouth.
- The person eats slowly, especially solid foods.
- The person complains that food will not go down or that the food is stuck.
- The person frequently coughs or chokes before, during, or after swallowing.
- The person regurgitates food after eating (Chapter 25).
- The person spits out food suddenly and almost violently.
- Food comes up through the person's nose.
- The person is hoarse—especially after eating.
- After swallowing, the person makes gargling sounds while talking or breathing.
- The person has a runny nose, sneezes, or has excessive drooling of saliva.
- The person complains of frequent heartburn.
- Appetite is decreased.

Safety and comfort are important when feeding a person with dysphagia. You must:

- Know the signs and symptoms of dysphagia (Box 24-5).
- Feed the person according to the care plan.
- Follow aspiration precautions (Box 24-6) and the care plan.
- Report changes in how the person eats.
- Observe for signs and symptoms of aspiration: choking, coughing, or difficulty breathing during or after meals, and abnormal breathing or respiratory sounds. Report these observations at once.

BOX 24-6 ASPIRATION PRECAUTIONS

- Help the person with meals and snacks.
- Position the person upright as the nurse and care plan direct. The person maintains this position for at least 1 hour after eating.
- Support the upper back, shoulders, and neck with a pillow.
- Observe for signs and symptoms of aspiration during meals and snacks (Chapter 25).
- Check the person's mouth after eating for pocketing. Check inside the cheeks, under the tongue, and on the roof of the mouth. Remove any food.
- Provide mouth care after eating.
- Report and record your observations.

BOX 24-7 COMMON CAUSES OF DEHYDRATION

- Bleeding
- Coma
- Dementia
- Diarrhea
- Drug therapy
- Fever
- Fluid intake: poor
- Fluid restriction
- Fluids: refusing
- Functional impairments: difficulty drinking, reaching fluids, communicating fluid needs
- Sweating: excess
- Urine production: increased
- Vomiting

FLUID BALANCE

Water is needed to live. Death can result from too much or too little water. Water is ingested through fluids and foods. Water is lost through urine, feces, and vomit. It is also lost through the skin (perspiration) and the lungs (exhalation).

Fluid balance is needed for health. *The amount of fluid taken in (intake)* and *the amount of fluid lost (output)* must be equal. When fluid intake exceeds fluid output *body tissues swell with water (edema)*. Edema is common in people with heart and kidney diseases. *Dehydration is a decrease in the amount of water in body tissues*. Fluid output exceeds intake. Common causes of dehydration are listed in Box 24-7.

Normal Fluid Requirements

An adult needs 1500 mL (milliliters) of water daily to survive. About 2000 to 2500 mL are needed for normal fluid balance. The water requirement increases with hot weather, exercise, fever, illness, and excess fluid losses.

See *Focus on Children and Older Persons: Normal Fluid Requirements*, p. 440.

Special Fluid Orders

The doctor may order the amount of fluid a person can have during a 24-hour period. This is done to maintain fluid balance. Found in the care plan and in the Kardex, common orders are:

- *Encourage fluids.* The person drinks an increased amount of fluid. The order states the amount to ingest. The person is given a variety of fluids allowed on the diet. They are kept within the person's reach. Offer fluids often to persons who cannot feed themselves.
- *Restrict fluids.* Fluids are limited to a certain amount. They are offered in small amounts and in small containers. The water pitcher is removed from the room or kept out of sight. Intake records are kept. The person needs frequent oral hygiene. It helps keep mucous membranes of the mouth moist.
- *Nothing by mouth.* The person cannot eat or drink anything. *NPO* stands for *non per os.* It means nothing *(non)* by *(per)* mouth *(os)*. NPO is ordered before and after surgery, before some laboratory tests and diagnostic procedures, and to treat certain illnesses. An NPO sign is posted above the bed. The water pitcher and glass are removed. Frequent oral hygiene is needed, but the person must not swallow any fluid. The person is NPO for 6 to 10 hours before surgery and before some laboratory tests and diagnostic procedures.
- *Thickened liquids.* All fluids are thickened, including water. The thickness depends on the person's ability to swallow (See Boxes 24-4 and 24-5). Thickener is added before fluids are served. Or thickened commercial fluids are used.

Intake and Output Records

The doctor or nurse may order intake and output (I&O) measurements. I&O records are kept. They are used to evaluate fluid balance and kidney function. They help in planning medical treatment. They also are kept when the person has special fluid orders.

All fluids taken by mouth are measured and recorded—water, milk, coffee, tea, juices, soups, and soft drinks. So are foods that melt at room temperature—ice cream, sherbet, custard, pudding, gelatin, and Popsicles. The nurse measures and records intravenous (IV) fluids and tube feedings (Chapter 25). Output includes urine, vomitus, diarrhea, and wound drainage.

Measuring Intake and Output. Intake and output are measured in milliliters (mL). You need to know these amounts:

- 1 oz equals 30 mL.
- 1 pint is about 500 mL.
- 1 quart is about 1000 mL.

You also need to know the serving sizes of bowls, dishes, cups, pitchers, glasses, and other containers. This information may be on the I&O record (Fig. 24-5).

A measuring container for fluid is called a graduate. It is used to measure left-over fluids, urine, vomitus, and drainage from suction. Like a measuring cup, the graduate is marked in ounces and milliliters (Fig. 24-6). Plastic urinals and kidney basins also have amounts marked. Hold the measuring device at eye level to read the amount.

An I&O record is kept at the bedside. When intake or output is measured, the amount is recorded in the correct column (see Fig. 24-5). Amounts are totaled at the end of the shift. The totals are recorded in the person's chart. They also are shared during the end-of-shift report.

The purpose of measuring I&O and how to help are explained to the person. Some persons measure and record their intake. Family members may help. The urinal, commode, bedpan, or specimen pan is used for voiding. Remind the person not to void in the toilet. Also remind the person not to put toilet tissue into the receptacle.

See *Delegation Guidelines: Intake and Output*, p. 442.
See *Promoting Safety and Comfort: Intake and Output*, p. 442.

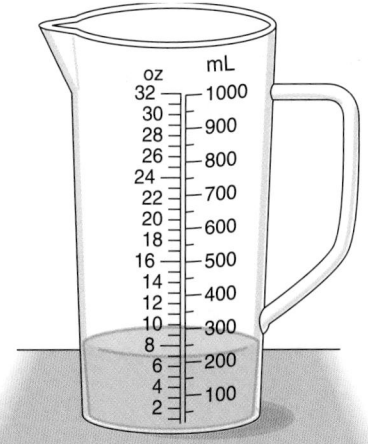

FLUID BALANCE CHART

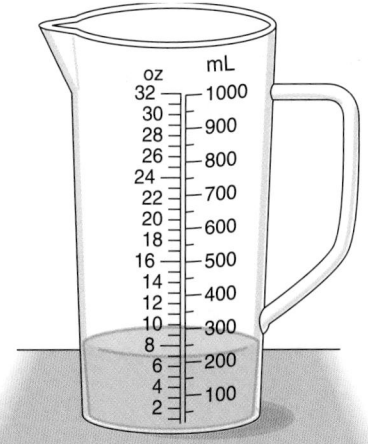

OSF
ST. JOSEPH MEDICAL CENTER
Bloomington, Illinois

DATE _6/15_

Water Glass	250mL	
Styrofoam Cup	180mL	
Cup (coffee)	250mL	
Milk Carton	240mL	
Pop (1 can)	360mL	
Broth-Soup	175mL	
Juice Carton	120mL	
Juice Glass	120mL	
Jello	120mL	

Ice Cream	120mL
Ice Chips	1/2 amt. of mL's in cup
Pitcher (Yellow)	1000mL

	INTAKE				OUTPUT					
					URINE		OTHER		CONT. IRRIGATION	
TIME	ORAL	Parenteral		Amt. mL Absbd.	Method Collected	Amt. (mL)	Method Collected	Amt. (mL)	In	Out
2400-0100		mL from previous shift			V	150				
0100-0200							Vom.	150		
0200-0300										
0300-0400										
0400-0500										
0500-0600	125				V	200				
0600-0700										
0700-0800										
	125	8 - hour Sub-total			8-hr T	350	8-hr T	150		
0800-0900	400	mL from previous shift			V	250				
0900-1000	100									
1000-1100										
1100-1200										
1200-1300	400				V	250				
1300-1400										
1400-1500	200									
1500-1600										
	1100	8 - hour Sub-total			8-hr T	500	8-hr T			
1600-1700		mL from previous shift			V	270				
1700-1800	350									
1800-1900	50									
1900-2000	200									
2000-2100					V	400				
2100-2200										
2200-2300										
2300-2400										
	600	8 - hour Sub-total			8-hr T	670	8-hr T			
	1825	24 - hour Sub-total			24-hr T	1520	24-hr T	150		

Source Key:
URINE

V — Voided
C — Catheter
INC — Incontinent
U.C. — Ureteral Catheter

Source Key:
OTHER

G.I.T. — Gastric Intestinal Tube
T.T. — T. Tube
Vom. — Vomitus
Liq S. — Liquid Stool
H.V. — Hemovac

310'   Marie Mills

Form No. MF36722 (Rev. 5/97)   **MFI**

Fig. 24-5 An intake and output record.

Fig. 24-6 A graduate marked in ounces and milliliters.

DELEGATION GUIDELINES
Intake and Output

When measuring I&O, you need this information from the nurse and the care plan:

- If the person has a special fluid order (p. 440)
- When to report measurements—hourly or end-of-shift
- What the person uses for voiding—urinal, bedpan, commode, or specimen pan (Chapter 22)
- If the person has a catheter
- What patient or resident concerns to report at once

PROMOTING SAFETY AND COMFORT
Intake and Output

Safety
Urine may contain microbes or blood. Microbes can grow in urinals, commodes, bedpans, specimen pans, and drainage systems. Follow Standard Precautions and the Bloodborne Pathogen Standard when handling such equipment. Thoroughly clean the item after it is used. Use a disinfectant for cleaning.

Comfort
Promptly measure the contents of urinals, bedpans, commodes, and specimen pans. This helps prevent or reduce odors. Odors can disturb the person.

MEASURING INTAKE AND OUTPUT

QUALITY OF LIFE

Remember to:
- Knock before entering the person's room.
- Address the person by name.
- Introduce yourself by name and title.

- Explain the procedure to the person before beginning and during the procedure.
- Protect the person's rights during the procedure.
- Handle the person gently during the procedure.

PRE-PROCEDURE

1 Follow *Delegation Guidelines: Intake and Output.* See *Promoting Safety and Comfort: Intake and Output.*
2 Practice hand hygiene.
3 Collect the following:
- I&O record
- Graduates
- Gloves

PROCEDURE

4 Put on gloves.
5 Measure intake:
- a Pour liquid remaining in the container into the graduate. Avoid spills and splashes on the outside of the graduate.
- b Measure the amount at eye level on a flat surface. Keep the container level.
- c Check the serving amount on the I&O record. Or check the serving size of each container.
- d Subtract the remaining amount from the full serving amount. Note the amount. (For example: a cup holds 250 mL. The amount in the graduate is 50 mL. 250 mL – 50 mL = 200 mL. You record 200 mL.)
- e Pour fluid in the graduate back into the container.
- f Repeat steps 5a through 5e for each liquid.
- g Add the amounts from each liquid together.
- h Record the time and amount on the I&O record.

6 Measure output as follows:
- a Pour the fluid into the graduate used to measure output. Avoid spills and splashes on the outside of the graduate.
- b Measure the amount at eye level on a flat surface. Keep the container level.
- c Dispose of fluid in the toilet. Avoid splashes.
7 Clean and rinse the graduates. Dispose of rinse into the toilet. Return the graduates to their proper place.
8 Clean, rinse, and disinfect the voiding receptacle or drainage container. Dispose of the rinse into the toilet. Return the item to its proper place.
9 Remove and discard the gloves. Practice hand hygiene.
10 Record the output amount on the person's I&O record.

POST-PROCEDURE

11 Provide for comfort. (See the inside of the front book cover.)
12 Make sure the signal light is within reach.
13 Complete a safety check of the room. (See the inside of the front book cover.)
14 Report and record your observations.

MEETING FOOD AND FLUID NEEDS

Weakness, illness, and confusion can affect appetite and ability to eat. So can unpleasant odors, sights, and sounds. An uncomfortable position, the need for oral hygiene, the need to eliminate, and pain also affect appetite.

See *Focus on Communication: Meeting Food and Fluid Needs.*

Preparing for Meals

Preparing patients and residents for meals promotes their comfort. To promote comfort:

- Assist with elimination needs.
- Provide oral hygiene. Make sure dentures are in place.
- Make sure eyeglasses and hearing aids are in place.
- Make sure incontinent persons are clean and dry.
- Position the person in a comfortable position.
- Assist the person with hand washing.
  See *Delegation Guidelines: Preparing for Meals.*
  See *Promoting Safety and Comfort: Preparing for Meals.*

DELEGATION GUIDELINES
Preparing for Meals

To prepare a person for a meal, you need this information from the nurse and the care plan:

- How much help the person needs
- Where the person will eat—room or dining room
- What the person uses for elimination—bathroom, commode, bedpan, urinal, or specimen pan
- What type of oral hygiene the person needs
- If the person wears dentures
- If the person wears eyeglasses or hearing aids
- How to position the person—in bed, a chair, or a wheelchair
- How the person gets to the dining room—by self or with help
- If the person uses a wheelchair, walker, or cane
- When to report observations
- What patient or resident concerns to report at once

FOCUS ON COMMUNICATION
Meeting Food and Fluid Needs

The person may not eat or drink all the food and fluids served. You need to find out why and tell the nurse. Ask the person to explain the answer.

- "Please tell me why you didn't eat everything."
- "Was there something wrong with your food?"
- "Did your food taste okay?"
- "Was there something you didn't like?"
- "Was your food too hot or too cold?"
- "Would you like something else?"
- "Weren't you hungry?"

PROMOTING SAFETY AND COMFORT
Preparing for Meals

Safety

Before meals, the person needs to eliminate and have oral hygiene. Follow Standard Precautions and the Bloodborne Pathogen Standard. Also follow them when cleaning equipment and the room.

Comfort

The meal setting must be free of unpleasant sights, sounds, and odors. Remove unpleasant equipment from the room.

PREPARING THE PERSON FOR A MEAL

QUALITY OF LIFE

Remember to:
- Knock before entering the person's room.
- Address the person by name.
- Introduce yourself by name and title.
- Explain the procedure to the person before beginning and during the procedure.
- Protect the person's rights during the procedure.
- Handle the person gently during the procedure.

PRE-PROCEDURE

1 Follow *Delegation Guidelines: Preparing for Meals.* See *Promoting Safety and Comfort: Preparing for Meals.*
2 Practice hand hygiene.
3 Collect the following:
  - Equipment for oral hygiene (Chapter 20)
  - Bedpan and cover, urinal, commode, or specimen pan
  - Toilet tissue
  - Wash basin
  - Soap
  - Washcloth
  - Towel
  - Gloves
4 Provide for privacy.

Continued

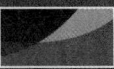 **PREPARING THE PERSON FOR A MEAL—cont'd**

PROCEDURE

5 Make sure eyeglasses and hearing aids are in place.
6 Assist with oral hygiene. Make sure dentures are in place. Wear gloves, and practice hand hygiene after removing and discarding them.
7 Assist with elimination. Make sure the incontinent person is clean and dry. Wear gloves, and practice hand hygiene after removing and discarding them.
8 Assist with hand washing. Wear gloves, and practice hand hygiene after removing and discarding them.

9 Do the following if the person will eat in bed:
  a Raise the head of the bed to a comfortable position.
  b Remove items from the overbed table. Clean the overbed table.
  c Adjust the overbed table in front of the person.
10 Do the following if the person will sit in a chair:
  a Position the person in a chair or wheelchair.
  b Remove items from the overbed table. Clean the table.
  c Adjust the overbed table in front of the person.
11 Assist the person to the dining area. (This step is for the person who eats in a dining area.)

POST-PROCEDURE

12 Provide for comfort. (See the inside of the front book cover.)
13 Place the signal light within reach.
14 Empty, clean, rinse, and disinfect equipment. Return equipment to its proper place. Wear gloves and practice hand hygiene after removing and discarding them.

15 Straighten the room. Eliminate unpleasant noise, odors, or equipment.
16 Unscreen the person.
17 Complete a safety check of the room. (See the inside of the front book cover.)
18 Practice hand hygiene.

Serving Meals

Food is served in containers that keep foods at the correct temperature. Hot food is kept hot. Cold food is kept cold.

You serve meals after preparing patients and residents for meals. You can serve meals promptly if they are ready to eat. Prompt serving keeps food at the correct temperature.

Some agencies have "room service" meal programs. A full menu (breakfast, lunch, dinner) is in the person's room. When ready to eat, the person calls the dietary department to place an order. Food is served a short while later. This program allows the person to eat when hungry. For a fee, visitors can also order food so they can dine with the person.

Serve meals in the assigned order. In nursing centers, residents seated at tables are served at the same time.

If food is not served within 15 minutes, re-check food temperatures. Follow agency policy. If not at the correct temperature, get fresh food. Temperature guides and food thermometers are in dining rooms and in nursing unit kitchens. Some agencies allow reheating in microwave ovens.

See *Focus on Long-Term Care and Home Care: Serving Meals.*
See *Delegation Guidelines: Serving Meals.*
See *Promoting Safety and Comfort: Serving Meals.*
See *Teamwork and Time Management: Serving Meals.*

FOCUS ON LONG-TERM CARE AND HOME CARE
Serving Meals

Long-Term Care
The following dining programs are common in nursing centers:
- *Social dining.* Four to six residents are seated at a dining room table (Fig. 24-7). Food is served as in a restaurant. This program is for persons who are oriented and can feed themselves. Sometimes quietly confused persons are included. They must be able to feed themselves and not disrupt others.
- *Family dining.* This is like social dining. However, food is served in bowls and on platters. Residents serve themselves as at home.
- *Low-stimulation dining.* Meal time distractions are prevented. The health team decides on the best place for each person to sit.
- *Restaurant-style menus.* The person selects food from a menu. This program allows more food choices. The person is served as in a restaurant.
- *Open dining.* A buffet is open for several hours. A breakfast buffet is an example. Residents can eat any time while the buffet is open.

Some centers have areas where residents can dine privately with guests. The person can have a meal with a partner, children, and other family or friends. They can celebrate holidays, birthdays, anniversaries, or other events. Food is provided by guests or the dietary department.

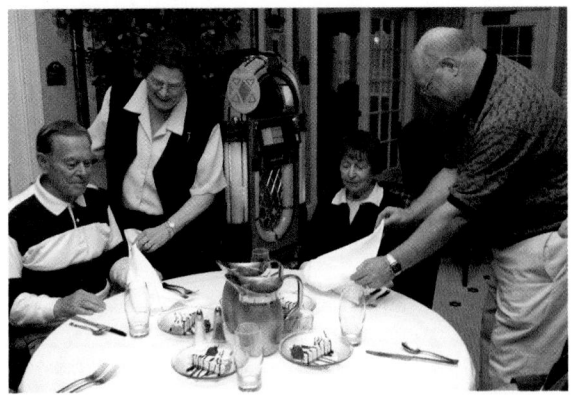
Fig. 24-7 These residents are eating in the dining room.

PROMOTING SAFETY AND COMFORT
Serving Meals

Safety
Always check food temperature after re-heating. Food that is too hot can cause burns.

Comfort
Check the person's position when serving a meal. The position may have changed after the person was prepared to eat. Provide other comfort measures as needed. See the inside of the front book cover for comfort measures.

DELEGATION GUIDELINES
Serving Meals

To serve meal trays, you need this information from the nurse and the care plan:
- The person's food allergies (if any)
- What assistive devices the person uses
- If the person needs help opening cartons, cutting food, buttering bread, and so on
- If the person's intake is measured (p. 440)
- If calorie counts are done (p. 448)
- When to report observations
- What patient or resident concerns to report at once

TEAMWORK AND TIME MANAGEMENT
Serving Meals

Meal trays are served in the order set by the health team. You will serve trays to your patients and residents and to those assigned to other nursing assistants. Your co-workers will do the same. The goal is to serve trays as fast as possible. This keeps food at the desired temperature.

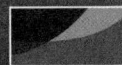 **SERVING MEAL TRAYS** `VIDEO`

QUALITY OF LIFE

Remember to:
- Knock before entering the person's room.
- Address the person by name.
- Introduce yourself by name and title.
- Explain the procedure to the person before beginning and during the procedure.
- Protect the person's rights during the procedure.
- Handle the person gently during the procedure.

PRE-PROCEDURE

1 Follow *Delegation Guidelines: Serving Meals.* See *Promoting Safety and Comfort: Serving Meals.*

2 Practice hand hygiene.

PROCEDURE

3 Make sure the tray is complete. Check items on the tray with the dietary card. Make sure assistive devices are included.
4 Identify the person. Check the ID (identification) bracelet against the dietary card. Also call the person by name.
5 Place the tray within the person's reach. Adjust the overbed table as needed.
6 Remove food covers. Open cartons, cut food into bite-size pieces, butter bread, and so on as needed (Fig. 24-8, p. 446). Season food as the person prefers and is allowed on the care plan.
7 Place the napkin, clothes protector, assistive devices, and eating utensils within reach.
8 Place the signal light within reach.

9 Do the following when the person is done eating:
  a Measure and record intake if ordered (p. 440).
  b Note the amount and type of foods eaten. (See "Calorie Counts" on p. 448.)
  c Check for and remove any food in the mouth (pocketing). Wear gloves. Practice hand hygiene after removing them.
  d Remove the tray.
  e Clean spills. Change soiled linen and clothing.
  f Help the person return to bed if needed.
  g Assist with oral hygiene and hand washing. Wear gloves. Practice hand hygiene after removing and discarding the gloves.

Continued

SERVING MEAL TRAYS—cont'd

VIDEO

POST-PROCEDURE

10 Provide for comfort. (See the inside of the front book cover.)

11 Place the signal light within reach.

12 Raise or lower bed rails. Follow the care plan.

13 Complete a safety check of the room. (See the inside of the front book cover.)

14 Follow agency policy for soiled linen.

15 Practice hand hygiene.

16 Report and record your observations.

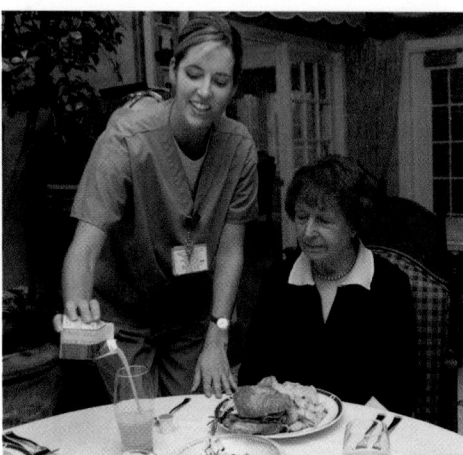

Fig. 24-8 Cartons and containers are opened for the person.

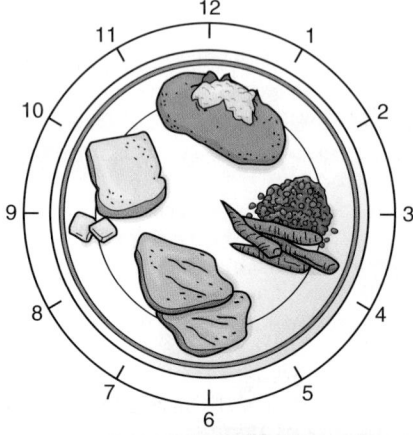

Fig. 24-9 The numbers on a clock are used to help a visually impaired person locate food.

Feeding the Person

Weakness, paralysis, casts, confusion, and other limits may make self-feeding impossible. These persons are fed.

Serve food and fluids in the order the person prefers. Offer fluids during the meal. Fluids help the person chew and swallow.

Use teaspoons to feed the person. They are less likely to cause injury than forks. The teaspoon should only be one-third full. This portion is chewed and swallowed easily. Some people need smaller portions. Follow the care plan.

Persons who need to be fed are often angry, humiliated, and embarrassed. Some are depressed, resentful, or refuse to eat. Let them do as much as possible. Some can manage "finger foods" (bread, cookies, crackers). If strong enough, let them hold milk or juice cups (never hot drinks). Do not exceed activity limits ordered by the doctor. Provide support. Encourage them to try, even if food is spilled.

Visually impaired persons are often very aware of food aromas. They may know the food served. Always tell the person what is on the tray. When feeding visually impaired persons, describe what you are offering. For persons who feed themselves, describe foods and fluids and their place on the tray. Use the numbers on a clock for the location of foods (Fig. 24-9).

Many people pray before eating. Allow time and privacy for prayer. This shows respect and caring.

Meals provide social contact with others. Engage the person in pleasant conversation. However, allow time for chewing and swallowing. Also, sit facing the person. Sitting is more relaxing. It shows that you have time for the person. By facing the person, you can see how well the person is eating. You can also see if the person has problems swallowing.

See *Focus on Children and Older Persons: Feeding the Person.*

See *Delegation Guidelines: Feeding the Person.*

See *Promoting Safety and Comfort: Feeding the Person.*

FOCUS ON CHILDREN AND OLDER PERSONS
Feeding the Person

Older Persons

Persons with dementia may become distracted during meals. Some cannot sit long enough for a meal. Others forget how to use eating utensils. Some persons resist your efforts to assist them with eating. A confused person may throw or spit food.

The Alzheimer's Disease Education and Referral Center (ADEAR) recommends the following. The measures may be part of the person's care plan.

- Provide a calm, quiet setting for eating. Limit noise and other distractions. This helps the person focus on the meal.
- Limit the number of food choices.
- Offer several small meals throughout the day instead of larger ones.
- Use straws or cups with lids. These make drinking easier.
- Provide finger foods if the person has problems with utensils. A bowl may be easier to use than a plate.
- Provide healthy snacks. Keep snacks where the person can see them.

You must be patient. Talk to the nurse if you feel upset or impatient. Remember, the person has the right to be treated with dignity and respect.

DELEGATION GUIDELINES
Feeding the Person

Before feeding a person, you need this information from the nurse and the care plan:
- The person's food allergies (if any)
- Why the person needs help
- How much help the person needs
- How to position the person
- If the person can manage finger foods
- What the person's activity limits are
- What the person's dietary restrictions are
- What size portion to feed the person—⅓ teaspoonful or less
- What safety measures are needed if the person has dysphagia
- If the person can use a straw
- What observations to report and record:
  - The amount and kind of food eaten
  - Complaints of nausea or dysphagia
  - Signs and symptoms of dysphagia
  - Signs and symptoms of aspiration
- When to report observations
- What patient or resident concerns to report at once

PROMOTING SAFETY AND COMFORT
Feeding the Person

Safety

Check food temperature. Very hot foods and fluids can burn the person.

Prevent aspiration. Check the person's mouth before offering more food or fluids. The person's mouth must be empty between bites and swallows.

Comfort

The person will eat better if not rushed. Sit to show the person that you have time for him or her. Standing communicates that you are in a hurry.

Wipe the person's hands, face, and mouth as needed during the meal. Use the napkin. If necessary, use a wet washcloth. Then dry the person with a towel.

FEEDING THE PERSON

| VIDEO | VIDEO CLIP | NNAAP® Skill | |

QUALITY OF LIFE

Remember to:
- Knock before entering the person's room.
- Address the person by name.
- Introduce yourself by name and title.
- Explain the procedure to the person before beginning and during the procedure.
- Protect the person's rights during the procedure.
- Handle the person gently during the procedure.

PRE-PROCEDURE

1 Follow *Delegation Guidelines: Feeding the Person.* See *Promoting Safety and Comfort: Feeding the Person.*
2 Practice hand hygiene.
3 Position the person in a comfortable position for eating— usually sitting or high-Fowler's. (NOTE: Some state competency tests require that the person sit upright at least 75 to 90 degrees.)
4 Get the tray. Place the tray on the overbed table or dining table where the person can see it.

Continued

FEEDING THE PERSON—cont'd

 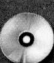

PROCEDURE

5 Identify the person. Check the ID bracelet against the dietary card. Also call the person by name.
6 Drape a napkin across the person's chest and underneath the chin. Clean the person's hands with a hand wipe.
7 Tell the person what foods and fluids are on the tray.
8 Prepare food for eating. Cut food into bite-size pieces. Season foods as the person prefers and is allowed on the care plan.
9 Place the chair where you can sit comfortably. Sit facing the person.
10 Serve foods in the order the person prefers. Identify foods as you serve them. Alternate between solid and liquid foods. Use a spoon for safety (Fig. 24-10). Allow enough time for chewing and swallowing. Do not rush the person. Also offer water, coffee, tea, or other beverage on the tray.
11 Check the person's mouth before offering more food or fluids. Make sure the person's mouth is empty between bites and swallows. Ask if the person is ready for the next bite or drink.
12 Use straws for liquids if the person cannot drink out of a glass or cup. Have one straw for each liquid. Provide short straws for weak persons.

13 Wipe the person's hands, face, and mouth as needed during the meal. Use the napkin or a hand wipe.
14 Follow the care plan if the person has dysphagia. (Some persons with dysphagia do not use straws.) Give thickened liquid with a spoon.
15 Converse with the person in a pleasant manner.
16 Encourage him or her to eat as much as possible.
17 Wipe the person's mouth with a napkin or a hand wipe. Discard the napkin or hand wipe.
18 Note how much and which foods were eaten. See "Calorie Counts."
19 Measure and record intake if ordered (p. 440).
20 Remove the tray.
21 Take the person back to his or her room (if in a dining area).
22 Assist with oral hygiene and hand washing. Provide for privacy. Wear gloves. Practice hand hygiene after removing and discarding the gloves.

POST-PROCEDURE

23 Provide for comfort. (See the inside of the front book cover.)
24 Place the signal light within reach.
25 Raise or lower bed rails. Follow the care plan.
26 Complete a safety check of the room. (See the inside of the front book cover.)

27 Return the food tray to the food cart.
28 Practice hand hygiene.
29 Report and record your observations.

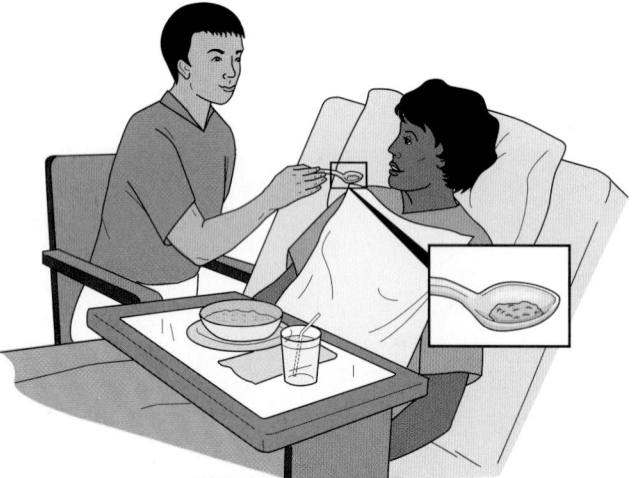

Fig. 24-10 A spoon is used to feed the person. The spoon is one-third full.

Between-Meal Snacks

Many special diets involve between-meal snacks. Common snacks are crackers, milk, juice, a milkshake, cake, wafers, a sandwich, gelatin, and custard.

Snacks are served upon arrival on the nursing unit. Provide needed utensils, a straw, and a napkin. Follow the same considerations and procedures for serving meals and feeding persons.

Calorie Counts

Calorie records are kept for some people. On a flow sheet, note what the person ate and how much. For example, a chicken breast, rice, beans, a roll, pudding, and 2 pats of butter were served. The person ate all the chicken, half the rice, and the roll. One pat of butter was used. The beans and pudding were not eaten. Note these on the flow sheet. A nurse or dietitian converts these portions into calories. The nurse tells you which persons need calorie counts.

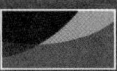 Providing Drinking Water

Patients and residents need fresh drinking water each shift. They also need water whenever the pitcher is empty.

Some agencies do not use the procedure that follows. Each person's pitcher is filled as needed. The pitcher is taken to an ice and water dispenser. If so, fill the pitcher with ice first. Then add water to the pitcher. Follow the agency's procedure for providing fresh drinking water.

See *Focus on Communication: Providing Drinking Water.*
See *Delegation Guidelines: Providing Drinking Water.*
See *Promoting Safety and Comfort: Providing Drinking Water.*

FOCUS ON COMMUNICATION
Providing Drinking Water

Some persons do not like ice in their water. Others like mostly ice with little water. Ask about the person's preferences. You can say:
- "How much ice do you want in your water?"
- "Do you like more ice or more water?"

Also ask the person where to place the drinking water. Be sure the person can reach the water.

DELEGATION GUIDELINES
Providing Drinking Water

To provide water, you need this information from the nurse and the care plan:
- The person's fluid orders
- If the person can have ice
- If the person uses a straw

PROMOTING SAFETY AND COMFORT
Providing Drinking Water

Safety

Water cups and pitchers can spread microbes. To prevent the spread of microbes:
- Make sure the pitcher is labeled with the person's name and room and bed number.
- Do not touch the rim or inside of the cup, pitcher, or lid.
- Do not let the ice scoop touch the cup, pitcher, or lid.
- Do not put the ice scoop in the ice container or dispenser. Place it in the scoop holder or on a towel for the scoop.
- Make sure the pitcher and cup are clean. Also check for cracks and chips. Provide a new pitcher or cup as needed.

PROVIDING DRINKING WATER

QUALITY OF LIFE

Remember to:
- Knock before entering the person's room.
- Address the person by name.
- Introduce yourself by name and title.

- Explain the procedure to the person before beginning and during the procedure.
- Protect the person's rights during the procedure.
- Handle the person gently during the procedure.

PRE-PROCEDURE

1 Follow *Delegation Guidelines: Providing Drinking Water.* See *Promoting Safety and Comfort: Providing Drinking Water.*
2 Obtain a list of persons who have special fluid orders from the nurse. Or use your assignment sheet.
3 Practice hand hygiene.
4 Collect the following:
   - Cart
   - Ice chest filled with ice
   - Cover for the ice chest

- Scoop
- Water cups
- Straws
- Paper towels
- Water pitchers for patient and resident use
- Large water pitcher filled with cold water (optional, depending on agency procedure)
- Towel for the scoop
5 Cover the cart with paper towels. Arrange equipment on top of the paper towels.

PROCEDURE

6 Take the cart to the person's room door. Do not take the cart into the room.
7 Check the person's fluid orders. Use the list from the nurse.
8 Identify the person. Check the ID bracelet against the fluid orders sheet or your assignment sheet. Also call the person by name.
9 Take the pitcher from the person's overbed table. Empty it into the bathroom sink.
10 Determine if a new pitcher is needed.

11 Use the scoop to fill the pitcher with ice (Fig. 24-11, p. 450). Do not let the scoop touch the pitcher or lid.
12 Place the ice scoop on the towel.
13 Fill the pitcher with water. Get water from the bathroom or use the larger water pitcher on the cart.
14 Place the pitcher, cup, and straw (if used) on the overbed table. Fill the cup with water. Do not let the water pitcher touch the cup.
15 Make sure the pitcher, cup, and straw (if used) are within the person's reach.

Continued

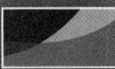 **PROVIDING DRINKING WATER—cont'd**

POST-PROCEDURE

16 Provide for comfort. (See the inside of the front book cover.)

17 Place the signal light within reach.

18 Complete a safety check of the room. (See the inside of the front book cover.)

19 Practice hand hygiene.

20 Repeat steps 6 through 19 for each person.

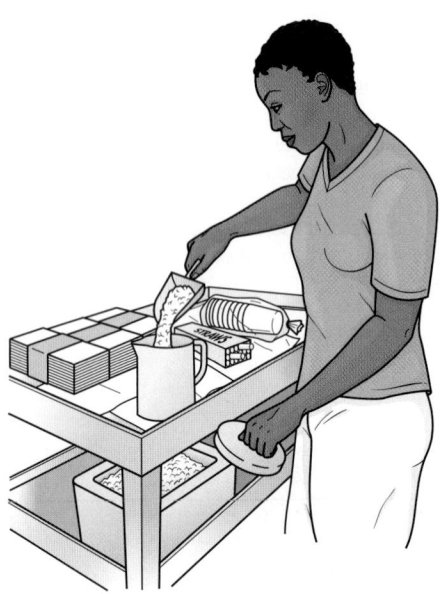

Fig. 24-11 Providing drinking water.

BOX 24-8	SIGNS AND SYMPTOMS OF FOODBORNE ILLNESSES

- Abdominal cramps or pain
- Backache
- Breathing problems
- Chills
- Diarrhea (may be bloody)
- Eyelids: droopy
- Fever
- Headache
- Muscle pain
- Nausea
- Speaking problems
- Swallowing problems
- Vision: double
- Vomiting

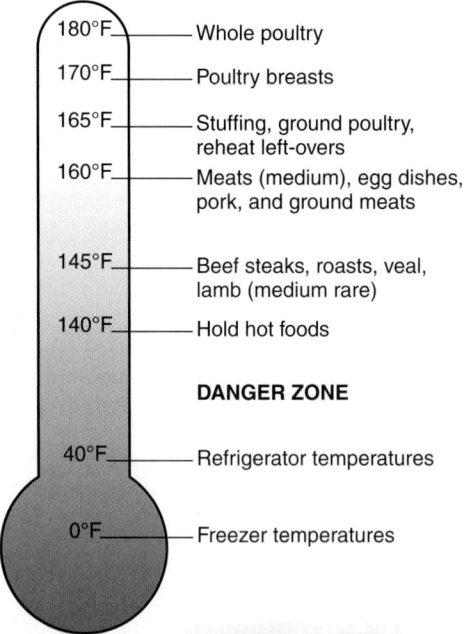

Fig. 24-12 Food temperature guide.

FOODBORNE ILLNESSES

A foodborne illness (food poisoning) is caused by pathogens in food and fluids. Report the signs and symptoms listed in Box 24-8 to the nurse at once.

Food is not sterile. Therefore pathogens are present in food. Cooked and ready-to-eat foods can become contaminated from other food. For example, meat juices can spill or splash onto other food. Food handlers with poor hygiene can contaminate the food.

Pathogens grow rapidly between 40°F and 140°F (Fahrenheit). This range is called the "danger zone" by the USDA. You must keep food out of the "danger zone." To do so, keep cold food cold and hot food hot.

To keep food safe, the USDA recommends these 4 safety tips:

- *Clean*. Wash hands, utensils, and counter tops often.
- *Separate*. Avoid cross-contamination. Do not let raw meat, poultry, or their juices touch other foods that will not be cooked.
- *Cook*. Cook food to a safe internal temperature (Fig. 24-12). Use a food thermometer to check the internal temperature. When re-heating cooked food, re-heat to 165°F.
- *Chill*. Refrigerate or freeze food within 2 hours. If the air is 90°F or above, chill food within 1 hour.

See *Focus on Long-Term Care and Home Care: Foodborne Illnesses.*

FOCUS ON LONG-TERM CARE AND HOME CARE
Foodborne Illnesses

Home Care

You need to protect the patient and family from foodborne illnesses. Follow the *clean, separate, cook,* and *chill* safety tips.

Clean

- Wash your hands with soap and warm water:
  - Before and after preparing food. Do so especially after handling raw seafood, meat, poultry, and eggs.
  - Before eating.
  - After elimination.
  - After changing diapers.
  - After coughing or sneezing.
  - Before and after providing care.
  - After touching animals.
  - After handling garbage.
- Wash surfaces with hot, soapy water. Use a solution of 1 tablespoon of unscented, liquid chlorine bleach in 1 gallon of water to sanitize surfaces.
  - Tables and counter tops.
  - Sinks.
  - Utensils.
  - Cutting boards.
  - The inside and outside of appliances and microwave ovens. This includes buttons and handles.
- Discard refrigerated foods:
  - Cooked left-overs after 4 days
  - Raw poultry and ground meats after 1 or 2 days
- Wipe up spills at once.
- Clean food contact surfaces often.
- Rinse all fruits and vegetables thoroughly. Products labeled as "pre-washed" or "ready-to-eat" do not need further rinsing.
  - Rinse under running water before eating, peeling, cutting, or cooking.
  - Do not use soap or detergent.
  - Scrub firm produce (melons, cucumbers, potatoes, and so on) with a clean produce brush while rinsing.
  - Dry produce with a clean towel or paper towel.
- Do not rinse raw seafood, meat, and poultry. Bacteria in the raw juices can spread to other foods, utensils, and surfaces.

Separate

- Place raw seafood, meat, and poultry in plastic bags. Separate them from other foods in the grocery cart and in bags.
- Store raw seafood, meat, and poultry in the refrigerator. Store them below ready-to-eat foods.

Separate—cont'd

- Clean re-usable grocery bags.
  - Wash canvas and cloth bags in the washing machine.
  - Wash plastic bags with hot, soapy water.
- Use a clean cutting board for fresh produce.
- Use a separate cutting board for raw seafood, meat, and poultry.
- Use a clean plate to serve and eat food.
- Do not place cooked food back on a plate or cutting board that held raw food.

Cook and Chill

- Cook seafood, meat, poultry, and egg dishes to the correct internal temperature.
- Use a food thermometer to make sure that:
  - Food is safely cooked.
  - Cooked food is held at safe temperatures until eaten.
- Place the food thermometer in the thickest part of the food. It should not touch bone, fat, or gristle.
- Follow the manufacturer's instructions for using the food thermometer.
- Clean food thermometers with hot, soapy water before and after each use.
- Stir, rotate, or flip foods for even cooking in a microwave oven. Follow package instructions.
- Keep foods at a safe temperature:
  - Keep cold foods at 40°F or below.
  - Keep hot foods at 140°F or above.
  - Do not eat or serve foods when they have been in the "danger zone" (see Fig. 24-12) of 40°F to 140°F for more than 2 hours. Or 1 hour if the temperature is above 90°F. This time frame includes:
    - The amount of time food is in the grocery cart, car, and at home.
    - When frozen foods begin to thaw and become warmer than 40°F.
- Thaw foods in one of these ways:
  - In the refrigerator.
  - In a leak-proof bag in cold water. Change the water every 30 minutes.
  - In the microwave.
- Never thaw food on the counter.
- Keep the refrigerator at 40°F or below. Keep the freezer at 0°F or below.

Modified from U.S. Department of Agriculture and U.S. Department of Health and Human Services. *Dietary Guidelines for Americans, 2010*. 7th Edition. Washington, DC: U.S. Government Printing Office, December 2010.

FOCUS ON PRIDE

The Person, Family, and Yourself

Personal and Professional Responsibility

Many agencies are serving food in new ways. The purpose is to allow freedom and personal choice. For example:

- *24-hour catering.* Meals and snacks are provided 24 hours a day. This is for persons who cannot or do not want to eat at the usual meal times. The person orders food directly from the food service department. The person orders desired foods within his or her ordered diet.
- *Mobile food carts.* Food service staff bring a food cart to the nursing unit. The patient selects food and a tray is prepared.

With such systems, you may have new responsibilities. For example, you may need to watch for the arrival of food trays more often. Or you may need to assist persons with reading or filling out menus. Know your agency's food ordering and delivery system and your role in that system. Take pride in helping others meet their nutritional needs.

Rights and Respect

The right to personal choice is important in meeting food and fluid needs. Everyone has a life-time of likes and dislikes. Cultural, social, religious, medical, and personal factors affect food choices. These do not change when in a hospital or nursing center. People often comment about food likes and dislikes. A person may say that the food is cold. Or it is bland. Or the food tastes bad.

People have the right to express their preferences. Do not become angry or upset. The person should not feel as if he or she is complaining or being picky. Learning the person's likes and dislikes can improve nutrition. It also shows interest and concern for the person. Respect the person's right to express personal food choices.

Independence and Social Interaction

Meals can provide a time for social contact with others. A friendly, social setting is important. Some nursing centers have areas where residents can dine with a partner, family, or friends. They can enjoy holidays, birthdays, anniversaries, and other special events together.

Sometimes families and friends bring food from home. This helps meet love and belonging needs. Sometimes the agency cannot provide everything the person likes. The person is usually pleased to receive home-made food. Tell the nurse when the person receives food. The food must not interfere with the person's diet.

Delegation and Teamwork

In some agencies, meal trays arrive on the nursing unit in a meal cart. Each tray is in a slot. Trays are served in the order that they appear in the cart. The entire nursing team serves trays. You may serve trays to patients or residents of other staff members. They do the same for you. The team works together to serve food promptly.

Ethics and Laws

Proper food and fluid intake are needed to live. The person must be closely observed for changes in nutrition and hydration. The following case is a real example of how poor hydration resulted in harm.

Mr. Caruso was admitted to a nursing center on January 22 after needing hospital care for about 5 weeks. He had nervous and urinary system disorders. A doctor examined him on January 23. The doctor found him to be in stable condition. He showed signs of adequate hydration and responded to the doctor's commands.

The nursing center did not keep a chart of Mr. Caruso's intake or output of fluids. According to the center nurses, Mr. Caruso received the following:

- Three meals a day.
- Three snacks [a day] with juice or milk.
- Drugs four times a day. He was given 4 ounces of water with the drugs.
- Offers of something to drink every two hours during the night.

Seven days after being admitted to the nursing center (January 29), Mr. Caruso was taken to the hospital. The emergency room doctor diagnosed severe dehydration. He was weak, confused, had tremors, and had dry skin with poor turgor. (Author note: poor skin turgor means that the skin slowly returns to its normal position after being grasped between two fingers.) In the hospital, Mr. Caruso was treated with IV fluids and a catheter. He was also treated for a urinary tract infection caused by the catheter.

Mr. Caruso returned to the nursing center on February 19. He died on May 14.

His family sued the nursing center. They charged the nursing center with negligence and with abuse and neglect because of failing to give Mr. Caruso enough water. They claimed that the dehydration led to declines in his physical and mental condition.

The jury found in favor of Mr. Caruso's family. The jury awarded the family $195,000 and attorney fees. The nursing home appealed the case. Because of a legal technicality, a judge ordered a new trial.

(I. Caruso v Pine Manor Nursing Center, IL 1989.)

You can do your part to promote good nutrition and fluid intake. Follow the person's care plan and dietary preferences. Carefully record intake and output as ordered. Tell the nurse if you notice a change in the person's intake.

REVIEW QUESTIONS

Circle the BEST answer.

1 Nutrition is
   a Fats, proteins, carbohydrates, vitamins, and minerals
   b The many processes involved in the ingestion, digestion, absorption, and use of food and fluids by the body
   c The MyPlate symbol
   d The balance between calories taken in and used by the body

2 MyPlate encourages the following *except*
   a The same diet for everyone
   b Balancing calories
   c Increasing the amount of fruits and vegetables
   d Choosing low-sodium foods

REVIEW QUESTIONS—cont'd

3 On a 2000 calorie diet, what is the amount of grains needed for an adult woman?
   a 5 to 6 oz
   b 4 to 5 oz
   c 3 to 4 oz
   d 2 oz

4 On a 2000 calorie diet, what is the amount of protein foods needed for an adult man?
   a 2½ oz
   b 3 to 4 oz
   c 4 to 5 oz
   d 5½ to 6½ oz

5 Which food group contains the *most* cholesterol?
   a Grains
   b Vegetables
   c Fruit
   d Protein foods

6 These statements are about oils. Which is *false?*
   a Oils are high in calories.
   b The best oil choices come from fish, nuts, and vegetable oils.
   c Oils from plant sources contain cholesterol.
   d Mayonnaise is mainly oil.

7 Protein is needed for
   a Tissue growth and repair
   b Energy and the fiber for bowel elimination
   c Body heat and to protect organs from injury
   d Improving the taste of food

8 Which foods provide the *most* protein?
   a Butter and cream
   b Tomatoes and potatoes
   c Meats and fish
   d Corn and lettuce

9 The sodium-controlled diet involves
   a Omitting high-sodium foods
   b Adding salt to food at the table
   c Using 2400 mg of salt in cooking
   d A sodium-intake flow sheet

10 A person on a sodium-controlled diet wants a salt shaker. You should
   a Provide the salt
   b Salt the person's food
   c Explain that added salt is not allowed on the diet
   d Ignore the request

11 Diabetes meal planning involves the following *except*
   a Food the person likes
   b Eating the same amount of carbohydrates, protein, and fat each day
   c Eating at regular times
   d Sodium control

12 OBRA requires the following *except*
   a Offering 24-hour meal service
   b Serving hot food hot; serving cold food cold
   c Providing needed eating devices
   d Serving food promptly

13 OBRA requires
   a 2 regular meals
   b 3 regular meals
   c 3 regular meals and a bedtime snack
   d Meals every 6 hours

14 Adult fluid requirements are about
   a 1000 to 1500 mL daily
   b 1500 to 2000 mL daily
   c 2000 to 2500 mL daily
   d 2500 to 3000 mL daily

15 A person is NPO. You should
   a Provide a variety of fluids
   b Offer fluids in small amounts and in small containers
   c Remove the water pitcher and cup from the room
   d Remove oral hygiene equipment from the room

16 Which are *not* counted as liquid foods?
   a Coffee, tea, juices, and soft drinks
   b Butter, sauces, and melted cheese
   c Ice cream, sherbet, custard, pudding
   d Jell-O, Popsicles, and creamed cereals

17 Residents serve themselves from bowls and platters on their tables. This is
   a A social dining program
   b A family dining program
   c A low-stimulation feeding program
   d An open-dining program

18 Persons with dysphagia
   a Use straws for all liquids
   b Have a regular diet
   c Are fed according to the care plan
   d Eat alone in their rooms

19 Which is *not* a sign of a swallowing problem?
   a Drooling
   b Coughing while eating
   c Pocketing
   d Edema

20 You are feeding a person. Which action is *not correct?*
   a Ask if he or she wants to pray before eating.
   b Use a fork to feed the person.
   c Ask the person the order in which to serve food and fluids.
   d Engage the person in a pleasant conversation.

21 Before providing fresh drinking water, you need to know the person's
   a I&O
   b Diet
   c Fluid orders
   d Preferred beverages

22 You are re-heating cooked food. The food temperature should be
   a 40°F
   b 90°F
   c 140°F
   d 165°F

Circle T if the statement is TRUE or F if it is FALSE.

23 T F You should wash vegetables and fruits before serving them.

24 T F Pre-washed fruits need further rinsing.

25 T F Raw meat can touch other foods.

26 T F Refrigerated left-over foods should be eaten within 4 days.

27 T F Poultry is washed and rinsed before cooking.

28 T F A cutting board can be used for all foods.

29 T F Raw meat, poultry, and seafood are stored on the top shelf of the refrigerator.

30 T F Ground beef can be placed on a counter top to thaw.

31 T F Left-over foods should be refrigerated within 2 hours.

32 T F Hot, soapy water is used to clean kitchen surfaces.

Answers to these questions are on p. 833.

25 Nutritional Support and IV Therapy

OBJECTIVES

- Define the key terms and key abbreviations listed in this chapter.
- Identify the reasons for nutritional support and IV therapy.
- Explain how tube feedings are given.
- Describe scheduled and continuous feedings.
- Explain how to prevent aspiration.
- Describe the comfort measures for the person with a feeding tube.
- Describe parenteral nutrition.

- Describe the IV therapy sites.
- Identify the equipment used in IV therapy.
- Describe how to assist with the IV flow rate.
- Identify the safety measures for IV therapy.
- Identify the observations to report when a person has nutritional support or IV therapy.
- Explain how to assist with nutritional support and IV therapy.
- Explain how to promote PRIDE in the person, the family, and yourself.

KEY TERMS

aspiration Breathing fluid, food, vomitus, or an object into the lungs

enteral nutrition Giving nutrients into the gastro-intestinal (GI) tract *(enteral)* through a feeding tube

flow rate The number of drops per minute *(gtt/min)* or milliliters per hour *(mL/hr)*

gastrostomy tube A feeding tube inserted through a surgically created opening *(stomy)* in the stomach *(gastro)*; stomach tube

gavage The process of giving a tube feeding

intravenous (IV) therapy Giving fluids through a needle or catheter inserted into a vein; IV and IV infusion

jejunostomy tube A feeding tube inserted into a surgically created opening *(stomy)* in the *jejunum* of the small intestine

naso-enteral tube A feeding tube inserted through the nose *(naso)* into the small bowel *(enteral)*

naso-gastric (NG) tube A feeding tube inserted through the nose *(naso)* into the stomach *(gastro)*

parenteral nutrition Giving nutrients through a catheter inserted into a vein; *para* means *beyond*; *enteral* relates to the *bowel*

percutaneous endoscopic gastrostomy (PEG) tube A feeding tube inserted into the stomach *(gastro)* through a small incision *(stomy)* made through *(per)* the skin *(cutaneous)*; a lighted instrument *(scope)* is used to see inside a body cavity or organ *(endo)*

regurgitation The backward flow of stomach contents into the mouth

KEY ABBREVIATIONS

GI	Gastro-intestinal	**NG**	Naso-gastric
gtt	Drops	**NPO**	Nothing by mouth
gtt/min	Drops per minute	**oz**	Ounce
IV	Intravenous	**PEG**	Percutaneous endoscopic gastrostomy
mL	Milliliter	**TPN**	Total parenteral nutrition
mL/hr	Milliliters per hour		

Many persons cannot eat or drink because of illness, surgery, or injury. They may have chewing or swallowing problems. Aspiration is a risk. *Aspiration is breathing fluid, food, vomitus, or an object into the lungs.*

Some persons have problems eating or refuse to eat or drink. Others cannot eat enough to meet their nutritional needs. The doctor may order nutritional support or intravenous (IV) therapy to meet food and fluid needs.

ENTERAL NUTRITION

Some persons cannot or will not ingest, chew, or swallow food. Or food cannot pass from the mouth into the esophagus and into the stomach or small intestine. Poor nutrition results. Common causes are:

- Cancer, especially cancers of the head, neck, and esophagus
- Trauma to the face, mouth, head, or neck
- Coma
- Dysphagia
- Dementia
- Eating disorders
- Nervous system disorders (Chapter 41)
- Prolonged vomiting
- Major trauma or surgery
- Acquired immunodeficiency syndrome (AIDS)
- Illnesses and disorders affecting eating and nutrition

Enteral nutrition is giving nutrients into the gastrointestinal (GI) tract (enteral) through a feeding tube. Gavage is the process of giving a tube feeding. Tube feedings replace or supplement normal nutrition.

Types of Feeding Tubes

These feeding tubes are common:

- *Naso-gastric (NG) tube. A feeding tube is inserted through the nose (naso) into the stomach (gastro)* (Fig. 25-1). A doctor or an RN inserts the tube.
- *Naso-enteral tube. A feeding tube is inserted through the nose (naso) into the small bowel (enteral)* (Fig. 25-2). A doctor or RN inserts the tube.
- *Gastrostomy tube. A feeding tube is inserted through a surgically created opening (stomy) in the stomach (gastro).* It is also called a *stomach tube.* See Figure 25-3.
- *Jejunostomy tube. A feeding tube is inserted into a surgically created opening (stomy) in the jejunum of the small intestine* (Fig. 25-4, p. 456).
- *Percutaneous endoscopic gastrostomy (PEG) tube. A* doctor inserts *a feeding tube into the stomach (gastro) through a small incision (stomy) made through (per) the skin (cutaneous).* See Fig. 25-5, p. 456. *A lighted instrument (scope) is used to see inside a body cavity or organ (endo).*

NG and naso-enteral tubes are used for short-term nutritional support—usually less than 6 weeks. Gastrostomy, jejunostomy, and PEG tubes are used for long-term nutritional support—usually longer than 6 weeks.

Formulas

The doctor orders the type of formula, the amount to give, and when to give tube feedings. Most formulas contain proteins, carbohydrates, fats, vitamins, and minerals. Commercial formulas are common.

Formula is given at room temperature. Cold fluids can cause cramping. Opened formula can remain at room temperature for about 8 hours. Microbes can grow in warm formula.

See *Teamwork and Time Management: Formulas*, p. 456.

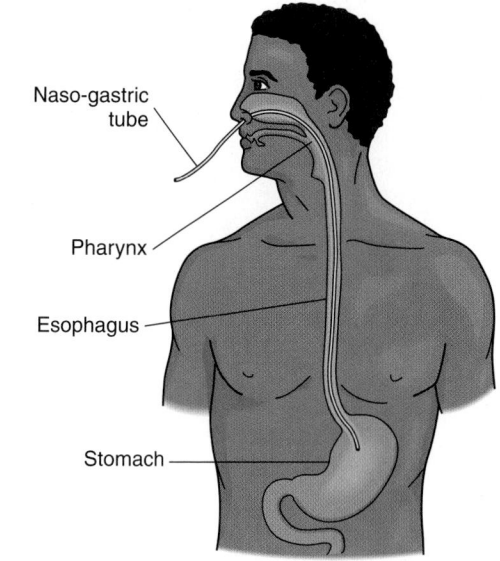

Fig. 25-1 A naso-gastric (NG) tube is inserted through the nose and esophagus and into the stomach.

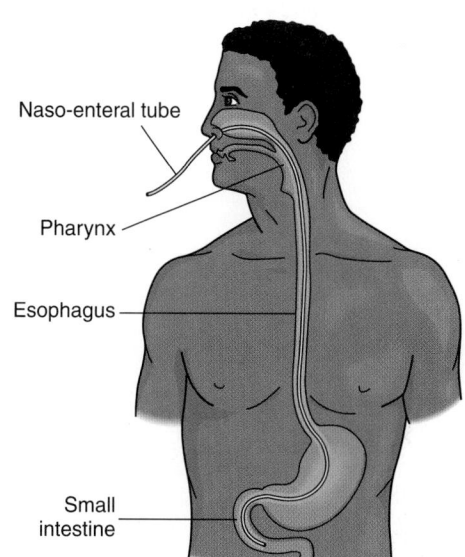

Fig. 25-2 A naso-enteral tube is inserted through the nose and into the small intestine.

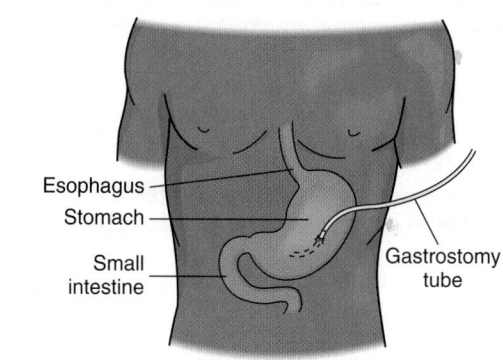

Fig. 25-3 A gastrostomy tube.

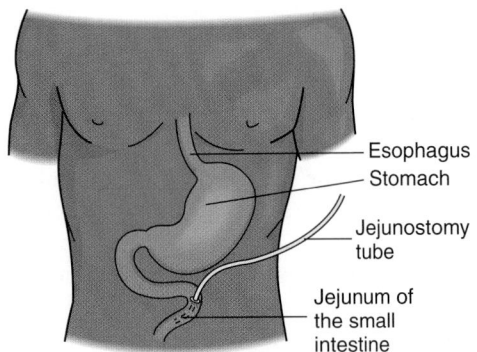

Fig. 25-4 A jejunostomy tube.

Esophagus
Stomach
Jejunostomy tube
Jejunum of the small intestine

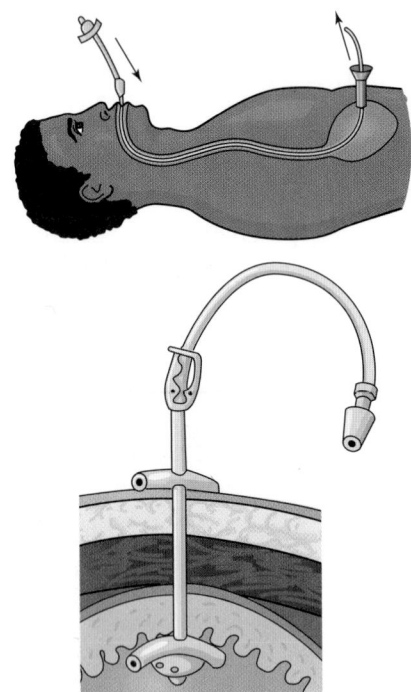

Fig. 25-5 A percutaneous endoscopic gastrostomy (PEG) tube.

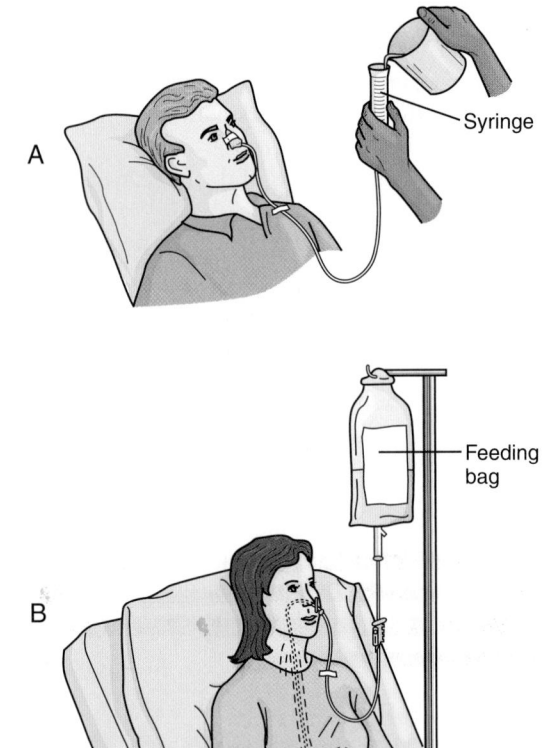

Fig. 25-6 **A,** A tube feeding is given with a syringe. **B,** Formula drips from a feeding bag into the feeding tube.

Syringe

A

Feeding bag

B

Feeding Times

Tube feedings are given at certain times (scheduled feedings). Or they are given over a 24-hour period (continuous feedings).

Scheduled Feedings. Such feedings also are called intermittent feedings. (*Intermittent* means to *start, stop, and then start again.*) Feeding times are scheduled. At least 4 feedings are given each day. Usually 8 to 12 ounces (oz) (240 to 360 milliliters [mL]) are given over about 30 minutes. The frequency, amount, and time are like a normal eating pattern.

The nurse uses a syringe or a feeding bag (Fig. 25-6). The syringe attaches to the feeding tube. Connecting tubing connects the feeding bag to the tube. Formula is added to the syringe or to the feeding bag. Then it slowly flows through the feeding tube into the stomach.

The nurse removes the syringe or connecting tubing after the feeding. Then the nurse clamps and covers the end of the feeding tube with a cap or gauze. Gauze is secured in place with a rubber band. Clamping prevents air from entering the tube. It also prevents fluid from leaking out of the tube. Covering the end of the tube also prevents leaking.

TEAMWORK AND TIME MANAGEMENT

Formulas

Refrigerated formula needs to warm to room temperature. To warm formula, place the container in a wash basin filled with warm water. If warmed in the sink, other staff cannot use the sink. They must go elsewhere. They waste time and energy. Or someone may remove the container to use the sink. The container does not warm in a timely manner. That affects you, the nurse, and the patient or resident.

The nurse and manufacturer's instructions tell you how long formula can hang. Check the time that the feeding started. Remind the nurse when the time limit is near. For example, a feeding started at 0800. The formula can hang for 8 hours. At 1530 or 1545, tell the nurse how much time is left. Also report the amount of formula left.

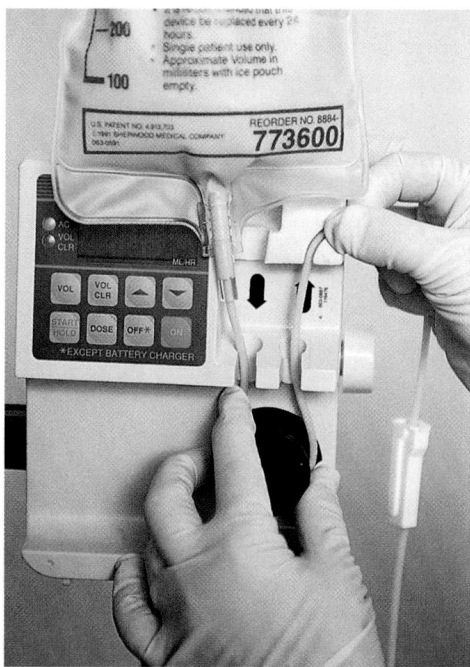

Fig. 25-7 Feeding pump.

Continuous Feedings. These feedings are usually given over 24 hours. A feeding pump is used (Fig. 25-7). Formula drips into the feeding tube at a certain rate per minute. The person receives a certain amount each hour.

A pump alarm sounds if something is wrong. When you hear an alarm, tell the nurse.

Observations

Diarrhea, constipation, delayed stomach emptying, and aspiration are risks. Report the following at once:
* Nausea
* Discomfort during the feeding
* Vomiting
* Distended (enlarged and swollen) abdomen
* Coughing
* Complaints of indigestion or heartburn
* Redness, swelling, drainage, odor, or pain at the ostomy site
* Fever
* Signs and symptoms of respiratory distress (Chapter 36)
* Increased pulse rate
* Complaints of flatulence (Chapter 23)
* Diarrhea (Chapter 23)

Preventing Aspiration

Aspiration is a major risk from tube feedings. It can cause pneumonia and death. Aspiration can occur:
* *During insertion.* NG tubes and naso-enteral tubes are passed through the nose into the esophagus and then into the stomach or small intestine. The tube can slip into the airway. An x-ray is taken after insertion to check tube placement.
* *From tube movement out of place.* Coughing, sneezing, vomiting, suctioning, and poor positioning are common causes. A tube can move from the stomach or intestines into the esophagus and then into the airway. The RN checks tube placement before every scheduled tube feeding. With continuous feedings, the RN checks tube placement every 4 hours. To do so, the RN attaches a syringe to the tube. GI secretions are withdrawn through the syringe. Then the pH of the secretions is measured (Chapter 31). *You never check feeding tube placement.*
* *From regurgitation.* Regurgitation *is the backward flow of stomach contents into the mouth.* Delayed stomach emptying and over-feeding are common causes.

To help prevent regurgitation and aspiration:
* Position the person in Fowler's or semi-Fowler's position before the feeding. Follow the care plan and the nurse's directions.
* Maintain Fowler's or semi-Fowler's position after the feeding. This allows formula to move through the GI tract. The position is required for 1 to 2 hours after the feeding or at all times. Follow the care plan and the nurse's directions.
* Avoid the left side-lying position. When the person lies on the left side, the stomach cannot empty into the small intestine.

Persons with NG or gastrostomy tubes are at great risk for regurgitation. The risk is less with intestinal tubes. Formula passes directly into the small intestine. Also, formula is given at a slow rate. During digestion, food slowly passes from the stomach into the small intestine. The stomach handles larger amounts of food at one time than does the small intestine.

See *Focus on Children and Older Persons: Preventing Aspiration.*

> **FOCUS ON CHILDREN AND OLDER PERSONS**
> **Preventing Aspiration**
>
> **Older Persons**
> Digestion slows with aging. Stomach emptying also slows. Older persons are at risk for regurgitation and aspiration. Less formula and longer feeding times prevent over-feeding.

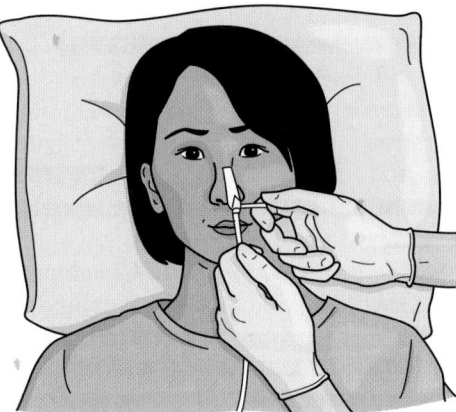

Fig. 25-8 The feeding tube is secured to the nose.

Comfort Measures

Persons with feeding tubes usually are not allowed to eat or drink. They are NPO—nothing by mouth (Chapter 24). Dry mouth, dry lips, and sore throat cause discomfort. Sometimes hard candy or gum is allowed. These measures are common:

• Oral hygiene every 2 hours while the person is awake
• Lubricant for the lips every 2 hours while the person is awake
• Mouth rinses every 2 hours while the person is awake

Feeding tubes can irritate and cause pressure on the nose. They can change the shape of the nostrils or cause pressure ulcers. These measures are common:

• Clean the nose and nostrils every 4 to 8 hours.
• Secure the tube to the nose (Fig. 25-8). Use tape or a tube holder. Tube holders have foam cushions that prevent pressure on the nose. Re-taping is not needed. Re-taping irritates the nose. Do not use safety pins.
• Secure the tube to the person's garment at the shoulder area. This prevents the tube from pulling or dangling. Both can cause pressure on the nose. These methods are common. Follow agency policy.
  • Loop a rubber band around the tube. Then pin the rubber band to the garment with a safety pin.
  • Tape the tube to the garment.

Assisting With Tube Feedings

You assist the nurse with tube feedings. In some states and agencies, nursing assistants give tube feedings and remove NG tubes. *Remember, you never insert feeding tubes or check their placement. They are the RN's responsibility.*

See *Delegation Guidelines: Assisting With Tube Feedings.*

See *Promoting Safety and Comfort: Assisting With Tube Feedings.*

DELEGATION GUIDELINES
Assisting With Tube Feedings

Before giving tube feedings or removing an NG tube, make sure that:
• Your state allows you to perform the procedure.
• The procedure is in your job description.
• You have had the necessary education and training.
• You know how to use the agency's equipment and supplies.
• You review the procedure in the agency's procedure manual.
• You review the procedure with the nurse.
• A nurse is available to answer questions and to supervise you.
• An RN has identified and labeled all other tubes, catheters, and needles.
• An RN checks tube placement and residual stomach contents. *Residual* means *what remains.* For an NG tube or gastrostomy tube, the nurse aspirates stomach contents and measures the amount. Depending on the amount, the nurse decides if the feeding should be given or delayed. The intent is to prevent aspiration from regurgitation caused by over-feeding.

If the above conditions are met, you need this information from the nurse and the care plan:
• The type of tube—NG, naso-enteral, gastrostomy, PEG, or jejunostomy
• What feeding method to use—syringe, feeding bag, or feeding pump
• What size syringe to use—usually 30 or 60 mL for an adult
• How to position the person for the feeding—Fowler's or semi-Fowler's
• How to position the person after the feeding—Fowler's or semi-Fowler's
• What formula to use
• How much formula to give
• How high to raise the syringe or hang the feeding bag (usually 18 inches above the stomach or intestines)
• The amount of flushing solution to use—usually 30 to 60 mL (1 to 2 oz) of water for an adult
• How fast to give the feeding if using a syringe—usually over 30 minutes
• The flow rate if a feeding bag is used (Flow rate is the number of drops per minute. See p. 461.)
• The flow rate if a feeding pump is used
• If ice is kept around the bag for a continuous feeding
• If you are to remove an NG tube, when to remove the tube
• What observations to report and record—see p. 457
• When to report observations
• What patient or resident concerns to report at once

PARENTERAL NUTRITION

Parenteral nutrition is giving nutrients through a catheter inserted into a vein (Fig. 25-9). (*Para* means *beyond. Enteral* relates to the *bowel.*) A nutrient solution is given directly into the bloodstream. Nutrients do not enter the GI tract. Parenteral nutrition is often called *total parenteral nutrition (TPN)* or *hyperalimentation.* (*Hyper* means *high* or *excessive. Alimentation* means *nourishment.*)

PROMOTING SAFETY AND COMFORT
Assisting With Tube Feedings

Safety

The person may have an IV, a breathing tube (Chapter 37), and drainage tubes (Chapter 33). You must know the purpose of each tube. Ask the nurse to label each tube and its purpose. *Formula must enter only the feeding tube.* Otherwise, the person can die.

Before giving a tube feeding, always:

- Turn on the light if the room is dark. Do so even if the person is sleeping.
- Check and inspect the feeding tube and label with the nurse.
- Make sure an RN checks for tube placement.
- Make sure every tube, catheter, and needle is labeled.

- Trace the feeding tube back to the insertion site. Start at the end of the feeding tube. Trace the tube backward. For example, if the person has an NG tube, you will end at the nose. If the person has a gastrostomy tube, you will end at the abdomen. *If you do not end at the correct place, do not give the tube feeding. Call for the nurse.*

Nasal secretions may contain blood or microbes. So can drainage at an ostomy site. Wear gloves. Follow Standard Precautions and the Bloodborne Pathogen Standard.

Remind visitors to call for a nurse if any tube becomes disconnected. They could connect the wrong tubes together.

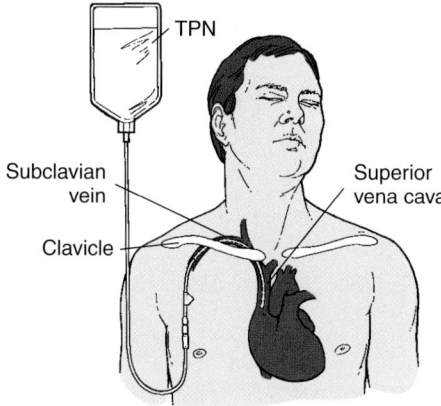

Fig. 25-9 Parenteral nutrition.

The solution contains water, proteins, carbohydrates, vitamins, and minerals. It drips through a catheter inserted into a large vein (p. 460). TPN is used when the person cannot receive oral or enteral feedings. Or it is used when oral or enteral feedings are not enough to meet the person's needs.

Common reasons for TPN include:

- Disease, injury, or surgery to the GI tract
- Severe trauma, infection, or burns
- Being NPO for more than 5 to 7 days
- GI side effects from cancer treatments (Chapter 40)
- Prolonged coma
- Prolonged anorexia (loss of appetite)

Observations

TPN risks include infection, fluid imbalances, and blood sugar imbalances. Report the following to the nurse at once:

- Fever, chills, and other signs and symptoms of infection (Chapter 15)
- Signs and symptoms of sugar imbalances (See "Diabetes" in Chapter 43.)

- Chest pain
- Difficulty breathing or shortness of breath
- Cough
- Nausea and vomiting
- Diarrhea
- Thirst
- Rapid heart rate or an irregular heartbeat
- Weakness or fatigue
- Sweating
- Pallor (pale skin)
- Trembling
- Confusion or behavior changes

Assisting With TPN

The nurse is responsible for all aspects of TPN. To assist, carefully observe the person. Also assist with the person's basic needs and activities of daily living. The person may be NPO. Provide frequent oral hygiene, lubricant to the lips, and mouth rinses as the nurse and care plan direct. Also follow other aspects of the person's care plan.

Many aspects of IV therapy apply to TPN.

IV THERAPY

Intravenous (IV) therapy is giving fluids through a needle or catheter inserted into a vein (Fig. 25-10, p. 460). Fluid flows directly into the bloodstream. *IV* and *IV infusion* also refer to IV therapy. Doctors order IV therapy to:

- Provide fluids when they cannot be taken by mouth.
- Replace minerals and vitamins lost because of illness or injury.
- Provide sugar for energy.
- Give drugs and blood.

RNs are responsible for IV therapy. They start and maintain the infusion as ordered. RNs also give IV drugs and administer blood. State laws vary about your role and that of LPNs/LVNs in IV therapy.

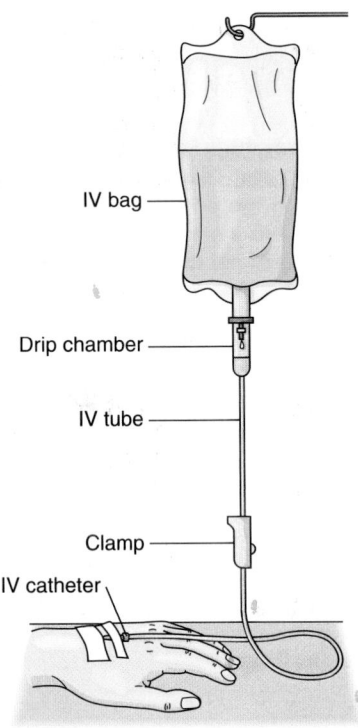

Fig. 25-10 Equipment for IV therapy.

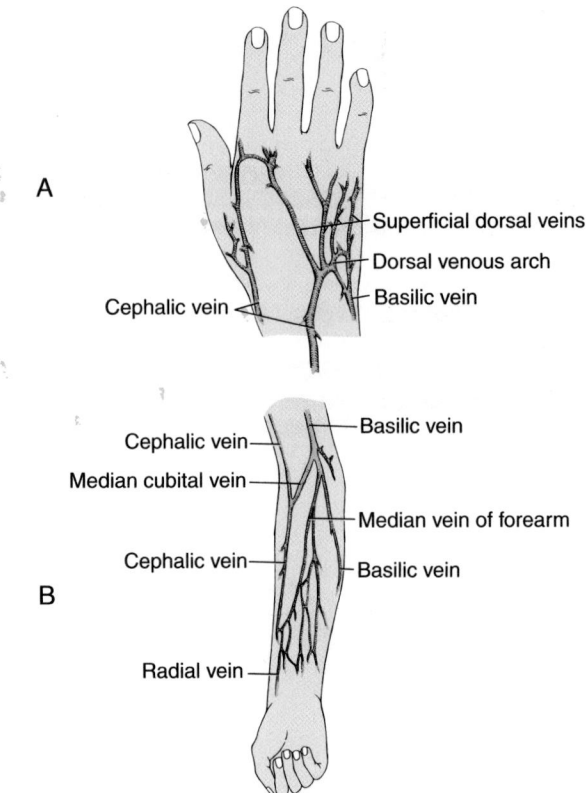

Fig. 25-11 Peripheral IV sites, **A,** Back of the hand. **B,** Inner forearm.

IV Sites

Peripheral and central venous sites are used. *Peripheral* means around *(peri)* a boundary *(pheral)*. The boundary is the center of the body near the heart. *Peripheral IV sites* are away from the center of the body. For adults, the back of the hand and inner forearm are useful sites (Fig. 25-11).

The subclavian vein and the internal jugular vein are *central venous sites*. They are close to the heart. A catheter is threaded into the superior vena cava or right atrium (Fig. 25-12, A and B). The catheter is called a *central venous catheter* or a *central line*. The cephalic and basilic veins in the arm also are used. Catheters inserted into these sites are called *peripherally inserted central catheters (PICCs)*. The catheter is threaded into the subclavian vein or the superior vena cava (Fig. 25-12, C).

Central venous sites are used:
* For parenteral nutrition
* To give large amounts of fluid
* For long-term IV therapy
* To give drugs that irritate peripheral veins
  See *Focus on Children and Older Persons: IV Sites.*
  See *Focus on Long-Term Care and Home Care: IV Sites.*

FOCUS ON CHILDREN AND OLDER PERSONS

IV Sites

Children
See Figure 25-13 for the IV sites in children. The hand, wrist, and inner arm sites are commonly used. The site selected depends on:
* The child's age. For example, scalp veins are sometimes used in infants. For a toddler, foot veins are avoided. IVs in foot veins prevent walking.
* The amount and kind of fluid ordered.
* How long the IV will be needed.

FOCUS ON LONG-TERM CARE AND HOME CARE

IV Sites

Home Care
Patients can receive IV therapy at home. They often have central venous catheters. The RN teaches the patient and family about giving drugs and managing the catheter.

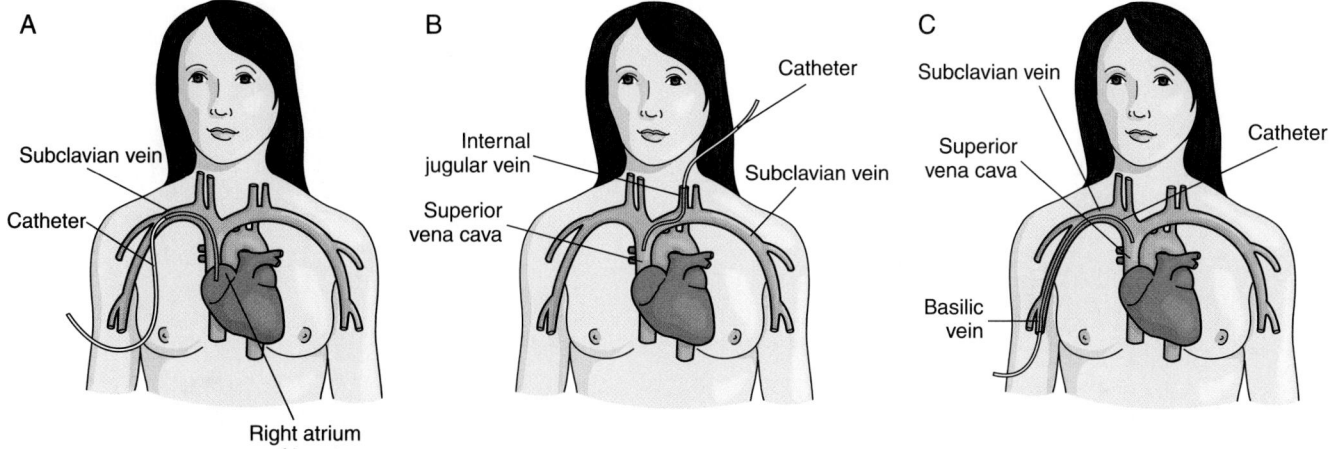

Fig. 25-12 Central venous sites. **A,** Subclavian vein. The catheter tip is in the right atrium. **B,** Internal jugular vein. The catheter tip is in the superior vena cava. **C,** Basilic vein. This is a peripherally inserted central catheter (PICC). The catheter tip is in the superior vena cava.

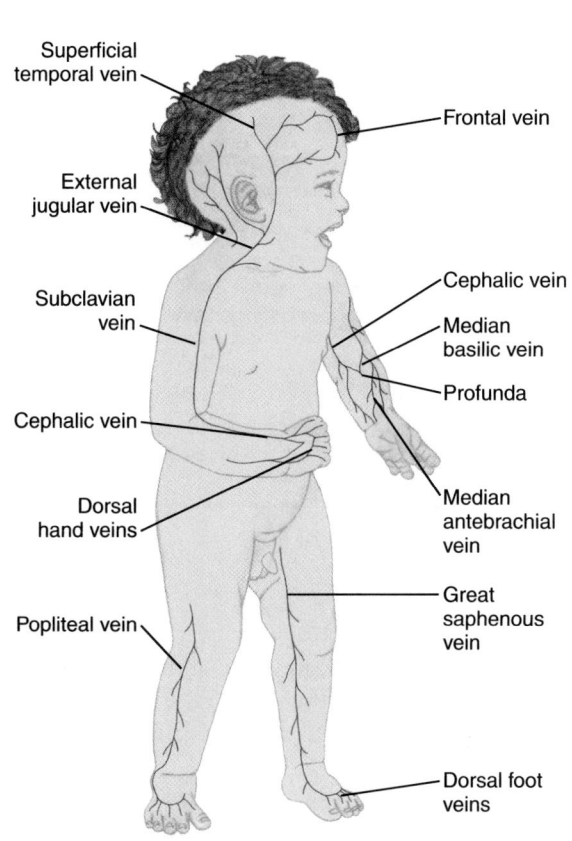

Fig. 25-13 IV sites in children.

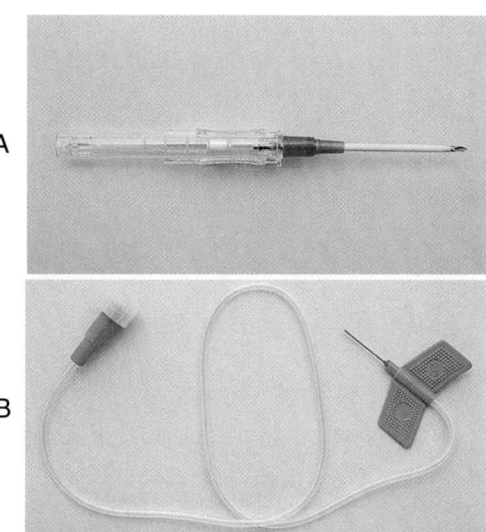

Fig. 25-14 **A,** Intravenous catheter. **B,** Butterfly needle.

IV Equipment

The basic equipment used in IV therapy is shown in Figure 25-10:

- The solution container is a plastic bag. It is called the *IV bag*.
- A *catheter* or *needle* is inserted into a vein (Fig. 25-14).
- The *IV tube* or *infusion tubing* connects the IV bag to the catheter or needle. Fluid drips from the bag into the *drip chamber*. The *clamp* is used to regulate the flow rate.
- The IV bag hangs from an IV pole (IV standard) or ceiling hook.

Flow Rate

The doctor orders the amount of fluid to give (infuse) and the amount of time to give it in. With this information, the RN figures the flow rate. The *flow rate is the number of drops per minute* (gtt/min) *or milliliters per hour* (mL/hr). The abbreviation *gtt* means *drops*. The Latin word *guttae* means *drops*.

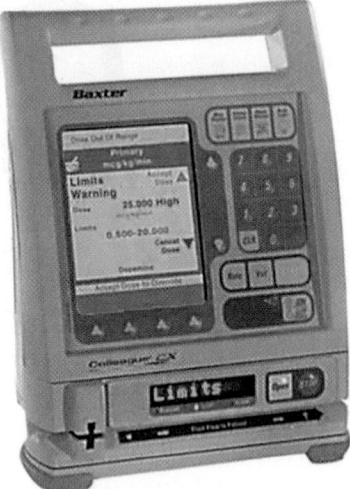

Fig. 25-15 Electronic IV pump.

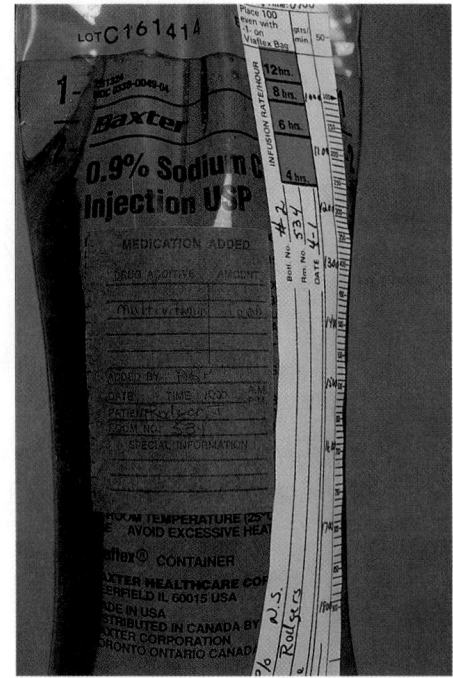

Fig. 25-17 Time tape applied to an IV bag.

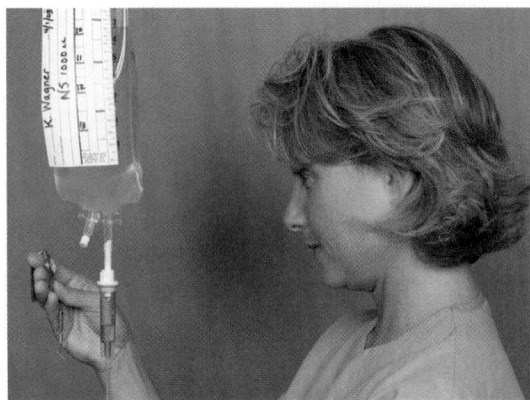

Fig. 25-16 The flow rate is checked by counting the number of drops per minute.

The RN sets the clamp for the flow rate. Or an electronic pump is used to control the flow rate (Fig. 25-15). The flow rate is displayed in mL/hr. An alarm sounds if something is wrong. Tell the nurse at once if you hear an alarm. *Never change the position of the clamp or adjust any controls on IV pumps.*

You can check the flow rate if a pump is not used. The RN tells you the number of drops per minute (gtt/min). To check the flow rate, count the number of drops in 1 minute (Fig. 25-16). Tell the RN at once if:

- No fluid is dripping.
- The rate is too fast.
- The rate is too slow.

The time tape shows how much fluid to give over a period of time (Fig. 25-17). For example, the doctor orders 1000 mL of fluid over 8 hours. The RN marks the tape in 8 one-hour intervals. To check if the infusion is on time, compare the fluid line with the time line on the tape. If the fluid line is above or below the time line, the flow rate is too slow or too fast. Tell the RN at once if too much or too little fluid was given.

See *Promoting Safety and Comfort: Flow Rate.*

PROMOTING SAFETY AND COMFORT
Flow Rate

Safety

The person can suffer serious harm if the flow rate is too fast or too slow. The flow rate can change from:

- Position changes
- Kinked tubes
- Lying on the tube

Never change the position of the clamp or adjust any controls on infusion pumps. Tell the nurse at once if there is a problem with the flow rate.

Assisting With IV Therapy

You help meet the safety, hygiene, and activity needs of persons with IVs. Follow the safety measures in Box 25-1. Report any of the signs and symptoms listed in Box 25-1 at once.

Your state and agency may allow you to change dressings at peripheral IV sites. They also may let you discontinue a peripheral IV.

You never start or maintain IV therapy. Nor do you regulate the flow rate or change IV bags. You never give blood or IV drugs.

See *Focus on Communication: Assisting With IV Therapy,* p. 464.

See *Delegation Guidelines: Assisting with IV Therapy,* p. 464.

See *Teamwork and Time Management: Assisting With IV Therapy,* p. 464.

BOX 25-1 SAFETY MEASURES FOR IV THERAPY

- Follow Standard Precautions and the Bloodborne Pathogen Standard.
- Do not move the needle or catheter. Needle or catheter position must be maintained. If the needle or catheter is moved, it may come out of the vein. Then fluid flows into tissues (infiltration). Or the flow stops.
- Follow the safety measures for restraints (Chapter 14). The nurse may splint or restrain the extremity to prevent movement (Fig. 25-18). Or the nurse may apply a protective device (Fig. 25-19). This helps prevent the needle or catheter from moving.
- Protect the IV bag, tubing, and needle or catheter when the person walks. Portable IV standards are rolled along next to the person (Fig. 25-20).
- Assist the person with turning and re-positioning. Move the IV bag to the side of the bed on which the person is lying. Always allow enough slack in the tubing. The needle or catheter can move from pressure on the tube.
- Tell the nurse at once if bleeding occurs from the insertion site. Follow Standard Precautions and the Bloodborne Pathogen Standard.

- Tell the nurse at once of any signs and symptoms of IV therapy complications:
  - Local—at the IV site
    - Bleeding
    - Blood backing up into the IV tube
    - Puffiness or swelling
    - Pale or reddened skin
    - Complaints of pain at or above the IV site
    - Hot or cold skin near the site
  - Systemic—involving the whole body
    - Fever
    - Itching
    - Drop in blood pressure
    - Pulse rate greater than 100 beats per minute
    - Irregular pulse
    - Cyanosis
    - Confusion or changes in mental function
    - Loss of consciousness
    - Difficulty breathing
    - Shortness of breath
    - Decreasing or no urine output
    - Chest pain
    - Nausea

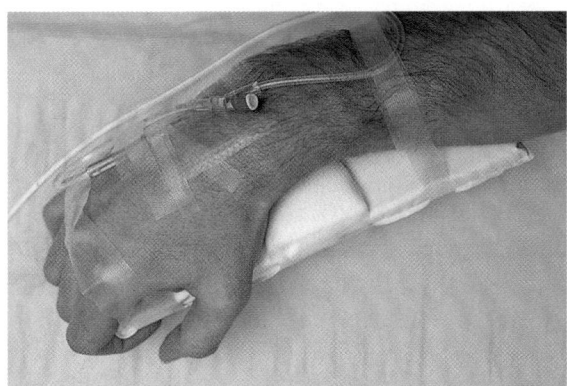

Fig. 25-18 An armboard prevents movement at an IV site.

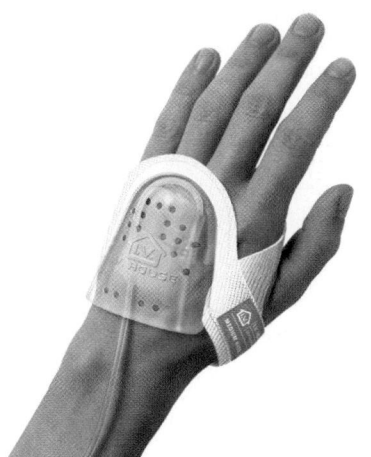

Fig. 25-19 I.V. House Protective Device.

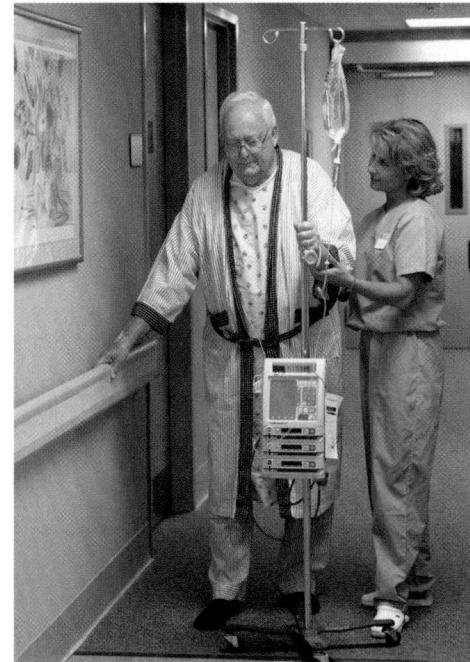

Fig. 25-20 A person walking with an IV.

FOCUS ON COMMUNICATION
Assisting With IV Therapy

The nurse may instruct the person how to position his or her arm during IV therapy. You may need to remind the person:

- To position his or her arm a certain way
- About position limits

For example, Mr. Winn has an IV in his arm. If he bends his arm, the tubing is kinked. The flow of fluid stops. You can say: "Mr. Winn, please keep your arm straight. The fluid will not flow through your IV when your arm is bent."

DELEGATION GUIDELINES
Assisting With IV Therapy

Before changing a peripheral IV dressing or discontinuing a peripheral IV, make sure that:

- Your state lets nursing assistants perform the procedure.
- The procedure is in your job description.
- You have the necessary education and training.
- You know how to use the agency's supplies and equipment.
- You review the procedure in the agency's procedure manual.
- You review the procedure with the nurse.
- A nurse is available to answer questions and to supervise you.
- An RN has identified and labeled all other tubes, catheters, and needles.

If the above conditions are met, you need this information from the nurse and the care plan:

- When to change the IV dressing
- If the person has an IV needle or catheter
- When to discontinue the IV
- If the person has more than one IV, which IV to discontinue
- What supplies to use
- What observations to report and record (see Box 25-1)
- When to report observations
- What patient or resident concerns to report at once

TEAMWORK AND TIME MANAGEMENT
Assisting With IV Therapy

If assigned to a person with an IV, you must know the flow rate. When you are with the person, always check the flow rate. Report any problems to the nurse at once.

Also check the amount of fluid in the bag. Tell the nurse at once if the bag is empty or almost empty.

Patients and residents cared for by other staff may have IVs. When you are near the person or walking past the person's room, always make sure the IV is dripping. Also, check the amount of fluid in the bag. Report any problems to a nurse at once.

FOCUS ON PRIDE
The Person, Family, and Yourself

Personal and Professional Responsibility

IV pump alarms can sound for many reasons:

- There is air in the tubing.
- The infusion is done.
- The pump's battery is low.
- Fluid flow is blocked. Kinks in the tubing and closed clamps are common reasons.

When you hear an IV pump alarm, tell the nurse. Do so even if you are not assigned to the person. If the battery is low, you may plug in the pump. If the person needs to reposition his or her arm for the fluid to flow, you may ask the person to do so. *You do not adjust controls on IV pumps or clamps on IV tubing.*

Know the limits of your role. If asked to do something outside those limits, politely refuse and explain why. Working within the limits of your role protects you and others from harm.

Rights and Respect

Persons needing nutritional support or IV therapy are often very ill. Sometimes decisions are made to stop the therapy. The person is allowed to die. The person may make the decision. Or the family does so after talking to the doctor. (See Chapter 52.)

You may agree or disagree with such choices. The choice may or may not be within your religious or cultural beliefs and values. Your beliefs must not interfere with the person's right to choose and to refuse treatment. The person's or family's wishes and doctor's orders must be followed. The person must receive quality care. Talk to the nurse if you have problems with the decision. The nurse may need to change your assignment.

Independence and Social Interaction

Some persons with IVs are allowed to shower or bathe in a tub. This promotes comfort and independence. IV sites must be kept clean and dry. The nurse may have you apply a bag, plastic wrap, or glove to protect the site. Follow agency policy and the nurse's instructions.

Delegation and Teamwork

Careful planning is needed before turning, repositioning, or transferring persons receiving IV therapy and tube feedings. You need to know what tubes are present and the purpose of each. You must protect tubes connected to the person.

When moving the person with a co-worker, plan and communicate how to protect tubes before moving the person. For example, move the IV pole before moving the person. Also, identify who will monitor the tubing during the move. If you notice a tube is being pulled, stop at once. If you continue, you may displace the feeding tube or IV. Fix the problem before moving the person farther.

Take the time to plan and coordinate moves and transfers when tubes are present. This increases the person's safety, comfort, and peace of mind.

Ethics and Laws

Caring for persons with nutritional support and IV therapy can be complex. The person's treatments may require you to change the way you give care. You have learned some safety measures in this chapter. For example, you learned to place a person receiving tube feedings in the semi-Fowler's or Fowler's position. If you lower the head of the bed, the person may regurgitate and aspirate. You will learn other safety measures in later chapters. For example, in Chapter 26, you will learn not to take a blood pressure in an arm with an IV infusion.

Each person is different. Consider what special care measures may be needed. If you do not know, ask the nurse. Neglecting safety measures is unethical. The person may be harmed. Legal action can be taken. You can lose your ability to work as a nursing assistant.

REVIEW QUESTIONS

Circle the BEST answer.

1 Enteral nutrition
   a Requires an NG tube
   b Is given into a central venous site
   c Is given into the GI tract
   d Requires an IV

2 The process of giving a tube feeding is called
   a Gavage   c Aspiration
   b Parenteral nutrition   d Regurgitation

3 For a tube feeding, the person is positioned in
   a Fowler's or semi-Fowler's position
   b The left side-lying position
   c The right side-lying position
   d The supine position

4 Formula for a tube feeding is given
   a At body temperature   c Hot
   b At room temperature   d Cold

5 Continuous feedings are given with a
   a Syringe   c PEG tube
   b Feeding bag   d Feeding pump

6 The nurse checks feeding tube placement to prevent
   a Aspiration   c Over-feeding
   b Bleeding   d Cramping

7 Which position prevents regurgitation after a tube feeding?
   a Fowler's or semi-Fowler's position
   b The supine position
   c The left or right side-lying position
   d The prone position

8 The risk of regurgitation is the greatest with
   a NG and gastrostomy tubes
   b A PEG tube
   c Naso-enteral tubes
   d A jejunostomy tube

9 A person with a feeding tube is NPO. You should do the following *except*
   a Give the person hard candy or gum
   b Provide oral hygiene
   c Provide mouth rinses
   d Apply lubricant to the lips

10 A person has an NG tube. The care plan includes these measures to prevent nasal irritation. Which measure should you question?
   a Clean the nose and nostrils every 4 hours.
   b Tape the tube to the nose.
   c Remove the tube every 4 hours.
   d Secure the tube to the person's gown.

11 A nurse asks you to give a tube feeding. The procedure is not in your job description. What should you do?
   a Refuse to perform the task.
   b Give the tube feeding.
   c Tell the director of nursing.
   d Ask another nurse what you should do.

12 A person is receiving TPN. The person complains of chest pain and difficulty breathing. What should you do?
   a Position the person in Fowler's position.
   b Call for the nurse.
   c Stop the TPN.
   d Provide oral hygiene.

13 A person is receiving TPN. You know that TPN
   a Involves a nutrient solution
   b Is given through a feeding tube
   c Can cause pressure ulcers on the nose
   d Requires that the person be NPO

14 Which is a peripheral IV site?
   a Subclavian vein
   b Superior vena cava
   c Jugular vein
   d A vein on the back of the hand

15 A nurse asks you to check an IV flow rate. A pump is not used. What should you do?
   a Count the drops in 30 seconds; multiply the number by 2.
   b Count the drops for 1 minute.
   c Check if the fluid is dripping too fast or slow.
   d Measure the amount of fluid.

16 The IV flow rate is
   a The number of gtt/mL
   b The number of gtt/min or mL/hr
   c The amount of fluid given in 1 minute
   d The amount of fluid in the IV bag

17 You note that an IV bag is almost empty. What should you do?
   a Clamp the IV tubing.   c Discontinue the IV.
   b Tell the nurse.   d Adjust the flow rate.

18 You note bleeding from an IV insertion site. What should you do?
   a Tell the nurse.
   b Move the needle or catheter.
   c Discontinue the IV.
   d Clamp the IV tubing.

Answers to these questions are on p. 833.

26 Measuring Vital Signs

OBJECTIVES

- Define the key terms and key abbreviations listed in this chapter.
- Explain why vital signs are measured.
- List the factors affecting vital signs.
- Identify the normal ranges for each temperature site.
- Explain when to use each temperature site.
- Explain how to use thermometers.
- Identify the pulse sites.

- Describe a normal pulse and normal respirations.
- Describe the practices to follow when measuring blood pressure.
- Perform the procedures described in this chapter.
- Know the normal vital signs for the different age-groups.
- Explain how to promote PRIDE in the person, the family, and yourself.

KEY TERMS

apical-radial pulse Taking the apical and radial pulses at the same time

blood pressure (BP) The amount of force exerted against the walls of an artery by the blood

body temperature The amount of heat in the body that is a balance between the amount of heat produced and the amount lost by the body

bradycardia A slow *(brady)* heart rate *(cardia)*; less than 60 beats per minute

diastole The period of heart muscle relaxation; the heart is at rest

diastolic pressure The pressure in the arteries when the heart is at rest

fever Elevated body temperature

hypertension When the systolic pressure is 140 mm Hg or higher *(hyper)*, or the diastolic pressure is 90 mm Hg or higher

hypotension When the systolic pressure is below *(hypo)* 90 mm Hg, or the diastolic pressure is below 60 mm Hg

pulse The beat of the heart felt at an artery as a wave of blood passes through the artery

pulse deficit The difference between the apical and radial pulse rates

pulse rate The number of heartbeats or pulses felt in 1 minute

respiration Breathing air into *(inhalation)* and out of *(exhalation)* the lungs

sphygmomanometer A cuff and measuring device used to measure blood pressure

stethoscope An instrument used to listen to sounds produced by the heart, lungs, and other body organs

systole The period of heart muscle contraction; the heart is pumping blood

systolic pressure The pressure in the arteries when the heart contracts

tachycardia A rapid *(tachy)* heart rate *(cardia)*; more than 100 beats per minute

thermometer A device used to measure *(meter)* temperature *(thermo)*

vital signs Temperature, pulse, respirations, and blood pressure; and pain in some agencies

KEY ABBREVIATIONS

BP	Blood pressure	**ID**	Identification
C	Centigrade	**IV**	Intravenous
DUS	Doppler ultrasound stethoscope	**mm**	Millimeter
F	Fahrenheit	**mm Hg**	Millimeters of mercury
Hg	Mercury		

Vital signs reflect the function of 3 body processes essential for life: regulation of body temperature, breathing, and heart function. The four *vital signs of body function are:*

* *Temperature*
* *Pulse*
* *Respirations*
* *Blood pressure*

Vital signs are often called TPR (temperature, pulse, and respirations) and BP (blood pressure). Some agencies include "pain" as a vital sign (p. 489 and Chapter 28).

MEASURING AND REPORTING VITAL SIGNS

A person's vital signs vary within certain limits. See Box 26-1 for the factors affecting vital signs.

Vital signs are measured to detect changes in normal body function. They tell about treatment response. They often signal life-threatening events. Vital signs are part of the assessment step in the nursing process. Vital signs are measured:

* During physical exams
* When the person is admitted to a health care agency
* As often as the person's condition requires
* Before and after surgery, complex procedures, and diagnostic tests
* After some care measures, such as ambulation (walking)
* After a fall or other injury
* When drugs affect the respiratory or circulatory system
* When the person complains of pain, dizziness, light-headedness, feeling faint, shortness of breath, a rapid heart rate, or not feeling well
* As stated on the care plan (usually daily, twice a day, or weekly in nursing centers)

Vital signs show even minor changes in the person's condition. Accuracy is essential when you measure, record, and report vital signs. If unsure of your measurements, promptly ask the nurse to take them again. Unless otherwise ordered, take vital signs with the person at rest—lying or sitting. Report the following at once:

* Any vital sign that is changed from a prior measurement
* Vital signs above the normal range
* Vital signs below the normal range

BOX 26-1	FACTORS AFFECTING VITAL SIGNS
• Activity	• Fear
• Anger	• Illness
• Anxiety	• Noise
• Drugs	• Pain
• Eating	• Sleep
• Exercise	• Weather

FOCUS ON COMMUNICATION
Measuring and Reporting Vital Signs

Patients and residents like to know their measurements. If agency policy allows, tell the person the measurements. With the person's consent, you can tell family members if they ask. Remember, this information is private and confidential. Roommates and visitors must not hear what you are saying.

A measurement may be abnormal. Or you may not be able to feel a pulse or hear a blood pressure. Do not alarm the person. You can say:

* "I'm not sure that I counted your pulse correctly. I'll ask the nurse to take it."
* "I'm not sure that I heard your blood pressure correctly. I'll ask the nurse to take it again."
* "Your pulse is a little slow (or fast). I'll ask the nurse to check it."
* "Your temperature is higher than normal. I'm going to use another thermometer. I'll also ask the nurse to check you."

FOCUS ON CHILDREN AND OLDER PERSONS
Measuring and Reporting Vital Signs

Older Persons

Measuring vital signs on persons with dementia may be difficult. The person may move about, hit at you, and grab equipment. This is not safe for the person or for you. Two staff may be needed. One uses touch and a soothing voice to calm and distract the person. The other measures the vital signs.

Trying the procedure when the person is calmer may help. Or take the pulse and respirations at one time. Then take the temperature and blood pressure at another time.

Always approach the person calmly. Use a soothing voice. Tell the person what you are going to do. Do not rush the person. Follow the care plan. If you cannot measure vital signs, tell the nurse right away.

Vital signs are recorded in the person's medical record. If measured often, a flow sheet is used. The doctor or nurse compares past and current measurements.

See *Focus on Communication: Measuring and Reporting Vital Signs.*

See *Focus on Children and Older Persons: Measuring and Reporting Vital Signs.*

BODY TEMPERATURE

Body temperature is the amount of heat in the body. It is a balance between the amount of heat produced and the amount lost by the body. Heat is produced as cells use food for energy. It is lost through the skin, breathing, urine, and feces. Body temperature stays fairly stable. It is lower in the morning and higher in the afternoon and evening. Body temperature is affected by the factors listed in Box 26-1, pregnancy, and the menstrual cycle.

You use thermometers to measure temperature. Temperature is measured using the Fahrenheit (F) and centigrade (C) scales.

BOX 26-2   TEMPERATURE SITES

Oral Site
Oral temperatures are *not* taken if the person:
- Is under 4 or 5 years of age.
- Is unconscious.
- Has had surgery or an injury to the face, neck, nose, or mouth.
- Is receiving oxygen.
- Breathes through the mouth.
- Has a naso-gastric tube.
- Is delirious, restless, confused, or disoriented.
- Is paralyzed on one side of the body.
- Has a sore mouth.
- Has a convulsive (seizure) disorder.

Rectal Site
The rectal site is used for infants and children under 3 years old. Rectal temperatures are taken when the oral site cannot be used. Rectal temperatures are *not* taken if the person:
- Has diarrhea.
- Has a rectal disorder or injury.
- Has heart disease.
- Had rectal surgery.
- Is confused or agitated.

Tympanic Membrane Site
The site has fewer microbes than the mouth or rectum. The risk of spreading infection is reduced. This site is *not* used if the person has:
- An ear disorder
- Ear drainage

Temporal Artery Site
Measures body temperature at the temporal artery in the forehead. The site is non-invasive.

Axillary Site
Less reliable than the other sites. It is used when the other sites cannot be used.

TABLE 26-1   NORMAL BODY TEMPERATURES

Site	Baseline	Normal range
Oral	98.6°F (37.0°C)	97.6°F to 99.6°F (36.5°C to 37.5°C)
Rectal	99.6°F (37.5°C)	98.6°F to 100.6°F (37.0°C to 38.1°C)
Axillary	97.6°F (36.5°C)	96.6°F to 98.6°F (35.9°C to 37.0°C)
Tympanic membrane	98.6°F (37.0°C)	98.6°F (37.0°C)
Temporal artery	99.6°F (37.5°C)	99.6°F (37.5°C)

FOCUS ON COMMUNICATION
Temperature Sites

Checking a rectal temperature can be embarrassing and uncomfortable. Be professional. Tell the person what you are going to do. Explain why you must use the rectal route. For example: "Mr. Presney, I need to check your temperature. I must check a rectal temperature because your oxygen changes the temperature in your mouth. The thermometer has to stay in place for 2 minutes. Please tell me if you feel pain."

A glass thermometer remains in the rectum for at least 2 minutes. This can cause discomfort. To promote comfort, talk the person through the procedure. You can say: "I'm almost done. There's about 1 minute left. Are you doing okay?"

FOCUS ON CHILDREN AND OLDER PERSONS
Temperature Sites

Children
The oral site is not used for infants and children younger than 4 to 5 years. Use other routes as directed by the nurse and the care plan. See Box 26-2.

Older Persons
Older persons have lower body temperatures than younger persons. An oral temperature of 98.6°F (37.0°C) may signal fever in an older person.

PROMOTING SAFETY AND COMFORT
Temperature Sites

Safety
Rectal temperatures are dangerous for persons with heart disease. The thermometer can stimulate the vagus nerve. This nerve affects the heart. Stimulation of the vagus nerve slows the heart rate. The heart rate can slow to dangerous levels in some persons.

Temperature Sites

Temperature sites are the mouth, rectum, axilla (underarm), tympanic membrane (ear), and temporal artery (forehead) (Box 26-2). Each site has a normal range (Table 26-1). *Fever means an elevated body temperature.* Always report temperatures that are above or below the normal range.

- See *Focus on Communication: Temperature Sites.*
- See *Focus on Children and Older Persons: Temperature Sites.*
  See *Promoting Safety and Comfort: Temperature Sites.*

Thermometers

A *thermometer is a device used to measure* (meter) *temperature* (thermo). Follow the manufacturer's instructions and agency procedures to use, clean, and store these devices.

- *Glass thermometer*—a hollow glass tube with a bulb tip (Fig. 26-1, A). The device is filled with a substance. When heated, the substance expands and rises in the tube. When cooled, the substance contracts and moves down the tube. See "Glass Thermometers" on p. 473.
- *Standard electronic thermometer*—is battery operated. The temperature is shown on the front of the device. See Figure 26-1, B. See "Electronic Thermometers" on p. 471.
- *Tympanic membrane thermometer*—measures body temperature at the tympanic membrane in the ear (Fig. 26-1, C).
- *Temporal artery thermometer*—measures body temperature at the temporal artery in the forehead (Fig. 26-1, D).
- *Digital thermometer*—shows the temperature on the front of the thermometer (Fig. 26-1, E). Depending on the type, the temperature is measured in 6 to 60 seconds.
- *Disposable oral thermometer*—has small chemical dots (Fig. 26-1, F, p. 470). The dots change color when heated. Each dot is heated to a certain temperature before it changes color. These thermometers are used once. They measure temperatures in 45 to 60 seconds.
- *Temperature-sensitive tape*—changes color in response to body heat (Fig. 26-1, G, p. 470). The tape is applied to the forehead. The measurement takes about 15 seconds.
- *Pacifier thermometer*—looks like a baby's pacifier (Fig. 26-1, H, p. 470). The baby sucks on the device for 90 seconds. The temperature is displayed on the front.

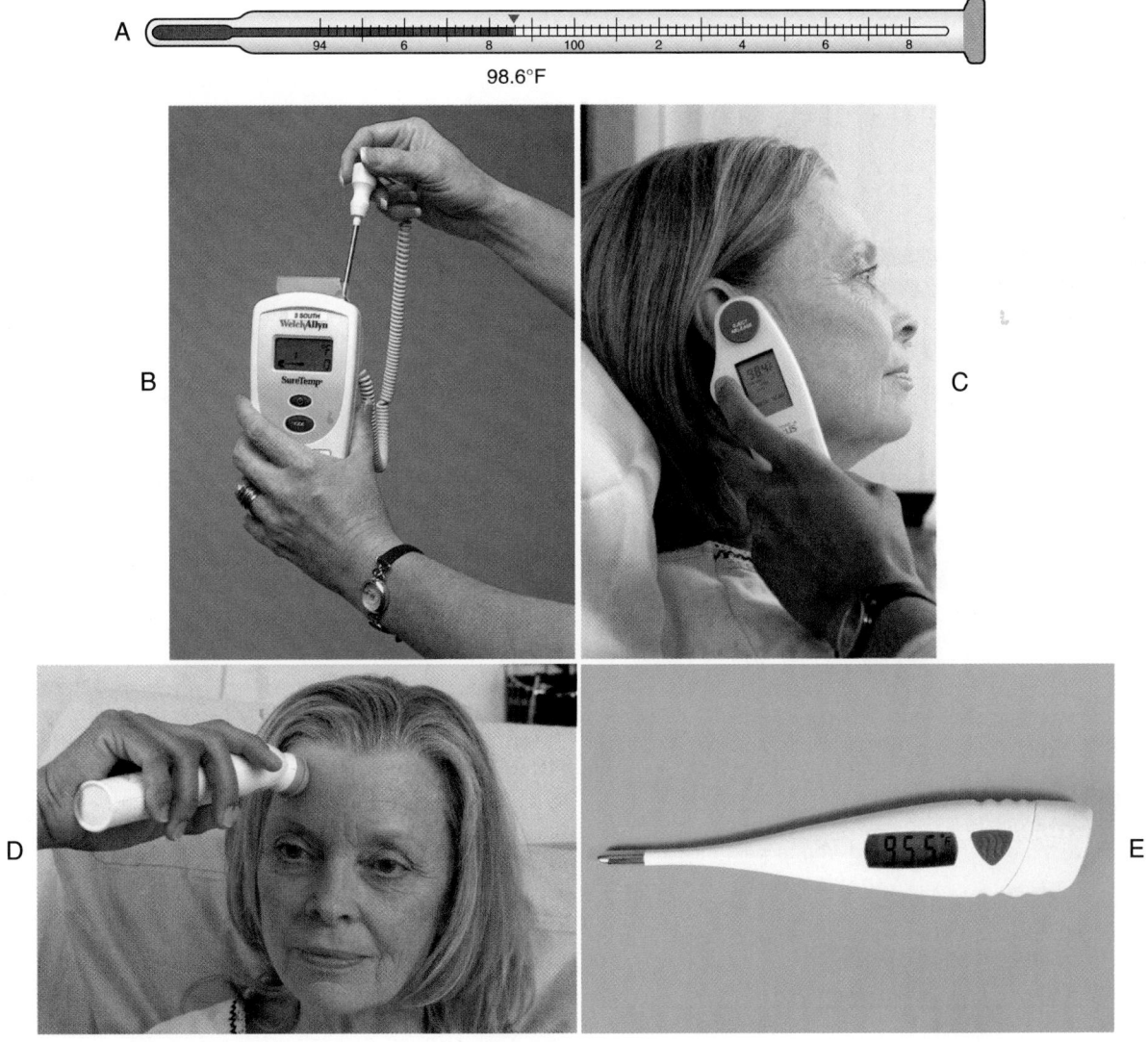

98.6°F

Fig. 26-1 Types of thermometers. **A,** Glass thermometer. **B,** Standard electronic thermometer. **C,** Tympanic membrane thermometer. **D,** Temporal artery thermometer. **E,** Digital thermometer.   *Continued*

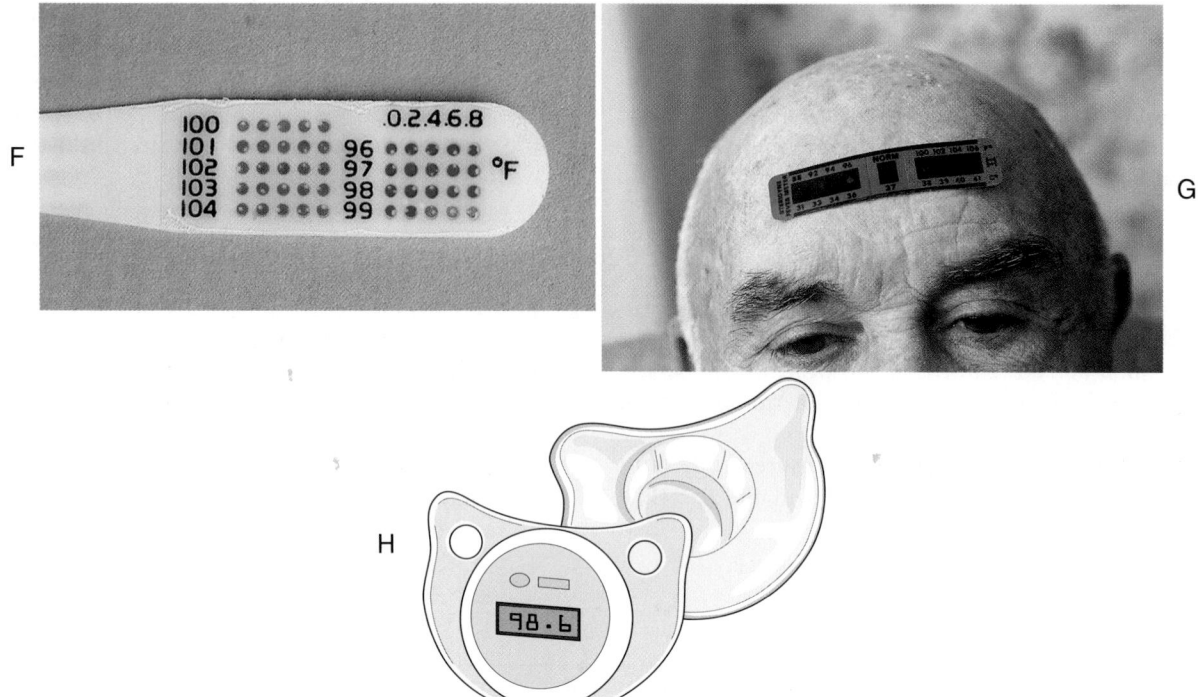

Fig. 26-1, cont'd   F, Disposable oral thermometer with chemical dots. **G,** Temperature sensitive tape. **H,** Pacifier thermometer.

Taking Temperatures

The nurse and care plan tell you:
- When to take the person's temperature
- What site to use
- What thermometer to use
    See *Delegation Guidelines: Taking Temperatures.*
    See *Promoting Safety and Comfort: Taking Temperatures.*

DELEGATION GUIDELINES
Taking Temperatures

Before taking temperatures, you need this information from the nurse and the care plan:
- What site to use for each person—oral, rectal, axillary, tympanic membrane, or temporal artery
- What thermometer to use for each person
- How long to leave a glass thermometer in place (p. 474)
- When to take temperatures
- Which persons are at risk for elevated temperatures
- What observations to report and record:
  - A temperature that is changed from a past measurement
  - A temperature above or below the normal range for the site used
- When to report observations
- What patient or resident concerns to report at once

PROMOTING SAFETY AND COMFORT
Taking Temperatures

Safety
Thermometers are inserted into the mouth, rectum, axilla, and ear. Each area has many microbes. The area may contain blood. Therefore each person has his or her own glass or digital thermometer. This prevents the spread of microbes and infection. Follow Standard Precautions and the Bloodborne Pathogen Standard when taking temperatures.

With rectal temperatures, your gloved hands may have contact with feces. If so, remove gloves and practice hand hygiene. Then note the temperature on your notepad or assignment sheet. Put on clean gloves to complete the procedure.

Comfort
Remove the thermometer in a timely manner. Do not leave it in place longer than needed. This affects the person's comfort. For example, an oral glass thermometer is left in place for 2 to 3 minutes. Do not leave it in place longer than that.

Electronic Thermometers

Electronic thermometers are commonly used. Probe covers are used to prevent the spread of infection.

Some electronic thermometers have batteries. Others are kept in battery chargers when not in use.

- Standard electronic thermometers (see Fig. 26-1, B) measure temperature in a few seconds. They have oral (blue) and rectal (red) probes. The oral (blue) probe is used for axillary temperatures. A disposable cover (sheath) protects the probe.
- Tympanic membrane thermometers measure temperature in 1 to 3 seconds. They are comfortable and not invasive like rectal thermometers and probes. There are fewer microbes in the ear than in the mouth or rectum. The risk of spreading infection is reduced. These devices are not used if there is ear drainage. To use one, gently insert the covered probe into the ear (see Fig. 26-1, C).

- Temporal artery thermometers measure body temperature in 3 to 4 seconds. Non-invasive, they measure the temperature of the blood in the temporal artery. It is the same temperature of the blood coming from the heart. To use one:
  - Use the side of the head that is exposed. Do not use the side covered by hair, a dressing, hat, or other covering. Do not use the side that was on a pillow.
  - Place a disposable cap or cover on the thermometer.
  - Place the device in the center of the forehead.
  - Press the scan button.
  - Slide the device across the forehead and across the temporal artery (see Fig. 26-1, D).
  - Release the scan button.
  - Read the temperature display.

See *Focus on Children and Older Persons: Electronic Thermometers.*

See *Teamwork and Time Management: Electronic Thermometers.*

FOCUS ON CHILDREN AND OLDER PERSONS
Electronic Thermometers

Older Persons

Tympanic membrane and temporal artery thermometers are used for persons who are confused and resist care. They are fast and comfortable. Oral and rectal thermometers are unsafe because:

- A glass thermometer can easily break if the person moves, resists care, or bites down on it. Serious injury can occur.
- A standard electronic thermometer can injure the mouth and teeth if the person bites down on it. It also can cause injury if the person moves quickly and without warning.

TEAMWORK AND TIME MANAGEMENT
Electronic Thermometers

The standard electronic, tympanic membrane, and temporal artery thermometers are shared with your co-workers. When using these devices, tell your co-workers what thermometer you have. Work quickly, but carefully. Return the device to the charging unit in a timely manner.

TAKING A TEMPERATURE WITH AN ELECTRONIC THERMOMETER

QUALITY OF LIFE

Remember to:
- Knock before entering the person's room.
- Address the person by name.
- Introduce yourself by name and title.

- Explain the procedure to the person before beginning and during the procedure.
- Protect the person's rights during the procedure.
- Handle the person gently during the procedure.

PRE-PROCEDURE

1 Follow *Delegation Guidelines: Taking Temperatures*. See *Promoting Safety and Comfort: Taking Temperatures.*
2 For an oral temperature, ask the person not to eat, drink, smoke, or chew gum for at least 15 to 20 minutes before the measurement or as required by agency policy.
3 Practice hand hygiene.
4 Collect the following:
   - Thermometer—electronic or tympanic membrane
   - Probe (blue for an oral or axillary temperature; red for a rectal temperature)

   - Probe covers
   - Toilet tissue (rectal temperature)
   - Water-soluble lubricant (rectal temperature)
   - Gloves
   - Towel (axillary temperature)
5 Plug the probe into the thermometer if using a standard electronic thermometer.
6 Practice hand hygiene.
7 Identify the person. Check the identification (ID) bracelet against the assignment sheet. Also call the person by name.

Continued

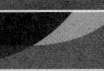

TAKING A TEMPERATURE WITH AN ELECTRONIC THERMOMETER— cont'd

  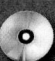

PROCEDURE

8 Provide for privacy. Position the person for an oral, rectal, axillary, or tympanic membrane temperature. The Sims' position is used for a rectal temperature.

9 Put on gloves if contact with blood, body fluids, secretions, or excretions is likely.

10 Insert the probe into a probe cover.

11 For an *oral temperature:*
   a Ask the person to open the mouth and raise the tongue.
   b Place the covered probe at the base of the tongue and to one side (Fig. 26-2).
   c Ask the person to lower the tongue and close the mouth.

12 For a *rectal temperature:*
   a Place some lubricant on toilet tissue.
   b Lubricate the end of the covered probe.
   c Expose the anal area.
   d Raise the upper buttock.
   e Insert the probe ½ inch into the rectum (Fig. 26-3).
   f Hold the probe in place.

13 For an *axillary temperature:*
   a Help the person remove an arm from the gown. Do not expose the person.
   b Dry the axilla with the towel.
   c Place the covered probe in the center of the axilla (Fig. 26-4).

   d Place the person's arm over the chest.
   e Hold the probe in place.

14 For a *tympanic membrane temperature:*
   a Ask the person to turn his or her head so the ear is in front of you.
   b Pull up and back on the adult's ear to straighten the ear canal (Fig. 26-5).
   c Insert the covered probe gently.

15 Start the thermometer.

16 Hold the probe in place until you hear a tone or see a flashing or steady light.

17 Read the temperature on the display.

18 Remove the probe. Press the eject button to discard the cover.

19 Note the person's name, temperature, and temperature site on your notepad or assignment sheet.

20 Return the probe to the holder.

21 Help the person put the gown back on (axillary temperature). For a rectal temperature:
   a Wipe the anal area with toilet tissue to remove lubricant.
   b Cover the person.
   c Dispose of used toilet tissue.
   d Remove and discard the gloves. Practice hand hygiene.

POST-PROCEDURE

22 Provide for comfort. (See the inside of the front book cover.)

23 Place the signal light within reach.

24 Unscreen the person.

25 Complete a safety check of the room. (See the inside of the front book cover.)

26 Return the thermometer to the charging unit.

27 Practice hand hygiene.

28 Report and record the temperature. Note the temperature site when reporting and recording. Report an abnormal temperature at once.

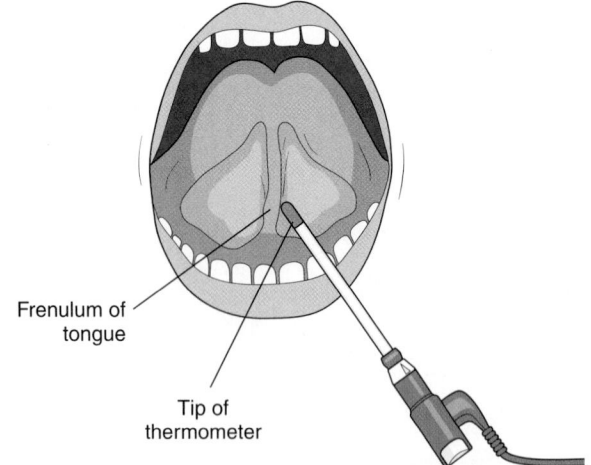

Frenulum of tongue

Tip of thermometer

Fig. 26-2 The thermometer is textced at the base of the tongue and to one side.

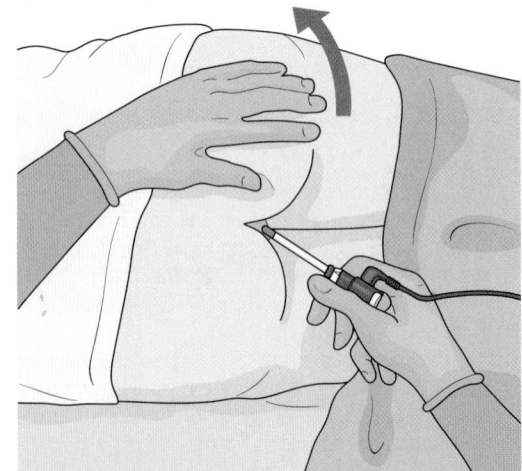

Fig. 26-3 The rectal temperature is taken with the person in Sims' position. The buttock is raised to expose the anus.

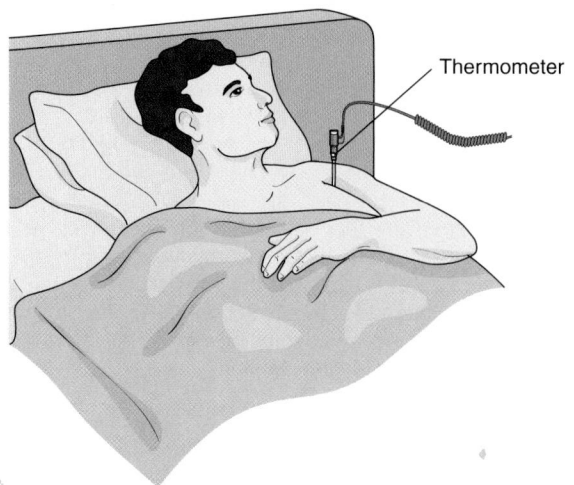

Fig. 26-4 The thermometer is held in place in the axilla by bringing the person's arm over the chest.

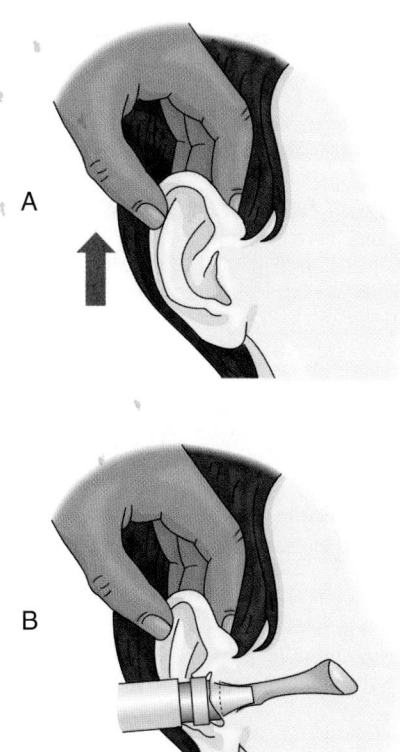

Fig. 26-5 Using a tympanic membrane thermometer. **A,** The ear is pulled up and back. **B,** The probe is inserted into the ear canal.

Glass Thermometers

Long- or slender-tip thermometers are used for oral and axillary temperatures. So are thermometers with stubby and pear-shaped tips. Rectal thermometers have stubby tips. See Figure 26-6.

Glass thermometers are color-coded:
- Blue—oral and axillary thermometers
- Red—rectal thermometers

Glass thermometers are re-usable. However, the following are problems:
- They take a long time to register—3 to 10 minutes depending on the site (p. 474).
- They break easily. Broken rectal thermometers can injure the rectum and colon.

- The person may bite down and break an oral thermometer. Cuts in the mouth are risks. If the thermometer contains mercury, swallowed mercury can cause mercury poisoning.

See Box 26-3, p. 474 for how to use and read glass thermometers.

See *Focus on Long-Term Care and Home Care: Glass Thermometers*, p. 474.

See *Promoting Safety and Comfort: Glass Thermometers*, p. 475.

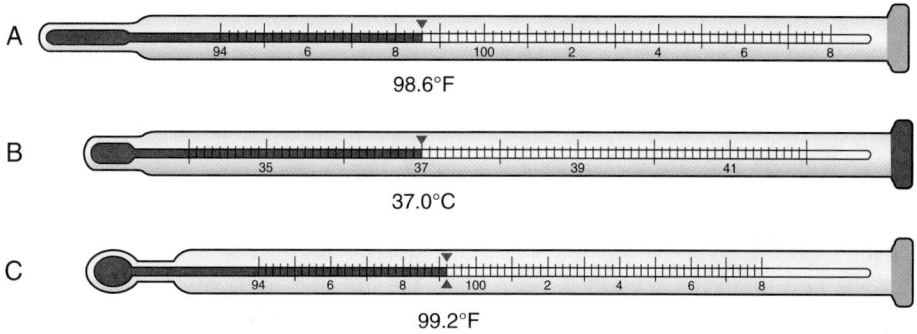

Fig. 26-6 Glass thermometers. **A,** A Fahrenheit thermometer with a long or slender tip. The temperature measurement is 98.6°F. **B,** Centigrade thermometer with a stubby tip (rectal thermometer). The temperature measurement is 37.0°C. **C,** Fahrenheit thermometer with a pear-shaped tip. The temperature measurement is 99.2°F.

BOX 26-3 **GLASS THERMOMETERS**

Reading a Glass Thermometer

- Fahrenheit thermometers (see Fig. 26-6, A and C):
  - Every other long line is an even degree from 94°F to 108°F.
  - The short lines mean 0.2 (two-tenths) of a degree.
- Centigrade thermometers (see Fig. 26-6, B):
  - Each long line means 1 degree. Degrees range from 34°C to 42°C.
  - Each short line means 0.1 (one-tenth) of a degree.
- To read a glass thermometer:
  - Hold it at the stem (Fig. 26-7). Bring it to eye level.
  - Turn it until you can see the numbers and the long and short lines.
  - Turn it back and forth slowly until you can see the silver or red line.
  - Read the nearest degree (long line).
  - Read the nearest tenth of a degree (short line)—an even number on a Fahrenheit thermometer.

Using a Glass Thermometer

- Follow Standard Precautions and the Bloodborne Pathogen Standard.
- Use the person's thermometer.
- Use a rectal thermometer only for rectal temperatures.
- Rinse the thermometer under cold, running water if it was soaking in a disinfectant. Dry it from the stem to the bulb end with tissues.
- Check the thermometer for breaks, cracks, and chips. Discard it following agency policy if it is broken, cracked, or chipped.

Using a Glass Thermometer—cont'd

- Shake down the thermometer to move the substance down in the tube. Hold it at the stem, stand away from walls, tables, or other hard surfaces. Flex and snap your wrist until the substance is below 94°F or 34°C. See Figure 26-8.
- Insert the thermometer into a plastic cover (Fig. 26-9). Remove the cover to read the device. Discard the cover after use.
- Clean and store the thermometer following agency policy. Wipe it with tissues first to remove mucus, feces, or sweat. Do not use hot water. It causes the substance to expand so much that the thermometer could break. After cleaning, rinse the thermometer under cold, running water. Then store it in a container with a disinfectant solution.

Taking Temperatures

- The oral site:
  - The glass thermometer remains in place 2 to 3 minutes or as required by agency policy.
- The rectal site:
  - Provide for privacy. The buttocks and anus are exposed. The procedure embarrasses many people.
  - Lubricate the bulb end of the rectal thermometer for easy insertion and to prevent injury.
  - Hold the device in place so it is not lost into the rectum or broken.
  - Leave the thermometer in the rectum for 2 minutes or as required by agency policy.
- The axillary site:
  - Make sure the axilla (underarm) is dry. Do not use this site right after bathing.
  - Leave the thermometer in place for 5 to 10 minutes or as required by agency policy.

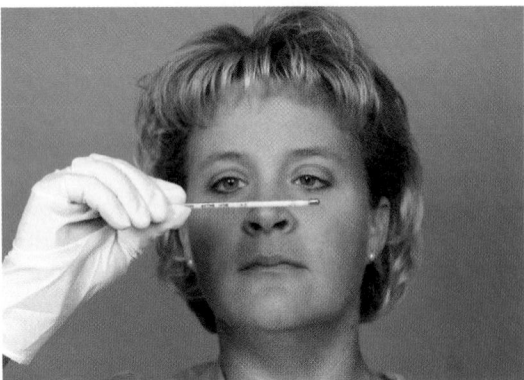

Fig. 26-7 The thermometer is held at the stem. It is read at eye level.

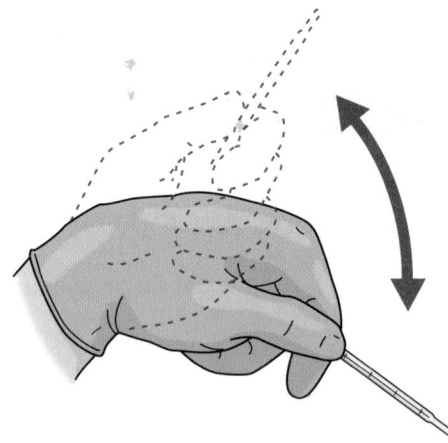

Fig. 26-8 The wrist is snapped to shake down the thermometer.

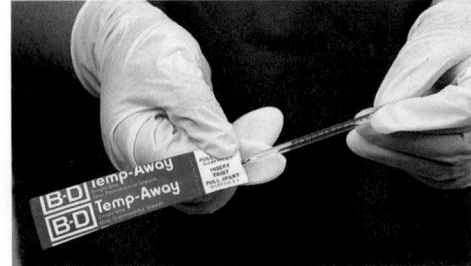

Fig. 26-9 The thermometer is inserted into a plastic cover.

FOCUS ON LONG-TERM CARE AND HOME CARE
Glass Thermometers

Home Care

Your home care agency may supply you with a digital thermometer. However, patients in home settings may have mercury-glass thermometers. If so, tell the nurse. The nurse can suggest that the person buy a digital thermometer.

You may care for children in home settings. Do not use a mercury-glass thermometer to measure a child's temperature.

Safety

Mercury-glass thermometers are rarely used today. However, do not assume that a glass thermometer contains a mercury-free mixture. If a thermometer breaks, tell the nurse at once.

Mercury is a hazardous substance. Do not touch the substance. Do not let the person do so. The agency follows special procedures for handling all hazardous materials. See Chapter 12.

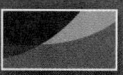

TAKING A TEMPERATURE WITH A GLASS THERMOMETER

QUALITY OF LIFE

Remember to:

- Knock before entering the person's room.
- Address the person by name.
- Introduce yourself by name and title.

- Explain the procedure to the person before beginning and during the procedure.
- Protect the person's rights during the procedure.
- Handle the person gently during the procedure.

PRE-PROCEDURE

1 Follow *Delegation Guidelines: Taking Temperatures,* p. 470. See *Promoting Safety and Comfort:*
  a *Taking Temperatures,* p. 470
  b *Glass Thermometers*
2 For an *oral temperature,* ask the person not to eat, drink, smoke, or chew gum for at least 15 to 20 minutes before the measurement or as required by agency policy.
3 Practice hand hygiene.
4 Collect the following:
  • Oral or rectal thermometer and holder
  • Tissues

  • Plastic covers if used
  • Gloves
  • Toilet tissue (rectal temperature)
  • Water-soluble lubricant (rectal temperature)
  • Towel (axillary temperature)
5 Practice hand hygiene.
6 Identify the person. Check the ID bracelet against the assignment sheet. Also call the person by name.
7 Provide for privacy.

PROCEDURE

8 Put on the gloves.
9 Rinse the thermometer under cold running water if it was soaking in a disinfectant. Dry it with tissues.
10 Check for breaks, cracks, or chips.
11 Shake down the thermometer below the lowest number. Hold the device by the stem.
12 Insert it into a plastic cover if used.
13 For an *oral temperature:*
  a Ask the person to moisten his or her lips.
  b Place the bulb end of the thermometer under the tongue and to one side (see Fig. 26-2).
  c Ask the person to close the lips around the thermometer to hold it in place.
  d Ask the person not to talk. Remind the person not to bite down on the thermometer.
  e Leave it in place for 2 to 3 minutes or as required by agency policy.
14 For a *rectal temperature:*
  a Position the person in Sims' position.
  b Put a small amount of lubricant on a tissue.
  c Lubricate the bulb end of the thermometer.
  d Fold back top linens to expose the anal area.
  e Raise the upper buttock to expose the anus (see Fig. 26-3).
  f Insert the thermometer 1 inch into the rectum. Do not force the thermometer.
  g Hold the thermometer in place for 2 minutes or as required by agency policy. Do not let go of it while it is in the rectum.

15 For an *axillary temperature:*
  a Help the person remove an arm from the gown. Do not expose the person.
  b Dry the axilla with the towel.
  c Place the bulb end of the thermometer in the center of the axilla.
  d Ask the person to place the arm over the chest to hold the thermometer in place (see Fig. 26-4). Hold it and the arm in place if he or she cannot help.
  e Leave the thermometer in place for 5 to 10 minutes or as required by agency policy.
16 Remove the thermometer.
17 Use tissues to remove the plastic cover. Discard the cover and tissues. Wipe the thermometer with a tissue if no cover was used. Wipe from the stem to the bulb end. Discard the tissue.
18 Read the thermometer.
19 Note the person's name and temperature on your notepad or assignment sheet.
20 For a *rectal temperature:*
  a Place used toilet tissue on several thicknesses of clean toilet tissue.
  b Place the thermometer on clean toilet tissue.
  c Wipe the anal area to remove excess lubricant and any feces.
  d Cover the person.

Continued

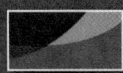

TAKING A TEMPERATURE WITH A GLASS THERMOMETER—cont'd

PROCEDURE—cont'd

21 For an *axillary temperature:* Help the person put the gown back on.
22 Shake down the thermometer.

23 Clean the thermometer according to agency policy. Return it to the holder.
24 Discard tissues and dispose of toilet tissue.
25 Remove and discard the gloves. Practice hand hygiene.

POST-PROCEDURE

26 Provide for comfort. (See the inside of the front book cover.)
27 Place the signal light within reach.
28 Unscreen the person.
29 Complete a safety check of the room. (See the inside of the front book cover.)

30 Practice hand hygiene.
31 Report and record the temperature. Note the temperature site when reporting and recording. Report an abnormal temperature at once.

BODY STRUCTURE AND FUNCTION REVIEW: THE HEART AND BLOOD VESSELS

The heart is a muscle. It pumps blood through the blood vessels to the tissues and cells. The heart lies in the middle to lower part of the chest cavity toward the left side (Fig. 26-10).

The heart has four chambers (Chapter 9). Upper chambers receive blood and are called the *atria.* The *right atrium* receives blood from body tissues. The *left atrium* receives blood from the lungs. Lower chambers are called *ventricles.* Ventricles pump blood. The *right ventricle* pumps blood to the lungs for oxygen. The *left ventricle* pumps blood to all parts of the body.

There are two phases of heart action. *Diastole* is the resting phase. Heart chambers fill with blood. *Systole* is the working phase. The heart contracts. Blood is pumped through the blood vessels when the heart contracts.

Blood flows to body tissues and cells through the blood vessels. *Arteries* carry blood away from the heart. Arterial blood is rich in oxygen. The *aorta* is the largest artery. The aorta receives blood directly from the left ventricle. The aorta branches into other arteries that carry blood to all parts of the body (Fig. 26-11). *Veins* return blood to the heart.

See Chapter 9 for more detailed information.

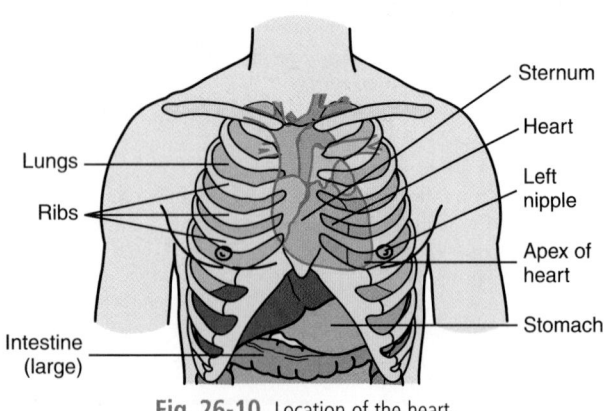

Fig. 26-10 Location of the heart.

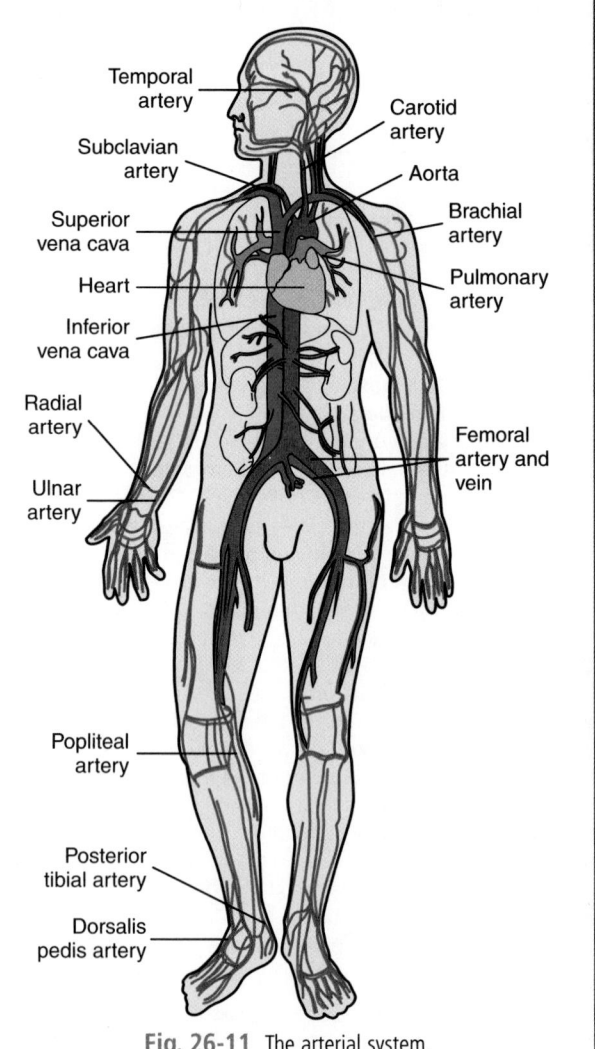

Fig. 26-11 The arterial system.

PULSE

Arteries carry blood from the heart to all parts of the body. The *pulse is the beat of the heart felt at an artery as a wave of blood passes through the artery.* A pulse is felt every time the heart beats.

> See *Body Structure and Function Review: The Heart and Blood Vessels.*

Pulse Sites

The temporal, carotid, brachial, radial, femoral, popliteal, posterior tibial, and dorsalis pedis (pedal) pulses are on each side of the body (Fig. 26-12). The arteries are close to the body surface and lie over a bone. Therefore they are easy to feel.

The radial pulse is used most often. It is easy to reach and find. The person is not exposed. The carotid pulse is taken during cardiopulmonary resuscitation (CPR) and other emergencies (Chapter 51).

The apical pulse is felt over the heart. The apex *(apical)* of the heart is at the tip of the heart, just below the left nipple (p. 480). This pulse is taken with a stethoscope.

> See *Focus on Children and Older Persons: Pulse Sites.*

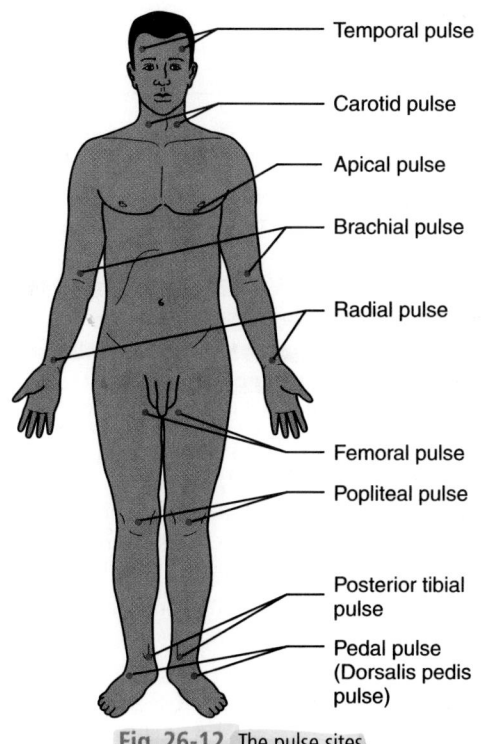

Fig. 26-12 The pulse sites.

- Temporal pulse
- Carotid pulse
- Apical pulse
- Brachial pulse
- Radial pulse
- Femoral pulse
- Popliteal pulse
- Posterior tibial pulse
- Pedal pulse (Dorsalis pedis pulse)

FOCUS ON CHILDREN AND OLDER PERSONS
Pulse Sites

Children
The apical pulse is used for infants and children under 2 years. The nurse may ask you to use the radial site for children older than 2 years.

Using a Stethoscope

A *stethoscope is an instrument used to listen to the sounds produced by the heart, lungs, and other body organs* (Fig. 26-13). It is used for apical pulses and blood pressures. The device makes sounds louder for easy hearing.

To use a stethoscope:
- Wipe the ear-pieces and diaphragm with antiseptic wipes before and after use.
- Place the ear-piece tips in your ears. The bend of the tips points forward. Ear-pieces should fit snugly to block out noises. They should not cause pain or ear discomfort.
- Tap the diaphragm gently. You should hear the tapping. If not, turn the chest piece at the tubing. Gently tap the diaphragm again. Proceed if you hear the tapping sound. Check with the nurse if you do not hear the tapping.
- Place the diaphragm over the pulse site. Hold it in place as in Figure 26-14, p. 478.
- Prevent noise. Do not let anything touch the tubing. Ask the person to be silent.

> See *Focus on Communication: Using a Stethoscope*, p. 478.
> See *Promoting Safety and Comfort: Using a Stethoscope*, p. 478.

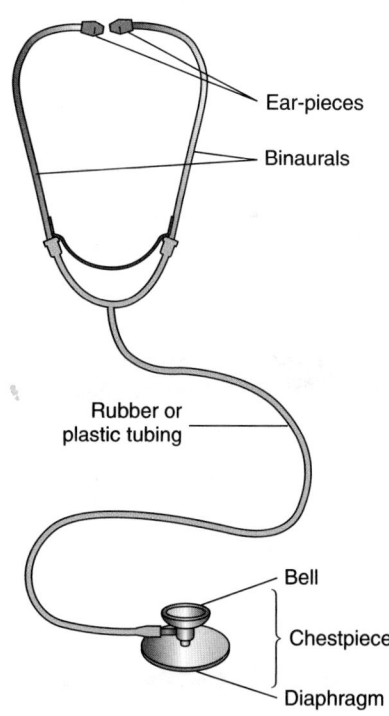

Fig. 26-13 Parts of a stethoscope.

- Ear-pieces
- Binaurals
- Rubber or plastic tubing
- Bell
- Chestpiece
- Diaphragm

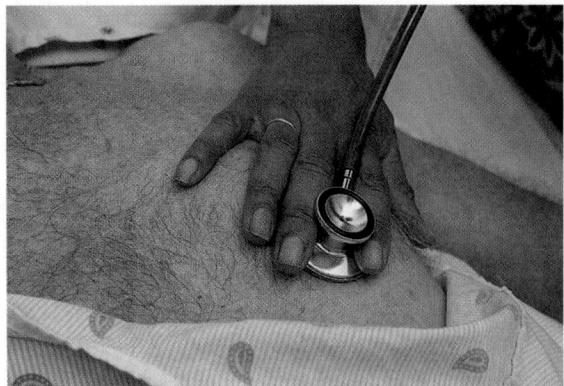

Fig. 26-14 The stethoscope is held in place with the fingertips of the index and middle fingers.

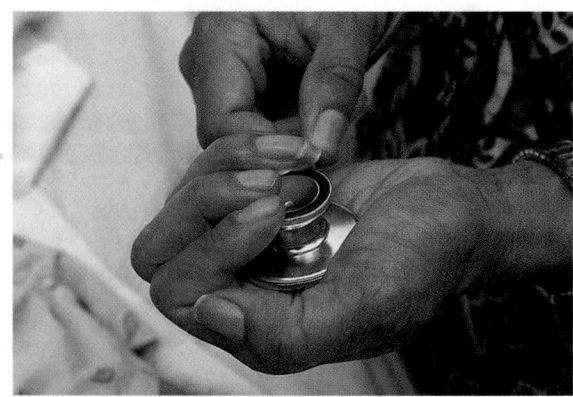

Fig. 26-15 The diaphragm of the stethoscope is warmed in the palm of the hand.

FOCUS ON COMMUNICATION

Using a Stethoscope

Hearing through the stethoscope is hard if the person is talking. Politely ask the person to be silent. Explain the procedure. Tell the person when and for how long he or she must remain silent. You can say:

"Mr. Bradley, I am going to check your pulse with a stethoscope. It is hard for me to hear your heart beat when you talk. Please do not talk when my stethoscope is on your chest. It will take about 1 minute."

The person may forget and begin talking. You can politely say: "I am almost finished. Please stay quiet for just a little longer." Thank the person when you are done.

PROMOTING SAFETY AND COMFORT

Using a Stethoscope

Safety

Stethoscopes are in contact with many persons and staff. You must prevent infection. Wipe the ear-pieces and diaphragm with antiseptic wipes before and after use.

Comfort

Stethoscope diaphragms tend to be cold. Warm the diaphragm in your hand before applying it to the person (Fig. 26-15). Cold diaphragms can startle the person.

Pulse Rate

The *pulse rate is the number of heartbeats or pulses felt in 1 minute.* The rate varies for each age-group (Table 26-2). The pulse rate is affected by the factors listed in Box 26-1. Some drugs increase the pulse rate. Other drugs slow down the pulse.

TABLE 26-2	PULSE RANGES BY AGE
Age	**Pulse Rate per Minute**
Birth to 1 year	80–190
2 years	80–160
6 years	75–120
10 years	70–110
12 years and older	60–100

The adult pulse rate is between 60 and 100 beats per minute. A rate of less than 60 or more than 100 is considered abnormal. Report abnormal pulses to the nurse at once.

- *Tachycardia is a rapid* (tachy) *heart rate* (cardia). *The heart rate is more than 100 beats per minute.*
- *Bradycardia is a slow* (brady) *heart rate* (cardia). *The heart rate is less than 60 beats per minute.*

Rhythm and Force of the Pulse

The pulse *rhythm* should be regular. That is, pulses are felt in a pattern. The same interval occurs between beats. An irregular pulse occurs when the beats are not evenly spaced or beats are skipped (Fig. 26-16).

Force relates to pulse strength. A forceful pulse is easy to feel. It is described as *strong, full,* or *bounding.* Hard-to-feel pulses are described as *weak, thready,* or *feeble.*

Electronic blood pressure equipment (p. 485) can also count pulses. The pulse rate and blood pressures are shown. Some show if the pulse is regular or irregular. However, you need to feel the pulse to determine its force.

Taking Pulses

You will take radial, apical, and apical-radial pulses. You must count, report, and record accurately.

See *Delegation Guidelines: Taking Pulses.*
See *Promoting Safety and Comfort: Taking Pulses.*

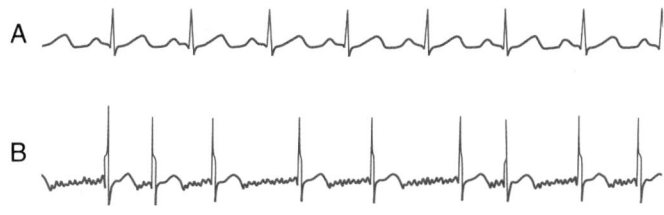

Fig. 26-16 **A,** The electrocardiogram shows a regular pulse. The beats occur at regular intervals. **B,** These beats are at irregular intervals.

Taking a Radial Pulse. The radial pulse is used for routine vital signs. Place the first 2 or 3 fingertips of one hand against the radial artery. The radial artery is on the thumb side of the wrist (Fig. 26-17). Count the pulse for 30 seconds. Then multiply the number by 2. This gives the number of beats per minute. If the pulse is irregular, count it for 1 minute.

In some agencies, all radial pulses are taken for 1 minute. Follow agency policy.

DELEGATION GUIDELINES
Taking Pulses

Before taking a pulse, you need this information from the nurse and the care plan:
- What pulse to take for each person—radial, apical, or apical-radial
- When to take the pulse
- What other vital signs to measure
- How long to count the pulse—30 seconds or 1 minute
- If the nurse has concerns about certain patients or residents
- What observations to report and record:
  - The pulse site
  - The pulse rate—report a pulse rate less than 60 (bradycardia) or more than 100 beats (tachycardia) per minute at once
  - Pulse deficit for an apical-radial pulse (p. 480)
  - If the pulse is regular or irregular
  - Pulse force—strong, full, bounding, weak, thready, or feeble
- When to report the pulse rate
- What patient or resident concerns to report at once

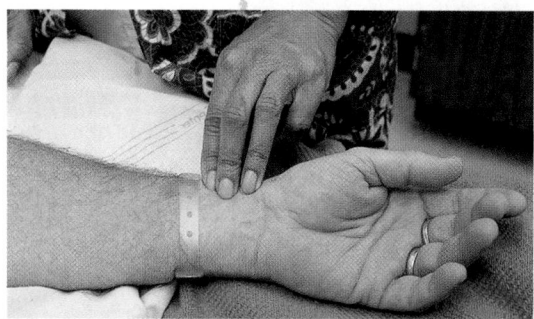

Fig. 26-17 The middle 3 fingertips are used to take the radial pulse.

TAKING A RADIAL PULSE

VIDEO | VIDEO CLIP | NNAAP® Skill

QUALITY OF LIFE

Remember to:
- Knock before entering the person's room.
- Address the person by name.
- Introduce yourself by name and title.

- Explain the procedure to the person before beginning and during the procedure.
- Protect the person's rights during the procedure.
- Handle the person gently during the procedure.

PRE-PROCEDURE

1 Follow *Delegation Guidelines: Taking Pulses.* See *Promoting Safety and Comfort: Taking Pulses.*
2 Practice hand hygiene.
3 Identify the person. Check the ID bracelet against the assignment sheet. Also call the person by name.
4 Provide for privacy.

PROCEDURE

5 Have the person sit or lie down.
6 Locate the radial pulse on the thumb side of the person's wrist. Use your first 2 or 3 middle fingertips (see Fig. 26-17).
7 Note if the pulse is strong or weak, and regular or irregular.
8 Count the pulse for 30 seconds. Multiply the number of beats by 2. Or count the pulse for 1 minute if:
  a Directed by the nurse and care plan.
  b Required by agency policy.

  c The pulse was irregular.
  d Required for your state competency test.
9 Note the person's name and pulse on your notepad or assignment sheet. Note the strength of the pulse. Note if it was regular or irregular.

Continued

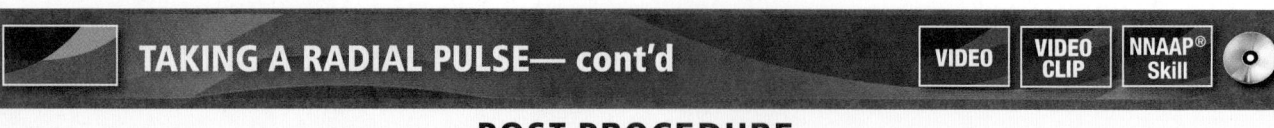

TAKING A RADIAL PULSE— cont'd | VIDEO | VIDEO CLIP | NNAAP® Skill |

POST-PROCEDURE

10 Provide for comfort. (See the inside of the front book cover.)
11 Place the signal light within reach.
12 Unscreen the person.
13 Complete a safety check of the room. (See the inside of the front book cover.)

14 Practice hand hygiene.
15 Report and record the pulse rate and your observations. Report an abnormal pulse at once.

Taking an Apical Pulse. The apical pulse is on the left side of the chest slightly below the nipple (Fig. 26-18). It is taken with a stethoscope. Apical pulses are taken on persons who:

- Have heart disease.
- Have irregular heart rhythms.
- Take drugs that affect the heart.

Count the apical pulse for 1 minute. The heartbeat normally sounds like a *lub-dub*. Count each *lub-dub* as one beat. Do not count the *lub* as one beat and the *dub* as another.

Taking an Apical-Radial Pulse. The apical and radial pulse rates should be the same. Sometimes heart contractions are not strong enough to create pulses in the radial artery. Then the radial rate is less than the apical rate. Heart disease is a common cause.

To see if the apical and radial pulses are equal, two staff members are needed. One takes the radial pulse; the other takes the apical pulse. *Taking the apical and radial pulses at the same time is called the apical-radial pulse.*

The *pulse deficit is the difference between the apical and radial pulse rates.* That is, you subtract the radial rate from the apical rate. (The radial rate is never greater than the apical rate.) For example:

- The apical rate is 84 beats per minute. The radial rate is 84 beats per minute. The pulse deficit is zero (0).
- The apical rate is 90 beats per minute. The radial rate is 86 beats per minute. The pulse deficit is 4.

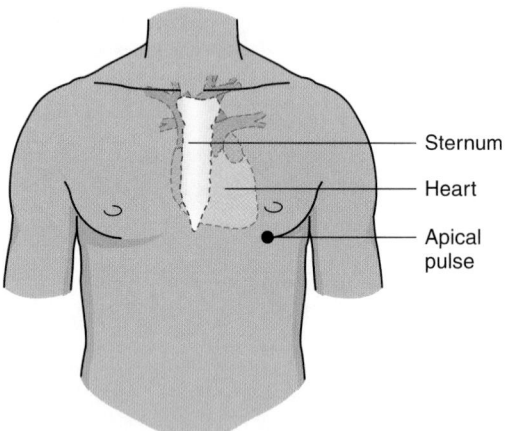

Sternum

Heart

Apical pulse

Fig. 26-18 The apical pulse is located 2 to 3 inches to the left of the sternum (breastbone) and below the left nipple.

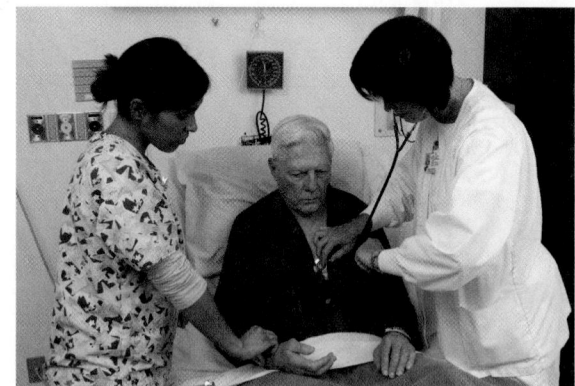

Fig. 26-19 Taking an apical-radial pulse. One worker takes the apical pulse. The other takes the radial pulse.

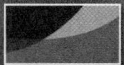

TAKING AN APICAL PULSE

VIDEO

QUALITY OF LIFE

Remember to:
- Knock before entering the person's room.
- Address the person by name.
- Introduce yourself by name and title.

- Explain the procedure to the person before beginning and during the procedure.
- Protect the person's rights during the procedure.
- Handle the person gently during the procedure.

PRE-PROCEDURE

1 Follow *Delegation Guidelines: Taking Pulses*, p. 479. See *Promoting Safety and Comfort: Using a Stethoscope*, p. 478.
2 Practice hand hygiene.
3 Collect a stethoscope and antiseptic wipes.

4 Practice hand hygiene.
5 Identify the person. Check the ID bracelet against the assignment sheet. Also call the person by name.
6 Provide for privacy.

PROCEDURE

7 Clean the ear-pieces and diaphragm with the wipes.
8 Have the person sit or lie down.
9 Expose the nipple area of the left chest. Expose a woman's breasts only to the extent necessary.
10 Warm the diaphragm in your palm.
11 Place the ear-pieces in your ears.

12 Find the apical pulse. Place the diaphragm 2 to 3 inches to the left of the breastbone and below the left nipple (see Fig. 26-18).
13 Count the pulse for 1 minute. Note if it was regular or irregular.
14 Cover the person. Remove the ear-pieces.
15 Note the person's name and pulse on your notepad or assignment sheet. Note if the pulse was regular or irregular.

POST-PROCEDURE

16 Provide for comfort. (See the inside of the front book cover.)
17 Place the signal light within reach.
18 Unscreen the person.
19 Complete a safety check of the room. (See the inside of the front book cover.)

20 Clean the ear-pieces and diaphragm with the wipes.
21 Return the stethoscope to its proper place.
22 Practice hand hygiene.
23 Report and record your observations. Record the pulse rate with *Ap* for apical. Report an abnormal pulse rate at once.

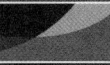

TAKING AN APICAL-RADIAL PULSE

QUALITY OF LIFE

Remember to:
- Knock before entering the person's room.
- Address the person by name.
- Introduce yourself by name and title.

- Explain the procedure to the person before beginning and during the procedure.
- Protect the person's rights during the procedure.
- Handle the person gently during the procedure.

PRE-PROCEDURE

1 Follow *Delegation Guidelines: Taking Pulses*, p. 479. See *Promoting Safety and Comfort:*
  a *Using a Stethoscope*, p. 478
  b *Taking Pulses*, p. 479
2 Ask a co-worker to help you.
3 Practice hand hygiene.

4 Collect a stethoscope and antiseptic wipes.
5 Practice hand hygiene.
6 Identify the person. Check the ID bracelet against the assignment sheet. Also call the person by name.
7 Provide for privacy.

PROCEDURE

8 Clean the ear-pieces and diaphragm with the wipes.
9 Have the person sit or lie down.
10 Expose the nipple area of the left chest. Expose a woman's breasts only to the extent necessary.
11 Warm the diaphragm in your palm.
12 Place the ear-pieces in your ears.
13 Find the apical pulse. Your helper finds the radial pulse (Fig. 26-19).

14 Give the signal to begin counting.
15 Count the pulse for 1 minute.
16 Give the signal to stop counting.
17 Cover the person. Remove the stethoscope ear-pieces.
18 Note the person's name and the apical and radial pulses on your notepad or assignment sheet. Subtract the radial pulse from the apical pulse for the pulse deficit. Note whether the pulse was regular or irregular.

Continued

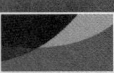

TAKING AN APICAL-RADIAL PULSE—cont'd

POST-PROCEDURE

19 Provide for comfort. (See the inside of the front book cover.)
20 Place the signal light within reach.
21 Unscreen the person.
22 Complete a safety check of the room. (See the inside of the front book cover.)
23 Clean the ear-pieces and diaphragm with the wipes.

24 Return the stethoscope to its proper place.
25 Practice hand hygiene.
26 Report and record your observations. (Report an abnormal pulse at once.) Include:
   • The apical and radial pulse rates
   • The pulse deficit

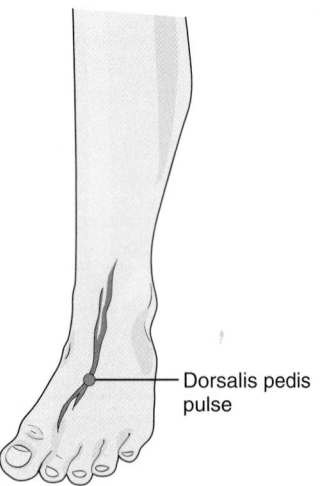

Fig. 26-20 The pedal pulse.

Dorsalis pedis pulse

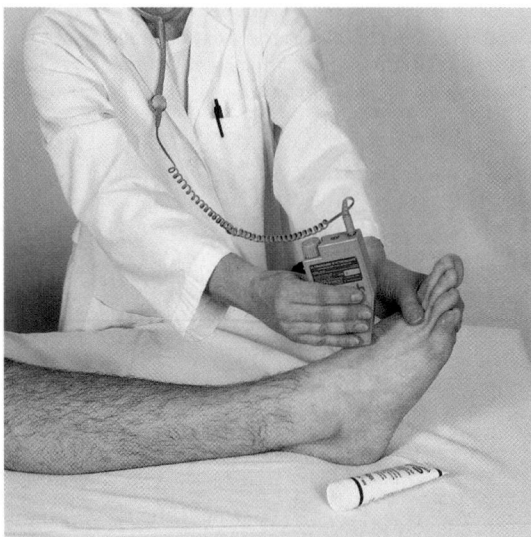

Fig. 26-21 A Doppler ultrasound stethoscope is used to check a pedal pulse.

Checking Pedal Pulses

The pedal (dorsalis pedis) pulse is used to check circulation in the foot. The dorsalis pedis artery is over a foot bone (Fig. 26-20). Often a nurse will mark the skin with an X where the pulse is found. This is so that all staff use the same site. When the pedal pulse cannot be felt, a *Doppler ultrasound stethoscope (DUS)* is used (Fig. 26-21).

• Doppler—the device is named after Christian J. Doppler. He developed the ultrasound method.
• Ultrasound—*ultra* means *beyond* or *farther*. *Sound* relates to *sound waves*. Blood flowing in an artery creates sound waves.

Your role may include using a DUS. If so, make sure that you:
• Have received the necessary training.
• Follow the nurse's directions.
• Follow the manufacturer's instructions.

RESPIRATIONS

Respiration means breathing air into (inhalation) *and out of* (exhalation) *the lungs.* Oxygen enters the lungs during inhalation. Carbon dioxide leaves the lungs during exhalation. Each respiration involves 1 inhalation and 1 exhalation. The chest rises during inhalation. It falls during exhalation.

See *Body Structure and Function Review: The Respiratory System*.

BODY STRUCTURE AND FUNCTION REVIEW: THE RESPIRATORY SYSTEM

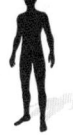

Oxygen is needed for life. Every cell needs oxygen. The respiratory system (Fig. 26-22) brings oxygen into the lungs and rids the body of carbon dioxide. *Respiration* is the process of supplying the cells with oxygen and removing carbon dioxide from them. Respiration involves *inhalation* (breathing in) and *exhalation* (breathing out). The terms *inspiration* (breathing in) and *expiration* (breathing out) are also used.

Air enters the body through the *nose.* The air then passes into the *pharynx* (throat), a tube-shaped passage-way for both air and food. Air passes from the pharynx into the *larynx* (the voice box). Air passes from the larynx into the *trachea* (the windpipe). The trachea divides at its lower end into the *right bronchus* and *left bronchus.* Each bronchus enters a lung.

On entering the lungs, the bronchi divide many times into smaller branches called *bronchioles.* Eventually the bronchioles further divide. They end in tiny one-celled air sacs called *alveoli.* They are supplied by capillaries.

Oxygen and carbon dioxide are exchanged between the alveoli and capillaries. Blood in the capillaries picks up oxygen from the alveoli. Then the blood returns to the left side of the heart and is pumped to the rest of the body. Alveoli pick up carbon dioxide from the capillaries for exhalation.

Each lung is divided into lobes. The right lung has three lobes, the left lung has two. The lungs are separated from the abdominal cavity by a muscle called the *diaphragm.* A bony framework made up of the ribs, sternum, and vertebrae protects the lungs.

See Chapter 9 for more detailed information.

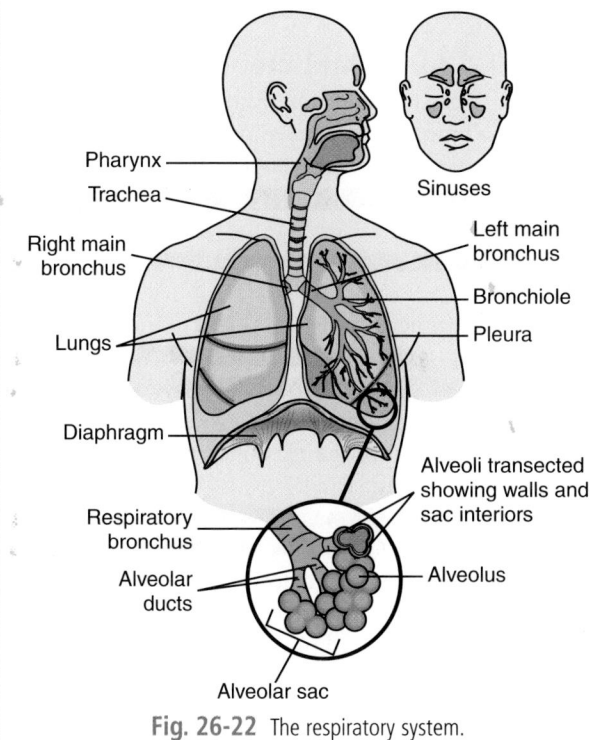

Fig. 26-22 The respiratory system.

Counting Respirations

The healthy adult has 12 to 20 respirations per minute. See Box 26-1 for the factors affecting vital signs. Heart and respiratory diseases often increase the respiratory rate.

Respirations are normally quiet, effortless, and regular. Both sides of the chest rise and fall equally. See Chapter 36 for abnormal respiratory patterns.

Count respirations when the person is at rest. Position the person so you can see the chest rise and fall. To some extent, a person can control the rate and depth of breathing. People tend to change their breathing patterns when they know their respirations are being counted. Therefore do not tell the person that you are counting them.

Count respirations right after taking a pulse. Keep your fingers or stethoscope over the pulse site. (The person assumes you are taking the pulse.) To count respirations, watch the chest rise and fall. Count them for 30 seconds. Multiply the number by 2 for the number of respirations in 1 minute. If you note an abnormal pattern, count the respirations for 1 minute.

In some agencies, respirations are counted for 1 minute. Follow agency policy.

See *Focus on Children and Older Persons: Respirations.*
See *Delegation Guidelines: Respirations*, p. 484.

FOCUS ON CHILDREN AND OLDER PERSONS
Respirations

Children

Infants and children have higher respiratory rates than adults (Table 26-3). Count an infant's respirations for 1 minute.

TABLE 26-3	NORMAL RESPIRATORY RATES FOR CHILDREN
Age	**Respirations per Minute**
Newborn	35
1 year	30
2 years	25
4 years	23
6 years	21
8 years	20
10 years	19
12 years	19
14 years	18
16 years	17
18 years	16–18

Modified from Hockenberry MJ, Wilson D: *Wong's nursing care of infants and children*, ed 9, St Louis, 2011, Mosby.

COUNTING RESPIRATIONS

VIDEO | VIDEO CLIP | NNAAP® Skill

PROCEDURE

1 Follow *Delegation Guidelines: Respirations*.
2 Keep your fingers or stethoscope over the pulse site.
3 Do not tell the person you are counting respirations.
4 Begin counting when the chest rises. Count each rise and fall of the chest as 1 respiration.
5 Note the following:
  a If respirations are regular
  b If both sides of the chest rise equally
  c The depth of respirations
  d If the person has any pain or difficulty breathing
  e An abnormal respiratory pattern

6 Count respirations for 30 seconds. Multiply the number by 2. Count respirations for 1 minute if:
  a Directed by the nurse and care plan.
  b Required by agency policy.
  c They are abnormal or irregular.
  d Required for your state competency test.
7 Note the person's name, respiratory rate, and other observations on your notepad or assignment sheet.

POST-PROCEDURE

8 Provide for comfort. (See the inside of the front book cover.)
9 Place the signal light within reach.
10 Unscreen the person.
11 Complete a safety check of the room. (See the inside of the front book cover.)

12 Practice hand hygiene.
13 Report and record the respiratory rate and your observations. Report abnormal respirations at once.

BLOOD PRESSURE

Blood pressure (BP) is the amount of force exerted against the walls of an artery by the blood. Blood pressure is controlled by:
- The force of heart contractions
- The amount of blood pumped with each heartbeat
- How easily the blood flows through the blood vessels

Systole is the period of heart muscle contraction. The heart is pumping blood. Diastole is the period of heart muscle relaxation. The heart is at rest.

You measure systolic and diastolic pressures. The *systolic pressure is the pressure in the arteries when the heart contracts.* It is the higher pressure. The *diastolic pressure is the pressure in the arteries when the heart is at rest.* It is the lower pressure.

Blood pressure is measured in millimeters (mm) of mercury (Hg). The systolic pressure is recorded over the diastolic pressure. A systolic pressure of 120 mm Hg (millimeters of mercury) and a diastolic pressure of 80 mm Hg are written as 120/80 mm Hg.

Normal and Abnormal Blood Pressures

Blood pressure can change from minute to minute. Factors affecting blood pressure are listed in Box 26-4.

Blood pressure has normal ranges:
- *Systolic pressure*—90 mm Hg or higher but lower than 120 mm Hg
- *Diastolic pressure*—60 mm Hg or higher but lower than 80 mm Hg

Treatment is indicated for:
- *Hypertension—When the systolic pressure is 140 mm Hg or higher* (hyper), *or the diastolic pressure is 90 mm Hg or higher.* Report any systolic measurement at or above 120 mm Hg. Also report a diastolic pressure at or above 80 mm Hg.
- *Hypotension—when the systolic pressure is below* (hypo) *90 mm Hg, or the diastolic pressure is below 60 mm Hg.* Report a systolic pressure below 90 mm Hg. Also report a diastolic pressure below 60 mm Hg. Some people normally have low blood pressures. However, hypotension can signal a life-threatening problem.

See *Focus on Communication: Normal and Abnormal Blood Pressures.*

See *Focus on Children and Older Persons: Normal and Abnormal Blood Pressures.*

BOX 26-4	**FACTORS AFFECTING BLOOD PRESSURE**

- *Age.* BP increases with age. It is lowest in infants and children. It is highest in adults.
- *Gender (male or female).* Women usually have lower blood pressures than men do. Blood pressures rise in women after menopause.
- *Blood volume.* This is the amount of blood in the system. Severe bleeding lowers the blood volume. Therefore BP lowers. Giving IV (intravenous) fluids rapidly increases the blood volume. The BP rises.
- *Stress.* Stress includes anxiety, fear, and emotions. BP increases as the body responds to stress.
- *Pain.* Pain generally increases BP. However, severe pain can cause *shock.* BP is seriously low in the state of shock (Chapter 51).
- *Exercise.* BP increases. Do not measure BP right after exercise.
- *Weight.* BP is higher in over-weight persons. It lowers with weight loss.

- *Race.* Black persons generally have higher blood pressures than white persons do.
- *Diet.* A high-sodium diet increases the amount of water in the body. The extra fluid volume increases BP.
- *Drugs.* Drugs can be given to raise or lower BP. Other drugs have the side effects of high or low BP.
- *Position.* BP is higher when lying down. It is lower in the standing position. Sudden changes in position can cause a sudden drop in BP (orthostatic hypotension). When standing suddenly, the person may have a sudden drop in BP. Dizziness and fainting can occur.
- *Smoking.* BP increases. Nicotine in cigarettes causes blood vessels to narrow. The heart must work harder to pump blood through narrowed vessels.
- *Alcohol.* Excessive alcohol intake can raise BP.

FOCUS ON COMMUNICATION
Normal and Abnormal Blood Pressures

Many persons want to know their blood pressures. If agency policy allows, tell the person the blood pressure. If the blood pressure is high or low, the person may worry. He or she may say: "That is higher (lower) than normal for me." Respond in a calm and professional manner. You can say: "Yes, I noticed it was a little high (low). I will tell your nurse." Report abnormal blood pressures to the nurse.

You must report some concerns at once. For example, you take Mr. Turner's blood pressure. It is 82/58. Mr. Turner says he is dizzy. You assist him to a lying position. You need to stay with Mr. Turner and report the concern. You press the signal light and identify yourself. You say: "Please have Mr. Turner's nurse come to room 216 right away." When the nurse arrives, you say: "I checked Mr. Turner's blood pressure. It was 82/58. He said he was dizzy. Would you please check him?"

FOCUS ON CHILDREN AND OLDER PERSONS
Normal and Abnormal Blood Pressures

Children
Age, sex, and height are used to determine a child's normal blood pressure. Young children can have high blood pressure. Over-weight children usually have higher blood pressures than do children with a normal weight. Children 3 years of age and older are screened for high blood pressure.

Older Persons
Older persons also are at risk for orthostatic hypotension (Chapter 27).

Equipment

You use a stethoscope and a sphygmomanometer to measure blood pressure. The *sphygmomanometer has a cuff and a measuring device.*

- The *aneroid type* has a round dial and a needle that points to the numbers (Fig. 26-23, A, p. 486).
- The *mercury type* has a column of mercury within a calibrated tube (Fig. 26-23, B, p. 486).
- The *electronic type* shows the systolic and diastolic blood pressures on the front of the device (Fig. 26-23, C, p. 486). It also shows the pulse rate. To use the device, follow the manufacturer's instructions.
- The *wrist monitor* (Fig. 26-23, D, p. 486) measures blood pressure at the wrist. This type is sometimes used for persons with bariatric needs. This type is very sensitive to body position. To use the device, follow the manufacturer's instructions.

You wrap the blood pressure cuff around the upper arm. Tubing connects the cuff to the manometer. Another tube connects the cuff to a small, hand-held bulb (aneroid and mercury types). To inflate the cuff, turn the valve on the bulb clockwise to close the valve and then squeeze the bulb. The inflated cuff causes pressure over the brachial artery. Turn the valve counter-clockwise to open the valve to deflate the cuff. Measure BP as the cuff deflates.

Blood flowing through the arteries produces sounds. Use the stethoscope to listen to the sounds in the brachial artery as you deflate the cuff. You do not need a stethoscope for an electronic manometer or wrist monitor.

See *Focus on Children and Older Persons: Equipment,* p. 486.

See *Promoting Safety and Comfort: Equipment,* p. 486.

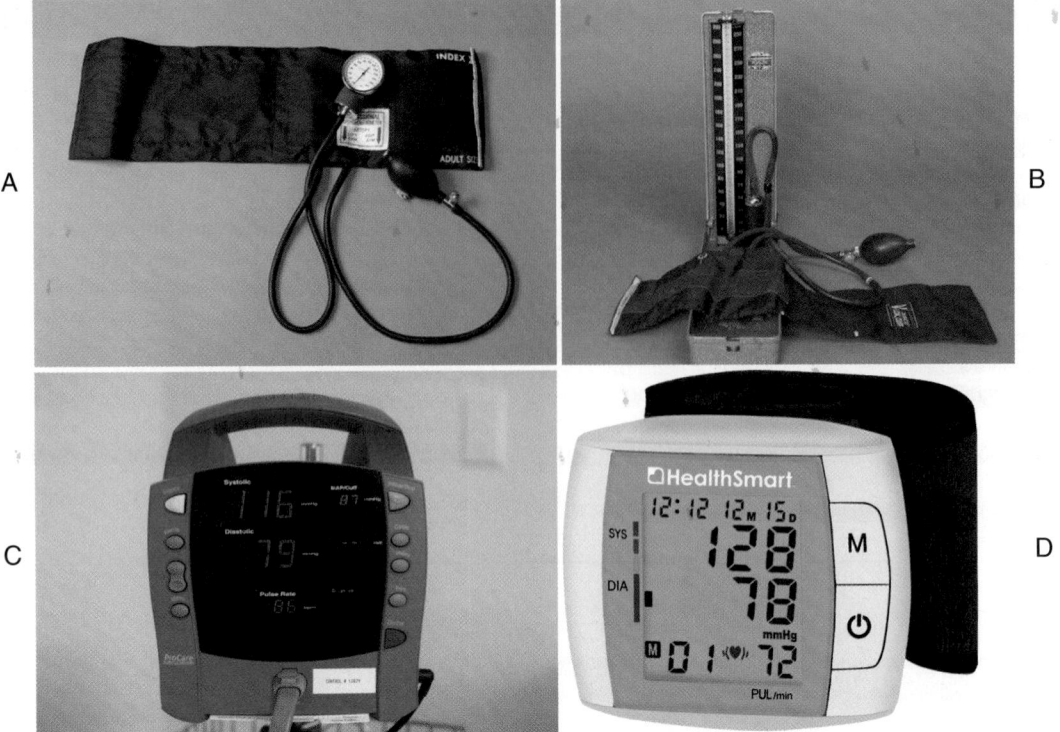

Fig. 26-23 Blood pressure equipment. **A,** Aneroid manometer and cuff. **B,** Mercury manometer and cuff. **C,** Electronic sphygmomanometer. **D,** Wrist monitor.

FOCUS ON CHILDREN AND OLDER PERSONS

Equipment

Children
Pediatric blood pressure cuffs are used for children. Infant and child sizes are available. The nurse tells you what size to use.

PROMOTING SAFETY AND COMFORT

Equipment

Safety
Mercury is a hazardous substance. Mercury manometers are being phased out of health care. Some agencies may still use them. Handle mercury manometers carefully. If one breaks, call for the nurse at once. Do not touch the mercury. Do not let the person touch it. The agency follows special procedures for handling all hazardous substances. See Chapter 12.

Comfort
Inflate the cuff only to the extent necessary (see procedure: *Measuring Blood Pressure*). The inflated cuff causes discomfort. The higher the inflation, the greater the discomfort.

Measuring Blood Pressure
You measure blood pressure in the brachial artery. Box 26-5 lists the guidelines for measuring blood pressure.
See *Delegation Guidelines: Measuring Blood Pressure.*

DELEGATION GUIDELINES

Measuring Blood Pressure

Before measuring BP, you need this information from the nurse and the care plan:
- When to measure BP
- What arm to use
- The person's normal blood pressure range
- If the nurse has concerns about certain patients or residents
- If the person needs to be lying down, sitting, or standing
- What size cuff to use—regular, child-size, extra large, bariatric
- What observations to report and record
- When to report the BP measurement
- What patient or resident concerns to report at once

BOX 26-5 GUIDELINES FOR MEASURING BLOOD PRESSURE

- Do not take BP on an arm:
  - With an IV infusion
  - With an arm cast
  - With a dialysis access site
  - On the side of breast surgery
  - On an injured arm
- Ask the nurse if you are not sure which arm to use.
- Let the person rest for 10 to 20 minutes before measuring BP.
- Measure BP with the person sitting or lying. Sometimes the doctor orders BP measured in the standing position.
- Apply the cuff to the bare upper arm. Clothing can affect the measurement.
- Make sure the cuff is snug. The reading will be wrong if the cuff is loose.
- Use a larger cuff if the person is obese or has a large arm. Use a small cuff if the person has a very small arm. Ask the nurse what size to use. Also check the care plan.

- Make sure the room is quiet. Talking, TV, radio, and sounds from the hallway can affect an accurate measurement.
- Place the diaphragm of the stethoscope firmly over the brachial artery. The entire diaphragm must have contact with the skin.
- Have the manometer where you can clearly see it.
- Measure the systolic and diastolic pressures.
  - Expect to hear the first BP sound at the point where you last felt the radial or brachial pulse. The first sound is the systolic pressure.
  - The point where the sound disappears is the diastolic pressure.
- Take the BP again if you are not sure of an accurate measurement. Wait 30 to 60 seconds to repeat the measurement. Ask the nurse to take the BP if you are unsure of the measurement.
- Tell the nurse at once if you cannot hear the blood pressure.

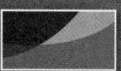 **MEASURING BLOOD PRESSURE** VIDEO | VIDEO CLIP | NNAAP® Skill

QUALITY OF LIFE

Remember to:
- Knock before entering the person's room.
- Address the person by name.
- Introduce yourself by name and title.

- Explain the procedure to the person before beginning and during the procedure.
- Protect the person's rights during the procedure.
- Handle the person gently during the procedure.

PRE-PROCEDURE

1 Follow *Delegation Guidelines: Measuring Blood Pressure.* See *Promoting Safety and Comfort:*
  a *Using a Stethoscope,* p.478
  b *Equipment*
2 Practice hand hygiene.
3 Collect the following:
- Sphygmomanometer
- Stethoscope
- Antiseptic wipes

4 Practice hand hygiene.
5 Identify the person. Check the ID bracelet against the assignment sheet. Also call the person by name.
6 Provide for privacy.

PROCEDURE

7 Wipe the stethoscope ear-pieces and diaphragm with the wipes. Warm the diaphragm in your palm.
8 Have the person sit or lie down.
9 Position the person's arm level with the heart. The palm is up.
10 Stand no more than 3 feet away from the manometer. The mercury type is vertical, on a flat surface, and at eye level. The aneroid type is directly in front of you.
11 Expose the upper arm.
12 Squeeze the cuff to expel any remaining air. Close the valve on the bulb.

13 Find the brachial artery at the inner aspect of the elbow. (The brachial artery is on the little finger side of the arm.) Use your fingertips.
14 Locate the arrow on the cuff (Fig. 26-24, A, p. 488). Place the arrow on the cuff over the brachial artery (Fig. 26-24, B, p. 488). Wrap the cuff around the upper arm at least 1 inch above the elbow. It is even and snug.
15 Place the stethoscope ear-pieces in your ears. Place the diaphragm over the brachial artery (Fig. 26-24, C, p. 488). Do not place it under the cuff.
16 Find the radial pulse. This step is for Methods 1 and 2 on p. 488.

Continued

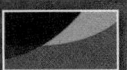
PROCEDURE—cont'd

17 *Method 1:*
  a Inflate the cuff until you can no longer feel the pulse. Note this point.
  b Inflate the cuff 30 mm Hg beyond the point where you last felt the pulse.

18 *Method 2:*
  a Inflate the cuff until you can no longer feel the pulse. Note this point.
  b Inflate the cuff 30 mm Hg beyond the point where you last felt the pulse.
  c Deflate the cuff slowly. Note the point when you feel the pulse.
  d Wait 30 seconds.
  e Inflate the cuff again, 30 mm Hg beyond the point where you felt the pulse return.

19 *Method 3:*
  a Inflate the cuff 160 mm Hg to 180 mm Hg.
  b Deflate the cuff if you hear a blood pressure sound. Re-inflate the cuff to 200 mm Hg.

20 Deflate the cuff at an even rate of 2 to 4 millimeters per second. Turn the valve counter-clockwise to deflate the cuff.

21 Note the point where you hear the first sound (Fig. 26-25). This is the systolic reading. It is near the point where the pulse disappeared.

22 Continue to deflate the cuff. Note the point where the sound disappears. This is the diastolic reading.

23 Deflate the cuff completely. Remove it from the person's arm. Remove the stethoscope ear-pieces from your ears.

24 Note the person's name and blood pressure on your notepad or assignment sheet.

25 Return the cuff to the case or wall holder.

POST-PROCEDURE

26 Provide for comfort. (See the inside of the front book cover.)

27 Place the signal light within reach.

28 Unscreen the person.

29 Complete a safety check of the room. (See the inside of the front book cover.)

30 Clean the ear-pieces and diaphragm with the wipes.

31 Return the equipment to its proper place.

32 Practice hand hygiene.

33 Report and record the BP (Fig. 26-26). Note which arm was used. Report an abnormal blood pressure at once.

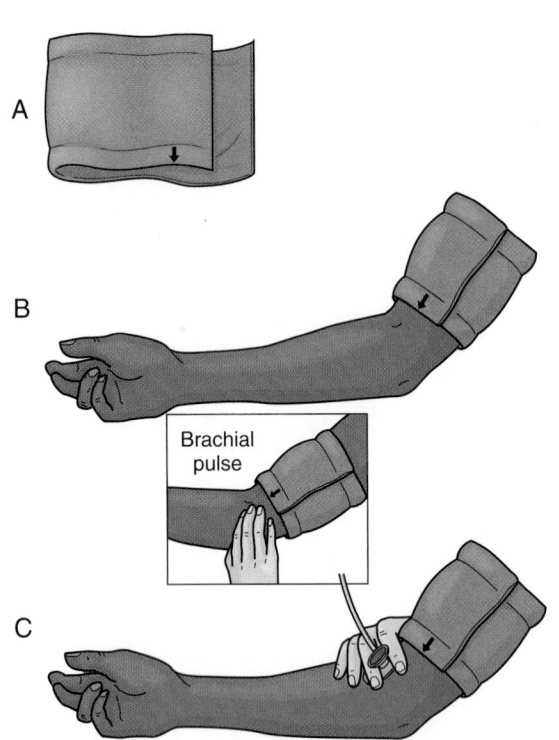

Fig. 26-24 Measuring blood pressure. **A,** The arrow is used for correct cuff alignment. **B,** The cuff is placed so the arrow is aligned with the brachial artery. **C,** The diaphragm of the stethoscope is over the brachial artery.

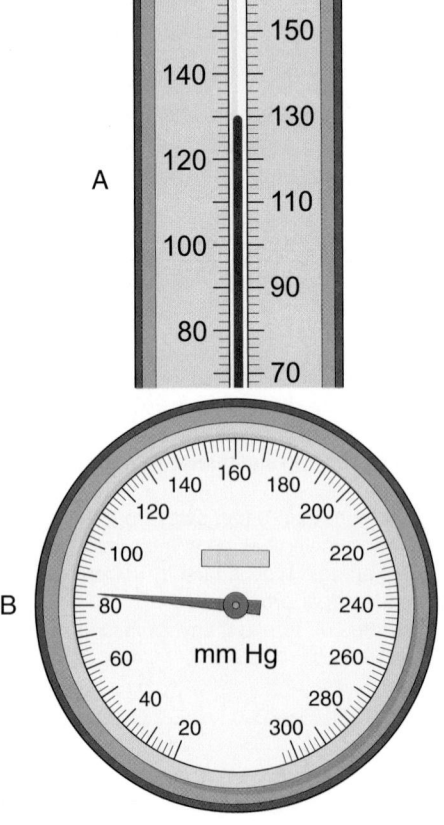

Fig. 26-25 Reading the manometer. Long lines mark 10 mm Hg values. Short lines mark 2 mm Hg values. **A,** This mercury manometer is at 130 mm Hg. **B,** This aneroid manometer is at 84 mm Hg.

DAILY SUMMARY AND GRAPHIC

DATE	6/12					
HOUR	2400	0400	0800	1200	1600	2000
BP	118/72	124/76	122/78			
BP SITE	R arm	R arm	L arm			

T E M P E R A T U R E	104	40						
	102.2	39						
	100.4	38						
	98.6	37						
	96.6	36						

TEMP ROUTE	Oral	Oral	Oral			
PULSE	76	74	78			
RESPIRATION	16	16	18			

Fig. 26-26 Charting sample.

PAIN

Pain is a warning sign from the body. It signals tissue damage. Therefore many agencies consider it to be a vital sign. See "Pain" in Chapter 28.

FOCUS ON P R I D E

The Person, Family, and Yourself

Personal and Professional Responsibility

Measurements and observations about the person are important for the nursing process. They help the nurse plan for and evaluate the person's care. You are responsible for knowing normal measurements and observations. For example, you must know normal vital sign ranges. You are responsible for reporting abnormal values. The person is at risk if you do not.

Report abnormal measurements and observations to the nurse. If you are unsure, tell the nurse. Take pride in safely assisting the nurse with the nursing process.

Rights and Respect

When you report an abnormal blood pressure, the nurse may ask you to repeat the measurement. The nurse may ask you to use different equipment, use the person's other arm, or change the person's position. Or the nurse may want to recheck the blood pressure himself or herself.

Do not be offended. Follow the nurse's directions. Show respect. Avoid negative thoughts or statements about the nurse or yourself. The nurse's request does not mean you have done something wrong. It does not mean the nurse cannot trust you. The nurse needs to check such measurements to be sure the person receives safe care.

Independence and Social Interaction

Personal choices help the person feel independent. The person may prefer that you use the right or left arm for pulses and blood pressures. If safe to do so, use the arm the person prefers. Unless orders direct otherwise, allow the person to choose to sit or lie when vital signs are measured.

Delegation and Teamwork

Hospitals, nursing centers, and home health agencies care for persons needing Transmission-Based Precautions (Chapter 15). You may be delegated care of such persons. Know your agency's policy for measuring vital signs on persons with isolation precautions.

Some agencies have isolation carts or kits that contain equipment. A stethoscope, blood pressure cuff, and thermometer are common. The equipment is taken into the person's room or home and left there. You use that equipment when measuring vital signs. You do not use your own stethoscope or bring other equipment into the room or home. If equipment must be brought in, it is cleaned after use. Special cleansers may be needed. Follow agency policy to protect others from infection.

Ethics and Laws

Your measurements must be accurate. Tell the nurse if you are unsure of any measurement. For example, you cannot feel a pulse or hear a blood pressure. Never make up a measurement. Reporting or recording false measurements is wrong. The person can be harmed. Take pride in doing the right thing by honest reporting and recording.

REVIEW QUESTIONS

Circle the BEST answer.

1 Which statement is *false?*
   a The vital signs are temperature, pulse, respirations, and blood pressure.
   b Vital signs detect changes in body function.
   c Vital signs change only during illness.
   d Sleep, exercise, drugs, emotions, and noise affect vital signs.

2 Which should you report at once?
   a An oral temperature of 98.4°F
   b A rectal temperature of 101.6°F
   c An axillary temperature of 97.6°F
   d An oral temperature of 99.0°F

3 A rectal temperature is taken when the person
   a Is unconscious
   b Has heart disease
   c Is confused
   d Has diarrhea

4 Which gives the *least* accurate measurement of body temperature?
   a Oral site
   b Rectal site
   c Axillary site
   d Tympanic membrane site

5 Which site is used to take an infant's temperature?
   a Oral site
   b Rectal site
   c Axillary site
   d Tympanic membrane site

6 Which is usually used to take an adult's pulse?
   a The radial pulse
   b The apical pulse
   c The apical-radial pulse
   d The brachial pulse

7 Which do you report to the nurse at once?
   a An adult has a pulse of 124 beats per minute.
   b An adult has a pulse of 90 beats per minute.
   c An adult has a pulse of 86 beats per minute.
   d An adult has a pulse of 64 beats per minute.

8 Which statement about the apical-radial pulse is *true?*
   a The radial pulse can be greater than the apical pulse.
   b The apical pulse can be greater than the radial pulse.
   c The apical and radial pulses are always equal.
   d The pulse deficit is always 0.

9 In an adult, normal respirations are
   a 10 to 18 per minute
   b 12 to 20 per minute
   c Less than 20 per minute
   d More than 20 per minute

10 Normal respirations
   a Are heard as the person inhales
   b Are heard as the person exhales
   c Are quiet
   d Sound like wheezing with inhalation and exhalation

11 Respirations are usually counted
   a After taking the temperature
   b After taking the pulse
   c Before taking the pulse
   d After taking the blood pressure

12 Which blood pressure is normal for an adult?
   a 88/54 mm Hg
   b 140/90 mm Hg
   c 100/58 mm Hg
   d 112/78 mm Hg

13 When measuring BP, you should do the following *except*
   a Use the arm with an IV infusion
   b Apply the cuff to a bare upper arm
   c Turn off the TV
   d Locate the brachial artery

14 The systolic pressure is the point
   a Where the pulse is no longer felt
   b Where the first sound is heard
   c Where the last sound is heard
   d 30 mm Hg above where the pulse was felt

15 You are not sure of hearing an accurate BP measurement. What should you do?
   a Record what you think that you heard.
   b Measure the BP again after 60 seconds.
   c Use the bell part of the stethoscope.
   d Ask another nursing assistant to take the BP.

Answers to these questions are on p. 833.

Exercise and Activity 27

OBJECTIVES

- Define the key terms and key abbreviations listed in this chapter.
- Describe bedrest.
- Explain how to prevent the complications from bedrest.
- Describe the devices used to support and maintain body alignment.
- Explain the purpose of a trapeze.
- Describe range-of-motion exercises.
- Describe four walking aids.
- Perform the procedures described in this chapter.
- Explain how to promote PRIDE in the person, the family, and yourself.

KEY TERMS

abduction Moving a body part away from the mid-line of the body

adduction Moving a body part toward the mid-line of the body

ambulation The act of walking

atrophy The decrease in size or the wasting away of tissue

contracture The lack of joint mobility caused by abnormal shortening of a muscle

deconditioning The loss of muscle strength from inactivity

dorsiflexion Bending the toes and foot up at the ankle

extension Straightening a body part

external rotation Turning the joint outward

flexion Bending a body part

footdrop The foot falls down at the ankle; permanent plantar flexion

hyperextension Excessive straightening of a body part

internal rotation Turning the joint inward

orthostatic hypotension Abnormally low (hypo) blood pressure when the person suddenly stands up (ortho and static); postural hypotension

plantar flexion The foot (plantar) is bent (flexion); bending the foot down at the ankle

postural hypotension See "orthostatic hypotension"

pronation Turning the joint downward

range of motion (ROM) The movement of a joint to the extent possible without causing pain

rotation Turning the joint

supination Turning the joint upward

syncope A brief loss of consciousness; fainting

KEY ABBREVIATIONS

ADL	Activities of daily living	**OBRA**	Omnibus Budget Reconciliation Act of 1987
CMS	Centers for Medicare & Medicaid Services	**PT**	Physical therapist
ID	Identification	**ROM**	Range of motion

Being active is important for physical and mental well-being. Most people move about and function without help. Illness, surgery, injury, pain, and aging cause weakness and some activity limits. Some people are in bed for a long time. Some are paralyzed. Some disorders worsen over time. They cause decreases in activity. Examples include arthritis and nervous system and muscular disorders (Chapter 41). Inactivity, whether mild or severe, affects every body system. It also affects mental well-being.

Nurses use the nursing process to promote exercise and activity in all persons to the extent possible. The person works closely with physical and occupational therapists to improve strength and endurance. Care plan goals for exercise and ambulation (p. 501) may change daily. The goal may be to improve the person's independence so he or she can go home. Or the goal may be to attain the highest level of function possible. The care plan and your assignment sheet include the person's activity level and needed exercises.

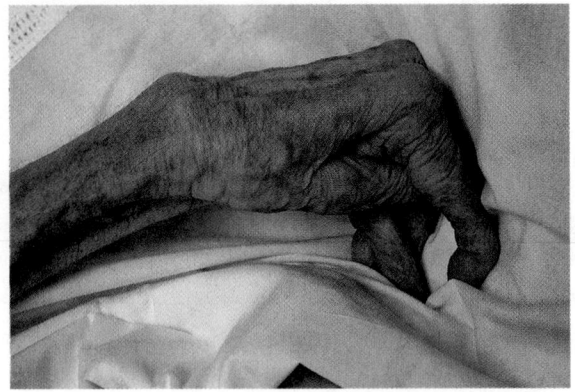

Fig. 27-1 A contracture.

To help promote exercise and activity, you need to understand:

- Bedrest
- How to prevent complications from bedrest
- How to help with exercise
  See *Focus on Children and Older Persons: Exercise and Activity.*

BEDREST

The doctor orders bedrest to treat a health problem. Or it is a nursing measure if the person's condition changes. Generally bedrest is ordered to:

- Reduce physical activity.
- Reduce pain.
- Encourage rest.
- Regain strength.
- Promote healing.
  These types of bedrest are common:
- *Strict bedrest.* Everything is done for the person. No activities of daily living (ADL) are allowed.
- *Bedrest.* Some ADL are allowed. Self-feeding, oral hygiene, bathing, shaving, and hair care are often allowed.
- *Bedrest with commode privileges.* The person uses the commode for elimination.
- *Bedrest with bathroom privileges (bedrest with BRP).* The person uses the bathroom for elimination.

The person's care plan and your assignment sheet tell you the activities allowed. Always ask the nurse what bedrest means for each person. Check with the nurse if you have questions about a person's activity limits.

Complications From Bedrest

Bedrest and lack of exercise and activity can cause serious complications. Every system is affected. Pressure ulcers, constipation, and fecal impaction can result. Urinary tract infections and renal calculi (kidney stones) can occur. So can blood clots (thrombi) and pneumonia (inflammation and infection of the lung).

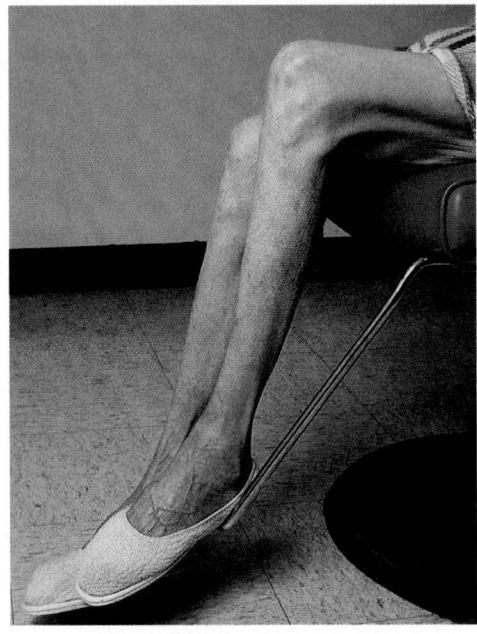

Fig. 27-2 Muscle atrophy.

The musculo-skeletal system is affected by lack of exercise and activity. You must help prevent the following to maintain normal movement:

- A *contracture is the lack of joint mobility caused by abnormal shortening of a muscle.* The contracted muscle is fixed into position, is deformed, and cannot stretch (Fig. 27-1). Common sites are the fingers, wrists, elbows, toes, ankles, knees, and hips. They can also occur in the neck and spine. The person is permanently deformed and disabled.
- *Atrophy is the decrease in size or the wasting away of tissue.* Tissues shrink in size. *Muscle atrophy* is a decrease in size or a wasting away of muscle (Fig. 27-2).
- Orthostatic hypotension and blood clots (Chapter 32) occur in the circulatory system.

BOX 27-1	PREVENTING ORTHOSTATIC HYPOTENSION

- Measure blood pressure, pulse, and respirations with the person supine.
- Position the person in Fowler's position. Raise the head of the bed slowly.
  - Ask the person about weakness, dizziness, or spots before the eyes. Lower the head of the bed if symptoms occur.
  - Measure blood pressure, pulse, and respirations.
  - Keep the person in Fowler's position for a short while. Ask about weakness, dizziness, or spots before the eyes.
- Help the person sit on the side of the bed (Chapter 17).
  - Ask about weakness, dizziness, or spots before the eyes. Help the person to Fowler's position if symptoms occur.
  - Measure blood pressure, pulse, and respirations.
  - Have the person sit on the side of the bed for a short while.
- Help the person stand.
  - Ask about weakness, dizziness, or spots before the eyes. Help the person sit on the side of the bed if any symptoms occur.
  - Measure blood pressure, pulse, and respirations.
- Help the person sit in a chair or walk as directed by the nurse.
  - Ask about weakness, dizziness, or spots before the eyes. If the person is walking, help the person to sit if symptoms occur.
  - Measure blood pressure, pulse, and respirations.
- Report blood pressure, pulse, and respirations to the nurse. Also report other symptoms or complaints.

FOCUS ON COMMUNICATION
Complications of Bedrest

Orthostatic hypotension can occur when the person moves from lying to sitting or standing. Fainting is a risk. To check for orthostatic hypotension, ask these questions:
- "Do you feel weak?"
- "Do you feel dizzy?"
- "Do you see spots before your eyes?"
- "Do you feel like fainting?"

Orthostatic hypotension is abnormally low (hypo) *blood pressure when the person suddenly stands up* (ortho *and* static). When a person moves from lying or sitting to a standing position, the blood pressure drops. The person is dizzy and weak and has spots before the eyes. Syncope can occur. *Syncope (fainting) is a brief loss of consciousness.* (Syncope comes from the Greek word *synkoptein.* It means *to cut short.*) *Orthostatic hypotension also is called postural hypotension.* (*Postural* relates to *posture or standing.*) Box 27-1 lists the measures that prevent orthostatic hypotension. Slowly changing positions is key.

Good nursing care prevents complications from bedrest. Good alignment, range-of-motion exercises (p. 495), and frequent position changes are important measures. These are part of the care plan.

See *Focus on Communication: Complications of Bedrest.*

Positioning

Body alignment and positioning were discussed in Chapter 16. Supportive devices are often used to support and maintain the person in a certain position:

- *Bed-boards*—are placed under the mattress. They prevent the mattress from sagging (Fig. 27-3, p. 494). Usually made of plywood, they are covered with canvas or other material. There are two sections so the head of the bed can be raised. One section is for the head of the bed. The other is for the foot of the bed.
- *Foot-boards*—are placed at the foot of mattresses (Fig. 27-4, p. 494). They prevent plantar flexion that can lead to footdrop. In *plantar flexion, the foot* (plantar) *is bent* (flexion). *Footdrop is when the foot falls down at the ankle* (permanent plantar flexion). The foot-board is placed so the soles of the feet are flush against it. The feet are in good alignment as when standing. Foot-boards also serve as bed cradles. They prevent pressure ulcers by keeping top linens off the feet and toes.
- *Trochanter rolls*—prevent the hips and legs from turning outward (external rotation) (Fig. 27-5, p. 494). A bath blanket is folded to the desired length and rolled up. The loose end is placed under the person from the hip to the knee. Then the roll is tucked alongside the body. Pillows or sandbags also keep the hips and knees in alignment.
- *Hip abduction wedges*—keep the hips abducted (apart) (Fig. 27-6, p. 494). The wedge is placed between the person's legs. These are common after hip replacement surgery.
- *Hand rolls or hand grips*—prevent contractures of the thumb, fingers, and wrist (Fig. 27-7, p. 494). Foam rubber sponges, rubber balls, and finger cushions (Fig. 27-8, p. 494) also are used.
- *Splints*—keep the elbows, wrists, thumbs, fingers, ankles, and knees in normal position. They are usually secured in place with Velcro (Fig. 27-9, p. 495).
- *Bed cradles*—keep the weight of top linens off the feet and toes (Fig. 27-10, p. 495). The weight of top linens can cause footdrop and pressure ulcers.

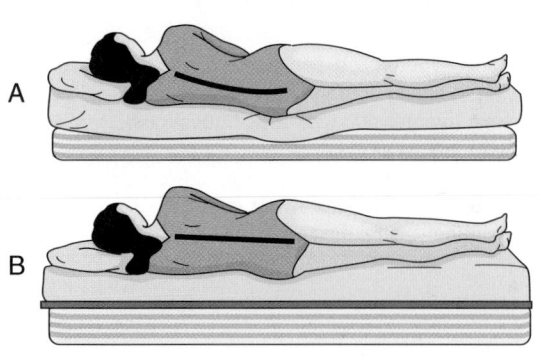

Fig. 27-3 Bed-boards. **A,** Mattress sagging without bed-boards. **B,** Bed-boards are under the mattress. No sagging occurs.

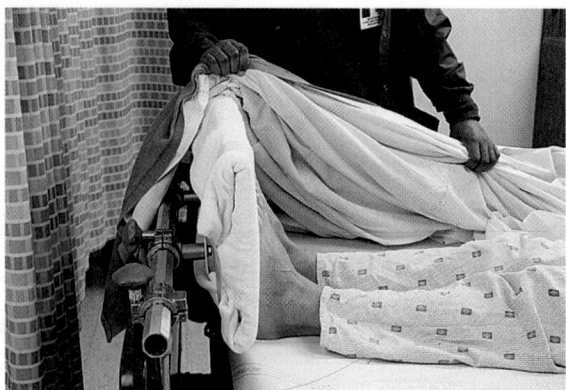

Fig. 27-4 A foot-board. Feet are flush with the board to keep them in normal alignment.

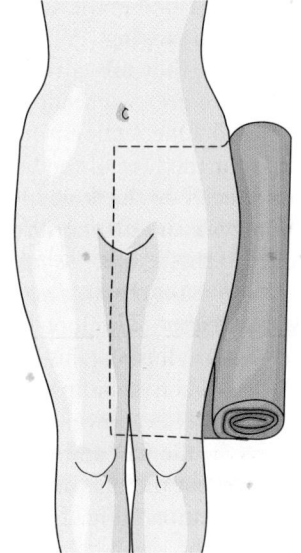

Fig. 27-5 A trochanter roll is made from a bath blanket. It extends from the hip to the knee.

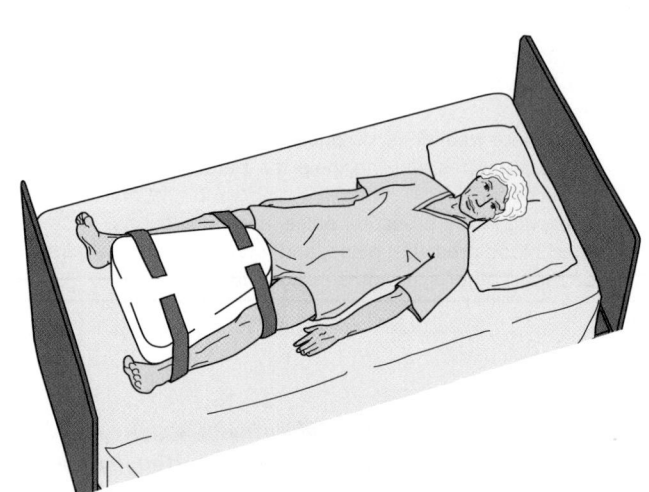

Fig. 27-6 Hip abduction wedge.

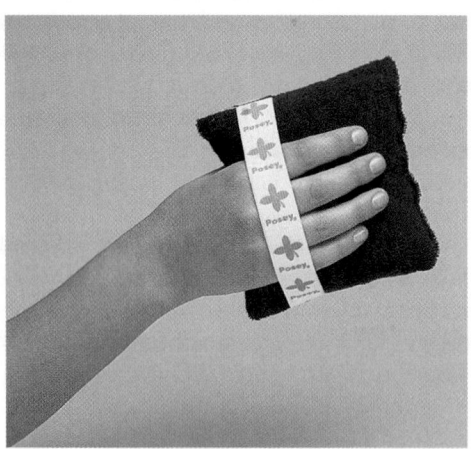

Fig. 27-7 Hand grip.

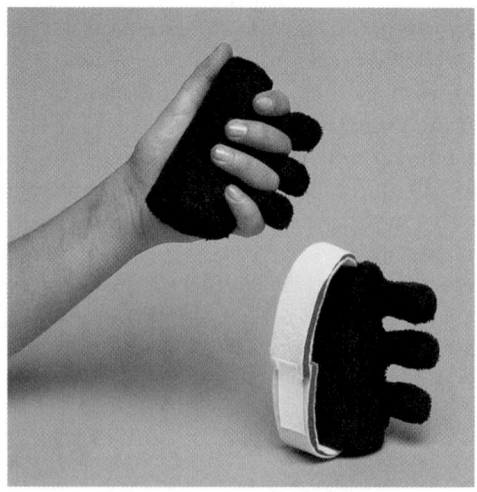

Fig. 27-8 Finger cushion.

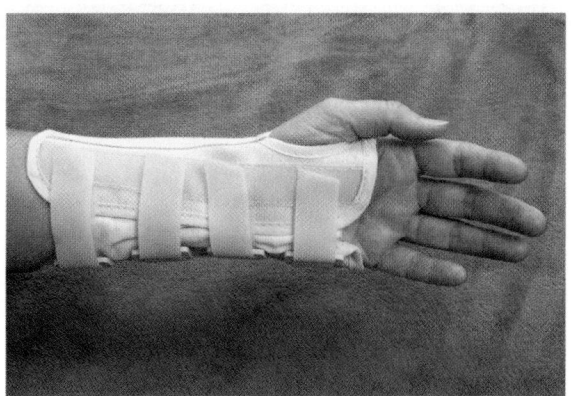

Fig. 27-9 A splint.

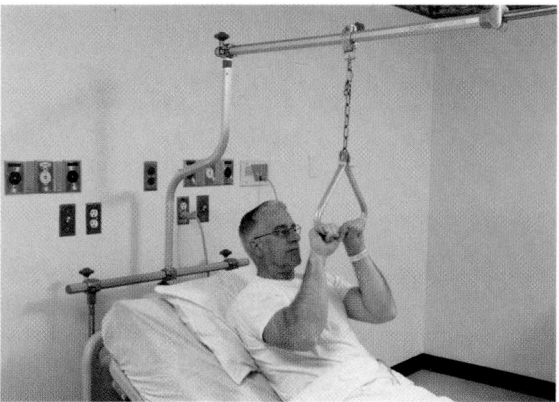

Fig. 27-11 A trapeze is used to strengthen arm muscles.

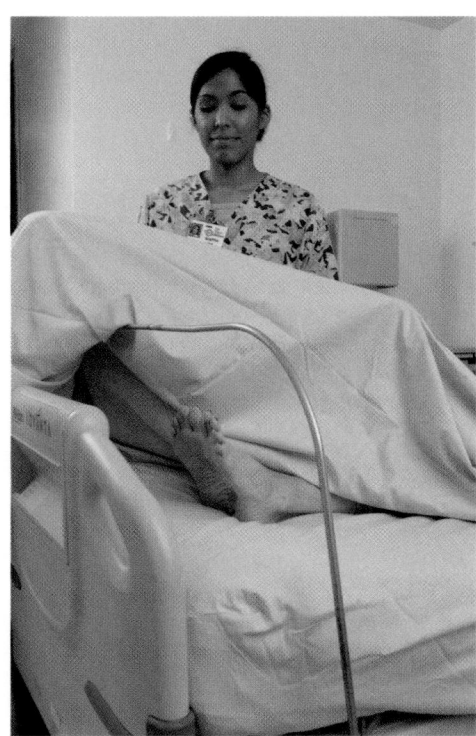

Fig. 27-10 A bed cradle.

Exercise

Exercise helps prevent contractures, muscle atrophy, and other complications from bedrest. Some exercise occurs with ADL and when turning and moving in bed without help. Other exercises are needed for muscles and joints. (See "Range-of-Motion Exercises" and "Ambulation," p. 501.)

A trapeze is used for exercises to strengthen arm muscles. The trapeze hangs from an overbed frame (Fig. 27-11). The person grasps the bar with both hands to lift the trunk off the bed. The trapeze is also used to move up and turn in bed.

◼ RANGE-OF-MOTION EXERCISES

The movement of a joint to the extent possible without causing pain is the range of motion (ROM) of that joint. Range-of-motion exercises involve moving the joints through their complete range of motion (Box 27-2, p. 496). They are usually done at least 2 times a day.

- *Active* range-of-motion exercises—are done by the person.
- *Passive* range-of-motion exercises—you move the joints through their range of motion.
- *Active-assistive* range-of-motion exercises—the person does the exercises with some help.

Bathing, hair care, eating, reaching, dressing and undressing, and walking all involve joint movements. Persons on bedrest need more frequent ROM exercises. So do those who cannot walk, turn, or transfer themselves because of illness or injury. The doctor or nurse may order ROM exercises.

See *Focus on Children and Older Persons: Range-of-Motion Exercises,* p. 496.

See *Focus on Long-Term Care and Home Care: Range-of-Motion Exercises,* p. 496.

See *Focus on Communication: Range-of-Motion Exercises,* p. 496.

See *Delegation Guidelines: Range-of-Motion Exercises,* p. 497.

See *Promoting Safety and Comfort: Range-of-Motion Exercises,* p. 497.

Text continued on p. 501

BOX 27-2	RANGE-OF-MOTION EXERCISES

Joint Movements

- *Abduction*—moving a body part away from the mid-line of the body
- *Adduction*—moving a body part toward the mid-line of the body
- *Flexion*—bending a body part
- *Extension*—straightening a body part
- *Hyperextension*—excessive straightening of a body part
- *Dorsiflexion*—bending the toes and foot up at the ankle
- *Plantar flexion*—bending the foot down at the ankle
- *Rotation*—turning the joint
- *Internal rotation*—turning the joint inward
- *External rotation*—turning the joint outward
- *Pronation*—turning the joint downward
- *Supination*—turning the joint upward

Safety Measures

- Cover the person with a bath blanket for warmth and privacy.
- Exercise only the joints the nurse tells you to exercise.
- Expose only the body part being exercised.
- Use good body mechanics.
- Support the part being exercised.
- Move the joint slowly, smoothly, and gently.
- Do not force a joint beyond its present range of motion.
- Do not force a joint to the point of pain.
- Ask the person if he or she has pain or discomfort.

FOCUS ON CHILDREN AND OLDER PERSONS
Range-of-Motion Exercises

Children

Depending on the child's activity limits, most play activities promote active range-of-motion exercises. For example:

- Kicking a Mylar balloon or foam ball.
- Touching a Mylar balloon that is held or hung in different places. For example, if a child is in traction you can hang a Mylar balloon from the trapeze.
- Playing basketball with bean-bags, wadded paper, or foam balls. Use a hoop or wastebasket as the target.
- Playing "pat-a-cake" or "Simon Says" (clap, kick, jump, and other motions).
- Having the child act like a bird, butterfly, spider, monkey, horse, and other animals.
- Playing video or computer games for finger and hand movements.
- Playing with finger paints, clay, or play dough.
- Having tricycle or wheelchair races.
- Playing "hide and seek." Hide a toy in the bed or room.

Always check with the nurse and care plan for the child's activity limits. Make sure the nurse approves of the play activity.

Modified from Hockenberry MJ and others: *Wong's nursing care of infants and children*, ed 8, St Louis, 2007, Mosby.

FOCUS ON LONG-TERM CARE AND HOME CARE
Range-of-Motion Exercises

Long-Term Care

The Omnibus Budget Reconciliation Act of 1987 (OBRA) and the Centers for Medicare & Medicaid Services (CMS) require an assessment and care planning process focused on the person's ROM. The intent is to reach or maintain the person's highest level of ROM. Or the focus is on preventing a decline in ROM. The goal may be one of the following:

- Prevent loss in range of motion.
- Increase range of motion.
- Prevent further decrease in range of motion.

During a survey, CMS surveyors may observe you performing ROM exercises.

FOCUS ON COMMUNICATION
Range-of-Motion Exercises

You must not force a joint beyond its present range of motion or to the point of pain. Ask the person to tell you if he or she:

- Feels that the joint cannot move any farther.
- Feels pain or discomfort in the joint.
- Needs to stop or rest.

The person may not be able to tell you about discomfort or limited joint movement. Observe for signs of pain (Chapter 28). Restlessness and grimacing are examples. Stop if you suspect pain or meet resistance. Tell the nurse.

When delegated range-of-motion exercises, you need this information from the nurse and the care plan:
- The kind of ROM exercises ordered—active, passive, active-assistive
- Which joints to exercise
- How often the exercises are done
- How many times to repeat each exercise
- What observations to report and record:
  - The time the exercises were performed
  - The joints exercised
  - The number of times the exercises were performed on each joint
  - Complaints of pain or signs of stiffness or spasm
  - The degree to which the person took part in the exercises
- When to report observations
- What patient or resident concerns to report at once

Safety

ROM exercises can cause injury if not done properly. Muscle strain, joint injury, and pain are possible. Practice the measures in Box 27-2 when performing or assisting with ROM exercises. Remind the person to tell you if he or she has pain during the procedure.

Range-of-motion exercises to the neck can cause serious injury if not done properly. Some agencies provide nursing assistants with special training before doing such exercises. Other agencies do not let nursing assistants do them. Know your agency's policy. *Perform ROM exercises to the neck only if allowed by your agency and if the nurse instructs you to do so.* In some agencies, only physical or occupational therapists do neck exercises.

Comfort

To promote physical comfort during ROM exercises, see Box 27-2. Provide privacy to promote mental comfort.

PERFORMING RANGE-OF-MOTION EXERCISES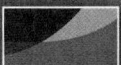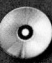

QUALITY OF LIFE

Remember to:
- Knock before entering the person's room.
- Address the person by name.
- Introduce yourself by name and title.

- Explain the procedure to the person before beginning and during the procedure.
- Protect the person's rights during the procedure.
- Handle the person gently during the procedure.

PRE-PROCEDURE

1 Follow *Delegation Guidelines: Range-of-Motion Exercises.* See *Promoting Safety and Comfort: Range-of-Motion Exercises.*
2 Practice hand hygiene.
3 Identify the person. Check the ID (identification) bracelet against the assignment sheet. Also call the person by name.
4 Obtain a bath blanket.
5 Provide for privacy.
6 Raise the bed for body mechanics. Bed rails are up if used.

PROCEDURE

7 Lower the bed rail near you if up.
8 Position the person supine.
9 Cover the person with a bath blanket. Fan-fold top linens to the foot of the bed.
10 Exercise the neck *if allowed by your agency and if the nurse instructs you to do so* (Fig. 27-12, p. 499):
   a Place your hands over the person's ears to support the head. Support the jaws with your fingers.
   b Flexion—bring the head forward. The chin touches the chest.
   c Extension—straighten the head.
   d Hyperextension—bring the head backward until the chin points up.
   e Rotation—turn the head from side to side.
   f Lateral flexion—move the head to the right and to the left.
   g Repeat flexion, extension, hyperextension, rotation, and lateral flexion 5 times—or the number of times stated on the care plan.

11 Exercise the shoulder (Fig. 27-13, p. 499):
   a Grasp the wrist with one hand. Grasp the elbow with the other hand.
   b Flexion—raise the arm straight in front and over the head.
   c Extension—bring the arm down to the side.
   d Hyperextension—move the arm behind the body. (Do this if the person sits in a straight-backed chair or is standing.)
   e Abduction—move the straight arm away from the side of the body.
   f Adduction—move the straight arm to the side of the body.
   g Internal rotation—bend the elbow. Place it at the same level as the shoulder. Move the forearm down toward the body.
   h External rotation—move the forearm toward the head.
   i Repeat flexion, extension, hyperextension, abduction, adduction, and internal and external rotation 5 times— or the number of times stated on the care plan.

Continued

PERFORMING RANGE-OF-MOTION EXERCISES—cont'd

VIDEO | VIDEO CLIP | NNAAP® Skill

PROCEDURE—cont'd

12 Exercise the elbow (Fig. 27-14):
   a Grasp the person's wrist with one hand. Grasp the elbow with your other hand.
   b Flexion—bend the arm so the same-side shoulder is touched.
   c Extension—straighten the arm.
   d Repeat flexion and extension 5 times—or the number of times stated on the care plan.

13 Exercise the forearm (Fig. 27-15):
   a Continue to support the wrist and elbow.
   b Pronation—turn the hand so the palm is down.
   c Supination—turn the hand so the palm is up.
   d Repeat pronation and supination 5 times—or the number of times stated on the care plan.

14 Exercise the wrist (Fig. 27-16):
   a Hold the wrist with both of your hands.
   b Flexion—bend the hand down.
   c Extension—straighten the hand.
   d Hyperextension—bend the hand back.
   e Radial flexion—turn the hand toward the thumb.
   f Ulnar flexion—turn the hand toward the little finger.
   g Repeat flexion, extension, hyperextension, radial flexion, and ulnar flexion 5 times—or the number of times stated on the care plan.

15 Exercise the thumb (Fig. 27-17):
   a Hold the person's hand with one hand. Hold the thumb with your other hand.
   b Abduction—move the thumb out from the inner part of the index finger.
   c Adduction—move the thumb back next to the index finger.
   d Opposition—touch each fingertip with the thumb.
   e Flexion—bend the thumb into the hand.
   f Extension—move the thumb out to the side of the fingers.
   g Repeat abduction, adduction, opposition, flexion, and extension 5 times—or the number of times stated on the care plan.

16 Exercise the fingers (Fig. 27-18):
   a Abduction—spread the fingers and the thumb apart.
   b Adduction—bring the fingers and thumb together.
   c Flexion—make a fist.
   d Extension—straighten the fingers so the fingers, hand, and arm are straight.
   e Repeat abduction, adduction, flexion, and extension 5 times—or the number of times stated on the care plan.

17 Exercise the hip (Fig. 27-19, p. 500):
   a Support the leg. Place one hand under the knee. Place your other hand under the ankle.
   b Flexion—raise the leg.
   c Extension—straighten the leg.
   d Hyperextension—move the leg behind the body.
   e Abduction—move the leg away from the body.
   f Adduction—move the leg toward the other leg.
   g Internal rotation—turn the leg inward.
   h External rotation—turn the leg outward.
   i Repeat flexion, extension, hyperextension, abduction, adduction, and internal and external rotation 5 times—or the number of times stated on the care plan.

18 Exercise the knee (Fig. 27-20, p. 500):
   a Support the knee. Place one hand under the knee. Place your other hand under the ankle.
   b Flexion—bend the knee.
   c Extension—straighten the knee.
   d Repeat flexion and extension of the knee 5 times—or the number of times stated on the care plan.

19 Exercise the ankle (Fig. 27-21, p. 500):
   a Support the foot and ankle. Place one hand under the foot. Place your other hand under the ankle.
   b Dorsiflexion—pull the foot upward. Push down on the heel at the same time.
   c Plantar flexion—turn the foot down. Or point the toes.
   d Repeat dorsiflexion and plantar flexion 5 times—or the number of times stated on the care plan.

20 Exercise the foot (Fig. 27-22, p. 500):
   a Continue to support the foot and ankle.
   b Pronation—turn the outside of the foot up and the inside down.
   c Supination—turn the inside of the foot up and the outside down.
   d Repeat pronation and supination 5 times—or the number of times stated on the care plan.

21 Exercise the toes (Fig. 27-23, p. 500):
   a Flexion—curl the toes.
   b Extension—straighten the toes.
   c Abduction—spread the toes apart.
   d Adduction—pull the toes together.
   e Repeat flexion, extension, abduction, and adduction 5 times—or the number of times stated on the care plan.

22 Cover the leg. Raise the bed rail if used.
23 Go to the other side. Lower the bed rail near you if up.
24 Repeat steps 11 through 21.

POST-PROCEDURE

25 Provide for comfort. (See the inside of the front book cover.)
26 Remove the bath blanket.
27 Place the signal light within reach.
28 Lower the bed to its lowest level.
29 Raise or lower bed rails. Follow the care plan.
30 Fold and return the bath blanket to its proper place.
31 Unscreen the person.
32 Complete a safety check of the room. (See the inside of the front book cover.)
33 Practice hand hygiene.
34 Report and record your observations.

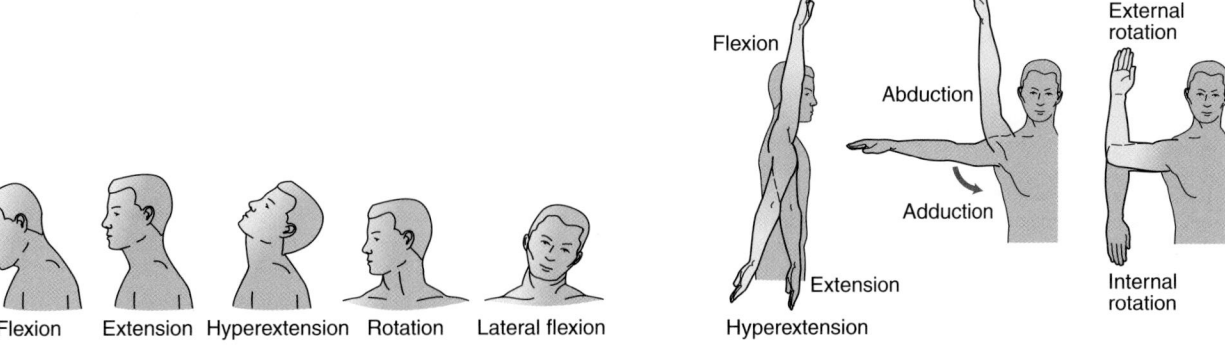

Fig. 27-12 Range-of-motion exercises for the neck.

Fig. 27-13 Range-of-motion exercises for the shoulder.

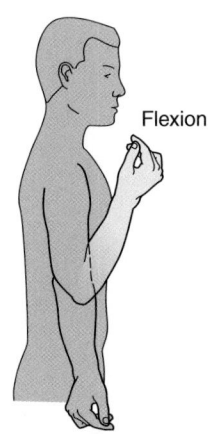

Fig. 27-14 Range-of-motion exercises for the elbow.

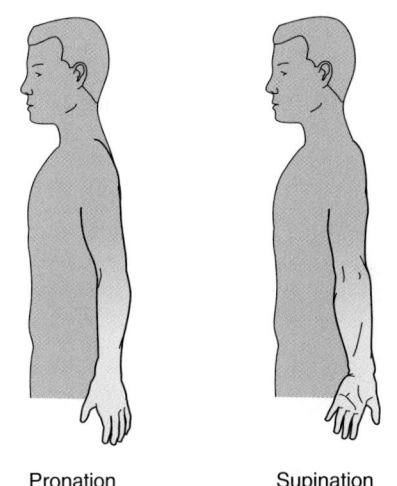

Fig. 27-15 Range-of-motion exercises for the forearm.

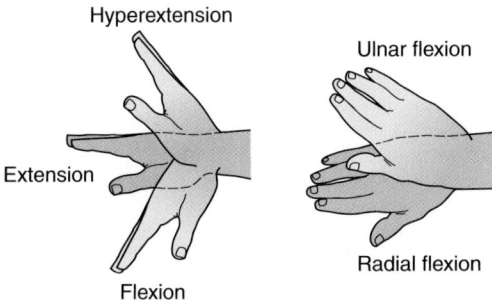

Fig. 27-16 Range-of-motion exercises for the wrist.

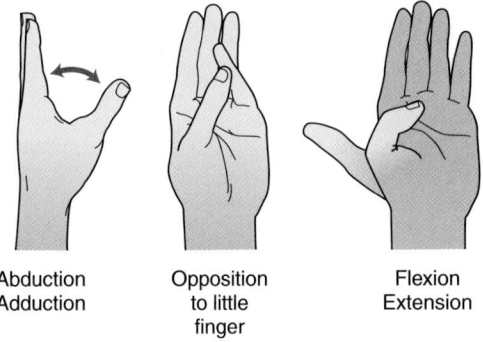

Fig. 27-17 Range-of-motion exercises for the thumb.

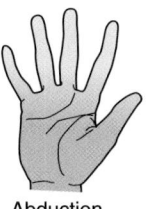
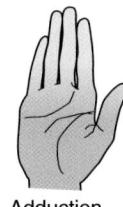
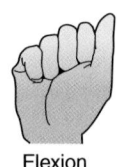
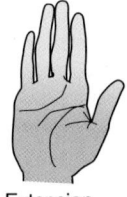

Fig. 27-18 Range-of-motion exercises for the fingers.

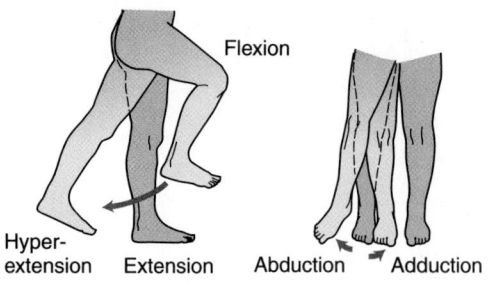

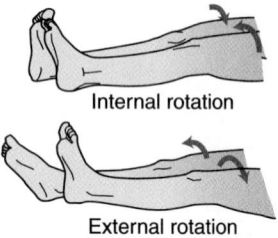

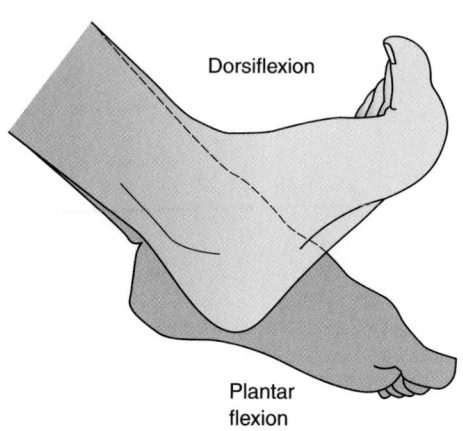

Fig. 27-19 Range-of-motion exercises for the hip.

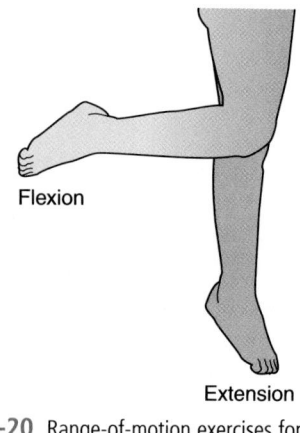

Fig. 27-20 Range-of-motion exercises for the knee.

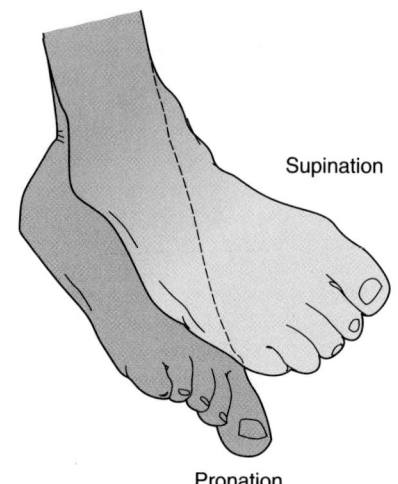

Fig. 27-21 Range-of-motion exercises for the ankle.

Fig. 27-22 Range-of-motion exercises for the foot.

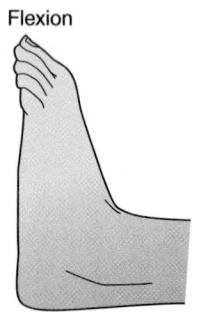

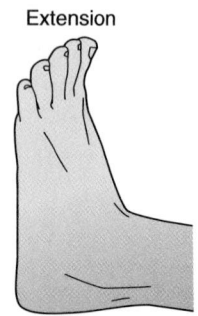

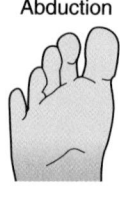

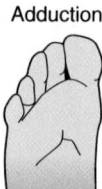

Fig. 27-23 Range-of-motion exercises for the toes.

AMBULATION

Ambulation is the act of walking. Some people are weak and unsteady from bedrest, illness, surgery, or injury. They need help walking. Some become strong enough to walk alone. Others will always need help.

After bedrest, activity increases slowly and in steps. First the person sits on the side of the bed (dangles). Sitting in a bedside chair follows. Next the person walks in the room and then in the hallway. To walk, contractures and muscle atrophy must be prevented. Proper positioning and exercises are needed during bedrest.

Regular walking helps prevent deconditioning. Some persons who use wheelchairs can walk with help. Follow the care plan when helping a person walk. Use a gait (transfer) belt if the person is weak or unsteady. The person also uses hand rails along the wall. Always check for orthostatic hypotension (p. 493).

See *Focus on Communication: Ambulation.*
See *Delegation Guidelines: Ambulation.*
See *Promoting Safety and Comfort: Ambulation.*

FOCUS ON COMMUNICATION
Ambulation

Before ambulating, talk with the person about the activity. Doing so promotes comfort and reduces fear. Explain to the person:
- How far to walk
- What assistive devices are used
- How you will assist
- What the person is to report to you
- How you will help if the person begins to fall
  For example, you can say:

  "Mr. Owens, I am going to help you walk from your bed to the doorway and back. This belt helps support you while you walk. I will be at your side and hold the belt at all times. Tell me right away if you feel unsteady, dizzy, or weak. Also tell me if you feel any pain or discomfort. If you begin to fall, I will use the belt to pull you close to me and gently lower you to the floor. Do you have any questions?"

DELEGATION GUIDELINES
Ambulation

Before helping with ambulation, you need this information from the nurse and the care plan:
- How much help the person needs
- If the person uses a cane, walker, crutches, or a brace
- Areas of weakness—right arm or leg, left arm or leg
- How far to walk the person
- What observations to report and record:
  - How well the person tolerated the activity
  - Shuffling, sliding, limping, or walking on tip-toes
  - Complaints of pain or discomfort
  - Complaints of orthostatic hypotension—weakness, dizziness, spots before the eyes, feeling faint
  - The distance walked
- When to report observations
- What patient or resident concerns to report at once

PROMOTING SAFETY AND COMFORT
Ambulation

Safety
Practice the safety measures to prevent falls (Chapter 13). Use a gait belt to help the person stand. Also use it during ambulation.

Comfort
The fear of falling affects mental comfort. Explain the purpose of the gait belt. Also explain how you will help the person if he or she starts to fall (Chapter 13).

HELPING THE PERSON WALK

QUALITY OF LIFE

Remember to:
- Knock before entering the person's room.
- Address the person by name.
- Introduce yourself by name and title.

- Explain the procedure to the person before beginning and during the procedure.
- Protect the person's rights during the procedure.
- Handle the person gently during the procedure.

PRE-PROCEDURE

1 Follow *Delegation Guidelines: Ambulation*, p. 501. See *Promoting Safety and Comfort: Ambulation*, p. 501.
2 Practice hand hygiene.
3 Collect the following:
   - Robe and non-skid shoes
   - Paper or sheet to protect bottom linens
   - Gait (transfer) belt

4 Identify the person. Check the ID bracelet against the assignment sheet. Also call the person by name.
5 Provide for privacy.

PROCEDURE

6 Lower the bed to its lowest position. Lock the bed wheels. Lower the bed rail if up.
7 Fan-fold top linens to the foot of the bed.
8 Place the paper or sheet under the person's feet. Put the shoes on the person. Fasten the shoes.
9 Help the person sit on the side of the bed. (See procedure: *Sitting on the Side of the Bed [Dangling]*, Chapter 17.)
10 Make sure the person's feet are flat on the floor.
11 Help the person put on the robe.
12 Apply the gait belt at the waist and over clothing. (See procedure: *Applying a Transfer/Gait Belt*, Chapter 13.)
13 Help the person stand. (See procedure: *Transferring the Person to a Chair or Wheelchair*, Chapter 17.) Grasp the gait belt at each side. If no gait belt, place your arms under the person's arms around to the shoulder blades.
14 Stand at the person's weak side while he or she gains balance. Hold the belt at the side and back. If not using a gait belt, have one arm around the back and the other at the elbow to support the person.

15 Encourage the person to stand erect with the head up and back straight.
16 Help the person walk. Walk to the side and slightly behind the person on the person's weak side. Provide support with the gait belt (Fig. 27-24). If not using a gait belt, have one arm around the back and the other at the elbow to support the person. Encourage the person to use the hand rail on his or her strong side.
17 Encourage the person to walk normally. The heel strikes the floor first. Discourage shuffling, sliding, or walking on tip-toes.
18 Walk the required distance if the person tolerates the activity. Do not rush the person.
19 Help the person return to bed. Remove the gait belt. (See procedure: *Transferring the Person From a Chair or Wheelchair to Bed*, Chapter 17.)
20 Lower the head of the bed. Help the person to the center of the bed.
21 Remove the shoes. Remove the paper or sheet over the bottom sheet.

POST-PROCEDURE

22 Provide for comfort. (See the inside of the front book cover.)
23 Place the signal light within reach.
24 Raise or lower bed rails. Follow the care plan.
25 Return the robe and shoes to their proper place.

26 Unscreen the person.
27 Complete a safety check of the room. (See the inside of the front book cover.)
28 Practice hand hygiene.
29 Report and record your observations (Fig. 27-25).

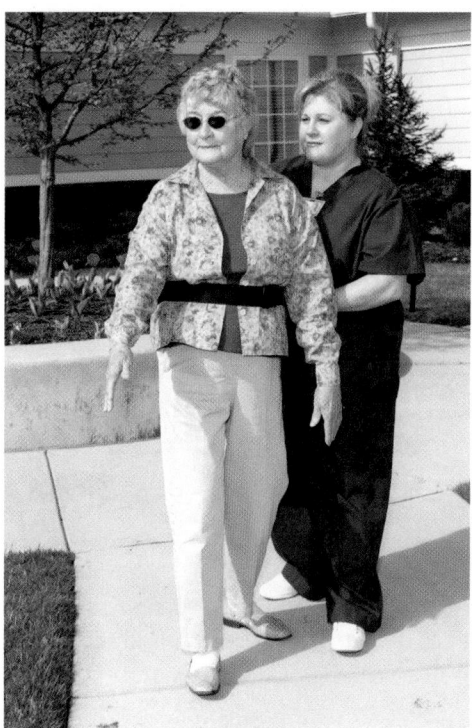

Fig. 27-24 Assist with ambulation. The nursing assistant uses a gait belt for the person's safety.

Walking Aids

Walking aids support the body. The doctor, nurse, or physical therapist (PT) orders them. The need may be temporary or permanent. The type ordered depends on the person's condition, the amount of support needed, and the type of disability. Older persons often need walkers or canes for safety. The PT measures and teaches the person to use the device.

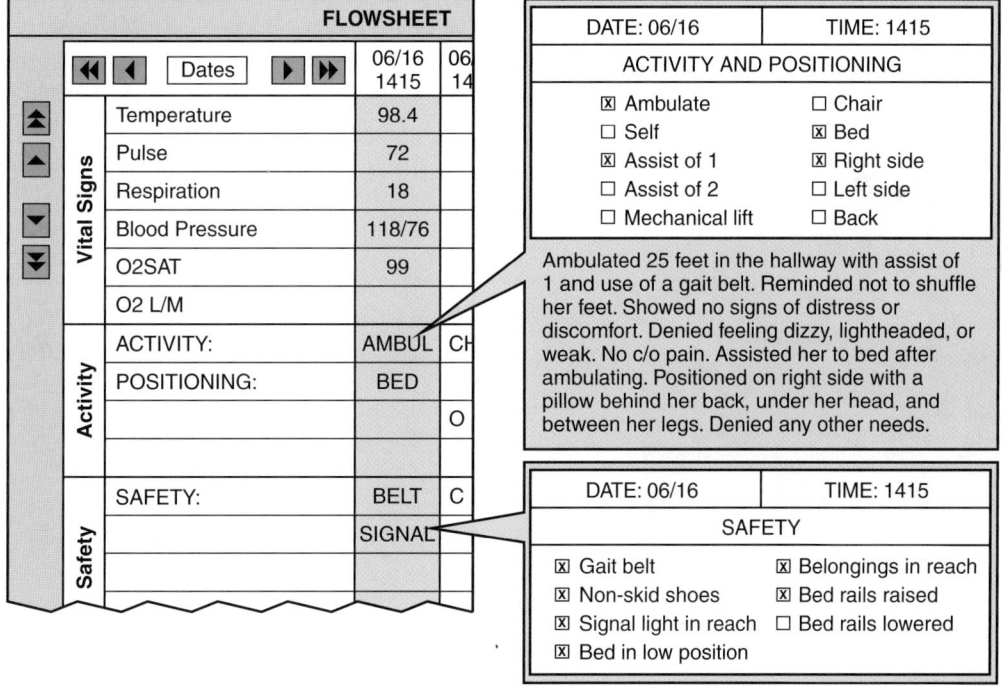

Fig. 27-25 Charting sample.

Crutches. Crutches are used when the person cannot use one leg or when one or both legs need to gain strength. Some persons with permanent leg weakness can use crutches. They usually use forearm crutches (Fig. 27-26). Underarm crutches extend from the underarm to the ground (Fig. 27-27).

The person learns to crutch walk, use stairs, and sit and stand. Safety is important. The person on crutches is at risk for falls. Follow these safety measures:

- Check the crutch tips. They must not be worn down, torn, or wet. Replace worn or torn crutch tips. Dry wet tips with a towel or paper towels.
- Check crutches for flaws. Check wooden crutches for cracks and metal crutches for bends.
- Tighten all bolts.
- Have the person wear street shoes. They must be flat and have non-skid soles.
- Make sure clothes fit well. Loose clothes may get caught between the crutches and underarms. Loose clothes and long skirts can hang forward and block the person's view of the feet and crutch tips.
- Practice safety rules to prevent falls (Chapter 13).
- Keep crutches within the person's reach. Put them by the person's chair or against a wall.
- Know which crutch gait the person uses:
  - Four-point gait (Fig. 27-28)
  - Three-point gait (Fig. 27-29)
  - Two-point gait (Fig. 27-30)
  - Swing-to gait (Fig. 27-31)
  - Swing-through gait (Fig. 27-32)

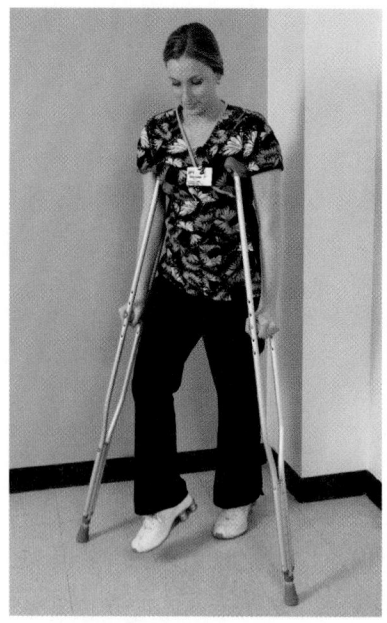

Fig. 27-27 Underarm crutches.

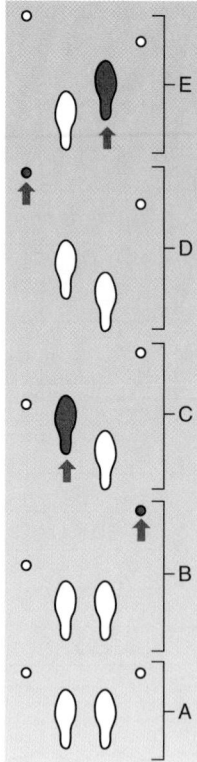

Fig. 27-28 The four-point gait. The person uses both legs. The right crutch is moved forward and then the left foot. Then the left crutch is moved forward followed by the right foot.

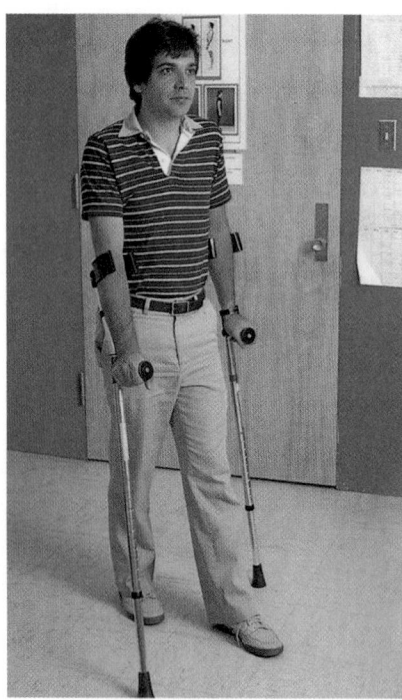

Fig. 27-26 Forearm crutches.

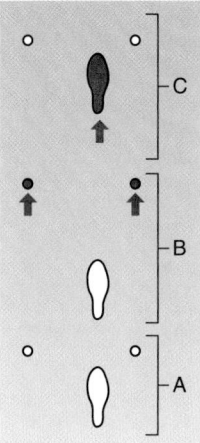

Fig. 27-29 The three-point gait. One leg is used. Both crutches are moved forward. Then the good foot is moved forward.

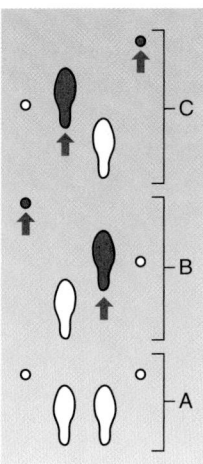

Fig. 27-30 The two-point gait. The person bears some weight on each foot. The left crutch and right foot are moved forward at the same time. Then the right crutch and left foot are moved forward.

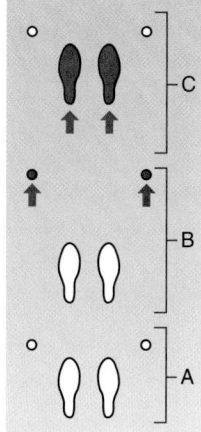

Fig. 27-31 Swing-to gait. The person bears some weight on each leg. Both crutches are moved forward. Then the person lifts both legs and *swings to* the crutches.

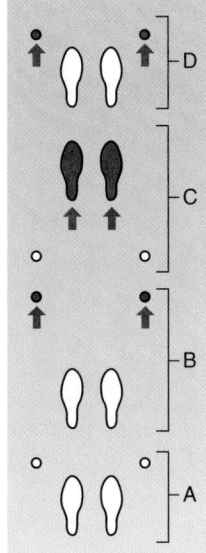

Fig. 27-32 Swing-through gait. The person bears some weight on each leg. Both crutches are moved forward. Then the person lifts both legs and *swings through* the crutches.

Canes. Canes are used for weakness on one side of the body. They help provide balance and support. Single-tip and four-point (quad) canes are common (Fig. 27-33). A cane is held on the *strong side* of the body. (If the left leg is weak, the cane is held in the right hand.) Four-point canes give more support than single-tip canes. However, they are harder to move.

The cane tip is about 6 to 10 inches to the side of the foot. It is about 6 to 10 inches in front of the foot on the strong side. The grip is level with the hip. The person walks as follows:

- *Step A:* The cane is moved forward 6 to 10 inches (Fig. 27-34, A, p. 506).
- *Step B:* The weak leg (opposite the cane) is moved forward even with the cane (Fig. 27-34, B, p. 506).
- *Step C:* The strong leg is moved forward and ahead of the cane and the weak leg (Fig. 27-34, C, p. 506).

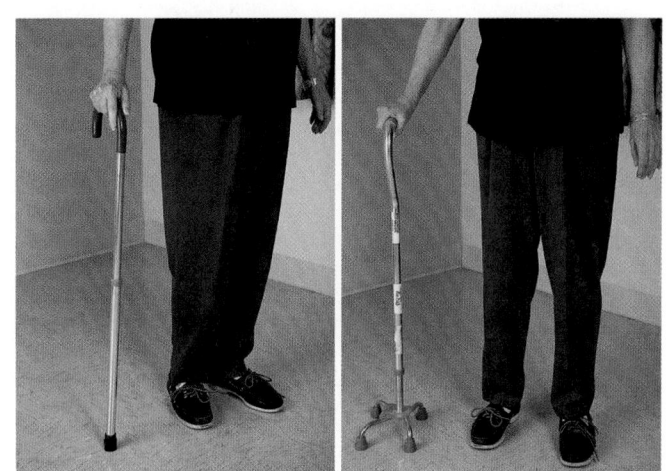

Fig. 27-33 A, Single-tip cane. **B,** Four-point cane.

A   B   C

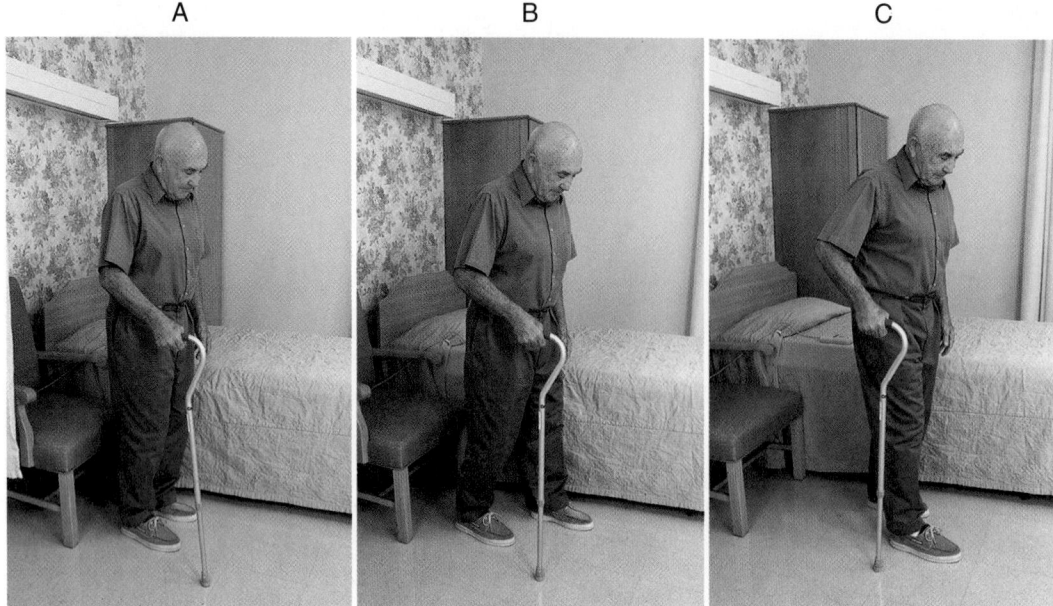

Fig. 27-34 Walking with a cane. **A,** The cane is moved forward about 6 to 10 inches. **B,** The leg opposite the cane (weak leg) is brought forward even with the cane. **C,** The leg on the cane side (strong side) is moved ahead of the cane and the weak leg.

Walkers. A walker gives more support than a cane. Wheeled walkers are common (Fig. 27-35). They have wheels on the front legs and rubber tips on the back legs. The person pushes the walker about 6 to 8 inches in front of his or her feet. Rubber tips on the back legs prevent the walker from moving while the person is standing. Some have a braking action when weight is applied to the walker's back legs.

Baskets, pouches, and trays attach to the walker. They are used for needed items. This allows more independence. They also free the hands to grip the walker.

See *Promoting Safety and Comfort: Walkers.*

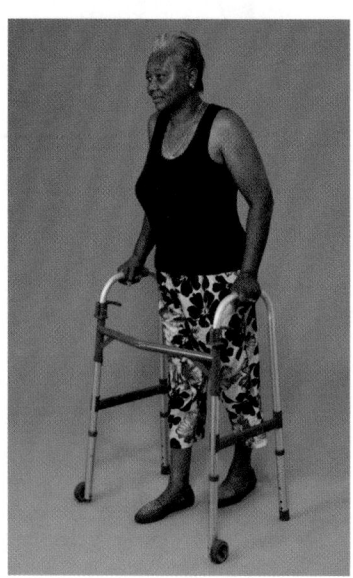

Fig. 27-35 Wheeled walker.

PROMOTING SAFETY AND COMFORT
Walkers

Safety

Walker wheels are usually on the outside of the walker (see Fig. 27-35). With the wheels on the outside, the walker may be too wide for some doorways. The wheels can be moved to the inside of the walker. This reduces the width of the walker. It will be easier for the person to go through some doorways.

Some walkers have seats. The person sits when he or she needs to rest. Never push the walker when the person is seated. Use a wheelchair instead.

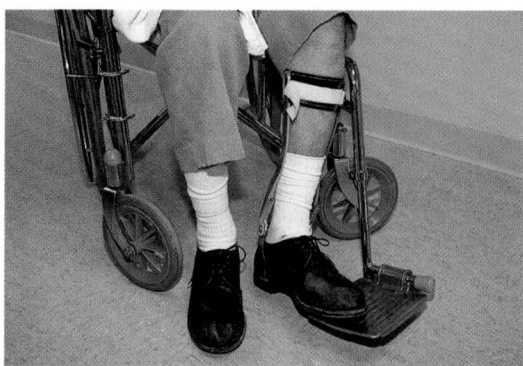

Fig. 27-36 Leg brace.

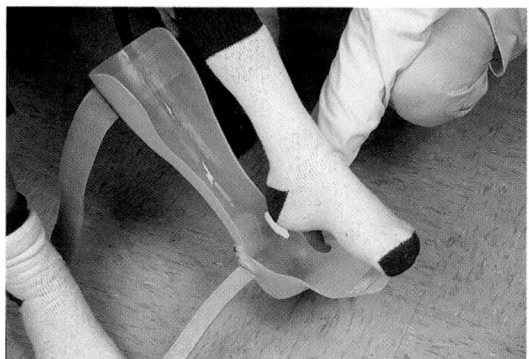

Fig. 27-37 Ankle-foot orthosis (AFO).

Braces. Braces support weak body parts. They also prevent or correct deformities or prevent joint movement. Metal, plastic, or leather is used for braces. A brace is applied over the ankle, knee, or back (Fig. 27-36). An ankle-foot orthosis (AFO) is placed in the shoe (Fig. 27-37). Then the foot is inserted. The AFO is secured in place with a Velcro strap. This type of brace is common after a stroke.

Keep skin and bony points under braces clean and dry. This prevents skin breakdown. Report redness or signs of skin breakdown at once. Also report complaints of pain or discomfort. The nurse assesses the skin under braces every shift. The care plan tells you when to apply and remove a brace.

FOCUS ON PRIDE

The Person, Family, and Yourself

Personal and Professional Responsibility

Exercise and activity help maintain normal joint and muscle function. They also promote normal function of all body systems. Good conditioning has long-term effects. The more active a person is in the present, the more likely that he or she will remain active in the future.

Every person has a responsibility to do his or her best to be active. Disease, injury, pain, and aging affect a person's ability to do daily activities. Even with such limits, you can promote activity, exercise, and well-being. You can:

- Encourage the person to be as active as possible.
- Resist the urge to do things for the person that he or she can safely do alone or with some assistance.
- Focus on the person's abilities.
- Tell the person when you notice he or she is doing well or making progress.
- Tell the person you are proud of what he or she did or tried to do.

Rights and Respect

Make sure the person's garments provide needed privacy during exercise and activity. When ambulating, the person must not walk in the room or hallway with a gown open in the back. During range-of-motion exercises, cover the person with a bath blanket. Expose only the body part being exercised. Protect the person's right to privacy. Privacy promotes dignity and mental comfort.

Independence and Social Interaction

The Omnibus Budget Reconciliation Act of 1987 requires activity programs for nursing center residents. The programs are important for physical and mental well-being. Joints and muscles are exercised. Circulation is stimulated. Social interaction is mentally stimulating.

Activities must meet the interests and physical, mental, and social needs of each resident. Bingo, movies, dances, exercise groups, shopping and museum trips, concerts, and guest speakers are often arranged. Some centers have gardening activities. Residents may share ideas with you or tell you about favorite pastimes. Or you may have ideas. Share these with the health team. They are given to the resident group that plans activities.

Encourage residents to be involved in activities. Listen to the person's interests. Suggest options that the person may like. Allow personal choice in selecting activities. Independence and well-being are promoted when the person attends activities that he or she chooses. Do not force the person to take part in activities that do not interest him or her.

Delegation and Teamwork

You must know the person's activity limits. The person's care plan and your assignment sheet tell you the activities allowed. Always ask the nurse what bedrest means for each person. Ask the nurse if you have questions about a person's activity limits. Take pride in providing safe care by knowing and following the person's activity level.

Continued

FOCUS ON PRIDE—cont'd

Ethics and Laws

Persons with contractures must be moved slowly and carefully. Pain and injury can occur if the person is moved carelessly. The following case shows the result of a nursing assistant's disregard for safe care.

A licensed nursing assistant (LNA) cared for a person with Alzheimer's disease. The resident was severely contracted. Her ability to communicate was poor. And she could not make decisions. The LNA admitted to:

- Being observed pulling the resident's arms away from her body and allowing them to snap back
- Being observed pulling the resident's legs upward from the bed and allowing them to fall back down
- Failing to remove a bowel movement while cleaning the resident

The Board found that the LNA abused and improperly cared for the resident. The unprofessional conduct violated the Administrative Rules of the Board of Nursing because of:

- Abusing or improperly caring for a patient
- Performing unsafe or unacceptable patient care
- Failing to conform to acceptable standards of practice
- Engaging in conduct likely to harm the public

The LNA's license was suspended indefinitely. (State of Vermont Board of Nursing in regard to A. Willard, 2000.) Suspend indefinitely means that the LNA:

- Had to give her license to the Board.
- Could ask the Board to re-instate her license but had to prove that:
  - She posed no danger to the public or practice of nursing.
  - She would safely and competently perform an LNA's duties.
  - She meets the requirements for license renewal and re-instatement.

You can lose your ability to work as a nursing assistant for handling persons in ways that can cause harm. Always work carefully. Move patients and residents in a way that shows you care for their comfort, safety, and well-being.

REVIEW QUESTIONS

Circle the BEST answer.

1. The purpose of bedrest is to
   a. Prevent orthostatic hypotension
   b. Reduce pain and promote healing
   c. Prevent pressure ulcers, constipation, and blood clots
   d. Cause contractures and muscle atrophy
2. Which helps prevent plantar flexion?
   a. Bed-boards
   b. A foot-board
   c. A trochanter roll
   d. Hand rolls
3. Which prevents the hip from turning outward?
   a. A cane
   b. A foot-board
   c. A trochanter roll
   d. A leg brace
4. A contracture is
   a. The loss of muscle strength from inactivity
   b. The lack of joint mobility from shortening of a muscle
   c. A decrease in the size of a muscle
   d. A blood clot in the muscle
5. A trapeze is used to
   a. Prevent footdrop
   b. Prevent contractures
   c. Strengthen arm muscles
   d. Strengthen leg muscles
6. Passive ROM exercises are performed by
   a. The person
   b. You
   c. The person with the help of another
   d. The person with the use of a trapeze
7. ROM exercises are ordered. You do the following *except*
   a. Support the part being exercised
   b. Move the joint slowly, smoothly, and gently
   c. Force the joint though its full range of motion
   d. Exercise only the joints indicated by the nurse
8. Flexion involves
   a. Bending the body part
   b. Straightening the body part
   c. Moving the body part toward the body
   d. Moving the body part away from the body
9. Turning the joint downward is called
   a. Dorsiflexion
   b. Rotation
   c. Pronation
   d. Supination
10. When ambulating a person
    a. A gait belt is used if the person is weak or unsteady
    b. The person can shuffle or slide when walking after bedrest
    c. Walking aids are needed
    d. You walk on the person's strong side
11. You are getting a person ready to crutch walk. You should do the following *except*
    a. Check the crutch tips
    b. Have the person wear non-skid shoes
    c. Get a pair of crutches from physical therapy
    d. Tighten the bolts on the crutches
12. A single-tip cane is used
    a. At waist level
    b. On the strong side
    c. On the weak side
    d. On either side

Circle T if the statement is TRUE or F if it is FALSE.

13. T F A walker and a four-point cane give the same support.
14. T F When using a cane, the feet are moved first.
15. T F When using a walker, the walker is pushed in front of the person's feet.
16. T F A person has a brace. Bony areas need protection from skin breakdown.

Answers to these questions are on p. 833.

Comfort, Rest, and Sleep

OBJECTIVES

- Define the key terms and key abbreviations listed in this chapter.
- Explain why comfort, rest, and sleep are important.
- List the OBRA room requirements for comfort, rest, and sleep.
- Describe four types of pain and the factors affecting pain.
- Explain why pain is personal.
- List the signs and symptoms of pain.
- List the nursing measures that relieve pain.
- Explain why meeting basic needs is important for rest.

- Identify when rest is needed.
- Explain how circadian rhythm affects sleep.
- Describe the stages of sleep.
- Know the sleep requirements for each age-group.
- Describe the factors that affect sleep.
- Describe the common sleep disorders.
- List the nursing measures that promote rest and sleep.
- Explain how dementia affects sleep.
- Explain how to promote PRIDE in the person, the family, and yourself.

KEY TERMS

acute pain Pain that is felt suddenly from injury, disease, trauma, or surgery

chronic pain Pain that continues for a long time (months or years) or occurs off and on; persistent pain

circadian rhythm Daily rhythm based on a 24-hour cycle; the day-night cycle or body rhythm

comfort A state of well-being; the person has no physical or emotional pain and is calm and at peace

discomfort See "pain"

distraction To change the person's center of attention

enuresis Urinary incontinence in bed at night

guided imagery Creating and focusing on an image

insomnia A chronic condition in which the person cannot sleep or stay asleep all night

NREM sleep The phase of sleep when there is *no rapid eye movement;* non-REM sleep

pain To ache, hurt, or be sore; discomfort

persistent pain See "chronic pain"

phantom pain Pain felt in a body part that is no longer there

radiating pain Pain felt at the site of tissue damage and in nearby areas

relaxation To be free from mental and physical stress

REM sleep The phase of sleep when there is *rapid eye movement*

rest To be calm, at ease, and relaxed with no anxiety or stress

sleep A state of unconsciousness, reduced voluntary muscle activity, and lowered metabolism

KEY ABBREVIATIONS

CMS	Centers for Medicare & Medicaid Services	**OBRA**	Omnibus Budget Reconciliation Act of 1987
F	Fahrenheit	**REM**	Rapid eye movement
NREM	No rapid eye movement		

Comfort, rest, and sleep are needed for well-being. The total person—the physical, emotional, social, and spiritual—is affected by comfort, rest, and sleep problems. Discomfort and pain can be physical or emotional. Whatever the cause, they affect rest and sleep. They also decrease function and quality of life.

Rest and sleep restore energy and well-being. Illness and injury increase the need for rest and sleep. The body needs more energy for healing and repair. And more energy is needed for daily functions.

See *Focus on Long-Term Care and Home Care: Comfort, Rest, and Sleep.*

COMFORT

Comfort is a state of well-being. The person has no physical or emotional pain. He or she is calm and at peace. Age, illness, and activity affect comfort. So do temperature, ventilation, noise, odors, and lighting. Such factors are controlled to meet the person's needs (Chapter 18).

See *Focus on Communication: Comfort.*

PAIN

Pain or *discomfort means to ache, hurt, or be sore.* It is unpleasant. Comfort and discomfort are subjective (Chapter 7). That is, you cannot see, hear, touch, or smell pain or discomfort. You must rely on what the person says. Report complaints to the nurse for the nursing process.

Pain is personal. It differs for each person. What *hurts* to one person may *ache* to another. What one person calls *sore*, another may call *aching*. If a person complains of pain or discomfort, the person *has* pain or discomfort. Believe the person. You cannot see, hear, feel, or smell the person's pain or discomfort.

Pain is a warning from the body. Often called the fifth vital sign (Chapter 26), it signals tissue damage. Pain often causes the person to seek health care.

See *Focus on Communication: Pain.*

Types of Pain

The doctor uses the type of pain when diagnosing. The nurse uses the type for the nursing process.
- *Acute pain is felt suddenly from injury, disease, trauma, or surgery.* It may signal a new injury or a life-threatening event. There is tissue damage. Acute pain lasts a short time. It lessens with healing.
- *Chronic pain (persistent pain) continues for a long time (months or years) or occurs off and on.* There is no longer tissue damage. Chronic pain remains long after healing. Arthritis is a common cause.
- *Radiating pain is felt at the site of tissue damage and in nearby areas.* Pain from a heart attack is often felt in the left chest, left jaw, left shoulder, and left arm. Gallbladder disease can cause pain in the right upper abdomen, the back, and the right shoulder (Fig. 28-1).
- *Phantom pain is felt in a body part that is no longer there.* A person with an amputated leg may still sense leg pain.

Factors Affecting Pain

A person may handle pain well one time and poorly the next time. Many factors affect reactions to pain.
Past Experience. We learn from past experiences. They help us know what to do or what to expect. Whether it is going to school, driving, taking a test, shopping, having a baby, or caring for children, the past prepares us for like

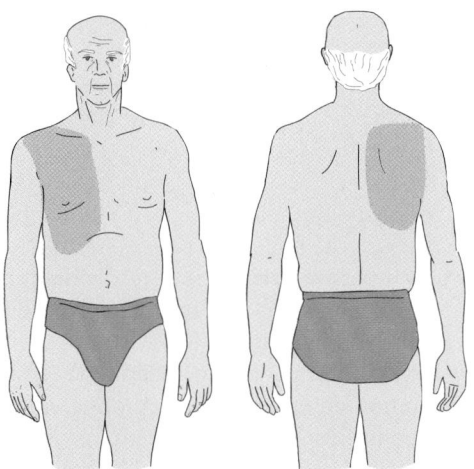

Fig. 28-1 Gallbladder pain may radiate to the right upper abdomen, the back, and the right shoulder.

events at another time. We also learn from the experiences of family and friends.

A person may have had pain before. The severity of pain, its cause, how long it lasted, and if relief occurred all affect the current response to pain. Knowing what to expect can help or hinder how the person handles pain.

Some people have not had pain. When it occurs, pain can cause fear and anxiety. They can make pain worse.

Anxiety. Anxiety relates to feelings of fear, dread, worry, and concern. The person is uneasy and tense. The person may feel troubled or threatened. Or the person may sense danger. Something is wrong but the person does not know what or why.

Pain and anxiety are related. Pain can cause anxiety. Anxiety increases how much pain is felt. Reducing anxiety helps lessen pain. For example, the nurse explains to Mr. Smith about pain after surgery. The nurse also explains that drugs are given for pain relief. Mr. Smith knows the cause of pain and what to expect. This helps lessen anxiety and therefore the amount of pain felt.

Rest and Sleep. Rest and sleep restore energy. They reduce body demands. The body repairs itself. Lack of needed rest and sleep affects thinking and coping with daily life. Sleep and rest needs increase with illness and injury. Pain seems worse when tired or restless. Also, the person tends to focus on pain when tired and unable to rest or sleep.

Attention. The more a person thinks about the pain, the worse it seems. Sometimes severe pain is all the person thinks about. Even mild pain can seem worse if the person thinks about it all the time.

Pain often seems worse at night. Activity is less, and it is quiet. There are no visitors. The music or TV is off. Others are asleep. When unable to sleep, the person has time to think about the pain.

Personal and Family Duties. Personal and family duties affect pain responses. Often pain is ignored when there are children to care for. Some people go to work with pain. Others deny pain if a serious illness is feared. The illness can interfere with a job, going to school, or caring for children, a partner, or ill parents.

The Value or Meaning of Pain. To some people, pain is a sign of weakness. It may mean a serious illness and the need for painful tests and treatments. Therefore pain is ignored or denied. Sometimes pain gives pleasure. The pain of childbirth is one example.

For some persons, pain means not having to work or assume daily routines. Pain is used to avoid certain people or things. The pain is useful. Some people like doting and pampering by others. The person values and wants such attention.

Support From Others. Dealing with pain is often easier when family and friends offer comfort and support. The pain of childbirth is easier when a loving father gives support and encouragement. A child bears pain much better when comforted by a caring parent or family member. The use of touch by a valued person is very comforting. Just being nearby also helps.

Some people do not have caring family or friends. They deal with pain alone. Being alone can increase anxiety. The person has more time to think about the pain. Facing pain alone is hard for everyone, especially children and older persons.

Culture. Culture affects pain responses. In some cultures, the person in pain is *stoic*. To be stoic means to show no reaction to joy, sorrow, pleasure, or pain. Strong verbal and nonverbal reactions to pain are seen in other cultures. See *Caring About Culture: Pain Reactions*.

Non-English-speaking persons may have problems describing pain. The agency must know who these persons are. Someone must be available to interpret the person's needs. All persons have the right to be comfortable and as pain-free as possible.

🌀 CARING ABOUT CULTURE
Pain Reactions

People of *Mexico* and the *Philippines* may appear stoic in reaction to pain. In the *Philippines*, pain is viewed as the will of God. It is believed that God will give strength to bear the pain.

In *Vietnam*, pain may be severe before pain relief measures are requested. The people of *India* accept pain quietly. They accept pain-relief measures.

In *China*, showing emotion is a weakness of character. Therefore pain is often suppressed.

From D'Avanzo CE, Geissler EM: *Pocket guide to cultural health assessment,* ed 4, St Louis, 2008, Mosby.

Children

Children know that pain feels bad. They have fewer pain experiences. They do not understand pain or know what to expect.

Children do not have many ways to deal with pain. They may restrict play, school, and sports to lessen pain. Adults can buy some pain drugs. They can go to a doctor. They know that heat or cold applications help relieve pain. They can distract attention away from the pain with music, working, reading, and hobbies. Children do not know how to relieve their own pain. They rely on adults for help.

You must be alert to behaviors and situations that signal a child's pain. Infants cry, fuss, and are restless. Such behaviors also mean hunger and needing a diaper changed. Toddlers and pre-schoolers may not have the words to express pain.

Older Persons

Some older persons have many painful health problems. Chronic pain may mask new pain. Older persons may ignore or deny new pain. They may think it relates to a known health problem. Older persons often deny or ignore pain because of what it may mean.

Thinking and reasoning are affected in some older persons. Some cannot tell you about pain. Changes in usual behavior may signal pain. Increased confusion, grimacing, restlessness, and loss of appetite are examples. A person who normally moans and groans may become quiet and withdrawn. A person who is friendly and outgoing may become agitated and aggressive. One who is nonverbal and quiet may become restless and cry easily.

You must be alert for the signs of pain. Always report changes in the person's behavior.

All persons have the right to correct pain management. The nurse does a pain assessment when behavior changes.

Illness. Some diseases decrease pain sensations. Central nervous system disorders are examples. The person may not feel pain. Or it may not feel severe. The person is at risk for undetected disease or injury. Pain occurs with tissue damage. The pain signals illness or injury. If pain is not felt, the person does not know to seek health care.

Age. See *Focus on Children and Older Persons: Factors Affecting Pain.*

Signs and Symptoms

You cannot see, hear, feel, or smell the person's pain. You must rely on what the person tells you. Promptly report any information you collect about pain. Write down what the person says. Use the person's exact words to report and record. The nurse needs this information to assess the person's pain:

- *Location.* Where is the pain? Ask the person to point to the area of pain (Fig. 28-2). Pain can radiate. Ask the person if the pain is anywhere else and to point to those areas.

- *Onset and duration.* When did the pain start? How long has it lasted?

- *Intensity.* Does the person complain of mild, moderate, or severe pain? Ask the person to rate the pain on a scale of 0 to 10, with 10 as the most severe (Fig. 28-3). Or use the Wong-Baker Faces Pain Rating Scale (Fig. 28-4). Designed for children, the scale is useful for persons of all ages. To use the scale, tell the person that each face shows how a person is feeling. Read the description for each face. Then ask the person to choose the face that best describes how he or she feels.

- *Description.* Ask the person to describe the pain. If the person cannot describe the pain, offer some of the words listed in Box 28-1.

- *Factors causing pain.* These are called *precipitating* factors. To *precipitate* means *to cause.* Such factors include moving or turning in bed, coughing or deep breathing, and exercise. Ask what the person was doing before the pain started and when it started.

- *Factors affecting pain.* Ask the person what makes the pain better. Also ask what makes it worse.

- *Vital signs.* Measure the person's pulse, respirations, and blood pressure (Chapter 26). Increases in these vital signs often occur with acute pain. Vital signs may be normal with chronic pain.

- *Other signs and symptoms.* Does the person have other symptoms—dizziness, nausea, vomiting, weakness, numbness or tingling, or others? Box 28-2 lists the signs and symptoms that often occur with pain.

See *Focus on Communication: Signs and Symptoms.*

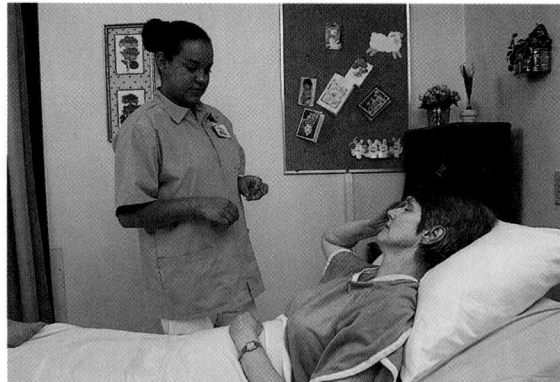

Fig. 28-2 The person points to the area of pain.

PAIN: Ask patient to rate pain on scale of 0-10										
No pain									Worst pain imaginable	
0	1	2	3	4	5	6	7	8	9	10

Fig. 28-3 Pain rating scale.

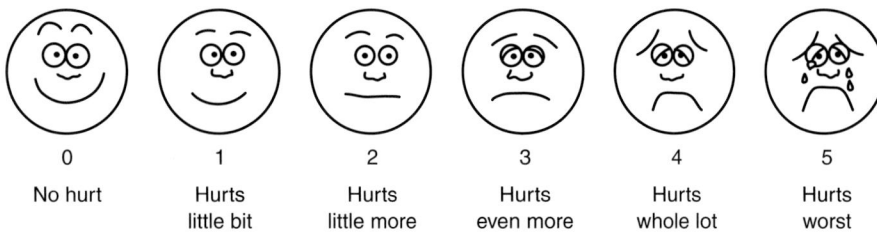

Fig. 28-4 Wong-Baker Faces Pain Rating Scale.

0	1	2	3	4	5
No hurt	Hurts little bit	Hurts little more	Hurts even more	Hurts whole lot	Hurts worst

---

BOX 28-1 **WORDS USED TO DESCRIBE PAIN**

- Aching
- Burning
- Cramping
- Crushing
- Discomfort
- Dull
- Gnawing
- Heaviness
- Hurting
- Knife-like
- Numbness
- Piercing
- Pins and needles
- Pressure
- Radiating
- Ripping
- Sharp
- Shooting
- Soreness
- Spasms
- Squeezing
- Stabbing
- Tearing
- Tenderness
- Throbbing
- Tingling
- Vise-like

FOCUS ON COMMUNICATION

Signs and Symptoms

A person may use words like "hurt" or "discomfort" instead of "pain." Children may use "owie" or "boo boo" when referring to pain. Use words that the person uses.

Some persons have trouble rating pain intensity on a 0 to 10 scale. Instead, you can ask if the pain is mild, moderate, or severe.

BOX 28-2 **SIGNS AND SYMPTOMS OF PAIN**

Body Responses
- Appetite: changes in
- Dizziness
- Nausea
- Numbness
- Skin: pale (pallor)
- Sleep: difficulty with
- Sweating (diaphoresis)
- Tingling
- Vital signs (pulse, respirations, and blood pressure): increased
- Vomiting
- Weakness
- Weight loss

Behaviors
- Clenching of the jaw
- Crying
- Frowning
- Gait: changes in; limping
- Gasping

Behaviors—cont'd
- Grimacing
- Groaning
- Grunting
- Holding the affected body part (splinting; guarding)
- Irritability
- Moaning
- Mood: changes in; depressed
- Pacing
- Positioning: maintaining one position; refusing to move; frequent position changes
- Quietness
- Resisting care
- Restlessness
- Rubbing a body part or area
- Screaming
- Speech: slow or rapid; loud or quiet
- Whimpering

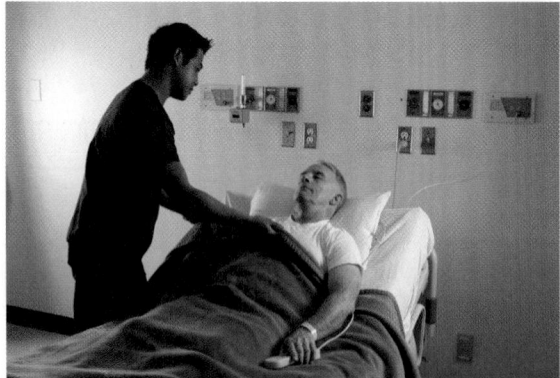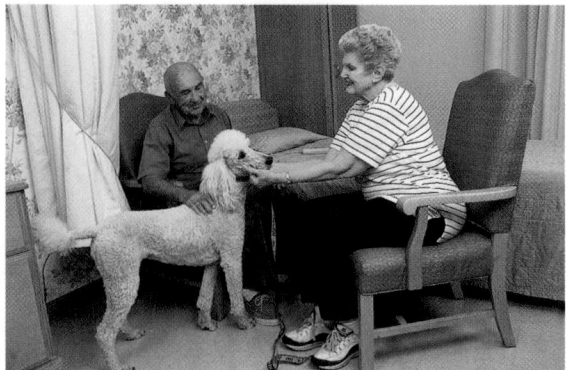

BOX 28-3 NURSING MEASURES TO PROMOTE COMFORT AND RELIEVE PAIN

- Position the person in good alignment. Use pillows for support.
- Keep bed linens tight and wrinkle-free.
- Make sure the person is not lying on tubes.
- Assist with elimination needs.
- Adjust the room temperature to meet the person's needs.
- Provide blankets for warmth and to prevent chilling.
- Use correct handling, moving, and turning procedures.
- Wait 30 minutes after pain-relief drugs are given before giving care or starting activities.
- Give a back massage.
- Provide soft music to distract the person.
- Talk softly and gently.
- Use touch to provide comfort.
- Allow family and friends at the bedside as requested by the person.
- Avoid sudden or jarring movements of the bed or chair.
- Handle the person gently.
- Practice safety measures if the person takes strong pain-relief drugs or sedatives:
  - Keep the bed in the low position.
  - Raise bed rails as directed. Follow the care plan.
  - Check on the person every 10 to 15 minutes.
  - Provide help when the person needs to get up and when he or she is up and about.
- Apply warm or cold applications as directed by the nurse (Chapter 35).
- Provide a calm, quiet, darkened setting.

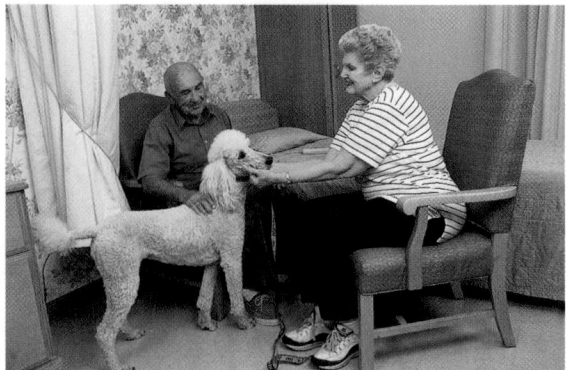
Fig. 28-6 A comforting pet can distract attention away from pain.

FOCUS ON CHILDREN AND OLDER PERSONS
Nursing Measures

Children
Pacifiers and favorite toys and blankets can comfort infants and young children. So can holding, rocking, touching, and talking or singing to them. Always check with the nurse before picking up and holding a child. Sometimes children are not held for treatment reasons.

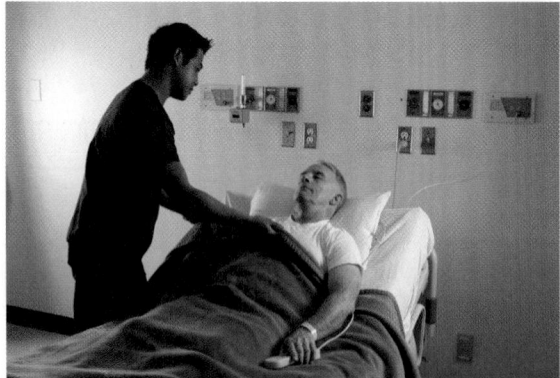
Fig. 28-5 Measures are implemented to relieve pain. The person is positioned in good alignment with pillows used for comfort. The room is darkened. Blankets provide warmth.

Nursing Measures

The nurse uses the nursing process to promote comfort and relieve pain. The care plan may include the measures in Box 28-3. See Figure 28-5.

Other measures are often needed. They include distraction, relaxation, and guided imagery. If asked to assist, the nurse tells you what to do.

Distraction means to change the person's center of attention. Attention is moved away from the pain. Music, games, singing, praying, TV, and needlework can distract attention (Fig. 28-6).

Relaxation means to be free from mental and physical stress. This state reduces pain and anxiety. The person is taught relaxation methods. The person is taught to breathe deeply and slowly and to contract and relax muscle groups. A comfortable position is important. So is a quiet room.

Guided imagery is creating and focusing on an image. The person is asked to create a pleasant scene. This is noted on the care plan so all staff use the same image with the person. A calm, soft voice is used to help the person focus on the image. Soft music, a blanket for warmth, and a darkened room may help. The person is coached to focus on the image and then to practice relaxation exercises.

Doctors often order drugs to control or relieve pain. Nurses give these drugs. Such drugs can cause orthostatic hypotension (Chapter 27). They also can cause drowsiness, dizziness, and coordination problems. Protect the person from injury, falls, and fractures. The nurse and care plan alert you to needed safety measures.

See *Focus on Children and Older Persons: Nursing Measures.*

REST

Rest means to be calm, at ease, and relaxed with no anxiety or stress. Rest may involve inactivity. Or the person does things that are calming and relaxing. Examples include reading, music, TV, needlework, and prayer. Some people garden, bake, golf, walk, or do woodworking.

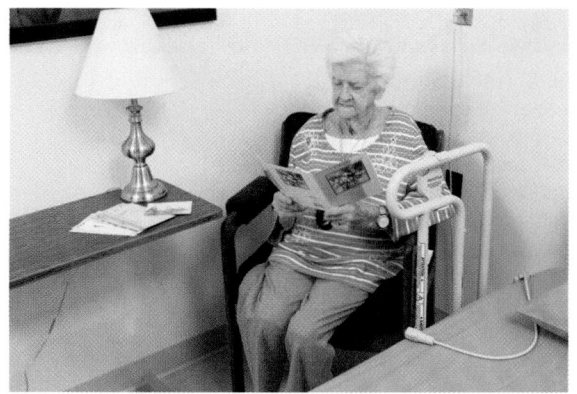

Fig. 28-7 The resident reads cards and letters from family and friends.

Promote rest by meeting physical needs. Thirst, hunger, and elimination needs can affect rest. So can pain or discomfort. A comfortable position and good alignment are important. A quiet setting promotes rest. So does a clean, dry, and wrinkle-free bed. Some people rest easier in a clean, neat, and uncluttered room.

Meet safety and security needs. The person must feel safe from falling or other injuries. The person is secure with the signal light within reach. Understanding the reasons for care also helps the person feel safe. So does knowing how care is given. That is why you always explain procedures before doing them.

Many people have rituals or routines before resting. These may include going to the bathroom, brushing teeth, and washing the face and hands. Some people pray. Some have a snack or beverage, lock doors, or make sure loved ones are safe at home. The person may want a certain blanket or afghan. Follow routines and rituals whenever possible.

Love and belonging promote rest. Visits or calls from family and friends may relax the person. The person knows that others care and are concerned. Reading cards and letters may also help the person relax and rest (Fig. 28-7).

Self-esteem needs relate to feeling good about oneself. Hospital gowns embarrass some people. Others fear exposure. Many persons rest better in their own sleepwear. Hygiene and grooming also affect self-esteem. This includes hair care and being clean and odor-free. Hygiene and grooming measures help people feel good about themselves. If esteem needs are met, the person may rest easier.

A 15- or 20-minute rest refreshes some people. Others need more time. Health care routines usually allow time for afternoon rest.

Ill or injured persons need to rest more often. Some rest during or after a procedure. For example, a bath tires a person. So does getting dressed. The person needs to rest before you make the bed. Some people need a few hours

for hygiene and grooming. Others need to rest after meals. Do not push the person beyond his or her limits. Allow rest when needed.

Distraction, relaxation, and guided imagery also promote rest. So does a back massage. Plan and organize care to allow uninterrupted rest.

The doctor may order bedrest for a person. Bedrest is presented in Chapter 27.

SLEEP

Sleep is a state of unconsciousness, reduced voluntary muscle activity, and lowered metabolism. An unconscious person is not aware of his or her setting. He or she cannot respond to people and things. There are no voluntary arm or leg movements. *Metabolism* is the burning of food to produce energy for the body. Less energy is needed during sleep. Thus metabolism is reduced during sleep. The sleep state is temporary. People wake up from sleep.

Sleep is a basic need. It lets the mind and body rest. The body saves energy. Body functions slow. Vital signs are lower than when awake. Tissue healing and repair occur. Sleep lowers stress, tension, and anxiety. It refreshes and renews the person. The person regains energy and mental alertness. The person thinks and functions better after sleep.

Circadian Rhythm

Sleep is part of circadian rhythm. (*Circa* means *about*. *Dies* means *day.*) *Circadian rhythm is a daily rhythm based on a 24-hour cycle.* It is called the *day-night cycle* or *body rhythm*. It affects functioning. Some people function better in the morning. They are more alert and active. They think and react better. Others do better in the evening.

Circadian rhythm includes a sleep-wake cycle. The person's *biological clock* signals when to sleep and when to wake up. You sleep and wake up at certain times. You may awaken before the alarm clock goes off. That is part of your biological clock. Health care often interferes with a person's circadian rhythm and the sleep-wake cycle. Sleep problems easily occur.

Many people work evening and night shifts. Their bodies must adjust to changes in the sleep-wake cycle.

Sleep Cycle

There are two phases of sleep (Box 28-4, p. 516). *NREM sleep (non-REM sleep) is the phase of sleep where there is "no rapid eye movement."* NREM sleep has 4 stages. Sleep goes from light to deep as the person moves through the 4 stages.

The "rapid eye movement" phase is called REM sleep. The person is hard to arouse. Mental restoration occurs. Events and problems of the day are thought to be reviewed. The person prepares for the next day.

There are usually 4 to 6 cycles of NREM and REM sleep during 7 to 8 hours of sleep. Stage 1 of NREM is usually not repeated (Fig. 28-8, p. 516).

BOX 28-4   SLEEP CYCLE

Stage 1: NREM Sleep
- Lightest sleep level
- Lasts a few minutes
- Gradual decrease in vital signs
- Gradual lowering of metabolism
- Person feels drowsy and relaxed
- Person is easily aroused
- Daydreaming feeling after being aroused

Stage 2: NREM Sleep
- Sound sleep
- Relaxation increases
- Still easy to arouse
- Lasts 10 to 20 minutes
- Body functions continue to slow

Stage 3: NREM Sleep
- First stage of deep sleep
- Hard to arouse the person
- Person rarely moves
- Muscles relax completely
- Vital signs decrease
- Lasts 15 to 30 minutes

Stage 4: NREM Sleep
- Deepest stage of sleep
- Hard to arouse the person
- Body rests and is restored
- Vital signs much lower than when awake
- Lasts about 15 to 30 minutes
- Sleepwalking may occur
- *Enuresis (urinary incontinence in bed at night)* may occur

REM Sleep
- Vivid, full-color dreaming
- Usually starts 50 to 90 minutes after sleep has begun
- Rapid eye movements
- Blood pressure, pulse, and respirations may fluctuate (increase and decrease)
- Voluntary muscles are relaxed
- Mental restoration occurs
- Hard to arouse the person
- Lasts about 20 minutes

Modified from Potter PA, Perry AG: *Fundamentals of nursing*, ed 7, St Louis, 2009, Mosby.

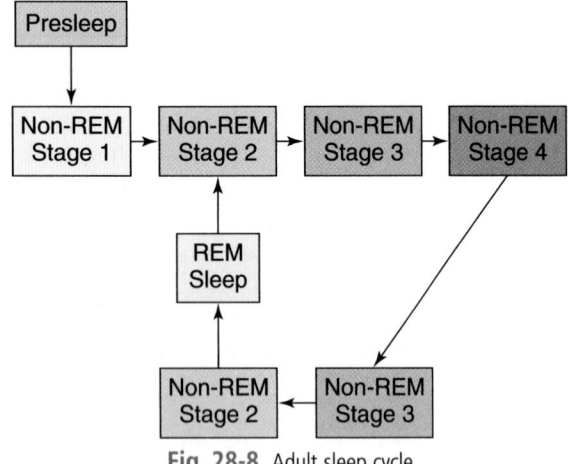

Fig. 28-8 Adult sleep cycle.

TABLE 28-1   AVERAGE SLEEP REQUIREMENTS

Age-Group	Hours per Day
Newborns (birth to 4 weeks)	14 to 18
Infants (4 weeks to 1 year)	12 to 14
Toddlers (1 to 3 years)	11 to 12
Pre-schoolers (3 to 6 years)	11 to 12
Middle and late childhood (6 to 12 years)	10 to 11
Adolescents (12 to 18 years)	8 to 9
Young adults (18 to 40 years)	7 to 8
Middle-age adults (40 to 65 years)	7
Older adults (65 years and older)	5 to 7

Sleep Requirements

Sleep needs vary for each age-group. The amount needed decreases with age (Table 28-1). Infants need more sleep than toddlers. Toddlers need more than pre-school children. School-age children need more than teenagers. Older persons often get less sleep than middle-age adults.

Factors Affecting Sleep

Many factors affect the amount and quality of sleep. Quality relates to how well the person slept. It also involves getting needed amounts of NREM and REM sleep.

- *Illness.* Illness increases the need for sleep. However, signs and symptoms of illness can interfere with sleep. They include pain, nausea, vomiting, coughing, difficulty breathing, diarrhea, frequent voiding, and itching. Treatments and therapies can also interfere with sleep. Often patients and residents are awakened for treatments or drugs. Care devices can cause uncomfortable positions. The emotional effects of illness can affect sleep. These include fear, anxiety, and worry.

- *Nutrition.* Sleep needs increase with weight gain. They decrease with weight loss. Some foods affect sleep. Those with caffeine (chocolate, coffee, tea, or colas) prevent sleep. The protein *tryptophan* tends to help sleep. It is found in protein sources—milk, cheese, red meat, fish, poultry, and peanuts.
- *Exercise.* Exercise improves health and fitness. Exercise requires energy. People usually feel good after exercising. Eventually they tire. Being tired helps them sleep well. Exercise before bedtime interferes with sleep. Exercise causes the release of substances into the bloodstream that stimulate the body. Exercise is avoided 2 hours before bedtime.
- *Environment.* People adjust to their usual sleep settings. They get used to such things as the bed, pillows, noises, lighting, and a sleeping partner. Any change in the usual setting can affect the amount and quality of sleep.
- *Drugs and other substances.* Sleeping pills promote sleep. Drugs for anxiety, depression, and pain may cause sleep. However, these drugs and sleeping pills reduce the length of REM sleep. Mental restoration occurs during REM sleep. Behavior problems and sleep deprivation can occur. Alcohol is a drug. It causes drowsiness and sleep. However, it interferes with REM sleep. Those under the influence of alcohol may awaken during sleep. Difficulty returning to sleep is common. Some drugs contain caffeine. Caffeine is a stimulant and prevents sleep. Besides drugs, caffeine is found in coffee, tea, chocolate, and colas. The side effects of some drugs cause frequent voiding and nightmares.
- *Life-style changes.* Life-style relates to a person's daily routines and way of living. Work, school, play, and social events are all part of life-style. Life-style changes can affect sleep. Travel, vacation, and social events often affect usual sleep and wake times. Children are usually up later and may sleep later during school holidays. If work hours change, so may sleep hours. Such changes affect normal sleep-wake cycles and the circadian rhythm.
- *Emotional problems.* Fear, worry, depression, and anxiety affect sleep. Causes include work, personal, or family problems. Loss of a loved one or friend is another cause. Money problems are stressful. People may have problems falling asleep, or they awaken often. Some have problems getting back to sleep.

Sleep Disorders

Sleep disorders involve repeated sleep problems. The amount and quality of sleep are affected. Sleep disorders affect life-style. See Box 28-5 for the signs and symptoms.

Insomnia. *Insomnia is a chronic condition in which the person cannot sleep or stay asleep all night.* There are three forms of insomnia:

- Cannot fall asleep
- Cannot stay asleep
- Early awakening and cannot fall back asleep

BOX 28-5	SIGNS AND SYMPTOMS OF SLEEP DISORDERS

- Agitation
- Attention: decreased
- Coordination: problems with
- Disorientation
- Eyes: red, puffy, dark circles under the eyes
- Fatigue
- Hallucinations (Chapters 45 and 46)
- Irritability
- Memory: reduced word memory; problems finding the right word
- Mood: moodiness; mood swings
- Pulse: irregular
- Reasoning and judgment: decreased
- Responses to questions, conversations, or situations: slowed
- Restlessness
- Sleepiness
- Speech: slurred
- Tremors: in the hands

TEAMWORK AND TIME MANAGEMENT
Sleepwalking

You may find a person sleepwalking. Help him or her back to bed even if you are not assigned to provide the person's care. Provide for the person's comfort. Then tell the nurse what happened and what you did.

Emotional problems are common causes of insomnia. The fear of dying during sleep is another cause. Some people are afraid of not waking up. This may occur with heart disease or when told of a terminal illness. The fear of not being able to sleep is another cause. The physical and emotional discomforts of illness can also cause insomnia.

The nurse plans measures to promote sleep. However, the emotional or physical problems causing the insomnia also are treated.

Sleep Deprivation. With sleep deprivation, the amount and quality of sleep are decreased. Sleep is interrupted. NREM and REM sleep stages are not completed. Illness, pain, and hospital care are common causes. Factors that affect sleep can also lead to sleep deprivation. The signs and symptoms in Box 28-5 may occur.

Sleepwalking. The person leaves the bed and walks about. The person is not aware of sleepwalking and has no memory of the event on awakening. Children sleepwalk more than adults. The event may last 3 to 4 minutes or longer.

Stress, fatigue, and some drugs are common causes. Protect the person from injury. Falling is a risk. Care tubings (intravenous, catheters, naso-gastric) can cause injury. They can be pulled out of the body when the person gets out of bed. Guide sleepwalkers back to bed. They startle easily. Awaken them gently.

See *Teamwork and Time Management: Sleepwalking.*

BOX 28-6   NURSING MEASURES TO PROMOTE SLEEP

- Plan care for uninterrupted rest.
- Avoid physical activity before bedtime.
- Encourage the person to avoid business or family matters before bedtime.
- Allow a flexible bedtime. Bedtime is when the person is tired, not a certain time.
- Provide a comfortable room temperature.
- Let the person take a warm bath or shower.
- Provide a bedtime snack.
- Avoid caffeine (coffee, tea, colas, chocolate).
- Avoid alcoholic beverages.
- Have the person void before going to bed.
- Make sure incontinent persons are clean and dry. Change a baby's diaper.
- Follow bedtime routines.
- Have the person wear loose-fitting sleepwear.
- Provide for warmth (blankets, socks) for those who tend to be cold.
- Reduce noise.
- Darken the room—close window coverings and the privacy curtain. Shut off or dim lights.
- Dim lights in hallways and the nursing unit.
- Make sure linens are clean, dry, and wrinkle-free.
- Position the person in good alignment and in a comfortable position.
- Support body parts as ordered.
- Give a back massage.
- Provide measures to relieve pain.
- Let the person read. Read to children. You can read to an adult if he or she prefers.
- Let the person listen to music or watch TV.
- Assist with relaxation exercises as ordered.
- Sit and talk with the person.

Promoting Sleep

The nurse assesses the person's sleep patterns. Report any of the signs and symptoms listed in Box 28-5. Measures are planned to promote sleep (Box 28-6). Follow the care plan. Also report your observations about how the person slept. This helps the nurse assess if the person has a regular sleep pattern.

Many people have bedtime rituals and routines. They are important to the person. They are allowed if safe. The person may have a bedtime snack or perform personal hygiene in a certain order. Some watch certain TV shows in bed. Others read religious writings, pray, or say a rosary before going to sleep.

The person is involved in planning care. The person chooses when to nap or go to bed. The person chooses the measures that promote comfort, rest, and sleep. Follow the care plan and the person's wishes.

See *Focus on Children and Older Persons: Promoting Sleep.*

See *Focus on Long-Term Care and Home Care: Promoting Sleep.*

FOCUS ON CHILDREN AND OLDER PERSONS
Promoting Sleep

Older Persons

Older persons have less energy than younger people. They may nap during the day. You need to let the person sleep. Plan care to allow uninterrupted naps.

Sleep problems are common in persons with Alzheimer's disease and other dementias. Night wandering is common. Restlessness and confusion often increase at night. This increases the risk of falls. It may help to quietly and calmly direct the person to his or her room. Night-time wandering in a safe and supervised setting is the best approach for some persons. The measures listed in Box 28-6 are tried. Follow the care plan.

FOCUS ON LONG-TERM CARE AND HOME CARE
Promoting Sleep

Long-Term Care

Some persons like to check on other residents before going to bed. Some have the duty of turning off lights at bedtime. These actions promote the person's dignity and mental comfort.

FOCUS ON PRIDE
The Person, Family, and Yourself

Personal and Professional Responsibility

Patients and residents have the right to have pain assessed and managed. Untreated pain decreases quality of life. You have an important role in assisting the nurse with pain control. You spend a lot of time with patients and residents. You observe them. You talk with them and listen to their needs.

You are responsible for reporting signs and symptoms of pain. Report what the person said and what you observed. The nurse uses this information to assess, plan, and evaluate pain relief.

Rights and Respect

OBRA and the CMS protect the right to quality of life. These agencies require measures that promote comfort, rest, and sleep. They relate to the bed, mattress, room temperature, noise level, lighting, linens, odors, and the number of persons in each room (Chapter 18). The right to personal choice and taking part in planning care also promote the person's comfort.

Your care of the person and his or her setting affects quality of life and well-being. You can either cause comfort and relaxation or stress, discomfort, and worry. Take pride in providing care that gives the person comfort and peace of mind.

Independence and Social Interaction

A person's comfort involves more than physical needs alone. Emotional, spiritual, and social needs must also be met. Try not to focus only on physical needs. Consider the person's thoughts, feelings, values, and beliefs.

Time spent with friends and family often provides comfort for patients and residents. For some, religious ceremonies or rituals promote peace and healing. Allow time and privacy for these needs. Small gestures show that you care. You can:

- Ask: "How are you feeling today?"
- Give the person time to pray before meals or at bedtime if this is something he or she values.
- While giving care, ask about the person's friends and family.

Emotional, spiritual, and social needs all interact and affect the person's well-being. Take pride in providing care that focuses on the person as a whole.

Delegation and Teamwork

You and other staff work as a team to promote comfort and rest. The health team coordinates care and therapies with pain-relief measures and rest periods. It is common to wait about 30 minutes after a pain-relief drug is given to perform procedures and provide care. The nurse tells you how long to wait. The person is allowed to rest after tiring activities, procedures, and therapies. Planning and communication are needed for effective teamwork and quality care.

Ethics and Laws

You may question what the person tells you about his or her pain. For example, Mrs. Watson says she has a headache. She rates the pain as 9 on the 0 to 10 pain rating scale. You observe that she is working a crossword puzzle and listening to music. When you have a headache that severe, you need to rest in a dark, quiet room. You doubt that her pain is really a 9 on the scale. You decide not to tell the nurse. Mrs. Watson's pain really was severe. She was trying to distract herself from the pain. She did not receive prompt pain relief because the pain was not reported to the nurse.

Pain is subjective, and it is handled in different ways. Ignoring a person's pain is wrong. Reporting a different pain rating is wrong. Avoid making judgments about the person's pain. Accurate reporting is needed for proper pain management.

REVIEW QUESTIONS

Circle the BEST answer.

1 These statements are about pain. Which is *false?*
   a Pain can be seen, heard, smelled, or felt.
   b Pain is a warning from the body.
   c Pain differs for each person.
   d Doctors use the type of pain to make diagnoses.

2 A person has pain in the left chest, the left jaw, and the left shoulder and arm. This is
   a Acute pain   c Radiating pain
   b Chronic pain   d Phantom pain

3 A person complains of pain. You should ask the person to do the following *except*
   a Point to where the pain is felt
   b Tell you when the pain started
   c Describe the pain
   d Let you look at the pain

4 The nurse gave a person a drug for pain relief. When should you give scheduled care?
   a Before the drug is given
   b Right after the drug is given
   c 30 minutes after the drug was given
   d The next day

5 A drug was given for pain relief. To promote safety, you should do the following *except*
   a Keep the bed in the high position
   b Raise bed rails as directed
   c Check on the person every 10 to 15 minutes
   d Provide help if the person needs to get up

6 Which measure will *not* help relieve pain?
   a Providing blankets as needed
   b Keeping lights on in the room
   c Providing soft music
   d Giving a back massage

7 A person's care plan has these measures. Which will *not* promote rest or sleep?
   a Voiding before rest or sleep
   b Positioning in a comfortable position
   c Having the person walk before rest or sleep
   d Letting the person choose sleepwear

8 A person tires easily. Morning care includes a bath, hair care, getting dressed, and making the bed. When should the person rest?
   a After you complete morning care
   b After the bath and before hair care
   c After you make the bed
   d When the person needs to

9 These statements are about sleep. Which is *false?*
   a Tissue healing and repair occur during sleep.
   b Voluntary muscle activity increases during sleep.
   c Sleep refreshes and renews the person.
   d Sleep lowers stress, tension, and anxiety.

10 A person was awake several nights. Which is *false?*
   a Circadian rhythm may be affected.
   b NREM and REM sleep are affected.
   c The person's biological clock still tells when to sleep and wake up.
   d Functioning may be affected.

11 A healthy 70-year-old person needs about
   a 12 to 14 hours of sleep per day
   b 8 to 9 hours of sleep per day
   c 7 to 8 hours of sleep per day
   d 5 to 7 hours of sleep per day

12 Which prevents sleep?
   a Chocolate   c Milk
   b Cheese   d Beef

13 These measures for sleep are in the person's care plan. Which should you question?
   a Let the person choose the bedtime.
   b Provide hot tea and a cheese sandwich at bedtime.
   c Position the person in good alignment.
   d Follow the person's bedtime rituals.

Circle T if the statement is TRUE or F if it is FALSE.

14 T F Changes in usual behavior may signal pain.

15 T F Persons with dementia usually sleep well at night.

16 T F A person's culture may affect how he or she reacts to pain.

Answers to these questions are on p. 833.

29 Admissions, Transfers, and Discharges

OBJECTIVES

- Define the key terms and key abbreviations listed in this chapter.
- Describe your role during admissions, transfers, discharges, and when moving the person to a new room.
- Explain how you can help the person and family feel comfortable in the health care setting.
- Identify the rules for measuring weight and height.
- Explain the reasons for moving a person to a new room within the agency.
- Perform the procedures described in this chapter.
- Explain how to promote PRIDE in the person, the family, and yourself.

KEY TERMS

admission Official entry of a person into a health care setting

discharge Official departure of a person from a health care setting

transfer Moving the person to another health care setting; moving the person to a new room

KEY ABBREVIATIONS

CMS	Centers for Medicare & Medicaid Services	**lb**	Pound
ID	Identification	**OBRA**	Omnibus Budget Reconciliation Act of 1987

*A*dmission *is the official entry of a person into a health care setting.* It causes anxiety and fear in patients, residents, and families. Worries and fears about serious health problems, treatments, surgeries, and pain are common.

Patients, residents, and families are in a new, strange setting. They may have concerns and fears about:
- Where to go, what to do, and what to expect
- Never returning home
- Who gives care, how care is given, and if the correct care is given
- Getting meals
- Finding the bathroom
- How to get help
- Being abused
- Strange sights and sounds
- Being apart from family and friends
- Making new friends
- Leaving homes and possessions behind

Moving to another room may cause similar concerns. So may transfer to another health care setting—hospital or nursing center. Discharge to a home setting is usually a happy time. However, the person may need home care.

Discharge and transfer are defined as follows:
- *Discharge is the official departure of a person from a health care setting.*
- *Transfer is moving the person to another health care setting.* In some agencies *it also means moving the person to a new room within the agency.*

Admission, transfer, and discharge are critical events. So is moving the person to a new room. Sometimes the new room is on another nursing unit. These events involve:
- Privacy and confidentiality
- Reporting and recording
- Understanding and communicating with the person
- Communicating with the health team
- Respect for the person and the person's property
- Being kind, courteous, and respectful

See *Focus on Long-Term Care and Home Care: Admissions, Transfers, and Discharges.*

See *Delegation Guidelines: Admissions, Transfers, and Discharges.*

See *Promoting Safety and Comfort: Admissions, Transfers, and Discharges.*

See *Teamwork and Time Management: Admissions, Transfers, and Discharges.*

FOCUS ON LONG-TERM CARE AND HOME CARE
Admissions, Transfers, and Discharges

Long-Term Care

The Omnibus Budget Reconciliation Act of 1987 (OBRA) and the Centers for Medicare & Medicaid Services (CMS) have standards for nursing center transfers and discharges. The person's rights are protected. Reasons for the transfer or discharge are part of the person's medical record. The person and family are informed in advance of the transfer or discharge plans. A procedure is followed if the person objects. An ombudsman protects the person's interests.

According to OBRA and the CMS, reasons for a transfer or discharge are:

- The measure is necessary to meet the person's welfare. The person's welfare cannot be met in the center.

- The person's health has improved to the extent that he or she no longer needs the center's services.
- The health or safety of other people in the center is in danger.
- The person has failed to pay for his or her stay in the center.
- The center closes.

The person and family are told of the date and time of the transfer or discharge. And they are given the name and location of the hospital or nursing center where the person will be going.

DELEGATION GUIDELINES
Admissions, Transfers, and Discharges

To admit, transfer, or discharge a person, you need this information from the nurse. You also need the same information when moving a person to a new room.

- If you need to admit, transfer, or discharge the person or move the person to a new room
- If moving to a new room, the person's new room and bed number
- The person's method of transportation to or from the agency—car, ambulance, or wheelchair van
- How the person will move about within the agency—walking, wheelchair, stretcher, or bed
- The person's room and bed number
- What equipment and supplies are needed
- If the person stays dressed or needs to wear a gown or sleepwear
- If the person stays in bed or can be in a chair
- When to report observations
- What patient or resident concerns to report at once

PROMOTING SAFETY AND COMFORT
Admissions, Transfers, and Discharges

Safety

The person may develop pain or become distressed during admission, transfer, discharge, or when moving to a new room. If so, call for the nurse at once. Stay with the person. When the nurse arrives, assist as needed.

Comfort

Admission, transfer, or discharge may be stressful for the person. So may moving to a new room. Some persons are happy. Others are sad and fearful. Some anxiety is normal. To provide for the person's mental comfort:

- Explain what you are doing and why.
- Do not rush the person.
- Be sensitive to the person's needs and feelings.

TEAMWORK AND TIME MANAGEMENT
Admissions, Transfers, and Discharges

Transfers and discharges are easier if a co-worker helps you. So is moving the person to a new room. When asking for help, politely tell your co-worker:

- The procedure you need help with
- When you plan to do the procedure
- What you need the person to do
- How much time it will take

Remember to thank the person for helping you.

ADMISSIONS

The admission process usually starts in the admitting office. In hospitals, it may start in the emergency room (ER). Admitting staff or a nurse obtains information for the admission record. This includes the person's:

- Full name
- Age and birth date
- Doctor's name
- Medicare or insurance number
- Religion

The person is given an identification (ID) number and ID bracelet (Chapter 12). Admitting papers and a general consent for treatment are signed by the person or legal representative.

The admitting office tells the nursing unit when there is a new patient or resident. The person's room and bed number are given. In some agencies, the person can walk to the room if able. Most persons require transport by wheelchair or stretcher.

See *Focus on Long-Term Care and Home Care: Admissions,* p. 522.

FOCUS ON LONG-TERM CARE AND HOME CARE
Admissions

Long-Term Care

Nursing centers have admission coordinators. They make the admission simple and easy. Often admission procedures are done 2 or 3 days before the person enters the center. Needed information is obtained from the person or family member.

The room assignment is made before the person arrives. Some residents arrive by ambulance or wheelchair van. The attendants take them to their rooms. Some arrive by car. Nurses or nursing assistants take them to their rooms. Often a family member is present.

A nurse or social worker explains the resident's rights to the person and family. They also get a booklet explaining them.

The person's photo is taken. Then the person may receive an ID bracelet. The photo and ID bracelet are used to identify the person (Chapter 12).

Persons with dementia and their families may need extra help during the admission process. Often confusion increases in a new setting. Fear, agitation, and wanting to leave are common. The family also is fearful. Many feel guilty about the need for nursing center care. The health team helps the person and family feel safe and welcome.

Admission is often a hard time for the person and family. They do not part until ready to do so. Remember, the center is now the person's home.

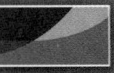 **Preparing the Room**

You prepare the room before the person arrives. Figure 29-1 shows a room ready for a new resident.

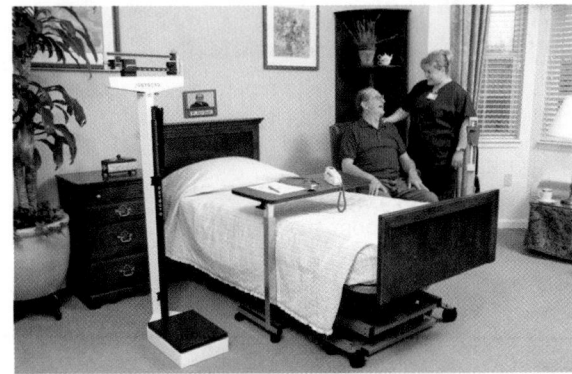

Fig. 29-1 The room is ready for a new resident.

PREPARING THE PERSON'S ROOM

PROCEDURE

1. Follow *Delegation Guidelines: Admissions, Transfers, and Discharges*, p. 521.
2. Practice hand hygiene.
3. Collect the following:
   - Admission kit—wash basin, soap, toothpaste, toothbrush, water pitcher and cup, and so on
   - Bedpan and urinal (for a man)
   - Admission form (Fig. 29-2)
   - Thermometer
   - Sphygmomanometer
   - Stethoscope
   - Gown or pajamas (if needed)
   - Towels and washcloth
   - IV (intravenous) pole (if needed)
   - Other items requested by the nurse
4. Place the following on the overbed table:
   - Thermometer
   - Sphygmomanometer
   - Stethoscope
   - Admission form
5. Place the water pitcher and cup on the bedside stand or overbed table.
6. Place the following in the bedside stand:
   a. Admission kit
   b. Bedpan and urinal
   c. Gown or pajamas
   d. Towels and washcloth
7. *If the person arrives by stretcher:*
   a. Make a surgical bed (Chapter 19).
   b. Raise the bed to its highest level.
8. *If the person is ambulatory or arrives by wheelchair:*
   a. Leave the bed closed.
   b. Lower the bed to its lowest position.
9. Attach the signal light to the bed linens.
10. Practice hand hygiene.

ADMISSION NURSING ASSESSMENT
STATUS UPON ADMISSION

Admission Notes

Date of admission ____/____/____   Time _____ a.m.
p.m.

Transported by _____

Accompanied by _____

Age _____ Sex _____ Weight _____ Height:_____ Ft. _____In.

Vitals: T _____ P _____ (❑ Reg ❑ Irreg) R _____ B/P _____/

Attending physician notified? ❑ No ❑ Yes, date/time ____/____/____ _____ a.m.
p.m.

Diagnosis: _____ Date last chest x-ray or PPD ____/____/____

Allergies

Meds _____

Food _____

_____

Other _____

Skin Condition

Using the diagrams provided, indicate all body marks such as old/recent scars (surgical and other), bruises, discolorations, abrasions, pressure ulcers, or questionable markings. Indicate size, depth (in cms), color and drainage.

PAIN

(As described by resident/representative)

Frequency:
❑ No pain
❑ Less than daily
❑ Daily, but not constant
❑ Constant

Location: _____

Intensity:
❑ No pain
❑ Mild pain
❑ Distressing pain
❑ Severe pain
❑ Horrible pain
❑ Excruciating pain

Pain on admission:
❑ No ❑ Yes, describe _____
_____

RIGHT   LEFT

COMMENTS: _____
_____
_____
_____

SPECIAL TREATMENTS & PROCEDURES:
_____
_____
_____
_____

CURRENT STATUS

General Skin Condition

Check all that apply.
❑ Reddened ❑ Pale ❑ Jaundiced
  ❑ Cyanotic ❑ Ashen
❑ Dry ❑ Moist ❑ Oily ❑ Warm ❑ Cold
❑ Edema, site _____

Physical Status (describe if applicable otherwise indicate NA)

Paralysis/paresis-site, degree _____
Contracture(s)-site, degree _____
Congenital anomalies _____
Prosthesis _____
Other _____

Functional Status

TRANSFERS-ABLE TO TRANSFER
❑ Independently
❑ 1 person assist
❑ 2 person assist
❑ Total assist

WEIGHT BEARING-ABLE TO BEAR
❑ Full weight
❑ Partial weight
❑ Non-weight bearing

AMBULATION-ABLE TO AMBULATE
❑ Independently
❑ 1 person assist
❑ 2 person assist
❑ With device
  Type _____
❑ Wheelchair only
❑ Wheelchair/propels self
❑ Bedrest

SUPPORTIVE DEVICES USED:
❑ Elastic hose   ❑ Footboard
❑ Bed cradle   ❑ Air mattress
❑ Sheepskin   ❑ Eggcrate
❑ Hand rolls ❑ Sling ❑ Trapeze
❑ Other _____

❑ Other _____
_____

Drug Therapy

	DRUG	DOSE/FREQUENCY		DRUG	DOSE/FREQUENCY
1			6		
2			7		
3			8		
4			9		
5			10		

NAME–Last	First	Middle	Attending Physician	Record No.	Room/Bed

CFS 5-3HH   © 1992 Briggs Corporation, Des Moines, IA 50306 (800) 247-2343
R1001   PRINTED IN U.S.A.

ADMISSION NURSING ASSESSMENT
❑ Continued on Reverse

Fig. 29-2 Admission form.

Continued

CURRENT STATUS - CONTINUED

Hearing	Right	Left	R & L	Vision	Right	Left	R & L	Communication
Adequate				Adequate				❏ Clear
Adequate w/aid				Adequate w/glasses				❏ Aphasic ❏ Dysphasic
Poor				Poor				Language(s) Spoken:
Deaf				Blind				_____

Oral Assessment / Eating/Nutrition

Oral Assessment

Complete oral cavity exam: ❏ Yes ❏ No
  If yes, condition _____

Own teeth: ❏ Yes ❏ No
  If yes, condition _____

Dentures: Upper ❏ Comp ❏ Part
      Lower ❏ Comp ❏ Part
Do dentures fit? ❏ Yes ❏ No

Eating/Nutrition

❏ Dependent ❏ Independent ❏ Needs assist
❏ Dysphagic; reason _____
❏ Adaptive equipment (specify) _____
_____
Type/consistency of diet _____

Food likes _____
Food dislikes _____
Bev. preference _____
HS snack preferred: ❏ Yes ❏ No

Sleep Patterns / Bathing/Oral Hyg. / General Grooming

Sleep Patterns	Bathing/Oral Hyg.	Indep.	Assist	Dep.	General Grooming	Indep.	Assist	Dep.
Usual bed time _____ a.m./p.m.	Tub				Shave			
Usual arising time _____ a.m./p.m.	Shower				Grooming			
Usual nap time _____ a.m./p.m.	Bed bath				Dressing			
Other _____	Oral hygiene				Shampoo			

Psychosocial Functioning

FAMILY RELATIONSHIPS:
  Members visit (frequency) _____
_____
  Closest relationship with _____
_____

ORIENTED: ❏ Yes ❏ No, if No,
DISORIENTED TO: ❏ Time ❏ Place
  ❏ Person
RESIDENT GIVEN EXPLANATION OF/OR INVOLVED IN PLAN OF CARE? ❏ Yes ❏ No
RESIDENT ORIENTED TO FACILITY? ❏ Call light ❏ Bathroom ❏ Mealtime ❏ Activities

WHICH WORDS BEST DESCRIBE RESIDENT? ❏ Alert ❏ Angry ❏ Fearful
  ❏ Noisy ❏ Friendly ❏ Cooperative ❏ Lethargic ❏ _____
  ❏ Non-questioning ❏ Combative
ANSWERS QUESTIONS: ❏ Readily ❏ Reluctantly ❏ Inappropriately
MOOD: ❏ Passive ❏ Depressed ❏ Elated ❏ Quiet ❏ Secure
  ❏ Questioning ❏ Talkative ❏ Homesick ❏ Wanders mentally
  ❏ Hyperactive ❏ _____
COMPREHENSION: ❏ Slow ❏ Quick ❏ Unable to understand
MOTIVATION: ❏ Good ❏ Fair ❏ Poor
PERSONAL HABITS: Smokes? ❏ Yes ❏ No Uses alcohol? ❏ Yes ❏ No

Bowel and Bladder Evaluation

Uses: ❏ Toilet ❏ Urinal ❏ Bedpan ❏ Bedside commode
BOWEL HABITS: Continent? ❏ Yes ❏ No Constipated? ❏ Yes ❏ No Laxative used? ❏ Yes ❏ No
  Enemas used? ❏ Yes ❏ No Last bowel movement _____ a.m./p.m.
BLADDER HABITS: Continent? ❏ Yes ❏ No Dribbles? ❏ Yes ❏ No Catheter? ❏ Yes, type _____ ❏ No
  Urine color _____ Consistency _____ Time last voiding _____ a.m./p.m.

Restorative Programs Indicated / Therapy Indicated

Restorative Programs Indicated

Based on the foregoing assessment, check all that apply:

❏ ROM
❏ Splint or brace assistance
❏ Bed mobility training & skill practice
❏ Transfer training & skill practice
❏ Walking training & skill practice

❏ Dressing/grooming training & skill practice
❏ Eating/swallowing training & skill practice
❏ Appliance/prosthesis training & skill practice
❏ Communication training & skill practice
❏ Scheduled tolieting
❏ Bladder retraining

Comments: _____
_____

Therapy Indicated

❏ Physical
❏ Occupational
❏ Speech
Comments: _____
_____
_____
_____
_____

Completed by:
Signature/Title _____ Date _____

NAME-Last	First	Middle	Attending Physician	Record No.	Room/Bed

ADMISSION NURSING ASSESSMENT

Fig. 29-2—cont'd Admission form.

Admitting the Person

A nurse usually greets and escorts the person and family to the room. The nurse may ask you to do so if the person has no discomfort or distress.

Admission is your first chance to make a good impression. You must:

- Greet the person by name and title. Use the admission form to find out the person's name.
- Introduce yourself by name and title to the person, family, and friends (Fig. 29-3).
- Make roommate introductions.
- Act in a professional manner.
- Treat the person with dignity and respect.
    See *Focus on Long-Term Care and Home Care: Admitting the Person.*

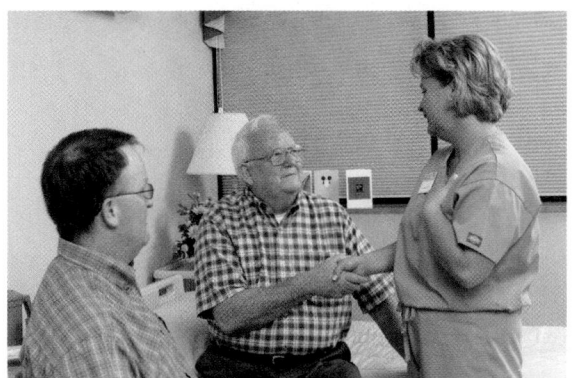

Fig. 29-3 The nursing assistant introduces herself to the person and family member.

FOCUS ON LONG-TERM CARE AND HOME CARE
Admitting the Person

Long-Term Care

Physical and mental comfort are important. So is feeling safe and secure. Do not rush the admission procedures. Rather, treat the person and family as guests in your home. Offer them a beverage. Visit with them. Tell them some of the good things about the center.

Introduce residents in nearby rooms. This way the person knows other residents. They can provide comfort and support. They understand, better than anyone else, what a nursing center is like.

The center is the person's home. Help make the room as home-like as possible. Also help the person unpack. Perhaps the person needs help putting clothes away. The person may want to hang pictures or display photos. Show caring and compassion. Help the person feel safe, comfortable, and secure.

The Admission Procedure. During the admission procedure the nurse may ask you to:

- Collect some information for the admission form.
- Measure the person's weight and height.
- Measure the person's vital signs.
- Obtain a urine specimen (if needed).
- Complete a clothing and personal belongings list.
- Orient the person to the room, the nursing unit, and the agency.

ADMITTING THE PERSON

QUALITY OF LIFE

Remember to:
- Knock before entering the person's room.
- Address the person by name.
- Introduce yourself by name and title.

- Explain the procedure to the person before beginning and during the procedure.
- Protect the person's rights during the procedure.
- Handle the person gently during the procedure.

PRE-PROCEDURE

1 Follow *Delegation Guidelines: Admissions, Transfers, and Discharges,* p. 521. See *Promoting Safety and Comfort: Admissions, Transfers, and Discharges,* p. 521.

2 Practice hand hygiene.
3 Prepare the room. See procedure: *Preparing the Person's Room,* p. 522.

PROCEDURE

4 Check the person's name on the admission form and ID bracelet.
5 Greet the person by name. Ask if he or she prefers a certain name.

6 Introduce yourself to the person and others present. Give your name and title. Explain that you assist the nurses in giving care.
7 Introduce the roommate.

Continued

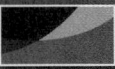

ADMITTING THE PERSON—cont'd

PROCEDURE—cont'd

8 Provide for privacy. Ask family or friends to leave the room. Tell them how much time you need, and direct them to the waiting area. Let a family member or friend stay if the person prefers.

9 Let the person stay dressed if his or her condition permits. Or help the person change into a gown or pajamas.

10 Provide for comfort. The person is in bed or in a chair as directed by the nurse.

11 Assist the nurse with assessment:
    a Measure vital signs (Chapter 26).
    b Measure weight and height.
    c Collect information for the admission form as requested by the nurse.

12 Explain ordered activity limits.

13 Orient the person and family to the area:
    a Give names of the nurses and nursing assistants.
    b Identify items in the bedside stand. Explain the purpose of each.
    c Explain how to use the overbed table.
    d Show how to use the signal light.
    e Show how to use the bed, TV, and light controls.
    f Explain how to make phone calls. Place the phone within reach.
    g Show the person the bathroom. Also show how to use the signal light in the bathroom.
    h Explain visiting hours and policies.
    i Explain where to find the nurses' station, lounge, chapel, dining room, and other areas.
    j Identify staff—housekeeping, dietary, physical therapy, and others. Also identify students who are in the agency.
    k Explain when meals and snacks are served.

14 Fill the water pitcher and cup if oral fluids are allowed.

15 Place the signal light within reach.

16 Place other controls and needed items within reach.

17 Provide a denture container if needed. Label it with the person's name and room and bed number.

18 Label the person's property and personal care items with his or her name (if not done by the family).

19 Complete a clothing and personal belongings list (Chapter 12).

20 Help the person put away clothes and personal items. Put them in the closet, drawers, and bedside stand. (The family may wish to help with this step.)

POST-PROCEDURE

21 Provide for comfort. (See the inside of the front book cover.)

22 Lower the bed to its lowest position.

23 Raise or lower bed rails. Follow the care plan.

24 Complete a safety check of the room. (See the inside of the front book cover.)

25 Practice hand hygiene.

26 Report and record your observations.

Weight and Height

Weight and height are measured on admission to the agency. Then the person is weighed daily, weekly, or monthly. This is done to measure weight gain or loss.

Standing, chair, wheelchair, bed, and lift scales are used (Fig. 29-4). Chair, wheelchair, bed, and lift scales are used for persons who cannot stand. Follow the manufacturer's instructions and agency procedures.

When measuring weight and height, follow these guidelines:

- The person only wears a gown or pajamas. Clothes add weight. No footwear is worn. Footwear adds to the weight and height measurements.
- The person voids before being weighed. A full bladder adds weight.
- A dry incontinence product is worn. A wet product adds weight.
- Weigh the person at the same time of day. Before breakfast is the best time. Food and fluids add weight.
- Use the same scale for daily, weekly, and monthly weights. Scales weigh differently.
- Balance the scale at zero (0) before weighing the person. For balance scales, move the weights to zero. A digital scale should read at zero.

See *Focus on Communication: Weight and Height.*
See *Delegation Guidelines: Weight and Height.*
See *Promoting Safety and Comfort: Weight and Height,* p. 528.
See *Teamwork and Time Management: Weight and Height,* p. 528.

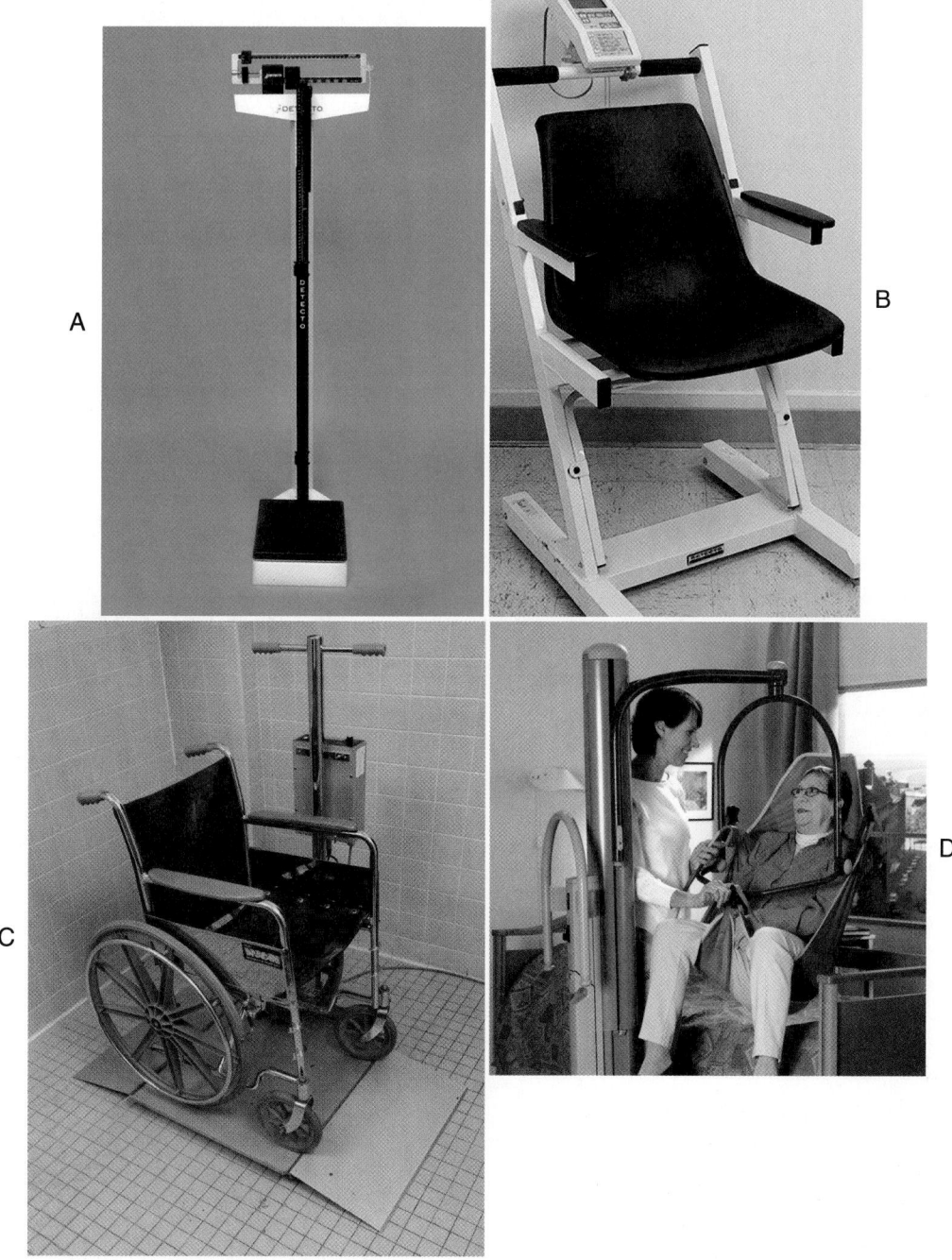

Fig. 29-4 Types of scales. **A,** Standing scale. **B,** Chair scale. **C,** Wheelchair scale. **D,** Lift scale.

FOCUS ON COMMUNICATION
Weight and Height

Accurate reporting and recording are needed for safe care. Agencies may use different scales for reporting and recording height and weight. For example, some use pounds (lb) for weight. Others use kilograms (kg). For height, some agencies use feet and inches. Others only use inches.

If you do not know what measurements to use, ask the nurse. Follow agency policy for reporting and recording height and weight.

DELEGATION GUIDELINES
Weight and Height

To measure weight and height, you need this information from the nurse and the care plan:
- When to measure weight and height
- What scale to use
- If height is measured with the person in bed
- When to report the measurements
- What patient or resident concerns to report at once

PROMOTING SAFETY AND COMFORT
Weight and Height

Safety

Follow the manufacturer's instructions when using chair, wheelchair, bed, or lift scales. Also follow the agency's procedures. Practice safety measures to prevent falls.

Comfort

The person wears only a gown or pajamas for the weight measurement. Prevent chilling and drafts (Chapter 18).

TEAMWORK AND TIME MANAGEMENT
Weight and Height

Nursing units usually have just one standing scale. In some agencies, chair, wheelchair, and lift scales are shared with other nursing units. Return the device to the storage area as quickly as possible. Do not have your co-workers wait or look for the scale.

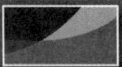 **MEASURING WEIGHT AND HEIGHT**

QUALITY OF LIFE

Remember to:
- Knock before entering the person's room.
- Address the person by name.
- Introduce yourself by name and title.

- Explain the procedure to the person before beginning and during the procedure.
- Protect the person's rights during the procedure.
- Handle the person gently during the procedure.

PRE-PROCEDURE

1 Follow *Delegation Guidelines: Weight and Height*, p. 527. See *Promoting Safety and Comfort: Weight and Height.*
2 Ask the person to void.
3 Practice hand hygiene.
4 Bring the scale and paper towels (for a standing scale) to the person's room.
5 Practice hand hygiene.
6 Identify the person. Check the ID bracelet against the assignment sheet. Also call the person by name.
7 Provide for privacy.

PROCEDURE

8 Place the paper towels on the scale platform.
9 Raise the height rod.
10 Move the weights to zero (0). The pointer is in the middle.
11 Have the person remove the robe and footwear. Assist as needed. (NOTE: For some state competency tests, shoes are worn.)
12 Help the person stand on the scale. The person stands in the center of the scale. Arms are at the sides. See Figure 29-5.
13 Move the lower and upper weights until the balance pointer is in the middle (Fig. 29-6).
14 Note the weight on your notepad or assignment sheet.
15 Ask the person to stand very straight.
16 Lower the height rod until it rests on the person's head (Fig. 29-7).
17 Read the height at the movable part of the height rod. Record the height in feet and inches to the nearest ¼ inch. See Figure 29-8.
18 Note the height on your notepad or assignment sheet.
19 Raise the height rod. Help the person step off of the scale.
20 Help the person put on a robe and non-skid footwear if he or she will be up. Or help the person back to bed.
21 Lower the height rod. Adjust the weights to zero (0) if this is your agency's policy.

POST-PROCEDURE

22 Provide for comfort. (See the inside of the front book cover.)
23 Place the signal light within reach.
24 Raise or lower bed rails. Follow the care plan.
25 Unscreen the person.
26 Complete a safety check of the room. (See the inside of the front book cover.)
27 Discard the paper towels.
28 Return the scale to its proper place.
29 Practice hand hygiene.
30 Report and record the measurements.

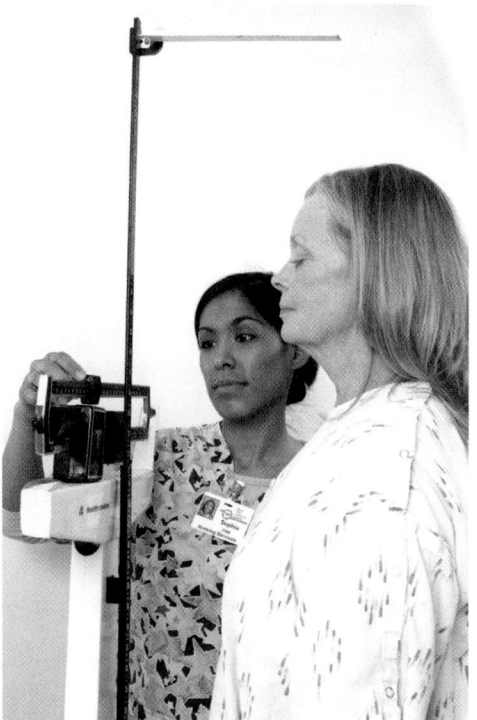

Fig. 29-5 The person is weighed.

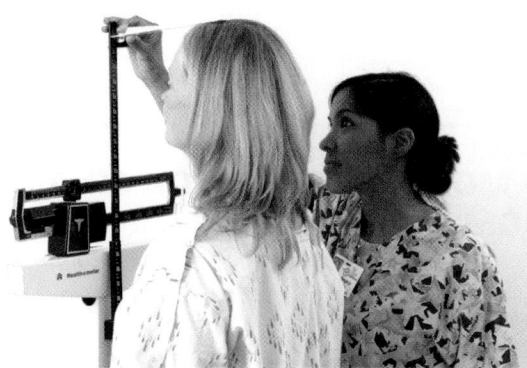

Fig. 29-7 The height rod rests on the person's head.

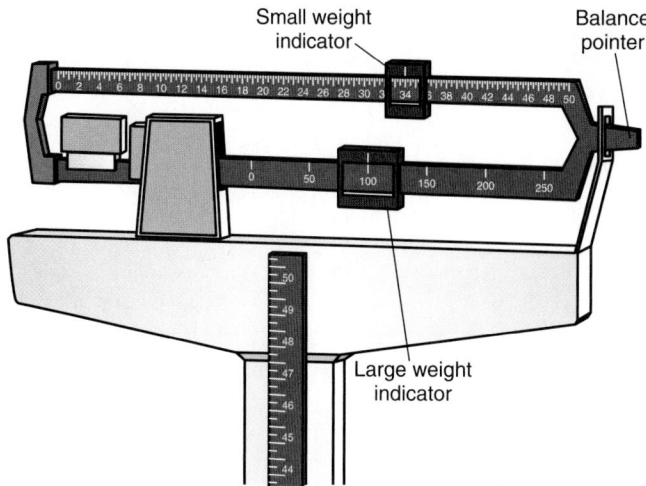

Fig. 29-6 Balance scale. The lower bar is divided into 50 lb values. The long lines on the upper bar are 1 lb values. The shorter lines are ¼, ½, and ¾ lb values. The lower and upper weights are moved until the balance pointer is in the middle. The values on the lower and upper bars are added for the weight. In this figure the lower bar is at 100 lb. The upper bar is at 34 lb. The weight is 134 lb (100 lb + 34 lb = 134 lb).

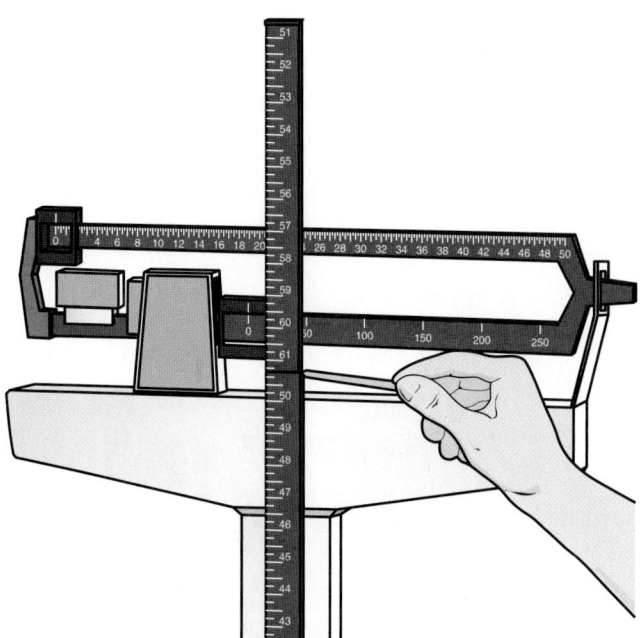

Fig. 29-8 The height is read at the movable part of the height rod. It is read at the nearest ¼ inch. This height rod measures 61 ¼ inches. (5 feet 1 ¼ inches).

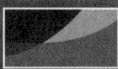 **MEASURING HEIGHT—THE PERSON IS IN BED**

QUALITY OF LIFE

Remember to:
- Knock before entering the person's room.
- Address the person by name.
- Introduce yourself by name and title.

- Explain the procedure to the person before beginning and during the procedure.
- Protect the person's rights during the procedure.
- Handle the person gently during the procedure.

PRE-PROCEDURE

1 Follow *Delegation Guidelines: Weight and Height*, p. 527. See *Promoting Safety and Comfort: Weight and Height*, p. 528.
2 Practice hand hygiene.
3 Ask a co-worker to help you.
4 Collect a measuring tape and ruler.

5 Practice hand hygiene.
6 Identify the person. Check the ID bracelet against the assignment sheet. Also call the person by name.
7 Provide for privacy.
8 Raise the bed for body mechanics. Bed rails are up if used.

PROCEDURE

9 Lower the bed rails (if up).
10 Position the person supine if the position is allowed.
11 Have your co-worker place and hold the beginning of the tape measure at the person's heel.
12 Pull the other end of tape measure along the person's body. Pull it until it extends a few inches past the person's head (Fig. 29-9).

13 Place the ruler flat across the top of the person's head. The ruler extends from the person's head to over the tape measure. Make sure the ruler is level.
14 Read the height measurement. This is the point where the lower edge of the ruler touches the tape measure.
15 Note the height measurement on your notepad or assignment sheet.

POST-PROCEDURE

16 Provide for comfort. (See the inside of the front book cover.)
17 Place the signal light within reach.
18 Lower the bed to its lowest position.
19 Raise or lower bed rails. Follow the care plan.

20 Complete a safety check of the room. (See the inside of the front book cover.)
21 Return equipment to its proper place.
22 Practice hand hygiene.
23 Report and record the height.

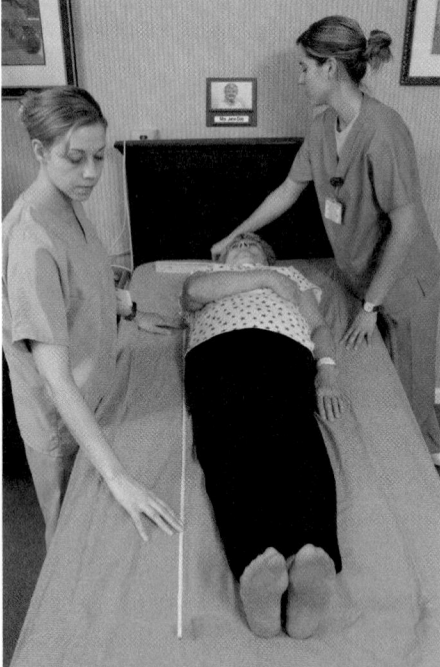

Fig. 29-9 The person's height is measured in bed. The tape measure extends from the heel to the top of the head. The ruler is flat across the top of the person's head.

MOVING THE PERSON TO A NEW ROOM

Sometimes a person is moved to a new room. Reasons include:
- A change in condition.
- The person requests a room change.
- Roommates do not get along.
- Changes in care needs.

The doctor, nurse, or social worker explains the reasons for the move. The family and business office are told. You assist with the move or perform the entire procedure. The person is transported by wheelchair, stretcher, or the bed.

Support and reassure the person. If the new room is on another nursing unit, the person does not know the staff. Use good communication skills.
- Avoid pat answers. "It will be OK" is an example.
- Use touch to provide comfort.
- Introduce the person to the staff and roommate.
- Wish the person well as you leave him or her.

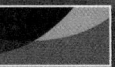 **MOVING THE PERSON TO A NEW ROOM**

QUALITY OF LIFE

Remember to:
- Knock before entering the person's room.
- Address the person by name.
- Introduce yourself by name and title.

- Explain the procedure to the person before beginning and during the procedure.
- Protect the person's rights during the procedure.
- Handle the person gently during the procedure.

PRE-PROCEDURE

1. Follow *Delegation Guidelines: Admissions, Transfers, and Discharges,* p. 521. See *Promoting Safety and Comfort: Admissions, Transfers, and Discharges,* p. 521.
2. Ask a co-worker to help you.
3. Practice hand hygiene.
4. Collect the following:
   - Wheelchair or stretcher
   - Utility cart
   - Bath blanket

5. Practice hand hygiene.
6. Identify the person. Check the ID bracelet against the assignment sheet. Call the person by name.
7. Provide for privacy.

PROCEDURE

8. Collect the person's belongings and care equipment. Place them on the cart.
9. Transfer the person to a wheelchair or stretcher (Chapter 17). Cover him or her with the bath blanket.
10. Transport the person to the new room. Your co-worker brings the cart.
11. Help transfer the person to the bed or chair. Help position the person (Chapters 16 and 17).

12. Help arrange the person's belongings and equipment.
13. Report the following to the receiving nurse:
    - How the person tolerated the transfer
    - Any observations made during the transfer
    - That the nurse will bring the medical record, care plan, Kardex, and drugs.

POST-PROCEDURE

14. Return the wheelchair or stretcher and the cart to the storage area.
15. Practice hand hygiene.
16. Report and record the following:
    - The time of the transfer
    - Who helped you with the transfer
    - Where the person was taken
    - How the person was transferred (bed, wheelchair, or stretcher)
    - How the person tolerated the transfer
    - Who received the person
    - Any other observations

17. Strip the bed and clean the unit. Practice hand hygiene and put on gloves for this step. (The housekeeping staff may do this step.)
18. Remove and discard the gloves. Practice hand hygiene.
19. Follow agency policy for dirty linen.
20. Make a closed bed.
21. Practice hand hygiene.

TRANSFERS AND DISCHARGES

When transferred or discharged, the person leaves the agency. He or she goes home or to another health care setting. Discharge is a happy time if the person is going home. Some persons need home care.

Transfers and discharges are usually planned in advance by the health team. If being discharged, they teach the person and family about diet, exercise, and drugs. They also teach them about procedures and treatments. They arrange for home care, equipment, and therapies as needed. A doctor's appointment is given.

The nurse tells you when to start the transfer or discharge procedure. The doctor must give the order before the person can leave. The nurse tells you when the person is ready to leave. Usually a wheelchair is used. If leaving by ambulance, a stretcher is used.

Use good communication skills when assisting with a transfer or discharge. Wish the person and family well as they leave the agency.

A person may want to leave the agency without the doctor's permission. Tell the nurse at once. The nurse or social worker handles the matter.

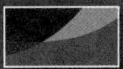

TRANSFERRING OR DISCHARGING THE PERSON

QUALITY OF LIFE

Remember to:
- Knock before entering the person's room.
- Address the person by name.
- Introduce yourself by name and title.

- Explain the procedure to the person before beginning and during the procedure.
- Protect the person's rights during the procedure.
- Handle the person gently during the procedure.

PRE-PROCEDURE

1 Follow *Delegation Guidelines: Admissions, Transfers, and Discharges*, p. 521. See *Promoting Safety and Comfort: Admissions, Transfers, and Discharges*, p. 521.
2 Ask a co-worker to help you.

3 Practice hand hygiene.
4 Identify the person. Check the ID bracelet against the assignment sheet. Also call the person by name.
5 Provide for privacy.

PROCEDURE

6 Help the person dress as needed.
7 Help the person pack. Check all drawers and closets. Make sure all items are collected.
8 Check off the clothing list and personal belongings list. Give the lists to the nurse.
9 Tell the nurse that the person is ready for the final visit. The nurse:
  a Gives prescriptions written by the doctor.
  b Provides discharge instructions.
  c Gets valuables from the safe.
  d Has the person sign the clothing and personal belongings lists.

10 *If the person will leave by wheelchair:*
  a Get a wheelchair and a utility cart for the person's items. Ask a co-worker to help you.
  b Help the person into the wheelchair.
  c Take the person to the exit area.
  d Lock the wheelchair wheels.
  e Help the person out of the wheelchair and into the car (Fig. 29-10).
  f Help put the person's items into the car.
11 *If the person will leave by ambulance:*
  a Raise the bed rails.
  b Place the signal light within reach.
  c Wait for the ambulance attendants.
  d Raise the bed to its highest level when the ambulance attendants arrive.

POST-PROCEDURE

12 Return the wheelchair and cart to the storage area.
13 Practice hand hygiene.
14 Report and record the following:
- The time of the discharge
- Who helped you with the procedure
- How the person was transported
- Who was with the person
- The person's destination
- Any other observations

15 Strip the bed and clean the unit. Practice hand hygiene and put on gloves for this step. (The housekeeping staff may do this step.)
16 Remove and discard the gloves. Practice hand hygiene.
17 Follow agency policy for dirty linen.
18 Make a closed bed.
19 Practice hand hygiene.

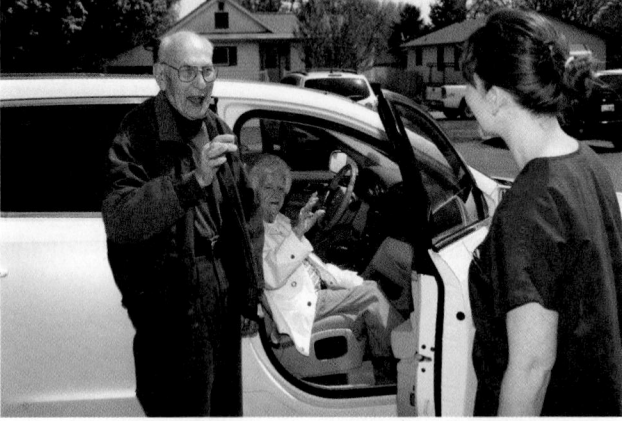

Fig. 29-10 This resident is being discharged to home with her husband.

FOCUS ON PRIDE

The Person, Family, and Yourself

Personal and Professional Responsibility

Admission to a hospital or nursing center is usually a hard time for the person and family. Transfers and discharges also can cause fear and worry. Discharge often is a happy and pleasant event. However, it may cause worry and concern if more care and treatment are needed. To help the person adjust:
- Be courteous, caring, efficient, and competent.
- Be sensitive to fears and concerns.
- Handle the person's property and valuables carefully and with respect. Protect them from loss or damage.
- Focus on the person and family. Do not seem rushed. Do not discuss other work you need to do.
- Treat the person and family like you want your loved ones treated.

Rights and Respect

Visitor policies provide rules for who can visit the person and when. Policies vary by agency or unit. For example, psychiatric, intensive care, and pediatric units often have special rules.

The person has the right to decide who is allowed to visit. Staff must respect the person's wishes. Tell the nurse about the person's requests.

Know your agency's rules for visitors. Do not assume that all units or agencies have the same rules. Give the person and visitors the correct information. If you do not know, ask the nurse.

Independence and Social Interaction

A new setting brings social challenges. A person admitted to a private hospital room may become lonely. A person with a roommate may not like sharing the room. The roommate may talk loudly, disturb the person's sleep, or invade the person's privacy by asking questions. Others like having a roommate. The person enjoys the company. Talking with the roommate helps pass the time. In a nursing center, the first hours and days can be lonely. The person can feel isolated and depressed.

You can help with these social challenges. In a nursing center, visit new residents often. Introduce them to other residents. Encourage them to take part in activities. In a hospital, observe for social isolation or roommate troubles. Tell the nurse what you observe. Always be kind and caring. Make sure your interactions are pleasant.

Delegation and Teamwork

The person's family often wants to be present during admissions, transfers, and discharges. They care about the person. They want to be sure the staff are caring, competent, and safe. The family may have questions. Or they may need to answer questions. If the person consents, the family may be present.

Some parts of admission, transfer, or discharge are best done privately. For example, the nurse may need to ask about personal or embarrassing topics. Or the person needs to undress. The nurse may ask you to manage and assist the family. The family is important. Treat them well. To show care and concern for the family at this time, you can:

- Take them to the waiting area.
- Offer them coffee or water while they wait.
- Show them where they can get food and drinks.
- Tell them where they can use a phone. Give them any special instructions for using the phone.
- Ask if there is anything they need.

Ethics and Laws

Before discharge, the person receives discharge instructions. The doctor tells the nurse what information the person needs. Common information includes drugs to continue or stop, new prescriptions, activity, diet, appointments with the doctor, and special care instructions. The nurse explains the information, provides teaching, and answers the person's questions. The information is given orally and in writing.

You may become very familiar with common discharge instructions. You may be tempted to give the person the information. The nurse has special training which allows him or her to give the information and answer the person's questions. Giving discharge teaching is beyond the scope of your role. You may provide wrong information. The person can be harmed.

If a person asks you about discharge instructions, you can say: "The nurse will give you information and answer your questions before you leave." Take pride in following the limits of your role.

REVIEW QUESTIONS

Circle T if the answer is TRUE or F if it is FALSE.

1   T   F   Identifying information is obtained when the person arrives in the room.

2   T   F   You are admitting a new resident. You must introduce yourself by name and title.

3   T   F   A person arrives at the center by ambulance. You transport the person to his or her room.

4   T   F   The person is greeted by name and title during the admission procedure.

5   T   F   Vital signs are measured during the admission procedure.

6   T   F   You explain the resident's rights to the person and family.

7   T   F   A person complains of pain. Report the complaint after completing the admission form.

8   T   F   The person arrives by stretcher. You make an occupied bed.

9   T   F   You help orient the person to the new setting.

10   T   F   A robe and footwear are worn when measuring weight.

11   T   F   A robe and footwear are worn when measuring height.

12   T   F   Clothing and personal belongings lists are made during the admission procedure.

13   T   F   A person's condition may require a transfer to another nursing unit.

14   T   F   A doctor's order is required for transfer or discharge from the center.

15   T   F   You teach the person about diet and drugs.

16   T   F   Starting with admission, the person's rights are protected.

17   T   F   A person with dementia may become more confused in a new setting.

18   T   F   A person objects to a transfer. An ombudsman makes sure the person's rights are protected.

Answers to these questions are on p. 833.

30 Assisting With the Physical Examination

OBJECTIVES

- Define the key terms listed in this chapter.
- Explain what to do before, during, and after an examination (exam).
- Identify the equipment used for an exam.
- Describe how to prepare and drape a person for an exam.
- Explain the rules for assisting with an exam.
- Perform the procedure described in this chapter.
- Explain how to promote PRIDE in the person, the family, and yourself.

KEY TERMS

dorsal recumbent position The supine position with the legs together; horizontal recumbent position

genupectoral position See "knee-chest position"

horizontal recumbent position See "dorsal recumbent position"

knee-chest position The person kneels and rests the body on the knees and chest; the head is turned to one side, the arms are above the head or flexed at the elbows, the back is straight, and the body is flexed about 90 degrees at the hips; genupectoral position

laryngeal mirror An instrument used to examine the mouth, teeth, and throat

lithotomy position The woman lies on her back with her hips at the edge of the exam table, her knees are flexed, her hips are externally rotated, and her feet are in stirrups

nasal speculum An instrument used to examine the inside of the nose

ophthalmoscope A lighted instrument used to examine the internal eye structures

otoscope A lighted instrument used to examine the external ear and the eardrum (tympanic membrane)

percussion hammer An instrument used to tap body parts to test reflexes; reflex hammer

tuning fork An instrument vibrated to test hearing

vaginal speculum An instrument used to open the vagina to examine it and the cervix

---

Doctors and many RNs perform physical exams. Exams are done to:
- Promote health.
- Determine fitness for work.
- Diagnose disease.

YOUR ROLE

Your role depends on agency policies and procedures. It also depends on what the examiner prefers. You may do some or all of the following:
- Collect needed linens.
- Collect equipment and supplies.
- Prepare the room for the exam.
- Provide lighting.
- Transport the person to and from the exam room.
- Measure vital signs, weight, and height.
- Position and drape the person.
- Hand equipment and supplies to the examiner.
- Label specimen containers.
- Discard used supplies.
- Clean equipment.
- Help the person dress or to a comfortable position after the exam.
- Follow agency policy for soiled linens.

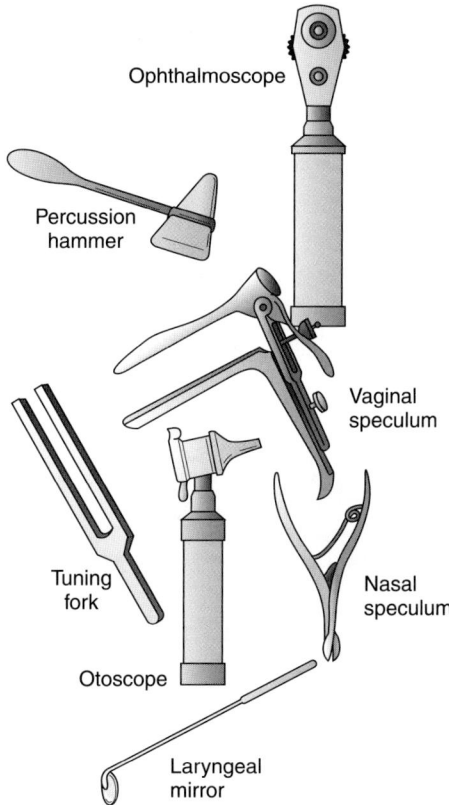

Fig. 30-1 Instruments used for a physical exam.

Labels on figure:
- Ophthalmoscope
- Percussion hammer
- Vaginal speculum
- Tuning fork
- Nasal speculum
- Otoscope
- Laryngeal mirror

EQUIPMENT

The instruments in Figure 30-1 are used in the exam:

- *Laryngeal mirror—is used to examine the mouth, teeth, and throat.*
- *Nasal speculum—is used to examine the inside of the nose.*
- *Ophthalmoscope—is a lighted instrument used to examine the internal eye structures.*
- *Otoscope—is a lighted instrument used to examine the external ear and the eardrum (tympanic membrane). Some scopes can be changed into an ophthalmoscope.*
- *Percussion hammer (reflex hammer)—is used to tap body parts to test reflexes.*
- *Tuning fork—is vibrated to test hearing.*
- *Vaginal speculum—is used to open the vagina to examine it and the cervix.*

Some agencies have exam trays in the supply department. If not, collect the items listed in the procedure: *Preparing the Person for an Examination,* p. 536. Arrange them on a tray or table.

◼ PREPARING THE PERSON

The physical exam concerns many people. They worry about the findings. Some are confused or fearful about the procedure. Discomfort, embarrassment, exposure, and not knowing the procedure cause anxiety. You must respect the person's feelings and concerns. To prepare the person physically and mentally, the nurse explains the exam's purpose and what to expect. The person must give informed consent for the exam.

You can assist the nurse by:
- Providing for privacy:
  - Screen the person and close the room door.
  - Help the person put on a patient gown. The person removes all clothes for the exam. The gown reduces the naked feeling and the fear of exposure.
  - Explain that only the part being examined is exposed.
- Having the person void to empty the bladder. This lets the examiner feel the abdominal organs. A full bladder can change the normal position and shape of organs. It also causes discomfort, especially when feeling the abdominal organs.
- Obtaining a urine specimen if one is needed. Explain how to collect the specimen (Chapter 31). Label the container.
- Measuring weight, height, and vital signs (Chapters 26 and 29). Record the measurements on the exam form.
- Draping the person. Use a paper drape, bath blanket, sheet, or drawsheet.
- Positioning the person for the exam.

See *Focus on Communication: Preparing the Person.*
See *Focus on Children and Older Persons: Preparing the Person.*
See *Delegation Guidelines: Preparing the Person,* p. 536.
See *Promoting Safety and Comfort: Preparing the Person,* p. 536.

FOCUS ON COMMUNICATION
Preparing the Person

When preparing a person for an exam, do not assume the person knows what to do. You need to tell him or her what clothing to remove, how to put on the gown (opening to the front or to the back), and where to sit. For example: "Mrs. Tucker, I need you to remove your clothes and put on this gown. The gown should open to the back. You may leave your undergarments on under the gown. Here is a blanket to cover yourself. Please have a seat on the exam table after you change. Do you have any questions?"

FOCUS ON CHILDREN AND OLDER PERSONS
Preparing the Person

Children
Babies are undressed for a physical exam. Leave diapers on baby boys to prevent urine sprays. Toddlers, pre-school children, and school-age children can wear underpants. The pants are lowered or removed as needed during the exam.

Older Persons
Nursing center residents have an exam at least once a year. The person has the right to personal choice. The doctor or nurse tells the person about the exam. Reasons for it are given. The person is told who will do the exam and when it will be done. The procedure is explained. The exam is done only with the person's consent. The person may want a different examiner. Or the person may want a family member present during the exam and when the results are explained.

DELEGATION GUIDELINES
Preparing the Person

To prepare a person for an exam, you need this information from the nurse and the care plan:
- When to prepare the person
- Where it will be done—an exam room or the person's room
- How to position the person
- What equipment and supplies are needed
- If a urine specimen is needed
- What patient or resident concerns to report at once

PROMOTING SAFETY AND COMFORT
Preparing the Person

Safety
Protect the person from falls and injury. Do not leave the person unattended.

Comfort
Warmth is a major concern during an exam. Protect the person from chilling. Have an extra bath blanket nearby. Also, take measures to prevent drafts.

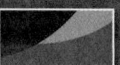 **PREPARING THE PERSON FOR AN EXAMINATION**

QUALITY OF LIFE

Remember to:
- Knock before entering the person's room.
- Address the person by name.
- Introduce yourself by name and title.
- Explain the procedure to the person before beginning and during the procedure.
- Protect the person's rights during the procedure.
- Handle the person gently during the procedure.

PRE-PROCEDURE

1. Follow *Delegation Guidelines: Preparing the Person.* See *Promoting Safety and Comfort: Preparing the Person.*
2. Practice hand hygiene.
3. Collect the following:
   - Flashlight
   - Sphygmomanometer
   - Stethoscope
   - Thermometer
   - Tongue depressors (blades)
   - Laryngeal mirror
   - Ophthalmoscope
   - Otoscope
   - Nasal speculum
   - Percussion (reflex) hammer
   - Tuning fork
   - Tape measure
   - Gloves
   - Water-soluble lubricant
   - Vaginal speculum
   - Cotton-tipped applicators
   - Specimen containers and labels
   - Disposable bag
   - Kidney basin
   - Towel
   - Bath blanket
   - Tissues
   - Drape (sheet, bath blanket, drawsheet, or paper drape)
   - Paper towels
   - Cotton balls
   - Waterproof pad
   - Eye chart (Snellen chart)
   - Slides
   - Gown
   - Alcohol wipes
   - Wastebasket
   - Container for soiled instruments
   - Marking pencils or pens
4. Practice hand hygiene.
5. Identify the person. Check the ID (identification) bracelet against the assignment sheet. Also call the person by name.
6. Provide for privacy.

PROCEDURE

7. Have the person put on the gown. Tell him or her to remove all clothes. Assist as needed.
8. Ask the person to void. Collect a urine specimen if needed. Provide for privacy.
9. Transport the person to the exam room. (This is not done for an exam in the person's room.)
10. Measure weight and height (Chapter 29). Record the measurements on the exam form.
11. Help the person onto the exam table. Provide a step stool if necessary. (Omit this step for an exam in the person's room.)
12. Raise the far bed rail (if used). Raise the bed to its highest level. (This step is not done if an exam table is used.)
13. Measure vital signs. Record them on the exam form.
14. Position the person as directed.
15. Drape the person.
16. Place a waterproof pad under the buttocks.
17. Raise the bed rail near you (if used).
18. Provide adequate lighting.
19. Put the signal light on for the examiner. Do not leave the person alone.

POSITIONING AND DRAPING

The examiner tells you how to position the person. Some positions are uncomfortable and embarrassing. Before helping the person assume and maintain the position, explain:

* Why the position is needed
* How to assume the position
* How the body is draped for warmth and privacy
* How long to expect to stay in the position

In the *dorsal recumbent position (horizontal recumbent position) the person is supine with the legs together.* The position is used to examine the abdomen, chest, and breasts. To examine the perineal area, the knees are flexed and hips externally rotated. Drape the person as in Figure 30-2, A.

In the *lithotomy position* (Fig. 30-2, B) *the woman lies on her back. Hips are at the edge of the exam table. Knees are flexed and her hips externally rotated. Feet are in stirrups.* The position is used to examine the vagina and cervix. Drape her as for perineal care (Chapter 20). Some agencies provide

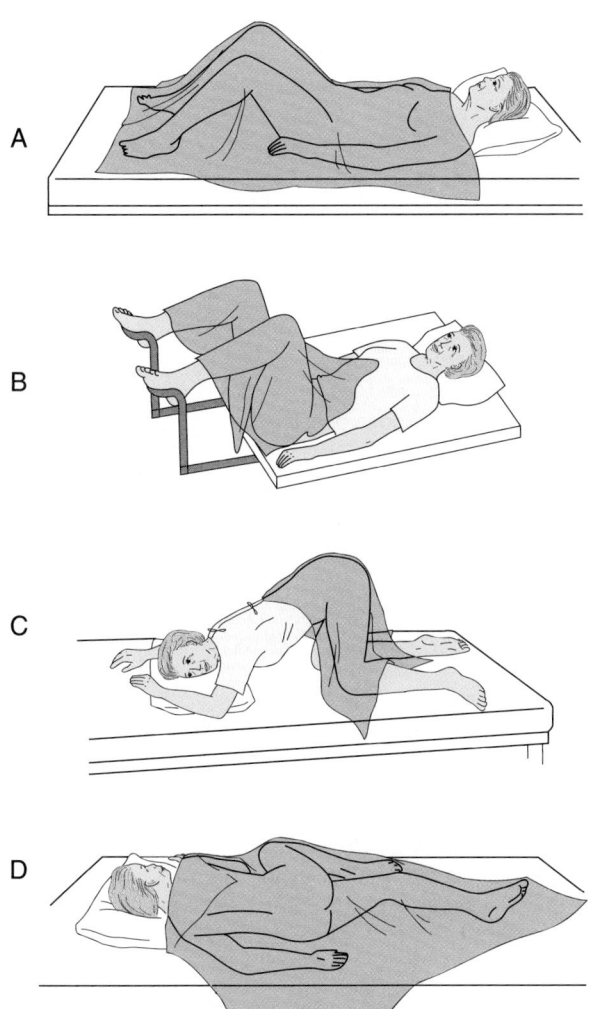

Fig. 30-2 Positioning and draping for the physical exam. **A,** Dorsal recumbent position. **B,** Lithotomy position. **C,** Knee-chest position. **D,** Sims' position.

> ### FOCUS ON CHILDREN AND OLDER PERSONS
> #### Positioning and Draping
>
> **Older Persons**
> The knee-chest position is rarely used for older persons. For them, the side-lying position is used to examine the rectum.

socks for the feet and calves. Some women cannot assume this position. If so, the examiner tells you how to position the woman.

In the *knee-chest position* (Fig. 30-2, C) *the person kneels and rests the body on the knees and chest. The head is turned to one side. The arms are above the head or flexed at the elbows. The back is straight. The body is flexed about 90 degrees at the hips.* The position is also called the *genupectoral position.* (*Genu* means *knee. Pectoral* relates to the *breast.*) The position is used to examine the rectum. Apply the drape in a diamond shape to cover the back, buttocks, and thighs.

The *Sims' position* (Fig. 30-2, D) is sometimes used to examine the rectum or vagina (Chapter 16). Apply the drape in a diamond shape. The examiner folds back the near corner to expose the rectum or vagina.

See *Focus on Children and Older Persons: Positioning and Draping.*

ASSISTING WITH THE EXAM

You may be asked to prepare, position, and drape the person. If assisting with the exam, follow the rules in Box 30-1.

See *Focus on Communication: Assisting With the Exam,* p. 538.

See *Focus on Children and Older Persons: Assisting With the Exam,* p. 538.

> ### BOX 30-1 RULES FOR ASSISTING WITH THE PHYSICAL EXAM
>
> * Practice hand hygiene before and after the exam.
> * Provide for privacy.
>   * Close doors and window coverings.
>   * Screen and drape the person.
>   * Expose only the body part being examined.
> * Position the person as directed by the examiner.
> * Place instruments and equipment near the examiner.
> * Stay in the room when a female is examined (unless you are a male). When a man examines a female, another female is in the room. This is for the legal protection of the female and the male examiner. A female attendant also adds to the woman's mental comfort. A female examiner may want a male attendant present when examining a male. This also is for their legal protection.
> * Protect the person from falling.
> * Re-assure the person throughout the exam.
> * Anticipate the examiner's need for equipment and supplies.
> * Place paper or paper towels on the floor if the person is asked to stand.
> * Follow Standard Precautions and the Bloodborne Pathogen Standard.

FOCUS ON COMMUNICATION
Assisting With the Exam

Each examiner has a routine. He or she does things in a certain order. To better assist, ask the examiner to explain the routine to you. Also ask him or her to tell you what equipment and supplies are needed. For example:

- "Dr. Weaver, I want to help in the best way that I can. Please tell me how you will start the exam and how you will proceed."
- "Ms. Carrigan, please ask for equipment and supplies as you need them. That way I can hand you the correct item."

TEAMWORK AND TIME MANAGEMENT
After the Exam

Make sure that the exam room is clean and that supplies and equipment are ready for the next exam. Otherwise you delay the patient or resident, examiner, and the staff member assisting.

You may find an exam room that is not clean. Or you may find that exam equipment and supplies are not ready. Call for the nurse before you start to prepare the room and ready supplies and equipment. The nurse needs to see the problem. The nurse can find out who last used the room or tray. The nurse can then talk to the staff members involved.

FOCUS ON CHILDREN AND OLDER PERSONS
Assisting With the Exam

Children

A parent is present when children are examined. If the child is uncooperative, the parent may need to hold him or her still during some parts of the exam. Being kept still may frighten an infant. The child may fear harm or separation from the parent. A calm, comforting manner helps the child and parent. The parent may have fears too.

The equipment used for children is like that for the adult exam. Toys are used to assess development. Vaginal speculums are not used.

Older Persons

Persons with dementia may resist the examiner's efforts. The person may be agitated and aggressive from confusion and fear. Do not restrain or force the person to have the exam. The exam is tried another time. Sometimes a family member can calm the person. The doctor may order drugs to help the person relax. The person's rights are always respected.

After the Exam

After the exam, the person dresses or returns to bed. Lubricant was used to examine the vagina or rectum. The area is wiped or cleaned before the person dresses or returns to the room. Assist as needed. You also need to:

- Discard disposable items.
- Replace supplies so the tray is ready for the next exam.
- Clean re-usable items. Follow agency policy. Return items to the tray or storage area. This includes the otoscope and ophthalmoscope tips and stethoscope.
- Send a re-usable speculum to the supply department. It needs to be sterilized.
- Cover the exam table with a clean drawsheet or paper.
- Label specimens. Take them to the designated area with a requisition slip. See Chapter 31.
- Clean and straighten the person's unit or exam room.
- Follow agency policy for soiled linens.
  See *Teamwork and Time Management: After the Exam.*

FOCUS ON PRIDE
The Person, Family, and Yourself

Personal and Professional Responsibility

Physical, mental, and social discomfort are common during the physical exam. Often only a gown is worn. Sometimes an uncomfortable position is required. Private body parts (breasts, vagina, penis, and rectum) may be examined. Anxiety and fear are common feelings.

The person needs to feel safe, secure, and protected from exposure. The person should feel comfortable with the examiner and the person assisting. Be professional and courteous at all times. Provide care in a way that promotes dignity, self-esteem, and well-being.

Rights and Respect

The person has the right to privacy. Protect the person from exposure. Only the examiner and the person assisting have the right to see the person's body. The person must consent for others to be present. This includes family. Proper draping and screening are needed. Keep the person covered. Expose only the body part being examined.

Independence and Social Interaction

Fears about the exam affect the person's well-being. These fears are common:

- Who will perform the exam? How will the exam be done?
- Why is the exam needed?
- Will an illness be found? Is it cancer?
- Will surgery be needed? Will more drugs be needed? Will I die?
  To ease the person's fears:
- Greet the person. Introduce yourself by name and title.
- Talk with the person. Be pleasant.
- Tell the person good things about the examiner or agency. For example: "Dr. Foster will examine you today. She is very kind and thorough."

Your interactions affect the person's mental comfort. Caring, kindness, and a positive attitude ease worries.

Delegation and Teamwork

When preparing for an exam, make sure needed supplies are in the room. Check that equipment works properly. If not, the examiner and person must wait while you get the supplies or new equipment. The person may be in an uncomfortable position. The delay causes more discomfort.

Know where to find supplies and equipment. If you need an item, you can get it quickly. If you do not know, ask a co-worker where to find the item. Thank your co-worker for helping you.

Ethics and Laws

Information discussed during the exam is confidential. Only staff involved in the person's care need to know the reason for the exam and its results. If the person consents, the doctor tells the family. The person can share the information with others if he or she wants to.

You must keep the person's information confidential. Talking about an exam with family, friends, or staff not involved in the person's care violates the Health Insurance Portability and Accountability Act of 1996 (HIPAA). HIPAA protects the privacy and security of the person's health information. Failure to follow HIPAA rules can result in fines, penalties, and criminal action.

REVIEW QUESTIONS

Circle the BEST answer.

1 The otoscope is used to examine
   a Internal eye structures
   b The external ear and the eardrum
   c Reflexes
   d The vagina

2 You are preparing a person for an exam. You should do the following *except*
   a Ask the person to void
   b Ask the person to undress
   c Drape the person
   d Go tell the nurse when the person is ready

3 Which part of an exam can you do?
   a Test reflexes.
   b Inspect the mouth, teeth, and throat.
   c Measure weight, height, and vital signs.
   d Observe the perineum and rectum.

4 A person is supine. The hips are flexed and externally rotated. The feet are supported in stirrups. The person is in the
   a Dorsal recumbent position
   b Lithotomy position
   c Knee-chest position
   d Sims' position

5 You will assist with Mrs. Janz's exam. Which is *false*?
   a Hand hygiene is practiced before and after the exam.
   b Instruments are placed near the examiner.
   c A male nursing team member stays in the room.
   d Privacy is provided by screening, closing the door, and proper draping.

Answers to these questions are on p. 833.

31 Collecting and Testing Specimens

OBJECTIVES

- Define the key terms and key abbreviations listed in this chapter.
- Explain why urine, stool, sputum, and blood specimens are collected.
- Explain the rules for collecting specimens.
- Describe the different types of urine specimens.
- Describe the equipment used for blood glucose testing.
- Identify the sites used for skin punctures.
- Perform the procedures described in this chapter.
- Explain how to promote PRIDE in the person, the family, and yourself.

KEY TERMS

acetone See "ketone"

glucosuria Sugar *(glucos)* in the urine *(uria);* glycosuria

glycosuria Sugar *(glycos)* in the urine *(uria);* glucosuria

hematoma A swelling *(oma)* that contains blood *(hemat)*

hematuria Blood *(hemat)* in the urine *(uria)*

hemoptysis Bloody *(hemo)* sputum *(ptysis means to spit)*

ketone A substance that appears in urine from the rapid breakdown of fat for energy; acetone, ketone body

ketone body See "ketone"

melena A black, tarry stool

sputum Mucus from the respiratory system that is expectorated *(expelled)* through the mouth

KEY ABBREVIATIONS

BM Bowel movement
ID Identification
I&O Intake and output

mL Milliliter
oz Ounce

Ordered by doctors, specimens *(samples)* are collected and tested to prevent, detect, and treat disease. Most specimens are tested in the laboratory. All specimens sent to the laboratory require requisition slips. The slip has the person's identifying information and the test ordered.

And the specimen container is labeled according to agency policy. Some tests are done at the bedside. When collecting specimens, follow the rules in Box 31-1.

See *Teamwork and Time Management: Collecting and Testing Specimens.*

BOX 31-1 RULES FOR COLLECTING SPECIMENS

- Follow the rules of medical asepsis.
- Follow Standard Precautions and the Bloodborne Pathogen Standard.
- Use a clean container for each specimen.
- Use the correct container.
- Do not touch the inside of the container or inside of the lid.
- Identify the person. Check the ID (identification) bracelet against the laboratory requisition slip or assignment sheet. Compare *all* information.
- Label the container in the person's presence. Provide clear, accurate information.
- Collect the specimen at the correct time.
- Ask a female if she is having a menstrual period. Tell the nurse. Menstruating may cause blood to be in the urine specimen.
- Ask the person not to have a bowel movement (BM) when collecting a urine specimen. The specimen must not contain stools.
- Ask the person to void before collecting a stool specimen. The specimen must not contain urine.
- Ask the person to put toilet tissue in the toilet or wastebasket. Urine and stool specimens must not contain tissue.
- Place the specimen container in a labeled *BIOHAZARD* plastic bag. Do not let the container touch the outside of the bag. Seal the bag.
- Take the specimen and requisition slip to the laboratory or storage area.

TEAMWORK AND TIME MANAGEMENT
Collecting and Testing Specimens

Nursing centers send specimens to a laboratory for study or analysis. The center has a storage area for specimens. A driver picks up specimens at a certain time and transports them to the laboratory.

Have ordered specimens collected and in the storage area by the pick-up time. If the specimen is not collected, results are delayed at least 1 day. This can cause the person harm. If the specimen was not collected in time, it may need to be discarded. If discarded, another is collected the next day. This also causes a results delay and can harm the person. Using more supplies and equipment costs more money.

URINE SPECIMENS

Urine specimens are collected for urine tests. Follow the rules in Box 31-1.

See *Delegation Guidelines: Urine Specimens.*
See *Promoting Safety and Comfort: Urine Specimens.*

DELEGATION GUIDELINES
Urine Specimens

To collect a urine specimen, you need this information from the nurse and the care plan:
- Voiding device used—bedpan, urinal, commode, or toilet with specimen pan
- The type of specimen needed
- What time to collect the specimen
- What special measures are needed
- If you need to test the specimen (p. 547)
- If measuring intake and output (I&O) is ordered (Chapter 24)
- What observations to report and record:
  - Problems obtaining the specimen
  - Color, clarity, and odor of urine
  - Blood in the urine
  - Particles in the urine
  - Complaints of pain, burning, urgency, difficulty voiding, or other problems
  - The time the specimen was collected
- When to report observations
- What patient or resident concerns to report at once

PROMOTING SAFETY AND COMFORT
Urine Specimens

Safety
Microbes can grow in urine. Urine also may contain blood. Follow Standard Precautions and the Bloodborne Pathogen Standard.

Comfort
Urine specimens may embarrass some people, including children. They do not like clear specimen containers that show urine. It may be helpful to place the specimen container in a paper bag.

The Random Urine Specimen

The random urine specimen is used for a routine urinalysis (UA). No special measures are needed. It is collected any time during a 24-hour period. Many people can collect the specimen themselves. Weak and very ill persons need help.

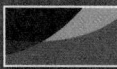 **COLLECTING A RANDOM URINE SPECIMEN**

QUALITY OF LIFE

Remember to:
- Knock before entering the person's room.
- Address the person by name.
- Introduce yourself by name and title.

- Explain the procedure to the person before beginning and during the procedure.
- Protect the person's rights during the procedure.
- Handle the person gently during the procedure.

PRE-PROCEDURE

1 Follow *Delegation Guidelines: Urine Specimens,* p. 541. See *Promoting Safety and Comfort: Urine Specimens,* p. 541.
2 Practice hand hygiene.
3 Collect the following before going to the person's room:
   - Laboratory requisition slip
   - Specimen container and lid
   - Voiding device—bedpan and cover, urinal, commode, or specimen pan (Fig. 31-1)
   - Specimen label
   - Plastic bag
   - *BIOHAZARD* label (if needed)
   - Gloves

4 Arrange collected items in the person's bathroom.
5 Practice hand hygiene.
6 Identify the person. Check the ID bracelet against the requisition slip. Also call the person by name.
7 Label the container in the person's presence.
8 Put on gloves.
9 Collect a graduate to measure output
10 Provide for privacy.

PROCEDURE

11 Ask the person to void into the device. Remind him or her to put toilet tissue into the wastebasket or toilet. Toilet tissue is not put in the bedpan or specimen pan.
12 Take the voiding device to the bathroom.
13 Pour about 120 mL (milliliters) (4 oz [ounces]) into the specimen container.
14 Place the lid on the specimen container. Put the container in the plastic bag. Do not let the container touch the outside of the bag. Apply a *BIOHAZARD* label.

15 Measure urine if I&O are ordered. Include the specimen amount.
16 Empty, rinse, clean, disinfect, and dry equipment. Return equipment to its proper place.
17 Remove and discard the gloves. Practice hand hygiene. Put on clean gloves.
18 Assist with hand washing.
19 Remove and discard the gloves. Practice hand hygiene.

POST-PROCEDURE

20 Provide for comfort. (See the inside of the front book cover.)
21 Place the signal light within reach.
22 Raise or lower bed rails. Follow the care plan.
23 Unscreen the person.
24 Complete a safety check of the room. (See the inside of the front book cover.)

25 Practice hand hygiene.
26 Take the specimen and requisition slip to the storage area. Wear gloves.
27 Remove and discard the gloves. Practice hand hygiene.
28 Report and record your observations.

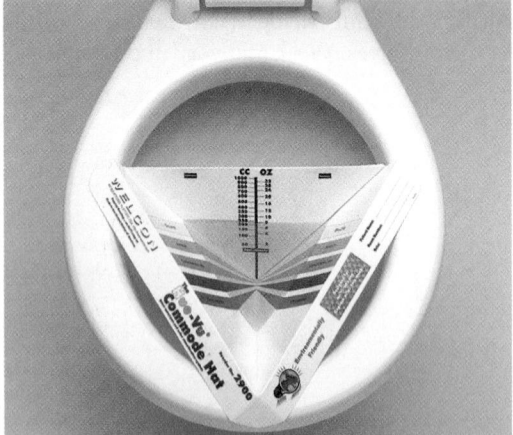

Fig. 31-1 The specimen pan is placed at the front of the toilet on the toilet rim. This pan has a color chart for urine.

The Midstream Specimen

The midstream specimen is also called a *clean-voided specimen* or *clean-catch specimen.* The perineal area is cleaned before collecting the specimen. This reduces the number of microbes in the urethral area. The person starts to void into a device. Then the person stops the urine stream, and a sterile specimen container is positioned. The person voids into the container until the specimen is obtained.

Stopping the urine stream is hard for many people. You may need to position and hold the specimen container in place after the person starts to void (Fig. 31-2).

See *Focus on Communication: The Midstream Specimen.*

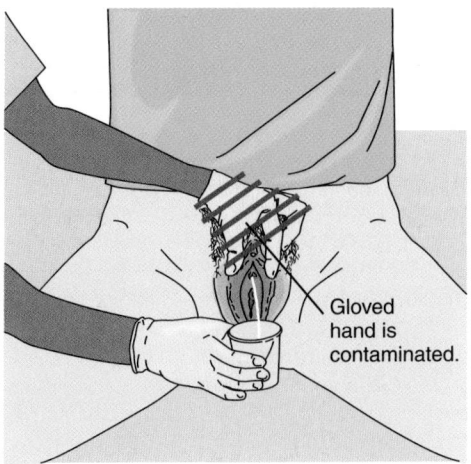

Gloved hand is contaminated.

Fig. 31-2 The labia are separated to collect a midstream specimen.

FOCUS ON COMMUNICATION
The Midstream Specimen

Some persons can collect the midstream specimen on their own. You may need to explain the procedure. Use words the person understands. Show what supplies to use. Also, ask if the person has any questions. For example:

"Ms. Jacobs, I need to collect a midstream urine specimen from you. This means I need urine from the middle of your urine stream. First, wipe well with this towelette (show the towelette). Wipe from front to back. The specimen goes in this cup (show the specimen cup). Please do not touch the inside of the cup. Start your urine stream and then stop. Position the cup to catch urine and begin your stream again. If you cannot stop your stream, just position the cup during the middle of the stream. I need at least this much urine in the cup if possible (point to the 30 mL measure on the cup). Remove the cup when it is about that full. Finish urinating. Secure the lid on top of the cup. Please do not touch the inside of the lid. I will take the specimen when you are done. Do you have any questions?"

COLLECTING A MIDSTREAM SPECIMEN

QUALITY OF LIFE

Remember to:
- Knock before entering the person's room.
- Address the person by name.
- Introduce yourself by name and title.

- Explain the procedure to the person before beginning and during the procedure.
- Protect the person's rights during the procedure.
- Handle the person gently during the procedure.

PRE-PROCEDURE

1 Follow *Delegation Guidelines: Urine Specimens*, p. 541. See *Promoting Safety and Comfort: Urine Specimens*, p. 541.
2 Practice hand hygiene.
3 Collect the following before going to the person's room:
   - Laboratory requisition slip
   - Midstream specimen kit—specimen container, label, towelettes, sterile gloves
   - Plastic bag
   - Sterile gloves (if not part of the kit)
   - Disposable gloves
   - *BIOHAZARD* label (if needed)

4 Arrange your work area.
5 Practice hand hygiene.
6 Identify the person. Check the ID bracelet against the requisition slip. Also call the person by name.
7 Put on disposable gloves.
8 Collect the following:
   - Voiding device—bedpan and cover, urinal, commode, or specimen pan if needed
   - Supplies for perineal care
   - Graduate to measure output
   - Paper towel
9 Provide for privacy.

PROCEDURE

10 Provide perineal care (Chapter 20). (Wear gloves for this step. Practice hand hygiene after removing and discarding them.)
11 Open the sterile kit.
12 Put on the sterile gloves.
13 Open the packet of towelettes.
14 Open the sterile specimen container. Do not touch the inside of the container or lid. Set the lid down so the inside is up.

15 *For a female*—clean the perineal area with towelettes.
   a Spread the labia with your thumb and index finger. Use your non-dominant hand. (This hand is now contaminated. It must not touch anything sterile.)
   b Clean down the urethral area from front to back. Use a clean towelette for each stroke.
   c Keep the labia separated to collect the urine specimen (steps 17 through 20).

Continued

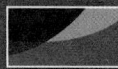

COLLECTING A MIDSTREAM SPECIMEN—cont'd

VIDEO

PROCEDURE—cont'd

16 *For a male*—clean the penis with towelettes.
- a Hold the penis with your non-dominant hand. (This hand is now contaminated. It must not touch anything sterile.)
- b Clean the penis starting at the meatus. (Retract the foreskin if the male is uncircumcised.) Clean in a circular motion. Start at the center and work outward.
- c Keep holding the penis (and the foreskin retracted in the uncircumcised male) until the specimen is collected (steps 17 through 20).

17 Ask the person to void into a device.
18 Pass the specimen container into the urine stream. Keep the labia separated (see Fig. 31-2).
19 Collect about 30 to 60 mL (1 to 2 oz) of urine.
20 Remove the specimen container before the person stops voiding. Release the foreskin of the uncircumcised male.
21 Release the labia or penis. Let the person finish voiding into the device.
22 Put the lid on the specimen container. Touch only the outside of the container and lid. Wipe the outside of the container. Set the container on a paper towel.
23 Provide toilet tissue when the person is done voiding.
24 Take the voiding device to the bathroom.
25 Measure urine if I&O are ordered. Include the specimen amount.
26 Empty, rinse, clean, disinfect, and dry equipment. Return equipment to its proper place.
27 Remove and discard the gloves. Practice hand hygiene. Put on clean disposable gloves.
28 Label the specimen container in the person's presence. Place the container in the plastic bag. Do not let the container touch the outside of the bag. Apply a *BIOHAZARD* label.
29 Assist with hand washing.
30 Remove and discard the gloves. Practice hand hygiene.

POST-PROCEDURE

31 Provide for comfort. (See the inside of the front book cover.)
32 Place the signal light within reach.
33 Raise or lower bed rails. Follow the care plan.
34 Unscreen the person.
35 Complete a safety check of the room. (See the inside of the front book cover.)
36 Practice hand hygiene.
37 Take the specimen and requisition slip to the laboratory or storage area. Wear gloves.
38 Remove and discard the gloves. Practice hand hygiene.
39 Report and record your observations.

The 24-Hour Urine Specimen

All urine voided during a 24-hour period is collected for a 24-hour urine specimen. Urine is chilled on ice or refrigerated during this time. This prevents the growth of microbes. For some tests, a preservative is added to the collection container.

The person voids to begin the test with an empty bladder. Discard this voiding. Save *all voidings* for the next 24 hours. The person and nursing staff must clearly understand the procedure and the test period. The test is restarted if:
- A voiding was not saved.
- Toilet tissue was discarded into the specimen.
- The specimen contains stools.

See *Promoting Safety and Comfort: The 24-Hour Urine Specimen.*

PROMOTING SAFETY AND COMFORT
The 24-Hour Urine Specimen

Safety

The urine container or preservative may contain an acid. Do not get the preservative or urine from the container on your skin or in your eyes. If you do, flush your skin or eyes with a large amount of water. Tell the nurse what happened and check the material safety data sheet (MSDS) (Chapter 12). Also complete an incident report.

Keep the specimen chilled to prevent the growth of microbes. If not refrigerated, place the urine container in a bucket with ice. Add ice to the bucket as needed.

Assist the person with hand washing after every voiding. This prevents the spread of microbes that may be in the urine.

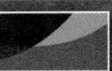 **COLLECTING A 24-HOUR URINE SPECIMEN**

QUALITY OF LIFE

Remember to:
- Knock before entering the person's room.
- Address the person by name.
- Introduce yourself by name and title.

- Explain the procedure to the person before beginning and during the procedure.
- Protect the person's rights during the procedure.
- Handle the person gently during the procedure.

PRE-PROCEDURE

1 Follow *Delegation Guidelines: Urine Specimens*, p. 541. See *Promoting Safety and Comfort:*
  a *Urine Specimens*, p. 541
  b *The 24-Hour Urine Specimen*
2 Practice hand hygiene.
3 Collect the following before going to the person's room:
  - Laboratory requisition slip
  - Urine container for a 24-hour collection
  - Specimen label
  - Preservative if needed
  - Bucket with ice if needed
  - Two 24-HOUR URINE labels
  - Funnel
  - *BIOHAZARD* label
  - Gloves

4 Arrange collected items in the person's bathroom.
5 Place one 24-HOUR URINE label in the bathroom. Place the other near the bed.
6 Practice hand hygiene.
7 Identify the person. Check the ID bracelet against the requisition slip. Also call the person by name.
8 Label the urine container in the person's presence. Apply the *BIOHAZARD* label. Place the labeled urine container in the person's bathroom.
9 Put on gloves.
10 Collect the following:
  - Voiding device—bedpan and cover, urinal, commode, or specimen pan
  - Graduate to measure output
11 Provide for privacy.

PROCEDURE

12 Ask the person to void. Provide a voiding device.
13 Measure and discard the urine. Note the time. This starts the 24-hour collection period.
14 Mark the time on the urine container.
15 Empty, rinse, clean, disinfect, and dry equipment. Return equipment to its proper place.
16 Remove and discard the gloves. Practice hand hygiene. Put on clean gloves.
17 Assist with hand washing.
18 Remove and discard the gloves. Practice hand hygiene.
19 Mark the time the test began and the time it ends on the room and bathroom labels.
20 Remind the person to:
  a Use the voiding device during the next 24 hours.
  b Not to have a BM when voiding.
  c Put toilet tissue in the toilet or wastebasket.
  d Put on the signal light after voiding.
21 Return to the room when the person signals for you. Knock before entering the room.

22 Do the following after every voiding:
  a Practice hand hygiene. Put on gloves.
  b Measure urine if I&O are ordered.
  c Use the funnel to pour urine into the urine container. Do not spill any urine. Re-start the test if you spill or discard the urine.
  d Empty, rinse, clean, disinfect, and dry equipment. Return equipment to its proper place.
  e Remove and discard the gloves. Practice hand hygiene. Put on clean gloves.
  f Assist with hand washing.
  g Remove and discard the gloves. Practice hand hygiene.
  h Follow "Post-Procedure" steps except for steps 28 and 33.
23 Ask the person to void at the end of the 24-hour period. Follow step 22, a–g.

POST-PROCEDURE

24 Provide for comfort. (See the inside of the front book cover.)
25 Place the signal light within reach.
26 Raise or lower bed rails. Follow the care plan.
27 Put on gloves.
28 Remove the labels from the room and bathroom.
29 Clean, rinse, dry, and return equipment to its proper place. Discard disposable items.

30 Remove and discard the gloves. Practice hand hygiene.
31 Unscreen the person.
32 Complete a safety check of the room. (See the inside of the front book cover.)
33 Take the specimen (labeled urine container) and requisition slip to the storage area. Wear gloves.
34 Remove and discard the gloves. Practice hand hygiene.
35 Report and record your observations.

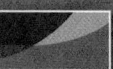 ### Collecting a Urine Specimen From an Infant or Child

Sometimes specimens are needed from infants and children who are not toilet-trained. A collection bag ("wee bag") is applied over the urethra (Fig. 31-3). A parent or another staff member assists if the child is upset.

Voiding on request is hard for toilet-trained toddlers and young children. Potty chairs and specimen pans are useful. Remember to use terms the child understands. "Pee pee," "wee wee," "potty," and "tinkle" are examples. Or ask the parent what term the child uses and understands.

The nurse may ask you to give the child water or other fluids when a urine specimen is needed. Usually the child needs to void about 30 minutes after drinking fluids.

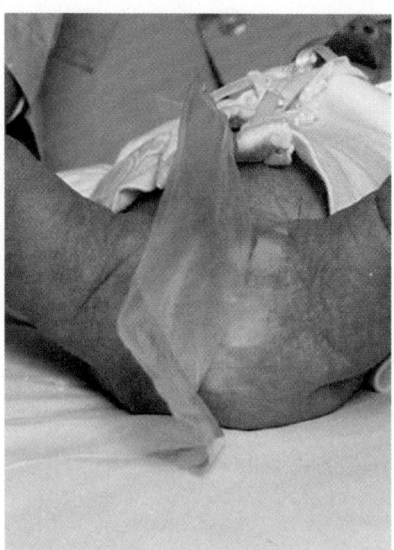

Fig. 31-3 A urine collection bag is applied to the female infant's perineum.

COLLECTING A URINE SPECIMEN FROM AN INFANT OR CHILD

QUALITY OF LIFE

Remember to:
- Knock before entering the person's room.
- Address the child by name.
- Introduce yourself by name and title.

- Explain the procedure to the child and parents before beginning and during the procedure.
- Protect the child's rights during the procedure.
- Handle the child gently during the procedure.

PRE-PROCEDURE

1 Follow *Delegation Guidelines: Urine Specimens*, p. 541. See *Promoting Safety and Comfort: Urine Specimens*, p. 541.
2 Practice hand hygiene.
3 Collect the following:
   - Collection bag ("wee bag")
   - *BIOHAZARD* label (if needed)
   - Cotton balls
   - Specimen container
   - Plastic bag

   - Scissors
   - Wash basin
   - Bath towel
   - Two diapers
   - Gloves
4 Arrange your work area.
5 Practice hand hygiene.
6 Identify the child. Check the ID bracelet against the requisition slip. Also call the child by name.
7 Provide for privacy.

PROCEDURE

8 Practice hand hygiene. Put on gloves.
9 Position the child on his or her back.
10 Remove and set aside the diaper.
11 Clean the perineal area with cotton balls. Use a new cotton ball for each stroke. Rinse and dry the area.

12 Remove and discard the gloves. Practice hand hygiene.
13 Put on clean gloves.
14 Flex the child's knees. Spread the legs.
15 Remove the adhesive backing from the collection bag.

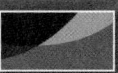

COLLECTING A URINE SPECIMEN FROM AN INFANT OR CHILD—cont'd

PROCEDURE—cont'd

16 Apply the bag to the perineum (see Fig. 31-3).
17 Cut a slit in the bottom of a new diaper.
18 Diaper the child.
19 Pull the collection bag through the slit in the diaper.
20 Remove and discard the gloves. Practice hand hygiene.
21 Raise the head of the crib if allowed. This helps urine collect in the bottom of the bag.
22 Make sure the crib rails are raised and locked before leaving the bedside.
23 Unscreen the child.
24 Dispose of the removed diaper. Follow agency policy. (Wear gloves for this step.)
25 Practice hand hygiene.
26 Check the child often. Check the bag for urine. (Provide for privacy and wear gloves for this step.)

27 Do the following if the child has voided:
  a Provide for privacy.
  b Practice hand hygiene. Put on clean gloves.
  c Remove the diaper.
  d Remove the collection bag gently.
  e Press the adhesive surfaces of the bag together. Make sure the seal is tight and there are no leaks. Or transfer the urine to the specimen container using the drainage tab.
  f Clean the perineal area. Rinse and dry well.
  g Diaper the child.
  h Remove and discard the gloves. Practice hand hygiene.
28 Put on clean gloves.
29 Label the collection bag or specimen container in the child's presence. Then place it in the plastic bag. Apply the BIOHAZARD label (if needed).

POST-PROCEDURE

30 Provide for comfort. (See the inside of the front book cover.)
31 Make sure the crib rails are raised and locked before leaving the bedside.
32 Unscreen the child.
33 Clean, rinse, dry, and return equipment to its proper place. Discard disposable items. (Wear gloves for this step.)

34 Complete a safety check of the room. (See the inside of the front book cover.)
35 Remove and discard the gloves. Practice hand hygiene.
36 Take the specimen and requisition slip to the laboratory or storage area. Wear gloves.
37 Remove and discard the gloves. Practice hand hygiene.
38 Report and record your observations.

Testing Urine

The doctor orders the type and frequency of urine tests. Random urine specimens are needed. The nurse may ask you to do these simple urine tests.

- *Testing for pH*—Urine pH measures if urine is acidic or alkaline. Changes in normal pH (4.6 to 8.0) occur from illness, food, and drugs.
- *Testing for glucose and ketones*—In diabetes, the pancreas does not secrete enough insulin (Chapter 43). The body needs insulin to use sugar for energy. If not used, sugar builds up in the blood. Some sugar appears in the urine. *Glucosuria (glycosuria) means sugar* (glucos, glycos) *in the urine* (uria). The diabetic person may also have ketones in the urine. *Ketones (ketone bodies, acetone) are substances that appear in urine from the rapid breakdown of fat for energy.* The body uses fat for energy if it cannot use sugar. Tests for glucose and ketones are usually done 4 times a day—30 minutes before each meal and at bedtime. The doctor uses the test to make drug and diet decisions.
- *Testing for blood*—Injury and disease can cause hematuria. *Hematuria means blood* (hemat) *in the urine* (uria). Sometimes blood is seen in the urine. At other times it is unseen (*occult*).

Reagent strips (dipsticks) are used to test urine. The strips have sections that change color when they react with urine. To use a reagent strip:

- Do not touch the test area on the strip.
- Dip the strip into urine.
- Compare the strip with the color chart on the bottle (Fig. 31-4).

See *Teamwork and Time Management: Testing Urine,* p. 548.
See *Delegation Guidelines: Testing Urine,* p. 548.
See *Promoting Safety and Comfort: Testing Urine,* p. 548.

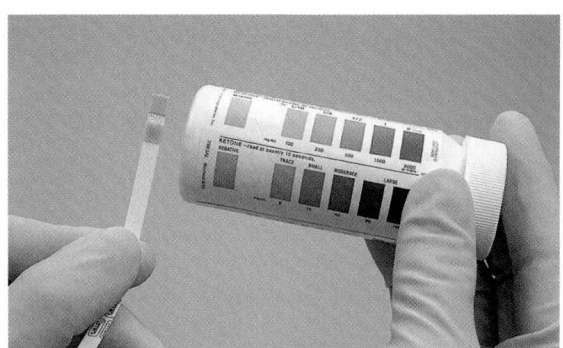

Fig. 31-4 Reagent strip for sugar and ketones.

TEAMWORK AND TIME MANAGEMENT
Testing Urine

Blood glucose testing is common for persons with diabetes (p. 555). However, the nurse may want urine tested for glucose and ketones. The nurse uses the test results to decide about giving the person diabetic drugs. The drugs are given at a certain time. The nurse needs the results before giving the drugs.

DELEGATION GUIDELINES
Testing Urine

When testing urine is delegated to you, you need this information from the nurse and the care plan:
- What test is needed
- What equipment to use
- When to test urine
- Instructions for the test ordered
- If the nurse wants to observe the results of each test
- What observations to report and record:
  - The time you collected and tested the specimen
  - Test results
  - Problems obtaining the specimen
  - Color, clarity, and odor of urine
  - Blood in the urine
  - Particles in the urine
  - Complaints of pain, burning, urgency, difficulty voiding, or other problems
- When to report test results and observations
- What patient or resident concerns to report at once

PROMOTING SAFETY AND COMFORT
Testing Urine

Safety
You must be accurate when testing urine. Promptly report the results to the nurse. Ordered drugs may depend on the results.

When using reagent strips:
- Check the color of the reagent strips. Do not use discolored strips.
- Check the expiration date on the bottle. Do not use the strips if the date has passed.
- Follow the manufacturer's instructions. Otherwise you could get the wrong result. The doctor uses the test results in diagnosing and treating the person. A wrong result could cause serious harm.

Urine may contain microbes and blood. Follow Standard Precautions and the Bloodborne Pathogen Standard.

Comfort
The person may want to know the test results. If allowed by agency policy, you can tell the person the results. This information is private and confidential. Only the person should hear what you are saying.

Straining Urine. A stone *(calculus)* can develop in the kidney, ureter, or bladder. Stones *(calculi)* vary in size (Chapter 44). They can be as small as grains of sand, pearl-size, or larger. Stones causing severe pain and urinary system damage may require removal by medical or surgical procedures. Some stones pass through urine. Therefore all urine is strained. Passed stones are sent to the laboratory.

The person drinks 8 to 12 glasses of water a day to help pass the stone. Expect the person to void in large amounts.

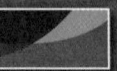

TESTING URINE WITH REAGENT STRIPS

QUALITY OF LIFE

Remember to:
- Knock before entering the person's room.
- Address the person by name.
- Introduce yourself by name and title.

- Explain the procedure to the person before beginning and during the procedure.
- Protect the person's rights during the procedure.
- Handle the person gently during the procedure.

PRE-PROCEDURE

1. Follow *Delegation Guidelines: Testing Urine.* See *Promoting Safety and Comfort: Testing Urine.*
2. Practice hand hygiene.
3. Collect gloves and the reagent strips ordered.
4. Practice hand hygiene.
5. Identify the person. Check the ID bracelet against the assignment sheet. Also call the person by name.
6. Put on gloves.
7. Collect equipment for the urine specimen. (See procedure: *Collecting a Random Urine Specimen*, p. 542.)
8. Provide for privacy.

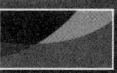

TESTING URINE WITH REAGENT STRIPS—cont'd

PROCEDURE

9 Collect the urine specimen. (See procedure: *Collecting a Random Urine Specimen,* p. 542.)

10 Remove the strip from the bottle. Put the cap on the bottle at once. It must be on tight.

11 Dip the strip test areas into the urine.

12 Remove the strip after the correct amount of time. See the manufacturer's instructions.

13 Tap the strip gently against the urine container. This removes excess urine.

14 Wait the required amount of time. See the manufacturer's instructions.

15 Compare the strip with the color chart on the bottle (see Fig. 31-4). Read the results.

16 Discard disposable items and the specimen.

17 Empty, rinse, clean, disinfect, and dry equipment. Return equipment to its proper place.

18 Remove and discard the gloves. Practice hand hygiene.

POST-PROCEDURE

19 Provide for comfort. (See the inside of the front book cover.)

20 Place the signal light within reach.

21 Raise or lower bed rails. Follow the care plan.

22 Unscreen the person.

23 Complete a safety check of the room. (See the inside of the front book cover.)

24 Practice hand hygiene.

25 Report and record the test results and other observations.

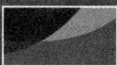

STRAINING URINE

QUALITY OF LIFE

Remember to:
- Knock before entering the person's room.
- Address the person by name.
- Introduce yourself by name and title.

- Explain the procedure to the person before beginning and during the procedure.
- Protect the person's rights during the procedure.
- Handle the person gently during the procedure.

PRE-PROCEDURE

1 Follow *Delegation Guidelines: Testing Urine.* See *Promoting Safety and Comfort: Testing Urine.*

2 Practice hand hygiene.

3 Collect the following before going to the person's room:
- Laboratory requisition slip
- Gauze or strainer
- Specimen container
- Specimen label
- Two STRAIN ALL URINE labels
- Plastic bag
- BIOHAZARD label (if needed)
- Gloves

4 Arrange collected items in the person's bathroom.

5 Place one STRAIN ALL URINE label in the bathroom. Place the other near the bed.

6 Practice hand hygiene.

7 Identify the person. Check the ID bracelet against the assignment sheet. Call the person by name.

8 Label the specimen container in the person's presence.

9 Put on gloves.

10 Collect the following:
- Voiding device—bedpan and cover, urinal, commode, or specimen pan
- Graduate

11 Provide for privacy.

PROCEDURE

12 Ask the person to use the voiding device for urinating. Ask the person to put on the signal light after voiding.

13 Remove and discard the gloves. Practice hand hygiene.

14 Return to the room when the person signals for you. Knock before entering the room.

15 Practice hand hygiene. Put on clean gloves.

16 Place the gauze or strainer into the graduate.

17 Pour urine into the graduate. Urine passes through the gauze or strainer (Fig. 31-5, p. 550).

18 Place the gauze or strainer in the specimen container if any crystals, stones, or particles appear.

19 Place the specimen container in the plastic bag. Do not let the container touch the outside of the bag. Apply a BIOHAZARD label.

20 Measure urine if I&O are ordered.

21 Empty, rinse, clean, disinfect, and dry equipment. Return equipment to its proper place.

22 Remove and discard the gloves. Practice hand hygiene. Put on clean gloves.

23 Assist with hand washing.

24 Remove and discard the gloves. Practice hand hygiene.

Continued

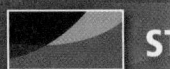

STRAINING URINE—cont'd

POST-PROCEDURE

25 Provide for comfort. (See the inside of the front book cover.)
26 Place the signal light within reach.
27 Raise or lower bed rails. Follow the care plan.
28 Unscreen the person.

29 Complete a safety check of the room. (See the inside of the front book cover.)
30 Practice hand hygiene.
31 Take the specimen container and requisition slip to the laboratory or storage area. Wear gloves.
32 Remove and discard the gloves. Practice hand hygiene.
33 Report and record your observations.

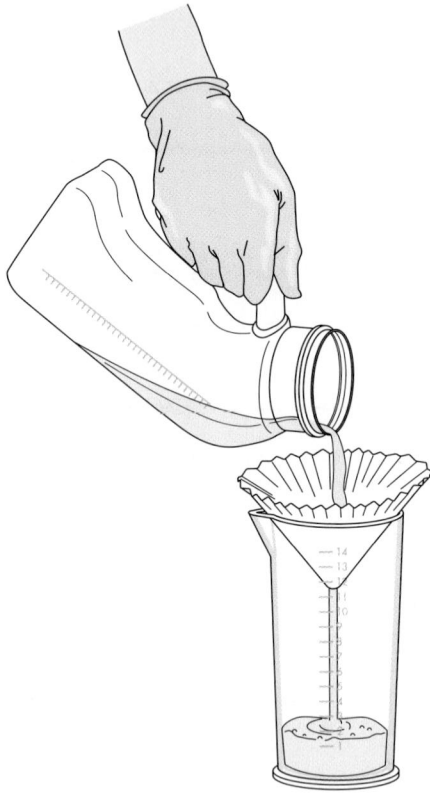

Fig. 31-5 A strainer is placed in the graduate. Urine is poured through the strainer into the graduate.

STOOL SPECIMENS

Stools also are studied for fat, microbes, worms, blood, and other abnormal contents. Ulcers, colon cancer, and hemorrhoids are common causes of bleeding. Often blood is seen if bleeding is low in the bowels. Stools are black and tarry from bleeding in the stomach or upper gastrointestinal tract. *Melena is a black, tarry stool.*

Sometimes bleeding occurs in very small amounts. Then stools are tested for *occult blood*. *Occult* means "hidden" or "not seen." The test is done to screen for colon cancer

and other digestive disorders. Occult blood test kits vary. Follow the manufacturer's instructions.

Urine must not contaminate the stool specimen. The person uses one device for voiding and another for a BM. Some tests require a warm stool. The specimen is taken at once to the laboratory or storage area. Follow the rules in Box 31-1.

See *Focus on Communication: Stool Specimens.*
See *Focus on Children and Older Persons: Stool Specimens.*
See *Delegation Guidelines: Stool Specimens.*
See *Promoting Safety and Comfort: Stool Specimens.*

FOCUS ON COMMUNICATION
Stool Specimens

Always explain the procedure before you begin. Explain what the person needs to do and what you will do. Also show what equipment and supplies you will use. For example:

"The doctor wants your stools tested. So, we need a specimen from a bowel movement. I'm going to place this specimen pan (show the specimen pan) at the back of the toilet seat. You will urinate into the toilet. Your bowel movement will collect in the specimen pan. Please put toilet tissue in the toilet, not in the specimen pan. After you have a bowel movement, put your signal light on right away. I'll put some stool in this specimen container (show the specimen container)."

After explaining the procedure, ask if the person has any questions. If you do not know the answer, refer questions to the nurse.

Also make sure the person understands what to do. You can say: "Mrs. Clark, please tell me what you're going to do, so I know you understand what I said."

FOCUS ON CHILDREN AND OLDER PERSONS
Stool Specimens

Children

If the child wears a diaper, you can obtain stool from the diaper. You may need to scrape the diaper.

DELEGATION GUIDELINES
Stool Specimens

Before collecting and testing a stool specimen, you need this information from the nurse:
- What time to collect and test the specimen
- What test is needed (if any)
- What equipment to use
- What special measures are needed
- Instructions for the test ordered
- If the nurse wants to observe the stool or test results
- What observations to report and record:
  - The time you collected and tested the specimen
  - Test results
  - Problems obtaining the specimen
  - Color, amount, consistency, and odor of stools
  - Blood in the stools
  - Complaints of pain or discomfort
- When to report observations
- What patient or resident concerns to report at once

PROMOTING SAFETY AND COMFORT
Stool Specimens

Safety

You must be accurate when testing stools. Follow the manufacturer's instructions for the test used. Promptly report the results to the nurse.

Stools contain microbes. And they may contain blood. Follow Standard Precautions and the Bloodborne Pathogen Standard.

Comfort

Stools normally have an odor. A person may be embarrassed that you need to collect a specimen. Complete the task quickly and carefully. Also act in a professional manner.

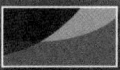 **COLLECTING AND TESTING A STOOL SPECIMEN**   VIDEO

QUALITY OF LIFE

Remember to:
- Knock before entering the person's room.
- Address the person by name.
- Introduce yourself by name and title.

- Explain the procedure to the person before beginning and during the procedure.
- Protect the person's rights during the procedure.
- Handle the person gently during the procedure.

PRE-PROCEDURE

1. Follow *Delegation Guidelines: Stool Specimens*. See *Promoting Safety and Comfort: Stool Specimens*.
2. Practice hand hygiene.
3. Collect the following before going to the person's room:
   - Laboratory requisition slip
   - Occult blood test kit (if needed)
   - Specimen pan for the toilet
   - Specimen container and lid
   - Specimen label
   - Tongue blades
   - Disposable bag
   - Plastic bag

   - *BIOHAZARD* label (if needed)
   - Gloves
4. Arrange collected items in the person's bathroom.
5. Practice hand hygiene.
6. Identify the person. Check the ID bracelet against the requisition slip. Also call the person by name.
7. Label the specimen container in the person's presence.
8. Put on gloves.
9. Collect the following:
   - Device for voiding—bedpan and cover, urinal, commode, or specimen pan
   - Toilet tissue
10. Provide for privacy.

PROCEDURE

11. Ask the person to void. Provide the voiding device if the person does not use the bathroom. Empty, rinse, clean, disinfect, and dry the device. Return it to its proper place.
12. Put the specimen pan on the toilet if the person will use the bathroom. Place it at the back of the toilet (Fig. 31-6, p. 552). Or provide a bedpan or commode.
13. Ask the person not to put toilet tissue into the bedpan, commode, or specimen pan. Provide a bag for toilet tissue.
14. Place the signal light and toilet tissue within reach. Raise or lower bed rails. Follow the care plan.

15. Remove and discard the gloves. Practice hand hygiene. Leave the room if the person can be left alone.
16. Return when the person signals. Or check on the person every 5 minutes. Knock before entering.
17. Practice hand hygiene. Put on clean gloves.
18. Lower the bed rail near you if up.
19. Remove the bedpan (if used). Note the color, amount, consistency, and odor of stools.
20. Provide perineal care if needed.

Continued

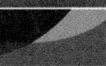

COLLECTING AND TESTING A STOOL SPECIMEN—cont'd

VIDEO

PROCEDURE—cont'd

21 Collect the specimen:
   a Use a tongue blade to take about 2 tablespoons of stool to the specimen container (Fig. 31-7). Take the sample from the middle of a formed stool.
   b Include pus, mucus, or blood present in the stool.
   c Take stool from 2 different places in the BM if required by agency policy.
   d Put the lid on the specimen container.
   e Place the container in the plastic bag. Do not let the container touch the outside of the bag. Apply a BIOHAZARD label according to agency policy.
   f Wrap the tongue blade in toilet tissue. Discard it into the disposable bag.
22 Remove and discard the gloves. Practice hand hygiene. Put on clean gloves.
23 Test the specimen (if ordered):
   a Open the test kit.
   b Use a tongue blade to obtain a small amount of stool.
   c Apply a thin smear of stool on *box A* on the test paper (Fig. 31-8, A).

   d Use another tongue blade to obtain stool from another part of the specimen.
   e Apply a thin smear of stool on *box B* on the test paper (Fig. 31-8, B).
   f Close the packet.
   g Turn the test packet to the other side. Open the flap. Apply developer (from the kit) to *boxes A* and *B*. Follow the manufacturer's instructions (Fig. 31-8, C).
   h Wait 10 to 60 seconds as required by the manufacturer.
   i Note the color changes on your assignment sheet (Fig. 31-8, D).
   j Dispose of the test packet.
   k Wrap the tongue blades with toilet tissue. Then discard them.
24 Empty, rinse, clean, disinfect, and dry equipment. Return equipment to its proper place.
25 Remove and discard the gloves. Practice hand hygiene. Put on clean gloves.
26 Assist with hand washing.
27 Remove and discard the gloves. Practice hand hygiene.

POST-PROCEDURE

28 Provide for comfort. (See the inside of the front book cover.)
29 Place the signal light within reach.
30 Raise or lower bed rails. Follow the care plan.
31 Unscreen the person.

32 Complete a safety check of the room. (See the inside of the front book cover.)
33 Deliver the specimen and requisition slip to the laboratory or storage area. Follow agency policy. Wear gloves.
34 Remove and discard the gloves. Practice hand hygiene.
35 Report and record your observations.

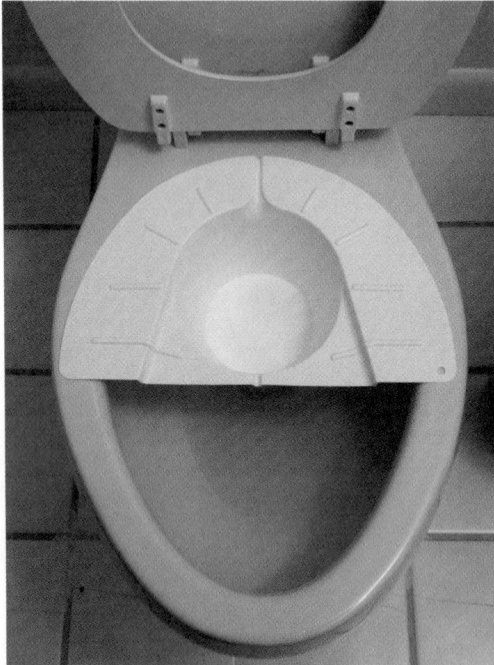

Fig. 31-6 The specimen pan is placed at the back of the toilet for a stool specimen.

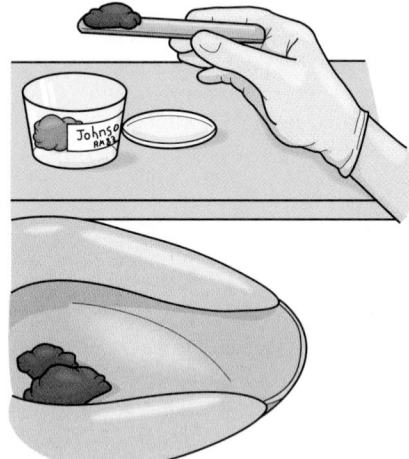

Fig. 31-7 A tongue blade is used to transfer a small amount of stool from the bedpan to the specimen container.

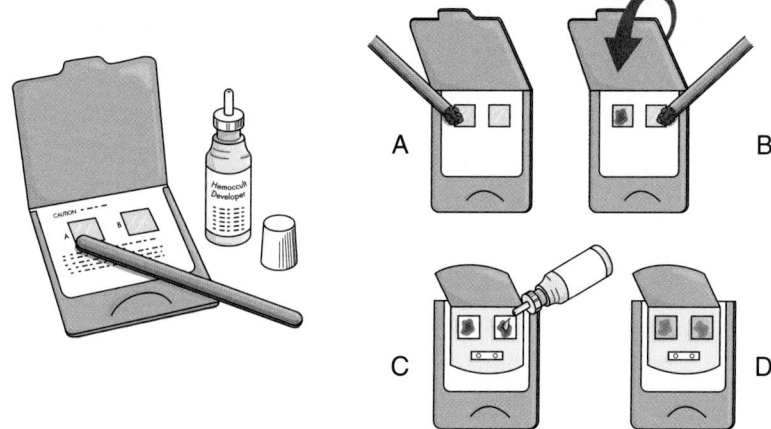

Fig. 31-8 Testing for occult blood. **A,** Stool is smeared on *box A.* **B,** Stool is smeared on *box B* and then the flap is closed. **C,** Developer is applied to *boxes A and B* on the back side of the test packet. **D,** Color changes are noted.

SPUTUM SPECIMENS

Respiratory disorders cause the lungs, bronchi, and trachea to secrete mucus. *Mucus from the respiratory system is called sputum when expectorated* (expelled) *through the mouth.* Sputum is not saliva. Saliva ("spit") is a thin, clear liquid produced by the salivary glands in the mouth.

Sputum specimens are studied for blood, microbes, and abnormal cells. The person coughs up sputum from the bronchi and trachea. This is often painful and hard to do. It is easier to collect a specimen in the morning. Secretions collect in the trachea and bronchi during sleep. They are coughed up on awakening.

To collect a specimen, follow the rules in Box 31-1. Also have the person rinse the mouth with water. Rinsing decreases saliva and removes food particles. Mouthwash is not used. It destroys some of the microbes in the mouth.

See *Focus on Children and Older Persons: Sputum Specimens.*
See *Delegation Guidelines: Sputum Specimens,* p. 554.
See *Promoting Safety and Comfort: Sputum Specimens,* p. 554.

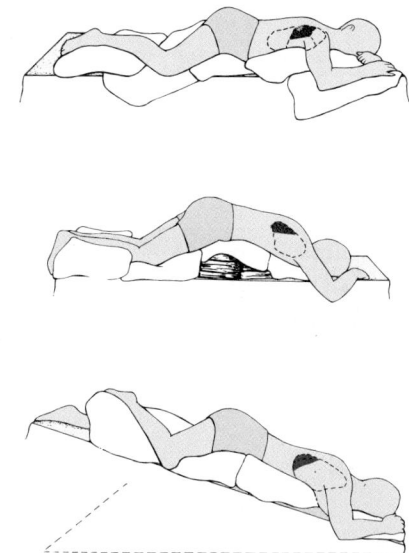

Fig. 31-9 Some positions for postural drainage.

FOCUS ON CHILDREN AND OLDER PERSONS

Sputum Specimens

Children
Breathing treatments and suctioning (Chapter 37) are often needed to produce sputum specimens in infants and small children. The RN or respiratory therapist gives the breathing treatment. The nurse suctions the trachea for the specimen. The infant or child is likely to be uncooperative during suctioning. You can assist by holding the child's head and arms still.

Older Persons
Older persons may lack the strength to cough up sputum. Coughing is easier after postural drainage. It drains secretions by gravity. Gravity causes fluids to flow down. The person is positioned so a lung part is higher than the airway (Fig. 31-9). The nurse or respiratory therapist does postural drainage. Assist as directed.

DELEGATION GUIDELINES
Sputum Specimens

To collect a sputum specimen, you need this information from the nurse:
- When to collect the specimen
- How much sputum is needed—usually 1 to 2 teaspoons
- If the person uses the bathroom
- If the person can hold the specimen container
- What observations to report and record:
  - The time the specimen was collected
  - The amount of sputum collected
  - How easily the person raised the sputum
  - Sputum color—clear, white, yellow, green, brown, or red
  - Sputum odor—none or foul odor
  - Sputum consistency—thick, watery, or frothy (with bubbles or foam)
  - *Hemoptysis*—*bloody* (hemo) *sputum* (ptysis, *meaning to spit*)
  - If the person was not able to produce sputum
  - Any other observations
- When to report observations
- What patient or resident concerns to report at once

PROMOTING SAFETY AND COMFORT
Sputum Specimens

Safety
Follow Standard Precautions and the Bloodborne Pathogen Standard to prevent contact with mucus. It may contain blood or microbes.

The doctor may order isolation precautions if the person has or may have tuberculosis (TB) (Chapter 42). Protect yourself by wearing a TB respirator (Chapter 15).

Comfort
The procedure can embarrass the person. Coughing and expectorating sounds can disturb others. Also, sputum is not pleasant to look at. For these reasons, privacy is important. Cover the specimen container and place it in a bag. Some sputum specimen containers are cloudy in color to hide the contents.

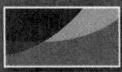 **COLLECTING A SPUTUM SPECIMEN** | **VIDEO**

QUALITY OF LIFE

Remember to:
- Knock before entering the person's room.
- Address the person by name.
- Introduce yourself by name and title.
- Explain the procedure to the person before beginning and during the procedure.
- Protect the person's rights during the procedure.
- Handle the person gently during the procedure.

PRE-PROCEDURE

1 Follow *Delegation Guidelines: Sputum Specimens*. See *Promoting Safety and Comfort: Sputum Specimens*.
2 Practice hand hygiene.
3 Collect the following before going to the person's room:
   - Laboratory requisition slip
   - Sputum specimen container and lid
   - Specimen label
   - Plastic bag
   - *BIOHAZARD* label (if needed)
4 Arrange collected items in the person's bathroom.
5 Practice hand hygiene.
6 Identify the person. Check the ID bracelet against the requisition slip. Also call the person by name.
7 Label the specimen container in the person's presence.
8 Collect gloves and tissues.
9 Provide for privacy. If able, the person uses the bathroom for the procedure.

PROCEDURE

10 Put on gloves.
11 Ask the person to rinse the mouth out with clear water.
12 Have the person hold the container. Only the outside is touched.
13 Ask the person to cover the mouth and nose with tissues when coughing. Follow agency policy for used tissues.
14 Ask him or her to take 2 or 3 deep breaths and cough up the sputum.
15 Have the person expectorate directly into the container (Fig. 31-10). Sputum should not touch the outside of the container.
16 Collect 1 to 2 teaspoons of sputum unless told to collect more.
17 Put the lid on the container.
18 Place the container in the plastic bag. Do not let the container touch the outside of the bag. Apply a *BIOHAZARD* label according to agency policy.
19 Remove and discard the gloves. Practice hand hygiene. Put on clean gloves.
20 Assist with hand washing.
21 Remove and discard the gloves. Practice hand hygiene.

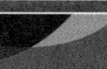

COLLECTING A SPUTUM SPECIMEN—cont'd

VIDEO

POST-PROCEDURE

22 Provide for comfort. (See the inside of the front book cover.)
23 Place the signal light within reach.
24 Raise or lower bed rails. Follow the care plan.
25 Unscreen the person.
26 Complete a safety check of the room. (See the inside of the front book cover.)

27 Practice hand hygiene.
28 Deliver the specimen and the requisition slip to the storage area. Follow agency policy. Wear gloves.
29 Remove and discard the gloves. Practice hand hygiene.
30 Report and record your observations.

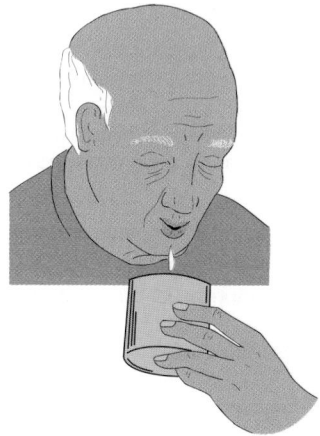

Fig. 31-10 The person expectorates into the center of the specimen container.

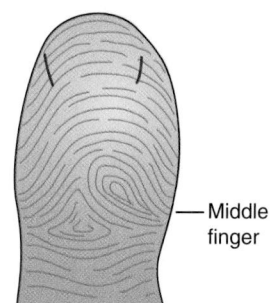

Fig. 31-11 Site for skin punctures.

Middle finger

BLOOD GLUCOSE TESTING

Blood glucose testing is used for persons with diabetes. The doctor uses the results to regulate the person's drugs and diet.

Capillary blood is obtained through a skin puncture. A drop of blood is collected. A fingertip is the most common site for skin punctures. This provides easy access and clothing is not removed.

Inspect the puncture site for signs of trauma and skin breaks. Do not use swollen, bruised, cyanotic (bluish color), scarred, or calloused sites. Such areas have poor blood flow. A *callus* is a thick, hardened area on the skin. Calluses often form over frequently used areas, such as the tips of the thumbs and index fingers. Therefore thumbs and index fingers are not good skin puncture sites.

Use the side toward the tip of the middle or ring finger (Fig. 31-11). Do not use the center, fleshy part of the fingertip. The site has many nerve endings making punctures painful.

You use a sterile, disposable lancet to puncture the skin (Fig. 31-12). The person feels a brief, sharp pinch. A *lancet* is a short, pointed blade. It punctures but does not cut the skin. The lancet is inside a protective cover. You do not touch the blade. Discard it into the sharps container after use.

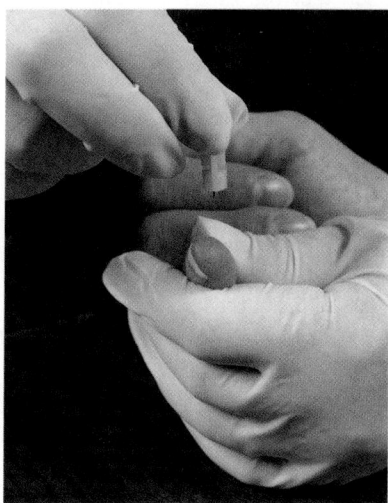

Fig. 31-12 A lancet.

Using a reagent strip, a *glucometer (glucose meter)* measures blood glucose. You apply a drop of blood to a reagent strip. The blood glucose level appears on the screen. Many types of glucometers are available. How fast results are displayed varies. Some take 5 seconds.

You will learn to use your agency's device. Always follow the manufacturer's instructions.

See *Teamwork and Time Management: Blood Glucose Testing,* p. 556.
See *Delegation Guidelines: Blood Glucose Testing,* p. 556.
See *Promoting Safety and Comfort: Blood Glucose Testing,* p. 556.

Perform blood glucose testing at times directed by the nurse and the care plan. The nurse uses the results to make decisions about the person's diet and drug dosages. The drugs are given at a certain time. The nurse needs the blood glucose results before giving the drugs.

Glucometers are shared with other staff. Tell your co-workers when you have one. Work quickly, but carefully. Return the device to the storage area in a timely manner.

If testing blood glucose is delegated to you, make sure that:
* Your state and agency allow you to perform the procedure.
* The procedure is in your job description.
* You have the necessary training.
* You know how to use the agency's equipment.
* You review the procedure with a nurse.
* The nurse is available to answer questions and to supervise you.

If the above conditions are met, you need this information from the nurse and the care plan:
* What sites to avoid for a skin puncture
* When to collect and test the specimen—usually before meals
* If the person receives drugs that affect blood clotting (NOTE: If yes, it may take a longer time to stop bleeding. Apply pressure until bleeding stops.)
* What to report and record:
  * The time the specimen was collected
  * The blood glucose test result
  * The site used for the skin puncture
  * The amount of bleeding at the skin puncture site
  * Any signs of a *hematoma* (a *swelling* [oma] *that contains blood* [hemat])
  * How the person tolerated the procedure
  * Complaints of pain at the skin puncture site
  * Other observations or patient or resident complaints
* When to report observations and the test result
* What patient or resident concerns to report at once

Safety
Accurate results are important. Inaccurate results can harm the person. Follow the rules in Box 31-2.

You must know how to use the equipment. Use only the type of reagent strip specified by the manufacturer. Otherwise you will get inaccurate results.

Disinfect the glucometer after testing a patient or resident. Follow the manufacturer's instructions for the disinfectant used. For example, if the instructions say to wait 2 minutes, you must wait 2 minutes. Always follow the time set by the manufacturer.

Contact with blood is likely. Follow Standard Precautions and the Bloodborne Pathogen Standard.

Comfort
The heel is used for skin punctures in infants who are not walking. The third finger (ring finger) is used for children. See Figure 31-13.

Older persons often have poor circulation in their fingers. To increase blood flow, apply a warm washcloth or wash the hands in warm water.

BOX 31-2	RULES FOR BLOOD GLUCOSE TESTING

* Follow the manufacturer's instructions for the glucometer and disinfectant.
* Know how to use the equipment. Request any necessary training.
* Make sure the glucometer was tested for accuracy. Check the testing log.
* Enter a code or user-ID if required by the glucometer. This is provided by the agency. Do not share your user-ID with others.
* Make sure you have the correct reagent strips for the glucometer you are using. Compare the code number on the strip with the code number on the glucometer. The code numbers should be the same.
* Scan the bar code on the bottle of reagent strips if needed (Fig. 31-14).
* Check the color of the reagent strips. Do not use discolored strips.
* Check the expiration date of the reagent strips. Do not use them if the date has passed.
* Report the result to the nurse at once.
* Record the result following agency policy.

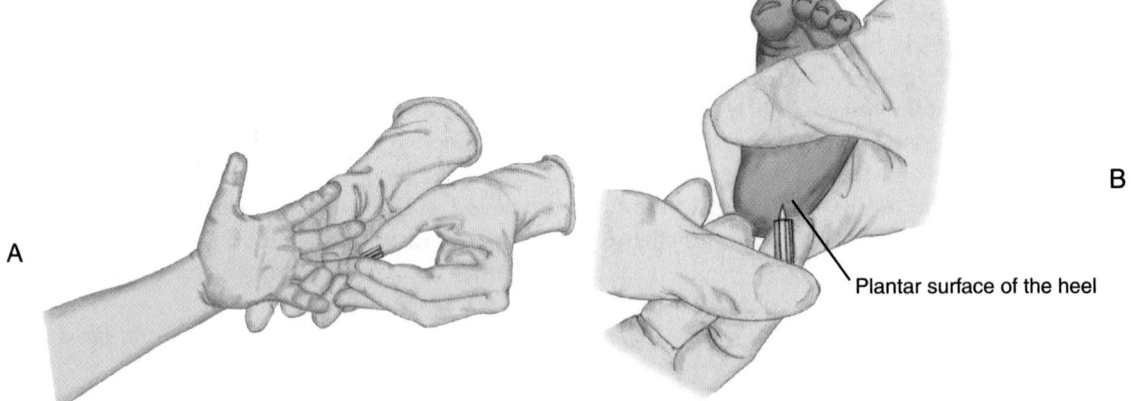

A

B

Plantar surface of the heel

Fig. 31-13 **A,** The third finger (ring finger) is used for skin punctures in children. **B,** Heel site is used for skin punctures in infants.

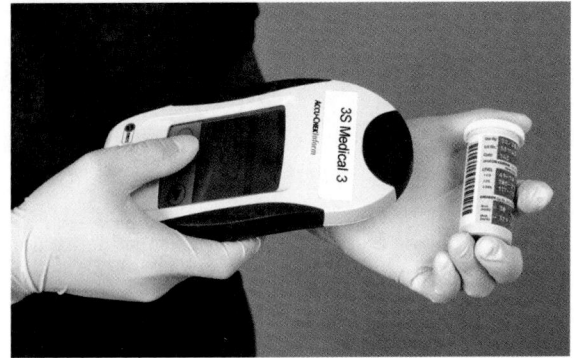

Fig. 31-14 The bar code on the bottle of reagent strips is scanned.

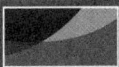

MEASURING BLOOD GLUCOSE

QUALITY OF LIFE

Remember to:
- Knock before entering the person's room.
- Address the person by name.
- Introduce yourself by name and title.

- Explain the procedure to the person before beginning and during the procedure.
- Protect the person's rights during the procedure.
- Handle the person gently during the procedure.

PRE-PROCEDURE

1 Follow *Delegation Guidelines: Blood Glucose Testing*. See *Promoting Safety and Comfort: Blood Glucose Testing*.
2 Practice hand hygiene.
3 Collect the following:
- Sterile lancet
- Antiseptic wipes
- Gloves
- 2 × 2 gauze squares
- Glucometer
- Reagent strips (Use the correct ones for the glucometer. Check the expiration date.)
- Disinfectant

- Paper towels
- Warm washcloth
4 Read the manufacturer's instructions for the lancet and glucometer.
5 Disinfect the glucometer. Follow the manufacturer's instructions for the disinfectant.
6 Arrange your work area.
7 Identify the person. Check the ID bracelet against the assignment sheet. Also call the person by name.
8 Provide for privacy.
9 Raise the bed for body mechanics. The far bed rail is up if used.

PROCEDURE

10 Help the person to a comfortable position.
11 Put on the gloves.
12 Prepare the supplies:
  a Open the antiseptic wipes.
  b Remove a reagent strip from the bottle. Place it on the paper towel. Place the cap securely on the bottle.
  c Prepare the lancet.
  d Turn on the glucometer.
  e Follow the prompts. You may need to enter a user-ID and the person's ID number. Scan the bar code on the bottle of reagent strips if needed.
  f Insert a reagent strip into the glucometer (Fig. 31-15, p. 558).

13 Perform a skin puncture to obtain a drop of blood:
  a Inspect the person's fingers. Select a puncture site.
  b Warm the finger. Rub it gently or apply a warm washcloth.
  c Massage the hand and finger toward the puncture site. And lower the finger below the person's waist. These actions increase blood flow to the site.
  d Hold the finger with your thumb and forefinger. Use your non-dominant hand. Hold the finger until step 14, c.
  e Clean the site with an antiseptic wipe. *Do not touch the site after cleaning.*
  f Let the site dry.
  g Pick up the sterile lancet.
  h Place the lancet against the puncture site.
  i Push the button on the lancet to puncture the skin. (Follow the manufacturer's instructions.)
  j Wipe away the first blood drop. Use a gauze square.
  k Apply gentle pressure below the puncture site.
  l Let a large drop of blood form.

Continued

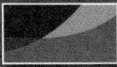

MEASURING BLOOD GLUCOSE—cont'd

PROCEDURE—cont'd

14 Collect and test the specimen. Follow the manufacturer's instructions and agency procedures for the glucometer used.

   a Hold the test area of the reagent strip close to the drop of blood.

   b Lightly touch the reagent strip to the blood drop (Fig. 31-16). Do not smear the blood. The glucometer will test the sample when enough blood is applied.

   c Apply pressure to the puncture site until bleeding stops. Use a gauze square. If able, let the person apply pressure to the site.

   d Read the result on the display (Fig. 31-17). Note the result on your notepad or assignment sheet. Tell the person the result.

   e Turn off the glucometer.

15 Discard the lancet into the sharps container.

16 Discard the gauze squares and reagent strip. Follow agency policy.

17 Remove and discard the gloves. Practice hand hygiene.

POST-PROCEDURE

18 Provide for comfort. (See the inside of the front book cover.)

19 Place the signal light within reach.

20 Lower the bed to its lowest position.

21 Raise or lower bed rails. Follow the care plan.

22 Unscreen the person.

23 Discard used supplies.

24 Complete a safety check of the room. (See the inside of the front book cover.)

25 Follow agency policy for soiled linen.

26 Disinfect the glucometer. (Wear gloves.) Follow the manufacturer's instructions. Return the device to its proper place.

27 Remove and discard the gloves. Practice hand hygiene.

28 Report and record the test result and your observations.

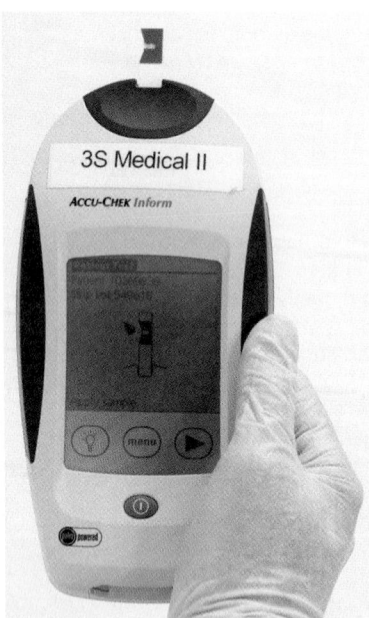

Fig. 31-15 A reagent strip is in the glucometer.

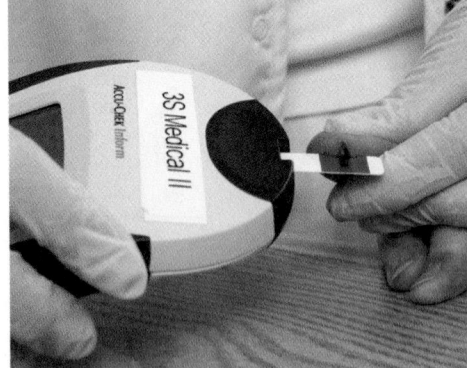

Fig. 31-16 A drop of blood is applied to the reagent strip.

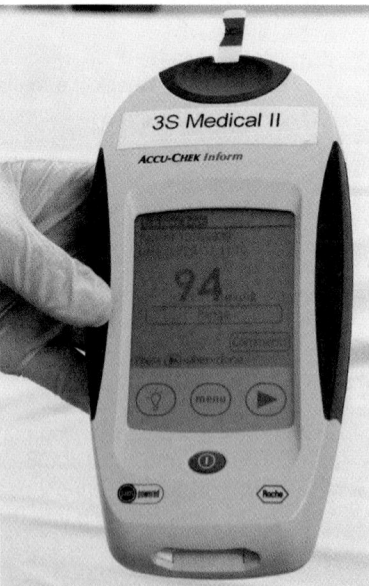

Fig. 31-17 The result is displayed on the glucometer.

FOCUS ON PRIDE

The Person, Family, and Yourself

Personal and Professional Responsibility

When collecting specimens, you are responsible for correctly identifying the person. You must collect and test specimens on the right person. Otherwise, one or both persons could be harmed. Before collecting or testing a specimen, carefully identify the person. Check the ID bracelet against the laboratory requisition slip or assignment sheet. Compare all information, not just the person's name.

Some agencies require placing collection information on the specimen container. Collection date, collection time, and the collector's name or initials are examples. Follow agency policy to label specimens. Take pride in promoting safety by collecting and labeling specimens properly.

Rights and Respect

Specimen collection embarrasses many people. Respect the person's right to privacy. To promote comfort and privacy:

- Politely ask visitors to leave the room.
- Close doors, privacy curtains, and window coverings.
- Leave the room if it is safe to do so. If you cannot leave, explain this to the person.
- Place the specimen container in a paper bag or wrap it in a paper towel or washcloth so others do not see the specimen.
- Always act professionally. Do not make statements that may embarrass the person.

Independence and Social Interaction

Some persons can collect their own urine and sputum specimens. Doing so promotes independence. It also helps reduce embarrassment.

Explain the procedure to the person. This helps the person know how to correctly collect the specimen. Show the person the specimen container and how it is used. Also, ask the person where you should place the container. When ready to collect the specimen, the person knows where to find the container.

Delegation and Teamwork

You may need to take a specimen to the laboratory. Before you go, tell the nurse and your co-workers that you are leaving the area. Also, ask if other staff need specimens taken to the laboratory. Doing so saves staff time. This also prevents having too many staff members off the unit at the same time. Return from the laboratory promptly.

Ethics and Laws

Ethics is concerned with right and wrong behavior. If you did not collect a specimen correctly, do not send it to the laboratory. Tell the nurse what happened. Then collect the specimen at the next opportunity. Test results must be accurate for correct diagnosis and treatment. Take pride in honestly reporting mistakes.

REVIEW QUESTIONS

Circle the BEST answer.

1 A random urine specimen is collected
   - a After sleep
   - c After meals
   - b Before meals
   - d Any time

2 Perineal care is given before collecting a
   - a Random specimen
   - b Midstream specimen
   - c 24-hour urine specimen
   - d Stool specimen

3 A 24-hour urine specimen involves
   - a Collecting all urine voided during a 24-hour period
   - b Collecting a random specimen every hour for 24 hours
   - c Testing urine for ketones every day
   - d Measuring output every hour for 24 hours

4 Urine is tested for ketones
   - a At bedtime
   - b 30 minutes after meals and at bedtime
   - c 30 minutes before meals and at bedtime
   - d Before breakfast

5 You need to strain a person's urine. Straining is done to find
   - a Blood
   - c Ketones
   - b Stones
   - d Acetone

6 You note a black, tarry stool. This is called
   - a Melena
   - c Hemostool
   - b Feces
   - d Occult blood

7 A stool specimen must be kept warm. After collecting the specimen,
   - a Put it in an oven
   - b Put it in a paper bag
   - c Cover it with a towel
   - d Take it to the laboratory or storage area

8 The best time to collect a sputum specimen is
   - a On awakening
   - c At bedtime
   - b After meals
   - d After oral hygiene

9 A sputum specimen is needed. You should ask the person to
   - a Use mouthwash
   - b Rinse the mouth with clear water
   - c Brush the teeth
   - d Remove dentures

10 Which is the *best* site for a skin puncture?
   - a The thumb
   - c The ring finger
   - b The index finger
   - d The little finger

11 Which is used to measure blood glucose?
   - a Glucometer
   - b Lancet
   - c Reagent strip
   - d Sphygmomanometer

12 Before using reagent strips for blood glucose testing, you need to
   - a Check the expiration date
   - b Make sure they are discolored
   - c Label each strip with the person's name
   - d Check the size of the test area

Answers to these questions are on p. 834.

32 The Person Having Surgery

OBJECTIVES

- Define the key terms and key abbreviations listed in this chapter.
- Describe the common fears and concerns of surgical patients.
- Explain how people are prepared for surgery.
- Describe how to prepare a room for the post-operative patient.

- List the signs and symptoms to report after surgery.
- Explain how to meet the person's needs after surgery.
- Perform the procedures described in this chapter.
- Explain how to promote PRIDE in the person, the family, and yourself.

KEY TERMS

anesthesia The loss of feeling or sensation produced by a drug
elective surgery Surgery done by choice to improve the person's life or well-being
embolus A blood clot that travels through the vascular system until it lodges in a blood vessel
emergency surgery Surgery done at once to save life or function
general anesthesia The loss of consciousness and all feeling or sensation
local anesthesia The loss of feeling or sensation in a small area

post-operative After surgery
pre-operative Before surgery
regional anesthesia The loss of feeling or sensation in a large area of the body
sedation A state of quiet, calmness, or sleep produced by a drug
thrombus A blood clot
urgent surgery Surgery needed for the person's health; it is done soon to prevent further damage or disease

KEY ABBREVIATIONS

AE	Anti-embolism, anti-embolic	**NG**	Naso-gastric
CBC	Complete blood count	**NPO**	Non per os; nothing by mouth
ECG	Electrocardiogram	**OR**	Operating room
EKG	Electrocardiogram	**PACU**	Post anesthesia care unit
ID	Identification	**SCD**	Sequential compression device
I&O	Intake and output	**TED**	Thrombo-embolic disease
IV	Intravenous		

The reasons for surgery are many. Surgery is done to:
- Remove a diseased or injured body part.
- Remove a tumor.
- Repair an injured body part.
- Make a diagnosis.
- Improve appearance.
- Relieve symptoms.
- Restore or improve function.
- Replace a body part.

Surgery often requires a hospital stay. Called *in-patients*, such persons are admitted the morning of surgery or 1 or 2 days before surgery. Some patients go directly to surgery from the emergency department. Patients stay for 1, 2, or more days after surgery.

Same-day surgery (out-patient, one-day, or ambulatory surgery) is common. Such surgeries are done in hospitals and *surgi-centers (surgery centers)*. Surgi-centers are designed and equipped for certain surgical and diagnostic procedures. The person goes home the same day or the next day.

Surgeries are described as:

- *Elective surgery—done by choice to improve the person's life or well-being.* It is not life-saving. Joint replacement surgery and cosmetic surgery are examples. The surgery is scheduled in advance.
- *Urgent surgery—needed for the person's health. It is done soon to prevent further damage or disease.* Cancer surgery and coronary artery bypass surgery are examples.
- *Emergency surgery—done at once to save life or function.* The need is sudden and not expected. Vehicle crashes, stabbings, and bullet wounds often require emergency surgery.

The person is prepared for what happens before, during, and after surgery. *Pre-operative refers to before surgery. Post-operative refers to after surgery.* Some people recover from surgery in nursing centers or rehabilitation centers. Some need home care.

PSYCHOLOGICAL CARE

Surgery causes many fears and concerns (Box 32-1). Past experiences affect feelings. Some persons have had surgery. Others have not. Patients are affected when family and friends talk about their own surgeries. Most people know about tragic events—surgery on the wrong person or body part, instruments left in the body, death during or after surgery. Some people do not share their fears and concerns. They may cry, be quiet or withdrawn, or talk about other things. Some pace. Others are very cheerful.

Mental preparation is important. Respect the person's fears and concerns. Show the person warmth, sensitivity, and caring.

BOX 32-1	COMMON FEARS AND CONCERNS OF SURGICAL PATIENTS

The fear of...
- Anesthesia and its effects
- Cancer
- Complications from surgery
- Disfigurement and scarring
- Disability
- Dying: during or after surgery
- Exposure
- Not waking up after surgery
- Pain: during surgery, after surgery
- Prolonged recovery
- Separation from family and friends
- Surgery on the wrong body part
- Tubes, needles, and other care equipment
- Waking up during surgery
- What happens after surgery—more surgery, treatments, care, and so on

Concern about...
- Caring for children and other family members
- Finances—monthly bills, loan payments, mortgages, hospital bills, doctor bills
- House, lawn, and garden
- Pets
- Plants

Patient Information

The doctor explains the need for surgery to the patient and family. They are told about:

- The surgical procedure, risks, and possible complications
- The risks from not having surgery
- Who will do the surgery
- The date and time of the surgery
- How long the surgery will take
  Questions are answered. Misunderstandings are cleared up. Care instructions are given.

After surgery, the doctor talks to the patient and family. The doctor decides what and when to tell them. Often the health team knows the results before the person.

See *Focus on Communication: Patient Information.*

FOCUS ON COMMUNICATION
Patient Information

Patients and families are anxious to know the results. They may ask you what the reports say. Refer such questions to the nurse. You never tell any results or diagnoses. You can say:
- "The doctor will tell you about the surgery and the reports. I'll tell the nurse that you are asking."
- "I'll get the nurse for you. She can answer your questions."

Your Role

You can assist in the person's psychological care. To assist in pre-operative and post-operative care:

- Listen. The person may talk about fears and concerns.
- Refer questions to the nurse.
- Explain the care you will give and why it is needed.
- Follow communication rules (Chapters 6 and 8).
- Use verbal and nonverbal communication (Chapter 8).
- Provide care with skill and ease.
- Report signs of fear or anxiety (Chapter 45).
- Report a request to see a member of the clergy.

PRE-OPERATIVE CARE

The pre-operative period may be many days or a few minutes. If time allows, the person is prepared mentally and physically for the effects of anesthesia and surgery. The goal is to prevent complications before, during, and after surgery.

See *Teamwork and Time Management: Pre-Operative Care.*

TEAMWORK AND TIME MANAGEMENT
Pre-Operative Care

The nurse has a limited amount of time for pre-operative care. Assist as directed. You must understand what to do, when to do it, and when to complete care.

The nurse may delegate several tasks to you. Tell the nurse when you complete each task. For example, the nurse asks you to assist with personal care (p. 563). Keep the nurse informed of your progress.

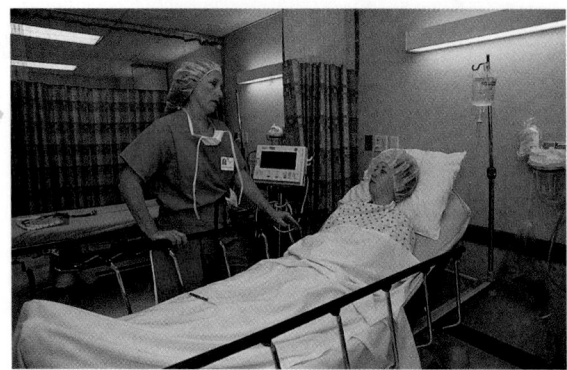

Fig. 32-1 The post anesthesia care unit (PACU).

Pre-Operative Teaching

The nurse explains what to expect before, during, and after surgery. Teaching includes:

- *Pre-operative care*—includes tests and their purpose, skin preparation, and personal care. The person learns about the purpose and effects of pre-operative drugs.
- *Deep breathing, coughing, and incentive spirometry*—are taught and practiced. After surgery, they are done every 1 or 2 hours when the person is awake. See Chapter 36.
- *Leg exercises*—are taught and practiced (p. 570). After surgery, they are done every 1 or 2 hours when the person is awake.
- *Post anesthesia care unit (PACU)*—is where the person wakes up after surgery (Fig. 32-1). Care given in the PACU is explained.
- *Vital signs*—are taken often until they are stable.
- *Food and fluids*—after surgery, the person is NPO (non per os; nothing by mouth) and has an IV (intravenous). The doctor orders food and oral fluids when the person's condition is stable.
- *Turning and re-positioning*—are done at least every 1 to 2 hours after surgery.
- *Early ambulation*—is done as soon as possible after surgery.
- *Pain*—relates to the type and amount of pain to expect. The nurse explains about pain-relief drugs and how they are given.
- *Treatments and equipment*—may involve a urinary catheter, NG (naso-gastric) tube, oxygen, wound suction, a cast, or traction.
- *Position restrictions*—are common after some surgeries. For example, the hip is abducted after hip replacement surgery (Chapter 41).

See *Focus on Children and Older Persons: Pre-Operative Care.*

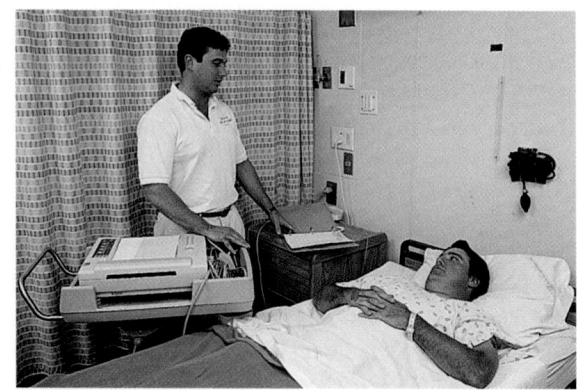

Fig. 32-2 An electrocardiogram is taken.

Special Tests

Before surgery, the doctor evaluates the person's health status. These tests are often ordered:

- Chest x-ray.
- Complete blood count (CBC).
- Urinalysis.
- Electrocardiogram (ECG; EKG). See Figure 32-2.

Other tests depend on the person's condition and surgery. For expected blood loss, the person's blood is tested for blood type and compatible blood. This is called *type and crossmatch.*

The person is prepared for the tests as needed. Test results must be on the chart by the time of surgery.

Nutrition and Fluids

A light meal usually is allowed. Then the person is NPO for 6 to 8 hours before surgery. These measures reduce the risk of vomiting and aspiration during anesthesia and after surgery. An NPO sign is placed in the person's room. The water pitcher and cup are removed.

Bowel Elimination

Bowel surgeries may require a *bowel prep*—cleansing the bowel of feces. Feces contain microbes. When the intestine is opened, feces can spill into the sterile abdominal cavity. The bowel prep prevents this contamination.

For the bowel prep, the doctor orders special fluids for the person to drink. Or enemas are ordered. Sometimes enemas are given to prevent constipation after surgery. The doctor orders what enema to give and when.

Urinary Elimination

The person voids before the nurse gives pre-operative drugs. If the person has a catheter, the drainage bag is emptied. The output is measured and recorded.

Often catheters are inserted in the OR. For pelvic and abdominal surgeries, the bladder must be empty. A full bladder is easily injured during surgery. Catheters also allow accurate output measurements during and after surgery.

Personal Care

Personal care before surgery involves:

- *A complete bath, shower, or tub bath.* A special soap or cleanser may be ordered. A shampoo is included. The bath and shampoo reduce the number of microbes on the body. This reduces the risk of a wound infection. A gown is worn after the bath.
- *Removing make-up, nail polish, and fake nails.* The skin, lips, and nail beds are observed for color and circulation. Observations are made during and after surgery.
- *Hair care.* All hairpins, clips, combs, and other items are removed. So are wigs and hairpieces. A surgical cap is worn to keep hair out of the face and the operative site.
- *Oral hygiene.* Being NPO causes thirst and a dry mouth. The person must not swallow any water during oral hygiene.
- *Removing dentures.* Provide denture care. Then store dentures following agency policy. Some people do not like being seen without their dentures. Let them wear dentures as long as possible. This promotes dignity and self-esteem.
- *Removing prostheses.* Eyeglasses, contact lenses, hearing aids, artificial eyes, and artificial limbs are examples. Sometimes hearing aids are left in if the surgeon needs to talk to or instruct the patient during surgery. Follow agency policy for storage and safe-keeping.
- *Other.* Often elastic stockings are put on before transport to the OR. So are sequential compression devices. See "Elastic Stockings" on p. 570. Also see "Sequential Compression Devices" on p. 573.

See *Promoting Safety and Comfort: Personal Care.*

> **PROMOTING SAFETY AND COMFORT**
> **Personal Care**
>
> **Safety**
> Check all patients for loose teeth. Loose teeth are common in children. Adults may have loose teeth from periodontal disease (Chapter 20). Report loose teeth to the nurse. The nurse notes this on the pre-operative checklist and tells the surgery staff. A loose tooth can fall out during anesthesia. The person can aspirate the tooth.

Jewelry

Jewelry is easily lost or broken in the OR and PACU. Transfers to and from the OR, PACU, and the person's room also present safety risks. And jewelry can cause pressure injuries (Chapter 34). Therefore all jewelry is removed and stored for safe-keeping. This includes body-piercing jewelry. Record jewelry removal and storage according to agency policy.

The person may want to wear a wedding ring or religious medal. Secure the item in place with gauze and tape according to agency policy. Hand, arm, shoulder, and breast surgeries can cause swelling of the fingers. Wedding rings are removed for such surgeries.

Skin Preparation

The skin and hair contain microbes that can enter the body through the surgical incision. To reduce the risk of infection, a *skin prep* is done. The doctor orders one or more of these for the skin prep at the operative site:

- Cleansing with an anti-microbial soap. *Anti* means *against*.
- Clipping the hair at and around the site.
- Removing hair at and around the site.

The incision site and a large area around it are *prepped* (Fig. 32-3, p. 564). The prep is done in the person's room or in the OR. To remove hair, a hair cream remover is used. Or the skin is shaved.

For shaving, a *skin prep kit* is used. The kit has a razor, a sponge filled with soap, a basin, a drape, and a towel (Fig. 32-4, p. 565). Lather the skin with soap. Then shave in the direction of hair growth (Fig. 32-5, p. 565).

See *Delegation Guidelines: Skin Preparation,* p. 565.
See *Promoting Safety and Comfort: Skin Preparation,* p. 565.

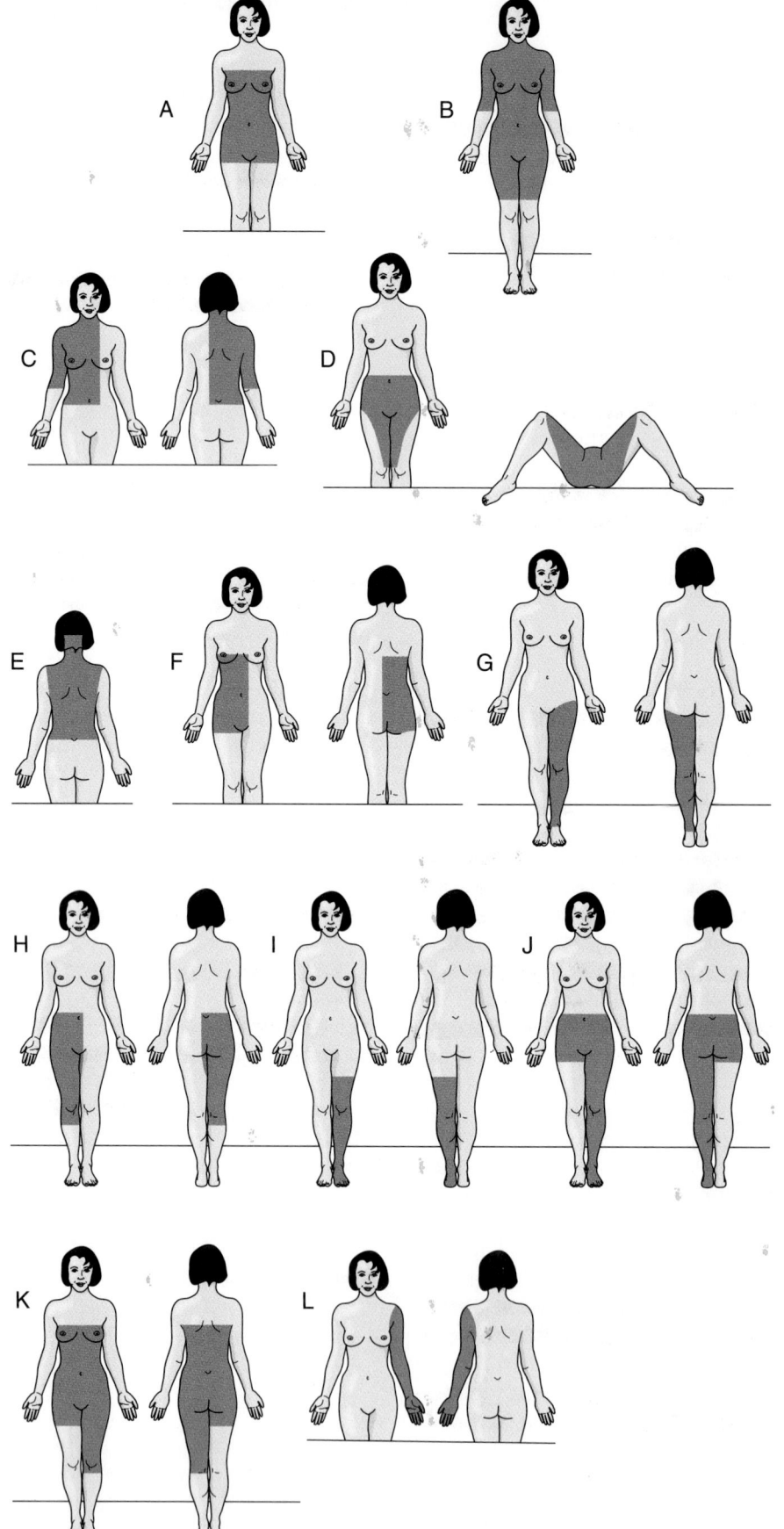

Fig. 32-3 Skin prep sites. The *shaded area* shows the area to prep. **A,** Abdominal surgery. **B,** Open-heart surgery. **C,** Chest, breast, and upper arm surgeries. **D,** Perineal surgery. **E,** Cervical spine surgery. **F,** Kidney surgery. **G,** Knee surgery. **H,** Hip and thigh surgery. **I,** Lower leg and foot surgery. **J,** Complete lower extremity surgery. **K,** Abdominal and leg surgery. **L,** Elbow and lower arm surgeries.

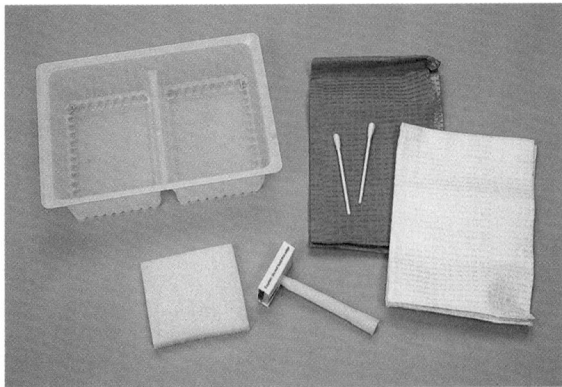

Fig. 32-4 Skin prep kit.

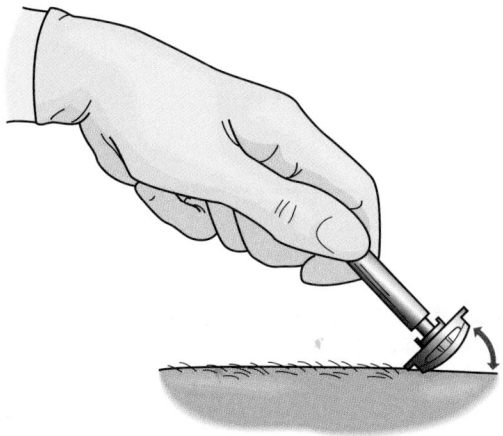

Fig. 32-5 Shave in the direction of hair growth.

THE SURGICAL SKIN PREP—SHAVING THE SKIN

QUALITY OF LIFE

Remember to:
- Knock before entering the person's room.
- Address the person by name.
- Introduce yourself by name and title.

- Explain the procedure to the person before beginning and during the procedure.
- Protect the person's rights during the procedure.
- Handle the person gently during the procedure.

PRE-PROCEDURE

1 Follow *Delegation Guidelines: Skin Preparation.* See *Promoting Safety and Comfort: Skin Preparation.*
2 Practice hand hygiene.
3 Collect the following:
- Skin prep kit
- Bath blanket
- Warm water

- Gloves
- Waterproof pad
- Bath towel
4 Identify the person. Check the identification (ID) bracelet against the assignment sheet. Also call the person by name.
5 Provide for privacy.

PROCEDURE

6 Make sure you have good lighting.
7 Raise the bed for body mechanics. Lower the bed rail near you (if up).

8 Cover the person with a bath blanket. Fan-fold top linens to the foot of the bed.
9 Place the waterproof pad under the area you will shave.

Continued

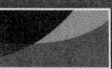

THE SURGICAL SKIN PREP—SHAVING THE SKIN—cont'd

PROCEDURE—cont'd

10 Open the skin prep kit.
11 Position the person for the skin prep.
12 Drape him or her with the drape.
13 Add warm water to the basin. Bed rails (if used) are up before you leave the bedside.
14 Put on the gloves.
15 Lather the skin with the sponge.
16 Hold the skin taut. Shave in the direction of hair growth (see Fig. 32-5).

17 Shave outward from the center using short strokes.
18 Rinse the razor often.
19 Make sure the entire area is free of hair. Check for cuts, scratches, or nicks.
20 Rinse the skin thoroughly. Pat dry.
21 Remove the drape and waterproof pad.
22 Remove and discard the gloves. Practice hand hygiene.
23 Return top linens. Remove the bath blanket.

POST-PROCEDURE

24 Provide for comfort. (See the inside of the front book cover.)
25 Place the signal light within reach.
26 Lower the bed to its lowest position. Lock the bed wheels.
27 Raise or lower bed rails. Follow the care plan.
28 Unscreen the person.

29 Return equipment to its proper place.
30 Discard supplies.
31 Complete a safety check of the room. (See the inside of the front book cover.)
32 Follow agency policy for dirty linen.
33 Practice hand hygiene.

The Surgery Consent

The person's consent is needed before surgery is done. A surgical consent is signed when the person understands the information given by the doctor. The person's spouse or nearest relative may be required to sign the consent. A parent or legal representative signs for a minor child. The legal representative signs for a person who is not mentally competent to sign.

The doctor is responsible for securing the written consent. Often this is delegated to an RN. *You do not obtain the person's written consent for surgery.*

The Pre-Operative Checklist

A pre-operative checklist (Fig. 32-6) is completed before surgery. The nurse may ask you to do some things on the list. Promptly report when you complete each task. Also report any observations. The checklist is completed before the nurse gives pre-operative drugs.

Marking the Surgical Site. The doctor marks the surgical site before the surgery. Sometimes the person marks the surgical site. Marking the site prevents surgery on the wrong body part or area.

Site marking may be part of the pre-operative checklist. It is done before the pre-operative drugs are given.

Pre-Operative Drugs

Pre-operative drugs are given before the person is transported to the OR. They are given to:
• Help the person relax and feel drowsy.

• Reduce respiratory secretions to prevent aspiration. A dry mouth also results.
• Prevent nausea and vomiting.

The person feels sleepy and light-headed. Falls and accidents are prevented after the drugs are given. Bed rails are raised. The person is not allowed out of bed. Therefore the person voids before the drugs are given. After they are given, the person uses the bedpan or urinal to void.

After the drugs are given, move furniture to make room for the stretcher. Also clean off the overbed table and the bedside stand. This prevents damage to equipment and valuables.

Transport to the Operating Room

An OR staff member brings a stretcher to the room. Identification checks are made. Then the patient is transferred to the stretcher and covered with a bath blanket. The blanket provides warmth and prevents exposure. Falls are prevented. Safety straps are secured and the side rails are raised. If allowed, a pillow is placed under the person's head for comfort.

The person's chart is given to the OR staff member. The person is transported to the OR. The family may be allowed to go as far as the OR entrance.

See *Focus on Children and Older Persons: Transport to the Operating Room.*

SURGICAL CHECK LIST

Patient's Name   Room

PATIENT STICKER ↑

I.D. Band on	
Surgical Permit Signed	
History & Physical	
Allergies	
Operative Area Prepped	
Pre-op Enema (if ordered)	
NPO after midnight	
Blood Work Done	
Urinalysis	
UCG on females age 12-50	
BP and TRP taken	
Voided and catheterized	
Jewelry removed and secured	
Hairpins, make up and nail polish removed	
Contact lenses and glasses removed	
Dentures removed	
Head cap and gown	
Premedication of _____	
_____	
_____	
Time given _____	
Date _____ Nurse _____	

IV20064   ©2005 133090 LKCS • www.lk-cs.com

Fig. 32-6 Pre-operative checklist.

FOCUS ON CHILDREN AND OLDER PERSONS

Transport to the Operating Room

Children

Some agencies allow a parent to be with the child while anesthesia is given. The parent stays in the OR until the child is asleep.

SEDATION AND ANESTHESIA

Some procedures only require sedation. *Sedation is a state of quiet, calmness, or sleep produced by a drug.* There are different levels of sedation—minimal, moderate (conscious), and deep.

Anesthesia is the loss of feeling or sensation produced by a drug.

- *General anesthesia is the loss of consciousness and all feeling or sensation.* A drug is given IV, or a gas is inhaled.
- *Regional anesthesia is the loss of feeling or sensation in a large area of the body.* The person is awake. A drug is injected into a body part.
- *Local anesthesia is the loss of feeling or sensation in a small area.* A drug is injected at the site.

Sedation and anesthesia are given by specially trained doctors and nurses. An *anesthesiologist* is a doctor who specializes in giving anesthetics. An *anesthetist* is an RN with advanced study in giving anesthetics.

POST-OPERATIVE CARE

After surgery the person is taken to the PACU. There the person recovers from the anesthesia. This takes 1 to 2 hours. The person is watched very closely. Vital signs are taken and observations are made often. The doctor allows the person to be transported to his or her room when:

- Vital signs are stable.
- Respiratory function is good.
- The person can respond and call for help.

Preparing the Person's Room

The room must be ready for the person. After the person is transported to the OR, you can:

- Make a surgical bed. Lower the bed rails and raise the bed to its highest position.
- Place equipment and supplies in the room:
  - Thermometer
  - Stethoscope
  - Sphygmomanometer
  - Kidney basin
  - Tissues
  - Waterproof bed protector
  - Vital signs flow sheet
  - I&O (intake and output) record
  - IV pole
  - Other items as directed by the nurse
- Move furniture out of the way for the stretcher.

Return From the PACU

The PACU staff calls the nursing unit when the person is ready for transfer. The transport is done by PACU nurses. A nurse meets them and the patient in the person's room. Then the person is transferred from the stretcher to bed. Assist as needed. Also help position the person.

Vital signs are measured and observations made. They are compared with those taken in the PACU. The nurse checks the incision for bleeding. Catheter, IV, and other tube placements and functions are checked. Bed rails are raised. The signal light is placed within the person's reach. Necessary care and treatments are given. Then the family can be with the person.

Measurements and Observations

Your role in post-operative care depends on the person's condition. Often you will measure vital signs and pulse oximetry and observe the person's condition:

- Every 15 minutes until the person's condition is stable
- Every 30 minutes for 1 to 2 hours
- Every hour for 4 hours
- Then every 4 hours

The nurse tells you how often to check the person. Many serious complications can result from surgery (Box 32-2). Be alert for the signs and symptoms in Box 32-2. Report them to the nurse at once.

| **BOX 32-2** | **POST-OPERATIVE COMPLICATIONS AND OBSERVATIONS** |

Complications
- Respiratory System
  - Pneumonia—an inflammation and infection of lung tissue
  - Atelectasis—the collapse of a portion of the lung
  - Pulmonary embolism—a blood clot from a vein that travels (embolus) in the bloodstream until it lodges in a lung
- Circulatory System
  - Hypovolemia—inadequate (hypo) amount (vol) of blood (emia)
  - Hemorrhage—the excessive loss (rrhage) of blood (hemo) in a short time
  - Hypovolemic shock—when organs and tissues do not get enough blood (shock) because of an inadequate (hypo) amount (vol) of blood (emia)
  - Thrombophlebitis—a blood clot (thrombo) causing inflammation (itis) of a vein (phleb)
  - Thrombus—a blood clot
  - Embolus—a blood clot that travels through the bloodstream until it lodges in a blood vessel
- Urinary System
  - Urinary retention—urine collects (retention) in the bladder from not being able to void
  - Urinary tract infection—inflammation and infection of the urinary structures (bladder, ureters, urethra)
- Gastro-Intestinal System
  - Nausea
  - Vomiting
  - Constipation
  - Flatulence
  - Post-operative ileus—the absence of normal intestinal (ileus) function from the lack of peristalsis after surgery
- Wound (Chapter 33)
  - Infection
  - Dehiscence—the separation of wound layers
  - Evisceration—the separation of the wound along with the protrusion of abdominal organs

Observations
- Abdominal: distention (swelling), pain
- Aching
- Anxiety
- Bleeding: from the incision, drainage tubes, suction tubes, or other sites
- Blood pressure: an increase or decrease
- Chest pain
- Choking
- Condition: any change in
- Confusion

Observations—cont'd
- Cough: weak
- Cramping: abdominal
- Discomfort in a leg
- Disorientation
- Drainage:
  - On or under dressings
  - On bed linens (including bottom linens and pillowcases)
  - Appearance from urinary catheter, NG tube, wound suction, and other tubes
- Hypoxia (Chapter 36)
- Intake and output
- IV flow rate
- Nausea
- Pain
- Pulse:
  - More than 100 beats per minute
  - Less than 60 beats per minute
  - Weak
  - Irregular
- Pulse oximetry measurement (Chapter 36)
- Respirations:
  - Shallow, slow breathing
  - Rapid
  - Gasping
  - Difficult (dyspnea)
  - Shortness of breath
  - Moist-sounding
  - Gurgling
- Restlessness
- Skin:
  - Moist or clammy
  - Pale (pallor)
  - Cyanosis (bluish color)
  - Cool
  - Warm or hot
- Sputum: clear, white, yellow, green, brown, or red; thick, watery, or frothy (with bubbles)
- Swelling in affected area
- Temperature: an increase or decrease
- Thirst
- Urinary complaints: inability to void, burning, urgency, lower abdominal pain
- Urine: amount, character, and time of first voiding after surgery
- Vomiting
- Wound drainage (Chapter 33)

Positioning

The person is positioned for comfort and to prevent complications. Depending on the surgery, position restrictions may be ordered. The person is usually positioned:

- For easy and comfortable breathing
- To prevent stress on the incision
- To prevent aspiration

When supine, the head of the bed is usually raised slightly. The person's head may be turned to the side.

The person is re-positioned at least every 1 to 2 hours. This prevents respiratory and circulatory complications. Turning may be painful. Provide support. Use smooth, gentle motions. Place pillows and positioning devices as the nurse directs (Chapters 16 and 27).

The nurse tells you when to re-position the person and the positions allowed. Usually you assist the nurse. The nurse may delegate these tasks when the person's condition is stable and care is simple.

See *Focus on Children and Older Persons: Positioning.*

Preventing Respiratory and Circulatory Complications

Coughing and deep breathing exercises help prevent respiratory complications (see Box 32-2). So does incentive spirometry. See Chapter 36.

Circulation must be stimulated for blood flow in the legs. If blood flow is sluggish, blood clots may form. They can form in the deep leg veins in the lower leg or thigh (Fig. 32-7, A). Many people do not have signs or symptoms. Report the following at once:

- Swollen area of a leg.
- Pain or tenderness in a leg. This may occur only when standing or walking.
- Warmth in the part of the leg that is swollen or painful.
- Red or discolored skin.

A blood clot (thrombus) can break loose and travel through the bloodstream. It then becomes an embolus. An *embolus is a blood clot that travels through the vascular system until it lodges in a blood vessel* (Fig. 32-7, B). An embolus from a vein lodges in the lungs (pulmonary embolism). A pulmonary embolus can cause severe respiratory problems and death. Report chest pain or shortness of breath at once.

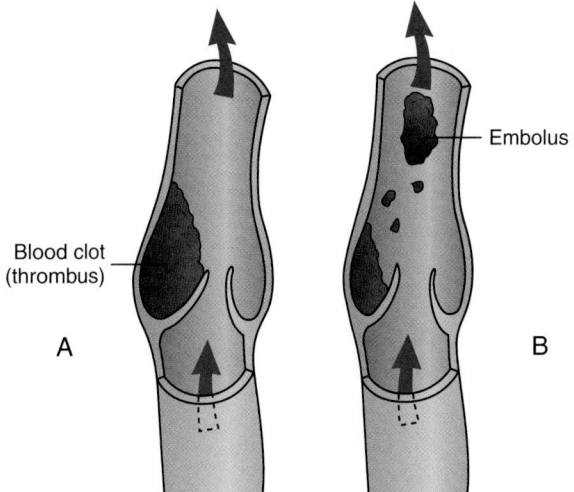

Fig. 32-7 A, A blood clot is attached to the wall of a vein. The arrow shows the direction of blood flow. **B,** Part of the thrombus breaks off and becomes an embolus. The embolus travels in the bloodstream until it lodges in a distant vessel.

After surgery, circulation is stimulated and thrombi prevented by:

- Leg exercises
- Ambulation as soon as possible
- Elastic stockings
- Elastic bandages
- Sequential compression devices (p. 573)
- No prolonged standing or sitting

See *Focus on Children and Older Persons: Preventing Respiratory and Circulatory Complications.*
See *Promoting Safety and Comfort: Preventing Respiratory and Circulatory Complications.*

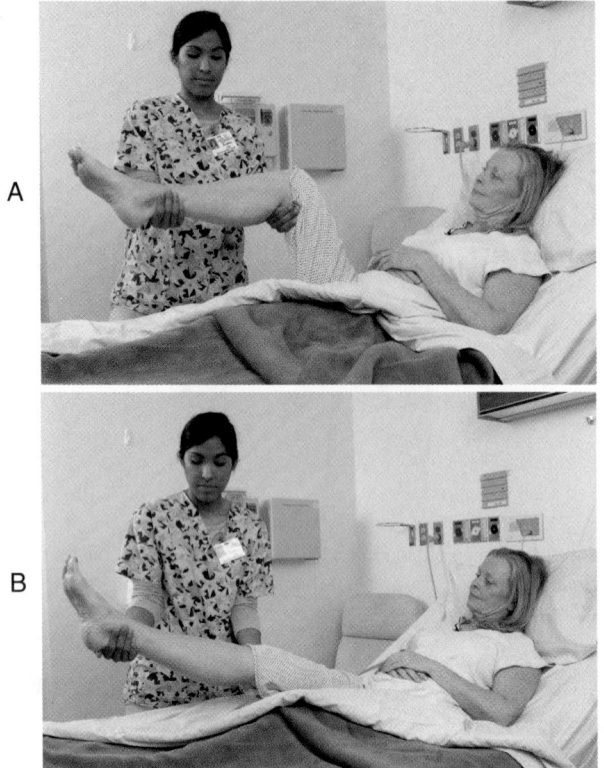

Fig. 32-8 Leg exercises to stimulate circulation. **A,** The knee is flexed and then extended. **B,** The leg is raised and lowered.

Stockings come in thigh-high and knee-high lengths. The nurse measures the person for the correct size. Most stockings have an opening near the toes. The opening is used to check circulation, skin color, and skin temperature.

The person usually has two pairs of stockings. Wash one pair while the other pair is worn. Wash them by hand with a mild soap. Hang them to dry.

See *Delegation Guidelines: Elastic Stockings.*

See *Promoting Safety and Comfort: Elastic Stockings.*

DELEGATION GUIDELINES
Elastic Stockings

To apply elastic stockings, you need this information from the nurse and the care plan:

- What size to use—small, medium, large, extra-large, or bariatric
- What length to use—thigh-high or knee-high
- When to remove them and for how long—usually every 8 hours for 30 minutes
- What observations to report and record:
  - The size and length of stockings applied
  - When you applied the stockings
  - Skin color and temperature
  - Leg and foot swelling
  - Skin tears, wounds, or signs of skin breakdown
  - Complaints of pain, tingling, or numbness
  - When you removed the stockings and for how long
  - When you re-applied the stockings
  - When you washed the stockings
- When to report observations
- What patient or resident concerns to report at once

Leg Exercises. Leg exercises increase venous blood flow and help prevent thrombi. After leg surgery, a doctor's order is needed for the exercises.

The nurse tells you when to do the exercises. They are done at least every 1 or 2 hours while the person is awake. Assist if the person is weak. These exercises are done 5 times:

- Make circles with the toes. This rotates the ankles.
- Dorsiflex and plantar flex the feet (Chapter 27).
- Flex and extend one knee and then the other (Fig. 32-8, A).
- Raise and lower the leg off the bed (Fig. 32-8, B). Repeat with the other leg.

Elastic Stockings. Elastic stockings exert pressure on the veins. The pressure promotes venous blood return to the heart. The stockings help prevent blood clots in leg veins. Elastic stockings also are called AE stockings (AE means *anti-embolism* or *anti-embolic*). They also are called TED hose (TED means *thrombo-embolic disease*). Persons at risk for thrombi include those who:

- Have heart and circulatory disorders.
- Are on bedrest.
- Have had surgery.
- Are older.
- Are pregnant.

PROMOTING SAFETY AND COMFORT
Elastic Stockings

Safety

Apply the stocking so the toe opening is over the top of the toes or under the toes. Follow the manufacturer's instructions. Use the opening to check circulation, skin color, and skin temperature in the toes.

Stockings should not have twists, creases, or wrinkles after you apply them. Twists can affect circulation. So can stockings that roll or bunch up. Creases and wrinkles can cause skin breakdown.

Loose stockings do not promote venous blood return to the heart. Stockings that are too tight can affect circulation. Tell the nurse if the stockings are too loose or too tight.

Comfort

Apply stockings before the person gets out of bed. Otherwise the person's legs can swell from sitting or standing. Stockings are hard to put on when the legs are swollen. The person lies in bed while they are off. This prevents the legs from swelling.

Gently handle and move the person's foot and leg. Do not force the joints (toes, foot, ankle, knee, and hip) beyond their range of motion or to the point of pain.

APPLYING ELASTIC STOCKINGS

QUALITY OF LIFE

Remember to:
- Knock before entering the person's room.
- Address the person by name.
- Introduce yourself by name and title.

- Explain the procedure to the person before beginning and during the procedure.
- Protect the person's rights during the procedure.
- Handle the person gently during the procedure.

PRE-PROCEDURE

1 Follow *Delegation Guidelines: Elastic Stockings.* See *Promoting Safety and Comfort: Elastic Stockings.*
2 Practice hand hygiene.
3 Obtain elastic stockings in the correct size and length. Note the location of the toe opening.

4 Identify the person. Check the ID bracelet against the assignment sheet. Also call the person by name.
5 Provide for privacy.
6 Raise the bed for body mechanics. Bed rails are up if used.

PROCEDURE

7 Lower the bed rail near you if up.
8 Position the person supine.
9 Expose the legs. Fan-fold top linens toward the thighs.
10 Turn the stocking inside out down to the heel.
11 Slip the foot of the stocking over the toes, foot, and heel (Fig. 32-9, A). Make sure the heel pocket is properly positioned on the person's heel. The toe opening is over or under the toes.

12 Grasp the stocking top. Pull the stocking up the leg. It turns right side out as it is pulled up. The stocking is even and snug (Fig. 32-9, B).
13 Remove twists, creases, or wrinkles.
14 Repeat steps 10 through 13 for the other leg.

POST-PROCEDURE

15 Cover the person.
16 Provide for comfort. (See the inside of the front book cover.)
17 Place the signal light within reach.
18 Lower the bed to its lowest position.
19 Raise or lower bed rails. Follow the care plan.

20 Unscreen the person.
21 Complete a safety check of the room. (See the inside of the front book cover.)
22 Practice hand hygiene.
23 Report and record your observations.

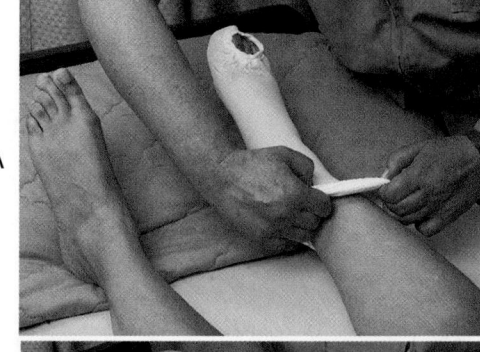

A

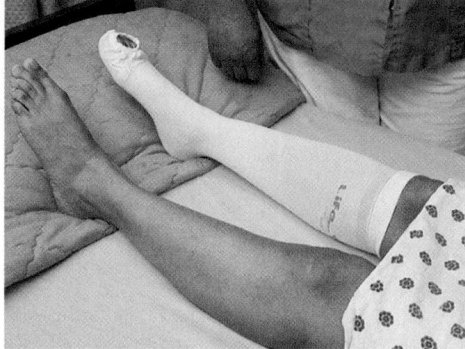

B

Fig. 32-9 Applying elastic stockings. **A,** The stocking is slipped over the toes, foot, and heel. **B,** The stocking turns right side out as it is pulled up over the leg. The heel is positioned in the heel pocket of the stocking.

Elastic Bandages. Elastic bandages have the same purposes as elastic stockings. They provide support and reduce swelling from injuries. Sometimes they are used to hold dressings in place. They are applied to arms and legs. When applying bandages:
- Use the correct size—length and width.
- Position the person in good alignment.
- Face the person during the procedure.
- Start at the lower *(distal)* part of the extremity. Work upward to the top *(proximal)* part.
- Expose fingers or toes if possible. This allows circulation checks.
- Apply the bandage with firm, even pressure.
- Check the color and temperature of the extremity every hour.
- Re-apply a loose or wrinkled bandage.
- Replace a moist or soiled bandage.
  See *Focus on Communication: Elastic Bandages,* p. 572.
  See *Delegation Guidelines: Elastic Bandages,* p. 572.
  See *Promoting Safety and Comfort: Elastic Bandages,* p. 572.

FOCUS ON COMMUNICATION
Elastic Bandages

Elastic bandages should promote comfort. To check for comfort, you can ask:
- "Does the bandage feel too tight?"
- "Do you feel pain, itching, tingling, or numbness?" If yes: "What do you feel?" "Where do you feel it?"

DELEGATION GUIDELINES
Elastic Bandages

To apply elastic bandages, you need this information from the nurse and the care plan:
- Where to apply the bandage
- What width and length to use
- When to remove the bandage and for how long—usually every 8 hours for 30 minutes
- What to do if the bandage is wet or soiled
- What observations to report and record:
  - The width and length applied
  - When you applied the bandage
  - Skin color and temperature
  - Swelling of the part
  - Skin tears, wounds, or signs of skin breakdown
  - Complaints of pain, itching, tingling, or numbness
  - When you removed the bandage and for how long
  - When you re-applied the bandage
- When to report observations
- What patient or resident concerns to report at once

PROMOTING SAFETY AND COMFORT
Elastic Bandages

Safety

Elastic bandages must be firm and snug, but not tight. A tight bandage can affect circulation.

Bandages are secured in place with clips, tape, or Velcro. Clips are made of metal or plastic. Clips can injure the skin if they become loose, fall off, or cause pressure. Use clips only if the nurse tells you to. Check the bandage often to make sure the clips are correctly in place.

Some agencies do not allow you to apply elastic bandages. Know your agency's policy.

Comfort

A tight bandage can cause pain and discomfort. Apply it with firm, even pressure. If the person complains of pain, tingling, or numbness, remove the bandage. Tell the nurse at once.

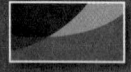 **APPLYING ELASTIC BANDAGES**

QUALITY OF LIFE

Remember to:
- Knock before entering the person's room.
- Address the person by name.
- Introduce yourself by name and title.

- Explain the procedure to the person before beginning and during the procedure.
- Protect the person's rights during the procedure.
- Handle the person gently during the procedure.

PRE-PROCEDURE

1. Follow *Delegation Guidelines: Elastic Bandages*. See *Promoting Safety and Comfort: Elastic Bandages*.
2. Practice hand hygiene.
3. Collect the following:
   - Elastic bandage as directed by the nurse
   - Tape or clips (unless the bandage has Velcro)
4. Identify the person. Check the ID bracelet against the assignment sheet. Also call the person by name.
5. Provide for privacy.
6. Raise the bed for body mechanics. Bed rails are up if used.

PROCEDURE

7. Lower the bed rail near you if up.
8. Help the person to a comfortable position. Expose the part you will bandage.
9. Make sure the area is clean and dry.
10. Hold the bandage so the roll is up. The loose end is on the bottom (Fig. 32-10, A).
11. Apply the bandage to the smallest part of the wrist, foot, ankle, or knee.

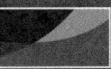

APPLYING ELASTIC BANDAGES—cont'd

PROCEDURE—cont'd

12 Make two circular turns around the part (Fig. 32-10, B).
13 Make overlapping spiral turns in an upward direction. Each turn overlaps about ½ to ⅔ of the previous turn (Fig. 32-10, C). Each overlap is equal.
14 Apply the bandage smoothly with firm, even pressure. It is not tight.
15 End the bandage with two circular turns.

16 Secure the bandage in place with Velcro, tape, or clips. Clips are not under the body part.
17 Check the fingers or toes for coldness or cyanosis (bluish color). Ask about pain, itching, numbness, or tingling. Remove the bandage if any are noted. Report your observations.

POST-PROCEDURE

18 Provide for comfort. (See the inside of the front book cover.)
19 Place the signal light within reach.
20 Lower the bed to its lowest position.
21 Raise or lower bed rails. Follow the care plan.

22 Unscreen the person.
23 Complete a safety check of the room. (See the inside of the front book cover.)
24 Practice hand hygiene.
25 Report and record your observations.

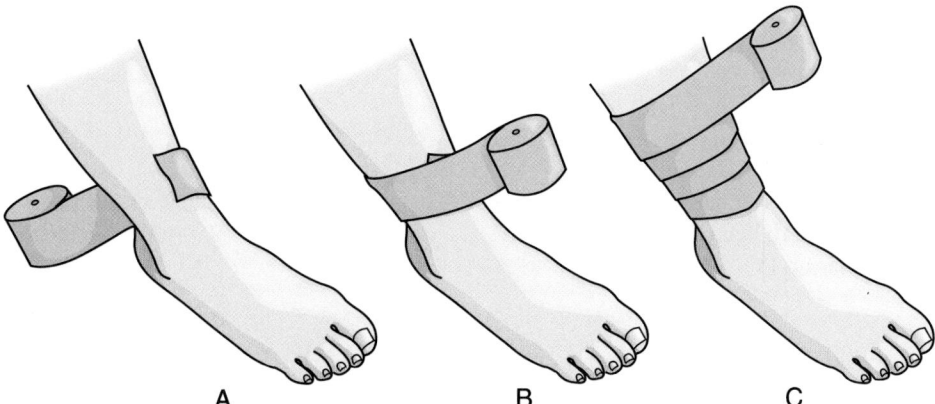

A   B   C

Fig. 32-10 Applying an elastic bandage. **A,** The roll of the bandage is up. The loose end is at the bottom. **B,** The bandage is applied to the smallest part with two circular turns. **C,** The bandage is applied with spiral turns in an upward direction.

Sequential Compression Devices. A sequential compression device (SCD) is a sleeve that wraps around the leg (Fig. 32-11). Made of cloth or plastic, the SCD is secured in place with Velcro.

The device is attached to a pump. The pump inflates the device with air. This promotes venous blood flow to the heart by causing pressure on the veins. Then the pump deflates the device.

SCDs are applied to both legs. After one side deflates, the other inflates. Applied pre-operatively, SCDs are worn post-operatively until the doctor orders their removal.

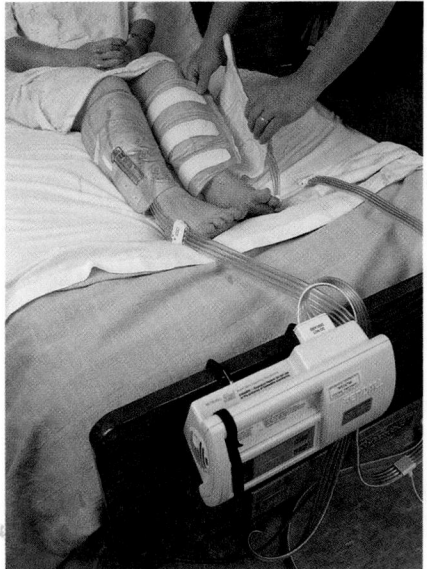

Fig. 32-11 Sequential compression device.

Early Ambulation

Early ambulation prevents complications such as thrombi, pneumonia, atelectasis, constipation, and urinary tract infections. The person usually walks the day of surgery. The person dangles (sits on the side of the bed) first. Blood pressure and pulse are measured. If they are stable, the person is assisted out of bed. The person does not walk very far, just in the room or into the hallway. Distance increases as the person gains strength.

The nurse tells you when the person can walk and how far to go. Usually you assist the nurse the first time.

Wound Healing

The incision needs protection. Healing is promoted and infection prevented. A dressing may be over the incision. Sterile dressing changes are done by the doctor or nurse. Your agency may let you do simple dressing changes. See Chapter 33 for wound care.

Nutrition and Fluids

The person returns from the OR with an IV. Continued IV therapy depends on the type of surgery and the person's condition. Anesthesia may cause nausea and vomiting. Diet progresses from NPO to clear liquids, to full liquids, to a regular diet. The doctor orders the diet. Frequent oral hygiene is important when the person is NPO.

Some patients have NG tubes (Chapter 25). Often the NG tube is attached to suction to keep the stomach empty. The person is NPO and has an IV.

Elimination

Anesthesia, the surgery, and being NPO affect normal bowel and urinary elimination. Pain-relief drugs can cause constipation. Provide measures to promote elimination as directed by the nurse and the care plan (Chapters 22 and 23).

Intake and output are measured. The person must void within 8 hours after surgery. Report the time and amount of the first voiding. If the person does not void within 8 hours, a catheter may be needed. Some patients have a catheter after surgery. See "Catheters" in Chapter 22.

Fluid intake and regular diet are needed for bowel elimination. Suppositories or enemas may be ordered for constipation.

Comfort and Rest

Pain is common after surgery. The degree of pain depends on:

- The extent of the surgery.
- The incision site and size.
- If drainage tubes, casts, or other devices are present.
- Positioning during surgery. The position can cause muscle strains and discomfort.

The doctor orders drugs for pain relief. The nurse uses the nursing process to promote comfort and rest. Many of the measures listed in Chapter 28 are part of the person's care plan.

Personal Hygiene

Personal hygiene is important for physical and mental well-being. Wound drainage and skin prep solutions can irritate the skin and cause discomfort. NPO causes a dry mouth and breath odors. Moist, clammy skin from blood pressure changes or fever also causes discomfort.

Frequent oral hygiene, hair care, and a complete bed bath after surgery help refresh and renew the person. The gown and linens are changed whenever wet or soiled.

FOCUS ON PRIDE

The Person, Family, and Yourself

Personal and Professional Responsibility

Surgery is a stressful time. The person can have many worries and fears. See Box 32-1. Imagine yourself in the person's situation. What if you needed surgery? Would you worry about pain or death? What if you are not able to function the same after surgery? Who will care for your children and home? Will you be able to support your family? Imagine having an accident. You wake up hours later. You are told that your right leg was amputated.

The person's fears and concerns are important. You can either ease worries or increase stress. Take time to listen. Avoid seeming rushed. Act professionally. Take pride in showing that you care.

Rights and Respect

Before surgery, the person will have many questions. The doctor and nurse explain what to expect before, during, and after surgery. Often the person is nervous and worried during pre-operative teaching. The person or family may forget to ask a question. Or they may need something explained again.

The person has the right to accurate and complete information. The person's questions are important. The person or family may ask you questions. You can answer questions that relate to the care you provide. If you do not know or are unsure of an answer, tell the person or family that you will notify the nurse. Some questions are best answered by the nurse. For example, "How long will the surgery last?" or "What will be done to relieve my pain after surgery?" Even if you think you know the answer, tell the person or family that you will ask the nurse to answer the question. Show good judgment. Only answer questions within the scope of your role.

Independence and Social Interaction

Some people prefer to be alone before and after surgery. The peaceful and quiet setting allows them to relax. Others want family and friends around. They like the support, and the conversation distracts from worries and pain. Each person is different. Ask the person which he or she prefers. Tell the nurse. The nurse can talk with the family about the person's wishes and needs.

Delegation and Teamwork

Post-operative observation is a critical time. You may be delegated parts of post-operative care. For example, you are asked to monitor vital signs every 15 minutes for an hour, then every 30 minutes for an hour, then hourly for 4 hours. Vital signs must be checked and reported or recorded promptly, as ordered. Delays risk missing critical changes early.

The patient and nurse rely on you. Complete post-operative vital signs on time. Report abnormal values, sudden changes, and any concerns to the nurse at once. Take pride in your role in post-operative care. You can make a difference in the safety and quality of the person's care.

Ethics and Laws

The pre-operative checklist contains items that must be completed before surgery. Some tasks are done by the nurse. Others you can do. See Figure 32-6. Know which tasks you are responsible for and which the nurse must do. For example, you do not obtain written consent for surgery or mark the person's surgical site.

Always follow agency policy and the limits of your role. Never accept a task outside those limits. You can lose your job or your ability to work as a nursing assistant. Take pride in safely assisting with pre-operative care by only performing the tasks you are trained and allowed to do.

REVIEW QUESTIONS

Circle the BEST answer.

1 Which is true of elective surgery?
  a It is done at once.
  b The need is sudden and not expected.
  c It is scheduled at a later date.
  d General anesthesia is always used.

2 A person states, "I'm afraid of the surgery." What should you do?
  a Call a member of the clergy.
  b Listen and use touch.
  c Change the subject.
  d Tell the family.

3 You can assist with pre-operative care by explaining
  a The reason for the surgery
  b The procedures you are doing
  c The risks and possible complications of surgery
  d What to expect during and after surgery

4 Before surgery, a person is
  a NPO
  b Allowed only water
  c Given a regular breakfast
  d Given a tube feeding

5 A bowel prep is ordered to
  a Clean the intestines of feces
  b Prevent bleeding
  c Relieve flatus
  d Prevent pain

6 A skin prep is done to
  a Completely bathe the body
  b Sterilize the skin
  c Reduce the amount of microbes on the skin
  d Destroy non-pathogens and pathogens

7 When shaving the skin
  a Shave in the direction opposite of hair growth
  b Shave toward the center of the operative site
  c Do not cut, scratch, or nick the skin
  d Use an electric shaver

8 Pre-operative drugs were given. The patient
  a Must stay in bed
  b Can use the bathroom
  c Can use the commode to void
  d Can have sips of water

9 General anesthesia
  a Is a specially educated nurse
  b Is the loss of consciousness and feeling or sensation
  c Is a specially educated doctor
  d Is the loss of sensation or feeling in a body part

10 Coughing and deep breathing after surgery prevent
  a Bleeding
  b A pulmonary embolus
  c Respiratory complications
  d Pain and discomfort

11 Leg exercises are ordered. Which is *false?*
  a They stimulate circulation.
  b They prevent thrombi.
  c They are done 5 times every 1 to 2 hours.
  d They are done only for leg surgery.

12 After surgery, a person's position is changed at least
  a Every 2 hours   c Every 4 hours
  b Every 3 hours   d Every shift

13 Elastic stockings
  a Hold dressings in place
  b Prevent blood clots
  c Reduce swelling after injury
  d Prevent pressure ulcers

14 Elastic stockings are applied
  a Before the person gets out of bed
  b When the person is standing
  c After the person's shower or bath
  d For 30 minutes and then removed

15 The purpose of an elastic bandage is to
  a Prevent infection
  b Absorb drainage
  c Provide moisture for wound healing
  d Reduce swelling

16 When applying an elastic bandage
  a Position the part in good alignment
  b Cover the fingers or toes if possible
  c Apply it from the large to small part of the extremity
  d Apply it from the upper to lower part of the extremity

Circle T if the statement is TRUE or F if it is FALSE.

17 T F Pins, clips, or combs are used to keep the hair out of the face.
18 T F Nail polish is removed before surgery.
19 T F Make-up can be worn to the OR.
20 T F Pajamas are worn to the OR.
21 T F Contact lenses are removed in the OR.
22 T F A surgical bed is made for the person's return from the PACU.
23 T F A decrease in blood pressure is reported at once.
24 T F The person walks for the first time 2 days after surgery.
25 T F Intake and output are measured after surgery.
26 T F The person should void within 8 hours after surgery.

Answers to these questions are on p. 834.

33 Wound Care

OBJECTIVES

- Define the key terms and key abbreviations listed in this chapter.
- Describe skin tears, circulatory ulcers, and diabetic foot ulcers.
- Identify the persons at risk for skin tears, circulatory ulcers, and diabetic foot ulcers.
- Explain how to assist in preventing skin tears, circulatory ulcers, and diabetic foot ulcers.
- Describe the process and complications of wound healing.
- Describe what to observe about wounds.
- Explain how to secure dressings.
- Explain the rules for applying dressings.
- Explain the purpose of binders and how to apply them.
- Describe how to meet the basic needs of persons with wounds.
- Perform the procedure described in this chapter.
- Explain how to promote PRIDE in the person, the family, and yourself.

KEY TERMS

abrasion A partial-thickness wound caused by the scraping away or rubbing of the skin

arterial ulcer An open wound on the lower legs or feet caused by poor arterial blood flow

chronic wound A wound that does not heal easily

circulatory ulcer An open sore on the lower legs or feet caused by decreased blood flow through the arteries or veins; vascular ulcer

clean-contaminated wound Occurs from the surgical entry of the reproductive, urinary, respiratory, or gastro-intestinal system

clean wound A wound that is not infected

closed wound Tissues are injured but the skin is not broken

contaminated wound A wound with a high risk of infection

contusion A closed wound caused by a blow to the body; a bruise

dehiscence The separation of wound layers

diabetic foot ulcer An open wound on the foot caused by complications from diabetes

dirty wound See "infected wound"

edema Swelling caused by fluid collecting in tissues

evisceration The separation of the wound along with the protrusion of abdominal organs

excoriation Loss of the epidermis (top skin layer) caused by scratching or when skin rubs against skin, clothing, or other material

full-thickness wound The dermis, epidermis, and subcutaneous tissue are penetrated; muscle and bone may be involved

gangrene A condition in which there is death of tissue

hematoma A swelling (*oma*) that contains blood (*hemat*)

hemorrhage The excessive loss of blood in a short time

incision A cut produced surgically by a sharp instrument; it creates an opening into an organ or body space

infected wound A wound containing large amounts of microbes that shows signs of infection; a dirty wound

intentional wound A wound created for therapy

laceration An open wound with torn tissues and jagged edges

open wound The skin or mucous membrane is broken

partial-thickness wound The dermis and epidermis of the skin are broken

penetrating wound An open wound that breaks the skin and enters a body area, organ, or cavity

phlebitis Inflammation (*itis*) of a vein (*phleb*)

puncture wound An open wound made by a sharp object

purulent drainage Thick green, yellow, or brown drainage

sanguineous drainage Bloody (*sanguis*) drainage

serosanguineous drainage Thin, watery drainage (*sero*) that is blood-tinged (*sanguineous*)

serous drainage Clear, watery fluid (*serum*)

shock Results when tissues and organs do not get enough blood

skin tear A break or rip in the outer layers of the skin; the epidermis (top skin layer) separates from the underlying tissues

stasis ulcer See "venous ulcer"

trauma An accident or violent act that injures the skin, mucous membranes, bones, and organs

ulcer A shallow or deep crater-like sore of the skin or a mucous membrane

unintentional wound A wound resulting from trauma

vascular ulcer See "circulatory ulcer"

venous ulcer An open sore on the lower legs or feet caused by poor venous blood flow; stasis ulcer

wound A break in the skin or mucous membrane

KEY ABBREVIATIONS

GI Gastro-intestinal
ID Identification

PPE Personal protective equipment

A wound is a break in the skin or mucous membrane. Wounds commonly result from:

- Surgery.
- *Trauma—an accident or violent act that injures the skin, mucous membranes, bones, and organs.* Falls, vehicle crashes, gun shots, stabbings, human and animal bites, burns, and frostbite are examples.
- Unrelieved pressure or friction (Chapter 34).
- Decreased blood flow through the arteries or veins.
- Nerve damage.

Wound causes and types are described in Box 33-1. Infection is a major threat. Wound care involves preventing infection and further injury to the wound and nearby tissues. Blood loss and pain also are prevented.

The nurse uses the nursing process to keep the person's skin healthy. Some agencies have wound therapists or skin care teams to manage all skin problems. The team includes an RN, physical therapist, and a dietitian.

BOX 33-1   WOUND CAUSES AND TYPES

Causes

- *Abrasion—a partial-thickness wound caused by the scraping away or rubbing of the skin* (Fig. 33-1, p. 578).
- *Excoriation—loss of the epidermis (top skin layer) caused by scratching or when skin rubs against skin, clothing, or other material* (Fig. 33-2, p. 578).
- *Contusion—a closed wound caused by a blow to the body (a bruise)* (Fig. 33-3, p. 578).
- *Incision—a cut produced surgically by a sharp instrument. It creates an opening into an organ or body space* (Fig. 33-4, p. 578).
- *Laceration—an open wound with torn tissues and jagged edges* (Fig. 33-5, p. 578).
- *Penetrating wound—an open wound that breaks the skin and enters a body area, organ, or cavity* (Fig. 33-6, p. 578).
- *Puncture wound—an open wound made by a sharp object* (knife, nail, metal, wood, glass). See Figure 33-7, p. 578.
- *Ulcer—a shallow or deep crater-like sore of the skin or a mucous membrane* (p. 579).

Types

- Intentional and unintentional wounds
  - *Intentional wound—is created for therapy.* Surgical incisions are examples. So are venipunctures for starting intravenous therapy and drawing blood specimens.
  - *Unintentional wound—results from trauma.*
- Open and closed wounds
  - *Open wound—the skin or mucous membrane is broken.* Intentional and most unintentional wounds are open.
  - *Closed wound—tissues are injured but the skin is not broken.* Bruises, twists, and sprains are examples.

Types—cont'd

- Clean and dirty wounds
  - *Clean wound—is not infected.* Microbes have not entered the wound. Closed wounds are usually clean. So are intentional wounds created under surgical asepsis. The reproductive, urinary, respiratory, and gastro-intestinal (GI) systems are not entered.
  - *Clean-contaminated wound—occurs from the surgical entry of the reproductive, urinary, respiratory, or GI system.* Some or all parts of these systems are not sterile and contain normal flora.
  - *Contaminated wound—has a high risk of infection.* Unintentional wounds are usually contaminated. Contamination occurs from breaks in surgical asepsis, spillage of intestinal contents, and trauma. Tissues may show signs of inflammation.
  - *Infected wound (dirty wound)—contains large amounts of microbes and shows signs of infection.* Examples include old wounds, surgical incisions into infected areas, and trauma that ruptures the bowel.
  - *Chronic wound—does not heal easily.* Pressure ulcers and circulatory ulcers are examples.
- Partial- and full-thickness wounds (describe wound depth)
  - *Partial-thickness wound—the dermis and epidermis of the skin are broken.*
  - *Full-thickness wound—the dermis, epidermis, and subcutaneous tissue are penetrated. Muscle and bone may be involved.*

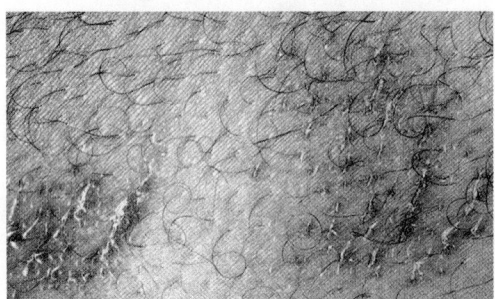

Fig. 33-1 An abrasion.

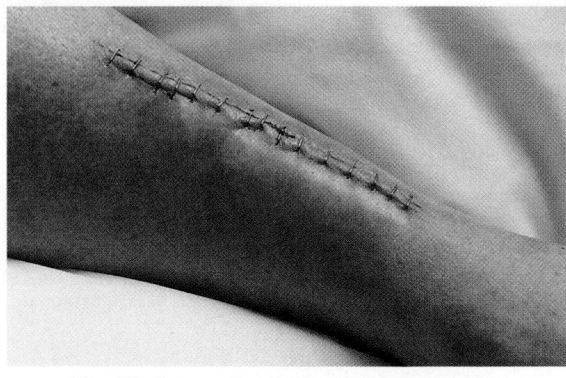

Fig. 33-4 A surgical incision closed with staples.

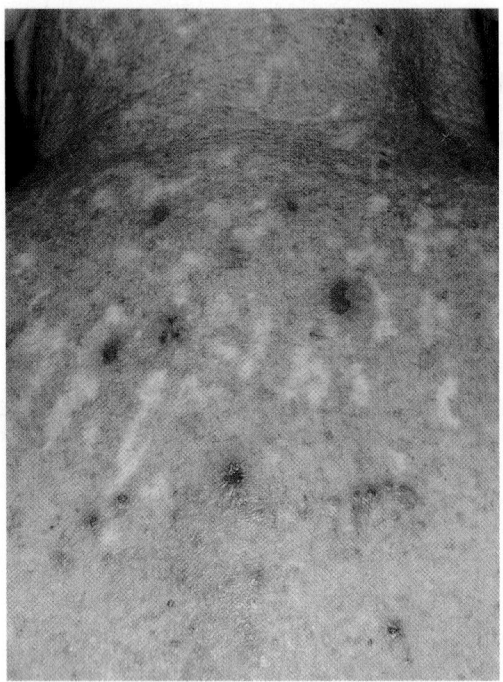

Fig. 33-2 Excoriation.

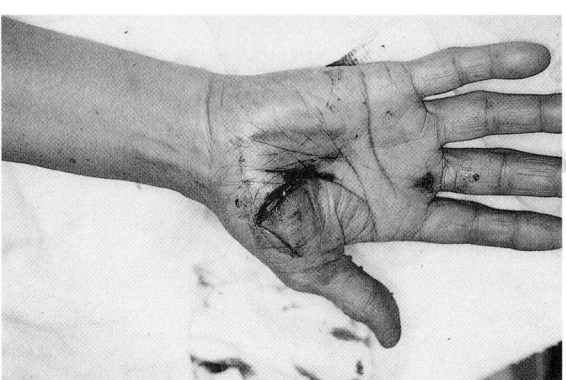

Fig. 33-5 Laceration.

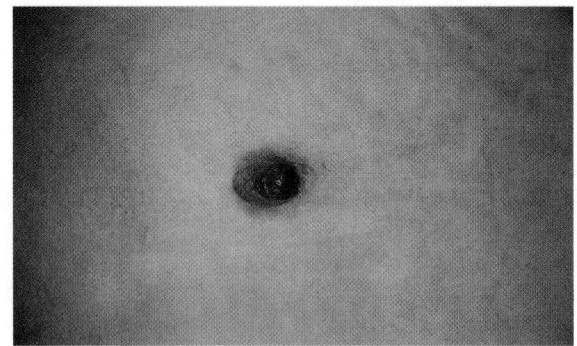

Fig. 33-6 Penetrating wound.

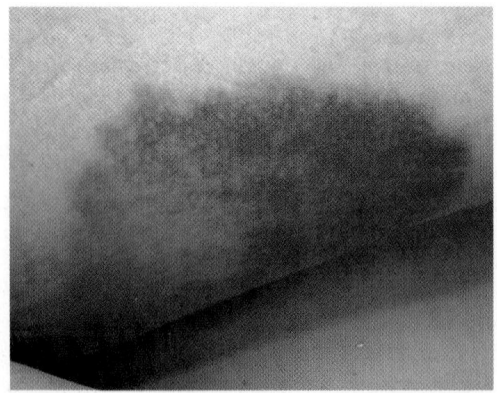

Fig. 33-3 Contusion.

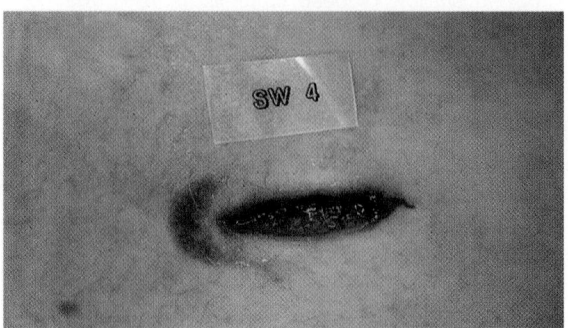

Fig. 33-7 Puncture wound.

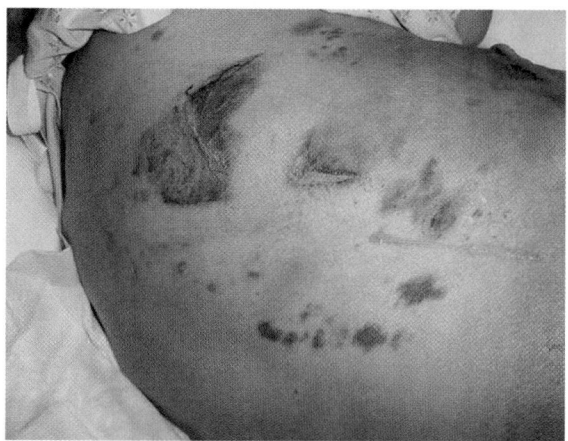

Fig. 33-8 Skin tear.

SKIN TEARS

A *skin tear is a break or rip in the outer layers of the skin* (Fig. 33-8). *The epidermis (top skin layer) separates from the underlying tissues* (Chapter 9). The skin is "peeled back." The hands, arms, and lower legs are common sites for skin tears. Very thin and fragile skin is common in older persons. Slight pressure can cause a skin tear.

Causes

Skin tears are caused by:

* Friction, shearing (Chapter 17), pulling, or pressure on the skin.
* Falls or bumping a hand, arm, or leg on any hard surface. Beds, bed rails, chairs, wheelchair footplates, and tables are dangers.
* Holding the person's arm or leg too tight.
* Removing tape or adhesives.
* Bathing, dressing, and other tasks.
* Pulling buttons and zippers across fragile skin.
* Jewelry—yours or the person's. Rings, watches, and bracelets are examples.
* Long or jagged fingernails (yours or the person's) and long or jagged toenails.

Skin tears are painful. They are portals of entry for microbes. Infection is a risk. Tell the nurse at once if you cause or find a skin tear.

Persons at Risk

Persons at risk for skin tears:

* Need help moving.
* Have poor nutrition.
* Have poor hydration.
* Have altered mental awareness.
* Are very thin.

See *Focus on Children and Older Persons: Persons at Risk (Skin Tears).*

FOCUS ON CHILDREN AND OLDER PERSONS
Persons at Risk (Skin Tears)

Older Persons

Some persons are confused and may resist care. They often move quickly and without warning. Or they pull away from you during care. Some try to hit or kick. These sudden movements can cause skin tears.

Never force care on a person. Chapter 46 describes how to care for persons who are confused and resist care. Always follow the care plan.

BOX 33-2   MEASURES TO PREVENT SKIN TEARS

* Follow the care plan and safety rules to:
  * Move, turn, position or transfer the person.
    * Prevent shearing and friction.
    * Use an assist device to move and turn the person in bed.
    * Use pillows to support arms and legs.
* Pad bed rails and wheelchair arms, footplates, and leg supports.
* Bathe the person.
* Keep the skin moisturized and apply lotion.
* Offer fluids.
* Keep your fingernails short and smoothly filed.
* Keep the person's fingernails short and smoothly filed. Report long, tough, or jagged toenails.
* Do not wear rings with large or raised stones. Do not wear bracelets.
* Be patient and calm when the person is confused, agitated, or resists care.
* Dress and undress the person carefully.
* Dress the person in soft clothes with long sleeves and long pants.
* Provide good lighting so the person can see. The person needs to avoid bumping into furniture, walls, and equipment.
* Provide a safe area for wandering (Chapter 46).
* Remove tape carefully (p. 587).
* Do not apply adhesive tape (p. 586).

Prevention and Treatment

Careful and safe care helps prevent skin tears and further injury. Follow the measures in Box 33-2. Also follow the care plan and the nurse's directions. They may include dressings (p. 586) and elastic bandages (Chapter 32) to protect the skin and promote healing.

CIRCULATORY ULCERS

Some diseases affect blood flow to and from the legs and feet. Such poor circulation can lead to pain, open wounds, and edema. *Edema is swelling caused by fluid collecting in tissues.* Infection and gangrene can result from the open wound and poor circulation. *Gangrene is a condition in which there is death of tissue* (Chapter 41).

| **BOX 33-3** | MEASURES TO PREVENT CIRCULATORY ULCERS |

- Remind the person not to sit with the legs crossed.
- Re-position the person according to the care plan—at least every 2 hours.
- Do not use elastic or rubber band–type garters to hold socks or hose in place.
- Do not dress the person in tight clothes.
- Provide good skin care daily. Keep the feet clean and dry. Clean and dry between the toes.
- Do not scrub or rub the skin during bathing and drying.
- Keep linens clean, dry, and wrinkle-free.
- Avoid injury to the legs and feet.
- Make sure shoes fit well.
- Keep pressure off the heels and other bony areas. Use pillows or other devices as the nurse and care plan direct.
- Check the person's legs and feet. Report skin breaks or changes in skin color.
- Do not massage over pressure points (Chapter 34). *Never rub or massage reddened areas.*
- Use protective devices as the nurse and care plan direct.
- Follow the care plan for walking and exercise.

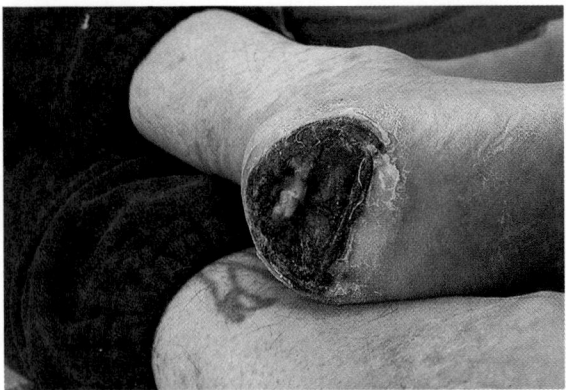

Fig. 33-9 Venous ulcer.

Circulatory ulcers (vascular ulcers) are open sores on the lower legs or feet. They are caused by decreased blood flow through the arteries or veins. Persons with diseases affecting the blood vessels are at risk. These wounds are painful and hard to heal.

The doctor orders drugs and treatments as needed. The nurse uses the nursing process to meet the person's needs (Box 33-3). You must help prevent skin breakdown on the legs and feet.

Venous Ulcers

Venous ulcers (stasis ulcers) are open sores on the lower legs or feet caused by poor venous blood flow (Fig. 33-9). *Stasis* means *stopped* or *slowed fluid flow*.

Venous ulcers can develop when valves in the leg veins do not close well. The veins do not pump blood back to the heart in a normal way. Blood and fluid collect in the legs and feet. Small skin veins rupture. This allows hemoglobin to enter the tissue causing the skin to turn brown. (Hemoglobin gives blood its red color.) The skin is dry, leathery, and hard. Itching is common.

The heels and inner part of the ankles are common sites for venous ulcers. They can occur from skin injury. Scratching is an example. Or they can occur without trauma.

Venous ulcers are painful and walking is difficult. Fluid may seep from the wound. Infection is a risk. Healing is slow.

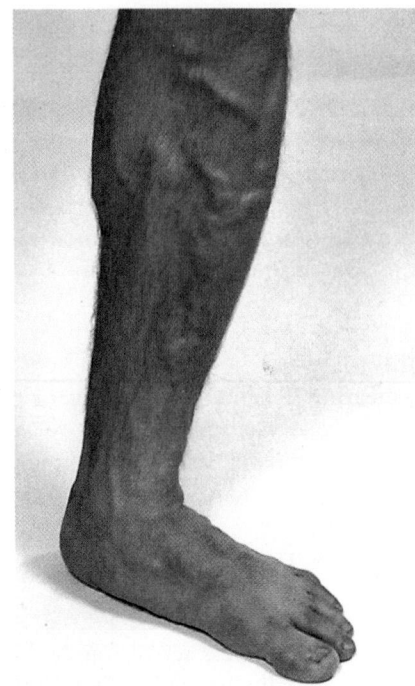

Fig. 33-10 Varicose veins. Veins under the skin are dilated (wide) and bulging.

Risk Factors. Risk factors for venous ulcers include:
- History of blood clots (Chapter 32)
- History of varicose veins (Fig. 33-10)
- Decreased mobility
- Obesity
- Leg or foot surgery
- Advanced age
- Surgery on the bones and joints
- *Phlebitis (inflammation* [itis] *of a vein* [phleb])

Prevention and Treatment. To prevent venous ulcers:

- Follow the care plan to prevent skin breakdown. See the measures in Box 33-3.
- Prevent injury. Do not bump the legs and feet.
- Move and transfer the person carefully and gently.

Persons at risk need professional foot care. Attention is given to toenails, corns, calluses, and other toe and foot problems. *You do not cut the toenails of persons with diseases affecting circulation.*

Venous ulcers are hard to heal. The doctor may order drugs for infection and to decrease swelling. Medicated bandages and other wound care products are often ordered. So are devices used for pressure ulcers. The doctor may order elastic stockings or elastic bandages (Chapter 32).

Arterial Ulcers

Arterial ulcers are open wounds on the lower legs or feet caused by poor arterial blood flow. They are found between the toes, on top of the toes, and on the outer side of the ankle (Fig. 33-11). The leg and foot may feel cold and look blue or shiny. The ulcer is very painful.

These ulcers are caused by diseases or injuries that decrease arterial blood flow to the legs and feet. High blood pressure and diabetes are common causes. So are narrowed arteries from aging. Smoking is a risk factor.

The doctor treats the disease causing the ulcer. Drugs, wound care, and a walking and exercise program are ordered. Professional foot care is important. Follow the care plan (see Box 33-3) and prevent further injury.

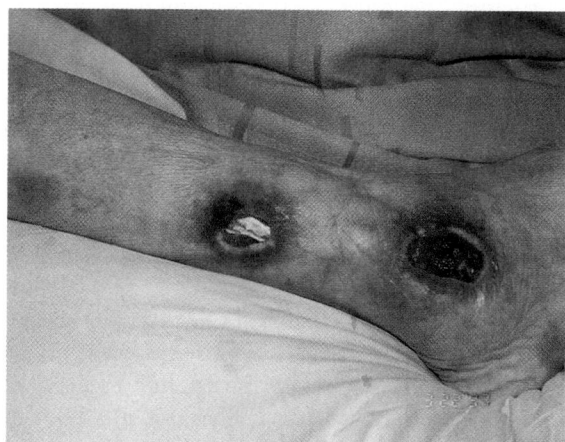

Fig. 33-11 Arterial ulcer.

Diabetic Foot Ulcers

A diabetic foot ulcer is an open wound on the foot caused by complications from diabetes. Diabetes (Chapter 43) can affect the nerves and blood vessels.

- *Nerves.* The person can lose sensation in a foot or leg. Loss of sensation can be complete or partial. The person may not feel pain, heat, or cold. Therefore the person may not feel a cut, blister, burn, or other trauma to the foot. Infection and a large sore can develop.
- *Blood vessels.* Blood flow decreases. Tissues and cells do not get needed oxygen and nutrients. Sores heal poorly. Tissue death (gangrene) can occur.

Some persons have both nerve and blood vessel damage. Both problems can lead to diabetic foot ulcers. Infection and gangrene are risks. Sometimes the affected part is amputated to prevent the spread of gangrene.

Check the person's feet every day. Look for the foot problems described in Box 33-4 (Fig. 33-12, p. 582). Report any sign of a foot problem to the nurse at once. Follow the care plan to prevent and treat diabetic foot ulcers.

BOX 33-4 FOOT PROBLEMS COMMON IN PERSONS WITH DIABETES

- *Corns and calluses* (see Fig. 33-12, A). These are thick layers of the skin caused by too much rubbing or pressure on the same spot. They occur over bony areas or the soles of the feet. Infection is a risk.
- *Blisters* (see Fig. 33-12, B). These form when shoes rub on the same spot. Shoes that do not fit well and wearing shoes without socks are causes. Infection is a risk.
- *Ingrown toenails* (see Fig. 33-12, C). An edge of a toenail grows into the skin. This occurs when the skin is cut while trimming toenails or from tight shoes. The skin becomes red and infected.
- *Bunions* (see Fig. 33-12, D). The big toe slants toward the small toes. The space between the bones near the base of the big toe grows larger. Bunions can occur on one or both feet. Heredity is a factor. Shoes that fit poorly and pointy shoes are causes. Bunions are removed by surgery.
- *Plantar warts* (see Fig. 33-12, E). *Plantar* means sole. Plantar warts occur on the soles (bottoms) of the feet. Caused by a virus, plantar warts are painful.
- *Hammer toes* (see Fig. 33-12, F). One or more toes are flexed. They form when a foot muscle weakens. Diabetic nerve damage can weaken foot muscles. The second toe is commonly affected. Because of deformed toes, the person has problems walking. Shoes do not fit well. Sores can develop on the tops of the toes and on the bottoms of the feet.
- *Dry and cracked skin* (see Fig. 33-12, G). Dry skin can occur from nerve damage in the legs and feet. These areas do not receive messages from the brain to keep the skin soft and moist. The dry skin can crack, causing portals of entry for microbes. Infection can occur.
- *Athlete's foot* (see Fig. 33-12, H). This is a fungus causing redness and cracked skin between the toes and on the bottoms of the feet. The cracks are portals of entry for microbes. The fungus can spread to the toenails. The toenails become thick, yellow, and hard to cut.

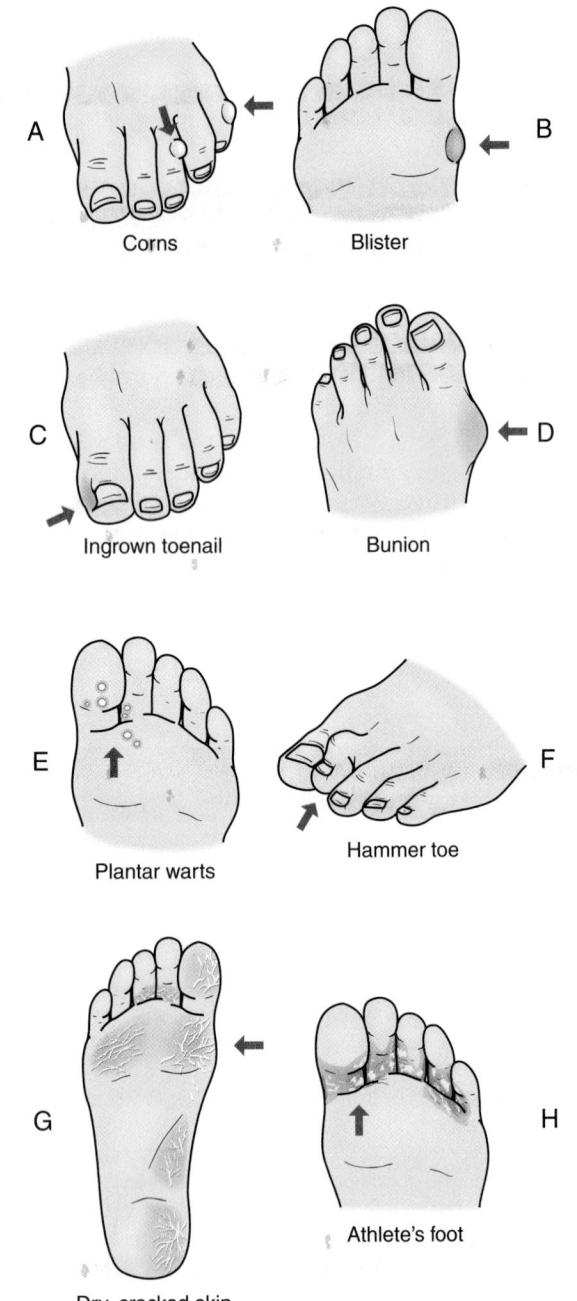

Fig. 33-12 Diabetic foot problems. **A,** Corns. **B,** A blister. **C,** An ingrown toenail. **D,** A bunion. **E,** Plantar warts. **F,** A hammer toe. **G,** Dry and cracked skin. **H,** Athlete's foot.

WOUND HEALING

The healing process has three phases:

- *Inflammatory phase* (3 days). Bleeding stops. A scab forms to protect against microbes entering the wound. Blood supply to the wound increases. The blood brings nutrients and healing substances. Because blood supply increases, signs and symptoms of inflammation appear—redness, swelling, heat or warmth, and pain. Loss of function may occur.

- *Proliferative phase* (day 3 to day 21). *Proliferate* means to multiply rapidly. Cells multiply to repair the wound.
- *Maturation phase* (day 21 to 2 years). The scar gains strength. The red, raised scar becomes thin and pale.

Types of Wound Healing

Healing occurs in three ways (Fig. 33-13).

- *First intention (primary intention, primary closure).* The wound is closed. Sutures (stitches), staples, clips, special glue, or adhesive strips hold the wound edges together.
- *Second intention (secondary intention).* This is for contaminated and infected wounds. Wounds are cleaned and dead tissue removed. Wound edges are not brought together. The wound gaps. Healing takes longer and leaves a larger scar. Infection is a great risk.
- *Third intention (delayed intention, tertiary intention).* The wound is left open and closed later. It combines first and second intention. Infection and poor circulation are common reasons for third intention.

Complications of Wound Healing

Many factors affect healing and the risk for complications. They include wound type and the person's age, health, nutrition, and life-style.

Good circulation is needed. Age, smoking, circulatory disease, and diabetes all affect circulation. Certain drugs (Coumadin and heparin) prolong bleeding.

Good nutrition is needed. Protein is needed for tissue growth and repair.

Infection is a risk for persons with immune system changes and for those taking antibiotics. Antibiotics kill pathogens. Specific antibiotics kill specific pathogens. In doing so, other pathogens may grow and multiply.

Hemorrhage and Shock. *Hemorrhage is the excessive loss of blood in a short time* (Chapter 51). The person can die.

- *Internal hemorrhage.* You cannot see internal hemorrhage. Bleeding occurs inside the body into tissues and body cavities. A hematoma may form. A *hematoma is a swelling* (oma) *that contains blood* (hemat). The area is swollen and reddish blue in color. Shock, vomiting blood, coughing up blood, and loss of consciousness signal internal hemorrhage.
- *External hemorrhage.* You can see external bleeding. Common signs are bloody drainage and dressings soaked with blood. Gravity causes fluid to flow down. Blood can flow down and collect under a body part. Check under the body part for pooling of blood. Shock can occur.

Shock results when tissues and organs do not get enough blood (Chapter 51). Blood pressure falls, the pulse is rapid and weak, and respirations are rapid. The skin is cold, moist, and pale. The person is restless and may complain of thirst. Confusion and loss of consciousness occur as shock worsens.

Hemorrhage and shock are emergencies. Alert the nurse at once. Assist as requested.

See *Promoting Safety and Comfort: Hemorrhage and Shock.*

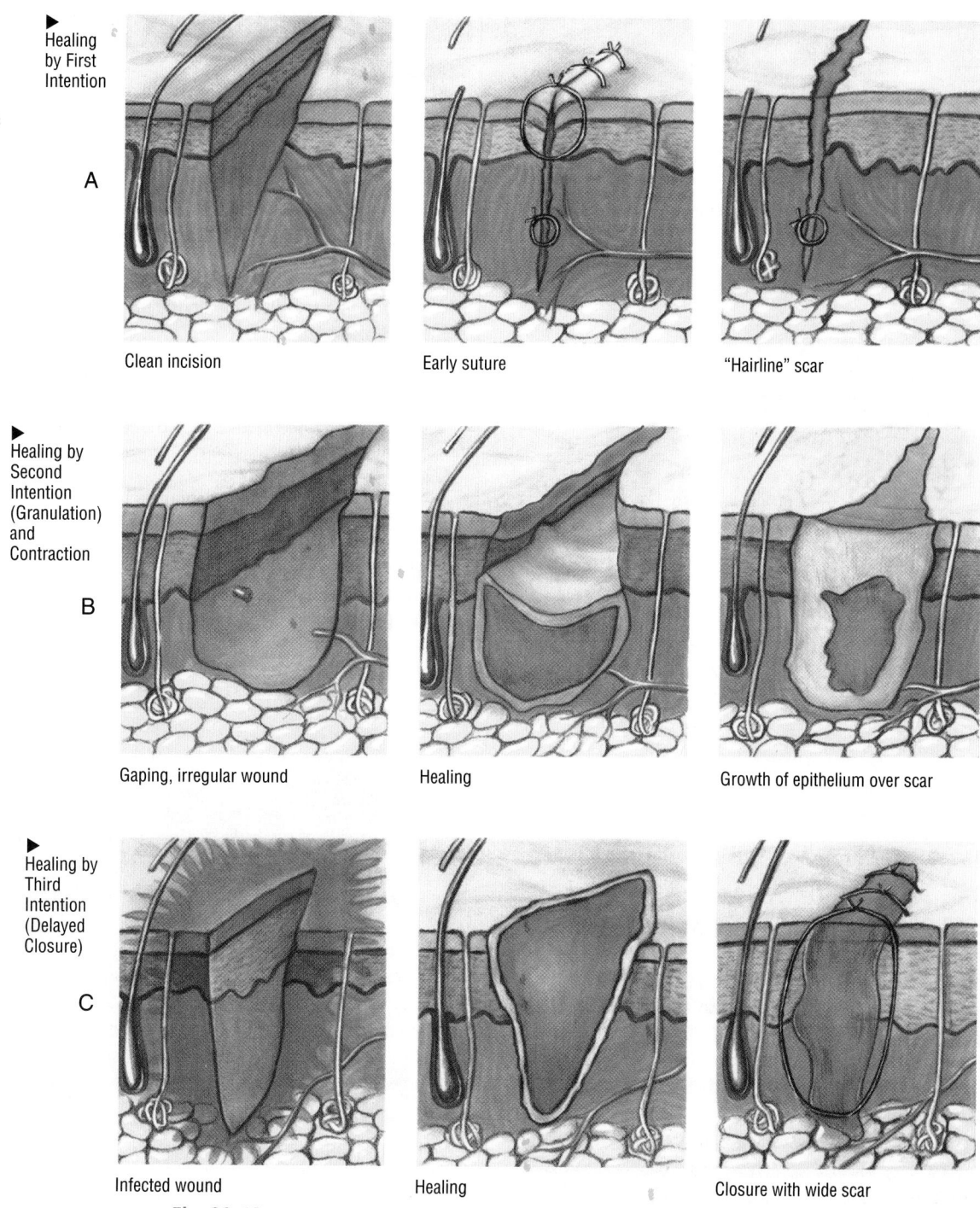

Fig. 33-13 Wound healing. **A,** First intention, **B,** Second intention. **C,** Third intention.

Infection. Contamination can occur during or after the injury. Trauma is a common cause. Surgical wounds can be contaminated during or after surgery. An infected wound appears inflamed (reddened) and has drainage (p. 585). The wound is painful and tender. The person has a fever.

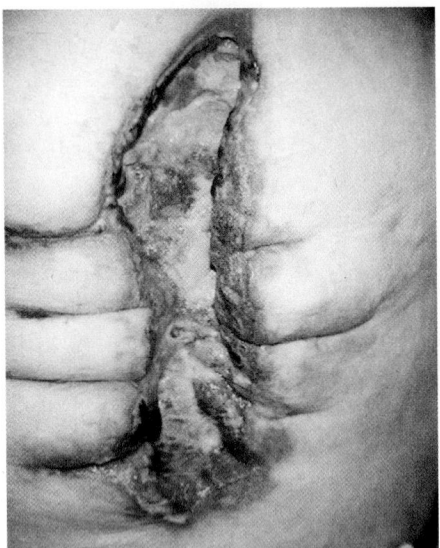

Fig. 33-14 Wound dehiscence.

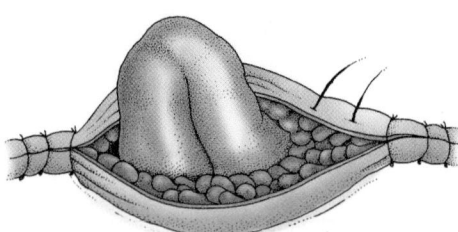

Fig. 33-15 Wound evisceration.

Dehiscence and Evisceration. *Dehiscence is the separation of wound layers* (Fig. 33-14). It may involve the skin layer or underlying tissues. Abdominal wounds are commonly affected. *Evisceration is the separation of the wound along with the protrusion of abdominal organs* (Fig. 33-15). Coughing, vomiting, and abdominal distention place stress on the wound. The person often describes the sensation of the wound "popping open."

Dehiscence and evisceration are surgical emergencies. Tell the nurse at once. The nurse covers the wound with large sterile dressings saturated with saline. Help prepare the person for surgery as directed.

Wound Appearance

Doctors and nurses observe the wound and its drainage. They observe for healing and complications. See Box 33-5 for observations to make when assisting with wound care. Report and record your observations according to agency policy.

See *Focus on Long-Term Care and Home Care: Wound Appearance.*

BOX 33-5	WOUND OBSERVATIONS

- Wound site:
  - Surgery or trauma result in multiple wounds.
- Wound size and depth are measured in centimeters (cm). The nurse uses a disposable ruler.
  - Size. The nurse measures from top to bottom and side to side (Fig. 33-16).
  - Depth. The nurse:
    - Inserts a sterile swab inside the deepest part of the wound.
    - Removes the swab.
    - Measures the distance on the swab.
- Wound appearance:
  - Is the wound red and swollen?
  - Is the area around the wound warm to touch?
  - Are sutures, staples, or clips intact or broken?
  - Are wound edges closed or separated?
  - Did the wound break open?
- Drainage:
  - Is the drainage serous, sanguineous, serosanguineous, or purulent?
  - What is the amount of drainage?
- Odor:
  - Does the wound or drainage have an odor?
- Surrounding skin:
  - Is surrounding skin intact?
  - What is the color of surrounding skin?
  - Are surrounding tissues swollen?

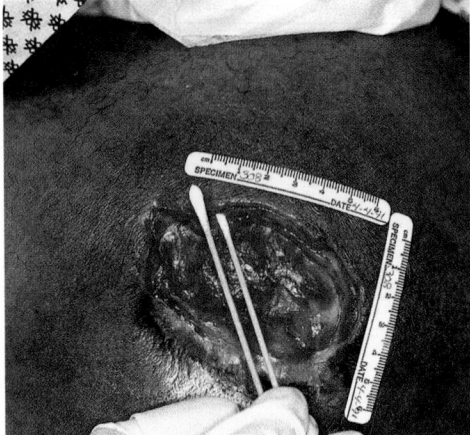

Fig. 33-16 The size and depth of the wound are measured.

FOCUS ON LONG-TERM CARE AND HOME CARE
Wound Appearance

Home Care

The nurse may ask you to take photos of wounds. The photos help the nurse assess the wound. Before taking a photo, make sure the person has signed a consent for photography. (The nurse obtains the consent.)

For a Polaroid camera, write the person's name, the date, and the time on the back of the photo. For regular film or digital camera, note the frame number, the person's name, and the date and time in the person's record.

The photo does not replace making accurate observations. See Box 33-5.

Wound Drainage

During injury and the inflammatory phase of wound healing, fluid and cells escape from the tissues. Drainage amounts may be large or small. This depends on wound size and site. Bleeding and infection also affect the amount and kind of drainage. Wound drainage is observed and measured. See Figure 33-17.

- *Serous drainage—clear, watery fluid.* *Serous* comes from the word *serum*. The fluid in a blister is serous. Serum is the clear, thin, fluid portion of blood. Serum does not contain blood cells or platelets.
- *Sanguineous drainage—bloody drainage.* The Latin word *sanguis* means *blood*. The amount and color of sanguineous drainage are important. Hemorrhage is suspected when large amounts are present. Bright drainage means fresh bleeding. Older bleeding is darker.
- *Serosanguineous drainage—thin, watery drainage* (sero) *that is blood-tinged* (sanguineous).
- *Purulent drainage—thick green, yellow, or brown drainage.*

Drainage must leave the wound for healing. Trapped drainage causes swelling of underlying tissues. The wound may heal at the skin level, but underlying tissues do not close. Infection and complications can occur.

When large amounts of drainage are expected, the doctor inserts a drain. A *Penrose drain* is a rubber tube that drains onto a dressing (Fig. 33-18). It opens onto the dressing. Therefore it is an open drain. Microbes can enter the drain and wound.

Closed drainage systems prevent microbes from entering the wound. A drain is attached to suction. The *Hemovac* (Fig. 33-19) and *Jackson-Pratt* (Fig. 33-20) systems are examples. Other systems are used depending on wound type, size, and site.

Drainage is measured in three ways:

- **Weighing dressings before applying them.** The weight of each new dressing is noted. Dressings are weighed after removal. The dry dressing weight is subtracted from the wet dressing weight. (Wet dressings weigh more.)
- **Noting the number and size of dressings with drainage.** What is the amount and kind of drainage? Are dressings saturated? Is drainage on just part of the dressing? If so, which part? Is drainage through some or all layers?
- **Measuring the amount of drainage in the collection container.** This is done for closed drainage.

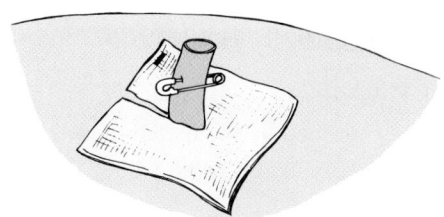

Fig. 33-18 Penrose drain.

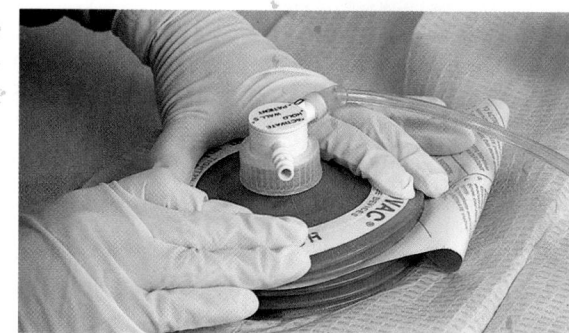

Fig. 33-19 Hemovac. Drains are sutured to the wound and connected to a reservoir.

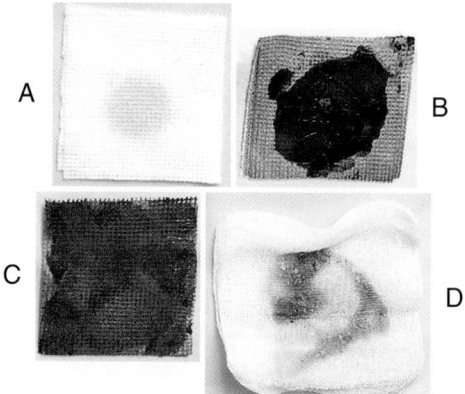

Fig. 33-17 Wound drainage. **A,** Serous drainage. **B,** Sanguineous drainage. **C,** Serosanguineous drainage. **D,** Purulent drainage.

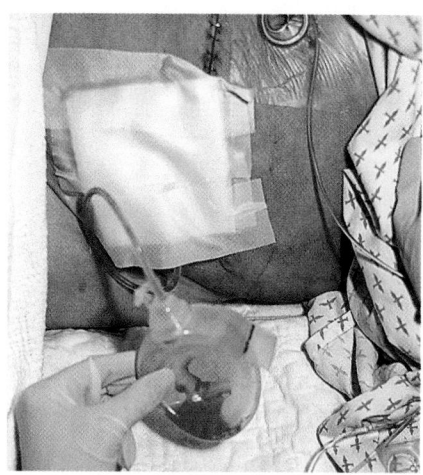

Fig. 33-20 Jackson-Pratt drainage system.

DRESSINGS

Wound dressings have many functions. They:
- Protect wounds from injury and microbes.
- Absorb drainage.
- Remove dead tissue.
- Promote comfort.
- Cover unsightly wounds.
- Provide a moist environment for wound healing.
- Apply pressure (pressure dressings) to help control bleeding.

Dressing type and size depend on many factors. These include the type of wound, its size and site, and amount of drainage. Infection is a factor. The dressing's function and the frequency of dressing changes are other factors. The doctor and nurse choose the dressing for each wound.

Types of Dressings

Dressings are described by the material used and how applied. There are many dressing products (Fig. 33-21). These are common:
- *Gauze.* It comes in squares, rectangles, pads, and rolls. Gauze dressings absorb drainage and moisture.
- *Non-adherent gauze.* This is a gauze dressing with a non-stick surface. It does not stick to the wound. It removes easily without injuring tissue.
- *Transparent adhesive film.* Air can reach the wound but fluids and microbes cannot. The wound is kept moist. Drainage is not absorbed. The transparent film allows for wound observation.

Some dressings contain special agents to promote wound healing. If you assist with a dressing change, the nurse explains its use to you.

Dressings are wet or dry:
- *Dry dressing.* A dry gauze dressing is placed over the wound. More dressings are placed on top of the first dressing as needed. Absorbed drainage is removed with the dressing. A dry dressing can stick to the wound. The dressing is removed carefully to prevent tissue injury and discomfort.

- *Wet-to-damp dressing.* This is used to remove dead tissue from the wound. Gauze dressings are saturated with a solution. The solution softens dead tissue. The dressing absorbs the dead tissue which is removed when the dressings are damp. The dressings do not dry completely.
- *Wet-to-wet dressing.* Gauze dressings are saturated with solution. The dressing is kept moist. It is not allowed to dry.

Securing Dressings

Dressings must be secured over wounds. Microbes can enter the wound and drainage can escape if the dressing is dislodged. Tape and Montgomery ties are used to secure dressings. Binders (p. 589) hold dressings in place.

Tape. Adhesive, paper, plastic, cloth, and elastic tapes are common. Adhesive tape sticks well. However, adhesive remaining on the skin is hard to remove. It can irritate the skin. An abrasion occurs if skin is removed with tape. Many people are allergic to adhesive tape. Paper, plastic, and cloth tapes usually do not cause allergic reactions. Elastic tape allows movement of the body part.

Tape comes in different sizes—½, ¾, 1, 2, and 3 inch widths. Tape is applied to the top, middle, and bottom parts of the dressing. The tape extends several inches beyond each side of the dressing (Fig. 33-22). *Do not apply tape to circle the entire body part. If swelling occurs, circulation to the part is impaired.*

See *Focus on Communication: Tape.*

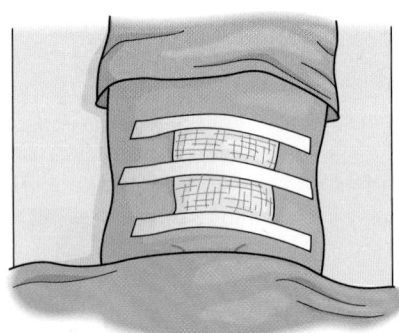

Fig. 33-22 Tape is applied at the top, middle, and bottom of the dressing. The tape extends several inches beyond both sides of the dressing.

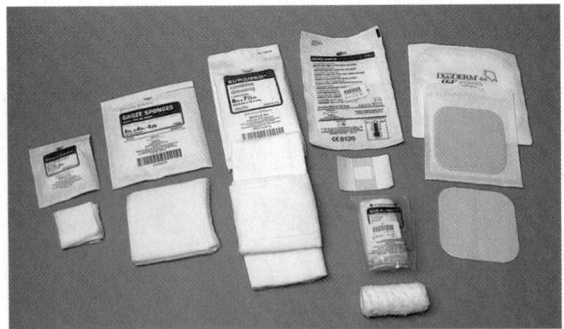

Fig. 33-21 Types of dressings.

FOCUS ON COMMUNICATION
Tape
Before applying tape, ask if the person has an allergy to tape. You can ask: • "Do any types of tape irritate your skin?" • "Do you have an allergy to tape?"

Montgomery Ties. Montgomery ties (Fig. 33-23) are used for large dressings and frequent dressing changes. A Montgomery tie has an adhesive strip and a cloth tie. When the dressing is in place, the adhesive strips are placed on both sides of the dressing. Then the cloth ties are secured over the dressing. A wound may need 2 or 3 Montgomery ties on each side. The ties are undone for the dressing change. The adhesive strips stay in place. They are not removed unless soiled. Montgomery ties protect the skin from frequent tape application and removal.

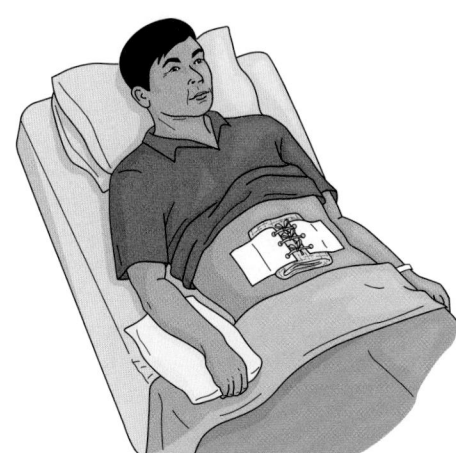

Fig. 33-23 Montgomery ties.

Applying Dressings

The nurse may ask you to assist with dressing changes. Some agencies let you apply simple, dry, non-sterile dressings to simple wounds. Follow the rules in Box 33-6.

See *Focus on Children and Older Persons: Applying Dressings.*

See *Teamwork and Time Management: Applying Dressings.*

See *Delegation Guidelines: Applying Dressings,* p. 588.

See *Promoting Safety and Comfort: Applying Dressings,* p. 588.

BOX 33-6 RULES FOR APPLYING DRESSINGS

- Let pain-relief drugs take effect, usually 30 minutes. The dressing change may cause discomfort. The nurse gives the drug and tells you how long to wait.
- Meet fluid and elimination needs before you begin.
- Collect equipment and supplies before you begin.
- Do not bend or reach over your work area.
- Control your nonverbal communication. Wound odors, appearance, and drainage may be unpleasant. Do not communicate your thoughts or reactions to the person.
- Remove soiled dressings so the person cannot see the soiled side. The drainage and its odor may upset the person.
- Do not force the person to look at the wound. A wound can affect body image and self-esteem. The nurse helps the person deal with the wound.
- Remove tape by pulling it toward the wound.
- Remove dressings gently. They may stick to the wound, drain, or surrounding skin. If the dressing sticks, the nurse may have you wet the dressing with a saline solution. A wet dressing is easier to remove.
- Touch only the outer edges of old and new dressings (Chapter 15).
- Report and record your observations. See *Delegation Guidelines: Applying Dressings,* p.588.

FOCUS ON CHILDREN AND OLDER PERSONS
Applying Dressings

Children
Children are often afraid of dressing changes. Tape removal is often painful. Wound appearance can be frightening. A calm, cooperative child helps prevent contamination of the sterile field. A parent or caregiver holds the child so the wound can be reached with ease. Holding or playing with a toy can comfort the child.

Older Persons
Older persons have thin, fragile skin. Skin tears must be prevented. Extreme care is necessary when removing tape.

TEAMWORK AND TIME MANAGEMENT
Applying Dressings

Collect all needed items before starting the procedure. Have extra dressings, tape, and other supplies on-hand. Leave unused items in the room for the next dressing change. Wound contamination can occur if you need to leave the room during the procedure.

DELEGATION GUIDELINES
Applying Dressings

When applying a dressing is delegated to you, make sure that:
- Your state allows you to perform the procedure.
- The procedure is in your job description.
- You have the necessary training.
- You know how to use the equipment.
- You review the procedure with the nurse.
- A nurse is available to answer questions and to supervise you.

If the above conditions are met, you need this information from the nurse:
- When to change the dressing
- When the person received a pain-relief drug; when it will take effect
- What to do if the dressing sticks to the wound
- How to clean the wound
- What dressings to use
- How to secure the dressing—tape or Montgomery ties
- What kind of tape to use—adhesive, paper, plastic, cloth, or elastic
- What size tape to use—½, ¾, 1, 2, or 3 inch width

- What observations to report and record:
  - What you used to dress the wound and secure the dressing
  - A red or swollen wound
  - An area around the wound that is warm to touch
  - If wound edges are closed or separated
  - A wound that has broken open
  - Drainage appearance—clear, bloody, or watery and blood-tinged; thick and green, yellow, or brown
  - The amount of drainage
  - Wound or drainage odor
  - Intactness and color of surrounding tissues
  - Swelling of surrounding tissues
  - Possible dressing contamination—urine; feces; other body fluids, secretions, or excretions; dislodged dressing
  - Pain
  - Fever
- When to report observations
- What patient or resident concerns to report at once

PROMOTING SAFETY AND COMFORT
Applying Dressings

Safety

Contact with blood, body fluids, secretions, or excretions is likely. Follow Standard Precautions and the Bloodborne Pathogen Standard. Wear personal protective equipment (PPE) as needed.

Do not apply tape to irritated, injured, or non-intact skin. Tape can further damage the skin.

Comfort

Wounds and dressing changes can cause discomfort or pain. The nurse may give a pain-relief drug before the dressing change. Allow time for the drug to take effect. Gently apply and remove tape and dressings.

The person may not report discomfort from a dressing. You should ask:
- "Is the dressing comfortable?"
- "Does the tape cause pain or itching?"

APPLYING A DRY, NON-STERILE DRESSING [VIDEO]

QUALITY OF LIFE

Remember to:
- Knock before entering the person's room.
- Address the person by name.
- Introduce yourself by name and title.

- Explain the procedure to the person before beginning and during the procedure.
- Protect the person's rights during the procedure.
- Handle the person gently during the procedure.

PRE-PROCEDURE

1 Follow *Delegation Guidelines: Applying Dressings.* See *Promoting Safety and Comfort: Applying Dressings.*
2 Practice hand hygiene.
3 Collect the following:
   - Gloves
   - PPE as needed
   - Tape or Montgomery ties
   - Dressings as directed by the nurse
   - Saline solution as directed by the nurse
   - Cleansing solution as directed by the nurse
   - Adhesive remover
   - Dressing set with scissors and forceps
   - Plastic bag
   - Bath blanket
4 Practice hand hygiene.
5 Identify the person. Check the ID (identification) bracelet against the assignment sheet. Also call the person by name.
6 Provide for privacy.
7 Arrange your work area. You should not have to reach over or turn your back on your work area.
8 Raise the bed for body mechanics. Bed rails are up if used.

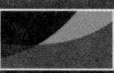

APPLYING A DRY, NON-STERILE DRESSING—cont'd | VIDEO

PROCEDURE

9 Lower the bed rail near you if up.
10 Help the person to a comfortable position.
11 Cover the person with a bath blanket. Fan-fold top linens to the foot of the bed.
12 Expose the affected body part.
13 Make a cuff on the plastic bag. Place the bag within reach.
14 Practice hand hygiene.
15 Put on needed PPE. Put on gloves.
16 Remove tape or undo Montgomery ties.
  a *Tape:* hold the skin down. Gently pull the tape toward the wound.
  b *Montgomery ties:* fold ties away from the wound.
17 Remove any adhesive from the skin. Wet a 4 × 4 gauze dressing with adhesive remover. Clean away from the wound.
18 Remove gauze dressings. Start with the top dressing, and remove each layer. Keep the soiled side away from the person's sight. Put dressings in the plastic bag. They must not touch the outside of the bag.

19 Remove the dressing over the wound very gently. It may stick to the wound or drain site. Moisten the dressing with saline if it sticks to the wound.
20 Observe the wound, drain site, and wound drainage.
21 Remove the gloves and put them in the bag. Practice hand hygiene.
22 Open the new dressings.
23 Cut the length of tape needed.
24 Put on clean gloves.
25 Clean the wound with saline as directed by the nurse. See Figure 33-24.
26 Apply dressings as directed by the nurse.
27 Secure the dressings. Use tape or Montgomery ties.
28 Remove the gloves. Put them in the bag.
29 Remove and discard PPE.
30 Practice hand hygiene.
31 Cover the person. Remove the bath blanket.

POST-PROCEDURE

32 Provide for comfort. (See the inside of the front book cover.)
33 Place the signal light within reach.
34 Lower the bed to its lowest position.
35 Raise or lower bed rails. Follow the care plan.
36 Return equipment and supplies to the proper place. Leave extra dressings and tape in the room.
37 Discard used supplies into the bag. Tie the bag closed. Discard the bag following agency policy. (Wear gloves for this step.)

38 Clean your work area. Follow the Bloodborne Pathogen Standard.
39 Unscreen the person.
40 Complete a safety check of the room. (See the inside of the front book cover.)
41 Remove and discard the gloves. Practice hand hygiene.
42 Report and record your observations.

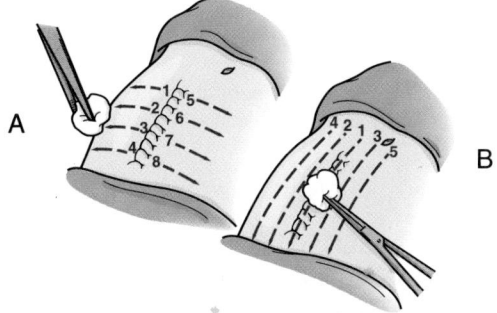

Fig. 33-24 Cleaning a wound. **A,** Clean starting at the wound and stroking out to the surrounding skin. Use new gauze for each stroke. **B,** Clean the wound from the top to bottom. Start at the wound. Then clean the surrounding areas. Use new gauze for each stroke.

BINDERS AND COMPRESSION GARMENTS

Binders are wide bands of elastic fabric. They are applied to the abdomen, chest, or perineal areas. Binders promote healing because they support wounds and hold dressings in place. They also prevent or reduce swelling, promote comfort, and prevent injury. These binders are common:

- *Abdominal binder*—provides abdominal support and holds dressings in place (Fig. 33-25, p. 590). The top part is at the person's waist. The lower part is over the hips. Binders are secured in place with Velcro or with hook and loop closures.
- *Breast binder*—supports the breasts after surgery (Fig. 33-26, p. 590). It is secured in place with Velcro or padded zippers.

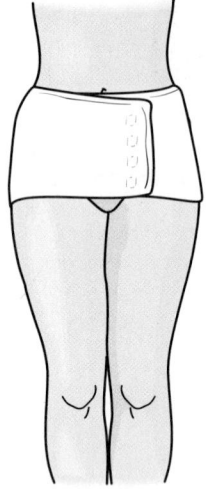

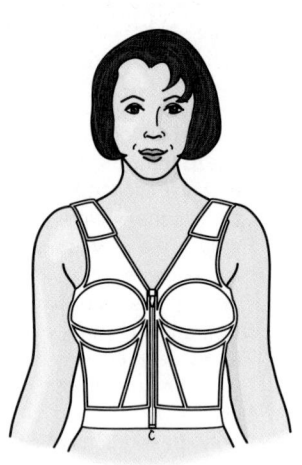

Fig. 33-25 Abdominal binder.   **Fig. 33-26** Breast binder.

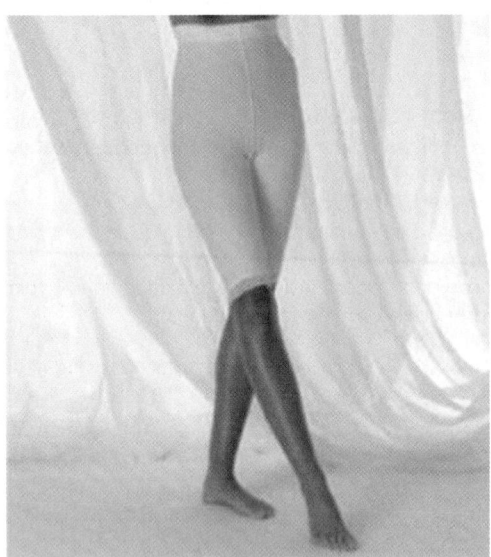

Fig. 33-27 Compression garment.

Compression garments are made of a tight, stretchy fabric (Fig. 33-27). They are commonly worn after plastic surgery. The doctor orders the type and size for the body part involved. They help:

- Reduce swelling.
- Prevent fluid buildup at the surgical site.
- Hold skin against the body.
- Achieve the desired shape.

Box 33-7 lists the rules for applying binders and compression garments.

   See *Focus on Communication: Binders and Compression Garments.*

   See *Promoting Safety and Comfort: Binders and Compression Garments.*

BOX 33-7	RULES FOR APPLYING BINDERS AND COMPRESSION GARMENTS

- Follow the manufacturer's instructions.
- Apply the device so there is firm, even pressure over the area.
- Apply the device so it is snug. It must not interfere with breathing or circulation.
- Position the person in good alignment.
- Re-apply the device if it is loose or wrinkled.
- Re-apply the device if it is out of position or causes discomfort.
- Secure safety pins, if used, so they point away from the wound.
- Change the device if it is moist or soiled. This prevents the growth of microbes.
- Tell the nurse at once if there is a change in the person's breathing.
- Check the person's skin under and around the device. Tell the nurse at once if there is redness, irritation, or other signs of a skin problem.

FOCUS ON COMMUNICATION

Binders and Compression Garments

The person may not tell you about pain or discomfort. Therefore you need to ask these questions:

- "Is the binder (or garment) too tight or too loose?"
- "Does the binder (or garment) cause pain?"
- "Do you feel pressure from the binder (or garment)?" If yes: "Where? Please show me."

PROMOTING SAFETY AND COMFORT

Binders and Compression Garments

Safety

Apply binders and compression garments properly. Otherwise, severe discomfort, skin irritation, and circulatory and respiratory problems can occur. Correct application is needed for safety and for the device to work effectively.

Comfort

A binder or compression garment should promote comfort. Tell the nurse if the device causes pain or discomfort.

HEAT AND COLD APPLICATIONS

Heat and cold applications promote healing and comfort. They also reduce tissue swelling. See Chapter 35.

MEETING BASIC NEEDS

The wound can affect basic needs. However, it is only one part of the person's care. Remember, the *person* has the wound.

The person is recovering from surgery or trauma. The wound causes pain and discomfort. These may affect breathing and moving. Turning, re-positioning, and walking may be painful. Handle the person gently. Allow pain-relief drugs to take effect before giving care.

Good nutrition is needed for healing. However, pain and discomfort can affect appetite. So can odors from wound drainage. Promptly remove soiled dressings from the room. Use room deodorizers as directed. Also keep drainage containers out of the person's sight. Tell the nurse if the person wants certain foods or drinks.

Infection is always a threat. Follow Standard Precautions and the Bloodborne Pathogen Standard. Carefully observe the wound for signs and symptoms of infection.

Delayed healing is a risk for persons who are older, obese, or have poor nutrition. Protein is needed for tissue growth and repair. Poor circulation and diabetes also affect healing. These conditions are risk factors for infection.

Many factors affect safety and security needs. The person fears scarring, disfigurement, delayed healing, and infection. Fears about the wound "popping open" are common. Medical bills are other concerns. The person may need care for a long time.

Victims of violence have many other concerns. Future attacks, finding and convicting the attacker, and fear for family members are common concerns. Victims of domestic, child, and elder abuse often hide the source of their injuries.

Wounds may be large or small. Others can see wounds on the face, arms, or legs. Clothing can hide some wounds. Wound drainage may have odors. Some wounds are disfiguring. They can affect sexual performance or feelings of sexual attraction. Amputation of a body part can affect function, everyday activities, and job. Eye injuries can affect vision. Abdominal trauma and surgery can affect eating and elimination.

Whatever the wound site or size, it affects function and body image. Love and belonging and self-esteem needs are affected. The person may be sad and tearful or angry and hostile. Adjustment may be hard and rehabilitation necessary. Be gentle and kind, give thoughtful care, and practice good communication. Other health team members—therapists, social workers, psychiatrists, and the clergy—may be involved in the person's care.

FOCUS ON PRIDE

The Person, Family, and Yourself

Personal and Professional Responsibility

You spend much of your time with patients and residents. You assist with hygiene and grooming. You help them dress and undress. You transfer and position them. These roles bring responsibilities for wound care.

If you are careless during a transfer, you can cause a skin tear. If you rush during a bath, you may not notice a wound between skin folds on a bariatric person. If you do not apply shoes properly on a diabetic person, a foot ulcer can develop.

The way you provide care affects the person's safety and well-being. Take pride in working safely and carefully. You have an impact on the person's health and quality of life.

Rights and Respect

Some wounds are large and disfiguring. Wound drainage may have odors. The person may feel embarrassed. Body image is often affected. Love, belonging, and self-esteem needs are also affected.

Do not judge the person by the size, site, odor, or cause of the wound. Be sensitive to the person's feelings. The person may be sad and tearful or angry and hostile. Treat the person with dignity and respect. Be gentle and kind, give thoughtful care, and practice good communication.

Independence and Social Interaction

Wounds and dressings may be disturbing to patients, residents, and visitors. Some wounds are connected to drainage devices. Drainage in the container or odors from wounds may disgust some persons. Family and friends may feel uncomfortable when visiting. To promote comfort and interaction with family and friends:

- Keep the wound or dressing covered if able.
- Ask visitors to leave the room during dressing changes or when exposing the wound or dressing.
- Remove soiled dressings from the room promptly.
- Keep drainage containers out of sight if able. Some large containers can be covered with a towel as directed by the nurse.
- Use a room deodorizer for odors as directed.

Delegation and Teamwork

Wound care can be painful and tiring. The team coordinates care to promote comfort and rest. To assist:

- Plan care with the nurse. Ask when drugs for pain will be given and when they will take effect. Allow rest periods before and after care that is tiring.
- Be prepared. Gather supplies. Leaving to get supplies causes delays. Care and procedures take longer than planned.
- Work with the nurse as instructed. You may need to position the person or raise a body part while the nurse changes a dressing. Teamwork reduces the amount of energy the person must use.

Ethics and Laws

Agencies have rules for charging for supplies used. Some are stored in a room or cart. Stickers on the items are removed and saved or a log is kept. A note is written in the log to document the person's name and the type and amount of items removed. Some agencies use an electronic cabinet. A code is used to open the cabinet. The person's name is chosen from a list on a screen. Then a button is pressed to select the type and amount of supplies needed.

Agency practices vary for charging supplies. Ethical practice involves honestly following agency rules. Not charging supplies correctly costs the nursing unit and agency money. Taking supplies home for your own use is unethical. This is stealing. Take pride in following agency rules and being an honest and reliable member of the nursing team.

REVIEW QUESTIONS

Circle the BEST answer.

1 A person has a laceration from a fall. The wound is
a Open, unintentional, and contaminated
b Open, unintentional, and infected
c Closed, intentional, and clean
d Closed, intentional, and chronic

2 A person had rectal surgery. The person has a
a Clean wound
b Dirty wound
c Clean-contaminated wound
d Contaminated wound

3 The skin and underlying tissues are pierced. This is
a A penetrating wound
b An incision
c A contusion
d An abrasion

4 Which can cause skin tears?
a Keeping your nails trimmed and smooth
b Dressing the person in soft clothing
c Wearing rings
d Padding wheelchair footplates

5 A person has a circulatory ulcer. Which measure should you question?
a Hold socks in place with elastic garters.
b Do not cut or trim toenails.
c Apply elastic stockings.
d Re-position the person every hour.

6 Diabetic foot ulcers are caused by
a Gangrene
b Amputation
c Infection
d Nerve and blood vessel damage

7 A person has diabetes. The person's feet are checked every
a 2 hours
b Day
c Week
d Month

8 A person with diabetes wears socks with shoes to prevent
a Corns
b Bunions
c Plantar warts
d Blisters

9 A wound is separating. This is called
a Primary intention
b Third intention
c Dehiscence
d Evisceration

10 Clear, watery drainage from a wound is called
a Purulent drainage
b Serous drainage
c Sero-purulent drainage
d Serosanguineous drainage

11 A dressing does the following *except*
a Protect the wound from injury
b Absorb drainage
c Provide moisture for wound healing
d Support the wound and reduce swelling

12 To secure a dressing, apply tape
a Around the entire part
b Along the sides of the dressing
c To the top, middle, and bottom of the dressing
d As the person prefers

13 A person has frequent dressing changes. The nurse will likely have the dressings secured with
a A binder
b Montgomery ties
c Paper or cloth tape
d An elastic bandage

14 A pain-relief drug is given before a dressing change. How long should you wait for the drug to take effect?
a 5 minutes
b 10 minutes
c 15 minutes
d 30 minutes

15 To remove tape
a Pull it toward the wound
b Pull it away from the wound
c Use an adhesive remover
d Use a saline solution

16 An abdominal binder is used to
a Prevent blood clots
b Prevent wound infection
c Provide support and hold dressings in place
d Decrease swelling and circulation

Answers to these questions are on p. 834.

Pressure Ulcers 34

OBJECTIVES

- Define the key terms and key abbreviations listed in this chapter.
- Describe the causes and risk factors for pressure ulcers.
- Identify the persons at risk for pressure ulcers.
- Describe the stages of pressure ulcers.

- Identify the sites for pressure ulcers.
- Explain how to prevent pressure ulcers.
- Identify the complications from pressure ulcers.
- Explain how to promote PRIDE in the person, the family, and yourself.

KEY TERMS

avoidable pressure ulcer A pressure ulcer that develops from the improper use of the nursing process
bedfast Confined to bed
bony prominence An area where the bone sticks out or projects from the flat surface of the body
chairfast Confined to a chair
colonized The presence of bacteria on the wound surface or in wound tissue; the person does not have signs and symptoms of an infection
epidermal stripping Removing the epidermis (outer skin layer) as tape is removed from the skin
eschar Thick, leathery dead tissue that may be loose or adhered to the skin; it is often black or brown
friction The rubbing of one surface against another

pressure ulcer A localized injury to the skin and/or underlying tissue usually over a bony prominence resulting from pressure or pressure in combination with shear and/or friction; any lesion caused by unrelieved pressure that results in damage to underlying tissues
shear When layers of the skin rub against each other; when the skin remains in place and underlying tissues move and stretch and tear underlying capillaries and blood vessels causing tissue damage
slough Dead tissue that is shed from the skin; it is usually light colored, soft, and moist; may be stringy at times
unavoidable pressure ulcer A pressure ulcer that occurs despite efforts to prevent one through proper use of the nursing process

KEY ABBREVIATIONS

CMS Centers for Medicare & Medicaid Services

TJC The Joint Commission

Before defining pressure ulcer, you need to understand these terms:

- *Bony prominence—an area where the bone sticks out or projects from the flat surface of the body.* The back of the head, shoulder blades, elbows, hips, spine, sacrum, knees, ankles, heels, and toes are bony prominences (Fig. 34-1, p. 594). These areas are sometimes called *pressure points.*
- *Shear—when layers of the skin rub against each other. Or shear is when the skin remains in place and underlying tissues move and stretch and tear underlying capillaries and blood vessels. Tissue damage occurs.* See Chapter 17.
- *Friction—the rubbing of one surface against another.* The skin is dragged across a surface. Friction is always present with shearing.

The National Pressure Ulcer Advisory Panel (NPUAP) defines a *pressure ulcer as a localized injury to the skin and/or underlying tissue usually over a bony prominence* (Fig. 34-2, p. 594). *It is the result of pressure or pressure in combination with shear and/or friction. Decubitus ulcer, bed sore,* or *pressure sore* are other terms for pressure ulcer.

The Centers for Medicare & Medicaid Services (CMS) defines a *pressure ulcer as any lesion caused by unrelieved pressure that results in damage to underlying tissues.* According to the CMS, friction and shear are not the main causes of pressure ulcers. However, friction and shear are important contributing factors.

See *Focus on Long-Term Care and Home Care: Pressure Ulcers,* p. 595.

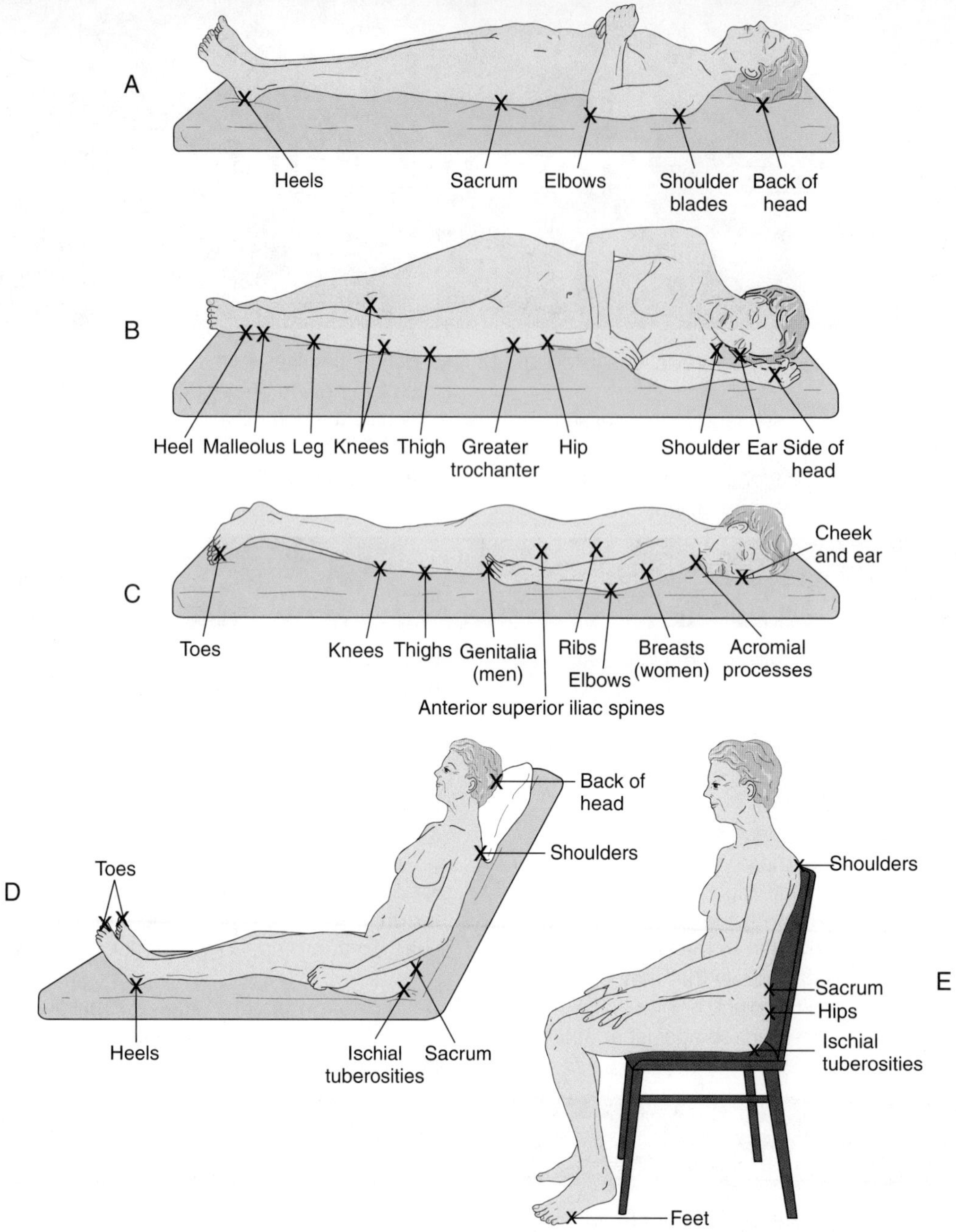

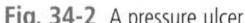

Fig. 34-1 Bony prominences (pressure points). **A,** The supine position. **B,** The lateral position. **C,** The prone position. **D,** Fowler's position. **E,** Sitting position.

A

Heels — Sacrum — Elbows — Shoulder blades — Back of head

B

Heel — Malleolus — Leg — Knees — Thigh — Greater trochanter — Hip — Shoulder — Ear — Side of head

C

Toes — Knees — Thighs — Genitalia (men) — Elbows — Ribs — Breasts (women) — Acromial processes — Cheek and ear — Anterior superior iliac spines

D

Toes — Heels — Ischial tuberosities — Sacrum — Back of head — Shoulders

E

Shoulders — Sacrum — Hips — Ischial tuberosities — Feet

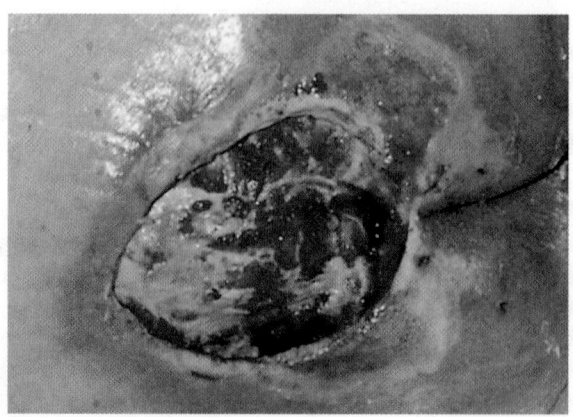

Fig. 34-2 A pressure ulcer.

FOCUS ON LONG-TERM CARE AND HOME CARE
Pressure Ulcers

Long-Term Care

Some persons are admitted to nursing centers with pressure ulcers. They come from hospitals or from home. The CMS requires nursing centers to ensure that:

- A person does not develop a pressure ulcer after entering the center. However, for some persons, a pressure ulcer cannot be avoided. An *unavoidable pressure ulcer occurs despite efforts to prevent one through proper use of the nursing process.* An *avoidable pressure ulcer is one that develops from the improper use of the nursing process.* The center must:
  - Evaluate the person's condition and pressure ulcer risk factors.
  - Identify and implement measures that meet the person's needs and goals.
  - Monitor and evaluate the effect of such measures.
  - Revise the measures as needed.

- A person with a pressure ulcer receives the necessary treatment and services to promote healing, prevent infection, and prevent new sores from developing.

Centers must identify persons at risk for pressure ulcers. A person's risk may increase during an illness (cold, flu) or when his or her condition changes. Many pressure ulcers occur within the first 4 weeks of admission to a nursing center. A person can develop a pressure ulcer within 2 to 6 hours after the onset of pressure. The person's care plan must include measures to reduce or remove risk factors.

BOX 34-1	**SKIN BREAKDOWN—COMMON CAUSES**

- Age-related changes in the skin
- Dryness
- Fragile and weak capillaries
- General thinning of the skin
- Loss of the fatty layer under the skin
- Decreased sensation to touch, heat, and cold
- Decreased mobility
- Sitting in a chair or lying in bed most or all of the day
- Chronic diseases (diabetes, high blood pressure)
- Diseases that decrease circulation
- Poor nutrition
- Poor hydration
- Incontinence (urinary, fecal)
- Moisture in dark body areas (skin folds, under breasts, perineal area)
- Pressure on bony parts
- Poor fingernail and toenail care
- Friction and shearing
- Edema

RISK FACTORS

Pressure is the major cause of pressure ulcers. Shearing and friction are important factors. They also cause skin breakdown (Box 34-1) that can lead to pressure ulcers. Risk factors include breaks in the skin, poor circulation to an area, moisture, dry skin, and irritation by urine and feces.

Unrelieved pressure squeezes tiny blood vessels. The skin does not receive oxygen and nutrients. Tissues die and a pressure ulcer forms when the skin is starved of oxygen and nutrients for too long. For example, pressure occurs

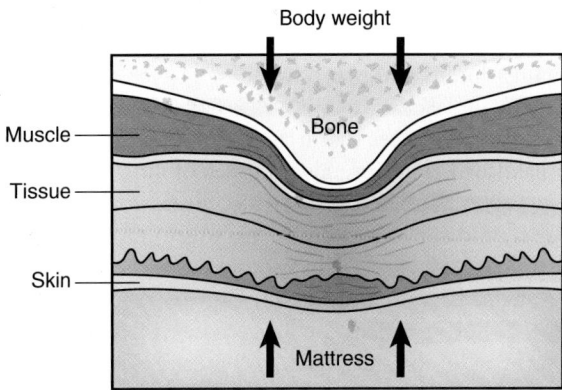

Fig. 34-3 Tissue under pressure. The skin is squeezed between two hard surfaces: the bone and the mattress.

when the skin over a bony area is squeezed between hard surfaces (Fig. 34-3). The bone is one hard surface. The other is usually the mattress or chair seat. Squeezing or pressure prevents blood flow to the skin and underlying tissues. Oxygen and nutrients cannot get to the cells. Skin and tissues die.

Friction scrapes the skin, causing an open area. The open area needs to heal. A good blood supply is needed. A poor blood supply or an infection can lead to a pressure ulcer.

Shear occurs when the person slides down in the bed or chair. Blood vessels and tissues are damaged. Blood flow to the area is reduced.

See *Teamwork and Time Management: Risk Factors*, p. 596.

PERSONS AT RISK

Persons at risk for pressure ulcers are those who:

- Are *bedfast (confined to a bed)* or *chairfast (confined to a chair)*. Pressure occurs from lying or sitting in the same position for too long.
- Need some or total help in moving. Coma, paralysis, or a hip fracture increases the risk for pressure ulcers.
- Are agitated or have involuntary muscle movements. The person's movements cause rubbing (friction) against linens and other surfaces.
- Have urinary or fecal incontinence. Urine and feces contain substances that irritate the skin and lead to skin breakdown. They are also sources of moisture.
- Are exposed to moisture. Urine, feces, wound drainage, sweat, and saliva expose the person to moisture. Moisture irritates the skin. It also increases the risk of damage from friction and shearing during re-positioning.
- Have poor nutrition. A balanced diet is needed to nourish the skin. Pressure ulcer risk increases when the skin is not healthy.
- Have poor fluid balance. Fluid balance is needed for healthy skin.
- Have lowered mental awareness. The person cannot act (move, change positions) to prevent pressure ulcers. Drugs and health problems affect mental awareness.
- Have problems sensing pain or pressure. These are symptoms of tissue damage. If unable to sense pain or pressure, the person does not know to alert the staff to the symptoms.
- Have circulatory problems. Good blood flow is needed to bring oxygen and nutrients to the cells. Cells and tissues die when starved of oxygen and nutrients.
- Are obese or very thin. Friction can damage the skin. Persons with bariatric needs are at great risk.
- Have a healed pressure ulcer. Areas of healed Stage 3 or 4 pressure ulcers are more likely to recur. See "Pressure Ulcer Stages."

See *Focus on Children and Older Persons: Persons at Risk.*

PRESSURE ULCER STAGES

In persons with light skin, a reddened bony area is the first sign of a pressure ulcer. In persons with dark skin, skin color may differ from surrounding areas. The color change remains after the pressure is relieved. The area may feel warm or cool. The person may complain of pain, burning, tingling, or itching in the area. Some persons do not feel anything unusual. Box 34-2 describes pressure ulcer stages.

- See *Focus on Communication: Pressure Ulcer Stages.*
- See *Focus on Long-Term Care and Home Care: Pressure Ulcer Stages.*

BOX 34-2 PRESSURE ULCER STAGES

Suspected deep tissue injury: A purple or maroon area of intact skin or a blood-filled blister. Pressure or shear has damaged underlying soft tissue. Involved tissue may be painful, firm, mushy, boggy, warm, or cool. This stage may be hard to detect in persons with dark skin. See Figure 34-4, A.

Stage 1: Intact skin with redness over a bony prominence. The color does not return to normal when the skin is relieved of pressure. In persons with dark skin, skin color may differ from surrounding areas. It may appear to be a persistent red, blue, or purple. See Figure 34-4, B.

Stage 2: Partial-thickness skin loss (Fig. 34-4, C). The wound may involve a blister or shallow ulcer. An ulcer may appear to be reddish-pink. A blister may be intact or open.

Stage 3: Full-thickness tissue loss (Fig. 34-4, D). The skin is gone. Subcutaneous fat may be exposed. Slough may be present. *Slough* is dead tissue that is shed from the skin. *It is usually light colored, soft, and moist. It may be stringy at times.*

Stage 4: Full-thickness tissue loss with muscle, tendon, and bone exposure (Fig. 34-4, E). Slough and eschar may be present. *Eschar is thick, leathery dead tissue that may be loose or adhered to the skin. It is often black or brown.*

Unstageable: Full-thickness tissue loss with the ulcer covered by slough and/or eschar (Fig. 34-4, F). Slough is yellow, tan, gray, green, or brown. Eschar is tan, brown, or black.

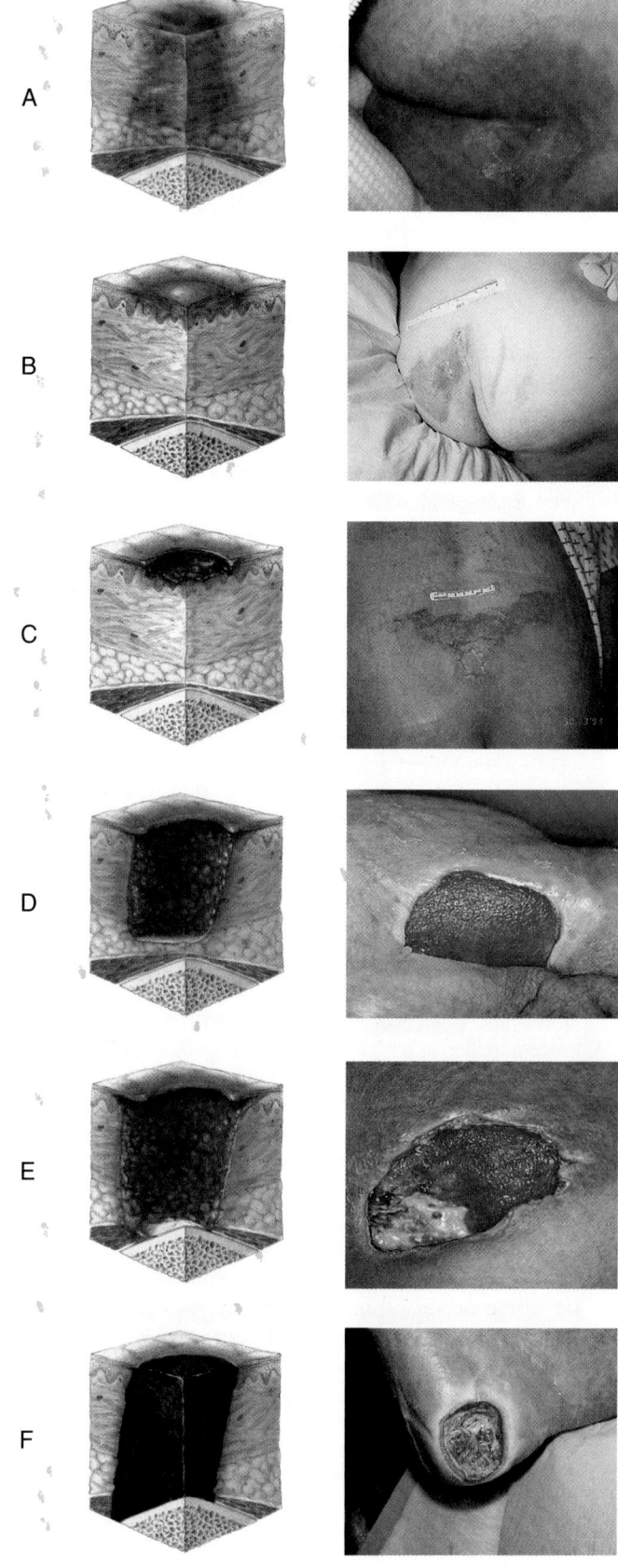

Fig. 34-4 Stages of pressure ulcers. **A,** Suspected deep tissue injury. **B,** Stage 1. **C,** Stage 2. **D,** Stage 3. **E,** Stage 4. **F,** Unstageable.

SITES

Pressure ulcers usually occur over bony prominences (*pressure points*). These areas bear the weight of the body in a certain position (see Fig. 34-1). Pressure from body weight can reduce the blood supply to the area. According to the CMS, the sacrum is the most common site for a pressure ulcer. However, pressure ulcers on the heels often occur.

The ears also are sites for pressure ulcers. This is from pressure on the ear from the mattress when in the side-lying position. Eyeglasses and oxygen tubing (Chapter 36) also can cause pressure on the ears. A urinary catheter can cause pressure and friction on the meatus. Tubes, casts, braces, and other devices can cause pressure on arms, hands, legs, and feet. A pressure ulcer can develop where medical equipment is attached to the skin.

In people who are obese, pressure ulcers can occur in areas where skin has contact with skin. Common sites are between abdominal folds, the legs, the buttocks, the thighs, and under the breasts. Friction occurs in these areas.

PREVENTION AND TREATMENT

Preventing pressure ulcers is much easier than trying to heal them. Good nursing care, cleanliness, and skin care are essential. The Joint Commission (TJC) and the CMS require pressure ulcer prevention programs. Pressure ulcer prevention involves:

- Identifying persons at risk. The nurse assesses the person when he or she is admitted to the agency. The person's risk factors and skin condition are assessed (p. 601).
- Implementing prevention measures for those at risk. Managing moisture, good nutrition and fluid balance, and relieving pressure are key measures. The measures in Box 34-3 may be part of the person's care plan to prevent skin breakdown and pressure ulcers. Always follow the person's care plan.

BOX 34-3   **MEASURES TO PREVENT PRESSURE ULCERS**

Moving and Positioning

- Follow the person's re-positioning schedule (Fig. 34-5). Re-position bedfast persons at least every 1 to 2 hours. Re-position chairfast persons every hour. Some persons are re-positioned every 15 minutes. Some persons are allowed to sit in a chair 3 times a day for 60 minutes or less.
- Position the person according to the care plan. Use pillows for support as directed. The 30-degree lateral position is recommended (Fig. 34-6).
- Do not position the person:
  - On a pressure ulcer
  - On a reddened area
  - On tubes or other medical devices
- Do not leave a person on a bedpan longer than needed.
- Prevent shearing and friction during moving and transfer procedures. Use assist devices as directed. See Chapter 17.
- Prevent friction in bed. Powder sheets lightly to prevent friction if directed to do so by the nurse.
- Prevent shearing. Do not raise the head of the bed more than 30 degrees. Follow the care plan for:
  - When to raise the head of the bed
  - How far to raise the head of the bed
  - How long (in minutes) to raise the head of the bed
- Use pillows, foam wedges, or other devices to prevent bony areas from contact with bony areas. The ankles, knees, hips, and sacrum are examples.
- Keep the heels and ankles off the bed. Use pillows or other devices as directed. Place the pillows or devices under the lower legs from mid-calf to the ankles.
- Use protective devices as directed.
- Remind persons sitting in chairs to shift their positions every 15 minutes.
- Support the person's feet properly. Use a footrest if the person's feet do not touch the floor when he or she is sitting in a chair. The body slides forward when the person's feet do not touch the floor. If the person is in a wheelchair, position the feet on the footrests.

Skin Care

- Inspect the skin every time you provide care. This includes during or after transfers, re-positioning, bathing, and elimination procedures. Report any concern at once.
- Follow the person's bathing schedule. Some persons do not need a bath every day.
- Do not use hot water to bathe or clean the skin. Hot water can irritate the skin.
- Use a cleansing agent as directed. Soap can dry and irritate the skin.
- Provide good skin care. The skin is clean and dry after bathing. The skin is free of moisture from a bath, urine, stools, perspiration, wound drainage, and other secretions.
- Follow measures to prevent incontinence.
- Prevent skin exposure to moisture. Check persons who are incontinent of urine or feces often. Provide good skin care and change linens and garments at the time of soiling. Use incontinence products as directed.
- Apply an ointment or moisture barrier if the person is incontinent of urine or feces.
- Check persons often who perspire heavily or have wound drainage. Change linens and garments as needed. Provide good skin care.
- Apply moisturizer to dry areas—hands, elbows, legs, ankles, heels, and so on. The nurse tells you what to use and what areas need attention.
- Give a back massage when re-positioning the person. *Do not massage bony areas.*
- Do not massage over pressure points. *Never rub or massage reddened areas.*
- Keep linens clean, dry, and wrinkle-free.
- Do not irritate the skin. Avoid scrubbing or vigorous rubbing when bathing or drying the person.
- Use pillows and blankets to prevent skin from being in contact with skin. They also reduce moisture and friction.
- Make sure socks and shoes are in good repair. Socks should not have wrinkles or creases. Make sure there is nothing in the shoes before the person puts them on.
- Do not apply heat or cold (Chapter 35) directly on a pressure ulcer.

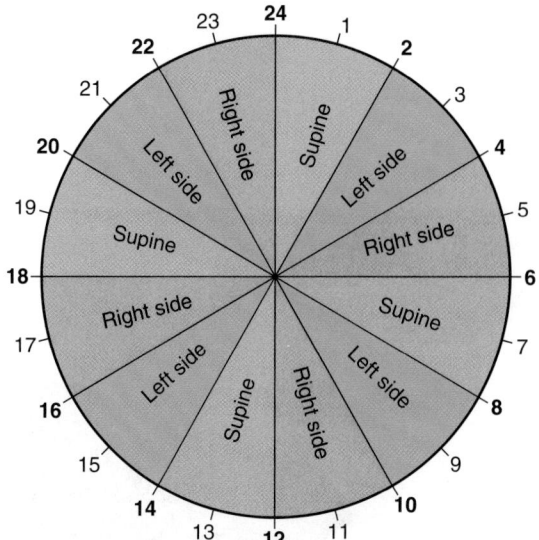

Fig. 34-5 Turn clock. The clock shows the times to turn the person and to what position.

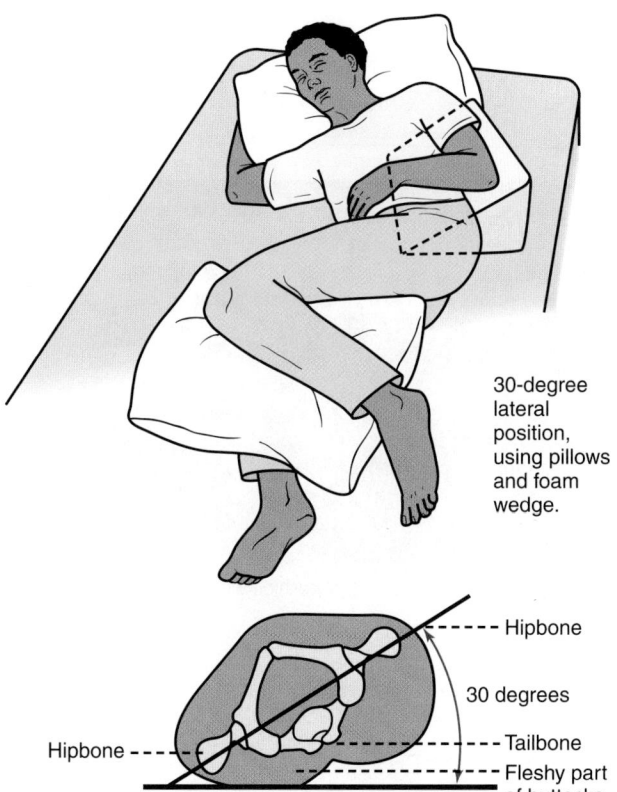

30-degree lateral position, using pillows and foam wedge.

Fig. 34-6 The 30 degree lateral position. Pillows are placed under the head, shoulder, and leg. This position inclines (lifts up) the hip to avoid pressure on the hip. The person does not lie on the hip as in the side-lying position.

Some agencies use symbols or colored stickers as pressure ulcer alerts. They are placed on the person's door or chart. They remind the staff that the person is at risk for a pressure ulcer.

Support surfaces are used to relieve or reduce pressure. Such surfaces include foam, air, alternating air, gel, or water mattresses. The best surface for the person is used.

Protective Devices

The doctor orders wound care products, drugs, treatments, and special equipment to promote healing. The nurse and care plan tell you what to do. Protective devices are often used to prevent and treat pressure ulcers and skin breakdown. These devices are common:

- *Bed cradle*—A bed cradle is a metal frame placed on the bed and over the person (Chapter 27). Top linens are brought over the cradle to prevent pressure on the legs, feet, and toes. Protect the person from drafts and chilling. To do so, tuck and miter linens at the bottom of the mattress. Also tuck them in under the mattress sides.
- *Heel and elbow protectors*—These devices are made of foam padding, pressure-relieving gel, sheepskin, and other cushion materials. They fit the shape of heels and elbows (Fig. 34-7, p. 600). Some are inserted inside sleeves or mesh. Others are secured in place with straps. These devices promote comfort. And they reduce shear and friction.
- *Heel and foot elevators*—These raise the heels and feet off of the bed (Fig. 34-8, p. 600). They prevent pressure. Some also prevent footdrop (Chapter 27).
- *Gel or fluid-filled pads and cushions*—These devices involve a pressure-relieving gel or fluid (Fig. 34-9, p. 600). They are used for chairs and wheelchairs to prevent pressure. The outer case is vinyl. The pad or cushion is placed in a fabric cover to protect the person's skin. Some covers are two colors (Fig. 34-10, p. 600). The colors remind the staff to re-position the person.
- *Eggcrate-type pads*—If used, these devices are placed on beds or in chairs or wheelchairs (Fig. 34-11, p. 601). The foam pad looks like an egg carton. Peaks in the pad distribute the person's weight more evenly. The pad is put in a special cover. The cover protects against heat, moisture, and soiling. Only a bottom sheet is used over the eggcrate-type pad and cover. No other bottom linens are used.
- *Special beds*—Some beds have air flowing through the mattresses (Fig. 34-12, p. 601). The person *floats* on the mattress. Body weight is distributed evenly. There is little pressure on body parts. Some beds allow re-positioning without moving the person. The person is turned to the prone or supine position or the bed is tilted various degrees. Alignment does not change. Pressure points change as the position changes. There is little friction. Some beds constantly rotate from side to side. They are useful for persons with spinal cord injuries.
- *Other equipment*—Pillows, trochanter rolls, foot-boards, and other positioning devices are used (Chapter 27). They help keep the person in good alignment.

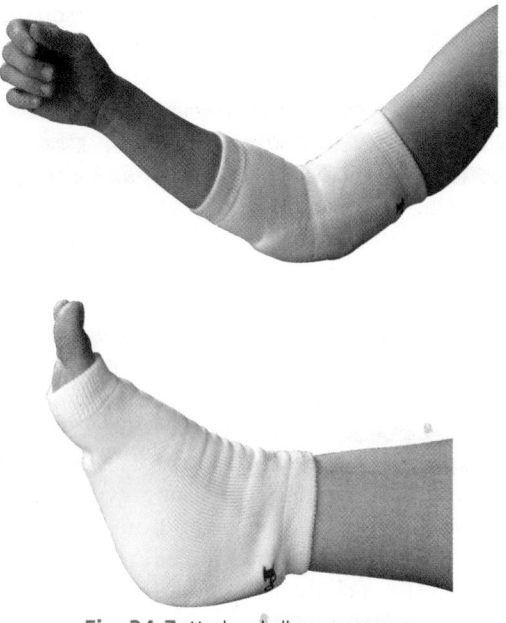

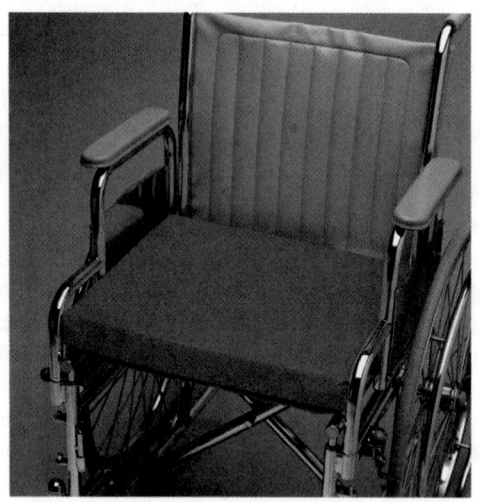

Fig. 34-7 Heel and elbow protectors.

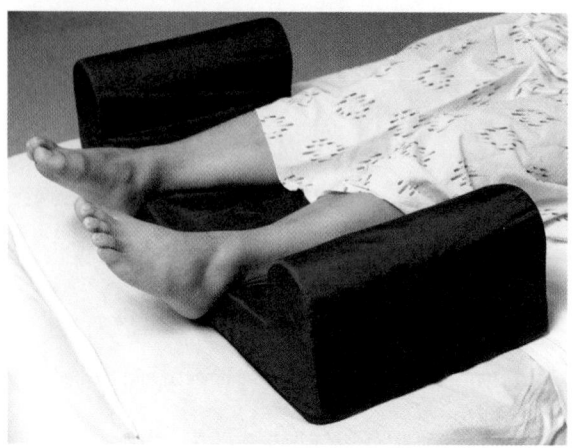

Fig. 34-8 Heel elevator.

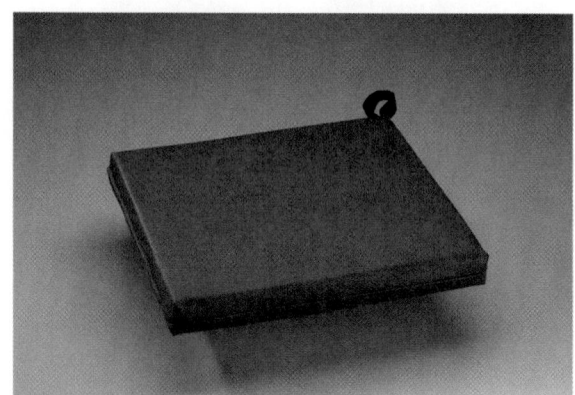

Fig. 34-9 Gel and foam cushion.

Fig. 34-10 Gel and foam cushion with a two-color cover.

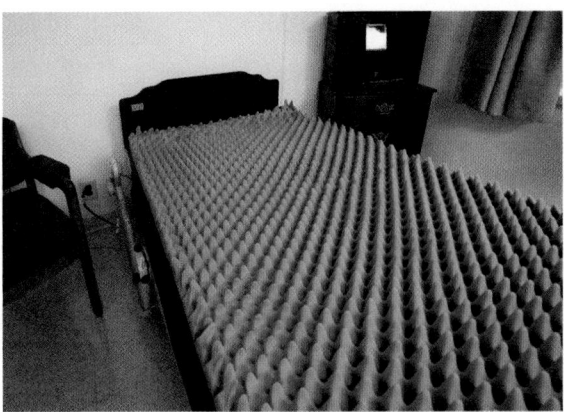

Fig. 34-11 Eggcrate-type pad on the bed.

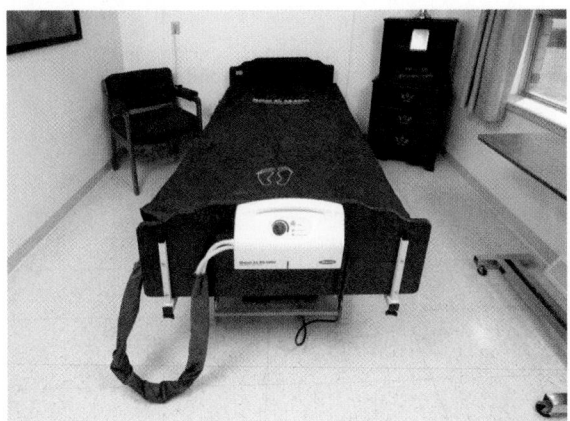

Fig. 34-12 Air flotation bed.

Dressings

The nurse decides what dressing to use (Chapter 33). Sometimes wet dressings are used. The wound must be moist enough to promote healing. However, it must not be too moist. If too moist, the dressing can interfere with healing.

A pressure ulcer may have drainage. A dressing that absorbs drainage is used. The dressing absorbs slough. The slough is removed when the dressing is removed.

Braden Scale

The Braden Scale for Predicting Pressure Sore Risk is a popular tool (Fig. 34-13, p. 602). Depending on the person's condition and risk factors, he or she is assessed daily or weekly.

You assist the nurse with the assessment step of the nursing process. Report signs and symptoms of a pressure ulcer at once. See Box 34-2.

COMPLICATIONS

Infection is the most common complication. According to the CMS, all Stage 2, 3, and 4 pressure ulcers are colonized with bacteria. *Colonized refers to the presence of bacteria on the wound surface or in wound tissue. The person does not have signs and symptoms of an infection.* Wounds are infected if the person has signs and symptoms of infection (Chapter 15). For some persons, pain and delayed healing signal an infection. For the pressure ulcer to heal, infection must be diagnosed and treated.

Osteomyelitis is a risk if the pressure ulcer is over a bony prominence. The risk is great if the ulcer is not healing. *Osteomyelitis* means inflammation *(itis)* of the bone *(osteo)* and bone marrow *(myel)*. The person has severe pain. The person is treated with bedrest and antibiotics. Careful and gentle positioning is needed. Surgery may be needed to remove dead bone and tissue.

Pressure ulcers can cause pain. Pain management is important (Chapter 28). Pain may affect movement and activity. Immobility is a risk factor for pressure ulcers. And it may delay healing of an existing pressure ulcer.

BRADEN SCALE FOR PREDICTING PRESSURE SORE RISK

Patient's name _____   Evaluator's name _____   Date of assessment

SENSORY PERCEPTION Ability to respond meaningfully to pressure-related discomfort	**1. Completely Limited** Unresponsive (does not moan, flinch, or grasp) to painful stimuli, due to diminished level of consciousness or sedation OR limited ability to feel pain over most of body.	**2. Very Limited** Responds only to painful stimuli. Cannot communicate discomfort except by moaning or restlessness OR has a sensory impairment which limits the ability to feel pain or discomfort over 1/2 of body.	**3. Slightly Limited** Responds to verbal commands, but cannot always communicate discomfort or the need to be turned OR has some sensory impairment which limits ability to feel pain or discomfort in 1 or 2 extremities.	**4. No Impairment** Responds to verbal commands. Has no sensory deficit which would limit ability to feel or voice pain or discomfort.
MOISTURE Degree to which skin is exposed to moisture	**1. Constantly Moist** Skin is kept moist almost constantly by perspiration, urine, etc. Dampness is detected every time patient is moved or turned.	**2. Very Moist** Skin is often, but not always moist. Linen must be changed at least once a shift.	**3. Occasionally Moist** Skin is occasionally moist, requiring an extra linen change approximately once a day.	**4. Rarely Moist** Skin is usually dry, linen only requires changing at routine intervals.
ACTIVITY Degree of physical activity	**1. Bedfast** Confined to bed.	**2. Chairfast** Ability to walk severely limited or non-existent. Cannot bear own weight and/or must be assisted into chair or wheelchair.	**3. Walks Occasionally** Walks occasionally during day, but for very short distances, with or without assistance. Spends majority of each shift in bed or chair.	**4. Walks Frequently** Walks outside room at least twice a day and inside room at least once every two hours during waking hours.
MOBILITY Ability to change and control body position	**1. Completely Immobile** Does not make even slight changes in body or extremity position without assistance.	**2. Very Limited** Makes occasional slight changes in body or extremity position but unable to make frequent or significant changes independently.	**3. Slightly Limited** Makes frequent though slight changes in body or extremity position independently.	**4. No Limitation** Makes major and frequent changes in position without assistance.
NUTRITION Usual food intake pattern	**1. Very Poor** Never eats a complete meal. Rarely eats more than 1/3 of any food offered. Eats 2 servings or less of protein (meat or dairy products) per day. Takes fluids poorly. Does not take a liquid dietary supplement OR is NPO and/or maintained on clear liquids or IVs for more than 5 days.	**2. Probably Inadequate** Rarely eats a complete meal and generally eats only about 1/2 of any food offered. Protein intake includes only 3 servings of meat or dairy products per day. Occasionally will take a dietary supplement OR receives less than optimum amount of liquid diet or tube feeding.	**3. Adequate** Eats over half of most meals. Eats a total of 4 servings of protein (meat, dairy products) per day. Occasionally will refuse a meal, but will usually take a supplement when offered OR is on a tube feeding or TPN regimen which probably meets most of nutritional needs.	**4. Excellent** Eats most of every meal. Never refuses a meal. Usually eats a total of 4 or more servings of meat and dairy products. Occasionally eats between meals. Does not require supplementation.
FRICTION & SHEAR	**1. Problem** Requires moderate to maximum assistance in moving. Complete lifting without sliding against sheets is impossible. Frequently slides down in bed or chair, requiring frequent re-positioning with maximum assistance. Spasticity, contractures or agitation leads to almost constant friction.	**2. Potential Problem** Moves feebly or requires minimum assistance. During a move skin probably slides to some extent against sheets, chair, restraints or other devices. Maintains relatively good position in chair or bed most of the time, but occasionally slides down.	**3. No Apparent Problem** Moves in bed and in chair independently and has sufficient muscle strength to lift up completely during move. Maintains good position in bed or chair.	

Total score

Fig. 34-13 Braden Scale for Predicting Pressure Sore Risk.

Date	Time	Nursing Margin	Other Depts Margin
8-27	0830	While assisting resident with a tub bath, a blister the size of a	
		quarter was noted on the outer aspect of the L heel. There is a $1/4$	
		inch reddened area around the blister. No drainage noted. Resident	
		states "It hurts a little." She said she thinks her shoes are rubbing	
		Asked Barabara Lane, RN to observe the area. Jean Hein, CNA	

Fig. 34-14 Charting sample.

REPORTING AND RECORDING

Report and record any signs of skin breakdown or pressure ulcers at once. See Figure 34-14. See "Wound Appearance" in Chapter 33.

See *Focus on Communication: Reporting and Recording.*

FOCUS ON COMMUNICATION
Reporting and Recording

You may be interviewed during a site survey. You might be asked about:
- How you are involved in the person's care.
- What measures the agency uses to prevent and treat pressure ulcers.
- What skin changes you should report and when.
- To whom you should report skin changes.
- Your knowledge of measures in a person's care plan.
  Answer questions honestly and completely. Respond in a professional manner.

FOCUS ON PRIDE
The Person, Family, and Yourself

Personal and Professional Responsibility

You have an important role in preventing and treating pressure ulcers. Tasks like positioning, applying protective devices, and skin care may be delegated to you. You must function in a way that improves the person's quality of life, health, and safety. Your attitude and the quality of your work affect the person. If you take your role seriously and believe you have a positive impact, the person will benefit. If you are careless and lack concern for the person's well-being, harm can result.

You are an important member of the nursing team. Take pride in your role. Work to the best of your ability. The person will benefit, and you will find joy in your work.

Rights and Respect

Observing and reporting skin problems to the nurse can prevent further skin breakdown. You have the right and responsibility to speak for your patients and residents. This is called being an *advocate*. When you see or suspect a problem, tell the nurse. You may be the first to notice a pressure ulcer. Telling the nurse can prevent further harm and result in prompt actions that promote healing. Take pride in being a voice for your patients and residents.

Independence and Social Interaction

A pressure ulcer is a serious matter. Infection, pain, amputation, and longer hospital or nursing center stays are complications. Healing can be a very long process. As time passes, family and friends may not be able to visit as often. Or the person may feel that he or she is a burden to others. Loneliness and depression can occur.

The person's physical needs are great. Do not neglect mental and social needs. Be kind. Show compassion. Take time to listen. Provide care in a way that improves the person's quality of life.

Delegation and Teamwork

Reporting and recording the completion of delegated tasks is an important part of your job. Be accurate and honest when reporting and recording. Never report or record something you did not do. Also, do not report or record before completing a task.

For example, Mrs. Scott was placed on the bedpan at 2250 (10:50 PM). The nursing assistant did not report this to the nurse. The next shift began at 2300 (11:00 PM). At 0700 (7:00 AM), the day shift found Mrs. Scott still on the bedpan. A pressure ulcer had developed. At risk for pressure ulcers, Mrs. Scott was to be re-positioned every 2 hours. Mrs. Scott's chart showed that she had been re-positioned every 2 hours from 2300 (11:00 PM) to 0700 (7:00 AM).

Poor communication, false recording, and negligence will cause harm. You must be thorough, honest, and careful when completing, reporting, and recording delegated tasks.

Continued

FOCUS ON P R I D E—cont'd

Ethics and Laws

Every year TJC develops National Patient Safety Goals for hospitals, nursing centers, and other agencies. The goals focus on ways to solve health care safety problems. Preventing pressure ulcers is an example. Agencies must have a plan to predict, prevent, and treat pressure ulcers early. Many agencies use a form or screening tool to identify persons at risk. Assessments are done on admission and regularly. The agency must take action to address risks. Know your agency's policies and procedures for identifying those at risk for pressure ulcers. Follow the measures in Box 34-3 to do your part to prevent pressure ulcers.

REVIEW QUESTIONS

Circle the BEST answer.

1 A pressure ulcer is
  a An open wound
  b A localized injury to the skin and/or underlying tissue
  c A bony prominence
  d Dead tissue

2 Pressure ulcers are the result of
  a Unrelieved pressure   c Medical devices
  b Moisture   d Aging

3 Which can contribute to the development of pressure ulcers?
  a Shear and friction   c Bony prominences
  b Slough and eschar   d CMS and TJC

4 A pressure ulcer can develop within
  a 2 to 6 hours   c 10 to 14 hours
  b 6 to 10 hours   d 14 to 18 hours

5 Which is *not* a risk factor for pressure ulcers?
  a Incontinence   c Moisture
  b Lowered mental awareness d Balanced diet

6 Which is the most common site for a pressure ulcer?
  a Back of the head   c Sacrum
  b Hip   d Heel

7 In a light-skinned person, the first sign of a pressure ulcer is
  a A blister   c Drainage
  b A reddened area   d Gangrene

8 A care plan includes the following. Which should you question?
  a Re-position the person every 2 hours.
  b Scrub and rub the skin during bathing.
  c Apply lotion to dry areas.
  d Keep linens clean, dry, and wrinkle-free.

9 You should position the person
  a On an existing pressure ulcer
  b On a reddened area
  c On tubes or other medical devices
  d Using assist devices

10 What is the preferred position for preventing pressure ulcers?
  a 30-degree lateral position c Prone position
  b Semi-Fowler's position   d Supine position

11 Which keep the heels and ankles off the bed?
  a Bed cradles   c Heel protectors
  b Pillows   d Eggcrate-type pads

12 Persons sitting in chairs should shift their positions every
  a 15 minutes   c Hour
  b 30 minutes   d Two hours

13 A person is sitting in a chair. The feet do not touch the floor. What should you do?
  a Have the person slide forward until the feet touch the floor.
  b Let the feet dangle.
  c Stack pillows under the person's feet.
  d Position the feet on a footrest.

14 Which are *not* used to treat pressure ulcers?
  a Special beds
  b Gel or fluid-filled pads and cushions
  c Plastic drawsheets and waterproof pads
  d Heel and elbow protectors

15 The following are sources of moisture *except*
  a Urine and feces
  b Wound drainage
  c Perspiration
  d Barrier ointment

16 You see a reddened area on the person's skin. What should you do?
  a Rub or massage the area.
  b Apply a moisturizer.
  c Apply a moisture barrier.
  d Tell the nurse.

17 A pressure ulcer is colonized. This means that
  a The wound is infected
  b Bacteria are present
  c The person has osteomyelitis
  d The person has a gauze dressing

Circle T if the statement is TRUE or F if it is FALSE.

18 T F All pressure ulcers are avoidable.
19 T F Skin breakdown can lead to a pressure ulcer.
20 T F Unrelieved pressure squeezes tiny blood vessels. Tissues do not receive needed oxygen and nutrients.
21 T F Persons who are bedfast or chairfast are at risk for pressure ulcers.
22 T F Pressure ulcers can develop on the ears.
23 T F Pressure ulcers can develop where medical devices are attached to the skin.
24 T F You are responsible for identifying persons at risk for pressure ulcers.
25 T F Pressure ulcers can involve muscles, tendons, and bones.
26 T F To prevent pressure ulcers, the head of the bed is raised higher than 30 degrees.
27 T F You should inspect the person's skin every time you provide care.
28 T F A person is at risk for pressure ulcers. A bath is needed every day.
29 T F You are giving a back massage. You should massage bony areas.
30 T F You can use pillows and blankets to prevent skin from being in contact with skin.

Answers to these questions are on p. 834.

Heat and Cold Applications

OBJECTIVES

- Define the key terms and key abbreviations listed in this chapter.
- Identify the purposes, effects, and complications of heat and cold applications.
- Identify the persons at risk for complications from heat and cold applications.
- Describe moist and dry heat applications.

- Describe moist and dry cold applications.
- Describe the rules for applying heat and cold.
- Explain how cooling and warming blankets are used.
- Perform the procedure described in this chapter.
- Explain how to promote PRIDE in the person, the family, and yourself.

KEY TERMS

compress A soft pad applied over a body area
constrict To narrow
cyanosis Bluish color
dilate To expand or open wider
hyperthermia A body temperature *(thermia)* that is much higher *(hyper)* than the person's normal range

hypothermia A very low *(hypo)* body temperature *(thermia)*
pack Wrapping a body part with a wet or dry application

KEY ABBREVIATIONS

C Centigrade
F Fahrenheit

ID Identification

Heat and cold applications promote healing and comfort. They also reduce tissue swelling. Heat and cold have opposite effects on body function. Severe injuries and changes in body function can occur. The risks are great.

In some agencies, only nurses apply heat and cold. Other agencies let nursing assistants do so. Before you perform these procedures, make sure that:

- Your state allows you to perform the procedure.
- The procedure is in your job description.
- You have the necessary training.
- You know how to use the equipment.
- You review the procedure with a nurse.
- A nurse is available to answer questions and to supervise you.

See *Focus on Children and Older Persons: Heat and Cold Applications.*

FOCUS ON CHILDREN AND OLDER PERSONS
Heat and Cold Applications

Children
Infants and young children have fragile skin. They are at risk for burns. They need careful attention. Always respond when a child cries. Crying is a way to communicate pain.

Older Persons
Older persons have thin and fragile skin. Burns are a risk. Changes from aging and health problems increase the risk for burns. They include circulatory and nervous system changes. Some drugs affect the ability to sense pain. Confused persons and those with dementia may not recognize pain. Look for behavior changes. Behavior changes can signal pain.

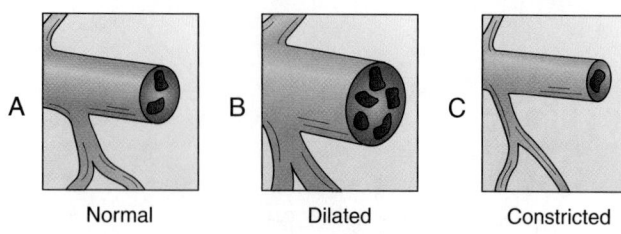

Normal   Dilated   Constricted

Fig. 35-1 A, Blood vessel under normal conditions. **B,** Dilated blood vessel. **C,** Constricted blood vessel.

HEAT APPLICATIONS

Heat applications can be applied to almost any body part. They are often used for musculo-skeletal injuries or problems (sprains, arthritis). Heat:

- Relieves pain.
- Relaxes muscles.
- Promotes healing.
- Reduces tissue swelling.
- Decreases joint stiffness.

When heat is applied to the skin, blood vessels in the area dilate. *Dilate means to expand or open wider* (Fig. 35-1). Blood flow increases. Tissues have more oxygen and nutrients for healing. Excess fluid is removed from the area faster. The skin is red and warm.

Complications

High temperatures can cause burns. Report pain, excessive redness, and blisters at once. Also observe for pale skin. When heat is applied too long, blood vessels *constrict (narrow)* (see Fig. 35-1). Blood flow decreases. Tissues receive less blood. Tissue damage occurs, and the skin is pale.

Older and fair-skinned persons have fragile skin that is easily burned. Persons with problems sensing heat and pain are also at risk. Nervous system damage, loss of consciousness, and circulatory disorders affect sensation. So do confusion and some drugs.

Metal implants pose risks. Metal conducts heat. Deep tissues can be burned. Pacemakers (cardiac devices) and joint replacements are made of metal. Do not apply heat to an implant area.

Heat is not applied to a pregnant woman's abdomen. The heat can affect fetal growth.

Moist and Dry Heat Applications

With a *moist heat application*, water is in contact with the skin. Water conducts heat. Moist heat has greater and faster effects than dry heat. Heat penetrates deeper with a moist application. To prevent injury, moist heat applications have lower (cooler) temperatures than dry heat applications. Moist heat applications (Fig. 35-2) include:

- *Hot compress.* A *compress is a soft pad applied over a body area.* It is usually made of cloth. Sometimes an aquathermia pad is applied over the compress. It maintains the temperature of the compress.
- *Hot soak.* A body part is put into water. This is usually used for smaller parts—a hand, lower arm, foot, or lower leg. A tub is used for larger areas.
- *Sitz bath.* The perineal and rectal areas are immersed in warm or hot water. (*Sitz* means *seat* in German.) Sitz baths are common for hemorrhoids, after rectal or female pelvic surgeries, and after childbirth. They are used to:
  - Clean perineal and anal wounds.
  - Promote healing.
  - Relieve pain and soreness.
  - Increase circulation.
  - Stimulate voiding.
- *Hot pack.* A *pack involves wrapping a body part with a wet or dry application.* There are single-use (disposable) and re-usable packs. Some are used for heat or cold. Follow the manufacturer's instructions to activate the heat or cold. Clean re-usable packs after use. Follow agency policy and the manufacturer's instructions.

With *dry heat applications*, water is not in contact with the skin. A dry heat application stays at the desired temperature longer. Dry heat does not penetrate as deeply as moist heat. Because water is not used, dry heat needs higher (hotter) temperatures for the desired effect. Therefore burns are still a risk.

Some *hot packs* and the *aquathermia pad* (Aqua-K, K-Pad) are dry heat applications (Fig. 35-3). The aquathermia pad is an electrical device. Tubes inside the pad are filled with distilled water. Heated water flows to the pad through a hose. Another hose returns water to the heating unit. The water is reheated and returned back into the pad.

See *Focus on Long-Term Care and Home Care: Moist and Dry Heat Applications.*

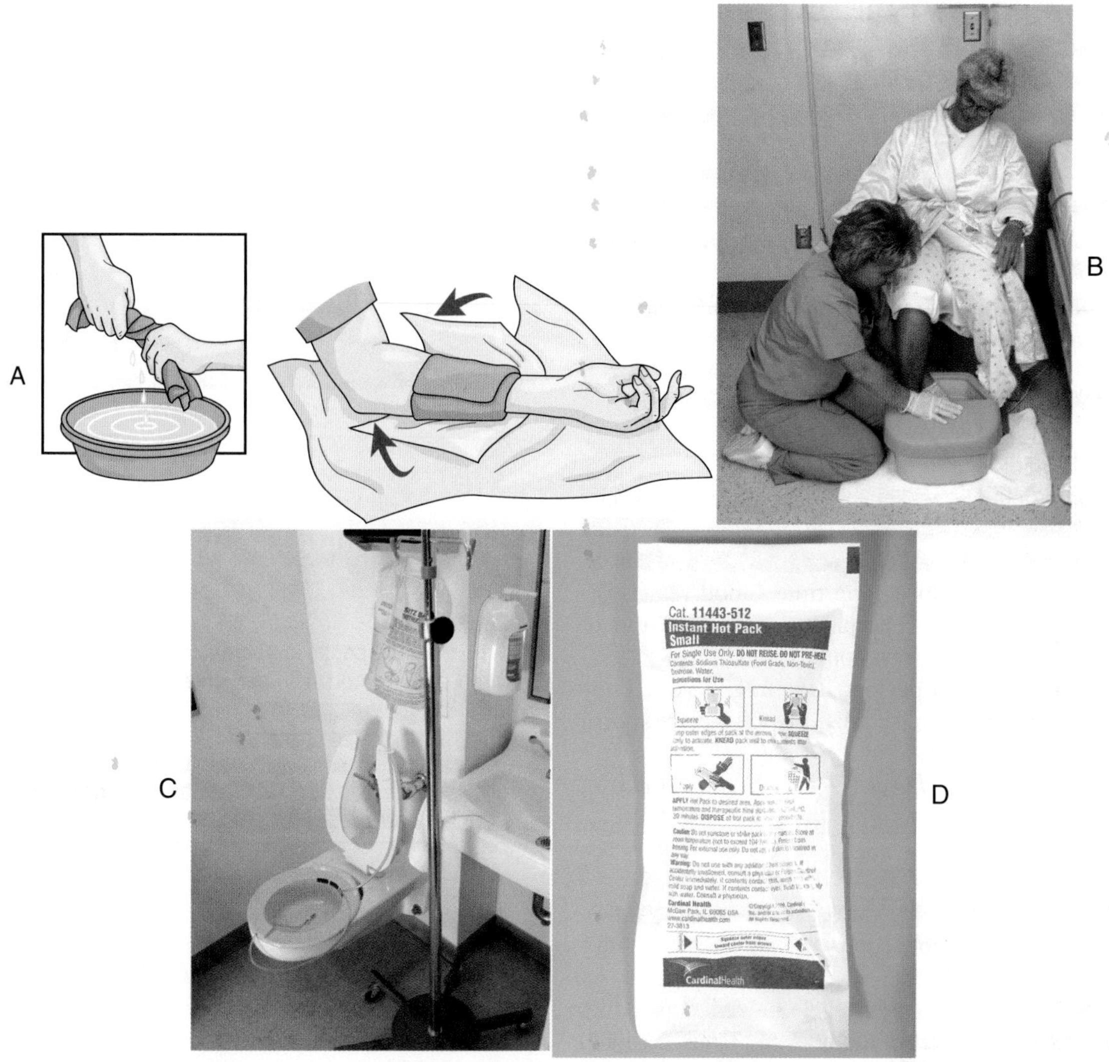

Fig. 35-2 Moist heat applications. **A,** Compress. **B,** Hot soak. **C,** Disposable sitz bath. **D,** Hot pack. (NOTE: Some hot packs can also be used as cold packs.)

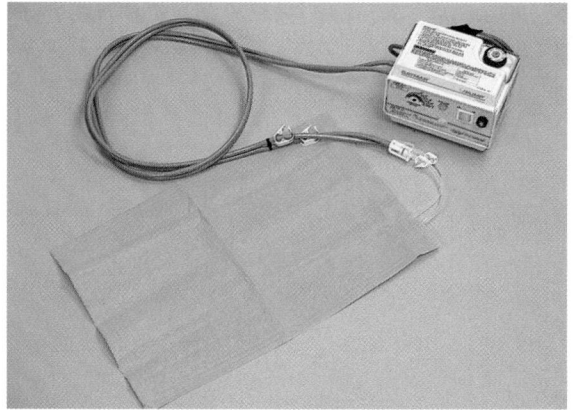

Fig. 35-3 The aquathermia pad.

FOCUS ON LONG-TERM CARE AND HOME CARE

Moist and Dry Heat Applications

Home Care

Heating pads may have electrical coils made of wire. The coils present fire hazards if they break. Always make sure the heating pad is in good repair.

The temperature of heating pads is easy to adjust. Burns are a great risk. Check the temperature often. Make sure the person has not changed it.

Some devices serve as heat and cold applications. They are filled with a special fluid. The pad is kept in the freezer until needed. For a heating pad, follow the manufacturer's instructions.

COLD APPLICATIONS

Cold applications are often used to treat sprains and fractures. They reduce pain, prevent swelling, and decrease circulation and bleeding. Cold cools the body when fever is present.

Cold has the opposite effect of heat. When cold is applied to the skin, blood vessels constrict (see Fig. 35-1). Blood flow decreases. Less oxygen and nutrients are carried to the tissues.

Cold applications are useful right after an injury. Decreased blood flow reduces the amount of bleeding. Less fluid collects in the tissues. Cold has a numbing effect on the skin. This helps reduce or relieve pain in the part.

Complications

Complications include pain, burns, blisters, and poor circulation. Burns and blisters occur from intense cold. They also occur when dry cold is in direct contact with the skin.

When cold is applied for a long time, blood vessels dilate. Blood flow increases. The prolonged application of cold has the same effect as heat applications.

Older and fair-skinned persons have fragile skin. They are at great risk for complications. So are persons with sensory impairments.

See *Focus on Children and Older Persons: Heat and Cold Applications*, p. 605.

Moist and Dry Cold Applications

Moist cold applications penetrate deeper than dry ones. Therefore moist cold applications are warmer than dry cold applications.

The cold compress is a moist cold application (see Fig. 35-2, A). Dry cold applications include ice bags, ice collars, and ice gloves (Fig. 35-4). The device is filled with crushed ice.

Cold packs can be moist or dry applications (see Fig. 35-2, D). Commercial cold packs are single-use (disposable) or re-usable. To activate the cold, follow the manufacturer's instructions. You will strike, knead, or squeeze the pack. Keep re-usable cold packs in the freezer. Clean them after use (see "Hot pack," p. 606). Discard single-use cold packs after use.

See *Focus on Long-Term Care and Home Care: Moist and Dry Cold Applications.*

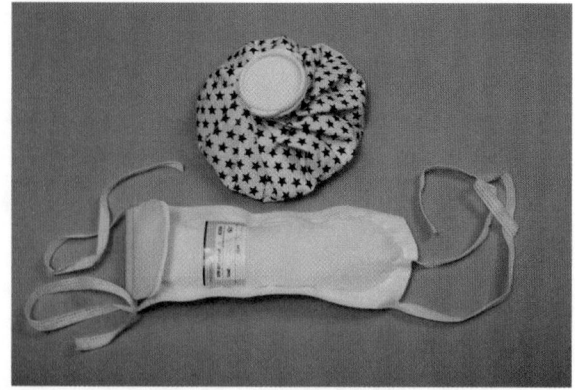

Fig. 35-4 Ice bags.

FOCUS ON LONG-TERM CARE AND HOME CARE
Moist and Dry Cold Applications

Home Care
Disposable ice packs are common in home settings. A bag of frozen peas or corn can serve as an ice bag. So can plastic bags. If using a plastic bag:
- Fill the plastic bag with ice.
- Close the bag securely to prevent leaks.
- Wrap the pack, bag of peas or corn, or plastic bag in a towel, dishcloth, or pillowcase.

APPLYING HEAT AND COLD

Protect the person from injury during heat and cold applications. Follow the rules in Box 35-1. See Table 35-1 for heat and cold temperature ranges.

See *Focus on Communication: Applying Heat and Cold.*
See *Teamwork and Time Management: Applying Heat and Cold.*
See *Delegation Guidelines: Applying Heat and Cold.*
See *Promoting Safety and Comfort: Applying Heat and Cold*, p. 610.

BOX 35-1 RULES FOR APPLYING HEAT AND COLD

- Know how to use the equipment. Follow the manufacturer's instructions for commercial devices.
- Measure the temperature of moist applications. Use a bath thermometer. Or follow agency policy for measuring temperature.
- Follow agency policies for safe temperature ranges. See Table 35-1.
- Do not apply *very hot* (above 106°F or 41.1°C) applications. Tissue damage can occur. A nurse applies *very hot* applications.
- Ask the nurse what the temperature should be.
  - Heat—cooler temperatures for persons at risk
  - Cold—warmer temperatures for persons at risk
- Know the exact site of the application. Have the nurse show you the site.
- Cover dry heat or cold applications before applying them. Use a flannel cover, towel, or other cover as directed.
- Provide for privacy. Properly screen and drape the person. Expose only the body part involved. Avoid unnecessary exposure.
- Maintain comfort and body alignment during the procedure.
- Observe the skin every 5 minutes for signs of complications. See *Delegation Guidelines: Applying Heat and Cold.*
- Do not let the person change the temperature of the application.
- Know how long to leave the application in place. See *Delegation Guidelines: Applying Heat and Cold.* Carefully watch the time. Heat and cold are applied no longer than 15 to 20 minutes.
- Follow the rules of electrical safety when using electrical appliances to apply heat.
- Place the signal light within the person's reach.
- Complete a safety check before leaving the room. (See the inside of the front book cover.)

TABLE 35-1 HEAT AND COLD TEMPERATURE RANGES

Temperature	Fahrenheit (F) Range	Centigrade (C) Range
Hot	98°F to 106°F	36.6°C to 41.1°C
Warm	93°F to 98°F	33.8°C to 36.6°C
Tepid	80°F to 93°F	26.6°C to 33.8°C
Cool	65°F to 80°F	18.3°C to 26.6°C
Cold	50°F to 65°F	10.0°C to 18.3°C

Modified from Perry AG, Potter PA: *Clinical nursing skills and techniques*, ed 7, St Louis, 2010, Mosby.

FOCUS ON COMMUNICATION
Applying Heat and Cold

The person may not tell you about pain or discomfort. The person may not know what symptoms to report. For heat and cold applications, you need to ask:
- "Does the application feel too hot or too cold?"
- "Do you feel any pain, numbness, or burning?"
- "Are you warm enough?"
- "Do you feel weak, faint, or drowsy?" If yes: "Tell me how you feel."

TEAMWORK AND TIME MANAGEMENT
Applying Heat and Cold

After applying heat or cold, check the person and the application every 5 minutes. Plan your work so you can stay in or near the person's room. For example, during the application:
- Make the bed and straighten the person's unit.
- Provide care to the person's roommate if you are assigned to him or her.
- Help the person complete his or her daily or weekly menu.
- Read cards and letters to the person, with his or her consent.
- Address envelopes and other correspondence for the person.
- Take time to visit with the person.

DELEGATION GUIDELINES
Applying Heat and Cold

To apply heat or cold, you need this information from the nurse and the care plan:
- The type of application—hot compress or pack, commercial compress, hot soak, sitz bath, aquathermia pad; ice bag, ice collar, ice glove, cold pack, or cold compress
- How to cover the application
- What temperature to use (see Table 35-1)
- The application site
- How long to leave the application in place
- What observations to report and record:
  - Complaints of pain or discomfort, numbness, or burning
  - Excessive redness
  - Blisters
  - Pale, white, or gray skin
  - *Cyanosis* (bluish color)
  - Shivering
  - Rapid pulse, weakness, faintness, and drowsiness (sitz bath)
  - Time, site, and length of application
- When to report observations
- What patient or resident concerns to report at once

PROMOTING SAFETY AND COMFORT
Applying Heat and Cold

Safety

Check the person every 5 minutes. Also follow these safety measures:

- *Sitz bath.* Blood flow increases to the perineum and rectum. Therefore less blood flows to other body parts. The person may become weak or feel faint. Drowsiness can occur from the bath's relaxing effect. Observe for signs of weakness, fainting, or fatigue. Also protect the person from injury. Check the person often. Keep the signal light within reach, and prevent chills and burns.
- *Commercial hot and cold packs.* Read warning labels and follow the manufacturer's instructions.
- *Aquathermia pad:*
  - Follow electrical safety precautions (Chapter 12).
  - Check the device for damage or flaws.
  - Follow the manufacturer's instructions.
  - Place the heating unit on an even, uncluttered surface. This prevents it from being knocked over or knocked off of the surface.
  - Make sure the hoses do not have kinks or bubbles. Water must flow freely.

Safety—cont'd

- Use a flannel cover to insulate the pad. It absorbs perspiration at the application site. (Some agencies use towels or pillowcases.)
- Secure the pad in place with ties, tape, or rolled gauze. Do not use pins. They can puncture the pad and cause leaks.
- Do not place the pad under the person or under a body part. This prevents the escape of heat. Burns can result if heat cannot escape.
- Give the key used to set the temperature to the nurse. This prevents anyone from changing the temperature. The temperature is usually set at 105°F (40.5°C) with a key.

Some persons have medicated patches or ointments applied to the skin. Do not apply heat over such areas.

Comfort

Cold applications can cause chills and shivering. Provide for warmth. Use bath blankets or other blankets as needed.

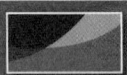

APPLYING HEAT AND COLD APPLICATIONS

`VIDEO`

QUALITY OF LIFE

Remember to:

- Knock before entering the person's room.
- Address the person by name.
- Introduce yourself by name and title.

- Explain the procedure to the person before beginning and during the procedure.
- Protect the person's rights during the procedure.
- Handle the person gently during the procedure.

PRE-PROCEDURE

1 Follow *Delegation Guidelines: Applying Heat and Cold,* p. 609. See *Promoting Safety and Comfort: Applying Heat and Cold.*
2 Practice hand hygiene.
3 Collect equipment.
- *For a hot compress:*
  - Basin
  - Bath thermometer
  - Small towel, washcloth, or gauze squares
  - Plastic wrap or aquathermia pad
  - Ties, tape, or rolled gauze
  - Bath towel
  - Waterproof pad
- *For a hot soak:*
  - Water basin or arm or foot bath
  - Bath thermometer
  - Waterproof pad
  - Bath blanket
  - Towel
- *For a sitz bath:*
  - Disposable sitz bath
  - Bath thermometer
  - Two bath blankets, bath towels, and a clean gown

- *For a hot or cold pack:*
  - Commercial pack
  - Pack cover
  - Ties, tape, or rolled gauze (if needed)
  - Waterproof pad
- *For an aquathermia pad:*
  - Aquathermia pad and heating unit
  - Distilled water
  - Flannel cover or other cover as directed by the nurse
  - Ties, tape, or rolled gauze
- *For an ice bag, ice collar, ice glove, or dry cold pack:*
  - Ice bag, collar, or glove or cold pack
  - Crushed ice (except for a cold pack)
  - Flannel cover or other cover as directed
  - Paper towels
- *For a cold compress:*
  - Large basin with ice
  - Small basin with cold water
  - Gauze squares, washcloths, or small towels
  - Waterproof pad
4 Identify the person. Check the ID (identification) bracelet against the assignment sheet. Also call the person by name.

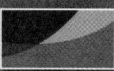 **APPLYING HEAT AND COLD APPLICATIONS—cont'd** | VIDEO |

PROCEDURE

5 Provide for privacy.
6 Position the person for the procedure.
7 Place the waterproof pad (if needed) under the body part.
8 *For a hot compress:*
  a Fill the basin ½ to ⅔ full with hot water as directed. Measure water temperature.
  b Place the compress in the water.
  c Wring out the compress.
  d Apply the compress over the area. Note the time.
  e Cover the compress as directed. Do one of the following:
    (1) Apply plastic wrap and then a bath towel. Secure the towel in place with ties, tape, or rolled gauze.
    (2) Apply an aquathermia pad.
9 *For a hot soak:*
  a Fill the container ½ full with hot water. Measure water temperature.
  b Place the part into the water. Pad the edge of the container with a towel. Note the time.
  c Cover the person with a bath blanket for warmth.
10 *For a sitz bath:*
  a Place the disposable sitz bath on the toilet seat.
  b Fill the sitz bath ⅔ full with water. Measure water temperature.
  c Secure the gown above the waist.
  d Help the person sit on the sitz bath. Note the time.
  e Provide for warmth. Place a bath blanket around the shoulders. Place another over the legs.
  f Stay with the person if he or she is weak or unsteady.
11 *For a hot or cold pack:*
  a Squeeze, knead, or strike the pack as directed by the manufacturer.
  b Place the pack in the cover.
  c Apply the pack. Note the time.
  d Secure the pack in place with ties, tape, or rolled gauze. Some packs are secured with Velcro straps.
12 *For an aquathermia pad:*
  a Fill the heating unit to the fill line with distilled water.
  b Remove the bubbles. Place the pad and tubing below the heating unit. Tilt the heating unit from side to side.
  c Set the temperature as the nurse directs (usually 105°F [40.5°C]). Remove the key.

  d Place the pad in the cover.
  e Plug in the unit. Let water warm to the desired temperature.
  f Set the heating unit on the bedside stand. Keep the pad and connecting hoses level with the unit. Hoses must not have kinks.
  g Apply the pad to the part. Note the time.
  h Secure the pad in place with ties, tape, or rolled gauze. Do not use pins.
13 *For an ice bag, collar, or glove:*
  a Fill the device with water. Put in the stopper. Turn the device upside down to check for leaks.
  b Empty the device.
  c Fill the device ½ to ⅔ full with crushed ice or ice chips.
  d Remove excess air. Bend, twist, or squeeze the device. Or press it against a firm surface.
  e Place the cap or stopper on securely.
  f Dry the device with paper towels.
  g Place the device in the cover.
  h Apply the device. Note the time.
  i Secure the device in place with ties, tape, or rolled gauze.
14 *For a cold compress:*
  a Place the small basin with cold water into the large basin with ice.
  b Place the compresses into the cold water.
  c Wring out a compress.
  d Apply the compress to the part. Note the time.
15 Place the signal light within reach. Unscreen the person.
16 Raise or lower bed rails. Follow the care plan.
17 Check the person every 5 minutes. Check for signs and symptoms of complications (see *Delegation Guidelines: Applying Heat and Cold,* p. 609). Remove the application if any occur. Tell the nurse at once.
18 Check the application every 5 minutes. Change the application if cooling (hot applications) or warming (cold applications) occurs.
19 Remove the application at the specified time. Heat and cold applications are left on for 15 to 20 minutes.

POST-PROCEDURE

20 Provide for comfort. (See the inside of the front book cover.)
21 Place the signal light within reach.
22 Raise or lower bed rails. Follow the care plan.
23 Unscreen the person.
24 Clean, rinse, dry, and return re-usable items to their proper place. Follow agency policy for soiled linen. Wear gloves for this step.

25 Complete a safety check of the room. (See the inside of the front book cover.)
26 Remove and discard the gloves. Practice hand hygiene.
27 Report and record your observations (Fig. 35-5, p. 612).

Date	Time	Nursing Margin	Other Depts Margin
3/6	1000	Aquathermia heating unit set at 105° F. The pad was placed in a flannel	
		cover and applied to the anterior R thigh. Secured in place with tape.	
		Resident positioned in semi-Fowler's position. States she is comfortable.	
		States the pad does not feel too hot. Overbed table with water pitcher and	
		water cup within reach. Bed in the low position. Signal light within	
		reach. Adam Aims, CNA	
3/6	1005	Aquathermia pad checked. Resident states she feels comfortable. States the	
		pad is not too hot. Denies pain or discomfort. There is no redness, swelling,	
		or blistering of the skin under the pad. Pad re-secured with tape. Overbed	
		table with water pitcher and cup within reach. Bed in the low position.	
		Signal light within reach. Adam Aims, CNA	

Fig. 35-5 Charting sample.

COOLING AND WARMING BLANKETS

Hyperthermia is a body temperature (thermia) *that is much higher* (hyper) *than the person's normal range.* Body temperature is greater than 103°F (39.4°C). It is often called *heat stroke* when caused by hot weather. Other causes include illness, dehydration, and not being able to perspire. Lowering the person's body temperature is necessary. Otherwise, death can occur. The doctor orders ice packs applied to the head, neck, underarms, and groin. Sometimes cooling blankets are used alone or with ice packs.

A cooling blanket is an electrical device. Made of rubber or plastic, the device has tubes filled with fluid. The fluid flows through the tubes. The blanket is placed on the bed and covered with a sheet. The blanket is turned on the cool setting and allowed to cool. The person lies on the blanket. Vital signs are measured often. Rapid and excess cooling is prevented.

Hypothermia is a very low (hypo) *body temperature* (thermia). Body temperature is less than 95°F (35°C). Cold weather is a common cause. The person is warmed to prevent death. Treatment may include a warming blanket. A warming blanket is like a cooling blanket except warm settings are used. Vital signs are checked often to prevent rapid or excess warming.

When used for cooling, the device is called a *hypothermia blanket.* When used for warming, it is called a *hyperthermia blanket.* The device has warm and cool settings.

See *Focus on Children and Older Persons: Cooling and Warming Blankets.*

FOCUS ON CHILDREN AND OLDER PERSONS
Cooling and Warming Blankets

Children
Rapid temperature changes can occur in infants and children. Observe them closely. Measure temperature as the nurse directs. Always report the measurement at once. Also report changes in other vital signs or in the child's condition.

FOCUS ON PRIDE
The Person, Family, and Yourself

Personal and Professional Responsibility
You are responsible for the tasks you perform. If unsure if you are allowed to apply heat or cold, ask the nurse. If you do not know how to use the equipment, tell the nurse. Never perform a task you are not comfortable doing. The person may be harmed. Do not be afraid, embarrassed, or ashamed to talk to the nurse about your concerns. Take pride in acting responsibly.

Rights and Respect
Heat and cold applications are used for many reasons. A person may ask about the need for a heat or cold application. Avoid answers like: "It's to help you get better." The person has the right to be informed of the reason for the application. Be kind, caring, and patient when the person asks questions. Refer questions to the nurse. Tell the person that you will ask the nurse to explain the reason for the application. Wait until the person's questions are answered before applying the heat or cold application.

Independence and Social Interaction

Remember to explain procedures to patients and residents. They can plan if they know what will happen. A person may want to make a phone call or finish an activity first. Or a person may want the procedure done by a certain time—before visitors arrive, before a TV program, or before an activity. You promote independence when you allow the person to plan procedure times.

Delegation and Teamwork

Completing tasks safely and in a way that promotes comfort requires time and planning. Heat and cold are usually applied for 15 to 20 minutes. You must also allow time for:

- Meeting elimination needs before the procedure.
- Positioning the person for comfort.
- Placing needed items within the person's reach. These include the signal light, water pitcher and cup, reading material, needlework, phone, and other items requested by the person.
- Checking the person often.
- Reporting and recording completion of the task and your observations.

Learning the amount of time needed for tasks comes with practice and experience. You can also ask for advice from co-workers who manage their work well. Take pride in learning to do your job well in a way that promotes the person's safety and comfort.

Ethics and Laws

Complications from heat and cold applications can be severe. Burns, blisters, circulation problems, and tissue damage are examples. Safety must be a priority. Harm and legal action can result if you:

- Apply a heat or cold application without an order.
- Use the equipment without training.
- Apply an application that is too hot or too cold.
- Do not cover an application as directed.
- Neglect to check the person often.
- Leave the application on longer than directed.
- Fail to report complications to the nurse.

Follow the rules in Box 35-1 for safely using heat and cold applications. Take pride in protecting the person from injury.

REVIEW QUESTIONS

Circle the BEST answer.

1 Heat applications have these effects *except*
a Pain relief   c Healing
b Muscle relaxation   d Decreased blood flow

2 The *greatest* threat from heat applications is
a Infection   c Chilling
b Burns   d Pressure ulcers

3 Who is at *greatest* risk for complications from heat applications?
a An older person with dark skin
b An older person with nerve damage
c An adult with a circulatory disorder
d A child with fair skin

4 These statements are about moist heat applications. Which is *false?*
a Water is in contact with the skin.
b The effects from moist heat are less than from a dry heat application.
c Moist heat penetrates deeper than dry heat.
d A moist heat application has a lower temperature than a dry heat application.

5 A hot application is usually
a 80°F to 93°F
b 93°F to 98°F
c 98°F to 106°F
d Above 106°F

6 These statements are about sitz baths. Which is *false?*
a The perineal and rectal areas are immersed in warm water.
b Sitz baths last 25 to 30 minutes.
c They clean the perineum, relieve pain, increase circulation, or stimulate voiding.
d Weakness and fainting can occur.

7 A person uses an aquathermia pad. Which is *false?*
a It is a dry heat application.
b A flannel cover is used.
c Electrical safety precautions are practiced.
d Pins secure the pad in place.

8 Cold applications
a Reduce pain, prevent swelling, and decrease circulation
b Dilate blood vessels
c Prevent the spread of microbes
d Prevent infection

9 Which is *not* a complication of cold applications?
a Pain
b Burns
c Blisters
d Infection

10 Before applying an ice bag
a Place the bag in the freezer
b Measure the temperature of the bag
c Place the bag in a cover
d Provide perineal care

11 Moist cold compresses are left in place no longer than
a 20 minutes
b 30 minutes
c 45 minutes
d 60 minutes

12 A cooling blanket is used for
a Hypothermia
b Hyperthermia
c Cyanosis
d Shivering

Answers to these questions are on p. 834.

36 Oxygen Needs

OBJECTIVES

- Define the key terms and key abbreviations listed in this chapter.
- Describe the factors affecting oxygen needs.
- List the signs and symptoms of hypoxia and altered respiratory function.
- Describe the tests used to diagnose respiratory problems.
- Explain the measures that promote oxygenation.
- Describe the devices used to give oxygen.
- Explain how to safely assist with oxygen therapy.
- Perform the procedures described in this chapter.
- Explain how to promote PRIDE in the person, the family, and yourself.

KEY TERMS

allergy A sensitivity to a substance that causes the body to react with signs and symptoms

apnea The lack or absence (a) of breathing (pnea)

atelectasis The collapse of a portion of the lung

Biot's respirations Rapid and deep respirations followed by 10 to 30 seconds of apnea

bradypnea Slow (brady) breathing (pnea); respirations are fewer than 12 per minute

Cheyne-Stokes respirations Respirations gradually increase in rate and depth and then become shallow and slow; breathing may stop (apnea) for 10 to 20 seconds

cyanosis Bluish color to the skin, lips, mucous membranes, and nail beds

dyspnea Difficult, labored, or painful (dys) breathing (pnea)

hemoptysis Bloody (hemo) sputum (ptysis means to spit)

hyperventilation Breathing (ventilation) is rapid (hyper) and deeper than normal

hypoventilation Breathing (ventilation) is slow (hypo), shallow, and sometimes irregular

hypoxemia A reduced amount (hypo) of oxygen (ox) in the blood (emia)

hypoxia Cells do not have enough (hypo) oxygen (oxia)

Kussmaul respirations Very deep and rapid respirations

orthopnea Breathing (pnea) deeply and comfortably only when sitting (ortho)

orthopneic position Sitting up (ortho) and leaning over a table to breathe (pneic)

oxygen concentration The amount (percent) of hemoglobin containing oxygen

pollutant A harmful chemical or substance in the air or water

respiratory arrest When breathing stops

respiratory depression Slow, weak respirations at a rate of fewer than 12 per minute

sputum Mucus from the respiratory system that is expectorated (expelled) through the mouth

tachypnea Rapid (tachy) breathing (pnea); respirations are more than 20 per minute

KEY ABBREVIATIONS

CO_2	Carbon dioxide	O_2	Oxygen
ID	Identification	RBC	Red blood cell
L/min	Liters per minute	SpO_2	Saturation of peripheral oxygen (oxygen concentration)

Oxygen (O_2) is a gas. It has no taste, odor, or color. It is a basic need required for life. Death occurs within minutes if breathing stops. Brain damage and serious illness can occur without enough oxygen. Illness, surgery, and injuries affect the amount of oxygen in the body. Respiratory complications are risks after surgery.

You assist in the care of persons with oxygen needs. You must give safe and effective care.

See *Body Structure and Function Review: The Respiratory System.*

BODY STRUCTURE AND FUNCTION REVIEW: THE RESPIRATORY SYSTEM

Oxygen is needed to live. Every cell needs oxygen. The respiratory system (Fig. 36-1) brings oxygen into the lungs and removes carbon dioxide. *Respiration* is the process of supplying the cells with oxygen (O_2) and removing carbon dioxide (CO_2) from them. Respiration involves breathing in (*inhalation, inspiration*) and breathing out (*exhalation, expiration*).

Air enters the body through the nose. Then the air passes into the *pharynx* (throat). It is a tube-shaped passage-way for air and food. Air passes from the pharynx into the *larynx* (voice box). Air passes from the larynx into the *trachea* (windpipe).

The trachea divides at its lower end into the *right bronchus* and the *left bronchus*. Each bronchus enters a *lung*. Upon entering the lungs, the bronchi divide many times into smaller branches (*bronchioles*). Eventually the bronchioles subdivide. They end up in tiny one-celled air sacs called *alveoli*.

O_2 and CO_2 are exchanged between the alveoli and capillaries. Blood in the capillaries picks up O_2 from the alveoli. Then the blood is returned to the left side of the heart and pumped to the rest of the body. Alveoli pick up CO_2 from the capillaries for exhalation.

Each lung is divided into lobes. The right lung has 3 lobes; the left lung has 2. The lungs are separated from the abdominal cavity by a muscle called the *diaphragm*. A bony framework made up of the ribs, sternum, and vertebrae protects the lungs.

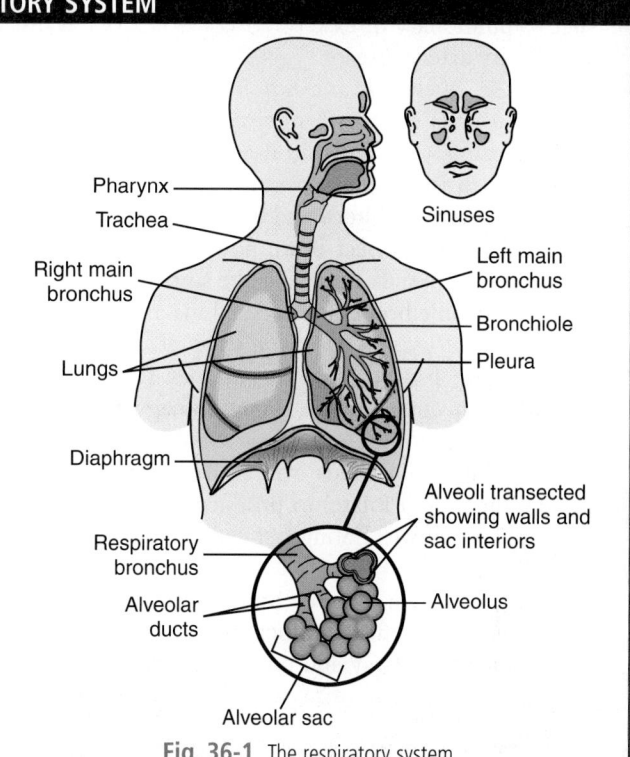

Fig. 36-1 The respiratory system.

FACTORS AFFECTING OXYGEN NEEDS

The respiratory and circulatory systems must function properly for cells to get enough O_2. Any disease, injury, or surgery involving these systems affects the intake and use of O_2. Body systems depend on each other. Altered function of any system (for example, the nervous, musculo-skeletal, or urinary system) affects oxygen needs. Oxygen needs are affected by:

- *Respiratory system function.* Structures must be intact and function properly. An open (*patent*) airway is needed. Alveoli (air sacs) must exchange O_2 and CO_2.
- *Circulatory system function.* Blood must flow to and from the heart. Narrowed vessels affect blood flow. Capillaries and cells must exchange O_2 and CO_2.
- *Red blood cell count.* Red blood cells (RBCs) contain hemoglobin. Hemoglobin picks up O_2 in the lungs and carries it to the cells. The bone marrow must produce enough RBCs. Poor diet, chemotherapy, and leukemia affect bone marrow function. Blood loss also reduces the number of RBCs.
- *Nervous system function.* Nervous system diseases and injuries can affect respiratory muscles. Breathing may be difficult or impossible. Brain damage affects respiratory rate, rhythm, and depth. Narcotics and depressant drugs affect the brain and slow respirations. O_2 and CO_2 blood levels also affect brain function. Respirations increase when O_2 is lacking to bring in more oxygen. They also increase when CO_2 increases to rid the body of CO_2.

- *Aging.* Respiratory muscles weaken. Lung tissue is less elastic. Strength for coughing decreases. The person must cough and remove secretions from the upper airway. Otherwise, *pneumonia* (inflammation and infection of the lung) can develop.
- *Exercise.* O_2 needs increase with exercise. Respiratory rate and depth increase to bring in O_2. Persons with heart and respiratory diseases may have enough oxygen at rest. However, even slight activity can increase O_2 needs. Their bodies may not be able to bring in O_2 and carry it to the cells. The doctor may limit activity.
- *Fever.* O_2 needs increase. Respiratory rate and depth increase to meet the body's needs.
- *Pain.* O_2 needs increase. Respirations increase to meet this need. Chest and abdominal injuries and surgeries often involve respiratory muscles. It hurts to breathe in and out.
- *Drugs.* Some drugs depress the respiratory center in the brain. *Respiratory depression means slow, weak respirations at a rate of fewer than 12 per minute.* Respirations are too shallow to bring enough O_2 into the lungs. *Respiratory arrest is when breathing stops.* Narcotics (morphine, Demerol, and others) can have these effects. (Narcotic comes from the Greek word *narkoun*. It means *stupor* or *to be numb.*) In safe amounts, these drugs relieve severe pain. Substance abusers are at risk for respiratory depression and respiratory arrest. They can over-dose on drugs.

- *Smoking.* Smoking causes lung cancer and chronic obstructive pulmonary disease (COPD). It is a risk factor for coronary artery disease.
- *Allergies.* An *allergy is a sensitivity to a substance that causes the body to react with signs and symptoms.* Runny nose, wheezing, and congestion are common. Mucous membranes in the upper airway swell. Severe swelling can close the airway. Shock and death are risks. Pollens, dust, foods, drugs, insect bites, powders, flowers, perfumes, sprays, animals, and cigarette smoke often cause allergies. Chronic bronchitis and asthma are risks.
- *Pollutants.* A *pollutant is a harmful chemical or substance in the air or water.* Examples are dust, fumes, toxins, asbestos, coal dust, and sawdust. They damage the lungs. Pollutants occur in home, work, and public settings.
- *Nutrition.* The body needs iron and vitamins (vitamin B_{12}, vitamin C, and folate) to produce RBCs. The person should eat slowly. Eating fast can cause shortness of breath.
- *Alcohol.* Alcohol depresses the brain. Excessive amounts reduce the cough reflex and increase the risk of aspiration. Obstructed airway and pneumonia are risks from aspiration.

ALTERED RESPIRATORY FUNCTION

Respiratory function involves three processes. Respiratory function is altered if even one process is affected.
- Air moves into and out of the lungs.
- O_2 and CO_2 are exchanged at the alveoli.
- The blood carries O_2 to the cells and removes CO_2 from them.

Hypoxia

Hypoxia means that cells do not have enough (hypo) *oxygen* (oxia). Without enough O_2, cells cannot function properly. Anything affecting respiratory function can cause hypoxia. The brain is very sensitive to inadequate O_2. Restlessness is an early sign. So are dizziness and disorientation. Report the signs and symptoms in Box 36-1 at once.

Hypoxia threatens life. All organs need O_2 to function. Oxygen is given (p. 624). The cause of hypoxia is treated.

BOX 36-1	SIGNS AND SYMPTOMS OF HYPOXIA
• Restlessness • Dizziness • Disorientation • Confusion • Behavior and personality changes • Concentrating and following directions: problems with • Apprehension • Anxiety • Fatigue • Agitation	• Pulse rate: increased • Respirations: increased rate and depth • Sitting position: often leaning forward • *Cyanosis (bluish color to the skin, lips, mucous membranes, and nail beds)* • Dyspnea

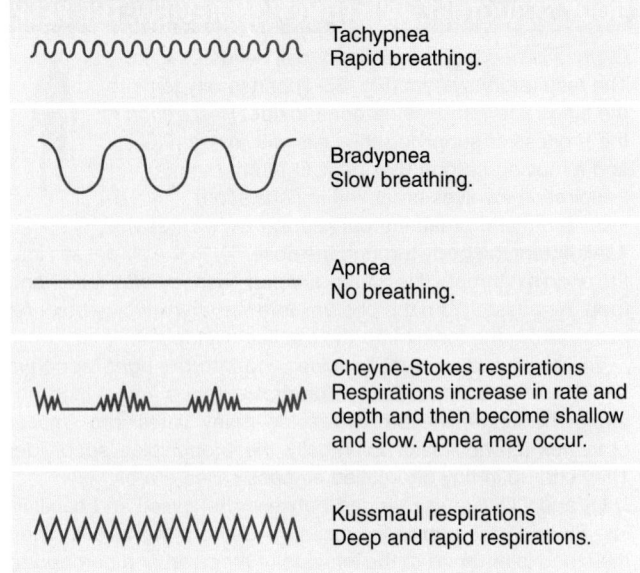

Fig. 36-2 Some abnormal breathing patterns.

Tachypnea
Rapid breathing.

Bradypnea
Slow breathing.

Apnea
No breathing.

Cheyne-Stokes respirations
Respirations increase in rate and depth and then become shallow and slow. Apnea may occur.

Kussmaul respirations
Deep and rapid respirations.

Abnormal Respirations

Normal adult respirations are 12 to 20 per minute. Infants and children have faster rates. Normal respirations are quiet, effortless, and regular. Both sides of the chest rise and fall equally. These breathing patterns are abnormal (Fig. 36-2):

- *Tachypnea—rapid* (tachy) *breathing* (pnea). *Respirations are more than 20 per minute.* Fever, exercise, pain, pregnancy, airway obstruction, and hypoxemia are common causes. *Hypoxemia is a reduced amount* (hypo) *of oxygen* (ox) *in the blood* (emia).
- *Bradypnea—slow* (brady) *breathing* (pnea). *Respirations are fewer than 12 per minute.* Drug over-dose and nervous system disorders are common causes.
- *Apnea—lack or absence* (a) *of breathing* (pnea). It occurs in sudden cardiac arrest and respiratory arrest. Sleep apnea is another type of apnea (Chapter 42).
- *Hypoventilation—breathing* (ventilation) *is slow* (hypo), *shallow, and sometimes irregular.* Lung disorders affecting the alveoli are common causes. Pneumonia is an example. Other causes include obesity, airway obstruction, and drug side effects. Nervous system and musculoskeletal disorders affecting the respiratory muscles also are causes.
- *Hyperventilation—breathing* (ventilation) *is rapid* (hyper) *and deeper than normal.* Causes include asthma, emphysema, infection, fever, nervous system disorders, hypoxia, anxiety, pain, and some drugs.
- *Dyspnea—difficult, labored, or painful* (dys) *breathing* (pnea). Heart disease and anxiety are common causes.

- *Cheyne-Stokes respirations—respirations gradually increase in rate and depth and then become shallow and slow. Breathing may stop (apnea) for 10 to 20 seconds.* Drug over-dose, heart failure, renal failure, and brain disorders are common causes. Cheyne-Stokes are common when death is near.
- *Orthopnea—breathing (pnea) deeply and comfortably only when sitting (ortho).* Common causes are emphysema, asthma, pneumonia, angina, and other heart and respiratory disorders.
- *Biot's respirations—rapid and deep respirations followed by 10 to 30 seconds of apnea.* They occur with nervous system disorders.
- *Kussmaul respirations—very deep and rapid respirations.* They signal diabetic coma.

ASSISTING WITH ASSESSMENT AND DIAGNOSTIC TESTS

Altered respiratory function may be an acute or chronic problem. Report your observations promptly and accurately (Box 36-2). Quick action is needed to meet the person's oxygen needs. Measures are taken to correct the problem and to prevent it from becoming worse.

The doctor may order these tests:

- *Chest x-ray (CXR).* An x-ray is taken of the chest to study lung changes.
- *Lung scan.* The lungs are scanned to see what areas are not getting air or blood. The person inhales radio-active gas. *Radio-active* means to give off radiation. A radio-isotope is injected into a vein. A *radio-isotope* is a substance that gives off radiation. Lung tissue getting air and blood flow "take up" the substance.
- *Bronchoscopy.* A scope *(scopy)* is passed into the trachea and bronchi *(broncho).* Airway structures are checked for bleeding and tumors. Tissue samples *(biopsies)* are taken. Or mucous plugs and foreign objects are removed. The nurse directs pre- and post-operative care.
- *Thoracentesis.* The pleura *(thora)* is punctured. Air or fluid is removed *(centesis)* from it. The doctor inserts a needle through the chest wall into the pleural sac (Fig. 36-3, p. 618). Injury or disease can cause the sac to fill with air, blood, or fluid.
- *Pulmonary function tests.* These measure the amount of air moving into and out of the lungs *(volume).* They also measure how much air the lungs can hold *(capacity).* The person takes as deep a breath as possible. Using a mouthpiece, the person blows into a machine (Fig. 36-4, p. 618).
- *Arterial blood gases (ABGs).* A radial, femoral, or brachial artery is punctured to obtain arterial blood. Laboratory tests measure the amount of O_2 in the blood.

See *Focus on Communication: Assisting With Assessment and Diagnostic Tests.*

BOX 36-2 | **SIGNS AND SYMPTOMS OF ALTERED RESPIRATORY FUNCTION**

- Hypoxia: signs and symptoms of (see Box 36-1)
- Breathing pattern: abnormal
- Shortness of breath or complaints of being "winded" or "short-winded"
- Cough (note frequency and time of day)
  - Dry and hacking
  - Harsh and barking
  - Productive (produces sputum) or non-productive
- Sputum (mucus from the respiratory system)
  - Color: clear, white, yellow, green, brown, or red
  - Odor: none or foul odor
  - Consistency: thick, watery, or frothy (with bubbles or foam)
  - *Hemoptysis: bloody* (hemo) *sputum* (ptysis *means* to spit); note if the sputum is bright red, dark red, blood-tinged, or streaked with blood
- Respirations: noisy
  - Wheezing
  - Wet-sounding
  - Crowing sounds
- Chest pain (note location)
  - Constant or comes and goes
  - Person's description (stabbing, knife-like, aching)
  - What makes it worse (movement, coughing, yawning, sneezing, sighing, deep breathing)
- Cyanosis (bluish color)
  - Skin
  - Mucous membranes
  - Lips
  - Nail beds
- Vital signs: changes in
- Position
  - Sitting upright
  - Leaning forward or hunched over a table

FOCUS ON COMMUNICATION

Assisting With Assessment and Diagnostic Tests

The questions you ask the person assist the nurse in the assessment step of the nursing process. For example:

- "Do you need more pillows?"
- "Do you want the head of your bed raised more?"
- "How often are you coughing?"
- "Are you coughing anything up?"
- "Are you coughing up any mucus? Please use a tissue when you cough up mucus, then put on your signal light. The nurse needs to observe the mucus."

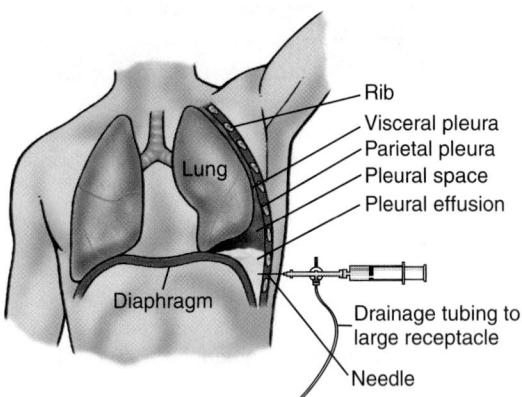

Rib
Visceral pleura
Parietal pleura
Pleural space
Pleural effusion

Lung

Diaphragm

Drainage tubing to
large receptacle

Needle

Fig. 36-3 Thoracentesis.

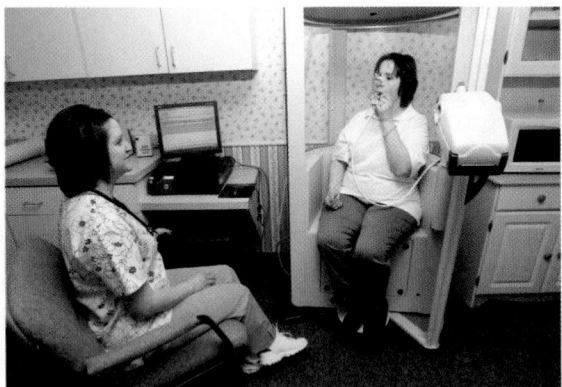

Fig. 36-4 Pulmonary function testing.

Pulse Oximetry

Pulse oximetry measures *(metry)* the oxygen *(oxi)* concentration in arterial blood. *Oxygen concentration is the amount (percent) of hemoglobin containing O_2.* Measurements are used to prevent and treat hypoxia. The normal range is 95% to 100%. For example, if 97% of all hemoglobin (100%) carries O_2, tissues get enough oxygen. If only 90% contains O_2, tissues do not get enough oxygen. As low as 85% may be normal for persons with some chronic diseases.

A sensor attaches to a finger, toe, earlobe, nose, or forehead (Fig. 36-5). Light beams on one side of the sensor pass through the tissues. A detector on the other side measures the amount of light passing through the tissues. With this information, the oximeter measures the O_2 concentration. The value and pulse rate are shown. Oximeter alarms are set when continuous monitoring is needed. An alarm sounds if:
- O_2 concentration is low.
- The pulse is too fast or slow.
- Other problems occur.

A good sensor site is needed. Avoid swollen sites and sites with skin breaks. Aging and vascular disease often cause poor circulation. Sometimes blood flow to the fingers or toes is poor. Then the earlobe, nose, and forehead sites are used.

Bright light, nail polish, fake nails, and movements affect measurements. Place a towel over the sensor to block bright light. Remove nail polish, or use another site. Do not use a finger site if the person has fake nails. Movements from shivering, seizures, or tremors affect finger sensors. The earlobe is a better site for such problems. Blood pressure cuffs affect blood flow. If using a finger site, do not measure blood pressure on that side.

Oxygen concentration is often measured with vital signs. Report and record oxygen concentration according to agency policy. An agency may use one of these terms:
- Pulse oximetry or pulse ox
- O_2 saturation or O_2 sat
- SpO_2 (saturation of peripheral oxygen)
  See *Focus on Children and Older Persons: Pulse Oximetry.*
  See *Delegation Guidelines: Pulse Oximetry.*
  See *Promoting Safety and Comfort: Pulse Oximetry.*

FOCUS ON CHILDREN AND OLDER PERSONS
Pulse Oximetry

Children
Different sensors may be used for children (Fig. 36-5, B). The sensor is attached to the sole of a foot, palm of a hand, toe, or earlobe. If the child moves a lot, the earlobe is a better site.

DELEGATION GUIDELINES
Pulse Oximetry

To assist with pulse oximetry, you need this information from the nurse and the care plan:
- What site to use
- How to use the equipment
- What sensor to use
- What type of tape to use
- The person's normal range of SpO_2
- Alarm limits for SpO_2 and pulse rate (if set)
- When to do the measurement
- What pulse site to use: apical or radial
- How often to check the sensor site (usually every 2 hours)
- What observations to report and record:
  - The date and time
  - The SpO_2 and display pulse rate
  - Apical or radial pulse rate
  - What the person was doing at the time
  - Oxygen flow rate (p. 627) and the device used (p. 626)
  - Reason for the measurement: routine or condition change
- When to report observations
- What patient or resident concerns to report at once:
  - An SpO_2 below the alarm limit (usually 95%)
  - A pulse rate above or below the alarm limit
  - The signs and symptoms listed in Boxes 36-1 and 36-2

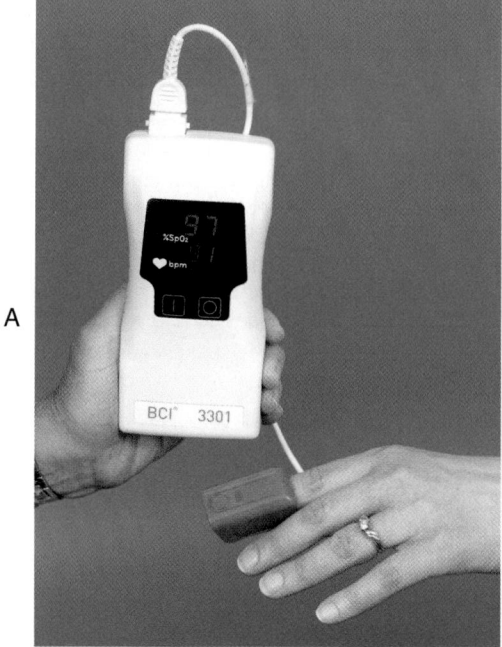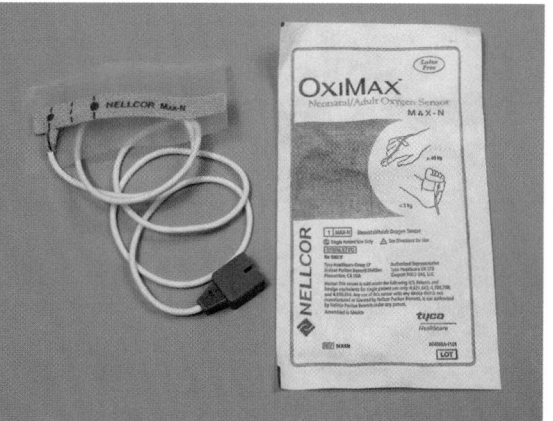

Fig. 36-5 **A,** A pulse oximetry sensor is attached to a finger. **B,** A pulse oximetry sensor for children.

PROMOTING SAFETY AND COMFORT
Pulse Oximetry

Safety

The person's condition can change rapidly. Pulse oximetry does not lessen the need for good observations. Observe for signs and symptoms of hypoxia (see Box 36-1) and altered respiratory system function (see Box 36-2).

Comfort

A clip-on sensor feels like a clothespin when applied. It should not hurt or cause discomfort. Ask the person to tell you at once if it causes pain, discomfort, or too much pressure. Change the sensor site when the nurse tells you to do so.

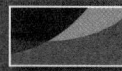 USING A PULSE OXIMETER `VIDEO`

QUALITY OF LIFE

Remember to:
- Knock before entering the person's room.
- Address the person by name.
- Introduce yourself by name and title.

- Explain the procedure to the person before beginning and during the procedure.
- Protect the person's rights during the procedure.
- Handle the person gently during the procedure.

PRE-PROCEDURE

1 Follow *Delegation Guidelines: Pulse Oximetry.* See *Promoting Safety and Comfort: Pulse Oximetry.*
2 Practice hand hygiene.
3 Collect the following before going to the person's room:
   - Oximeter and sensor
   - Tape
   - Towel

4 Arrange your work area.
5 Practice hand hygiene.
6 Identify the person. Check the identification (ID) bracelet against your assignment sheet. Also call the person by name.
7 Provide for privacy.

Continued

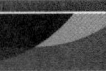

USING A PULSE OXIMETER—cont'd

VIDEO

PROCEDURE

8 Provide for comfort.
9 Dry the site with a towel.
10 Clip or tape the sensor to the site.
11 Turn on the oximeter.
12 Set the high and low alarm limits for SpO₂ and pulse rate. Turn on audio and visual alarms. (This step is for continuous monitoring.)

13 Check the person's pulse (apical or radial) with the pulse on the display. The pulse rates should be about the same. Note both pulses on your assignment sheet.
14 Read the SpO₂ on the display. Note the value on the flow sheet and your assignment sheet.
15 Leave the sensor in place for continuous monitoring. Otherwise, turn off the device and remove the sensor.

POST-PROCEDURE

16 Provide for comfort. (See the inside of the front book cover.)
17 Place the signal light within reach.
18 Unscreen the person.
19 Complete a safety check of the room. (See the inside of the front book cover.)

20 Return the device to its proper place (unless monitoring is continuous).
21 Practice hand hygiene.
22 Report and record the SpO₂, the pulse rates, and your other observations.

Sputum Specimens

Respiratory disorders cause the lungs, bronchi, and trachea to secrete mucus. *Mucus from the respiratory system is called sputum when expectorated* (expelled) *through the mouth*. Sputum specimens are studied for blood, microbes, and abnormal cells. See Chapter 31.

MEETING OXYGEN NEEDS

To get enough oxygen, air must move deep into the lungs. Air must reach the alveoli where O₂ and CO₂ are exchanged. Disease, injury, and surgery can prevent air from reaching the alveoli. Pain and immobility interfere with deep breathing and coughing. So do narcotics. Therefore secretions collect in the airway and lungs. They interfere with air movement and lung function. Secretions also provide a place for microbes to grow and multiply. Infection is a threat.

Oxygen needs must be met. The following measures are common in care plans.

Positioning

Breathing is usually easier in the semi-Fowler's and Fowler's positions. Persons with difficulty breathing often prefer *sitting up and leaning over a table to breathe. This is called the orthopneic position.* (*Ortho* means *sitting* or *standing.* *Pneic* means *breathing.*) Place a pillow on the table to increase the person's comfort (Fig. 36-6).

Frequent position changes are needed. Unless the doctor limits positioning, the person must not lie on one side for a long time. Secretions pool. The lungs cannot expand on that side. Position changes are needed at least every 2 hours. Follow the care plan.

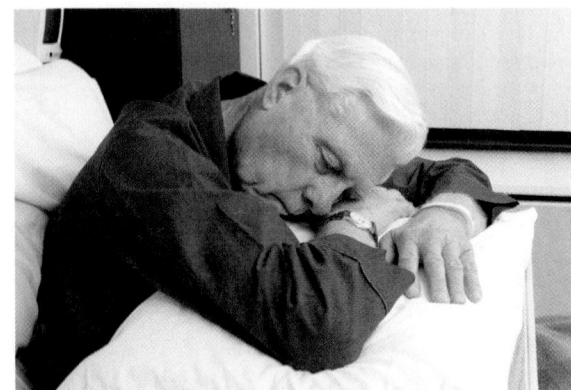

Fig. 36-6 The person is in the orthopneic position. A pillow is on the overbed table for the person's comfort.

Deep Breathing and Coughing

Deep breathing moves air into most parts of the lungs. Coughing removes mucus. Deep-breathing and coughing exercises promote oxygenation. They are done after surgery or injury and during bedrest. The exercises are painful after surgery or injury. Breaking an incision open while coughing is a fear.

Deep breathing and coughing are usually done every 1 to 2 hours while the person is awake. They help prevent pneumonia and atelectasis. *Atelectasis is the collapse of a portion of the lung.* It occurs when mucus collects in the airway. Air cannot get to a part of the lung. The lung collapses. Surgery, bedrest, lung diseases, and paralysis are risk factors.

See *Focus on Communication: Deep Breathing and Coughing.*

See *Focus on Children and Older Persons: Deep Breathing and Coughing.*

See *Delegation Guidelines: Deep Breathing and Coughing.*

See *Promoting Safety and Comfort: Deep Breathing and Coughing.*

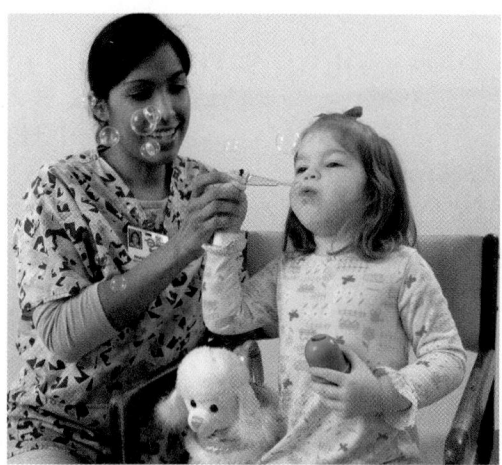

Fig. 36-7 The child blows bubbles for a deep-breathing exercise.

FOCUS ON COMMUNICATION
Deep Breathing and Coughing

To encourage cough etiquette (Chapter 15), you can say:

"Please remember to cover your nose and mouth when coughing. I'll put these tissues where you can reach them. Here is a waste container to dispose of your tissues. Where would you like me to place it? Also, please remember to wash your hands often. Let me know if you need help."

DELEGATION GUIDELINES
Deep Breathing and Coughing

When delegated deep-breathing and coughing exercises, you need this information from the nurse and the care plan:

- When to do them and how often
- How many deep breaths and coughs the person needs to do
- What observations to report and record:
  - The number of deep breaths and coughs
  - How the person tolerated the procedure
- When to report observations
- What patient or resident concerns to report at once

FOCUS ON CHILDREN AND OLDER PERSONS
Deep Breathing and Coughing

Children
Party favors are useful for helping children deep breathe. They include paper blowouts, horns, whistles, pinwheels, and others. They are fun and colorful. Blowing bubbles also can promote deep breathing. Before blowing bubbles, have the child take a deep breath (Fig. 36-7).

PROMOTING SAFETY AND COMFORT
Deep Breathing and Coughing

Safety
Respiratory hygiene and cough etiquette are needed if the person has a productive cough (Chapter 15). The person needs to:

- Cover the nose and mouth when coughing or sneezing.
- Use tissues to contain respiratory secretions.
- Dispose of tissues in the nearest waste container after use.
- Wash his or her hands after coughing or contact with respiratory secretions.

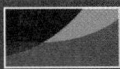

ASSISTING WITH DEEP-BREATHING AND COUGHING EXERCISES
VIDEO

QUALITY OF LIFE

Remember to:
- Knock before entering the person's room.
- Address the person by name.
- Introduce yourself by name and title.

- Explain the procedure to the person before beginning and during the procedure.
- Protect the person's rights during the procedure.
- Handle the person gently during the procedure.

PRE-PROCEDURE

1. Follow *Delegation Guidelines: Deep Breathing and Coughing*, p. 621. See *Promoting Safety and Comfort: Deep Breathing and Coughing*, p. 621.
2. Practice hand hygiene.
3. Identify the person. Check the ID bracelet against the assignment sheet. Also call the person by name.
4. Provide for privacy.

PROCEDURE

5. Lower the bed rail if up.
6. Help the person to a comfortable sitting position: sitting on the side of the bed, semi-Fowler's, or Fowler's.
7. Have the person deep breathe:
   a. Have the person place the hands over the rib cage (Fig. 36-8).
   b. Have the person take a deep breath. It should be as deep as possible. Remind the person to inhale through the nose.
   c. Ask the person to hold the breath for 2 to 3 seconds.

   d. Ask the person to exhale slowly through pursed lips (Fig. 36-9). Ask the person to exhale until the ribs move as far down as possible.
   e. Repeat this step 4 more times.
8. Ask the person to cough:
   a. Have the person place both hands over the incision. One hand is on top of the other (Fig. 36-10, A). The person can hold a pillow or folded towel over the incision (Fig. 36-10, B).
   b. Have the person take in a deep breath as in step 7.
   c. Ask the person to cough strongly twice with the mouth open.

POST-PROCEDURE

9. Provide for comfort. (See the inside of the front book cover.)
10. Place the signal light within reach.
11. Raise or lower bed rails. Follow the care plan.
12. Unscreen the person.
13. Complete a safety check of the room. (See the inside of the front book cover.)
14. Practice hand hygiene.
15. Report and record your observations (Fig. 36-11).

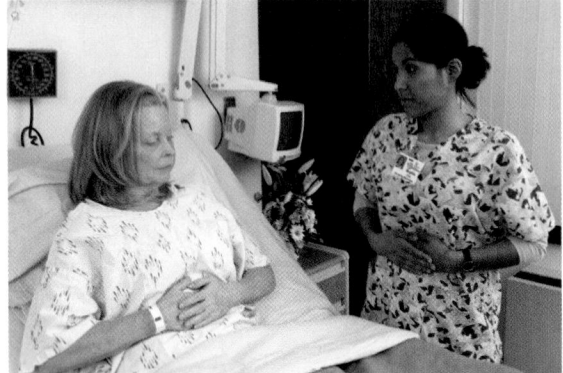

Fig. 36-8 The hands are over the rib cage for deep breathing.

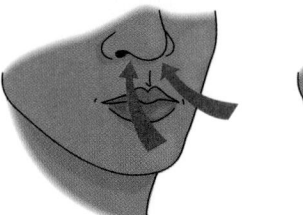 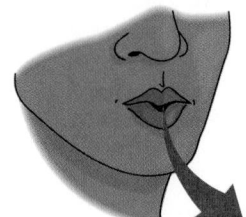

Fig. 36-9 The person inhales through the nose and exhales through pursed lips during the deep-breathing exercise.

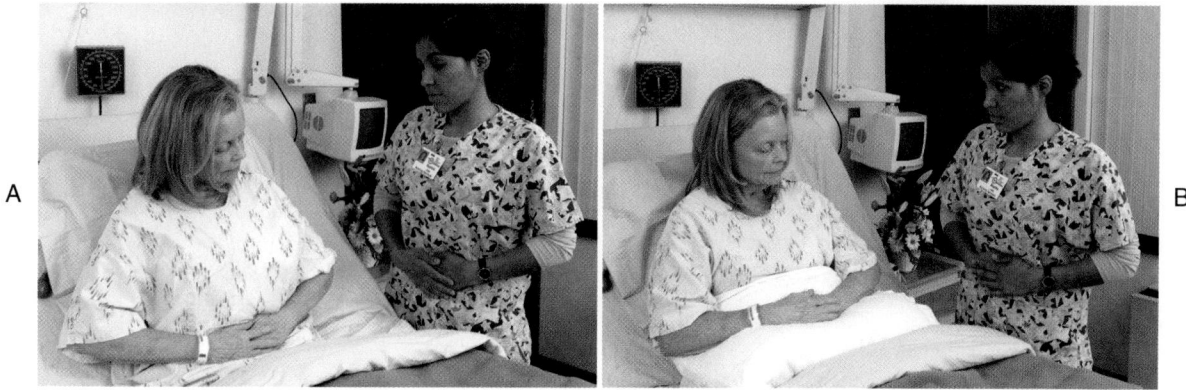

Fig. 36-10 The person supports an incision for the coughing exercises. **A,** The hands are over the incision. **B,** A pillow is held over the incision.

Date	Time	Nursing Margin / Other Depts Margin
3/15	0830	Assisted resident with deep-breathing (x5) and coughing (x2)
		exercises. He states "It is getting easier every day." Denied pain
		or discomfort. Requested to sit in his chair after the exercises.
		Tray table with water pitcher and cup, tissues, and a book
		within reach. Signal light within reach. Jean Hein, CNA

Fig. 36-11 Charting sample.

Incentive Spirometry

Incentive means to encourage. A *spirometer* is a machine that measures the amount *(volume)* of air inhaled. With incentive spirometry, the person inhales until reaching a pre-set volume of air. Balls or bars in the device move as the person inhales (Fig. 36-12).

Incentive spirometry also is called *sustained maximal inspiration (SMI)*. *Sustained* means constant. *Maximal* means the most or the greatest. And *inspiration* relates to breathing in. SMI means inhaling as deeply as possible and holding the breath for a certain time. The breath is usually held for at least 3 seconds.

The goal is to improve lung function. Atelectasis is prevented or treated. Like yawning or sighing, breathing is long, slow, and deep. This moves air deep into the lungs. Secretions loosen. O_2 and CO_2 exchange occurs between the alveoli and capillaries.

The device is used as follows:
1 The spirometer is placed upright.
2 The person exhales normally.
3 He or she seals the lips around the mouthpiece.
4 A slow, deep breath is taken until the balls rise to the desired height.

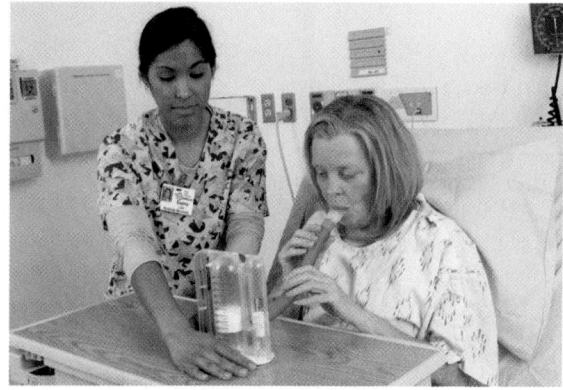

Fig. 36-12 The person uses a spirometer.

5 The breath is held for 3 to 6 seconds to keep the balls floating.
6 The person removes the mouthpiece and exhales slowly. The person may cough at this time.
7 After some normal breaths, the device is used again.
   See *Delegation Guidelines: Incentive Spirometry*, p. 624.

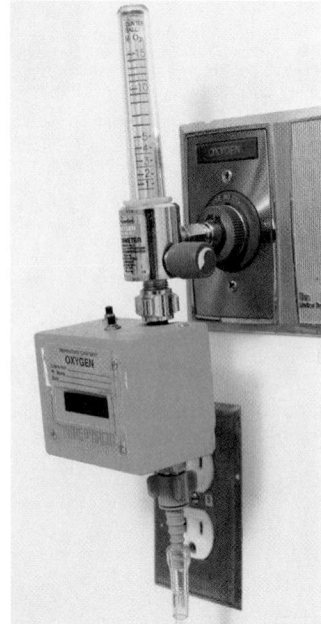

Fig. 36-13 Wall oxygen outlet.

ASSISTING WITH OXYGEN THERAPY

Disease, injury, and surgery often interfere with breathing. The amount of O_2 in the blood may be less than normal (hypoxemia). If so, the doctor orders oxygen therapy.

Oxygen is treated as a drug. The doctor orders when to give O_2, the amount, and the device to use. Some people need oxygen constantly. Others need it for symptom relief—chest pain or shortness of breath. Oxygen helps relieve chest pain. Persons with respiratory diseases may have enough oxygen at rest. With mild exercise or activity, they become short of breath. Oxygen helps to relieve shortness of breath.

You do not give oxygen. The nurse and respiratory therapist start and maintain oxygen therapy. You help provide safe care.

Oxygen Sources

Oxygen is supplied as follows:
- *Wall outlet.* O_2 is piped into each person's unit (Fig. 36-13).
- *Oxygen tank.* The oxygen tank is placed at the bedside. Small tanks are used for emergencies and transfers. They also are used by persons who walk or use wheelchairs (Fig. 36-14). A gauge tells how much oxygen is left (Fig. 36-15).
- *Oxygen concentrator.* The machine removes oxygen from the air (Fig. 36-16). A power source is needed. If the machine is not portable, the person stays near it. A portable oxygen tank is needed for power failures and mobility.
- *Liquid oxygen system.* A portable unit is filled from a stationary unit. The portable unit has enough O_2 for about 8 hours of use. A dial shows the amount of O_2 in the unit. The portable unit is worn over the shoulder (Fig. 36-17). This allows the person to be mobile.

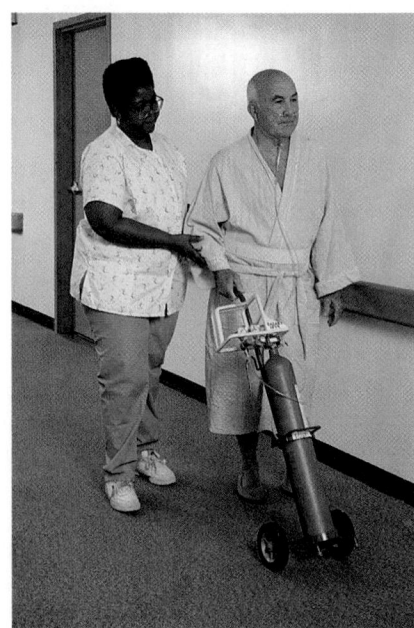

Fig. 36-14 A portable oxygen tank is used when walking.

See *Focus on Long-Term Care and Home Care: Oxygen Sources.*
See *Promoting Safety and Comfort: Oxygen Sources.*
See *Teamwork and Time Management: Oxygen Sources.*

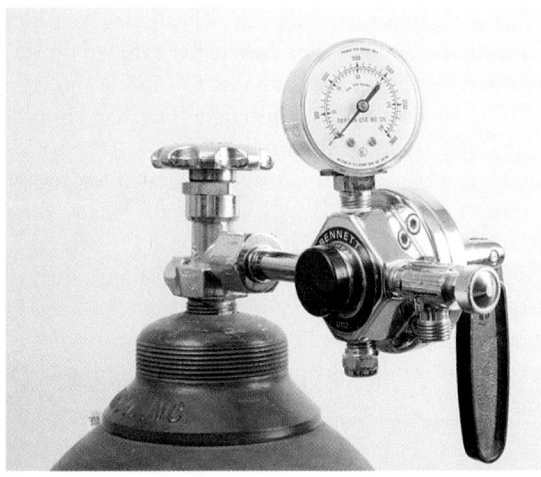

Fig. 36-15 The gauge shows the amount of oxygen in the tank.

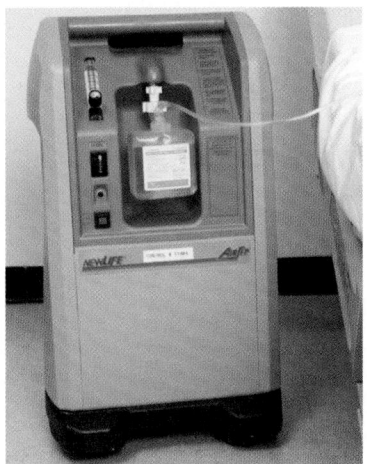

Fig. 36-16 Oxygen concentrator.

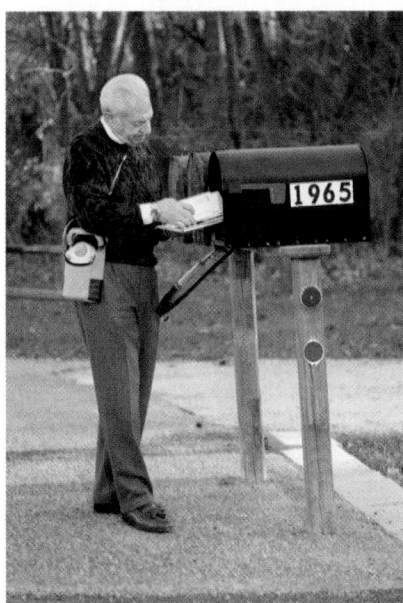

Fig. 36-17 A portable liquid oxygen unit is worn over the shoulder.

FOCUS ON LONG-TERM CARE AND HOME CARE
Oxygen Sources

Home Care

Oxygen tanks, oxygen concentrators, and liquid oxygen systems are used in home care. The type used depends on the person's needs. It is maintained by a medical supply company. Keep the company's name and phone number near the phone.

The patient and family must practice safety measures where oxygen is used and stored. This includes measures to prevent fires.

- Practice fire prevention measures. See Chapter 12.
- Keep a fire extinguisher in the room.
- Place NO SMOKING signs in the room and on the room door.
- Remove smoking materials—cigarettes, cigars, pipes, matches, and lighters.
- Remove materials that ignite easily—alcohol, nail polish remover, oils, greases.
- Keep O_2 sources and O_2 tubing away from heat sources and open flames. These include candles, stoves, heating ducts, radiators, heating pipes, space heaters, oil lamps, and kerosene heaters and lamps.
- Turn off electrical items before unplugging them.
- Use electrical items that are in good repair—shaver, radio, TV, music players, and others.
- Use only electrical items with three-prong plugs.
- Do not use materials that cause static electricity (wool and synthetic fabrics).
- Turn off the O_2 if a fire occurs. Get the person and family out of the home. Call 911 to report a fire.

PROMOTING SAFETY AND COMFORT
Oxygen Sources

Safety

Liquid oxygen is very cold. If touched, it can freeze the skin. Never tamper with the equipment. Doing so is unsafe and could damage the equipment. Follow agency procedures and the manufacturer's instructions when working with liquid oxygen.

Many activities can increase the need for O_2. This includes moving in bed, transfer procedures, and walking. Do not remove the person's device (p. 626). If necessary, ask the nurse for longer tubing. Or ask the nurse to change to a portable oxygen tank.

TEAMWORK AND TIME MANAGEMENT
Oxygen Sources

Oxygen tanks and liquid oxygen systems contain a certain amount of O_2. When the O_2 level is low, a new tank is needed or the liquid oxygen system is refilled. Always check the O_2 level when you are with or near persons using these oxygen sources. Report a low O_2 level at once.

Oxygen Devices

The doctor orders the device for giving O_2. These devices are common:

- *Nasal cannula* (Fig. 36-18). The prongs are inserted into the nostrils (Fig. 36-19). A band goes behind the ears and under the chin to keep the device in place. A cannula allows eating and drinking. Tight prongs can irritate the nose. Pressure on the ears and cheekbones is possible.
- *Simple face mask* (Fig. 36-20). It covers the nose and mouth. The mask has small holes in the sides. CO_2 escapes when exhaling.

- *Partial-rebreather mask* (Fig. 36-21). A bag is added to the simple face mask. The bag is for exhaled air. When breathing in, the person inhales O_2 and some exhaled air. Some room air also is inhaled. The bag should not totally deflate when inhaling.
- *Non-rebreather mask* (Fig. 36-22). Exhaled air and room air cannot enter the bag. Exhaled air leaves through holes in the mask. When inhaling, only O_2 from the bag is inhaled. The bag must not totally collapse during inhalation.
- *Venturi mask* (Fig. 36-23). Precise amounts of O_2 are given. Color-coded adapters show the amount of O_2 given.

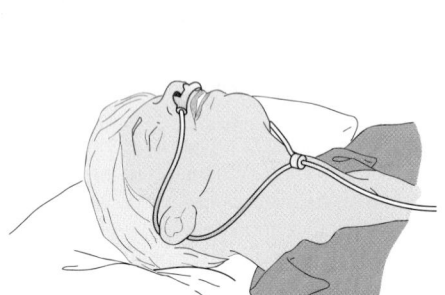

Fig. 36-18 Nasal cannula.

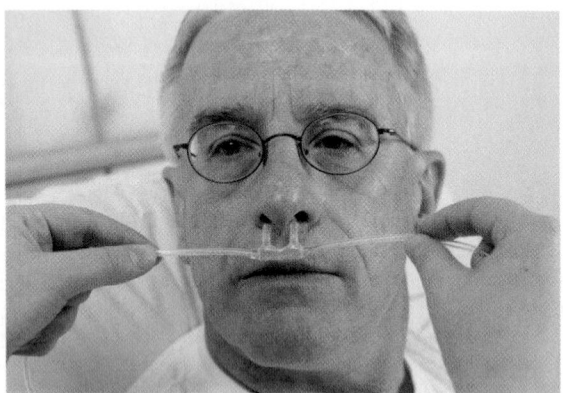

Fig. 36-19 Cannula prongs are inserted. The prong openings face downward.

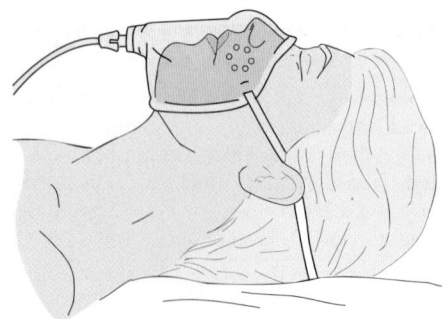

Fig. 36-20 Simple face mask.

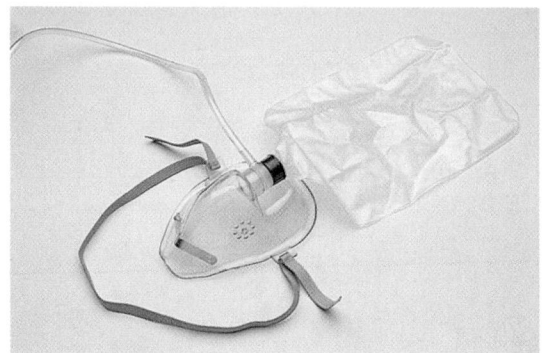

Fig. 36-21 Partial-rebreather mask.

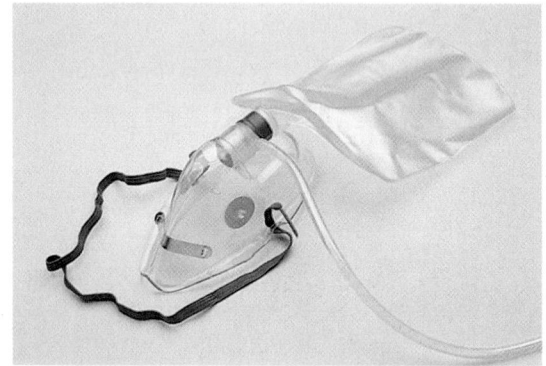

Fig. 36-22 Non-rebreather mask.

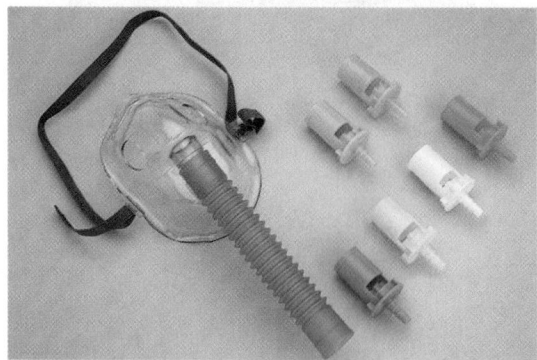

Fig. 36-23 Venturi mask.

Talking and eating are hard to do with a mask. Listen carefully. Moisture can build up under the mask. Keep the face clean and dry. This helps prevent irritation from the mask. For eating, the nurse changes the oxygen mask to a cannula.

See *Focus on Children and Older Persons: Oxygen Devices.*

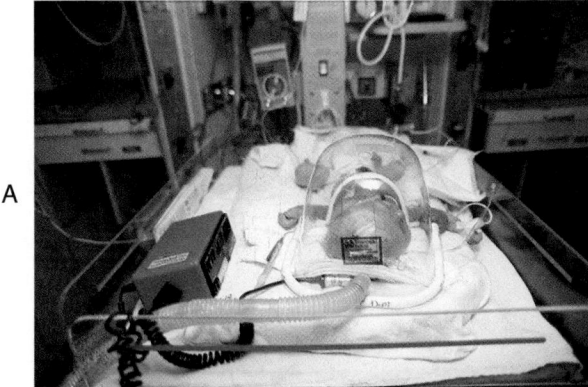

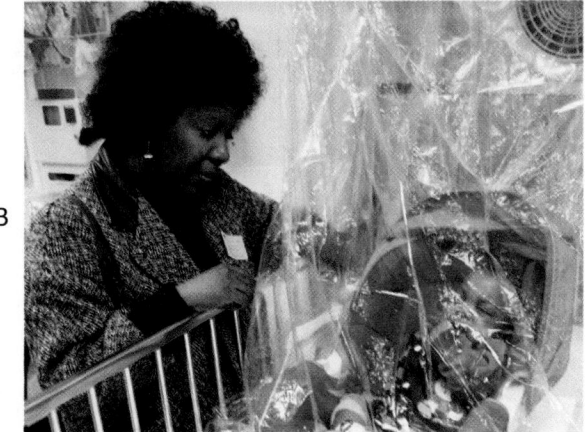

Fig. 36-24 A, Oxygen hood. **B,** Mist tent.

Oxygen Flow Rates

The *flow rate* is the amount of oxygen given. It is measured in liters per minute (L/min). The doctor orders 1 to 15 liters of O_2 per minute. The nurse or respiratory therapist sets the flow rate with a flowmeter (Fig. 36-25).

The nurse and care plan tell you the person's flow rate. When giving care and checking the person, always check the flow rate. Tell the nurse at once if it is too high or too low. A nurse or respiratory therapist will adjust the flow rate. Some states and agencies let nursing assistants adjust O_2 flow rates. Know your agency's policy.

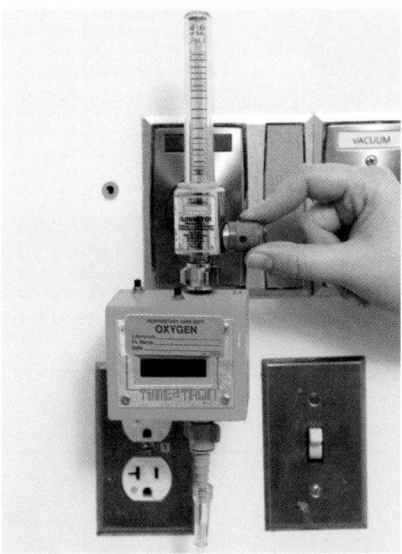

Fig. 36-25 The flowmeter is used to set the oxygen flow rate.

Oxygen Administration Set-Up

Oxygen is a dry gas. If not humidified (made moist), O_2 dries the airway's mucous membranes. Distilled water is added to the humidifier (Fig. 36-26, p. 628). (Distilled water is pure. Dissolved salts were removed by a chemical process.)

When added to the humidifier, the distilled water creates water vapor. Oxygen picks up the water vapor as it flows into the system. Bubbling in the humidifier means that water vapor is being produced. Low flow rates (1 to 2 L/min) by cannula are not usually humidified.

See *Delegation Guidelines: Oxygen Administration Set-Up,* p. 628.
See *Promoting Safety and Comfort: Oxygen Administration Set-Up,* p. 628.
See *Teamwork and Time Management: Oxygen Administration Set-Up,* p. 628.

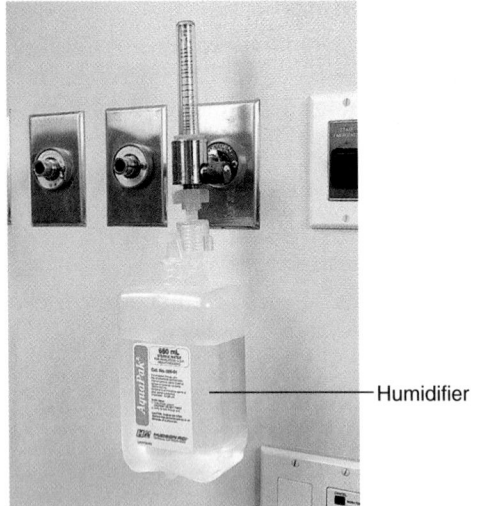

Fig. 36-26 Oxygen administration system with humidifier.

PROMOTING SAFETY AND COMFORT
Oxygen Administration Set-Up

Safety

You do not give oxygen. Tell the nurse when the O_2 administration system is set up. The nurse turns on the O_2, sets the flow rate, and applies the O_2 device.

Practice medical asepsis. Do not let the connecting tubing hang on the floor.

TEAMWORK AND TIME MANAGEMENT
Oxygen Administration Set-Up

As you walk past the room of any person receiving humidified O_2, always check the humidifier. Make sure the humidifier is bubbling. Also make sure it has enough water. Tell the nurse if:
- There is no bubbling.
- The water level is low.

DELEGATION GUIDELINES
Oxygen Administration Set-Up

If setting up O_2 is delegated to you, you need this information from the nurse:
- The person's name and room and bed numbers
- What oxygen device was ordered
- If you need a humidifier

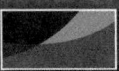 **SETTING UP FOR OXYGEN ADMINISTRATION**

QUALITY OF LIFE

Remember to:
- Knock before entering the person's room.
- Address the person by name.
- Introduce yourself by name and title.

- Explain the procedure to the person before beginning and during the procedure.
- Protect the person's rights during the procedure.
- Handle the person gently during the procedure.

PRE-PROCEDURE

1 Follow *Delegation Guidelines: Oxygen Administration Set-Up*. See *Promoting Safety and Comfort: Oxygen Administration Set-Up*.
2 Practice hand hygiene.
3 Collect the following before going to the person's room:
 - Oxygen device with connecting tubing
 - Flowmeter
 - Humidifier (if ordered)
 - Distilled water (if using a humidifier)
4 Arrange your work area.
5 Practice hand hygiene.
6 Identify the person. Check the ID bracelet against the assignment sheet. Also call the person by name.

PROCEDURE

7 Make sure the flowmeter is in the *OFF* position.
8 Attach the flowmeter to the wall outlet or to the tank.
9 Fill the humidifier with distilled water.
10 Attach the humidifier to the bottom of the flowmeter.
11 Attach the oxygen device and connecting tubing to the humidifier. *Do not set the flowmeter. Do not apply the O_2 device on the person.*

12 Place the cap securely on the distilled water. Store the water according to agency policy.
13 Discard the packaging from the O_2 device and connecting tubing.

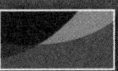 **SETTING UP FOR OXYGEN ADMINISTRATION—cont'd**

POST-PROCEDURE

14 Provide for comfort. (See the inside of the front book cover.)
15 Place the signal light within reach.
16 Complete a safety check of the room. (See the inside of the front book cover.)
17 Practice hand hygiene.
18 Tell the nurse when you are done. The nurse will:
   • Turn on the O₂ and set the flow rate.
   • Apply the O₂ device on the person.

Oxygen Safety

You assist the nurse with oxygen therapy. You do not give oxygen. You do not adjust the flow rate unless allowed by your state and agency. However, you must give safe care. Follow the rules in Box 36-3. Also follow the rules for fire and the use of oxygen (Chapter 12).

BOX 36-3 SAFETY RULES FOR OXYGEN THERAPY

• Do not remove the oxygen device.
• Make sure the oxygen device is secure but not tight.
• Check for signs of irritation from the device. Check behind the ears, under the nose (cannula), and around the face (mask). Also check the cheekbones.
• Keep the face clean and dry when a mask is used.
• Do not shut off the oxygen flow. *However, turn off the oxygen flow if there is a fire. And remove the oxygen device.*
• Do not adjust the flow rate unless allowed by your state and agency.
• Tell the nurse at once if the flow rate is too high or too low.
• Tell the nurse at once if the humidifier is not bubbling.
• Secure tubing in place. Tape or pin it to the person's garment following agency policy.
• Make sure there are no kinks in the tubing.
• Make sure the person does not lie on any part of the tubing.
• Make sure the oxygen tank is secure in its holder.
• Report signs and symptoms of hypoxia, respiratory distress, or abnormal breathing patterns to the nurse at once (see Boxes 36-1 and 36-2).
• Give oral hygiene as directed. Follow the care plan.
• Make sure the oxygen device is clean and free of mucus.
• Maintain an adequate water level in the humidifier.

FOCUS ON PRIDE

The Person, Family, and Yourself

Personal and Professional Responsibility

You are responsible for reporting patient and resident complaints to the nurse. A person may say: "I can't breathe" or "I'm not getting enough air." Yet you see the person breathing. Do not dismiss the person's complaint. Tell the nurse at once. You cannot feel what the person does. Trust what the person tells you.

Rights and Respect

People have the right to a safe setting. To protect the person, smoking is not allowed where oxygen is used and stored. NO SMOKING signs in the room and hallways are often used. You may need to remind the person or visitors not to smoke. Be polite and respectful. Direct the person to an area where smoking is allowed.

Independence and Social Interaction

The need for long-term oxygen therapy changes a person's life. Work, daily activities, and hobbies can become a challenge. The person may feel alone and depressed. Social support from family and friends is important.

Portable oxygen sources increase the person's independence. Small oxygen tanks and portable liquid oxygen units are examples. Such devices allow freedom and promote quality of life.

Delegation and Teamwork

Oxygen is treated as a drug. State nurse practice acts allow nurses to give drugs. You assist the nurse with oxygen therapy. You do not give oxygen. You do not adjust the flow rate unless allowed by your state and agency and instructed to do so by the nurse.

If you are asked to give oxygen or adjust a flow rate, politely refuse. Remember, refusing to perform a task is your right and duty when the task is beyond the legal limits of your role. Do not ignore the request. Tell the nurse that you are not trained to give oxygen. Offer to do what you can to assist. Gathering and setting up the supplies are examples. Or ask if you can help with another task instead.

Ethics and Laws

Safe use of oxygen is a serious issue. The following case shows how harm resulted from unsafe use of oxygen by a certified nursing assistant (CNA) who was not trained or qualified to handle oxygen.

A CNA took a group of residents outside to smoke. One resident, who used oxygen, was taken outside with her oxygen tank. Center policy stated that oxygen was only to be used and handled by nurses. The CNA tried to turn off the oxygen so the resident could smoke, but she did not turn it off completely. The resident's cigarette set fire to the oxygen and caused severe facial burns on her face.

The CNA lost her job at the center. The state's board of nursing asked the CNA to provide a written response to complaints against her. The CNA did not respond.

Continued

FOCUS ON PRIDE—cont'd

The CNA's conduct provided grounds for disciplinary action. The CNA was charged with:

- *Committing an act that deceives, defrauds, or harms the public*
- *Conduct or practice that is or may be harmful to the health of a patient or the public*
- *Failing to follow policies and procedures designed to protect the patient or resident*
- *Violating the rights or dignity of a patient or resident*
- *Neglecting or abusing a resident physically, verbally, emotionally, or financially*
- *Accepting patient or resident care tasks that the CNA lacks the education or competence to perform*
- *Failing to cooperate with the board during an investigation by:*
  - *Not providing a complete, written explanation of the matter*
  - *Not completing and returning a board-issued questionnaire within 30 days*

The CNA's certification was revoked.

(Arizona State Board of Nursing, 2010. NOTE: names withheld per request of the Arizona State Board of Nursing.)

Performing tasks that you are not trained to do can cause harm. You can lose your job and your ability to work as a nursing assistant. Take pride in following the limits of your role and providing safe care.

REVIEW QUESTIONS

Circle the BEST answer.

1 Alcohol and narcotics affect oxygen needs because they
   a Depress the brain
   b Are pollutants
   c Cause allergies
   d Cause infection

2 Hypoxia is
   a Not enough oxygen in the blood
   b The amount of hemoglobin that affects oxygen
   c Not enough oxygen in the cells
   d The lack of carbon dioxide

3 An early sign of hypoxia is
   a Cyanosis
   b Increased pulse and respiratory rates
   c Restlessness
   d Dyspnea

4 A person can breathe deeply and comfortably only while sitting. This is called
   a Biot's respirations
   b Orthopnea
   c Bradypnea
   d Kussmaul respirations

5 Tachypnea means that respirations are
   a Slow
   b Rapid
   c Absent
   d Difficult or painful

6 Which should you report to the nurse at once?
   a A respiratory rate of 18 per minute
   b An SpO_2 of 97%
   c Bubbling in a humidifier
   d Dyspnea

7 A person's SpO_2 is 98%. Which is *true*?
   a The pulse oximeter is wrong.
   b The pulse is 98 beats per minute.
   c The measurement is within normal range.
   d The person has respiratory depression.

8 Which is *not* a site for a pulse oximetry sensor?
   a Toe
   b Finger
   c Earlobe
   d Upper arm

9 You are assisting with deep breathing and coughing. Which is *false*?
   a The person inhales through pursed lips.
   b The person sits in a comfortable sitting position.
   c The person inhales deeply through the nose.
   d The person holds a pillow over an incision.

10 A person has a productive cough. You remind the person to
   a Cover the nose and mouth when coughing
   b Use a face mask
   c Cough and deep breathe twice daily
   d Inhale through the mouth

11 Liquid oxygen can freeze the skin.
   a True
   b False

12 Which is useful for deep breathing?
   a Pulse oximeter
   b Incentive spirometer
   c Simple face mask
   d Partial-rebreather mask

13 Which oxygen device allows for eating?
   a Nasal cannula
   b Simple face mask
   c Partial-rebreather mask
   d Venturi mask

14 Oxygen flow rate is measured in
   a mm/Hg
   b minutes
   c L/min
   d SpO_2

15 When assisting with oxygen therapy, you can
   a Turn the oxygen on and off
   b Start the oxygen
   c Decide what device to use
   d Keep connecting tubing secure and free of kinks

16 A person has humidified oxygen. The water level should move up with inspiration and down with expiration.
   a True
   b False

17 These statements are about oxygen safety. Which is *false*?
   a Smoking materials are removed.
   b Lit candles are allowed in the person's room.
   c Three-pronged plugs are used for electrical items.
   d NO SMOKING signs are posted.

18 A person is receiving oxygen therapy. Which measure should you question?
   a Provide oral hygiene.
   b Check for signs of irritation.
   c Adjust the flow rate if it is too high or too low.
   d Secure tubing in place.

Answers to these questions are on p. 834.

Respiratory Support and Therapies

37

OBJECTIVES

- Define the key terms and key abbreviations listed in this chapter.
- Explain how to assist in the care of persons with artificial airways.
- Describe the principles and safety measures for suctioning.

- Explain how to assist in the care of persons on mechanical ventilation.
- Explain how to assist in the care of persons with chest tubes.
- Explain how to promote PRIDE in the person, the family, and yourself.

KEY TERMS

hemothorax Blood *(hemo)* in the pleural space *(thorax)*

intubation Inserting an artificial airway

mechanical ventilation Using a machine to move air into and out of the lungs

patent Open and unblocked

pleural effusion The escape and collection of fluid *(effusion)* in the pleural space

pneumothorax Air *(pneumo)* in the pleural space *(thorax)*

suction The process of withdrawing or sucking up fluid *(secretions)*

tracheostomy A surgically created opening *(stomy)* into the trachea *(tracheo)*

KEY ABBREVIATIONS

CO_2	Carbon dioxide	O_2	Oxygen
ET	Endotracheal	RT	Respiratory therapist

BODY STRUCTURE AND FUNCTION REVIEW: THE RESPIRATORY SYSTEM

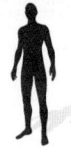

Oxygen is needed to live. Every cell needs oxygen. The respiratory system (Fig. 37-1) brings oxygen into the lungs and removes carbon dioxide. *Respiration* is the process of supplying the cells with oxygen (O_2) and removing carbon dioxide (CO_2) from them. Respiration involves breathing in *(inhalation, inspiration)* and breathing out *(exhalation, expiration)*.

Air enters the body through the nose. Then the air passes into the *pharynx* (throat). It is a tube-shaped passage-way for air and food. Air passes from the pharynx into the *larynx* (voice box). Air passes from the larynx into the *trachea* (windpipe).

The trachea divides at its lower end into the *right bronchus* and the *left bronchus*. Each bronchus enters a *lung*. Upon entering the lungs, the bronchi divide many times into smaller branches *(bronchioles)*. Eventually the bronchioles subdivide. They end up in tiny one-celled air sacs called *alveoli*.

O_2 and CO_2 are exchanged between the alveoli and capillaries. Blood in the capillaries picks up O_2 from the alveoli. Then the blood is returned to the left side of the heart and pumped to the rest of the body. Alveoli pick up CO_2 from the capillaries for exhalation.

Each lung is divided into lobes. The right lung has 3 lobes; the left lung has 2. The lungs are separated from the abdominal cavity by a muscle called the *diaphragm*. A bony framework made up of the ribs, sternum, and vertebrae protects the lungs.

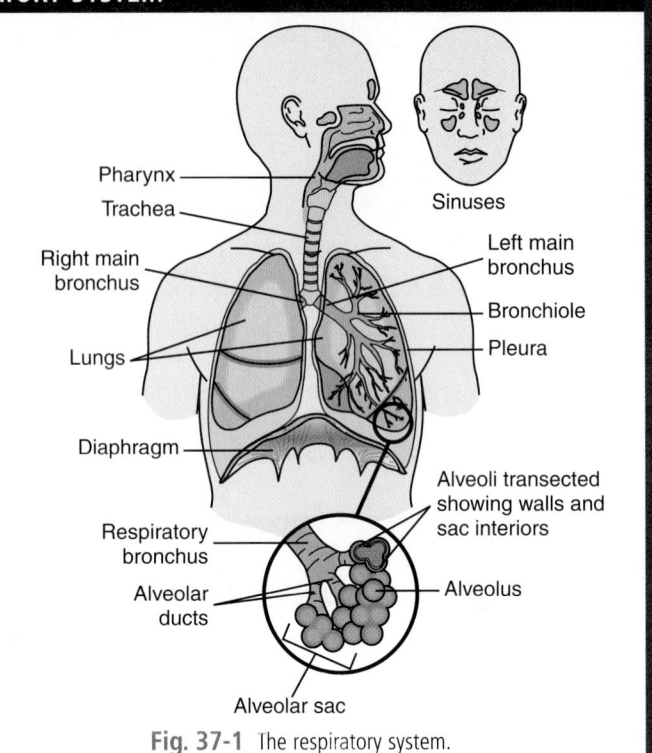

Fig. 37-1 The respiratory system.

Some persons need artificial airways, suctioning, mechanical ventilation, and chest tubes. Needing respiratory rehabilitation, often they are very ill. They need to recover from problems affecting the airway and lungs. They need complex procedures and equipment. The nurse may ask you to assist in their care.

See *Body Structure and Function Review: The Respiratory System.*

ARTIFICIAL AIRWAYS

Artificial airways keep the airway *patent (open and unblocked)*. They are needed:

* When disease, injury, secretions, or aspiration obstructs the airway
* For mechanical ventilation (p. 636)
* By some persons who are semi-conscious or unconscious
* When the person is recovering from anesthesia

Intubation means inserting an artificial airway. Such airways are usually plastic and disposable. They come in various sizes. These airways are common:

* *Oropharyngeal airway*—inserted through the mouth and into the pharynx (Fig. 37-2, A). A nurse or respiratory therapist (RT) inserts the airway.

* *Endotracheal (ET) tube*—inserted through the mouth or nose and into the trachea (Fig. 37-2, B). A doctor inserts it using a lighted scope. Some RNs and respiratory therapists are trained to insert ET tubes. A cuff is inflated to keep the airway in place.
* *Tracheostomy tube*—inserted through a surgically created opening *(stomy)* into the trachea *(tracheo)* (Fig. 37-2, C). Cuffed tubes are common. The cuff is inflated to keep the tube in place. Doctors perform tracheostomies.

Vital signs and pulse oximetry are measured often. Observe for hypoxia and other signs and symptoms. If an airway comes out or is dislodged, tell the nurse at once. Frequent oral hygiene is needed. Follow the care plan.

Gagging and choking feelings are common. Imagine something in your mouth, nose, or throat. Comfort and reassure the person. Remind the person that the airway helps breathing. Use touch to show you care.

See *Focus on Communication: Artificial Airways.*

FOCUS ON COMMUNICATION
Artificial Airways

Persons with ET tubes cannot speak. Some tracheostomy tubes allow speech. Paper and pencils, Magic Slates, and communication boards are ways to communicate. Hand signals, nodding the head, and hand squeezes are common for simple "yes" and "no" questions. Follow the care plan. *Always keep the signal light within reach.*

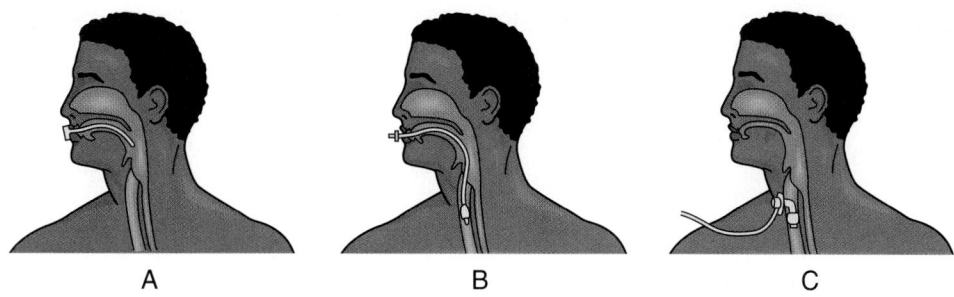

Fig. 37-2 Artificial airways. **A,** Oropharyngeal airway. **B,** Endotracheal tube. **C,** Tracheostomy tube.

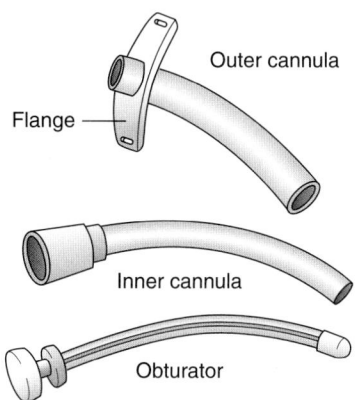

Fig. 37-3 Parts of a tracheostomy tube.

Tracheostomies

A *tracheostomy is a surgically created opening* (stomy) *into the trachea* (tracheo). Tracheostomies are temporary or permanent. They are permanent when airway structures are surgically removed. Cancer, severe airway trauma, or brain damage may require a permanent tracheostomy.

A tracheostomy tube has three parts (Fig. 37-3):

* The *obturator* has a round end. It is used to guide the insertion of the outer cannula (tube). Then it is removed. The obturator is placed within easy reach in case the tracheostomy tube falls out and needs re-insertion. It is taped to the wall or bedside stand.
* The *inner cannula* is inserted and locked in place. It fits inside the outer cannula. It is removed for cleaning and mucus removal. This keeps the airway patent. Some inner cannulas are disposable. Other tracheostomy tubes do not have inner cannulas.
* The *outer cannula* is secured in place with ties around the neck or a Velcro collar. The outer cannula is not removed. It keeps the tracheostomy patent. *Call for the nurse at once if the outer cannula comes out.*

The cuffed tracheostomy tube provides a seal between the cannula and the trachea (see Fig. 37-2, C). This prevents air from leaking around the tube. It also prevents aspiration. A nurse or respiratory therapist inflates and deflates the cuff.

The tube must not come out *(extubation)*. If not secure, it could come out with coughing or if pulled on. A loose tube moves up and down. It can damage the trachea.

The tube must remain patent. If able, the person coughs up secretions. Otherwise suctioning is needed (p. 634). *Call for the nurse if you note signs and symptoms of hypoxia or respiratory distress.*

Safety Measures. Nothing must enter the stoma. Otherwise the person can aspirate. These safety measures are needed:

* Dressings do not have loose gauze or lint.
* The stoma or tube is covered when outdoors. The person wears a stoma cover, scarf, or shirt or blouse that buttons at the neck. The cover prevents dust, insects, and other small particles from entering the stoma.
* The stoma is not covered with plastic, leather, or similar materials. They prevent air from entering the stoma. The person cannot breathe.
* Tub baths are taken. For showers, a shower guard is worn. A hand-held nozzle is used to direct water away from the stoma.
* The person is assisted with shampooing. Water must not enter the stoma.
* The stoma is covered when shaving.
* Swimming is not allowed. Water will enter the tube or stoma.
* Medical-alert jewelry is worn. The person carries a medical alert ID (identification) card.

Assisting With Tracheostomy Care. The nurse may ask you to assist with tracheostomy care (trach care). The care is done daily or every 8 to 12 hours. It also is done as needed for excess secretions, soiled ties or collar, or soiled or moist dressings. The care involves:

- Cleaning the inner cannula to remove mucus and keep the airway patent. Disposable inner cannulas are discarded after 1 use. A new one is inserted. Re-usable inner cannulas are cleaned with a small bottle brush or a pipe cleaner. The nurse tells you what cleaning agent is needed—usually hydrogen peroxide with normal saline or a mild soap.
- Cleaning the stoma to prevent infection and skin breakdown.
- Applying clean ties or a Velcro collar to prevent infection. Clean ties are applied before removing the dirty ones. Hold the outer cannula in place when the nurse changes the ties or collar. Continue to do so until the nurse secures the new ties or collar. The ties or collar must be secure but not tight. For an adult, a finger should slide under the ties or collar (Fig. 37-4, A).

See *Focus on Children and Older Persons: Tracheostomies.*
See *Promoting Safety and Comfort: Tracheostomies.*

FOCUS ON CHILDREN AND OLDER PERSONS
Tracheostomies

Children
Some children have congenital defects. (The Latin word *congenitus* means *to be born with*.) Congenital defects are present at birth. Tracheostomies are needed for some congenital defects affecting the neck and airway.

Some infections cause swelling of the airway structures. This obstructs air flow. So does foreign body aspiration. These problems may require emergency tracheostomies.

Tracheostomy ties must be secure but not tight. Only a fingertip should slide under the ties (Fig. 37-4, B). Ties are too loose if you can slide your whole finger under them.

Assist the nurse by holding the child still. Position the child's head as the nurse directs.

PROMOTING SAFETY AND COMFORT
Tracheostomies

Safety
Mucus may contain microbes or blood. Follow Standard Precautions and the Bloodborne Pathogen Standard.

SUCTIONING THE AIRWAY

Secretions can collect in the airway. Retained secretions:
- Obstruct air flow into and out of the airway.
- Provide an environment for microbes.
- Interfere with oxygen (O_2) and carbon dioxide (CO_2) exchange.

Hypoxia can occur. Usually coughing removes secretions. Some persons cannot cough, or the cough is too weak to remove secretions. They need suctioning.

Suction is the process of withdrawing or sucking up fluid (secretions). A suction source is needed—wall outlet or suction machine. A tube connects to a suction source at one end and to a suction catheter at the other end. The catheter is inserted into the airway. Secretions are withdrawn through the catheter.

The nose, mouth, and pharynx make up the upper airway. The trachea and bronchi make up the lower airway. These routes are used to suction the airway:

- *Oropharyngeal.* The mouth (*oro*) and pharynx (*pharyngeal*) are suctioned. A suction catheter is passed through the mouth and into the pharynx. The Yankauer suction catheter is often used for thick secretions (Fig. 37-5).
- *Nasopharyngeal.* The nose (*naso*) and pharynx (*pharyngeal*) are suctioned. The suction catheter is passed through the nose into the pharynx.
- *Lower airway.* The suction catheter is passed through an ET or tracheostomy tube (Fig. 37-6).

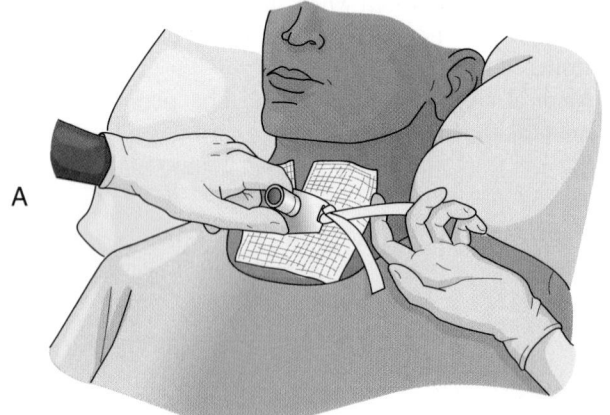
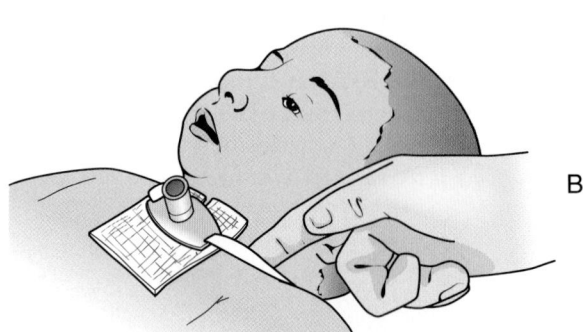

Fig. 37-4 A, For an adult, a finger is inserted under the ties. **B,** For children, only a fingertip is inserted under the ties.

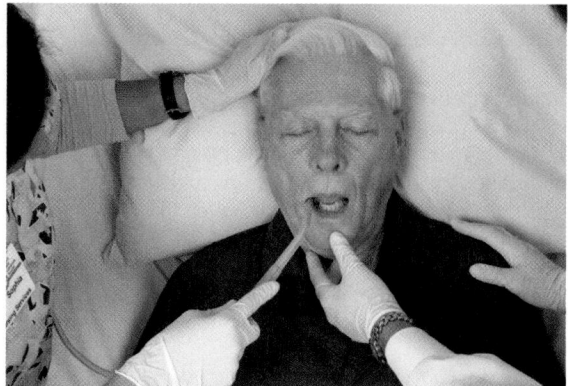

Fig. 37-5 The Yankauer suction catheter is often used when there are large amounts of thick secretions.

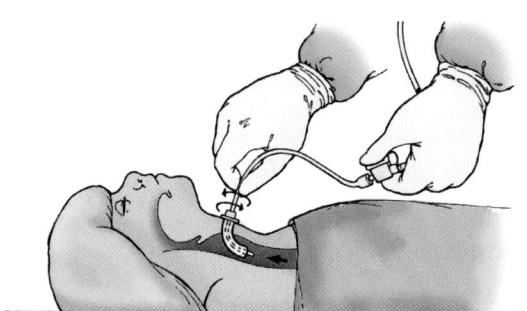

Fig. 37-6 A tracheostomy tube is suctioned.

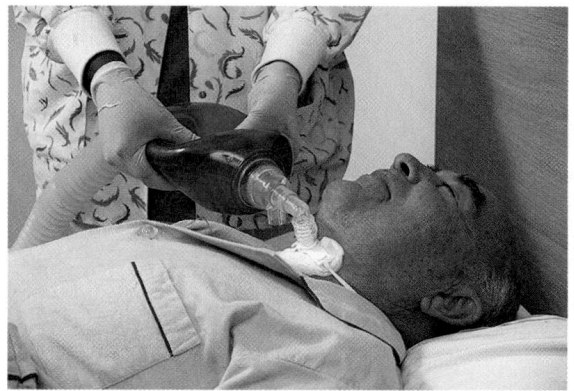

Fig. 37-7 The Ambu bag is squeezed with two hands.

The person's lungs are hyperventilated before suctioning an ET or a tracheostomy tube. *Hyperventilate* means to given extra *(hyper)* breaths *(ventilate)*. An Ambu bag is used (Fig. 37-7). The Ambu bag is attached to an oxygen source. Then the oxygen delivery device is removed from the ET or tracheostomy tube. The Ambu bag is attached to the ET or tracheostomy tube. To give a breath, the bag is squeezed with both hands. The nurse or respiratory therapist gives 3 to 5 breaths.

Oxygen is treated like a drug. You do not give drugs. Check if your state and agency allow you to use an Ambu bag attached to an oxygen source.

See *Focus on Children and Older Persons: Suctioning.*

See *Promoting Safety and Comfort: Suctioning.*

FOCUS ON CHILDREN AND OLDER PERSONS
Suctioning

Children
Suctioning may frighten children. They need clear, simple explanations about the procedure. You may need to hold the child still. To do so, control the child's head and arm movements.

PROMOTING SAFETY AND COMFORT
Suctioning

Safety
If not done correctly, suctioning can cause serious harm. Suctioning removes oxygen from the airway. The person does not get oxygen during suctioning. Hypoxia and life-threatening problems can occur. They arise from the respiratory, cardiovascular, and nervous systems. Cardiac arrest can occur. Infection and airway injury are possible.

You can assist the nurse with suctioning (Box 37-1, p. 636). However, you do not perform the suctioning procedure.

Always keep needed suction equipment and supplies at the bedside. When suctioning is needed, you do not have time to collect items from the supply area.

Mucus may contain microbes or blood. Follow Standard Precautions and the Bloodborne Pathogen Standard.

BOX 37-1   ASSISTING WITH SUCTIONING: SAFETY MEASURES

- Review the procedure with the nurse. Know what you are to do.
- Report coughing and the signs and symptoms of respiratory distress (Chapter 36). They signal the need for suctioning. Suctioning is done as needed, not on a schedule.
- Follow Standard Precautions and the Bloodborne Pathogen Standard. Secretions may contain blood and are potentially infectious.
- Sterile technique is used to suction ET and tracheostomy tubes (Chapter 15). This helps prevent microbes from entering the airway.
- The nurse tells you the catheter type and size needed. If too large, it can injure the airway.
- Needed suction supplies and equipment are kept at the bedside. They are ready when the person needs suctioning.
- Suction is *not* applied while inserting the catheter into the lower airway. When suction is applied, air is sucked out of the airway.
- The catheter is inserted smoothly. This helps prevent injury to mucous membranes.
- A suction cycle for adults takes no more than 10 to 15 seconds. For infants and children, the suction cycle is no more than 5 seconds. A suction cycle involves:
  - Inserting the catheter
  - Suctioning
  - Removing the catheter

- The catheter is cleared with sterile water or saline between suction cycles.
- The nurse waits 20 to 30 seconds between each suction cycle. Some agencies require waiting 60 seconds.
- The suction catheter is passed (inserted) no more than 3 times. Injury and hypoxia are risks when the suction catheter is passed.
- Check the pulse, respirations, and pulse oximeter measurements before, during, and after the procedure. Also observe level of consciousness. Tell the nurse at once if any of these occur:
  - A decrease in pulse rate or a pulse rate less than 60 beats per minute.
  - Irregular pulse rhythms.
  - An increase or decrease in blood pressure.
  - Respiratory distress.
  - A decrease in oxygen saturation. Normal range is 95% to 100%. See Chapter 36.

MECHANICAL VENTILATION

Weak muscle effort, obstructed airway, and damaged lung tissue cause hypoxia. Nervous system diseases and injuries can affect the respiratory center in the brain. Nerve damage interferes with messages between the lungs and the brain. Drug overdose depresses the brain. With severe problems, the person cannot breathe. Or normal blood oxygen levels are not maintained. Often mechanical ventilation is needed.

Mechanical ventilation is using a machine to move air into and out of the lungs (Fig. 37-8). O_2 enters the lungs. CO_2 leaves them. An ET or tracheostomy tube is needed.

Alarms sound when something is wrong. One alarm means the person is disconnected from the ventilator. The nurse shows you how to reconnect the ET or tracheostomy tube. *When any alarm sounds, first check to see if the tube is attached to the ventilator. If not, attach it to the ventilator. The person can die if not attached to the ventilator.* Then tell the nurse at once about the alarm. Do not reset alarms.

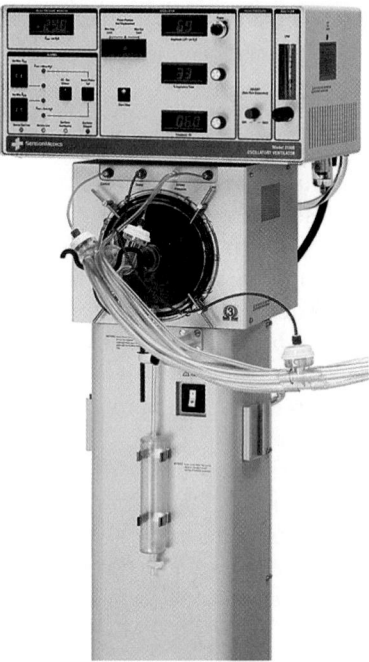

Fig. 37-8 A mechanical ventilator.

BOX 37-2	CARE OF PERSONS ON MECHANICAL VENTILATION

- Keep the signal light within reach.
- Answer signal lights promptly. The person depends on others for basic needs.
- Make sure hoses and connecting tubing have slack. They must not pull on the artificial airway.
- Explain who you are and what you are going to do. Do this whenever you enter the room.
- Give the day, date, and time every time you give care.
- Report signs of respiratory distress or discomfort at once.
- Do not change settings on the machine or reset alarms.
- Follow the care plan for communication. The person cannot talk. Use agreed-upon hand or eye signals for "yes" and "no." Everyone must use the same signals. Some persons can use paper and pencils, Magic Slates, communication boards, and hand signals.
- Ask questions that have simple answers. It may be hard to write long responses.
- Watch what you say and do. This includes when you are near and away from the person and family. They pay close attention to your verbal and nonverbal communication. Do not say or do anything that could upset the person.
- Use touch to comfort and reassure the person. Also tell the person about the weather, pleasant news events, and gifts and cards.
- Meet basic needs. Follow the care plan.
- Tell the person when you are leaving the room and when you will return.
- Complete a safety check before leaving the room. (See the inside of the front book cover.)

FOCUS ON LONG-TERM CARE AND HOME CARE
Mechanical Ventilation

Long-Term Care
Mechanical ventilation is started in the hospital. Some people need it for a few hours or days. Others require long-term care or subacute care. Often the person needs weaning from the ventilator. That is, the person needs to breathe without the machine. The respiratory therapist and RN plan the weaning process. Weaning can take many weeks.

Home Care
Home care is an option for some ventilator-dependent persons. The nurse teaches you how to care for the person. Family members learn how to assist with the person's care. Make sure you can reach the nurse by phone when in the person's home. Make sure delegated tasks are allowed by your state and agency.

Persons needing mechanical ventilation are often very ill. Other problems and injuries are common. Some persons are confused, disoriented, or cannot think clearly. The machine and fear of dying frighten many. Some are relieved to get enough oxygen. Many fear needing the machine for life. Mechanical ventilation can be painful for those with chest injuries or chest surgery. Tubes and hoses restrict movement. This causes more discomfort.

The nurse may ask you to assist with the person's care. See Box 37-2.

See *Focus on Long-Term Care and Home Care: Mechanical Ventilation.*

CHEST TUBES

Air, blood, or fluid can collect in the pleural space (sac or cavity). This occurs when the chest is entered because of injury or surgery.

- *Pneumothorax is air* (pneumo) *in the pleural space* (thorax).
- *Hemothorax is blood* (hemo) *in the pleural space* (thorax).
- *Pleural effusion is the escape and collection of fluid* (effusion) *in the pleural space.*

Pressure occurs when air, blood, or fluid collects in the pleural space. The pressure collapses the lung. Air cannot reach affected alveoli. O_2 and CO_2 are not exchanged. Respiratory distress and hypoxia result. Pressure on the heart affects the heart's ability to pump blood.

Hospital care is required. The doctor inserts chest tubes to remove the air, blood, or fluid (Fig. 37-9, p. 638). The sterile procedure is done in surgery, in the emergency room, or at the bedside. A nurse assists.

Chest tubes attach to a drainage system (Fig. 37-10, p. 638). The system must be airtight so air does not enter the pleural space. Water-seal drainage keeps the system airtight. The bottles in Figure 37-11, p. 638 show how the system works:

- A chest tube attaches to connecting tubing.
- Connecting tubing attaches to a tube in the drainage container.
- The tube in the drainage container extends under water. The water prevents air from entering the chest tube and then the pleural space.

See Box 37-3, p. 638 for care of the person with chest tubes.

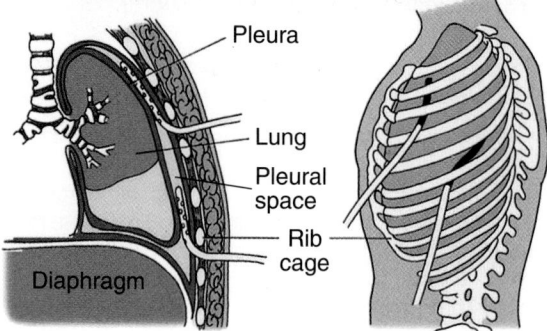

Fig. 37-9 Chest tubes inserted into the pleural space.

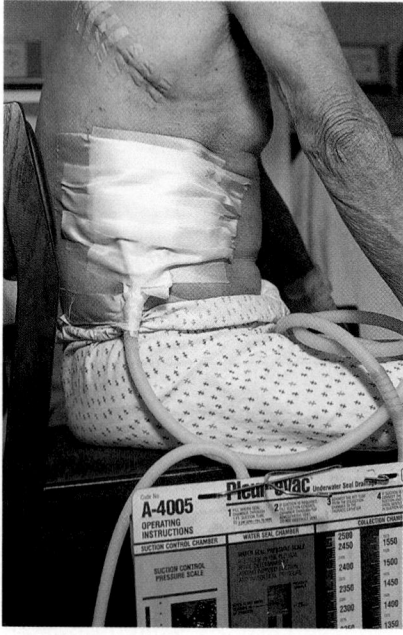

Fig. 37-10 Chest tubes attached to a disposable water-seal drainage system. Chest tubes are inserted into the pleural space.

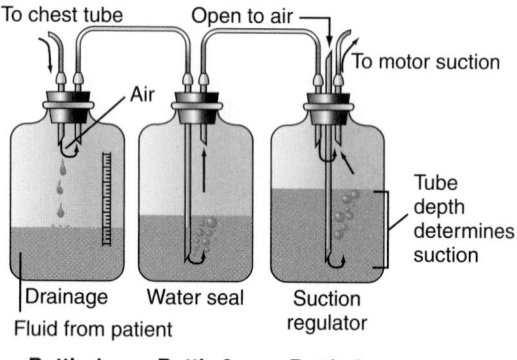

Fig. 37-11 Water-seal drainage system.

BOX 37-3 CARE OF THE PERSON WITH CHEST TUBES

- Keep the drainage system below the chest.
- Measure vital signs and pulse oximetry as directed. Report changes at once.
- Report signs and symptoms of hypoxia and respiratory distress at once. See Chapter 36.
- Report complaints of pain or difficulty breathing at once.
- Keep connecting tubing coiled on the bed. Allow enough slack so the chest tubes are not dislodged when the person moves. If tubing hangs in loops, drainage collects in the loops.
- Prevent tubing kinks. Kinks obstruct the chest tube. Air, blood, or fluid collects in the pleural space.
- Observe chest drainage. Report any change in chest drainage at once. This includes increases in drainage or the appearance of bright red drainage.
- Record chest drainage according to agency policy.
- Turn and position the person as directed. Be careful and gentle to prevent the chest tubes from dislodging.
- Assist with deep-breathing and coughing exercises as directed.
- Assist with incentive spirometry as directed.
- Note bubbling in the drainage system. Tell the nurse at once if bubbling increases, decreases, or stops.
- Tell the nurse at once if any part of the system is loose or disconnected.
- Keep sterile petrolatum gauze at the bedside. It is needed if a chest tube comes out.
- Call for help at once if a chest tube comes out. Cover the insertion site with sterile petrolatum gauze. Stay with the person. Follow the nurse's directions.
- Complete a safety check before leaving the room. (See the inside of the front book cover.)

FOCUS ON PRIDE

The Person, Family, and Yourself

Personal and Professional Responsibility

The person's airway must be clear for survival. You must know the signs and symptoms that signal the need for suctioning (Box 37-1 and Chapter 36). Tell the nurse right away if you suspect suctioning is needed. Delay can cause harm or death.

Observing the person and reporting concerns are important parts of your role. Take pride in safely assisting with respiratory support and therapies.

Rights and Respect

Persons with ET tubes cannot speak. Many cannot respond in any way. Coma (Chapter 12) and sedation (Chapter 32) are causes. However, the person may hear and understand. Show dignity and respect when providing care.

- Tell the person when he or she will be moved or touched.
- Explain what the person will feel. Also say where it will be felt.
- Talk to the person. Discuss pleasant things.
- Focus on the person. Do not ignore the person or talk with co-workers about personal matters.
- Use touch to show you care.

Every person has the right to dignified care. Take pride in providing care in a way that shows respect for the person.

Independence and Social Interaction

The need for mechanical ventilation brings fears and worries for the family. They may wonder how long the ventilator will be needed or if the person will die. The doctor and nurse answer the family's questions. You can provide social support. Allowing the family quality time with the person can bring peace and ease stress. You can:

- Encourage the family to talk to the person. For persons who cannot respond, tell the family that the person may hear and understand.
- Allow private time.
- Promote the use of touch. Provide chairs so the family can sit beside the person and hold a hand, stroke the hair, and so on.
- Allow family involvement in care measures. Brushing the person's hair, applying lotion, and performing nail care are examples.

Delegation and Teamwork

The health team involves many workers. The team works together to meet the person's needs. Some team members have one focus of care. For example, a respiratory therapist (RT) provides respiratory treatments and therapies. The RT is an important part of the team.

As with all team members, develop a good working relationship with the RT. Be polite. Offer to help as needed. The RT is a good source of knowledge and skill for respiratory issues. You can learn from the RT. Do not be afraid to ask questions. Thank the person for answering your questions.

Learn about other members of the health team. Learn their roles and how they provide care. Positive relationships with the health team make your work more enjoyable.

Ethics and Laws

Respiratory support and therapies involve complex care. Many in this chapter are outside the scope of your role. Serious problems can occur from the wrong care. Know your limits. Follow the nurse's directions when assisting with care measures. Remember your legal and ethical responsibilities. You have the right to refuse a function or task. Do not function beyond your legal scope, preparation, and skill level.

REVIEW QUESTIONS

Circle the BEST answer.

1 A person has a tracheostomy. Which is *false*?
   a The person must not cough.
   b The obturator is taped to the wall or bedside stand.
   c The nurse removes the inner cannula for cleaning.
   d The outer cannula must be secured in place.

2 A person with a tracheostomy *cannot*
   a Shampoo
   b Shave
   c Shower with a hand-held nozzle
   d Swim

3 The nurse is changing tracheostomy ties. You must
   a Remove the inner cannula
   b Clean the stoma
   c Remove the dressing
   d Hold the outer cannula in place

4 You cannot slide a finger under tracheostomy ties. This means that the ties
   a Are secure
   b Are too tight
   c Need to be replaced
   d Need to be removed

5 Which signals the need for suctioning?
   a A pulse rate of 90 beats per minute
   b Signs and symptoms of respiratory distress
   c The orthopneic position
   d Being unable to speak

6 Suctioning the lower airway requires
   a Sterile technique
   b Mechanical ventilation
   c An artificial airway
   d Chest tubes

7 You are assisting the nurse with suctioning. You must
   a Insert the catheter no more than 3 times
   b Suction for no more than 10 to 15 minutes
   c Clear the suction catheter with water
   d Keep needed suction supplies at the bedside

8 You note the following while assisting with suctioning. Which should you report at once?
   a A pulse rate of 82 beats per minute
   b A regular heart rhythm
   c Oxygen saturation of 92%
   d Thick secretions

9 A person requires mechanical ventilation. Which is *false*?
   a The person has an ET or tracheostomy tube.
   b The signal light must always be within reach.
   c Touch provides comfort and reassurance.
   d You can reset alarms on the ventilator.

10 A ventilator alarm sounds. What should you do *first*?
   a Reset the alarm.
   b Check to see if the airway is attached to the machine.
   c Call the nurse at once.
   d Ask the person what is wrong.

11 A person has a pneumothorax. This is
   a Fluid in the pleural space
   b Blood in the pleural space
   c Air in the pleural space
   d Secretions in the pleural space

12 Chest tubes are attached to water-seal drainage. You should do the following *except*
   a Tell the nurse if bubbling increases, decreases, or stops
   b Make sure tubing is not kinked
   c Keep the drainage system below the chest
   d Hang tubing in loops

Answers to these questions are on p. 834.

38 Rehabilitation and Restorative Nursing Care

OBJECTIVES

- Define the key terms and key abbreviations listed in this chapter.
- Describe how rehabilitation and restorative care involve the whole person.
- Identify the complications to prevent.
- Identify the common reactions to rehabilitation.
- List the common rehabilitation programs and services.
- Explain your role in rehabilitation and restorative care.
- Explain how to promote PRIDE in the person, the family, and yourself.

KEY TERMS

activities of daily living (ADL) The activities usually done during a normal day in a person's life
disability Any lost, absent, or impaired physical or mental function
prosthesis An artificial replacement for a missing body part

rehabilitation The process of restoring the person to his or her highest possible level of physical, psychological, social, and economic function
restorative aide A nursing assistant with special training in restorative nursing and rehabilitation skills
restorative nursing care Care that helps persons regain health, strength, and independence

KEY ABBREVIATIONS

ADL	Activities of daily living	**ROM**	Range of motion
OBRA	Omnibus Budget Reconciliation Act of 1987		

Disease, injury, and surgery can affect body function. So can birth injuries and birth defects (Chapter 47). Often more than one function is lost. Losses are temporary or permanent. Eating, bathing, dressing, and walking are hard or seem impossible. Some persons cannot work. Others cannot care for children or family.

A *disability is any lost, absent, or impaired physical or mental function*. Causes are acute or chronic (Box 38-1).
- An *acute problem* has a short course. Recovery is complete. A fracture is an acute problem with a short course. The person has a cast. Crutches are used until the bone heals.
- A *chronic problem* has a long course. The problem is controlled—not cured—with treatment. Diabetes and arthritis are chronic health problems. A spinal cord injury is long-term if paralysis results.

The person may depend totally or in part on others for basic needs. The degree of disability affects how much function is possible.

A goal of health care is to prevent and reduce the degree of disability. Helping the person adjust is another goal. *Rehabilitation is the process of restoring the person to his or her highest possible level of physical, psychological, social, and economic function*. The focus is on improving abilities. This promotes function at the highest level of independence. For some persons the goal is to return to work. For others, self-care is the goal. Sometimes improved function is not possible. Then the goal is to prevent further loss of function. This helps the person maintain the best possible quality of life.

Some persons return home after rehabilitation. The process may continue in home or community settings.

See *Focus on Long-Term Care and Home Care: Rehabilitation and Restorative Nursing Care.*

BOX 38-1	COMMON HEALTH PROBLEMS REQUIRING REHABILITATION

- Amputation
- Birth defects
- Brain tumor
- Burns
- Cerebral palsy
- Chronic obstructive pulmonary disease
- Fractures
- Head injury
- Myocardial infarction (heart attack)
- Spinal cord injury
- Spinal cord tumor
- Stroke
- Substance abuse—drug, alcohol

FOCUS ON LONG-TERM CARE AND HOME CARE
Rehabilitation and Restorative Nursing Care

Long-Term Care

Some nursing center residents have physical disabilities. Causes include strokes, fractures, amputations, and injuries. They need to regain function or adjust to a long-term disability. Often these residents return home.

Other residents have progressive illnesses. They become more and more disabled. The goals are to help them:
- Maintain their highest level of function.
- Prevent unnecessary decline in function.

RESTORATIVE NURSING

Some persons are weak. Many cannot perform daily functions. They need restorative nursing care. *Restorative nursing care is care that helps persons regain health, strength, and independence.* With progressive illnesses, the person becomes more and more disabled. Restorative nursing programs:
- Help maintain the highest level of function.
- Prevent unnecessary decline in function.

Restorative nursing may involve measures that promote:
- Self-care
- Elimination
- Positioning
- Mobility
- Communication
- Cognitive function

Many persons need restorative nursing and rehabilitation. Often it is hard to separate them. In many agencies, they mean the same thing. Both focus on the whole person.

Restorative Aides

Some agencies have restorative aides. A *restorative aide is a nursing assistant with special training in restorative nursing and rehabilitation skills.* These aides assist the nursing and health teams as needed. Required training varies among states. If there are no state requirements, the agency provides needed training.

REHABILITATION AND THE WHOLE PERSON

A health problem has physical, psychological, and social effects. So does a disability. Suppose an illness left you paralyzed from the waist down.
- Would you be angry, afraid, or depressed?
- How would you move about?
- How would you care for yourself?
- How would you care for your family?
- How would you worship, shop, or visit friends?
- What job could you do?
- How would you support yourself?

The person needs to adjust physically, psychologically, socially, and economically. Abilities—what the person can do—are stressed. Complications are prevented. They can cause further disability.

See *Focus on Children and Older Persons: Rehabilitation and the Whole Person.*

FOCUS ON CHILDREN AND OLDER PERSONS
Rehabilitation and the Whole Person

Children

Disabilities occur from birth defects or from illness, injury, or surgery. They can affect normal growth and development (Chapter 10). For normal growth and development, the child needs hand skills, mobility, communication, play, and relationships with parents, family, and peers. A disability can affect one or more of these factors.

Older Persons

Rehabilitation takes longer in older persons than in other age-groups. Changes from aging affect healing, mobility, vision, hearing, and other functions. Chronic health problems can slow recovery. Older persons also are at risk for injuries. Fast-paced rehabilitation programs are hard for them. Their programs usually are slower-paced.

Physical Aspects

Rehabilitation starts when the person first seeks health care. Complications are prevented. They can occur from bedrest, a long illness, or recovery from surgery or injury. Bowel and bladder problems are prevented. So are contractures and pressure ulcers. Good alignment, turning and re-positioning, range-of-motion (ROM) exercises, and supportive devices are needed (Chapters 16, 17, and 27). Good skin care also prevents pressure ulcers (Chapters 20 and 34).

Elimination. Some persons need bladder training (Chapter 22). The method depends on the person's problems, abilities, and needs. Some need bowel training (Chapter 23). Control of bowel movements and regular elimination are goals. Fecal impaction, constipation, and fecal incontinence are prevented. Follow the care plan and the nurse's instructions.

Self-care. Self-care is a major goal. *Activities of daily living (ADL) are the activities usually done during a normal day in a person's life.* ADL include bathing, oral hygiene, dressing, eating, elimination, and moving about. The health team evaluates the person's ability to perform ADL. The need for self-help devices is considered.

Sometimes the hands, wrists, and arms are affected. Self-help devices are often needed. Equipment is changed, made, or bought to meet the person's needs.

- Eating devices include glass holders, plate guards, and silverware with curved handles or cuffs (Chapter 24). Some devices attach to splints (Fig. 38-1).
- Electric toothbrushes are helpful. They have back-and-forth brushing motions for oral hygiene.
- Longer handles attach to combs, brushes, and sponges. Or the devices have long handles. See Chapters 20 and 21.
- Self-help devices are useful for cooking, dressing, writing, phone calls, and other tasks. Some are shown in Figure 38-2.

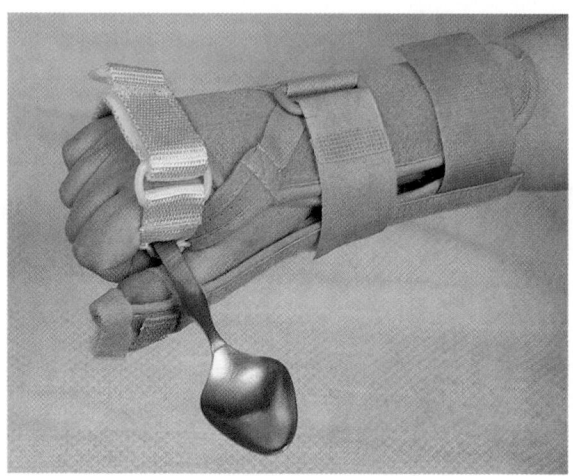

Fig. 38-1 Eating device attached to a splint.

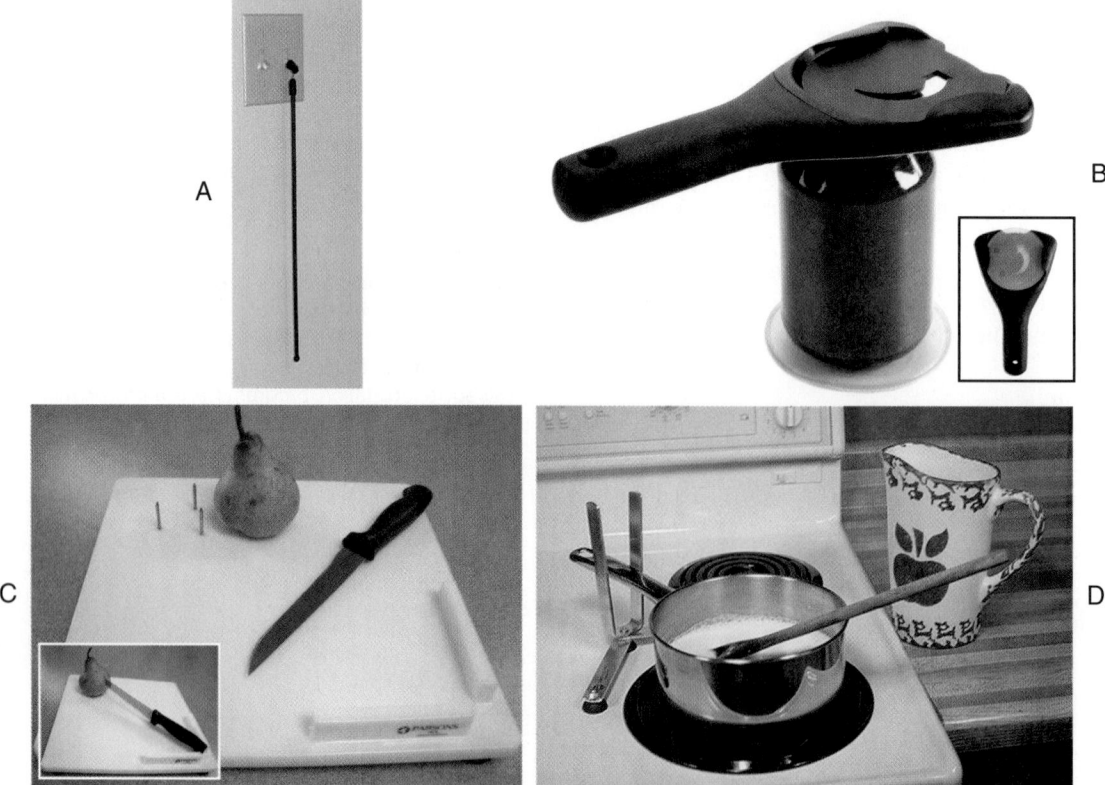

Fig. 38-2   A, Light switch extender. **B,** Jar opener. **C,** Cutting board. **D,** Pot stabilizer.

Mobility. The person may need crutches or a walker, cane, or brace. Physical and occupational therapies are common for musculo-skeletal and nervous system problems (Fig. 38-3). Some people need wheelchairs. If possible, they learn wheelchair transfers. Such transfers include to and from the bed, toilet, bathtub, sofa, and chair and in and out of vehicles (Figs. 38-4 and 38-5 below and 38-6, p. 644).

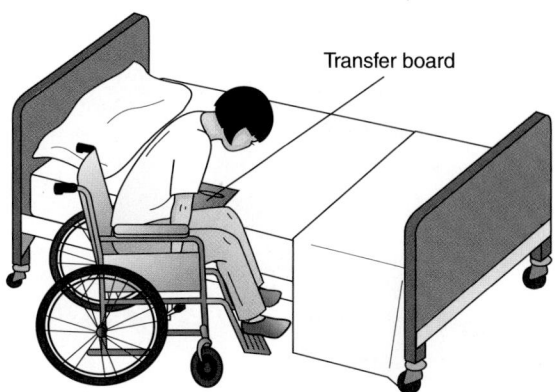

Fig. 38-4 The person uses a transfer board to transfer from the wheelchair to bed.

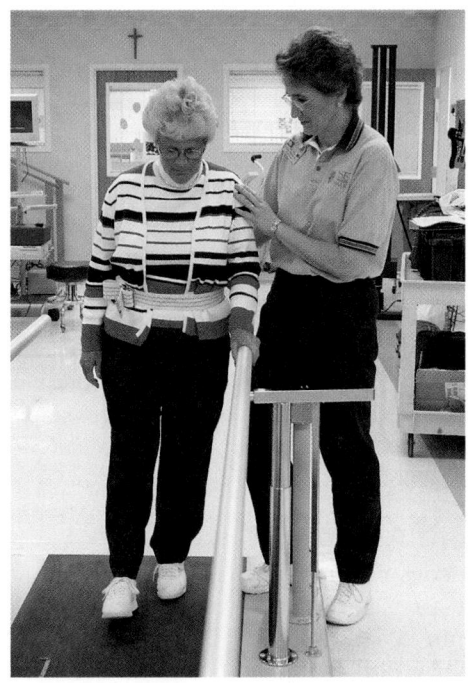

Fig. 38-3 The person is assisted with walking in physical therapy.

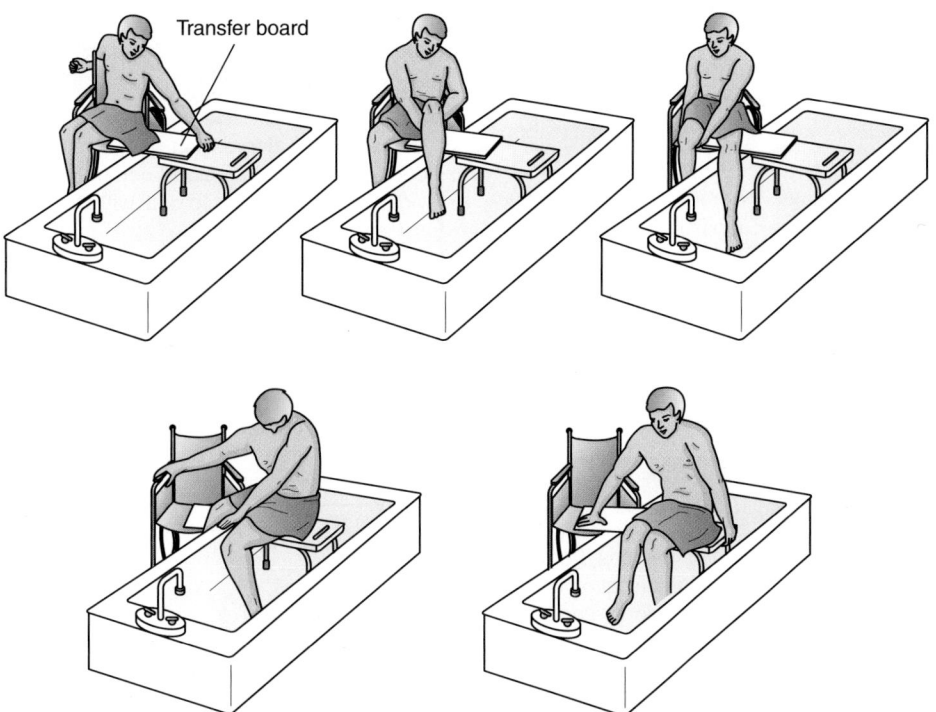

Fig. 38-5 The person transfers from the wheelchair to the bathtub. A transfer board is used.

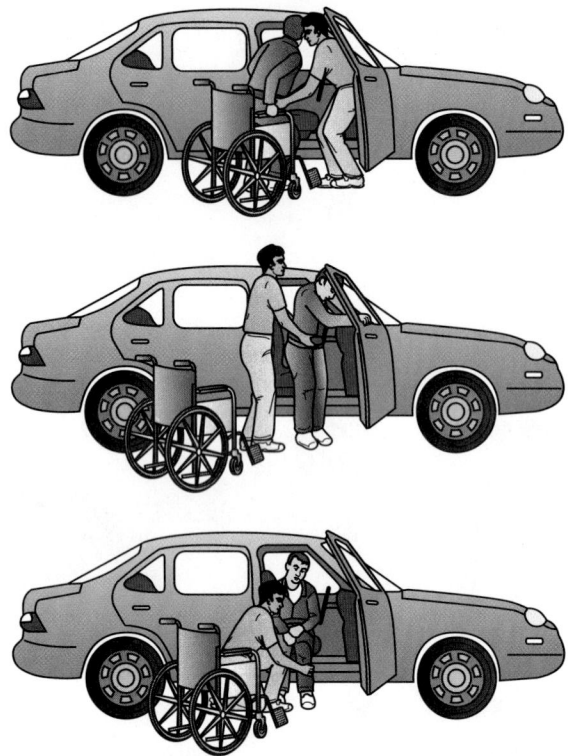

Fig. 38-6 The person transfers from the wheelchair to the car.

A *prosthesis is an artificial replacement for a missing body part.* The person learns how to use the artificial arm or leg (Chapter 41). The goal is for the device to be like the missing body part in function and appearance.

Nutrition. Difficulty swallowing *(dysphagia)* may occur after a stroke. The person may need a dysphagia diet (Chapter 24). When possible, the person learns exercises to improve swallowing. Some persons cannot swallow. They need enteral nutrition (Chapter 25).

Communication. *Aphasia* may occur from a stroke (Chapter 41). Aphasia is the total or partial loss *(a)* of the ability to use or understand language *(phasia)*. It is a language disorder resulting from damage to parts of the brain responsible for language. The person does not have normal speech. Speech therapy and communication devices are helpful (Chapter 8).

See *Focus on Communication: Communication.*

FOCUS ON COMMUNICATION

Communication

Speaking is difficult or impossible for some persons. Persons with speech disorders may need other communication methods. Pictures, reading, writing, facial expressions, and gestures are examples. The person and health team decide on the best method. All health team members and the family use the same method with the person. Changing methods can cause confusion and delay progress.

Mechanical Ventilation. Some persons need mechanical ventilation (Chapter 37). Some are weaned from the ventilator. That is, the person learns to breathe without the machine. The process may take many weeks. Other persons learn to live with life-long mechanical ventilation.

Psychological and Social Aspects

A disability can affect function and appearance. Self-esteem and relationships may suffer. Some persons may feel unwhole, useless, unattractive, unclean, or undesirable. They may deny the disability and expect therapy to correct the problem. Some persons are depressed, angry, and hostile.

Successful rehabilitation depends on the person's attitude. The person must accept his or her limits and be motivated. The focus is on abilities and strengths. Despair and frustration are common. Progress may be slow. Learning a new task is a reminder of the disability. Old fears and emotions may recur.

Remind persons of their *progress*. They need help accepting disabilities and limits. Give support, reassurance, and encouragement. Psychological and social needs are part of the care plan. Spiritual support helps some persons.

See *Focus on Communication: Psychological and Social Aspects.*

Economic Aspects

Some persons return to their jobs. Others cannot do so. They are assessed for work skills, work history, interests, and talents. A job skill may be restored or a new one learned. The goal is for the person to become gainfully employed. Help is given finding a job.

FOCUS ON COMMUNICATION

Psychological and Social Aspects

Denial, anger, depression, fear, and frustration are common during rehabilitation. Good communication and support provide encouragement. To deal with such emotions:

• Listen to the person.
• Show concern not pity.
• Focus on what the person can do. Point out even slight progress.
• Be polite but firm. Do not let the person control you.
• Do not shout at or insult the person. Such behaviors are abuse and mistreatment.
• Do not argue with the person.
• Tell the nurse. The person may need other support measures.

THE REHABILITATION TEAM

Rehabilitation is a team effort. The person is the key team member. The family, doctor, and nursing and health teams help the person set goals and plan care. The focus is on regaining function and independence.

The team meets often to discuss the person's progress. The rehabilitation plan is changed as needed. The person and family attend the meetings when possible. Families are important. They provide support and encouragement. Often they help with home care.

Your Role

Your job focuses on promoting the person's independence. Preventing decline in function also is a goal. The many procedures, care measures, and rules in this book apply. Safety, communication, legal, and ethical aspects apply. So do the measures in Box 38-2.

See *Focus on Communication: Your Role.*

See *Teamwork and Time Management: Your Role.*

FOCUS ON COMMUNICATION

Your Role

You may need to guide and direct the person during care measures. First, listen to how the nurse or therapist guides and directs the person. Use those words. Hearing the same thing helps the person learn and remember what to do.

TEAMWORK AND TIME MANAGEMENT

Your Role

Rehabilitation can frustrate the person, you, and the health team. Teamwork is about helping with care. But it is also about giving emotional support. Talking about your feelings may help. The team can help you control or express your feelings. You may need to assist with other patients or residents for a while.

BOX 38-2	**ASSISTING WITH REHABILITATION AND RESTORATIVE CARE**

- Follow the care plan and the nurse's instructions carefully.
- Follow the person's daily routine.
- Provide for safety.
- Protect the person's rights. Privacy and personal choice are very important.
- Report early signs and symptoms of complications. They include pressure ulcers, contractures, and bowel and bladder problems.
- Keep the person in good alignment at all times.
- Turn and re-position the person as directed.
- Use safe transfer methods.
- Practice measures to prevent pressure ulcers.
- Perform ROM exercises as instructed.
- Apply assistive devices as ordered.
- Provide needed self-help devices.
- Do not pity the person or give sympathy.
- Encourage the person to perform ADL to the extent possible.
- Give the person time to complete tasks. Do not rush the person.
- Give praise when even a little progress is made.
- Provide emotional support and reassurance.
- Try to understand and appreciate the person's situation, feelings, and concerns.
- Provide for spiritual needs.
- Practice the methods developed by the rehabilitation team. This helps you better assist the person.
- Practice the task that the person must do. This helps you guide and direct the person.
- Know how to apply the person's self-help devices.
- Know how to use the person's equipment.
- Stress what the person can do. Focus on abilities and strengths. Do not focus on disabilities and weaknesses.
- Remember that muscles will atrophy if not used. And contractures can develop.
- Have a hopeful outlook.

REHABILITATION PROGRAMS AND SERVICES

Rehabilitation begins when the person first needs health care. Often this is in the hospital. Common rehabilitation programs include:

- *Cardiac rehabilitation*—for heart disorders (Chapter 42)
- *Brain injury rehabilitation*—for nervous system disorders including traumatic brain injury (Chapter 41)
- *Spinal cord rehabilitation*—for spinal cord injuries (Chapter 41)
- *Stroke rehabilitation*—after a stroke (Chapter 41)
- *Respiratory rehabilitation*—for respiratory system disorders such as chronic obstructive pulmonary disease, after lung surgery, for respiratory complications from other health problems (Chapter 42), and for mechanical ventilation (Chapter 37)
- *Musculo-skeletal rehabilitation*—for fractures, joint replacement surgery, and so on (Chapter 41)
- *Rehabilitation for complex medical and surgical conditions*—for wound care (Chapters 33 and 34), diabetes (Chapter 43), burns (Chapter 51), and so on

The process may continue after hospital discharge. The person may transfer to a nursing center or to a rehabilitation agency. There are agencies for persons who are blind or deaf, have intellectual disabilities (formerly called mental retardation), are physically disabled, or have speech problems. Some agencies are for persons who are mentally ill. Substance abuse programs are common.

Home care agencies also provide rehabilitation services. So do some assisted living residences (Chapter 50) and adult day-care centers.

See *Focus on Children and Older Persons: Rehabilitation Programs and Services,* p. 646.

See *Focus on Long-Term Care and Home Care: Rehabilitation Programs and Services,* p. 646.

FOCUS ON CHILDREN AND OLDER PERSONS
Rehabilitation Programs and Services

Children
Federal laws require that schools provide needed therapies. In-school therapy is required to meet the child's learning needs.

FOCUS ON LONG-TERM CARE AND HOME CARE
Rehabilitation Programs and Services

Long-Term Care
The Omnibus Budget Reconciliation Act of 1987 (OBRA) requires that nursing centers provide rehabilitation services. If not provided by center staff, the service is obtained from another source. For example, a center does not have a speech therapist. Instead, the service is obtained from a hospital or other agency.

The center must provide services required by a person's care plan. If a person requires physical therapy, it must be provided. If occupational therapy is required, it must be provided. If speech therapy is required, it must be provided. Such services require a doctor's order.

Home Care
The rehabilitation team assesses the person's home setting (Box 38-3). Changes in the home are made as needed. Some persons require personal attendants 24 hours a day.

BOX 38-3 HOME ASSESSMENT

Outdoors
- Where is parking located? How far is the parking to the door?
- Where is the car parked?
- Where is the mailbox?
- How wide are the doors?
- Can the person turn a key? Or open and close doors?
- Are ramps or hand rails needed?
- Is private or public transportation available?
- Can the person drive a car?
- How wide and high are ramps and sidewalks?

Indoors
- Are there floor obstructions?
- Are there steps? Where are they? How many are there?
- How is furniture arranged? Can the person use the furniture?
- Where are phones located? Can the person use a phone?
- Can the person open and close windows?
- How are floors covered (wall-to-wall carpeting, tile, hardwood floors, throw rugs)?
- Can the person use a wheelchair throughout the home?
- Where is the fuse or circuit-breaker box located?
- Can the person control the heat?
- Are walkways, doors, and hallways wide enough for wheelchair use?
- Does the building have an elevator?

Kitchen
- Can the person access the stove, sink, cupboards, storage areas, work space, refrigerator, and other appliances?
- How high is the sink and counter top?
- Is there an opening under the sink for wheelchair access?
- Can the person turn faucets on and off?
- Can the person use the microwave and other appliances?
- Can the person reach stove knobs?

Bathroom
- How high are the sink, toilet, shower, and tub?
- Can the person turn the faucets on and off?
- Is there room for a wheelchair and other assistive devices?

Bathroom—cont'd
- Can the person get into and out of the tub or shower?
- Are there safety bars by the toilet, shower, and tub?

Bedroom
- How high is the person's bed?
- Can the person reach closet rods and shelves?
- Can the person transfer in and out of bed safely? Is there room around the bed for the person to move?
- How is furniture arranged? Does it allow for a wheelchair or assistive devices?

Safety
- Is the house number clearly visible and readable for an emergency?
- Are deadbolts and locks secure? Can the person use them?
- Can the person see and talk to a visitor at the door without being seen?
- Are steps, porch, and entrances lighted?
- Are the steps, porch, and entrances protected from rain, sleet, and snow?
- Is there a non-slip doormat?
- Are emergency phone numbers clearly posted?
- Can the person control water temperature?
- Do electrical outlets have childproof covers or plates?
- Where are the smoke detectors? Are they working?
- Are rooms and hallways well lighted?
- Can the person turn indoor and outdoor lighting on and off?
- Can the person exit the home in an emergency?
- Is oxygen used? Are safety measures for oxygen in place?
- Can the person reach the phone, TV, radio, and lights in bed?
- Are space heaters used? Are safety measures in place?
- Does the person have good judgment for cooking and stove use?
- Is there a safe play area for children?
- Can the person safely dispose of blood, body fluids, secretions, and excretions?
- Is there a pest-free method of trash storage?

Modified from Hoeman SP: *Rehabilitation nursing: process, application, and outcomes*, ed 4, St Louis, 2007, Mosby.

QUALITY OF LIFE

Successful rehabilitation and restorative care improves quality of life. The goal is independence to the greatest extent possible. A hopeful and winning outlook is needed. The more the person can do alone, the better his or her quality of life. To promote quality of life:

* Protect the right to privacy.
* Encourage personal choice.
* Protect the right to be free from abuse and mistreatment.
* Learn to deal with your anger and frustration.
* Encourage activities.
* Provide a safe setting.
* Show patience, understanding, and sensitivity.
  See *Focus on PRIDE: The Person, Family, and Yourself.*

FOCUS ON PRIDE

The Person, Family, and Yourself

Personal and Professional Responsibility

Some agencies have opportunities for nursing assistants to advance to restorative aides. In some states, special training is needed for certification. Such training teaches the knowledge and skills needed to assist with rehabilitation.

Often nursing assistants are promoted to restorative aide positions. Professional behaviors are highly valued when considering persons to promote. Restorative aides require patience, kindness, and good communication skills. Persons with a positive attitude, good work ethic, and excellent job performance are considered first.

Becoming a restorative aide is one rewarding option to advance as a nursing assistant. Seek out learning opportunities and practice positive work habits. Take pride in continuing to learn, improve, and grow as a nursing assistant.

Rights and Respect

Rehabilitation is challenging for the person, the family, and the nursing staff. No matter how difficult the situation, the person's rights must be protected.

Right to privacy—The person re-learns old skills or practices new skills in private. No one needs to watch. They do not need to see mistakes, falls, spills, or clumsiness. Nor do they need to see anger or tears. Privacy protects dignity and promotes self-respect.

Right to be free from abuse and mistreatment—Improvement may not be seen for weeks. Learning to use self-help devices and re-learning how to speak and dress take time. Simple things are often very hard to do. Repeated explanations and demonstrations may have no or little results. You, other staff, or the family may become upset and short-tempered. Protect the person from abuse and mistreatment. No one can shout at, scream at, yell at, or call the person names. They cannot hit or strike the person. Unkind remarks are not allowed. Report signs of abuse or mistreatment to the nurse.

Right to a safe setting—The setting must meet the person's needs. Needed changes are made. The overbed table, bedside stand, signal light, and other needed items are moved to the person's strong side. If unable to use the signal light, another form of communication is used. The rehabilitation team suggests these and other changes. They explain the need and purpose to the person and family.

Independence and Social Interaction

The more the person can do for himself or herself, the better his or her quality of life. Independence to the greatest extent possible is the goal of rehabilitation and restorative care. To promote independence:

* Focus on what the person can do. Stress the person's abilities and strengths. Do not show pity or sympathy.
* Encourage activities. Let the person do what interests him or her. The person usually chooses activities that he or she can do.
* Remain patient. Avoid rushing the person.
* Resist the urge to do things for the person that he or she can do. This hinders the person's ability to regain function. Remind the family to resist as well.
* Offer encouragement and support. The person may worry about how others view the disability. Remind the person that others have disabilities. They can give support and understanding. Persons who are sad and depressed may rely on others and not try to improve. Encourage them. Have a caring and positive attitude. This can help motivate them.
* Have the person use self-help devices as needed.
* Encourage personal choice. Not being able to control body movements or functions is very frustrating. Personal choice gives the person control.

Delegation and Teamwork

Disability affects the whole person. Many emotions are felt. Anger and frustration are common. Many are upset and discouraged. Some persons have trouble controlling such feelings. They may have outbursts.

You may feel short-tempered. You must learn to deal with your anger and frustration. The person does not choose loss of function. If the process upsets you, think how the person must feel. You must show patience, understanding, sensitivity, and respect. You must be calm and act in a professional manner. Control your words and actions. And give the person support and encouragement.

Managing your feelings can be a challenge. Rely on the nursing team for support. Share your feelings with the nurse. The nurse can suggest ways to help you control or express your feelings. You may need to assist with other persons for a while. Take pride in being a part of a strong, supportive team.

Ethics and Laws

The person may not want to practice rehabilitation procedures or methods. He or she may want you to provide care instead. Personal choice is important. However, the person needs to follow the rehabilitation plan. Otherwise, he or she will not make progress. Do not let the person control you. Letting the person control you is the wrong thing to do. Report any problems to the nurse.

REVIEW QUESTIONS

Circle the BEST answer.

1 Rehabilitation and restorative nursing care focus on
  a What the person cannot do
  b Self-care
  c The whole person
  d The person's rights

2 Rehabilitation begins with preventing
  a Angry feelings
  b Contractures and pressure ulcers
  c Illness and injury
  d Loss of self-esteem

3 A person has weakness on the right side. ADL are
  a Done by the person to the extent possible
  b Done by you
  c Postponed until the right side can be used
  d Supervised by a therapist

4 Persons with disabilities are likely to feel the following *except*
  a Undesirable
  b Angry and hostile
  c Depressed
  d Relief

5 During a therapy, a person wants music played. You should
  a Explain that music is not allowed
  b Choose some music
  c Ask the person to choose some music
  d Ask a therapist to choose some music

6 A person's right side is weak. You move the signal light to the left side. You have promoted quality of life by
  a Protecting the person from abuse and mistreatment
  b Allowing personal choice
  c Providing for safety
  d Taking part in activities

Circle T if the statement is TRUE and F if it is FALSE.

7 T F You should give praise for even slight progress.

8 T F Speech therapy should be done in private.

9 T F A person is not allowed dessert until exercises are done. This is abuse and mistreatment.

10 T F A person refuses to attend a concert at the nursing center. The person must attend. It is part of the rehabilitation plan.

11 T F Rehabilitation for older persons is usually slower paced than for younger persons.

12 T F You need to stress what the person can do.

13 T F Sympathy and pity help the person adjust.

14 T F You should know how to apply self-help devices.

15 T F You should know how to use the person's care equipment.

16 T F You need to convey hopefulness to the person.

Answers to these questions are on p. 834.

Hearing, Speech, and Vision Problems

39

OBJECTIVES

- Define the key terms and key abbreviations listed in this chapter.
- Describe the common ear disorders.
- Describe how to communicate with persons who have hearing loss.
- Explain the purpose of a hearing aid.
- Describe how to care for hearing aids.
- Describe the common speech disorders.
- Explain how to communicate with speech-impaired persons.

- Describe the common eye disorders.
- Explain how to assist persons who are visually impaired or blind.
- Explain how to protect an ocular prosthesis from loss or damage.
- Perform the procedure described in this chapter.
- Explain how to promote PRIDE in the person, the family, and yourself.

KEY TERMS

aphasia The total or partial loss *(a)* of the ability to use or understand language *(phasia);* a language disorder resulting from damage to parts of the brain responsible for language

blindness The absence of sight

braille A touch reading and writing system that uses raised dots for each letter of the alphabet; the first 10 letters also represent the numbers 0 through 9

Broca's aphasia See "expressive aphasia"

cerumen Earwax

deafness Hearing loss in which it is impossible for the person to understand speech through hearing alone

expressive aphasia Difficulty expressing or sending out thoughts; motor aphasia, Broca's aphasia

expressive-receptive aphasia Difficulty expressing or sending out thoughts and difficulty understanding language; global aphasia, mixed aphasia

global aphasia See "expressive-receptive aphasia"

hearing loss Not being able to hear the normal range of sounds associated with normal hearing

low vision Eyesight that cannot be corrected with eyeglasses, contact lenses, drugs, or surgery

mixed aphasia See "expressive-receptive aphasia"

motor aphasia See "expressive aphasia"

receptive aphasia Difficulty understanding language; Wernicke's aphasia

tinnitus A ringing, roaring, hissing, or buzzing sound in the ears or head

vertigo Dizziness

Wernicke's aphasia See "receptive aphasia"

KEY ABBREVIATIONS

AMD	Age-related macular degeneration	**ASL**	American Sign Language

Hearing, speech, and vision allow communication, learning, and moving about. They are important for self-care, work, and most activities. They also are important for safety and security needs. For example, you see dark clouds and hear tornado warning sirens. You know to seek shelter. With speech, you can alert others.

Many people have some degree of hearing or vision loss. Common causes are birth defects, accidents, infections, diseases, and aging.

BODY STRUCTURE AND FUNCTION REVIEW: THE EAR

The *ear* is a sense organ (Fig. 39-1). It functions in hearing and balance. It has three parts: the *external ear, middle ear,* and *inner ear.*

The external ear (outer part) is called the *pinna* or *auricle.* Sound waves are guided through the external ear into the *auditory canal.* Glands in the auditory canal secrete a waxy substance called *cerumen.* The auditory canal extends about 1 inch to the *eardrum.* The eardrum *(tympanic membrane)* separates the external and middle ear.

The middle ear is a small space. It contains the *eustachian tube* and three small bones called *ossicles.* The eustachian tube connects the middle ear and the throat. Air enters the eustachian tube so that there is equal pressure on both sides of the eardrum.

The ossicles amplify sound received from the eardrum and transmit the sound to the inner ear. The three ossicles are:

- The *malleus.* It looks like a hammer.
- The *incus.* It looks like an anvil.
- The *stapes.* It is shaped like a stirrup.

The inner ear consists of *semicircular canals* and the *cochlea.* The cochlea looks like a snail shell. It contains fluid. The fluid carries sound waves from the middle ear to the *acoustic nerve.* The acoustic nerve then carries the message to the brain.

The three semicircular canals are involved with balance. They sense the head's position and changes in position. They send messages to the brain.

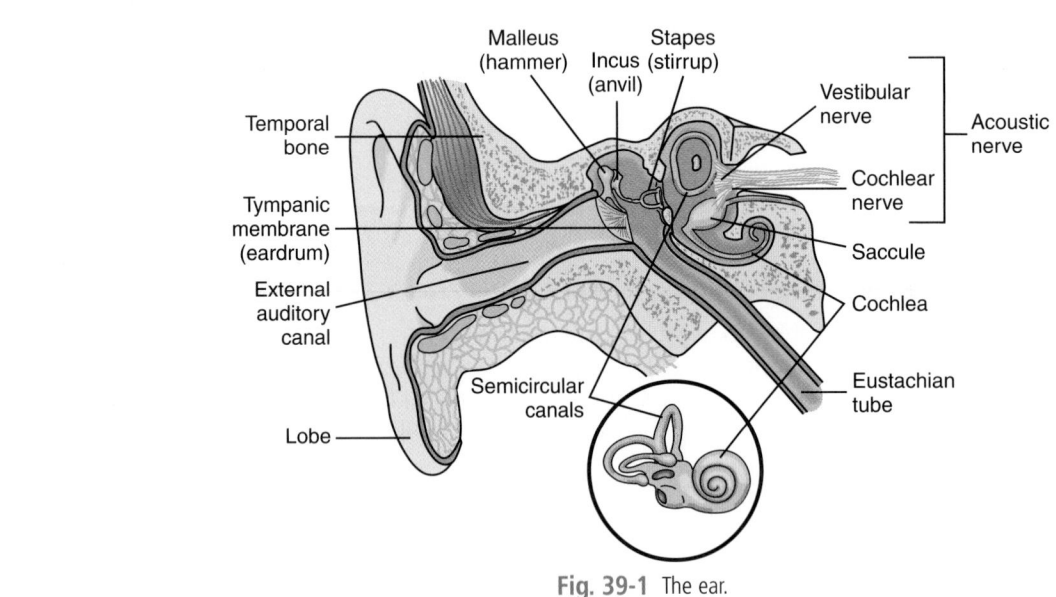

Fig. 39-1 The ear.

EAR DISORDERS

The ear functions in hearing and balance.

See *Body Structure and Function Review: The Ear.*

Otitis Media

Otitis media is infection *(itis)* of the middle *(media)* ear *(ot).* It often begins with infections that cause sore throats, colds, or other respiratory infections that spread to the middle ear. Viruses and bacteria are causes.

Otitis media is acute or chronic. Chronic otitis media can damage the tympanic membrane (eardrum) or the ossicles (see Fig. 39-1). The structures are needed for hearing. Permanent hearing loss can occur.

Fluid builds up in the ear. Pain (earache) and hearing loss occur. So do fever and tinnitus. *Tinnitus is a ringing, roaring, hissing, or buzzing sound in the ears or head.* An untreated infection can travel to the brain and other structures in the head. The doctor orders antibiotics, drugs for pain relief, or drugs to relieve congestion.

See *Focus on Children and Older Persons: Otitis Media.*

Meniere's Disease

Meniere's disease involves the inner ear. It is a common cause of hearing loss. Usually one ear is affected. Symptoms include:
- *Vertigo* (dizziness)
- Tinnitus
- Hearing loss
- Pain or pressure in the affected ear

With Meniere's disease, there is increased fluid in the inner ear. The increased fluid causes swelling and pressure in the inner ear. Symptoms are sudden. They can occur daily or just once a year. An attack can last several hours.

An attack usually involves vertigo, tinnitus, and hearing loss. Vertigo causes whirling and spinning sensations. The dizziness causes severe nausea and vomiting.

Drugs, fluid restriction, a low-salt diet, and no alcohol or caffeine decrease fluid in the inner ear. Safety is needed during vertigo. The person must lie down. Falls are prevented. Bed rails are used according to the care plan. The person's head is kept still. The person avoids turning the head. To talk to the person, stand directly in front of him or her. When movement is necessary, the person moves slowly. Sudden movements are avoided. So are bright or glaring lights. Assist with walking. The person should not walk alone in case vertigo occurs.

Hearing Loss

Hearing loss is not being able to hear the normal range of sounds associated with normal hearing. Losses are mild to severe. Deafness is the most severe form. *Deafness is hearing loss in which it is impossible for the person to understand speech through hearing alone.*

Hearing loss occurs in all age-groups. According to the National Institute on Deafness and Other Communication Disorders (NIDCD), about one third (33%) of persons over 60 years of age have hearing problems. About half (50%) of persons age 85 years and older have hearing loss. Hearing loss is more common in men than in women.

Common causes of hearing loss are:
- Damage to the outer, middle, or inner ear
- Damage to the acoustic nerve
  Risk factors that can damage ear structures include:
- Aging
- Exposure to very loud sounds and noises—job-related noises, loud music, loud engines from vehicles, firearms
- Drugs—antibiotics, too much aspirin
- Infections
- Reduced blood flow to the ear caused by high blood pressure, heart and vascular diseases, and diabetes
- Stroke
- Head injuries
- Tumors
- Heredity
- Birth defects

Temporary hearing loss can occur from *earwax (cerumen)*. Hearing improves after the earwax is removed.

Clear speech, responding to others, safety, and awareness of surroundings require hearing. Many people deny hearing problems. They relate hearing loss to aging.

See *Focus on Communication: Hearing Loss.*
See *Promoting Safety and Comfort: Hearing Loss.*

Effects on the Person. A person may not notice gradual hearing loss. Others may see changes in the person's behavior or attitude. They may not relate the changes to hearing loss. Obvious signs and symptoms of hearing loss in children and adults include:

- Speaking too loudly
- Leaning forward to hear
- Turning and cupping the better ear toward the speaker
- Answering questions or responding inappropriately
- Asking for words to be repeated
- Asking others to speak louder or to speak more slowly and clearly
- Having trouble hearing over the phone
- Problems following conversations when two or more people are talking
- Turning up the TV, radio, or music volume so loud that others complain
- Thinking that others are mumbling or slurring words
- Having problems understanding women and children

Psychological and social changes are less obvious. People may give wrong answers or responses. Therefore they tend to shun social events to avoid embarrassment. Often they feel lonely, bored, and left out. Only parts of conversations are heard. They may become suspicious. They think others are talking about them or are talking softly on purpose. Some control conversations to avoid responding or being labeled "senile" because of poor answers. Straining and working hard to hear can cause fatigue, frustration, and irritability.

Hearing is needed for speech. Pronouncing words and voice volume depend on how you hear yourself. Hearing loss may result in slurred speech. Words may be pronounced wrong. Some people have monotone speech or drop word endings. It may be hard to understand what the person says. Do not assume or pretend that you understand what the person says. Otherwise serious problems can result. See "Speech Disorders" on p. 655.

See *Focus on Children and Older Persons: Effects on the Person.*

FOCUS ON CHILDREN AND OLDER PERSONS
Effects on the Person

Children
Some babies are born with hearing problems. Others develop hearing problems as they grow older. Hearing is needed for language development. Children learn to talk by imitating sounds and voices.

Medical attention is needed if a child does not hear well or speak clearly. See Box 39-1 for a hearing checklist for children. Items checked "No" may signal hearing loss. Report concerns about a child's hearing to the nurse.

BOX 39-1	**HEARING CHECKLIST FOR CHILDREN**

Items marked "No" may signal hearing loss.

Yes	No	**Birth to 3 Months**
—	—	Reacts to loud sounds.
—	—	Calms down or smiles when spoken to.
—	—	Recognizes your voice and calms down if crying.
—	—	When feeding, starts or stops sucking in response to sound.
—	—	Coos and makes pleasure sounds.
—	—	Has a special way of crying for different needs.
—	—	Smiles when he or she sees you.
		4 to 6 Months
—	—	Follows sounds with his or her eyes.
—	—	Responds to changes in the tone of your voice.
—	—	Notices toys that make sounds.
—	—	Pays attention to music.
—	—	Babbles in a speech-like way and uses many different sounds, including sounds that begin with p, b, and m.
—	—	Laughs.
—	—	Babbles when excited or unhappy.
—	—	Makes gurgling sounds when alone or playing with you.
		7 Months to 1 Year
—	—	Enjoys playing peek-a-boo and pat-a-cake.
—	—	Turns and looks in the direction of sounds.
—	—	Listens when spoken to.
—	—	Understands words for common items such as "cup," "shoe," or "juice."
—	—	Responds to requests ("Come here" or "Want more?").
—	—	Babbles using long and short groups of sounds ("tata, upup, bibibi").
—	—	Babbles to get and keep attention.
—	—	Communicates using gestures such as waving or holding up arms.
—	—	Imitates different speech sounds.
—	—	Has one or two words ("Hi," "dog," "Dada," or "Mama") by first birthday.

Modified from National Institute on Deafness and Other Communication Disorders: *Your baby's hearing and communicative development checklist,* NIH Publication No. 10-4040, updated September, 2011, Bethesda, Md.

BOX 39-1	HEARING CHECKLIST FOR CHILDREN—cont'd

Yes	No	**1 to 2 Years**
—	—	Knows a few parts of the body and can point to them when asked.
—	—	Follows simple commands ("Roll the ball") and understands simple questions ("Where's your shoe?").
—	—	Enjoys simple stories, songs, and rhymes.
—	—	Points to pictures, when named, in books.
—	—	Acquires new words on a regular basis.
—	—	Uses some one- or two-word questions ("Where kitty?" or "Go bye-bye?").
—	—	Puts two words together ("More cookie" or "No juice").
—	—	Uses many different consonant sounds at the beginning of words.
		2 to 3 Years
—	—	Has a word for almost everything.
—	—	Uses two- or three-word phrases to talk about and ask for things.
—	—	Uses k, g, f, t, d, and n sounds.
—	—	Speaks in a way that is understood by family members and friends.
—	—	Names objects to ask for them or to direct attention to them.
		3 to 4 Years
—	—	Hears you when you call from another room.
—	—	Hears the television or radio at the same sound level as other family members.
—	—	Answers simple "Who?" "What?" "Where?" and "Why?" questions.
—	—	Talks about activities at daycare, preschool, or friends' homes.
—	—	Uses sentences with four or more words.
—	—	Speaks easily without having to repeat syllables or words.
		4 to 5 Years
—	—	Pays attention to a short story and answers simple questions about it.
—	—	Hears and understands most of what is said at home and in school.
—	—	Uses sentences that give many details.
—	—	Tells stories that stay on topic.
—	—	Communicates easily with other children and adults.
—	—	Says most sounds correctly except for a few (l, s, r, v, z, ch, sh, and th).
—	—	Uses rhyming words.
—	—	Names some letters and numbers.
—	—	Uses adult grammar.

Communication. Persons with hearing loss may wear hearing aids or lip-read (speech-read). They watch facial expressions, gestures, and body language. Some people learn American Sign Language (ASL) (Figs. 39-2 and 39-3, p. 654). ASL uses signs made with the hands and other movements such as facial expressions, gestures, and postures. To promote communication, practice the measures in Box 39-2, p. 655. (Different sign languages are used in different countries and regions. For example, British Sign Language is different from ASL.)

Some people have *hearing assistance dogs* (hearing dogs). The dog alerts the person to sounds. Phones, doorbells, smoke detectors, alarm clocks, sirens, and on-coming cars are examples.

Hearing Aids. *Hearing aids* fit inside or behind the ear (Fig. 39-4, p. 655). They make sounds louder. They do not correct, restore, or cure hearing problems. Hearing ability does not improve. The person hears better because the device makes sounds louder. Background noise and speech are louder. The measures in Box 39-2 apply.

Hearing aids are battery-operated. If the device does not seem to work properly:

- Check if the hearing aid is *on*. It has an *on* and *off* switch.
- Check the battery position.
- Insert a new battery if needed.
- Clean the hearing aid. *Follow the nurse's directions and the manufacturer's instructions.*

Hearing aids are turned off when not in use. And the battery is removed. These measures prolong battery life. The person should not use hair spray or other hair care products while wearing a hearing aid. They can damage the device.

Hearing aids are costly. Handle and care for them properly. When not in the ear, store a hearing aid in its case. Place the case in the top drawer of the bedside stand. Report lost or damaged hearing aids to the nurse at once.

Other Hearing Devices. Other devices can help the person with hearing loss.

- *Telephone amplifying devices.* Special telephone receivers make sounds louder. Some phones work with hearing aids.
- *TV and radio listening systems.* These are used with or without hearing aids. The person does not have to turn the volume up high.

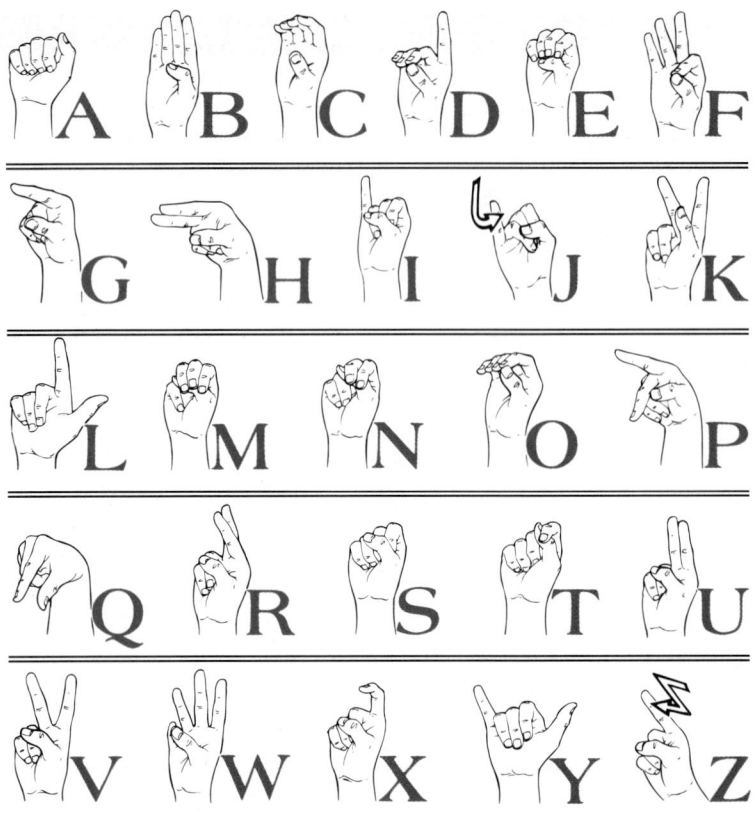

Fig. 39-2 Manual alphabet.

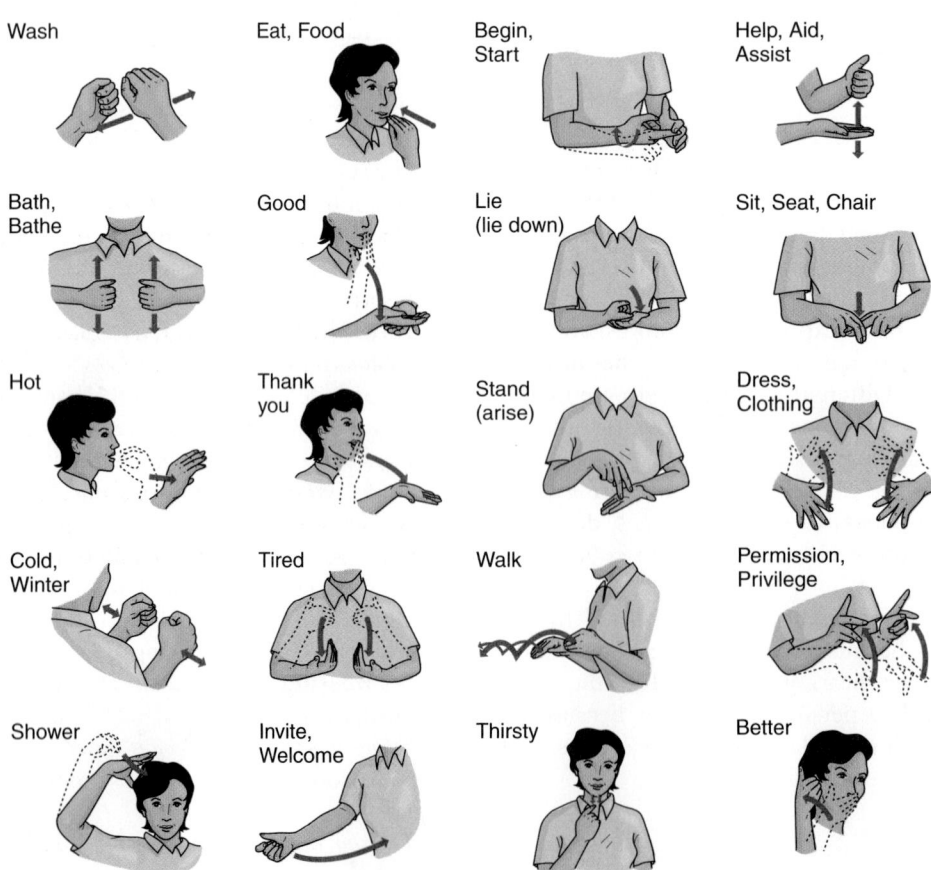

Fig. 39-3 American Sign Language examples.

The Environment
- Reduce or eliminate background noises. Turn off radios, stereos, music players, TVs, air conditioners, fans, and so on.
- Provide a quiet place to talk.
- Have the person sit in small groups or where he or she hears best.

The Person
- Have the person wear his or her hearing aid. It must be turned on and working.
- Have the person wear needed eyeglasses or contact lenses. The person needs to see your face to lip-read (speech-read).

You
- Gain attention. Alert the person to your presence. Raise an arm or hand, or lightly touch the person's arm. Do not startle or approach the person from behind.
- Position yourself at the person's level. Sit if the person is sitting. Stand if the person is standing.
- Face the person when speaking. Do not turn or walk away while you are talking. Do not talk to the person from the doorway or another room.
- Stand or sit in good light. Shadows and glares affect the person's ability to see your face clearly.
- Speak clearly, distinctly, and slowly.

You—cont'd
- Speak in a normal tone of voice. Do not shout.
- Adjust the pitch of your voice as needed. Ask if the person can hear you better:
  - If the person does not wear a hearing aid, lower the pitch if you are a female. Women's voices are higher-pitched and harder to hear than lower-pitched male voices.
  - If the person wears a hearing aid, raise the pitch slightly.
- Do not cover your mouth, smoke, eat, or chew gum while talking. Mouth movements are affected.
- Keep your hands away from your face. The person needs to see your face clearly.
- Stand or sit on the side of the better ear.
- State the topic of conversation first.
- Tell the person when you are changing the subject. State the new subject of conversation.
- Use short sentences and simple words.
- Use gestures and facial expressions to give useful clues.
- Write out important names and words.
- Say things in another way if the person does not seem to understand.
- Keep conversations and discussions short. This avoids tiring the person.
- Repeat and re-phrase statements as needed.
- Be alert to messages sent by your facial expressions, gestures, and body language.

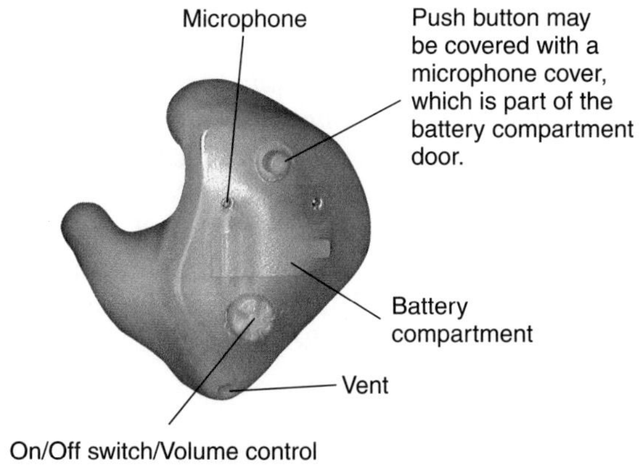

Fig. 39-4 A hearing aid.

SPEECH DISORDERS

Speech is used for communication. Speech disorders result in impaired or ineffective oral communication. Hearing loss, developmental disabilities (Chapter 47), and brain injury are common causes. These problems are common:
- *Aphasia*. See "Aphasia" on p. 656.
- *Apraxia* means not *(a)* to act, do, or perform *(praxia)*. The person with *apraxia of speech* cannot use the speech muscles for understandable speech. The person understands speech and knows what to say. However, the brain cannot coordinate the speech muscles to make the words. The motor speech area in the brain is damaged.
- *Dysarthria* means difficult or poor *(dys)* speech *(arthria)*. It is caused by nervous system damage. Mouth and face muscles are affected. Slurred speech, speaking slowly or softly, hoarseness, and drooling also can occur.

To communicate with the speech-impaired person, practice the measures in Box 39-3, p. 656.

BOX 39-3	MEASURES TO COMMUNICATE WITH THE SPEECH-IMPAIRED PERSON

The Person
- Ask the person to repeat or re-phrase statements as needed.
- Repeat what the person has said. Ask if you understood correctly.
- Ask the person to write down key words or the message.
- Ask the person to point, gesture, or draw key words.

You
- Follow the care plan. A consistent approach is needed.
- Provide a calm, quiet setting. Turn off the TV, radio, music, and other distractions.
- Include the person in conversations.
- Listen, and give the person your full attention.

You—cont'd
- Use short, simple sentences.
- Repeat what you are saying as needed.
- Write down key words as needed.
- Speak in a normal, adult tone. Do not treat or talk to an adult in a babyish or child-like way.
- Ask the person questions to which you know the answers. This helps you learn how the person speaks.
- Allow the person plenty of time to talk.
- Determine the topic being discussed. This helps you understand main points. Watch the person's lip movements.
- Watch facial expressions, gestures, and body language. They give clues about what is being said.
- Do not correct the person's speech.

Some persons need speech rehabilitation. The goal is to improve the ability to communicate. A speech/language pathologist and other health team members help the person:
- Improve affected language skills.
- Use remaining abilities.
- Restore language abilities to the extent possible.
- Learn other methods of communicating.
- Strengthen the muscles of speech.

The amount of improvement possible depends on many factors. They include the cause, amount, and area of brain damage and age and health. Willingness and ability to learn are other factors.

Aphasia

Aphasia is the total or partial loss (a) *of the ability to use or understand language* (phasia). *Aphasia is a language disorder. Parts of the brain responsible for language are damaged.* Stroke, head injury, brain infections, and cancer are common causes. Most people who have aphasia are middle-aged adults and older.

Expressive aphasia (motor aphasia, Broca's aphasia) relates to difficulty expressing or sending out thoughts. Thinking is clear. The person knows what to say but has difficulty or cannot speak the words. There are problems speaking, spelling, counting, gesturing, or writing. The person may:
- Omit small words such as "is," "and," "of," and "the."
- Speak in single words or short sentences. "Walk dog" can mean "I will take the dog for a walk" or "You take the dog for a walk."
- Put words in the wrong order. Instead of "bathroom," the person may say "room bath."
- Think one thing but say another. The person may want food but asks for a book.
- Call people by the wrong names.
- Make up words.
- Produce sounds and no words.
- Cry or swear for no reason.

Receptive aphasia (Wernicke's aphasia) is difficulty understanding language. The person has trouble understanding what is said or read. The person may speak in long sentences that have no meaning. Because of difficulty understanding speech, the person may not be aware of his or her mistakes. People and common objects are not recognized. The person may not know how to use a fork, toilet, cup, TV, phone, or other items.

Some people have both expressive and receptive aphasia. *Expressive-receptive aphasia (global aphasia, mixed aphasia) involves difficulty expressing or sending out thoughts (expressive aphasia) and difficulty understanding language (receptive aphasia).* The person has problems speaking and understanding language.

The person has many emotional needs. Frustration, depression, and anger are common. Communication is needed to function and relate to others. The person wants to communicate but cannot. Be patient and kind.

EYE DISORDERS

Vision loss occurs at all ages. Problems range from mild loss to complete blindness. *Blindness is the absence of sight.* Vision loss is sudden or gradual. One or both eyes are affected.

See *Body Structure and Function Review: The Eye.*

BODY STRUCTURE AND FUNCTION REVIEW: THE EYE

Receptors for vision are in the *eyes* (Fig. 39-5). Bones of the skull, eyelids and eyelashes, and tears protect the eyes from injury. The eye has three layers:

* The *sclera,* the white of the eye, is the outer layer. It is made of tough connective tissue.
* The *choroid* is the second layer. Blood vessels, the *ciliary muscle,* and the *iris* make up the choroid. The iris gives the eye its color. The opening in the middle of the iris is the *pupil.* Pupil size varies with the amount of light entering the eye. The pupil constricts (narrows) in bright light. It dilates (widens) in dim or dark places.
* The *retina* is the inner layer. It has receptors for vision and the nerve fibers of the *optic nerve.* The *macula* is near the center of the retina. This area contains cells that are sensitive to light, color, and fine detail needed for central vision (p. 659).

Light enters the eye through the *cornea.* It is the transparent part of the outer layer that lies over the eye. Light rays pass to the *lens,* which lies behind the pupil. The light is then reflected to the retina. Light is carried to the brain by the optic nerve.

The *aqueous chamber* separates the cornea from the lens. The chamber is filled with a fluid called *aqueous humor.* The fluid helps the cornea keep its shape and position. The *vitreous body* is behind the lens. It is a gelatin-like substance that supports the retina and maintains the eye's shape.

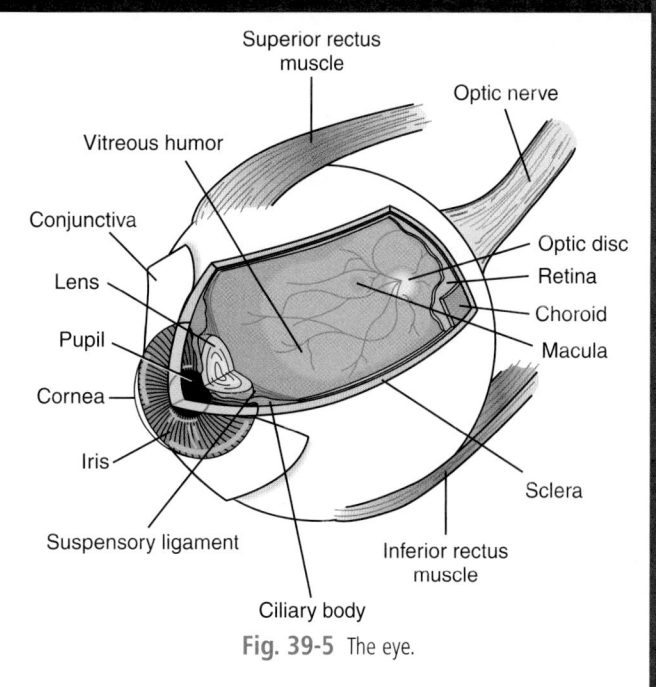

Fig. 39-5 The eye.

Cataracts

Cataract is a clouding of the lens (Fig. 39-6). The normal lens is clear. *Cataract* comes from the Greek word for *waterfall.* Trying to see is like looking through a waterfall. A cataract can occur in one or both eyes. Signs and symptoms include:

* Cloudy, blurry, or dimmed vision (Fig. 39-7).
* Colors seem faded. Blues and purples are hard to see.
* Sensitivity to light and glares.
* Poor vision at night.
* Halos around lights.
* Double vision in the affected eye.

Risk Factors. Most cataracts are caused by aging. A family history, diabetes, smoking, alcohol use, and prolonged exposure to sunlight are risk factors. So are high blood pressure, obesity, and eye injuries and surgeries.

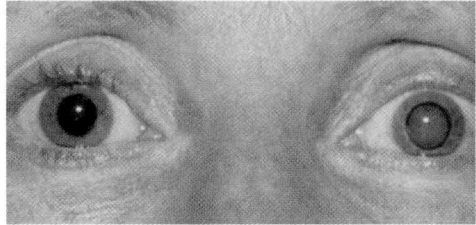

Fig. 39-6 One eye is normal. The other has a cataract.

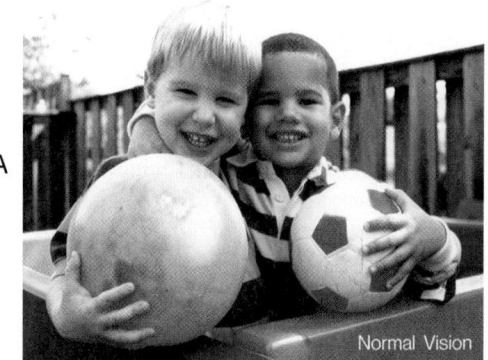

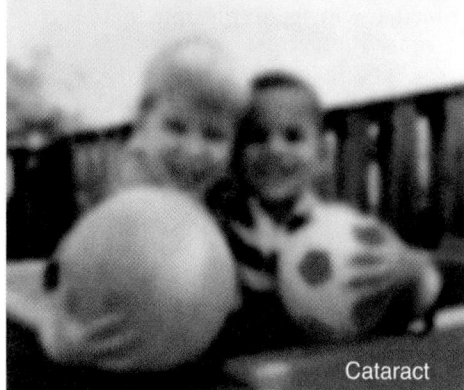

Fig. 39-7 Vision loss from a cataract. **A,** Normal vision. **B,** Scene viewed with a cataract.

Treatment. Surgery is the only treatment. The lens is removed, and a plastic lens is implanted. Surgery is done when the cataract starts to interfere with daily activities. Driving, reading, and watching TV are examples. Vision improves after surgery.

Post-operative care includes the following:

- Keep the eye shield in place as directed. The shield is worn for sleep, including naps.
- Follow measures for persons who are visually impaired or blind when an eye shield is worn (p. 660). The person may have vision loss in the other eye.
- Remind the person not to rub or press the affected eye.
- Do not bump the eye.
- Place the overbed table and the bedside stand on the un-operative side.
- Place the signal light within reach.
- Report eye drainage or complaints of pain at once.

Glaucoma

Glaucoma causes damage to the optic nerve. The eye produces a fluid that nourishes certain eye structures. The fluid normally drains from the eye. When the fluid cannot drain properly, it builds up in the eye causing pressure on the optic nerve. The optic nerve is damaged. Vision loss with eventual blindness occurs.

Glaucoma can occur in one or both eyes. Onset is sudden or gradual. Peripheral vision (side vision) is lost. The person sees through a tunnel (Fig. 39-8), has blurred vision, and sees halos around lights. Severe eye pain, nausea, and vomiting occur with sudden onset.

Risk Factors. Glaucoma is a leading cause of vision loss in the United States. Persons at risk include:

- African-Americans over 40 years of age
- Everyone over 60 years of age, especially Mexican-Americans
- Those with a family history of the disease

Treatment. Glaucoma has no cure. Prior damage cannot be reversed. Drugs and surgery can control glaucoma and prevent further damage to the optic nerve.

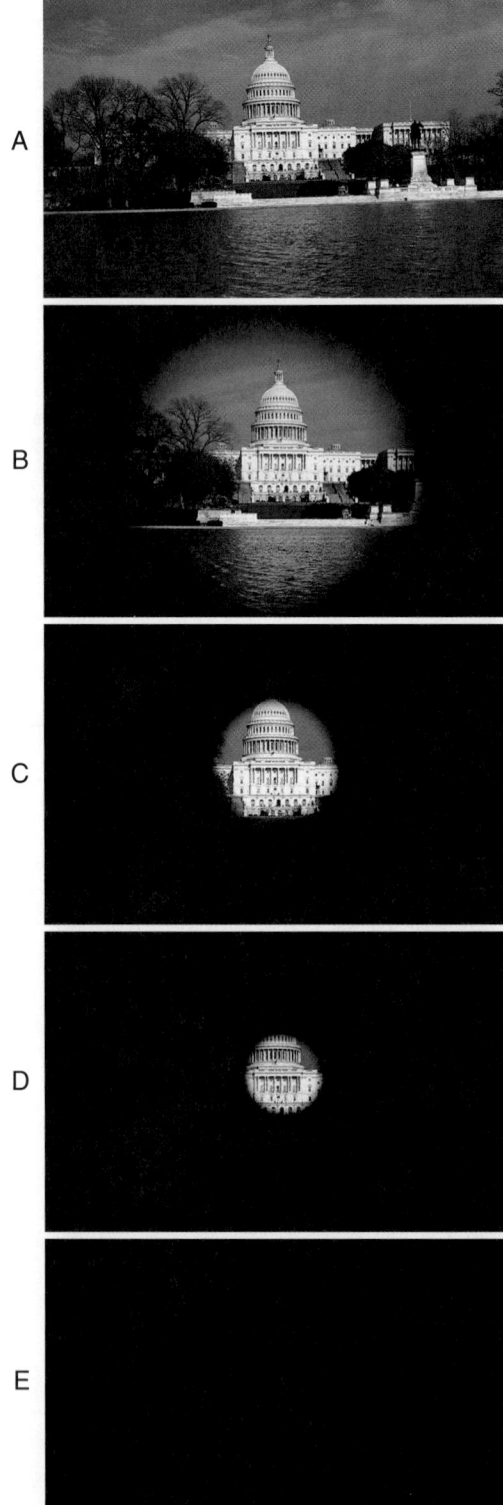

Fig. 39-8 Vision loss from glaucoma. **A,** Normal vision. **B,** Loss of peripheral vision begins. **C, D,** and **E,** Vision loss continues, with eventual blindness.

Diabetic Retinopathy

In diabetic retinopathy, the tiny blood vessels in the retina are damaged. A complication of diabetes, it is a leading cause of blindness. Usually both eyes are affected.

Vision blurs (Fig. 39-9). The person may see spots "floating." Often there are no early warning signs.

Risk Factors. Everyone with diabetes (Chapter 43) is at risk.

Treatment. The person needs to control diabetes, blood pressure, and blood cholesterol. Laser surgery may help. In another surgery, blood is removed from the center of the eye. The person may need low vision services.

Age-Related Macular Degeneration

Age-related macular degeneration (AMD) blurs central vision. *Central vision* is what you see "straight-ahead." AMD causes a blind spot in the center of vision (Fig. 39-10). Central vision is needed for reading, sewing, driving, and seeing faces and fine detail.

The disease damages the macula in the center of the retina. The retina receives light and sends messages to the brain through the optic nerve. Normal signals are not sent to the brain. Onset is gradual and painless. AMD is the leading cause of blindness in persons 60 years of age and older.

Risk Factors. AMD can occur during middle age. However, the risk increases with aging. Besides age, risk factors include:
* Smoking.
* Obesity.
* Race. Whites are at greater risk than any other group.
* Family history.
* Gender. Women are at greater risk than men.

Treatment. For advanced AMD, no treatment can prevent vision loss. Some treatments may stop or slow the disease progress. They may save what is left of central vision. Laser surgery is an example.

The following can reduce the risk of AMD:
* Eating a healthy diet high in green leafy vegetables and fish
* Not smoking
* Maintaining a normal blood pressure
* Maintaining a normal weight
* Exercising

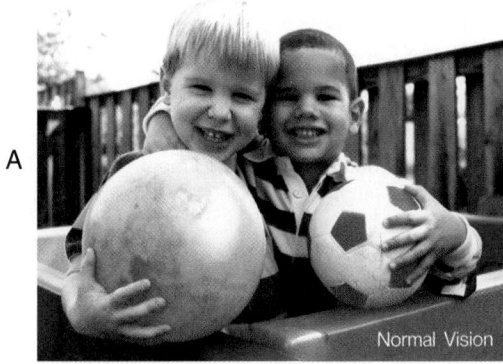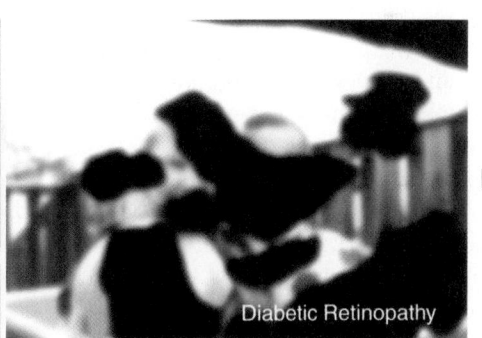

Fig. 39-9 Vision loss from diabetic retinopathy. **A,** Normal vision. **B,** Vision with diabetic retinopathy.

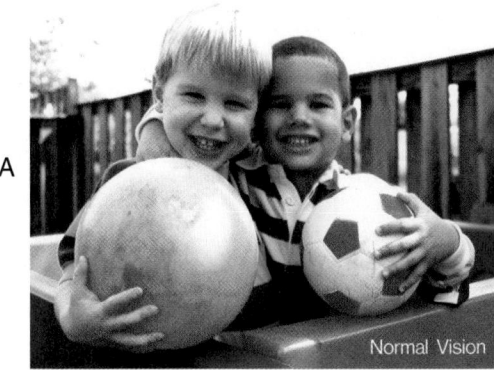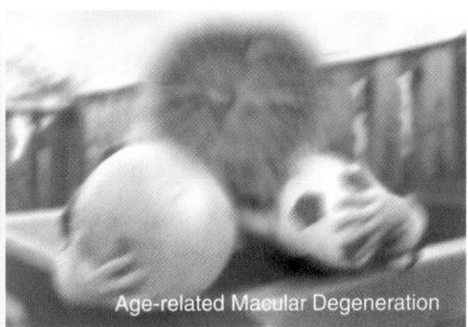

Fig. 39-10 Vision loss from macular degeneration. **A,** Normal vision. **B,** Central vision is blurred.

Low Vision

Low vision is eyesight that cannot be corrected with eyeglasses, contact lenses, drugs, or surgery. Reading, shopping, cooking, watching TV, writing, and other tasks are hard to do.

While wearing eyeglasses or contact lenses, the person has problems:

- Recognizing the faces of family and friends
- Doing tasks that require close vision—reading, cooking, sewing, and so on
- Picking out and matching the color of clothing
- Reading signs
- Doing things because lighting seems dimmer

Risk Factors. Persons at risk for low vision have:

- Eye diseases including glaucoma, cataracts, and AMD
- Diabetes
- Eye injuries
- Birth defects

Treatment. The person learns to use visual and adaptive devices. The devices used depend on the person's needs. Examples include:

- Prescription reading glasses
- Large-print reading materials
- Magnifying aids for close vision
- Telescopic aids for far vision
- A black felt-tip marker for writing
- Paper with bold lines for writing
- Audio tapes
- Electronic reading machines
- Computer systems using large print
- Computer systems that talk
- Closed-circuit TV
- Phones, clocks, and watches with large numbers
- Phones for people who have low vision, are visually impaired, or blind
- Lighting that can be adjusted
- Dark-colored light switches and electrical outlets against light-colored walls
- Motion lights that turn on when the person enters a room

Impaired Vision and Blindness

Birth defects, injuries, and eye diseases are among the causes of impaired vision and blindness. They also are complications of some diseases. Some people are totally blind. Others sense some light but have no usable vision. Others have some usable vision but cannot read newsprint. The legally blind person sees at 20 feet what a person with normal vision sees at 200 feet. See Box 39-4 for the signs and symptoms of vision problems.

Loss of sight is serious. Adjustments can be hard and long. Special education and training are needed. Moving about, performing daily tasks, reading and writing, communicating with others, and using a guide dog are among the tasks the person needs to learn. All are needed for quality of life. The person may need some of the devices used for low vision. When caring for blind or visually impaired persons, follow the practices in Box 39-5.

Rehabilitation programs help the person adjust to the vision loss and learn to be independent. The goal is for the person to be as active as possible and to have quality of life. The person learns to use visual and adaptive devices, braille, long canes, and dog guides.

See *Focus on Long-Term Care and Home Care: Impaired Vision and Blindness.*

FOCUS ON LONG-TERM CARE AND HOME CARE
Impaired Vision and Blindness

Home Care
The practices in Box 39-5 apply in the home setting. A safe setting is needed. Outdoor walks and stairs must be free of toys, ice, and snow. Furniture, closets, drawers, shelves, and other items are arranged to meet the person's needs. Always replace items where you found them. Do not re-arrange the person's belongings.

BOX 39-4	SIGNS AND SYMPTOMS OF VISION PROBLEMS

The Person Complains of:
- Halos or rings around lights
- Headaches with blurry vision
- Not being able to see at night
- Spots in front of the eyes
- Eyes hurting
- Seeing flashes of light
- Seeing double
- Things looking distorted
- Needing more light

You Observe the Person:
- Bumping into things
- Hesitating when moving
- Walking close to the wall

You Observe the Person—cont'd
- Groping for objects
- Touching things in an uncertain way
- Squinting to see
- Tilting the head to see
- Asking for more or different lighting
- Holding books, newspapers, and so on close to the face
- Dropping food when eating
- Having trouble making out faces
- Having trouble reading signs
- Not seeing stains on clothing
- Wearing clothes that do not match
- Acting disoriented or confused in strange settings
- Tripping on rugs

Modified from the American Foundation for the Blind.

BOX 39-5	CARING FOR BLIND AND VISUALLY IMPAIRED PERSONS

The Environment
- Report worn carpeting and other flooring.
- Keep furniture, equipment, and electrical cords out of areas where the person will walk.
- Keep chairs pushed in under the table or desk.
- Keep doors fully open or fully closed. This includes room, closet, and cabinet doors.
- Keep drawers fully closed.
- Report burnt out light bulbs.
- Provide lighting as the person prefers. Tell the person when the lights are on or off.
- Adjust window coverings to prevent glares. Sunny days and bright, snowy days cause glares.
- Keep the signal light and TV, light, and other controls within the person's reach.
- Turn on night-lights in the person's room and bathroom and in hallways.
- Practice safety measures to prevent falls (Chapter 13).
- Orient the person to the room. Describe the layout. Include the location and purpose of furniture and equipment.
- Let the person move about. Let him or her touch and find furniture and equipment.
- Do not re-arrange furniture and equipment.

The Environment—cont'd
- Provide a consistent meal time setting:
  - Avoid plates, napkins, placemats, and tablecloths with patterns and designs. Use solid colors and provide contrast. For example, place a white plate on a dark placemat or tablecloth.
  - Have the person sit in good light.
  - Keep place settings the same. The knife and spoon are to the right of the plate. The fork and napkin are to the left of the plate. The glass or cup is to the right of the plate if the person is right-handed. It is to the left of the plate if the person is left-handed.
  - Arrange main dishes, side dishes, seasonings, and condiments in a straight line or in a semi-circle just beyond the person's place setting. Arrange things in the same way for each meal.
  - Explain the location of food and beverages. Use the face of a clock (Chapter 24). Or guide the person's hand to each item on the tray or place setting.
  - Cut meat, open containers, butter bread, and perform other tasks as needed.
- Complete a safety check before leaving the room. (See the inside of the front book cover.)

Modified from American Foundation for the Blind.

Continued

BOX 39-5 CARING FOR BLIND AND VISUALLY IMPAIRED PERSONS—cont'd

The Person

- Have the person use railings when climbing stairs.
- Have the person wear comfortable shoes that fit correctly.
- Assist with walking as needed. Offer to guide the person. Ask if he or she would like help. Respect the person's answers. If your help is accepted:
  - Offer your arm. Tell the person which arm is offered. Tap the back of your hand against the person's hand.
  - Have the person hold on to your arm just above the elbow (Fig. 39-11). Do not grab the person's arm.
  - Walk at a normal pace. Walk one step ahead of the person. Stand next to the person at the top and bottom of stairs and when crossing streets.
  - Never push, pull, or guide the person in front of you.
  - Pause when changing direction, stepping up, and stepping down.
  - Tell the person about stairs, elevators, escalators, doors, turns, furniture, and other obstructions. State if steps are up or down.
  - Have the person hold on to a railing, the wall, or other strong surface if you need to leave his or her side. Tell the person that you are leaving and what to hold on to.
- Guide the person to a seat by placing your guiding arm on the seat. The person will move his or her hand down your arm to the seat.
- Let the person do as much for himself or herself as possible. Do not do things that the person can do. Cutting meat, seasoning food, getting dressed, and putting on shoes are examples.
- Provide visual and adaptive devices. Follow the care plan.

You

- Identify yourself when you enter the room. Give your name, title, and reason for being there. Do not touch the person until you have indicated your presence.
- Ask the person how much he or she can see. Do not assume the person is totally blind or that the person has some vision.
- Identify others. Explain where each person is located and what the person is doing.
- Offer to help. Simply say: "May I help you?" Respect the person's answer.
- Leave the person's belongings in the same place that you found them. Do not move or re-arrange things. If you have to move things, tell the person what you moved and where.

Communication

- Face the person when speaking. Speak slowly and clearly.
- Use a normal tone of voice. Do not shout or speak loudly. Vision loss does not mean the person has hearing loss.
- Address the person by name. This tells the person that you are directing a comment or question to him or her.
- Speak directly to the person. Do not just talk to family and friends who are present.
- Feel free to use words such as "see," "look," "read," or "watch TV." You also can use "blind" and "visually impaired."
- Feel free to refer to colors, sizes, shapes, patterns, designs, and so on.
- Describe people, places, and things thoroughly. Do not leave out a detail because you do not think it is important.
- Warn the person of dangers. Provide a calm and clear warning. You can say "wait" first. Then describe the danger. For example, "Wait, there is ice on the walk."
- Greet the person by name when he or she enters a room. This alerts the person to your presence in the room. Tell the person who you are. Also identify others in the room.
- Listen to the person. Give the person verbal cues that you are listening. Say "yes," "okay," "I see," "tell me more," "I don't understand," and so on.
- Answer the person's questions. Provide specific and descriptive responses.
- Give step-by-step explanations of procedures as you perform them. Say when the procedure is over.
- Give specific directions:
  - Say "right behind you," "on your left," or "in front of you." Avoid phrases like "over here" or "over there."
  - Tell the distance. For example, "Three steps in front of you" or "At the end of the hallway by the nurses' station."
  - Give landmarks if possible. Sounds and scents can serve as "landmarks." "By the kitchen" is an example.
- Tell the person when you are leaving the room or the area. If appropriate, tell the person where you are going. For example, "I'm going to go into your bathroom now."
- Tell the person when you are ending a conversation. For example, "I enjoyed hearing about your children. Thank you for sharing stories with me."

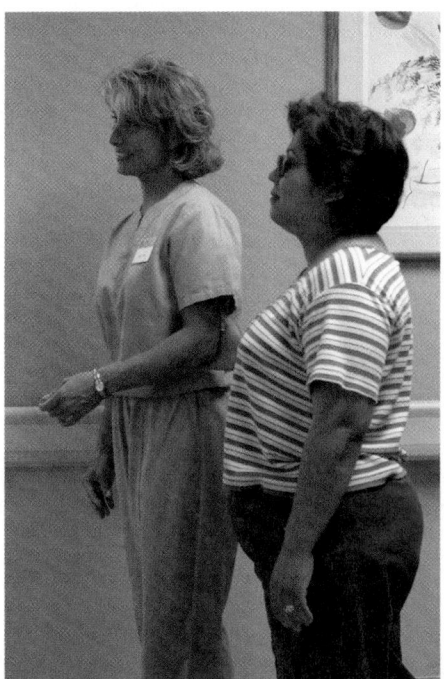

Fig. 39-11 The blind person walks slightly behind the nursing assistant. She touches the nursing assistant's arm lightly.

Braille. *Braille is a touch reading and writing system using raised dots for each letter of the alphabet* (Fig. 39-12). *The first 10 letters also represent the numbers 0 through 9.* Braille is read by moving the hands from left to right along each line of braille (Fig. 39-13).

Special devices allow computer access. A "braille display" sits on a desk. Using braille, the person reads information on the computer display. Braille printers allow printing computer information in braille. Braille keyboards also are available.

Mobility. Blind and visually impaired persons learn to move about using a long cane with a red tip or using a guide dog. Both are used worldwide.

- Long canes are white or silver-gray. Some are one piece. Others fold or collapse for storage. To assist a person, announce your presence first. Ask if you can assist before trying to help. Do not interfere with the arm holding the cane. The person stores the cane. If you store it, tell the person where to find the cane.

- The guide dog sees for the person. The dog moves in response to the master's commands. Commands are disobeyed to avoid danger. For example, the master wants to cross the street. The guide dog disobeys the command if a car is approaching. Do not pet, feed, or distract a guide dog. Such actions can place the person in danger.

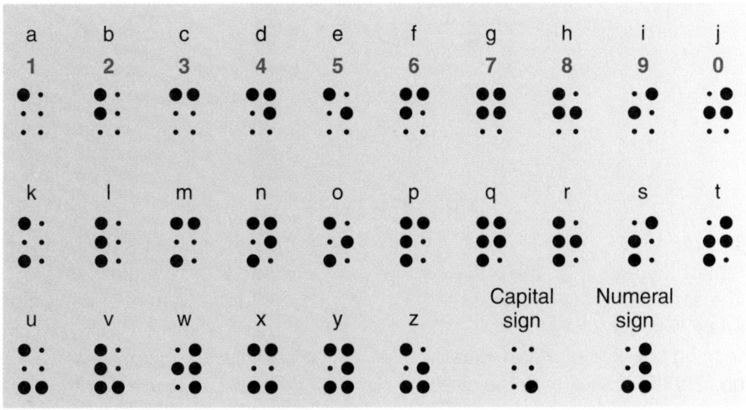

Fig. 39-12 Braille.

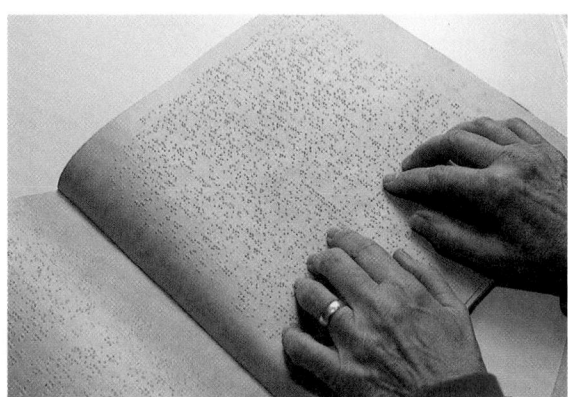

Fig. 39-13 Braille is read by moving the fingers left to right across the braille lines.

Corrective Lenses

Eyeglasses and contact lenses can correct many vision problems. Some people wear eyeglasses for reading or seeing at a distance. Others wear them for all activities. Contact lenses are usually worn while awake. Some contacts can be worn day and night for up to 30 days.

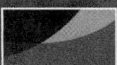 **Eyeglasses.** Lenses are hardened glass or plastic. Clean them daily and as needed. Wash glass lenses with warm water. Dry them with a lens cloth or cotton cloth. Plastic lenses scratch easily. Use special cleaning solutions and cloths.

See *Delegation Guidelines: Eyeglasses.*
See *Promoting Safety and Comfort: Eyeglasses.*

DELEGATION GUIDELINES
Eyeglasses

Cleaning eyeglasses is a routine care measure. Do not wait until the nurse tells you to clean them. Clean them daily and as needed.

To clean eyeglasses, find out if you need a special cleaning solution. Then follow the manufacturer's instructions.

PROMOTING SAFETY AND COMFORT
Eyeglasses

Safety
Eyeglasses are costly. Protect them from loss or damage. When not worn, put them in their case. Place the case in the top drawer of the bedside stand.

CARING FOR EYEGLASSES

QUALITY OF LIFE

Remember to:
- Knock before entering the person's room.
- Address the person by name.
- Introduce yourself by name and title.

- Explain the procedure to the person before beginning and during the procedure.
- Protect the person's rights during the procedure.
- Handle the person gently during the procedure.

PRE-PROCEDURE

1 Follow *Delegation Guidelines: Eyeglasses.* See *Promoting Safety and Comfort: Eyeglasses.*
2 Practice hand hygiene.

3 Collect the following:
- Eyeglass case
- Cleaning solution or warm water
- Disposable lens cloth or cotton cloth

PROCEDURE

4 Remove the eyeglasses.
   a Hold the frames in front of the ears (Fig. 39-14, A).
   b Lift the frames from the ears. Bring the eyeglasses down away from the face (Fig. 39-14, B).
5 Clean the lenses with cleaning solution or warm water. Clean in a circular motion. Dry the lenses with the cloth.
6 If the person will not wear the eyeglasses:
   a Open the eyeglass case.
   b Fold the glasses. Put them in the case. Do not touch the clean lenses.
   c Place the case in the top drawer of the bedside stand.

7 If the person wears the eyeglasses:
   a Unfold the eyeglasses.
   b Hold the frames at each side. Place them over the ears.
   c Adjust the eyeglasses so the nosepiece rests on the nose.
   d Return the case to the top drawer in the bedside stand.

POST-PROCEDURE

8 Provide for comfort. (See the inside of the front book cover.)
9 Place the signal light within reach.
10 Return the cleaning solution to its proper place.
11 Discard the disposable cloth.

12 Complete a safety check of the room. (See the inside of the front book cover.)
13 Practice hand hygiene.
14 Report and record your observations.

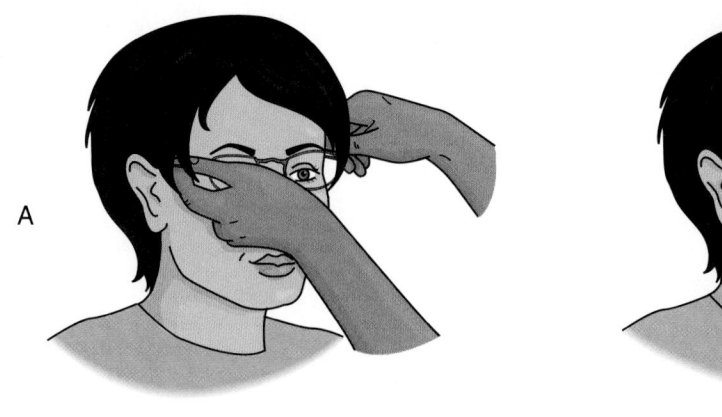
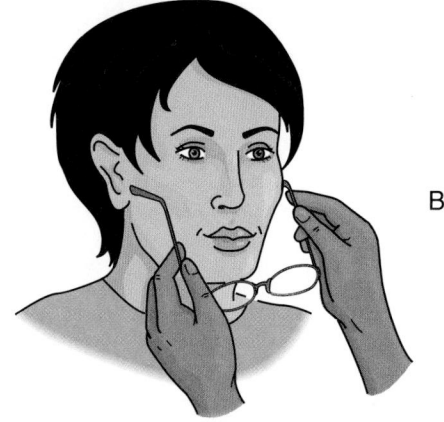

Fig. 39-14 Removing eyeglasses. **A,** Hold the frames in front of the ears. **B,** Lift the frames from the ears. Bring the glasses down away from the face.

> **PROMOTING SAFETY AND COMFORT**
> **Contact Lenses**
>
> **Safety**
> Some agencies let nursing assistants remove and insert contact lenses. Others do not. Know your agency's policy. If allowed to insert and remove contacts, follow agency procedures.

Contact Lenses

Contact lenses fit on the eye. There are hard and soft contacts. Disposable ones are discarded daily, weekly, or monthly. Contacts are cleaned, removed, and stored according to the manufacturer's instructions.

Report and record the following:
- Eye redness or irritation
- Eye drainage
- Complaints of eye pain, blurred or fuzzy vision, or uncomfortable lenses
  See *Promoting Safety and Comfort: Contact Lenses.*

Ocular Prostheses

Removal of an eyeball is sometimes done because of injury or disease. The person is fitted with an ocular (eye) prosthesis. See Figure 39-15, p. 666. This artificial eye does not provide vision. It matches the other eye in color and shape. The other eye may have normal, some, or no vision.

Some prostheses are permanent implants. Others are removable. If removable, the person is taught to remove, clean, and insert it. If the prosthesis is not inserted after removal:
- Wash it with mild soap and warm water. Rinse well.
- Line a container with a soft cloth or 4 × 4 gauze. This prevents scratches and damage.
- Fill the container with sterile water or saline (salt) solution.
- Place the eye in the container. Close the container.
- Label the container with the person's name and room and bed number.
- Place the labeled container in the top drawer of the bedside stand.
- Wash the eye socket with warm water or saline. Use a washcloth or gauze square. Remove excess moisture with a gauze square.
- Wash the eyelid and eyelashes with warm water. Clean from the inner to the outer aspect of the eye (Chapter 20). Dry the eyelid.
- Rinse the prosthesis with sterile water before the person inserts the eye.
  See *Promoting Safety and Comfort: Ocular Prostheses,* p. 666.

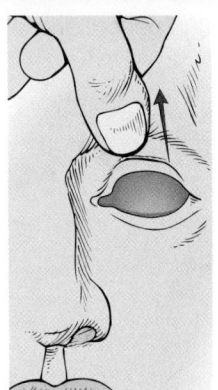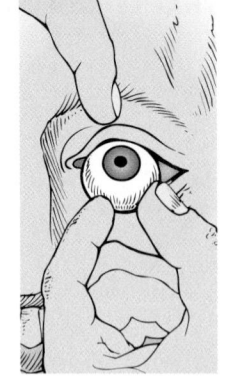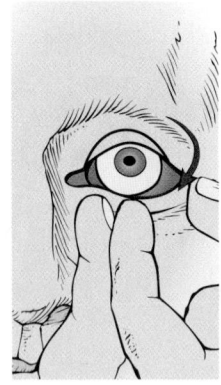

Fig. 39-15 An ocular prosthesis is inserted.

PROMOTING SAFETY AND COMFORT
Ocular Prostheses

Safety
When an ocular prosthesis is removed, you must prevent chips and scratches. It must not fall on the floor or other hard surface. Always hold the eye over a towel or other soft surface.

The prosthesis is the person's property. Protect it from loss or damage.

FOCUS ON PRIDE
The Person, Family, and Yourself

Personal and Professional Responsibility
Hearing aides, contact lenses, and glasses are common devices that improve hearing and vision. Such devices can be costly to repair or replace. Also the person will be without the device while it is fixed or replaced.

Always protect devices from loss or damage. Treat all of the person's belongings with care. If a device is lost or damaged, tell the nurse. Take pride in being a responsible and honest member of the nursing team.

Rights and Respect
Too often persons are defined by a disability. For example, you hear a person referred to as "the blind person" or "the deaf man." Or the person is treated like a child because others think that he or she cannot function.

Many persons with hearing, speech, and vision problems have overcome great challenges. They even take pride in how they have adapted. They deserve to be treated with dignity and respect. Do not pity the person. Treat the person like an adult, not like a child. Focus on the person's abilities, not disabilities.

When talking about the person, refer to the person first. Then state the person's disability if needed. For example, a nurse says: "Mrs. Jones needs a warm blanket. Please take one to her. She is blind, so knock and introduce yourself before entering her room. She will position the blanket as she prefers."

Independence and Social Interaction
Hearing, speech, and vision problems can interfere with quality of life. Adjusting is often long and hard. The person may show frustration and anger. Take time to listen. Be patient, understanding, and sensitive to the person's needs and feelings.

Focus on the person's abilities. Allow the person to be in control to the extent possible. This helps promote independence to improve quality of life.

Delegation and Teamwork
Communicating with persons with hearing problems can be difficult. You must adjust the setting and how you talk to the person. See Box 39-2. The health team must provide for the person's needs. Measures are included in the person's care plan. Using gestures, written notes, or an ASL interpreter are examples.

You must try to communicate with the person. Follow the care plan. These measures take time. Plan ahead. Do not be afraid to ask for help or advice. The nurse and other staff may have ideas for helping you communicate. Take pride in being a part of a supportive team that works together to meet the person's needs.

Ethics and Laws
The Americans with Disabilities Act (ADA) is a federal law. The law protects the rights of persons with disabilities. It includes persons with problems that limit hearing, speech, and vision. The ADA covers rights such as employment, access to public services and places, and the use of communication services.

Agencies comply with the ADA for persons with hearing, vision, and speech disabilities in many ways. Agencies often provide:

- Braille on signs for areas with public access. Offices, lobbies, restrooms, elevators, stairways, and cafeterias are examples.
- Communication devices for those with hearing and speech problems. For example, a device with a keyboard and small screen is connected to a phone line. The device is used instead of a phone.
- ASL interpreters. Some agencies have a person on staff or on call. Others use an outside agency.
- Information in a form the person can understand. Large print and braille are examples.

Know your agency's resources for persons with disabilities. Offer to help. If you are unsure how to help, ask the nurse. Take pride in helping others.

Circle the BEST answer.

1 A person with Meniere's disease has
  a A middle ear infection
  b Vertigo
  c A hearing aid to correct the problem
  d A speech problem

2 Care of the person with Meniere's disease includes preventing
  a Infection c Pain
  b Falls d Deafness

3 Which is *not* an obvious sign of hearing loss?
  a Loneliness and boredom
  b Speaking too loudly
  c Asking to repeat things
  d Answering questions poorly

4 You are talking to a person with hearing loss. You should do the following *except*
  a Speak clearly, distinctly, and slowly
  b Sit or stand in good light
  c Shout
  d Stand or sit on the side of the better ear

5 You are talking to a person with hearing loss. You can do the following *except*
  a State the topic
  b Change the subject if the person does not seem to understand
  c Use short sentences and simple words
  d Write out key words and names

6 A hearing aid
  a Corrects a hearing problem
  b Makes sounds louder
  c Makes speech clearer
  d Lowers background noise

7 A hearing aid does not seem to be working. Your *first* action is to
  a See if it is turned on
  b Wash it with soap and water
  c Have it repaired
  d Remove the batteries

8 A person has aphasia. You know that
  a The person cannot use the muscles of speech
  b Mouth and face muscles are affected
  c The person has a language disorder
  d The person cannot speak

9 A person with receptive aphasia has trouble
  a Talking
  b Writing
  c Understanding messages
  d Using gestures

10 A person has a speech disorder. You should do the following *except*
  a Correct the person's speech
  b Have the person write key words
  c Ask the person to repeat or rephrase as needed
  d Watch lip movements

11 A person has a cataract. Which is *false*?
  a Vision is cloudy, blurry, or dimmed.
  b Colors seem faded.
  c Central vision is lost.
  d The person is sensitive to light and glares.

12 A person had cataract surgery. You should do the following *except*
  a Follow measures for blind or visually impaired persons if an eye shield is worn
  b Let the person rub the eye
  c Place the overbed table on the un-operative side
  d Have the person wear an eye shield during naps

13 A person has age-related macular degeneration. Which is *true*?
  a There is a blind spot in the center of the eye.
  b Lost vision can be restored with surgery.
  c Peripheral (side) vision is lost.
  d Vision is blurry with spots.

14 These statements are about low vision. Which is *false*?
  a The person has usable vision.
  b Eyesight can be corrected.
  c The person needs visual or adaptive devices.
  d The person has problems doing things that require close vision.

15 Who is at risk for low vision?
  a The person with diabetic retinopathy
  b The person with global aphasia
  c The person with Meniere's disease
  d The person who is blind

16 Braille involves
  a A long cane for walking
  b Raised dots arranged for letters of the alphabet
  c A guide dog
  d Special computers and printers

17 Which are dangers to persons who are blind or visually impaired?
  a Drawers that are fully closed
  b Doors that are fully open
  c Burnt out bulbs
  d Night-lights

18 A person is blind. The meal time setting should
  a Be the same for every meal
  b Provide variety for mental stimulation
  c Include plates, napkins, and placemats with designs
  d Be arranged like the face of a clock

19 A person is blind. You should do the following *except*
  a Identify yourself
  b Move furniture to provide variety
  c Explain procedures step-by-step
  d Have the person walk behind you

20 You are talking to a person who is visually impaired. You should
  a Face the person when talking to him or her
  b Avoid words such as "see" and "look"
  c Avoid using colors when describing things
  d Assume that the person has no sight

21 A person is blind. To give directions you can say
  a "Over there" c "Across the room"
  b "Right here" d "On your left"

22 When eyeglasses are not worn they should be
  a Soaked in a cleansing solution
  b Kept within the person's reach
  c Put in the eyeglass case
  d Placed on the overbed table

Answers to these questions are on p. 834.

40 Cancer, Immune System, and Skin Disorders

OBJECTIVES

- Define the key terms and key abbreviations listed in this chapter.
- Explain the difference between benign tumors and cancer.
- Identify cancer risk factors.
- Identify the signs and symptoms of cancer.
- Explain the common cancer treatments.
- Describe the needs of a person with cancer.
- Explain how immune system disorders occur.
- Describe the common immune system disorders.
- Explain how the human immunodeficiency virus (HIV) is spread.
- Identify the signs and symptoms of acquired immunodeficiency syndrome (AIDS).
- Explain how to assist in the care of persons with AIDS.
- Describe the causes, signs and symptoms, and treatment of shingles.
- Explain how to promote PRIDE in the person, the family, and yourself.

KEY TERMS

benign tumor A tumor that does not spread to other body parts; it can grow to a large size

cancer See "malignant tumor"

malignant tumor A tumor that invades and destroys nearby tissues and can spread to other body parts; cancer

metastasis The spread of cancer to other body parts

stomatitis Inflammation *(itis)* of the mouth *(stomat)*

tumor A new growth of abnormal cells; tumors are benign or malignant

KEY ABBREVIATIONS

AIDS	Acquired immunodeficiency syndrome
HIV	Human immunodeficiency virus
IV	Intravenous

Understanding cancer, immune system, and skin disorders gives meaning to the required care. Refer to Chapter 9 while you study this chapter.

CANCER

Cells reproduce for tissue growth and repair. Cells divide in an orderly way. Sometimes cell division and growth are out of control. A mass or clump of cells develops. *This new growth of abnormal cells is called a tumor. Tumors are benign or malignant* (Fig. 40-1):

* *Benign tumors do not spread to other body parts. They can grow to a large size,* but rarely threaten life. They usually do not grow back when removed.
* *Malignant tumors (cancer) invade and destroy nearby tissues* (Fig. 40-2). *They can spread to other body parts.* They may be life-threatening. Sometimes they grow back after removal.

Metastasis is the spread of cancer to other body parts (Fig. 40-3). Cancer cells break off the tumor and travel to other body parts. New tumors grow in other body parts. This occurs if cancer is not treated and controlled.

Cancer can occur almost anywhere. If detected early, cancer can be treated and controlled (Box 40-1, p. 670).

See *Focus on Children and Older Persons: Cancer,* p. 671.

Text continued on p. 672

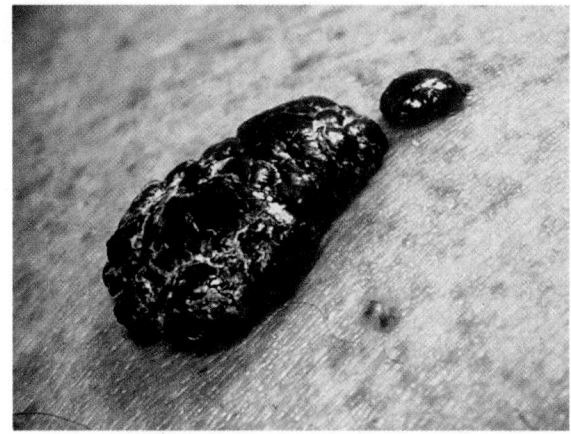

Fig. 40-2 Malignant tumor on the skin.

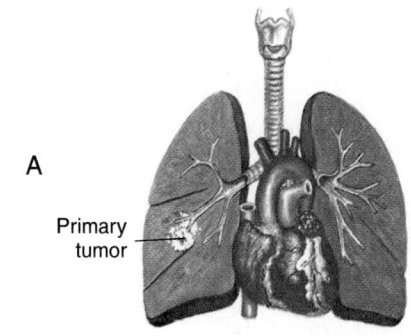

A

Primary tumor

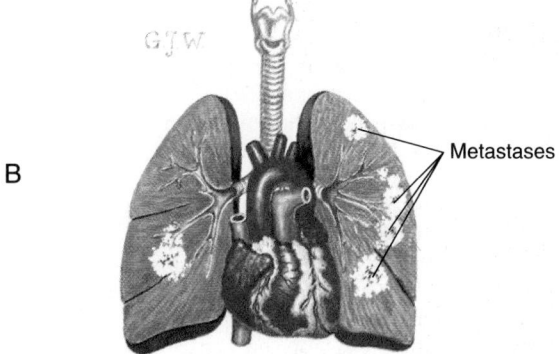

B

Metastases

Fig. 40-3 **A,** Tumor in the lung. **B,** Tumor has metastasized to the other lung.

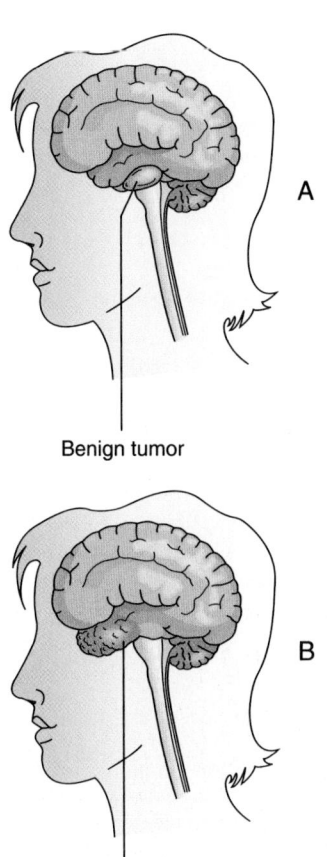

Benign tumor

A

Malignant tumor

B

Fig. 40-1 Tumors. **A,** A benign tumor grows within a local area. **B,** A malignant tumor invades other tissues.

BOX 40-1 SOME SIGNS AND SYMPTOMS OF CANCER

General Signs and Symptoms

- Thickening or lump in the breast or any other part of the body
- New mole or an obvious change in an existing mole
- A sore that does not heal
- Hoarseness or cough that does not go away
- Changes in bowel or bladder habits
- Discomfort after eating
- A hard time swallowing
- Weight gain or loss with no known reason
- Unusual bleeding or discharge
- Feeling weak or very tired *(fatigue)*

Signs and Symptoms of Cancer by Cancer Type

Brain Tumor

- Headaches (usually worse in the morning)
- Nausea and vomiting
- Changes in speech, vision, or hearing
- Problems with balance or walking
- Changes in mood, personality, or ability to concentrate
- Problems with memory
- Seizures or convulsions
- Numbness or tingling in the arms or legs

Cervix

- Abnormal vaginal bleeding
  - Between regular menstrual periods
  - After intercourse, douching, or pelvic exam
  - Longer or heavier menstrual periods
  - After menopause
- Increased vaginal discharge
- Pelvic pain
- Pain during sex

Breast

- A lump or thickening in or near the breast or underarm
- A change in breast size or shape
- Dimpling or puckering in the breast skin
- A nipple turned inward into the breast
- Discharge (fluid) from the nipple, especially if bloody
- Scaly, red, or swollen skin on any part of the breast or the skin looks like the skin of an orange

Bladder

- Hematuria (urine looks rusty or dark red)
- Urinary urgency
- Urinary frequency
- Feeling unable to empty the bladder
- Need to strain (bear down) to void
- Dysuria

Colon and Rectum

- Change in bowel habits
- Diarrhea or constipation

Colon and Rectum—cont'd

- Feeling that the bowel does not empty completely
- Blood (bright red or very dark) in the stool
- Stools are narrower than usual
- Frequent gas pains or cramps
- Full or bloated feeling
- Weight loss
- Fatigue
- Nausea or vomiting

Kidney

- Hematuria (urine looks rusty or dark red)
- Pain in the side that does not go away
- An abdominal lump or mass in the side
- Weight loss
- Fever
- Fatigue

Larynx

- A hoarse voice or other voice changes for more than 3 weeks
- A sore throat or trouble swallowing for more than 6 weeks
- A lump in the neck
- Dyspnea
- A cough that does not go away
- An earache that does not go away

Leukemia

- Painless, swollen lymph nodes in the neck or underarm
- Fevers or night sweats
- Frequent infections
- Fatigue
- Bleeding or bruising (bleeding gums, purple patches in the skin, tiny red spots under the skin)
- Abdominal swelling or discomfort
- Weight loss
- Bone or joint pain

Lung

- A cough that gets worse or does not go away
- Dyspnea
- Constant chest pain
- Coughing up blood (hemoptysis)
- Hoarse voice
- Frequent lung infections; pneumonia
- Fatigue
- Weight loss

Lymphoma

- Painless, swollen lymph nodes in the neck, underarm, or groin
- Weight loss
- Fever
- Night sweats
- Coughing, dyspnea, or chest pain
- Weakness and fatigue
- Pain, swelling, or full feeling in the abdomen

Modified from National Cancer Institute: *What you need to know about cancer: an overview*, NIH Publication No. 06-1566, Bethesda, Md., posted October 4, 2006; *What you need to know about brain tumors*, posted April 4, 2009; *What you need to know about cervical cancer*, posted November 20, 2008; *What you need to know about breast cancer*, posted October 15, 2009; *What you need to know about cancer of the colon and rectum*, posted May 26, 2006; *What you need to know about kidney cancer*, posted January 19, 2011; *What you need to know about leukemia*, posted November 25, 2008; *What you need to know about lung cancer*, posted July 26, 2007; *What you need to know about non-Hodgkin lymphoma*, posted February 12, 2008; *What you need to know about melanoma and other skin cancers*, posted January 11, 2011; *What you need to know about oral cancer*, posted December 23, 2009; *What you need to know about cancer of the pancreas*, posted July 14, 2010; *What you need to know tebout prostate cancer*, posted November 20, 2008; *What you need to know about thyroid cancer*, posted October 26, 2007; *What you need to know about cancer of the uterus*, posted October 25, 2010.

| **BOX 40-1** | **SOME SIGNS AND SYMPTOMS OF CANCER—cont'd** |

Melanoma
- Change in the shape, color, size, or feel of a mole (especially over the past few weeks or months)
- New mole
- Uneven mole shape: one half does not match the other half
- Mole edges are ragged, notched, or blurred
- Mole color is uneven (shades of black, brown, and tan; areas of white, gray, red, pink, or blue)
- Increase in mole size
- Mole surface breaks down or appears scraped
- Mole is hard or lumpy
- Mole surface may ooze or bleed
- Mole is itchy, tender, or painful

Mouth
- White or red patches inside the mouth or on the lips
- A mouth or lip sore that does not heal
- Bleeding in the mouth
- Loose teeth
- Dysphagia
- Problems wearing dentures
- A lump in the neck
- Earache that does not go away
- Numbness of the lower lip and chin

Pancreas
- Jaundice (dark urine, pale stools, yellow skin and eyes)
- Upper abdominal pain
- Middle back pain that does not subside with position change
- Nausea and vomiting
- Stools that float in the toilet
- Fatigue
- Anorexia or full feeling
- Weight loss

Skin
- A small, smooth, shiny, pale, or waxy lump
- A sore or lump that bleeds
- A sore or lump with a crust or scab
- A red or brown patch that is rough and scaly
- A firm or red lump
- A flat red spot that is rough, dry, or scaly; may be itchy or tender

Prostate
- Not being able to void
- Problems starting or stopping urine flow
- Urinary frequency
- Nocturia
- Weak urine flow
- Urine flow that starts and stops
- Dysuria
- Erection problems
- Hematuria
- Blood in semen
- Frequent pain in the lower back, hips, or upper thighs

Thyroid
- Lump in front of the neck
- Hoarseness or voice changes
- Swollen neck lymph nodes
- Dysphagia
- Dyspnea
- Throat or neck pain

Uterus
- Abnormal vaginal bleeding, spotting, or discharge
- Dysuria
- Problems emptying the bladder
- Pain during sex
- Pelvic pain

FOCUS ON CHILDREN AND OLDER PERSONS

Cancer

Children

Sites of cancer in children are the same as for adults. However, some cancers are more common in children. They include:
- Leukemia—a cancer of the blood. It develops in the bone marrow. The bone marrow is a spongy substance found inside bones. Blood cells are made in the bone marrow. Leukemia is the most common form of childhood cancer.
- Brain tumors.
- Lymphomas—tumors of the lymph tissue.
- Bone cancers.
- Liver cancers.
- Kidney cancers.
- Cancer of nerve cells.

  Childhood cancers often occur suddenly. Often there are no symptoms. Childhood cancers have a high cure rate.

Risk Factors

Cancer is the second leading cause of death in the United States. Certain factors increase the risk of cancer. The National Cancer Institute describes these risk factors:

- *Growing older.* Cancer occurs in all age-groups. However, most cancers occur in persons over 65 years of age.
- *Tobacco.* This includes using tobacco (smoking, snuff, and chewing tobacco) and being around tobacco (second-hand smoke). This risk can be avoided.
- *Sunlight.* Sun, sunlamps, and tanning booths cause early aging of the skin and skin damage. These can lead to skin cancer.
- *Ionizing radiation.* This can cause cell damage that leads to cancer. Sources are x-rays and radon gas that forms in the soil and some rocks. Miners are at risk for radon exposure. Radon is found in some homes. Radioactive fallout is another source. It can come from nuclear power plant accidents and from the production, testing, or use of atomic weapons.
- *Certain chemicals and other substances.* Painters, construction workers, and those in the chemical industry are at risk. Paint, pesticides, used engine oil, and other chemicals can be harmful.
- *Some viruses and bacteria.* Certain viruses increase the risk of these cancers—cervical, liver, lymphoma, leukemia, Kaposi's sarcoma (associated with AIDS, p. 675), stomach.
- *Certain hormones.* Hormone replacement for menopause may increase the risk of breast cancer. Some pregnant women received diethylstilbestrol (DES), a form of estrogen, between the early 1940s and 1971. They are at risk for breast cancer. Their daughters are at risk for a rare type of cervical cancer.
- *Family history of cancer.* Certain cancers tend to occur in families. They include melanoma and cancers of the breast, ovary, prostate, and colon.
- *Alcohol.* More than 2 drinks a day increases the risk of certain cancers—mouth, throat, esophagus, larynx, liver, and breast. Women should have only 1 drink a day. Men should have only 2 drinks a day.
- *Poor diet, lack of physical activity, and being over-weight.* A high-fat diet increases the risk of cancers of the colon, uterus, and prostate. Lack of physical activity and being over-weight increase the risk for cancers of the breast, colon, esophagus, kidney, and uterus.

Treatment

Treatment depends on the tumor type, its site and size, and if it has spread. The treatment goal may be to:

- Cure the cancer.
- Control the disease.
- Reduce symptoms for as long as possible.

Some cancers respond to 1 type of treatment. Others require 2 or more types. Cancer treatments also damage healthy cells and tissues. Side effects depend on the type and extent of the treatment.

Surgery. Surgery removes tumors. It is done to cure or control cancer or to relieve pain. See Chapter 32.

Radiation Therapy. Radiation therapy *(radiotherapy)* kills cells. X-ray beams are aimed at the tumor. Sometimes radioactive material is implanted in or near the tumor.

Cancer cells and normal cells receive radiation. Both are destroyed. Radiation therapy:

- Destroys certain tumors.
- Shrinks a tumor before surgery.
- Destroys cancer cells that remain after surgery.
- Controls tumor growth to prevent or relieve pain.

Burns, skin breakdown, and hair loss can occur at the treatment site. Special skin care measures are ordered. Extra rest is needed for fatigue. Discomfort, nausea, vomiting, diarrhea, and loss of appetite *(anorexia)* are other side effects.

See *Promoting Safety and Comfort: Radiation Therapy.*

PROMOTING SAFETY AND COMFORT
Radiation Therapy

Safety

Radiation implants are in the form of seeds, ribbons, and capsules. They are placed in the body in or near the tumor. Therefore the person's body gives off radiation. When near the person, you are exposed to radiation. Practice these safety measures:

- Tell the nurse if you are or may be pregnant. The nurse needs to change your assignment.
- Don protective gloves before entering the person's room.
- Work quickly.
- Stay as far away from the person as possible while still giving effective care.
- Leave trash, linens, and food trays in the room. These items will be removed by staff trained to do so.
- Remove and discard your gloves before leaving the room.
- Wash your hands after leaving the room.
- Talk to the person from the doorway if you do not need to enter the room. Radiation exposure decreases with distance.

Comfort

Other persons must be protected from radiation exposure. The person has a private room. A visitor may be limited to 30 minutes or less a day. Visitors may stand at the doorway rather than enter the room. Children under 18 years of age and pregnant women are not allowed to visit.

Therefore the person may feel sad, lonely, and depressed. Assure the person that care needs will be met. Treat the person with caring, kindness, and dignity.

Chemotherapy. Chemotherapy involves drugs that kill cells. It is used to:

* Shrink a tumor before surgery.
* Kill cells that break off the tumor. The goal is to prevent metastasis.
* Relieve symptoms caused by the cancer.

Cancer cells and normal cells are affected. Side effects depend on the drug used:

* Hair loss *(alopecia).*
* Gastro-intestinal irritation. Poor appetite, nausea, vomiting, and diarrhea can occur. *Stomatitis, an inflammation* (itis) *of the mouth* (stomat), may occur.
* Decreased blood cell production. Bleeding and infection are risks. The person may be weak and tired.

The drug usually stays in the person's body for 3 to 7 days. It is excreted in urine, feces, vomitus, semen, and vaginal secretions. Safety measures are listed in Box 40-2.

BOX 40-2 | **SAFETY MEASURES DURING CHEMOTHERAPY**

General Safety
* Wear gloves for any contact with the person's urine, stools, or vomit. Wash your hands after removing and discarding the gloves.
* Wash the hands or any body part or area that has contact with the person's urine, stools, or vomit. Do so at once. Use soap and water. This applies to you, the person, and others.

Elimination and Vomiting
* Wear gloves to handle bedpans, urinals, or emesis basins.
* Empty and rinse bedpans, urinals, and emesis basins after use.
* Flush after the person uses the toilet or you empty a bedpan, urinal, or emesis basin. Flush twice if young children or pets will have contact with the toilet.
* Wash bedpans, urinals, and emesis basins at least once a day with soap and water. Or provide the person with new items. Follow agency policy.
* Wear gloves when changing diapers, incontinence products, and waterproof pads.
* Double-bag diapers, incontinence products, and disposable waterproof pads. Follow agency policy.
* Double-bag ostomy products.

Laundry
* Follow agency policy for soiled linens and clothing. In the home setting:
  * Wash soiled items as soon as possible. Or place them in a plastic bag. Discard the plastic bag after washing the items.
  * Wash soiled items separately from other linens or garments.
  * Wash soiled items twice.

Modified from UPMC: *Patient education: safe handling of chemotherapy waste material,* 2011, Pittsburgh, Pa.

Hormone Therapy. Hormone therapy prevents cancer cells from getting or using hormones needed for their growth. Drugs are given to prevent the production of certain hormones. Organs or glands that produce a certain hormone are removed. For example, the ovaries are removed if a breast cancer needs estrogen. A prostate cancer may need testosterone. The testicles may be removed.

Side effects include fatigue, fluid retention, weight gain, hot flashes, nausea, vomiting, appetite changes, and blood clots. Fertility is affected in men and women. Men may experience impotence (Chapter 48) and loss of sexual desire.

Biological Therapy. Biological therapy *(immunotherapy)* helps the immune system fight the cancer. It also protects the body from the side effects of cancer treatments.

Side effects include flu-like symptoms—chills, fever, muscle aches, weakness, loss of appetite, nausea, vomiting, and diarrhea. Bleeding, bruising, swelling, and skin rashes may occur.

Other Therapies.

* Stem cell transplants. A *stem cell* is a cell from which new cell types develop. The new cells have certain functions—blood cells, brain cells, bone cells, and so on. Some persons with cancer need high doses of chemotherapy or radiation therapy. Such therapies kill cancer cells and blood cells in the bone marrow. Therefore fewer blood cells are produced. The person is given blood-forming stem cells. New blood cells develop from the stem cells.
* Complementary and alternative medicine (CAM). *Complementary medicine* is used along with standard cancer treatments. *Alternative medicine* is used instead of standard cancer treatments. Types of CAM include massage therapy, herbal products, vitamins, special diets, spiritual healing, and acupuncture. *Acupuncture* involves inserting small needles at certain points in the skin to control pain and other symptoms.

The Person's Needs

Persons with cancer have many needs. They include:

* Pain relief or control
* Rest and exercise
* Fluids and nutrition
* Preventing skin breakdown
* Preventing bowel problems (constipation from pain-relief drugs; diarrhea from some cancer treatments)
* Dealing with treatment side effects
* Psychological and social needs
* Spiritual needs
* Sexual needs

Psychological and social needs are great. Anger, fear, and depression are common. Some surgeries are disfiguring. The person may feel unwhole, unattractive, or unclean. The person and family need support.

BODY STRUCTURE AND FUNCTION REVIEW: THE IMMUNE SYSTEM

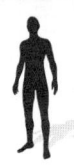

The immune system protects the body from disease and infection. Abnormal body cells can grow into tumors. Sometimes the body produces substances that cause the body to attack itself. Microorganisms (bacteria, viruses, and other germs) can cause an infection. The immune system defends against threats inside and outside the body.

The immune system gives the body *immunity*. Immunity means that a person has protection against a disease or condition. The person will not get or be affected by the disease:

- *Specific immunity* is the body's reaction to a certain threat.
- *Nonspecific immunity* is the body's reaction to anything it does not recognize as a normal body substance.

Special cells and substances function to produce immunity:

- *Antibodies*—normal body substances that recognize other substances. They are involved in destroying abnormal or unwanted substances.
- *Antigens*—substances that cause an immune response. Antibodies recognize and bind with unwanted antigens. This leads to the destruction of unwanted substances and the production of more antibodies.
- *Phagocytes*—white blood cells that digest and destroy microorganisms and other unwanted substances.
- *Lymphocytes*—white blood cells that produce antibodies. Lymphocyte production increases as the body responds to an infection.
- *B lymphocytes (B cells)*—cause the production of antibodies that circulate in the plasma. The antibodies react to specific antigens.
- *T lymphocytes (T cells)*—cells that destroy invading cells. *Killer T cells* produce poisons near the invading cells. Some T cells attract other cells. The other cells destroy the invaders.

When the body senses an antigen from an unwanted substance, the immune system acts. Phagocyte and lymphocyte production increases. Phagocytes destroy the invaders through digestion. The lymphocytes produce antibodies that identify and destroy the unwanted substances.

Spiritual needs are important. A spiritual leader may provide comfort. To many people, spiritual needs are just as important as physical needs.

Persons dying of cancer often receive hospice care (Chapters 1 and 52). Support is given to the person and family.

See *Focus on Communication: The Person's Needs.*

IMMUNE SYSTEM DISORDERS

The immune system protects the body from microbes, cancer cells, and other harmful substances. It defends against threats inside and outside the body. Immune system disorders occur from problems with the immune response. The response may be inappropriate, too strong, or lacking.

See *Body Structure and Function Review: The Immune System.*

Autoimmune Disorders

Autoimmune disorders can occur. The immune system attacks the body's own *(auto)* normal cells, tissues, or organs. One of these may occur:

- One or more types of body tissues are destroyed.
- An organ grows abnormally.
- There is a change in how an organ functions.

The organs and tissues commonly affected are:

- Red blood cells
- Blood vessels
- Connective tissue
- The endocrine glands (thyroid gland, pancreas)
- Muscles
- Joints
- Skin

Common autoimmune disorders include:

- Graves' disease. The immune system attacks the thyroid gland. The thyroid gland produces excess *(hyper)* amounts of the hormone thyroxine. The person has anxiety, problems sleeping, rapid heart rate, weight loss, and bulging of the eyeballs (Fig. 40-4).
- Lupus. This is an inflammatory disease affecting the blood cells, joints, skin, kidneys, lungs, heart, or brain. Lupus comes from the Latin word for *wolf*. It was thought that the lupus rash looked like a wolf bite (Fig. 40-5). Sometimes called the "butterfly rash," it may also look like a butterfly.
- Multiple sclerosis. See Chapter 41.
- Rheumatoid arthritis. See Chaper 41.
- Type 1 diabetes. See Chapter 43.

Signs and symptoms depend on the disease. Fatigue, dizziness, not feeling well, and fever are common.

Most autoimmune disorders are chronic. Treatment depends on the disorder and the tissues and organs affected. Treatment is aimed at:

- Reducing symptoms
- Controlling the autoimmune response
- Maintaining the body's ability to fight disease

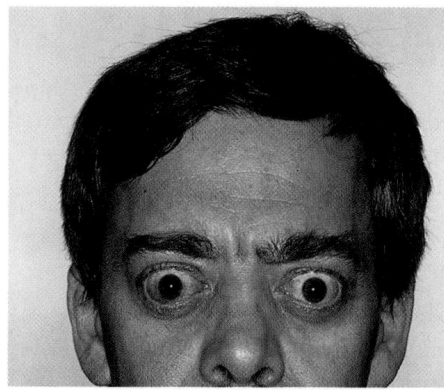

Fig. 40-4 Bulging of the eyes occurs in Graves' disease.

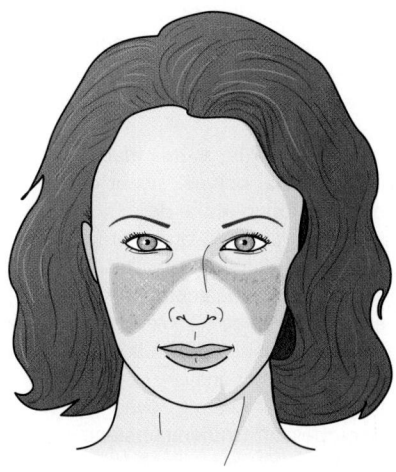

Fig. 40-5 The rash from lupus is across the nose and cheeks.

Acquired Immunodeficiency Syndrome

Acquired immunodeficiency syndrome (AIDS) is caused by the *human immunodeficiency virus (HIV)*. The virus attacks the immune system. Therefore it destroys the body's ability to fight infections and certain cancers. Some infections are life-threatening.

The virus is spread through body fluids—blood, semen, vaginal secretions, and breast milk. HIV is not spread by saliva, tears, sweat, sneezing, coughing, insects, or casual contact. HIV is transmitted mainly by:

- Unprotected anal, vaginal, or oral sex with an infected person. "Unprotected" is without a new latex or polyurethane condom. The virus enters the bloodstream through the rectum, vagina, penis, mouth, or skin breaks. Small breaks in the vagina or rectum may occur when the penis, finger, or other objects are inserted. Gum disease can cause breaks in the gums. The virus can enter the bloodstream through these mucous membrane breaks (mouth, vagina, rectum). Breaks in the skin pose a risk.

- Needle and syringe sharing among IV (intravenous) drug users. The virus is carried in contaminated blood left in needles or syringes. When the devices are shared, contaminated blood enters the bloodstream. Needle-sticks are a threat to the health team.

- HIV-infected mothers. Babies can become infected during pregnancy, shortly after birth, and through breast-feeding.

HIV cannot live outside the body. HIV is not spread by casual, everyday contact. Such contact includes using public phones, restrooms, swimming pools, hot tubs, or water fountains. Other casual contact includes talking to, hugging, or dancing with an infected person. HIV is not transmitted by food prepared by the infected person.

Box 40-3 lists the signs and symptoms of AIDS. Some HIV-infected persons have symptoms within a few months. Others are symptom-free for more than 10 years. However, they carry the virus. They can spread it to others.

The person with AIDS can develop other health problems. The immune system is damaged. Pneumonia, tuberculosis, Kaposi's sarcoma (a cancer), and nervous system damage are risks. Memory loss, loss of coordination, paralysis, mental health disorders, and dementia signal nervous system damage.

Many new drugs help slow the spread of HIV in the body. They also reduce complications and prolong life. AIDS has no vaccine and no cure at present. It is a life-threatening disease.

BOX 40-3 SIGNS AND SYMPTOMS OF AIDS

- Appetite: loss of
- Cough
- Depression
- Diarrhea
- Energy: lack of
- Fatigue
- Fever
- Headache
- Memory loss, confusion, and forgetfulness
- Mouth or tongue:
  - Brown, red, pink, or purple spots or blotches
  - Sores or white patches
- Night sweats
- Pneumonia
- Shortness of breath
- Skin:
  - Rashes or flaky skin
  - Brown, red, pink, or purple spots or blotches on the skin, eyelids, or nose
- Swallowing: painful or difficult
- Swollen glands: neck, underarms, and groin
- Vision loss
- Weight loss

You may care for persons with AIDS or for persons who are HIV carriers (Box 40-4). You may have contact with the person's blood or body fluids. Protect yourself and others. Follow Standard Precautions and the Bloodborne Pathogen Standard. A person may have the HIV virus but no symptoms. In some persons, HIV or AIDS is not yet diagnosed.

See *Focus on Children and Older Persons: Acquired Immunodeficiency Syndrome.*

BOX 40-4 | **CARING FOR THE PERSON WITH AIDS**

- Practice Standard Precautions.
- Follow the Bloodborne Pathogen Standard.
- Provide daily hygiene. Avoid irritating soaps.
- Provide oral hygiene according to the care plan. A toothbrush with soft bristles is best.
- Provide oral fluids as ordered.
- Measure and record intake and output.
- Measure weight daily.
- Encourage deep-breathing and coughing exercises as ordered.
- Prevent pressure ulcers.
- Assist with range-of-motion exercises and ambulation as ordered.
- Encourage self-care as able. The person may need assistive devices (walker, commode, eating devices).
- Encourage the person to be as active as possible.
- Change linens and garments as often as needed when fever or night sweats are present.
- Be a good listener. Provide emotional support.

FOCUS ON CHILDREN AND OLDER PERSONS

Acquired Immunodeficiency Syndrome

Older Persons

The Centers for Disease Control and Prevention (CDC) reported that through 2007, there were over 244,500 cases of AIDS in persons age 45 years and older. In 2009, the CDC reported that there were over 276,000 cases. This is an increase of 31,500 cases in 2 years.

- Ages 45 to 54—over 198,700 cases
- Ages 55 to 64—over 59,600 cases
- Ages 65 and older—17,700 cases

Older persons get and spread HIV through sexual contact and IV drug use. Many do not consider themselves at risk. Older persons tend to be less informed about the disease. They tend not to practice safe sex. A blood transfusion between 1978 and 1985 increases the HIV risk.

Aging and some diseases can mask the signs and symptoms of AIDS. Older persons are less likely to be tested for HIV/AIDS. Often the person dies without the disease being diagnosed. You must follow Standard Precautions and the Bloodborne Pathogen Standard.

SKIN DISORDERS

There are many types of skin disorders. Alopecia, hirsutism, dandruff, lice, and scabies are discussed in Chapter 21. Skin tears and pressure ulcers are discussed in Chapters 33 and 34. Burns are discussed in Chapter 51.

See *Body Structure and Function Review: The Integumentary System.*

BODY STRUCTURE AND FUNCTION REVIEW: THE INTEGUMENTARY SYSTEM

The Skin

The skin is the largest system. It is the body's natural covering. There are two layers (Fig. 40-6).

- The *epidermis* is the outer layer. It has living cells and dead cells. Dead cells constantly flake off and are replaced by living cells. Living cells also die and flake off. Living cells of the epidermis contain *pigment*. The epidermis has no blood vessels and few nerve endings.
- The *dermis* is the inner layer. It is made up of connective tissue. Blood vessels, nerves, sweat glands, oil glands, and hair roots are found in the dermis.

Sweat glands help regulate body temperature. Sweat is secreted through the skin's pores. The body is cooled as sweat evaporates. *Oil glands* secrete an oily substance into the space near the hair shaft. Oil travels to the skin surface. The oil helps keep the hair and skin soft and shiny.

The skin has many functions:

- Provides the body's protective covering.
- Prevents microbes and other substances from entering the body.
- Prevents excess amounts of water from leaving the body.
- Protects organs from injury.
- Contains sensory structures. Nerve endings in the skin sense both pleasant and unpleasant stimulation. They sense cold, pain, touch, and pressure to protect the body from injury.
- Helps regulate body temperature. Blood vessels dilate (widen) when temperature outside the body is high. More blood is brought to the body surface for cooling during evaporation. When blood vessels constrict (narrow), the body retains heat. This is because less blood reaches the skin.
- Stores fats and water.

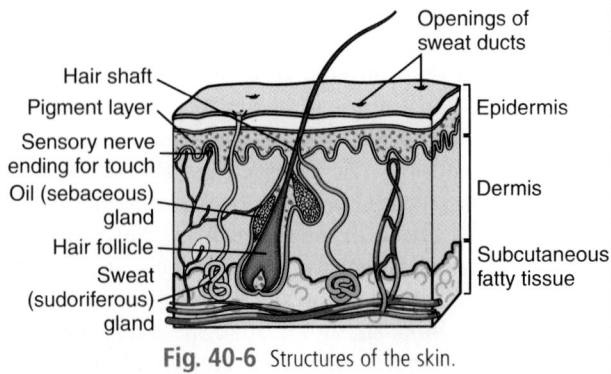

Fig. 40-6 Structures of the skin.

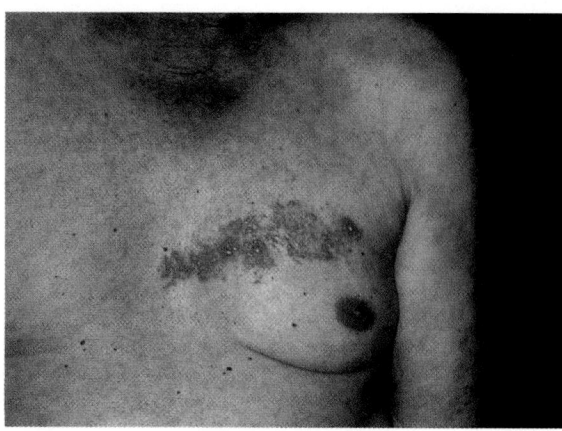

Fig. 40-7 Shingles.

Shingles

Shingles (herpes zoster) is caused by the same virus that causes chicken pox. The virus lies dormant in nerve tissue. (*Dormant* means to be *inactive*.) The virus can become active years later.

A rash or blisters occur on the skin. At first there is burning or tingling pain, numbness, or itching. This occurs in an area on one side of the body or one side of the face. After a few days or a week, a rash with fluid-filled blisters appears (Fig. 40-7). Pain is mild to intense. Itching is a common complaint.

Shingles is most common in persons over 50 years of age. Persons who have had chicken pox are at risk. So are persons with weakened immune systems from HIV infection, cancer treatments, transplant surgeries, and stress.

The doctor orders anti-viral drugs and drugs for pain relief. For many healthy people, blisters heal and pain is gone in 3 to 5 weeks. A vaccine is now available to prevent shingles.

According to the CDC, shingles lesions are infectious until they crust over. Avoid contact with an infected person if you:

- Are pregnant and have not had chicken pox.
- Are pregnant and have not had the vaccine to prevent chicken pox.
- Have a weakened immune system.

FOCUS ON PRIDE

The Person, Family, and Yourself

Personal and Professional Responsibility

Hospitals often have special units for cancer patients. They are called oncology units. *Oncology* is the study of cancer. Staff are experienced with the care and needs of persons with cancer. Some hospitals have oncology units for children.

Professional behavior is needed to work on oncology units. Staff and patients value a person who is kind, caring, patient, and compassionate. Such units want staff with a positive attitude, strong work ethic, and good communication skills.

Working on an oncology unit is challenging and rewarding. Professional qualities are needed to provide quality care and to work well with the team.

Rights and Respect

Without knowing it, people often form opinions about others. The opinion may be based on the person's life-style, appearance, or even a disease. Often this affects how the person is treated. For example, a staff member is more caring toward a person with cancer than a person with AIDS.

You cannot always control your opinions or feelings. However, they must not affect the care you give. Treat all persons with dignity and respect.

Independence and Social Interaction

Any illness affects the family. The person and family have many reactions. Fear, anger, worry, and guilt are common. This is especially true for persons with cancer, AIDS, and other immune system disorders. The person may have chronic health problems. Treatments require hospital stays and many appointments. Nursing center care or home care may be needed. Help and support are needed from the family.

Families respond in different ways. A helping and encouraging family provides motivation and support. Family bonds are stronger when the family shares responsibility and relies on each other during stress. The person's health and quality of life also benefit. Some families refuse to help. Or only 1 or 2 members help and support the person. This strains the family and places extra stress on the person.

Delegation and Teamwork

Some disorders are life-threatening. AIDS and some malignant tumors are examples. Chapter 52 explains how to care for persons at the end of life. Caring for patients or residents who will die soon is a challenge. This is harder when you have cared for the person many times and know the person well. You may have emotions and responses similar to the family.

You provide support for the family. But you need comfort as well. The nursing team can give this support. Share your feelings with the nursing team. Listen when others need to talk. Take pride in being a part of a caring and supportive team.

Ethics and Laws

Oncology staff often care for persons many times. Staff get to know the person well. They learn about likes, dislikes, and preferences. Staff learn about the person's family, school or work, hobbies, and so on. Interest in the person adds to quality of care.

However, staff must avoid crossing professional boundaries (Chapter 4). For example, a nursing assistant working on an oncology unit visits a patient during breaks and after work. She brings the person food from home. She trades assignments to care for the person and talks badly about care given by other nursing assistants. She also takes pictures of her and the patient and makes a scrapbook.

These actions signal the crossing of professional boundaries. Maintaining these boundaries can be hard when caring for persons you see often and get to know well. However, you must protect the person's privacy and rights. Watch your behavior closely to avoid crossing boundaries. Tell the nurse if you suspect a person is crossing boundaries.

REVIEW QUESTIONS

Circle the BEST answer.

1 A person has cancer. You know that
  a The tumor will not threaten life
  b The tumor can spread to other body parts
  c The tumor is benign
  d The person's mouth is inflamed

2 Who has the greatest risk for cancer?
  a The person who smokes
  b The person who is physically active
  c The person who limits time in the sun
  d The person who is 40 years old

3 Which is *not* a warning sign of cancer?
  a Painful, swollen joints
  b A sore that does not heal
  c Unusual bleeding or discharge
  d Discomfort after eating

4 Care after cancer surgery will likely include
  a Pain-relief measures
  b Mouth care for stomatitis
  c Skin care for burns at the treatment site
  d Measures to prevent hair loss

5 Chemotherapy will likely cause
  a Diarrhea
  b Burns
  c Skin breakdown
  d Weight gain

6 Mrs. Jones has cancer. She is telling you about her treatments and how she feels. What should you do?
  a Listen.
  b Change the subject.
  c Call for the nurse.
  d Ask about her feelings.

7 HIV is spread through
  a Body fluids
  b Coughing and sneezing
  c Using public phones and restrooms
  d Hugging or dancing with an infected person

8 HIV can enter the bloodstream in the following ways *except*
  a Through gum disease
  b Through the rectum, vagina, penis, mouth, or skin breaks
  c Through needle-sharing
  d Through swimming pools and hot tubs

9 HIV and AIDS are prevented by
  a Isolation precautions
  b Radiation therapy
  c Chemotherapy
  d Standard Precautions

10 A person has shingles. You assist the nurse with
  a Preventing diarrhea
  b Relieving pain
  c Preventing skin breakdown
  d Preventing weight loss

Circle T if the statement is TRUE and F if it is FALSE.

11 T F Cancer can occur suddenly in children without symptoms.
12 T F Cancer treatments damage healthy cells and tissues.
13 T F A person has a radiation implant. You are exposed to radiation when near the person.
14 T F For chemotherapy, agency policy may require double-bagging incontinence products.
15 T F A person has an autoimmune disorder. The person's body has attacked its own cells, tissues, or organs.
16 T F Autoimmune disorders commonly affect the heart.
17 T F Autoimmune disorders are usually chronic.
18 T F A person infected with HIV does not have signs and symptoms. The person can spread the virus to others.

Answers to these questions are on p. 834.

Nervous System and Musculo-Skeletal Disorders

41

OBJECTIVES

- Define the key terms and key abbreviations listed in this chapter.
- Describe stroke and the care required.
- Describe Parkinson's disease and the care required.
- Describe multiple sclerosis and the care required.
- Describe amyotrophic lateral sclerosis and the care required.
- Describe traumatic head injury and spinal cord injury and the care required.
- Describe autonomic dysreflexia and the care required.

- Describe arthritis and the care required.
- Explain how to assist in the care of persons after total joint replacement surgery.
- Describe the care required for osteoporosis.
- Explain how to assist in the care of persons in casts, in traction, and with hip pinnings.
- Describe the effects of amputation.
- Explain how to promote PRIDE in the person, the family, and yourself.

KEY TERMS

amputation The removal of all or part of an extremity

arthritis Joint *(arthr)* inflammation *(itis)*

arthroplasty The surgical replacement *(plasty)* of a joint *(arthro)*

closed fracture The bone is broken but the skin is intact; simple fracture

compound fracture See "open fracture"

fracture A broken bone

gangrene A condition in which there is death of tissue

hemiplegia Paralysis *(plegia)* on one side *(hemi)* of the body

open fracture The broken bone has come through the skin; compound fracture

paralysis Loss of muscle function, sensation, or both

paraplegia Paralysis in the legs and lower trunk *(para* means *beyond; plegia* means *paralysis)*

quadriplegia Paralysis in the arms, legs, and trunk *(quad* means *four; plegia* means *paralysis)*; tetraplegia

simple fracture See "closed fracture"

tetraplegia See "quadriplegia" *(tetra* means *four; plegia* means *paralysis)*

KEY ABBREVIATIONS

ADL	Activities of daily living	**PVS**	Persistent vegetative state
ALS	Amyotrophic lateral sclerosis	**RA**	Rheumatoid arthritis
CVA	Cerebrovascular accident	**ROM**	Range-of-motion
JRA	Juvenile rheumatoid arthritis	**TBI**	Traumatic brain injury
MS	Multiple sclerosis	**TIA**	Transient ischemic attack

Understanding nervous and musculo-skeletal disorders gives meaning to the required care. Refer to Chapter 9 while you study this chapter.

NERVOUS SYSTEM DISORDERS

Nervous system disorders can affect mental and physical function. They can affect the ability to speak, understand, feel, see, hear, touch, think, control bowels and bladder, and move.

See *Body Structure and Function Review: The Nervous System,* p. 680.

BODY STRUCTURE AND FUNCTION REVIEW: THE NERVOUS SYSTEM

The nervous system controls, directs, and coordinates body functions. It consists of the brain and spinal cord (Fig. 41-1) and *nerves* throughout the body.

Nerves connect to the spinal cord. Nerves carry messages or impulses to and from the brain. A stimulus causes a nerve impulse. A *stimulus* is anything that excites or causes a body part to function, become active, or respond. A *reflex* is the body's response (functioning or movement) to a stimulus. Reflexes are involuntary, unconscious, and immediate. The person cannot control reflexes.

Some nerve fibers have a protective covering called a *myelin sheath*. Nerve fibers covered with myelin conduct impulses faster than those fibers without it.

The Central Nervous System

The *brain* and *spinal cord* make up the central nervous system. The brain is covered by the skull. The three main parts of the brain are the *cerebrum*, the *cerebellum*, and the *brainstem* (Fig. 41-2).

The cerebrum is the center of thought and intelligence. The cerebrum is divided into the *right* and *left hemispheres*. The

The Central Nervous System—cont'd

right hemisphere controls movement and activities on the body's left side. The left hemisphere controls the right side.

The outside of the cerebrum is called the *cerebral cortex*. It controls reasoning, memory, consciousness, speech, voluntary muscle movement, vision, hearing, sensation, and other activities.

The cerebellum regulates and coordinates body movements. It controls balance and the smooth movements of voluntary muscles.

The brainstem contains the *midbrain, pons,* and *medulla*. The midbrain and pons relay messages between the medulla and the cerebrum. The medulla controls heart rate, breathing, blood vessel size, swallowing, coughing, and vomiting. The brain connects to the spinal cord at the lower end of the medulla.

The spinal cord lies within the spinal column. It contains pathways that conduct messages to and from the brain. The brain and spinal cord are covered and protected by three layers of connective tissue called *meninges*.

Cerebrospinal fluid circulates around the brain and spinal cord. Cerebrospinal fluid cushions shocks that could easily injure brain and spinal cord structures.

The Peripheral Nervous System

The peripheral nervous system has 12 pairs of *cranial nerves* and 31 pairs of *spinal nerves* (Chapter 9). The nerves conduct impulses between the brain and the head, neck, chest, and abdomen. They conduct impulses for smell, vision, hearing, pain, touch, temperature, and pressure. They also conduct impulses for voluntary and involuntary muscles. Spinal nerves carry impulses from the skin, extremities, and the internal structures not supplied by cranial nerves.

Some peripheral nerves form the *autonomic nervous system*. This system controls involuntary muscles and certain body functions—heartbeat, blood pressure, intestinal contractions, and glandular secretions. The autonomic nervous system is divided into the *sympathetic nervous system* and the *parasympathetic nervous system*. They balance each other. The sympathetic nervous system speeds up functions. The parasympathetic nervous system slows functions.

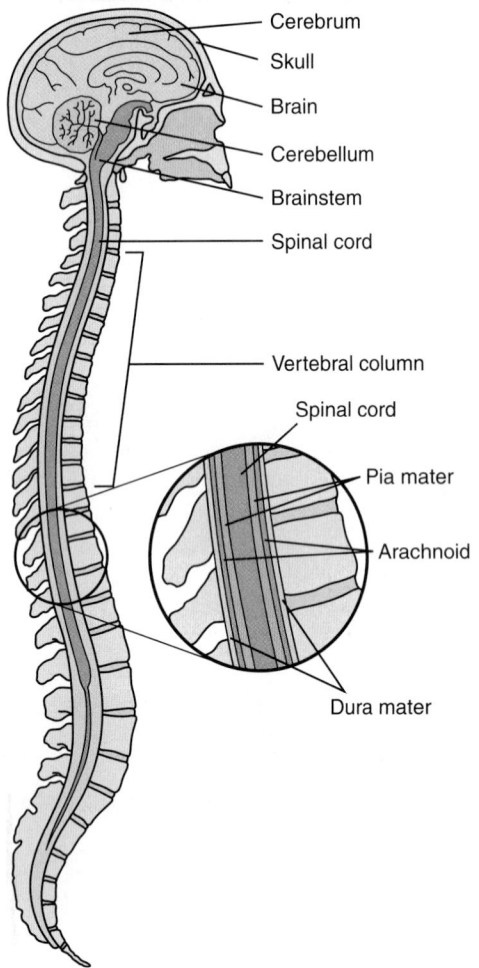

Fig. 41-1 Central nervous system.

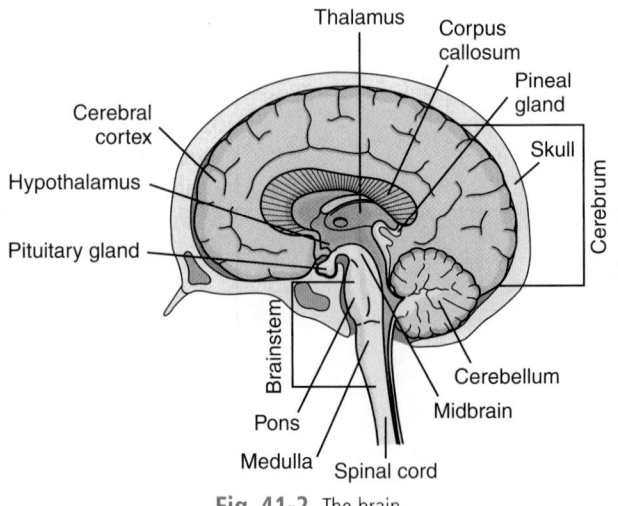

Fig. 41-2 The brain.

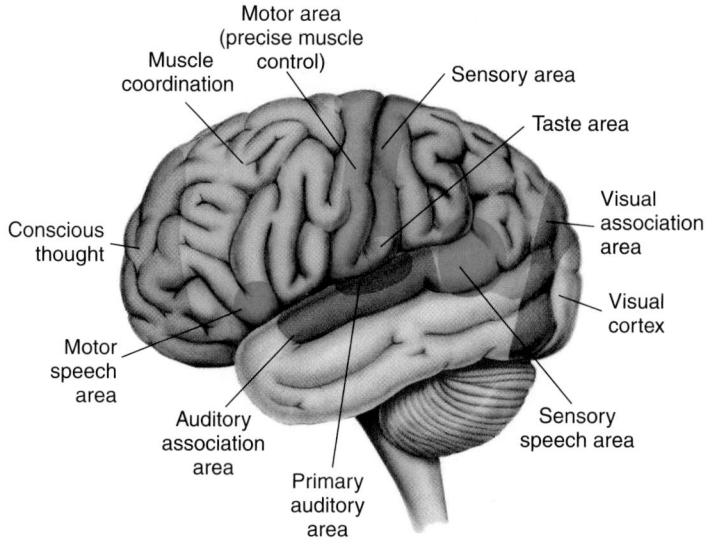

Fig. 41-3 Functions lost from a stroke depend on the area of brain damage.

Motor area (precise muscle control)

Muscle coordination

Sensory area

Taste area

Conscious thought

Visual association area

Visual cortex

Motor speech area

Auditory association area

Sensory speech area

Primary auditory area

Stroke

Stroke is a disease that affects the arteries that supply blood to the brain. It also is called a *brain attack* or *cerebrovascular accident (CVA)*. It occurs when one of these happens:

- A blood vessel in the brain bursts. Bleeding occurs in the brain (cerebral hemorrhage).
- A blood clot blocks blood flow to the brain.

Brain cells in the affected area do not get enough oxygen and nutrients. Brain damage occurs. Functions controlled by that part of the brain are lost (Fig. 41-3).

Stroke is the third leading cause of death in the United States. It is a leading cause of disability in adults. See Box 41-1 for warning signs. The person needs emergency care. Blood flow to the brain must be restored as soon as possible.

Warning signs may last a few minutes. This is called a *transient ischemic attack (TIA)*. (*Transient* means *temporary* or *short term*. *Ischemic* means to *hold back* [ischein] *blood* [hemic].) Blood supply to the brain is interrupted for a short time. A TIA may occur before a stroke. All stroke-like symptoms signal the need for emergency care.

Risk Factors. Risk factors include:

- High blood pressure
- Cigarette smoking; exposure to second-hand smoke
- Heart disease
- Diabetes
- TIAs
- Age 55 and older
- Being over-weight
- Lack of physical activity

Signs and Symptoms. Stroke can occur suddenly. The person may have warning signs (see Box 41-1). The person also may have nausea, vomiting, and memory loss. Unconsciousness, noisy breathing, high blood pressure, slow pulse, redness of the face, and seizures may occur. So can *hemiplegia—paralysis* (plegia) *on one side* (hemi) *of the body*. The person may lose bowel and bladder control and the ability to speak. (See "Aphasia" in Chapter 39.)

Effects on the Person. If the person survives, some brain damage is likely. Functions lost depend on the area of brain damage (see Fig. 41-3). They include:

- Loss of face, hand, arm, leg, or body control
- Hemiplegia
- Changing emotions (crying easily or mood swings, sometimes for no reason)
- Difficulty swallowing (dysphagia)
- Aphasia or slowed or slurred speech (Chapter 39)
- Changes in sight, touch, movement, and thought
- Impaired memory
- Urinary frequency, urgency, or incontinence
- Loss of bowel control or constipation
- Depression and frustration

Behavior changes occur. The person may forget about or ignore the weaker side. This is called *neglect*. It is from the loss of vision or movement and feeling on that side. Sometimes thinking is affected. The person may not recognize or know how to use common items. Activities of daily living (ADL) and other tasks are hard to do. The person may forget what to do and how to do it. If the person does know, the body may not respond.

Rehabilitation starts at once. The person may depend in part or totally on others for care. The health team helps the person regain the highest possible level of function (Box 41-2, p. 682).

See *Focus on Long-Term Care and Home Care: Stroke,* p. 682.

BOX 41-2 CARE OF THE PERSON WITH A STROKE

- Position the person in the lateral (side-lying) position to prevent aspiration.
- Keep the bed in semi-Fowler's position.
- Approach the person from the strong (unaffected) side. Place objects on the strong (unaffected) side. The person may have loss of vision on the affected side.
- Turn and re-position the person at least every 2 hours.
- Use assist devices to move, turn, re-position, and transfer the person.
- Encourage incentive spirometry and deep breathing and coughing.
- Prevent contractures.
- Meet food and fluid needs. The person may need a dysphagia diet (Chapter 24).
- Apply elastic stockings to prevent thrombi (blood clots) in the legs.
- Assist with range-of-motion (ROM) exercises to prevent contractures. They also strengthen affected extremities.
- Meet elimination needs. Follow the care plan for:
  - Catheter care or bladder training
  - Bowel training
- Practice safety precautions:
  - Keep the signal light within reach on the person's strong (unaffected) side.
  - Check the person often if he or she cannot use the signal light. Follow the care plan.
  - Use bed rails according to the care plan.
  - Prevent falls and other injuries.
- Have the person do as much self-care as possible. This includes turning, positioning, and transferring. The person uses assistive, self-help, and ambulation aids as needed.
- Do not rush the person. Movements are slower after a stroke.
- Follow established communication methods (Chapters 8 and 39).
- Give support, encouragement, and praise.
- Complete a safety check before leaving the room. (See the inside of the front book cover.)

FOCUS ON LONG-TERM CARE AND HOME CARE
Stroke

Long-Term Care
The person may need subacute or long-term care. Some persons return home after rehabilitation. For others, long-term care is often permanent. Many measures listed in Box 41-2 are part of the person's care.

Home Care
Many stroke survivors return home. The family assists with the person's care. Home health care services are often needed. The care measures in Box 41-2 continue in the home setting. The health team recommends changes in the home setting to help the person function.

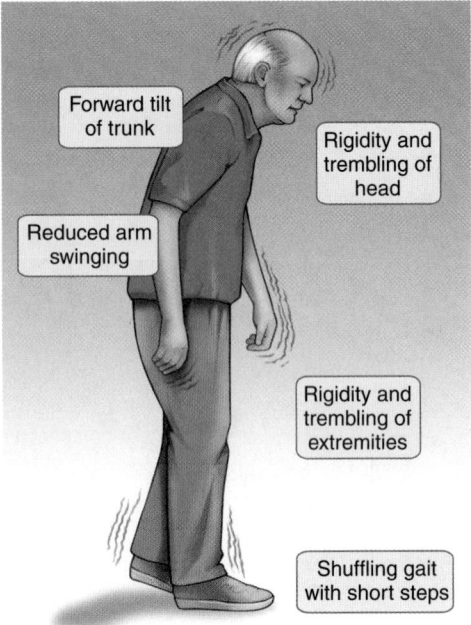

Fig. 41-4 Signs of Parkinson's disease.

Parkinson's Disease

Parkinson's disease is a slow, progressive disorder with no cure. Movement is affected. Persons over the age of 50 are at risk. Signs and symptoms become worse over time (Fig. 41-4). They include:

- *Tremors*—often start in a hand. Pill-rolling movements—rubbing the thumb and index finger—may occur. The person may have trembling in the hands, arms, legs, jaw, and face.
- *Rigid, stiff muscles*—in the arms, legs, neck, and trunk.
- *Slow movements*—the person has a slow, shuffling gait.
- *Stooped posture and impaired balance*—it is hard to walk. Falls are a risk.
- *Mask-like expression*—the person cannot blink and smile. A fixed stare is common.

Other signs and symptoms develop over time. They include swallowing and chewing problems, constipation, and bladder problems. Sleep problems, depression, and emotional changes (fear, insecurity) can occur. So can memory loss and slow thinking. The person may have slurred, monotone, and soft speech. Some people talk too fast or repeat what they say.

Drugs are ordered to treat and control the disease. Exercise and physical therapy help improve strength, posture, balance, and mobility. Therapy is needed for speech and swallowing problems. The person may need help with eating and self-care. Normal elimination is a goal. Safety measures are needed to prevent falls and injuries.

Multiple Sclerosis

Multiple sclerosis (MS) is a chronic disease. *Multiple* means *many*. *Sclerosis* means *hardening* or *scarring*. The myelin (which covers nerve fibers) in the brain and spinal cord is destroyed. Nerve impulses are not sent to and from the brain in a normal way. Functions are impaired or lost. There is no cure.

Symptoms usually start between the ages of 20 and 40. Women and whites are at greater risk than other groups. The risk increases if a family member has MS. Signs and symptoms may include:

- Blurred or double vision, blindness in one eye
- Muscle weakness in the arms and legs
- Balance and coordination problems
- Tingling, prickling, or numb sensations
- Partial or complete paralysis
- Pain
- Speech problems
- Tremors
- Dizziness
- Concentration, attention, memory, and judgment problems
- Depression
- Bowel and bladder problems
- Problems with sexual function
- Hearing loss
- Fatigue

MS can present in many ways. For example:

- The person's symptoms last for a few weeks or a few months. The symptoms gradually disappear with partial or complete recovery. The person is in *remission*. At some point, symptoms flare up again *(relapse)*.
- The person's condition gradually declines with more and more symptoms. There are no remissions.
- Symptoms become worse. More symptoms occur with each flare-up. The person's condition declines.

Persons with MS are kept active as long as possible and as independent as possible. The care plan reflects the person's changing needs. Skin care, hygiene, and ROM exercises are important. So are turning, positioning, and deep breathing and coughing. Bowel and bladder elimination is promoted. Injuries and complications from bedrest are prevented.

See *Focus on Long-Term Care and Home Care: Multiple Sclerosis.*

FOCUS ON LONG-TERM CARE AND HOME CARE
Multiple Sclerosis

Home Care
The person may need help with housekeeping to avoid fatigue. As mobility decreases, the person depends more on others. Occupational and physical therapists are often involved in the person's care.

Amyotrophic Lateral Sclerosis

Amyotrophic lateral sclerosis (ALS) is a disease that attacks the nerve cells that control voluntary muscles. Commonly called *Lou Gehrig's disease*, it is rapidly progressive and fatal. (Lou Gehrig was a New York Yankees baseball player. He died of the disease in 1941.)

More common in men, it usually strikes between 40 and 60 years of age. Most die 3 to 5 years after onset. Some live for 10 or more years.

Motor nerve cells in the brain, brainstem, and spinal cord are affected. These cells stop sending messages to the muscles. The muscles weaken, waste away (atrophy), and twitch. Over time, the brain cannot start voluntary movements or control them. The person cannot move the arms, legs, and body. Muscles for speaking, chewing and swallowing, and breathing also are affected. Eventually respiratory muscles fail. The person needs a ventilator to breathe (Chapter 37).

The disease usually does not affect the mind, intelligence, or memory. Sight, smell, taste, hearing, and touch are not affected. Usually bowel and bladder functions remain intact.

ALS has no cure. Some drugs can slow disease and improve symptoms. However, damage cannot be reversed. The person is kept active and independent to the extent possible. The care plan reflects the person's changing needs. It may include:

- Physical, occupational, and speech/language therapies
- ROM exercises
- Braces, a walker, or a wheelchair for mobility
- Comfort and pain-relief measures
- Communication methods
- Dysphagia diet or feeding tube
- Suctioning to remove excess fluids and saliva
- Mechanical ventilation
- Safety measures to prevent falls and injuries
- Psychological and social support
- Hospice care

Head Injury

Head injuries result from trauma to the scalp, skull, or brain. Some minor injuries do not need health care. Or the person needs some emergency treatment.

Traumatic brain injury (TBI) occurs when a sudden trauma damages the brain. Brain tissue is bruised or torn. Bleeding can be in the brain or in nearby tissues. Spinal cord injuries are likely. Motor vehicle crashes, falls, assaults, and firearms are common causes. So are sports and recreation injuries.

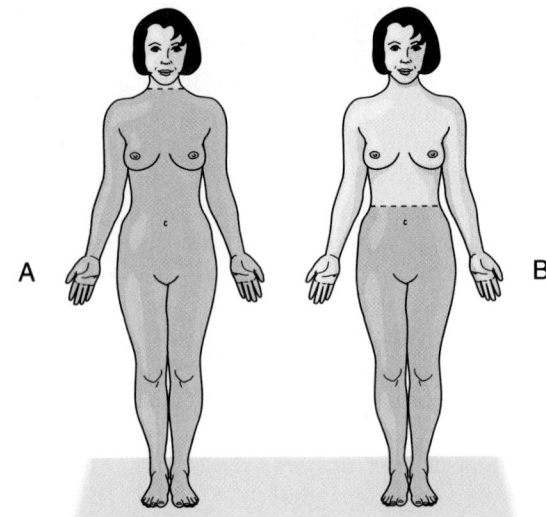

Fig. 41-5 The *shaded areas* show the area of paralysis. **A,** Quadriplegia (tetraplegia). **B,** Paraplegia.

Death can occur at the time of injury or later. If the person survives, some permanent damage is likely. Disabilities depend on the severity and site of the injury. They include:

- Cognitive problems—thinking, memory, and reasoning.
- Sensory problems—sight, hearing, touch, taste, and smell.
- Communication problems—expressing or understanding language.
- Behavior or mental health problems—depression, anxiety, personality changes, aggressive behavior, socially inappropriate behavior.
- Stupor—an unresponsive state; the person can be briefly aroused.
- Coma—the person is unconscious, does not respond, is unaware, and cannot be aroused.
- Vegetative state—the person is unconscious and unaware of surroundings. He or she has sleep-wake cycles and periods of being alert.
- Persistent vegetative state (PVS)—the person is in a vegetative state for more than 1 month.

Rehabilitation is required. Physical, occupational, speech/language, and mental health therapies depend on the person's needs. Nursing care depends on the person's needs and abilities.

See *Focus on Children and Older Persons: Head Injury.*

Spinal Cord Injury

Spinal cord injuries can permanently damage the nervous system. *Paralysis (loss of muscle function, sensation, or both)* can result. Young adult men have the highest risk. Common causes are stab or gunshot wounds, motor vehicle crashes, falls, and sports injuries.

Problems depend on the amount of damage to the spinal cord and the level of injury. Damage to the spinal cord may be incomplete or complete:

- Incomplete—some sensory (feeling) and muscle (movement) function below the level of the injury remains.
- Complete—no sensory or muscle function below the level of the injury remains.

The higher the level of injury, the more functions lost (Fig. 41-5):

- Lumbar injuries—sensory and muscle function in the legs is lost. The person has paraplegia. *Paraplegia is paralysis in the legs and lower trunk.* (*Para* means *beyond; plegia* means *paralysis.*)
- Thoracic injuries—sensory and muscle function below the chest is lost. The person has paraplegia.
- Cervical injuries—sensory and muscle function of the arms, legs, and trunk is lost. *Paralysis in the arms, legs, and trunk is called* quadriplegia *or* tetraplegia. (*Quad* and *tetra* mean *four. Plegia* means *paralysis.*)

Cervical traction with a special bed may be needed (p. 691). The spine is kept straight at all times. See Box 41-3 for care measures. Emotional needs are great. Reactions to paralysis and loss of function are often severe.

If the person lives, rehabilitation is needed. Some agencies focus on spinal cord injuries. The person learns to function at the highest possible level with self-help, assistive, and other devices. Some persons live independently at home or with home care. Others need long-term care or assisted-living settings.

BOX 41-3	**CARE OF PERSONS WITH PARALYSIS**

- Practice safety measures to prevent falls. Use bed rails as directed.
- Keep the bed in the low position.
- Keep the signal light within reach. If unable to use the signal light, check the person often.
- Prevent burns. Check bath water, heat applications, and food for proper temperature.
- Turn (logroll) and re-position the person at least every 2 hours.
- Prevent pressure ulcers. Follow the care plan.
- Use supportive devices to maintain good alignment.

- Follow bowel and bladder training programs.
- Keep intake and output records.
- Maintain muscle function and prevent contractures. Assist with ROM exercises.
- Assist with food and fluids as needed. Provide self-help devices as ordered.
- Give emotional and psychological support.
- Follow the person's rehabilitation plan.
- Complete a safety check of the room. (See the inside of the front book cover.)

BOX 41-4	**PREVENTING AUTONOMIC DYSREFLEXIA**

- Monitor urinary output.
- Follow measures for the person with an indwelling catheter. See "Catheters" in Chapter 22. Do not let the drainage bag get too full.
- Prevent urinary tract infections.
- Promote bowel elimination. Prevent constipation and fecal impaction.
- Prevent pressure ulcers.
- Prevent skin injuries—skin tears, cuts, bruises, blisters, and so on.

- Check the feet for ingrown toenails, blisters, pressure ulcers, and so on.
- Prevent burns. This includes burns from hot water.
- Have the person wear loose and comfortable clothing.
- Remove wrinkles from clothing and linens.
- Re-position the person at least every 2 hours. Avoid prolonged pressure from the bed or chair.
- Report menstrual cramps.

Autonomic Dysreflexia. This syndrome occurs with spinal cord injuries above the mid-thoracic level. There is uncontrolled stimulation of the sympathetic nervous system. If untreated, stroke, heart attack, and death are risks. Report any of the following at once:

- High blood pressure
- Throbbing or pounding headache
- Heart rate less than 60 beats per minute
- Blurred vision
- Sweating above the level of injury
- Flushing, reddening of the skin above the level of injury
- Cold, clammy skin below the level of injury
- "Goose bumps" below the level of injury
- Nasal congestion or stuffiness
- Nausea
- Anxiety

To treat the syndrome, the head of the bed is raised 45 degrees or the person sits upright if allowed. And the cause is treated. Common causes are a full bladder, constipation or fecal impaction, and skin disorders. See Box 41-4.

See *Promoting Safety and Comfort: Autonomic Dysreflexia.*

> **PROMOTING SAFETY AND COMFORT**
> **Autonomic Dysreflexia**
>
> **Safety**
> Constipation and fecal impaction can cause autonomic dysreflexia. So can checking for an impaction and enemas. Do not perform these procedures if the person is at risk for the syndrome. The procedures are best done by a nurse.

MUSCULO-SKELETAL DISORDERS
Musculo-skeletal disorders affect movement. Activities of daily living, social activities, and quality of life are affected. Injury and aging are common causes of musculo-skeletal disorders.

> See *Body Structure and Function Review: The Musculo-Skeletal System,* p. 686.

BODY STRUCTURE AND FUNCTION REVIEW: THE MUSCULO-SKELETAL SYSTEM

Bones

Bones are hard, rigid structures.
- *Long bones* bear the body's weight. Leg bones are long bones.
- *Short bones* allow skill and ease in movement. Bones in the wrists, fingers, ankles, and toes are short bones.
- *Flat bones* protect the organs. They include the ribs, skull, pelvic bones, and shoulder blades.
- *Irregular bones* are the vertebrae in the spinal column. They allow various degrees of movement and flexibility.

Joints

A *joint* is the point at which two or more bones meet (Fig. 41-6). Joints allow movement.
- *Ball-and-socket joint* allows movement in all directions. The rounded end of one bone fits into the hollow end of another bone. The joints of the hips and shoulders are ball-and-socket joints.
- *Hinge joint* allows movement in one direction. The elbow is a hinge joint.
- *Pivot joint* allows turning from side to side. A pivot joint connects the skull to the spine.

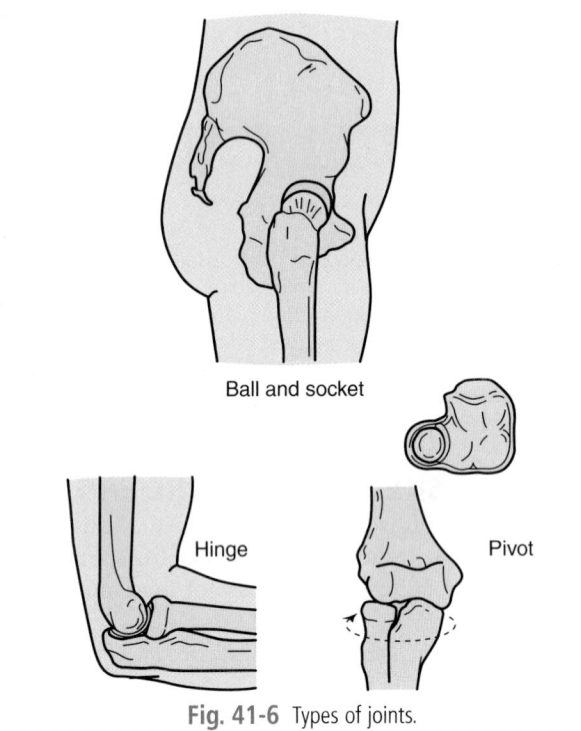

Ball and socket

Hinge

Pivot

Fig. 41-6 Types of joints.

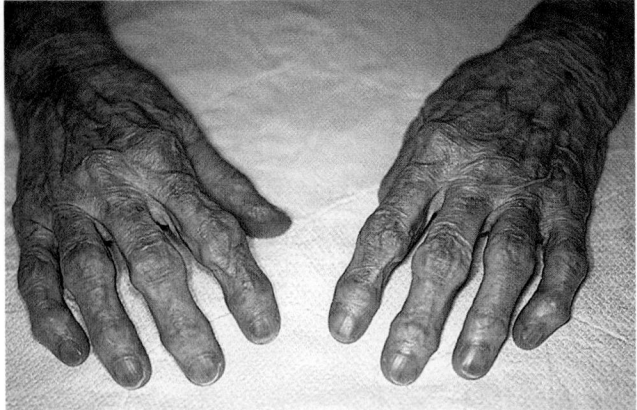

Fig. 41-7 Bony growths called *Heberden nodes* occur in the finger joints.

weakness, and heredity. The fingers, spine (neck and lower back), and weight-bearing joints (hips, knees, and feet) are often affected (Fig. 41-7).

The person has joint stiffness, pain, swelling, and tenderness. Joint stiffness occurs with rest and lack of motion. Pain occurs with weight-bearing and motion. Or pain is constant or occurs from lack of motion. Pain can affect rest, sleep, and mobility. Swelling is common after using the joint. Cold weather and dampness seem to increase symptoms.

There is no cure. Treatment involves:
- *Pain relief.* Drugs decrease swelling and inflammation and relieve pain.
- *Heat and cold.* Heat relieves pain, increases blood flow, and reduces swelling. Heat applications and warm baths or showers are helpful. So is water therapy in a heated pool. Sometimes cold applications are used after joint use.
- *Exercise.* Exercise decreases pain, increases flexibility, and improves blood flow. It helps with weight control and promotes fitness. Mental well-being improves. The person is taught what exercises to do.
- *Rest and joint care.* Good body mechanics, posture, and regular rest protect the joints. Relaxation methods are helpful. Canes and walkers provide support. Splints support weak joints and keep them in alignment. Adaptive and self-help devices for hands and wrists are useful.
- *Weight control.* Weight loss is stressed for persons who are over-weight. It reduces stress on weight-bearing joints. And it helps prevent further joint injury.
- *Healthy life-style.* Arthritis support programs can help the person develop a healthy outlook. Abilities and strengths are stressed. The focus is on fitness, exercise, rest, managing stress, and good nutrition.

Falls are prevented. Help is given with ADL as needed. Toilet seat risers are helpful when hips and knees are affected. So are chairs with higher seats and armrests. Some people need joint replacement surgery.

Arthritis

Arthritis means joint (arthr) *inflammation* (itis). Pain, swelling, and stiffness occur in the affected joints. The joints are hard to move.

Osteoarthritis (Degenerative Joint Disease).

This is the most common type of arthritis. Aging, being over-weight, and joint injury are causes. So are stress, muscle

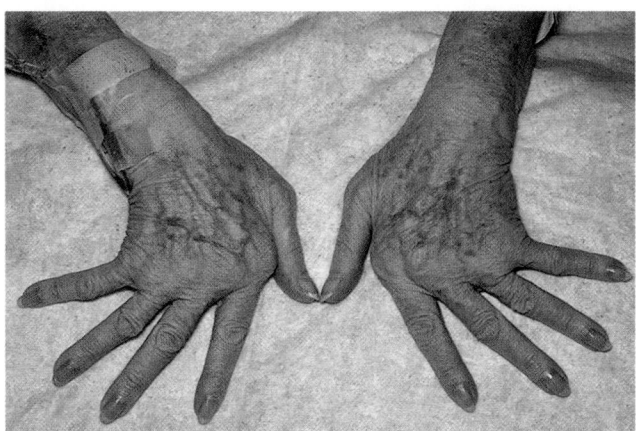

Fig. 41-8 Deformities caused by rheumatoid arthritis.

Rheumatoid Arthritis. Rheumatoid arthritis (RA) is a chronic inflammatory disease. It causes joint pain, swelling, stiffness, and loss of function. More common in women than in men, it usually develops between the ages of 20 and 50.

RA occurs on both sides of the body. For example, if the right wrist is involved, so is the left wrist. The wrist and finger joints near the hand are often affected (Fig. 41-8). Other joints affected are the neck, shoulders, elbows, hips, knees, ankles, and feet. Joints are tender, warm, and swollen. Fatigue and fever are common. The person does not feel well. Symptoms may last for many years.

Other body parts may be affected. Decreased production of red blood cells and dry eyes and mouth are common. Inflammation of the linings of the heart, blood vessels, and lungs can occur but are rare.

RA varies from person to person. Some people have flare-ups and then feel better. In others, the disease is active most of the time.

Treatment goals are to:
- Relieve pain.
- Reduce inflammation.
- Slow down or stop joint damage.
- Improve well-being and ability to function.

The person's care plan may include:
- *Rest balanced with exercise.* More rest is needed when RA is active. More exercise is needed when it is not. Short rest periods during the day are better than long times in bed. An exercise program is prescribed. ROM exercises are included. Exercise helps maintain healthy and strong muscles, joint mobility, and flexibility. It also promotes sleep, reduces pain, and helps weight control.
- *Proper positioning.* Contractures and deformities are prevented. Bed-boards, a bed cradle, trochanter rolls, and pillows are used.
- *Joint care.* Good body mechanics and body alignment, wrist and hand splints, and self-help devices reduce stress on the joints. Some need walking aids.

- *Weight control.* Excess weight places stress on the weight-bearing joints. Exercise and a healthy diet help control weight.
- *Measures to reduce stress.* Relaxation, distraction, exercise, and regular rest help reduce stress.
- *Measure to prevent falls.* See Chapter 13.

Drugs are given for pain relief and inflammation. Heat and cold applications may be ordered. Some persons need joint replacement surgery.

Emotional support is needed. A good outlook is important. Persons with RA need to stay as active as possible. The more they can do for themselves, the better off they are. Give encouragement and praise. Listen when the person needs to talk.

See *Focus on Children and Older Persons: Rheumatoid Arthritis.*

Total Joint Replacement Surgery. *Arthroplasty is the surgical replacement* (plasty) *of a joint* (arthro). The damaged joint is removed and replaced with an artificial joint *(prosthesis).* See Fig. 41-9.

Hip and knee replacements are common. Ankle, foot, shoulder, elbow, and finger joints also can be replaced. The surgery is done to relieve pain, restore joint function, or correct a deformed joint. See Box 41-5, p. 688.

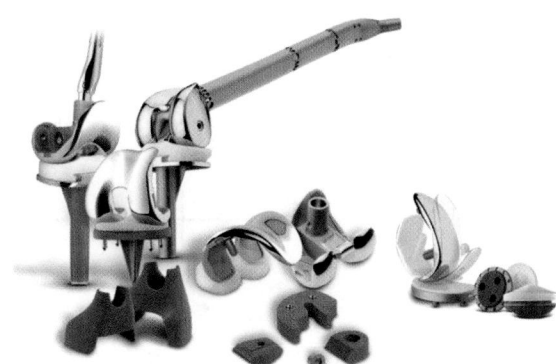

Fig. 41-9 Knee replacement prosthesis.

| **BOX 41-5** | **CARE OF THE PERSON AFTER TOTAL JOINT REPLACEMENT SURGERY—HIP AND KNEE** |

- Incentive spirometry and deep-breathing and coughing exercises to prevent respiratory complications.
- Elastic stockings to prevent thrombi (blood clots) in the legs.
- Exercises to strengthen the hip or knee. These are taught by a physical therapist.
- Measures to protect the hip as shown in Figure 41-10.
- Food and fluids for tissue healing and to restore strength.
- Safety measures to prevent falls.
- Measures to prevent infection. Wound, urinary tract, and skin infections must be prevented.
- Measures to prevent pressure ulcers.
- Assist devices for moving, turning, re-positioning, and transfers.
- Assistance with walking and a walking aid. The person may need a cane, walker, or crutches.

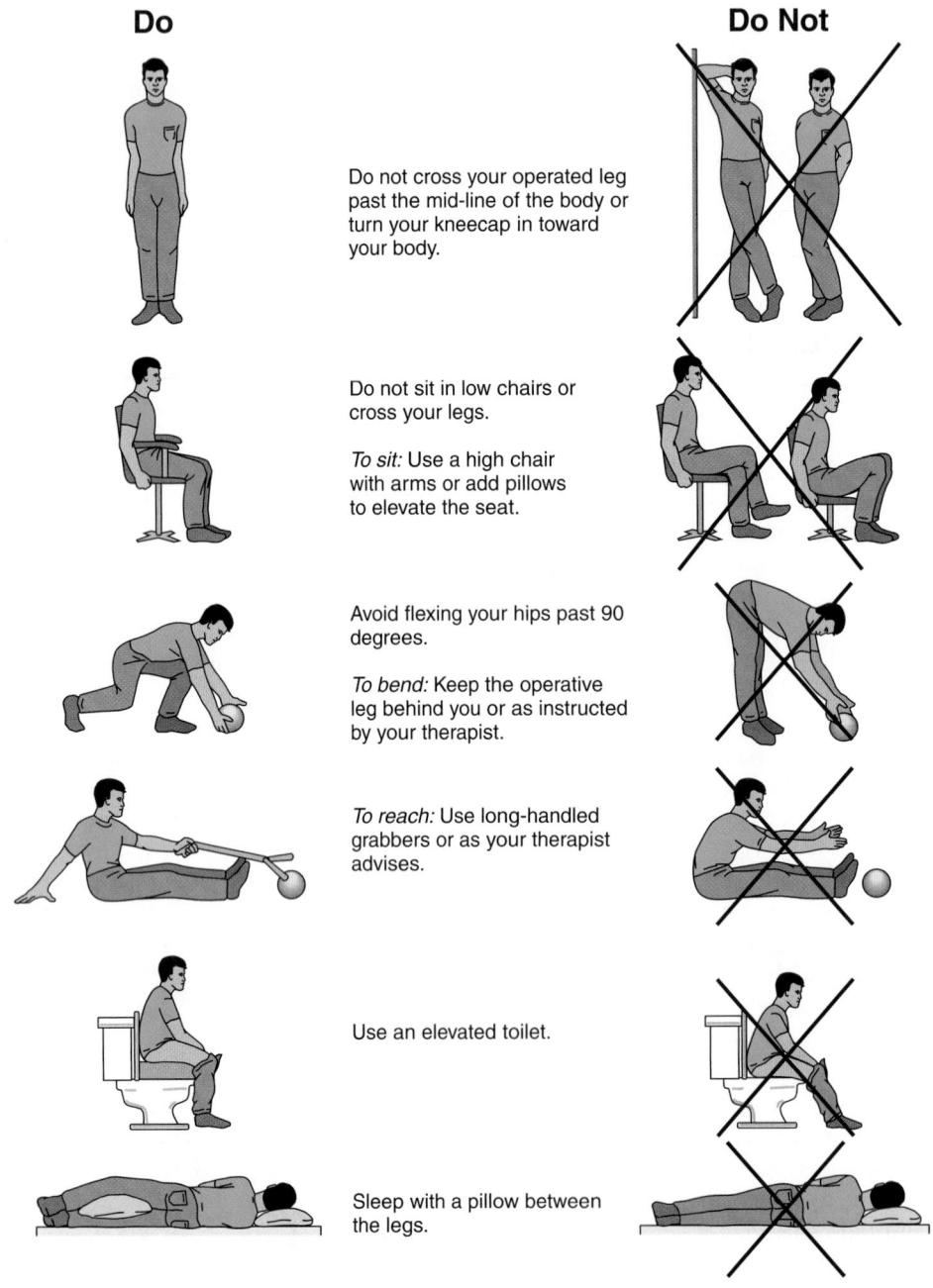

Fig. 41-10 Measures to protect the hip after total hip replacement surgery.

Osteoporosis

With osteoporosis, the bone *(osteo)* becomes porous and brittle *(porosis)*. Bones are fragile and break easily. Spine, hip, wrist, and rib fractures are common.

Older people are at risk. The risk for women increases after menopause because the ovaries do not produce estrogen. The lack of estrogen and low levels of dietary calcium cause bone changes.

All ethnic groups are at risk. Other risk factors include a family history of the disease, being thin or having a small frame, eating disorders (Chapter 45), tobacco use, alcoholism, lack of exercise, bedrest, and immobility. Exercise and activity are needed for bone strength. Bone must bear weight to form properly. If not, calcium is lost from the bone. The bone becomes porous and brittle.

Back pain, gradual loss of height, and stooped posture occur. Fractures are a major threat. Even slight activity can cause fractures. They can occur from turning in bed, getting up from a chair, or coughing. Fractures are great risks from falls and accidents.

Prevention is important. Doctors often order calcium and vitamin supplements. Estrogen is ordered for some women. Other preventive measures include:

* Exercising weight-bearing joints—walking, jogging, stair climbing
* Strength-training (lifting weights)
* No smoking
* Limiting alcohol and caffeine
* Back supports or corsets for good posture
* Walking aids if needed
* Safety measures to prevent falls and accidents
* Good body mechanics
* Safe moving, transfer, and turning and positioning procedures

Fractures

A *fracture is a broken bone.* Tissues around the fracture—muscles, blood vessels, nerves, and tendons—are injured. Fractures are open or closed (Fig. 41-11):

* *Closed fracture (simple fracture). The bone is broken but the skin is intact.*
* *Open fracture (compound fracture). The broken bone has come through the skin.*

Falls and accidents are causes. Bone tumors, metastatic cancer, and osteoporosis are other causes. Signs and symptoms of a fracture are:

* Pain
* Swelling
* Loss of function
* Limited or no movement of the part
* Movement where motion should not occur
* Deformity (the part is in an abnormal position)
* Bruising and skin color changes at the fracture site
* Bleeding (internal or external)

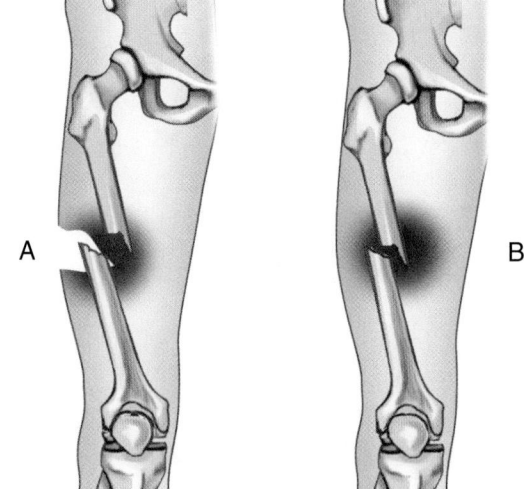

Fig. 41-11 A, Open fracture. **B,** Closed fracture.

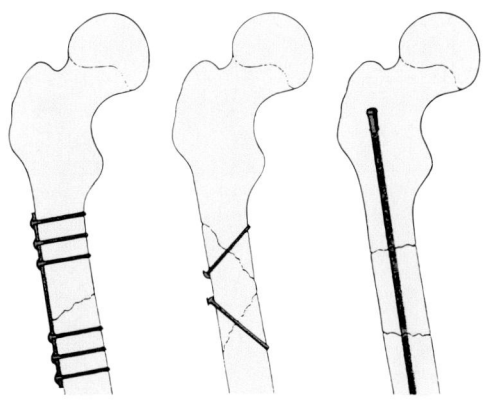

Fig. 41-12 Devices used for open reduction of a fracture.

For healing, bone ends are brought into and held in normal position. This is called *reduction* and *fixation:*

* *Closed reduction and external fixation.* The bone is moved back into place. The bone is not exposed.
* *Open reduction and internal fixation.* This requires surgery. The bone is exposed and moved into alignment. Nails, rods, pins, screws, plates, or wires keep the bone in place (Fig. 41-12).

After reduction, the bone ends must not move. The person has a cast or traction. Splints, walking boots, and external fixators also are used (Fig. 41-13, p. 690).

See *Focus on Children and Older Persons: Fractures,* p. 690.

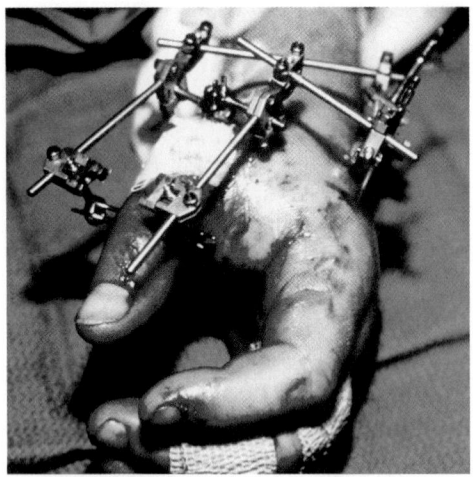

Fig. 41-13 External fixator.

Casts. Casts are made of plaster of Paris, plastic, or fiberglass (Fig. 41-14). Before casting, the part is protected with stockinette or cotton padding. Moistened cast rolls are wrapped around the part. Plastic and fiberglass casts dry quickly. A plaster of Paris cast dries in 24 to 48 hours. It is odorless, white, and shiny when dry. When wet, it is gray and cool and has a musty smell. The nurse may ask you to assist with care (Box 41-6).

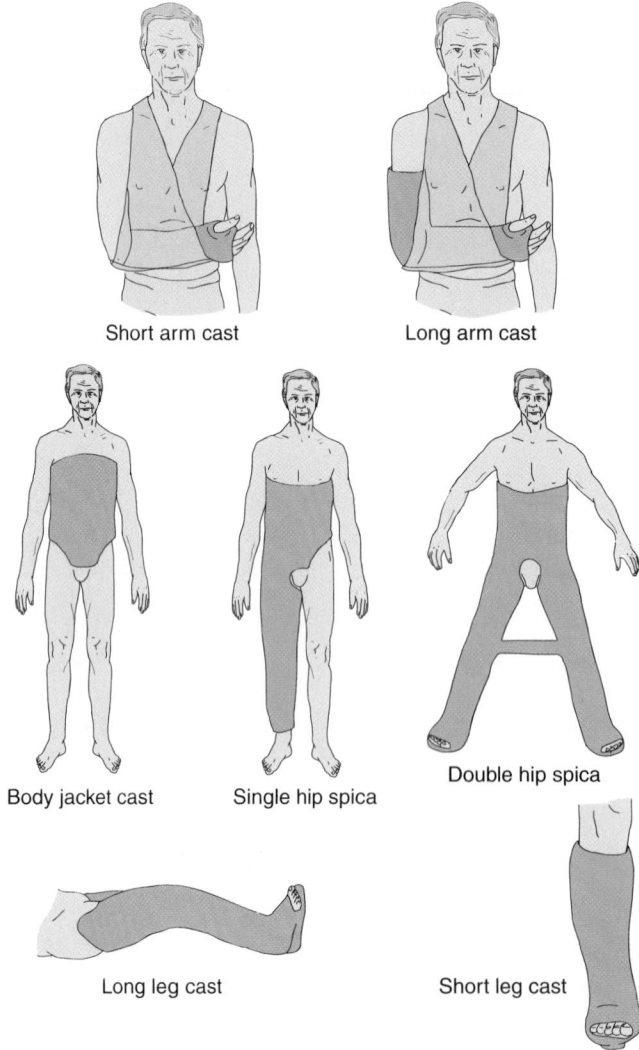

Short arm cast

Long arm cast

Body jacket cast

Single hip spica

Double hip spica

Long leg cast

Short leg cast

Fig. 41-14 Common casts.

BOX 41-6 RULES FOR CAST CARE

- Do not cover the cast with blankets, plastic, or other material. A cast gives off heat as it dries. Covers prevent the escape of heat. Burns can occur if heat cannot escape.
- Turn the person every 2 hours or as directed. All cast surfaces need exposure to air. Turning promotes even drying.
- Do not place a wet cast on a hard surface. It flattens the cast. The cast must keep its shape. Use pillows to support the entire length of the cast (Fig. 41-15).
- Support the wet cast with your palms to turn and position the person (Fig. 41-16). Fingertips can dent the cast. The dents can cause pressure areas and skin breakdown.
- Report rough cast edges. The nurse needs to cover the cast edges with tape.
- Keep the cast dry. A wet cast loses its shape. Some casts are near the perineal area. The nurse may apply a waterproof material around the perineal area after the cast dries.
- Do not let the person insert anything into the cast. Itching under the cast causes an intense desire to scratch. Items used for scratching (pencils, coat hangers, knitting needles, back scratchers, and so on) can open the skin. Infection is a risk. Scratching items can wrinkle the stockinette or cotton padding. Or they can be lost into the cast. Both can cause pressure and skin breakdown.

- Elevate a casted arm or leg on pillows. This reduces swelling.
- Have enough help to turn and re-position the person. Plaster casts are heavy and awkward. Balance is lost easily.
- Position the person as directed.
- Follow the care plan for elimination needs. Some persons use a fracture pan.
- Report these signs and symptoms at once:
  - *Pain*—pressure ulcer, poor circulation, nerve damage
  - *Swelling and a tight cast*—reduced blood flow to the part
  - *Pale skin*—reduced blood flow to the part
  - *Cyanosis (bluish skin color)*—reduced blood flow to the part
  - *Odor*—infection
  - *Inability to move the fingers or toes*—pressure on a nerve
  - *Numbness*—pressure on a nerve, reduced blood flow to the part
  - *Temperature changes*—cool skin means poor circulation; hot skin means inflammation
  - *Drainage on or under the cast*—infection or bleeding
  - *Chills, fever, nausea, and vomiting*—infection
- Complete a safety check before leaving the room. (See the inside of the front book cover.)

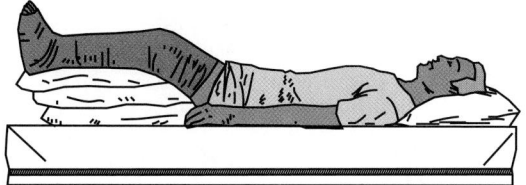

Fig. 41-15 Pillows support the entire length of the wet cast.

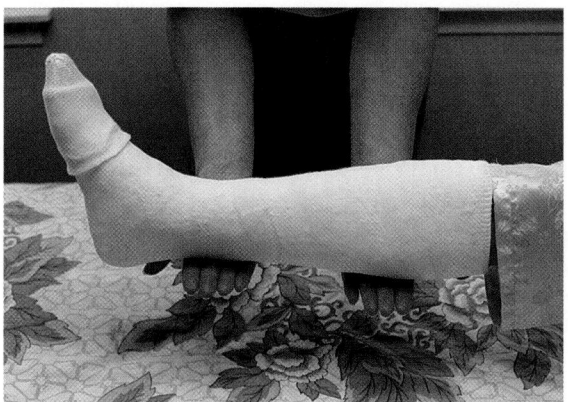

Fig. 41-16 The cast is supported with the palms.

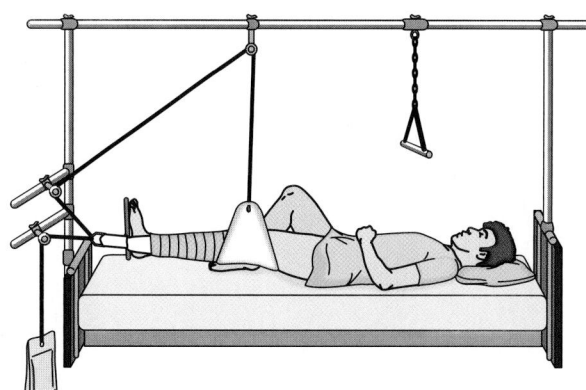

Fig. 41-17 Traction set-up. Note the weights, pulleys, and ropes.

Traction. With traction, a steady pull from two directions keeps the bone in place. Traction also is used for muscle spasms and to correct deformities or contractures. Weights, ropes, and pulleys are used (Fig. 41-17). Traction is applied to the neck, arms, legs, or pelvis.

Skin traction is applied to the skin. Boots, wraps, tape, or splints are used. Weights are attached to the device (see Fig. 41-17). For *skeletal traction*, wires or pins are inserted through the bone (Fig. 41-18, p. 692). For cervical traction, tongs are applied to the skull (Fig. 41-19, p. 692). Weights are attached to the device.

To assist with the person's care, see Box 41-7, p. 692.

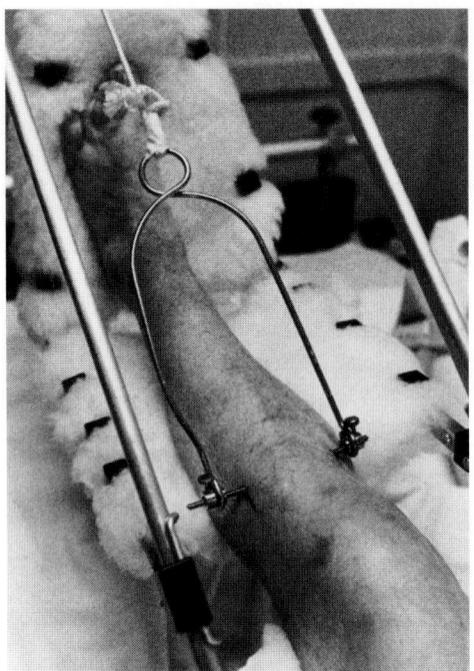

Fig. 41-18 Skeletal traction is attached to the bone.

Hip Fractures. Fractured hips are common in older persons (Fig. 41-20). Older women are at risk. Healing is slower in older people. Slow healing and other health problems affect the person's condition and care.

Post-operative problems present life-threatening risks. They include respiratory complications, urinary tract infections, and thrombi (blood clots) in the leg veins. Pressure ulcers, constipation, and confusion are other risks.

The fracture requires internal fixation (p. 689). Some hip fractures require partial or total hip replacement. Adduction, internal rotation, external rotation, and severe hip flexion are avoided after surgery. Rehabilitation is usually needed. If home care is not possible, the person needs subacute or long-term care. Recovery can take 6 months. Some persons return home after rehabilitation. Others stay in nursing centers. See Box 41-8 for the care required for a hip fracture.

See *Focus on Long-Term Care and Home Care: Hip Fractures.*

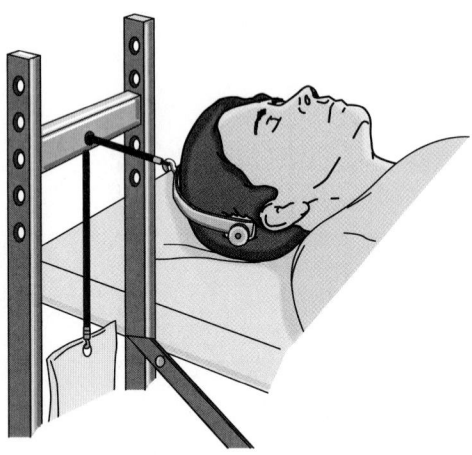

Fig. 41-19 Tongs are inserted into the skull for cervical spine traction.

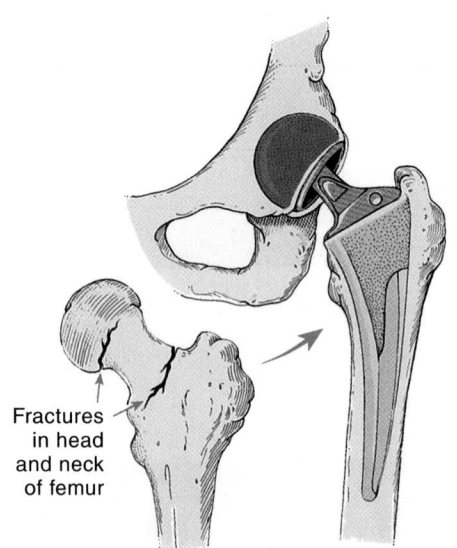

Fractures in head and neck of femur

Fig. 41-20 Hip fracture repaired with a prosthesis.

BOX 41-7	**CARING FOR PERSONS IN TRACTION**

- Keep the person in good alignment.
- Do not remove the traction.
- Keep the weights off the floor. Weights must hang freely from the traction set-up (see Fig. 41-17).
- Do not add or remove weights.
- Check for frayed ropes. Report fraying at once.
- Perform ROM exercises for the uninvolved joints as directed.
- Position the person as directed. Usually only the supine position is allowed. Slight turning may be allowed.

- Provide the fracture pan for elimination.
- Give skin care as directed.
- Put bottom linens on the bed from the top down. The person uses a trapeze to raise the body off the bed.
- Check pin, nail, wire, or tong sites for redness, drainage, and odors. Report observations at once.
- Observe for the signs and symptoms listed under cast care (see Box 41-6). Report them at once.
- Complete a safety check before leaving the room. (See the inside of the front book cover.)

BOX 41-8	CARE OF THE PERSON WITH A HIP FRACTURE

- Give good skin care. Skin breakdown can be rapid.
- Prevent pressure ulcers.
- Prevent wound, skin, and urinary tract infections.
- Encourage incentive spirometry and deep-breathing and coughing exercises as directed.
- Turn and position the person as directed. Turning and positioning depend on the type of fracture and the surgery. Usually the person is not positioned on the operative side.
- Prevent external rotation of the hip. Use trochanter rolls, pillows, or sandbags.
- Keep the leg abducted at all times. Use pillows (Fig. 41-21) or a hip abduction wedge (abductor splint). Do not exercise the affected leg.
- Provide a straight-back chair with armrests. The person needs a high, firm seat.
- Place the chair on the unaffected side.
- Use assist devices to move, turn, re-position, and transfer the person.
- Do not let the person stand on the operated leg unless allowed by the doctor.
- Elevate the leg following the care plan. With an internal fixation device, the leg is not elevated when the person sits in a chair. Elevating the leg puts strain on the device.
- Apply elastic stockings to prevent thrombi (blood clots) in the legs.
- Remind the person not to cross his or her legs.
- Assist with walking according to the care plan. The person uses a walker or crutches.
- Follow measures to protect the hip. See Box 41-5 and Figure 41-10.
- Practice safety measures to prevent falls.
- Complete a safety check before leaving the room. (See the inside of the front book cover.)

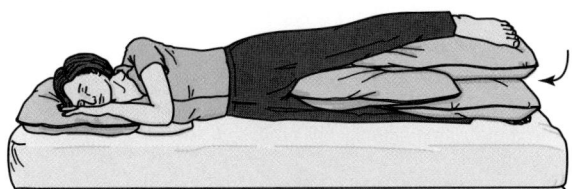

Fig. 41-21 Pillows are used to keep the hip in abduction.

FOCUS ON LONG-TERM CARE AND HOME CARE

Hip Fractures

Home Care

The prosthesis can dislocate (move out of place) with adduction, internal rotation, and severe hip flexion. Such movements are avoided. See Box 41-8.

An occupational therapist helps the person learn self-care activities. Self-help devices are used for dressing and bathing.

A physical therapist helps the person learn muscle-strengthening exercises. A walker is usually needed.

Loss of Limb

An *amputation is the removal of all or part of an extremity*. Most amputations involve a lower extremity. Severe injuries, tumors, severe infection, gangrene, and vascular disorders are common causes. Diabetes can cause vascular changes leading to amputation.

Gangrene is a condition in which there is death of tissue. Causes include infection, injuries, and vascular disorders. Blood flow is affected. Tissues do not get enough oxygen and nutrients. Poisonous substances and wastes build up in the tissues. Tissue death results. Tissues become black, cold, and shriveled (Fig. 41-22). Surgery is needed to remove dead tissue. If untreated, gangrene spreads throughout the body. For example, in diabetes the toes are often affected first. If the toes are not removed, gangrene spreads up the foot and leg. Gangrene can cause death.

Much support is needed. The amputation affects the person's life. Body image, appearance, daily activities, moving about, and work are some areas affected. Fear, shock, anger, denial, and depression are common emotions.

The person is fitted with a prosthesis—an artificial replacement for a missing body part (Fig. 41-23). The stump

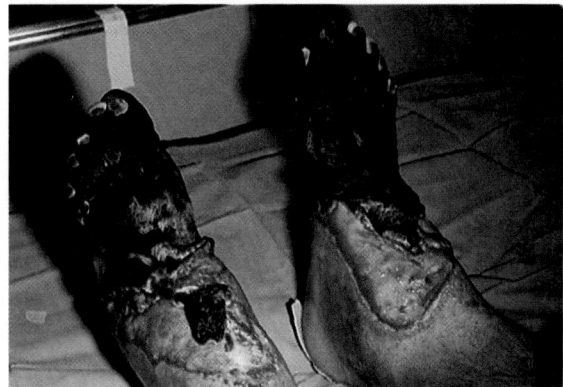

Fig. 41-22 Gangrene.

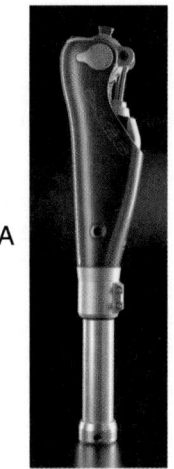
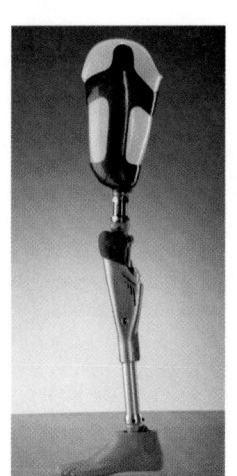

A   B

Fig. 41-23 Leg prostheses. **A,** Above-the-knee prosthesis. **B,** Below-the-knee prosthesis.

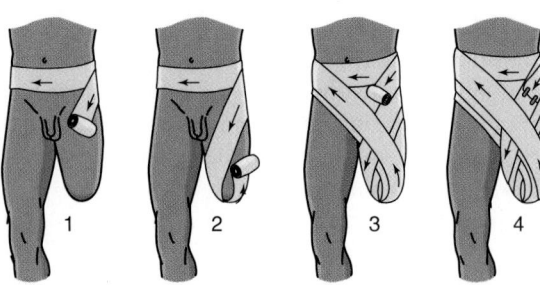

Fig. 41-24 A mid-thigh amputation is bandaged to shrink and shape the stump.

is conditioned for a proper fit. This involves shrinking and shaping the stump into a cone shape with bandages (Fig. 41-24). Exercises are done to strengthen other limbs. The person learns to use the prosthesis.

The person may feel that the limb is still there. Aching, tingling, and itching are common sensations. Or the person complains of pain in the amputated part *(phantom pain)*. This is a normal reaction. It may occur for a short time or for many years.

Lower limb amputations are common in older persons. Because of other health problems, many older persons cannot use a prosthesis. They need to use wheelchairs. After amputation, most older persons need long-term care on a temporary or permanent basis.

FOCUS ON PRIDE

The Person, Family, and Yourself

Personal and Professional Responsibility

Nervous system and musculo-skeletal system disorders affect the whole person. Social, psychological, physical, and spiritual needs must be addressed. You have a great impact on the person's quality of care. Provide care that focuses on the person as a whole.

Rights and Respect

With some disorders, the person does not improve. Function does not return. For some, function declines over time. The family watches the person struggle to move, perform ADL, or live. The person, family, and caregivers need support and encouragement. Treat the person with dignity, respect, and kindness.

Independence and Social Interaction

The disorders in this chapter affect the person's independence. The person relies on family and caregivers for support and daily needs. The person may feel useless, angry, and depressed. To promote independence:
- Focus on the person's abilities, not disabilities.
- Tell the person when you notice progress.
- Allow personal choice.
- Encourage the person for trying.

Delegation and Teamwork

Providing care for persons often requires teamwork. Work done as a team is safer and more time efficient than work done alone. Value your team members. Thank them for their help. Offer to help others. Take pride in being a good team member.

Ethics and Laws

The following is a real case in which two nursing assistants were accused of negligence.

A patient and her husband filed suit in a Louisiana court against a hospital and two nursing aides. The patient had a total hip replacement in March 1994. The patient claimed that the following occurred while she was recovering from surgery.
- *Two ladies came into her room to turn her.*
- *The ladies "raised her up high and then one of the ladies let go of the pad they were using to turn her and they dropped her."*
- *She was in severe pain when she was dropped and continued to have pain.*
- *She could not do any physical therapy or walk while in the hospital.*
- *She did not want to be discharged because of the severe pain after being dropped.*

During a May 1994 office visit, the doctor noted that the patient had an abnormal gait. An x-ray showed that the hip prosthesis was dislocated. Two days later she had another surgery. The patient claimed that the dislocated hip was the result of negligence by the two nursing aides.

The nursing aides would testify that:
- *They were in the process of transferring the patient from an orthopedic chair to bed.*
- *The hand of one nursing aide slipped. She let go of the sheet while they were pulling the patient onto the bed.*
- *The patient was already on the bed when the hand slipped.*
- *The patient was "not up in the air or dropped."*
- *The patient did not voice any complaints that she was hurting from the transfer.*

The doctor testified that:
- *The patient was "always in pain in all parts of her body before and after the first hip surgery."*
- *The patient did not tell him about being dropped until she was in the hospital for the second surgery.*
- *When she told him of the incident, she said that:*
  - *"Within 24 hours of the first hip surgery, the bed dropped about two feet."*
  - *She had "sudden onset of pain in her hip."*
- *She was complaining of pain before and after the bed dropped.*
- *The dislocated hip may have resulted from the hip prosthesis design.*
- *After the first surgery, physical therapy records showed that the patient was able to:*
  - *Walk with a walker.*
  - *Do several exercises.*

The trial judge ruled in favor of the hospital and the nursing aides. The lawsuit was dismissed. The judge ruled that the patient did not prove that the dislocation was caused by nursing aides. The decision was appealed to a higher court. The Appellate Court reached the same decision.

(F. Guillot wife of /and R. Guillot v East Jefferson General Hospital, Jane Doe and Mary Doe, 2003.)

Mistakes occur. Accidents happen. Mistakes do not always mean negligence. To be found negligent, evidence must show that you did not act in a reasonable and careful manner. And as a result, the person or the person's property was harmed.

Always work carefully. If an accident occurs, notify the nurse. Take pride in being honest and accountable.

Circle the BEST answer.

1 A stroke also is called
   a A cerebrovascular accident
   b Aphasia
   c Hemiplegia
   d A transient ischemic attack

2 Warning signs of stroke occur
   a With exertion
   b Suddenly
   c Between the ages of 20 and 40
   d At rest

3 A person had a stroke. Which should you question?
   a Semi-Fowler's position
   b Range-of-motion exercises every 2 hours
   c Turn, re-position, and give skin care every 2 hours
   d Bed in the highest horizontal position

4 A person has Parkinson's disease. Which is *false*?
   a The part of the brain controlling muscle movements is affected.
   b Mental function is affected first.
   c Tremors, slow movements, and a shuffling gait occur.
   d The person needs protection.

5 Parkinson's disease
   a Can be cured with drugs
   b Can be cured with surgery
   c Is a slow, progressive disorder
   d Progresses rapidly

6 A person has multiple sclerosis. Which is *false*?
   a There is no cure.
   b Only voluntary muscles are affected.
   c Symptoms begin in young adulthood.
   d Over time, the person depends on others for care.

7 A person has multiple sclerosis. Signs, symptoms, and the care required depend on the area of damage.
   a True
   b False

8 Amyotrophic lateral sclerosis affects nerve cells that control
   a Involuntary muscles   c The brain
   b Voluntary muscles   d The lungs

9 A person has amyotrophic lateral sclerosis. Which should you question?
   a Range-of-motion exercises
   b Dysphagia diet
   c Walker for mobility
   d Measures to prevent confusion

10 Persons with head or spinal cord injuries require
   a Rehabilitation   c Long-term care
   b Speech therapy   d Chemotherapy

11 A person has tetraplegia from a spinal cord injury. Which should you question?
   a Keep the bed in the low position.
   b Assist with active ROM exercises.
   c Follow the bowel training program.
   d Turn and re-position every hour.

12 Autonomic dysreflexia occurs
   a After spinal cord injures
   b In Parkinson's disease
   c With Lou Gehrig's disease
   d Following stroke

13 Autonomic dysreflexia is usually triggered by
   a High blood sugar
   b High blood pressure
   c A full bladder
   d A virus

14 Arthritis affects
   a The joints
   b The bones
   c The muscles
   d The hips and knees

15 A person has arthritis. Care includes the following *except*
   a Preventing contractures
   b Range-of-motion exercises
   c A cast or traction
   d Assisting with ADL

16 A person had hip replacement surgery. Which should you question?
   a Provide a chair with a low seat.
   b Do not cross the legs.
   c Keep a hip abduction wedge between the legs.
   d Provide a long-handled brush for bathing.

17 A person with osteoporosis is at risk for
   a Fractures
   b An amputation
   c Phantom pain
   d Paralysis

18 A cast needs to dry. Which is *false*?
   a The cast is covered with blankets and plastic.
   b The person is turned so the cast dries evenly.
   c The entire cast is supported with pillows.
   d The cast is supported by the palms when lifted.

19 A person has a cast. You report the following at once *except*
   a Pain, numbness, or inability to move the fingers
   b Chills, fever, nausea, or vomiting
   c Odor, cyanosis, or temperature changes of the skin
   d Pulse rate of 76 and a respiratory rate of 18

20 A person is in traction. Care includes the following *except*
   a Performing ROM exercises as directed
   b Keeping the weights off the floor
   c Removing the weights if the person is uncomfortable
   d Giving skin care at frequent intervals

21 After a hip pinning, the operated leg is
   a Abducted at all times
   b Adducted at all times
   c Externally rotated at all times
   d Flexed at all times

22 After an amputation, the person
   a Is fitted with a prosthesis
   b Needs a wheelchair
   c Has quadriplegia
   d Needs arthroplasty

Answers to these questions are on p. 834.

42 Cardiovascular, Respiratory, and Lymphatic Disorders

OBJECTIVES

- Define the key terms and key abbreviations listed in this chapter.
- Describe congenital heart defects.
- Describe hypertension, its risk factors, signs and symptoms, complications, and treatment.
- Describe coronary artery disease, its risk factors, and complications.
- Describe cardiac rehabilitation.
- Describe angina, its signs and symptoms, and treatment.
- Describe myocardial infarction, its signs and symptoms, and treatment.
- Describe heart failure, its signs and symptoms, and treatment.
- Explain dysrhythmia, its signs and symptoms, and treatment.
- Describe chronic obstructive pulmonary disease, its signs and symptoms, and treatment.

- Describe asthma, its signs and symptoms, and treatment.
- Describe sleep apnea, its signs and symptoms, and treatment.
- Explain the difference between a cold and influenza.
- Explain how influenza is treated.
- Describe pneumonia, its signs and symptoms, and treatment.
- Describe tuberculosis, its signs and symptoms, and treatment.
- Describe lymphedema, its signs and symptoms, and treatment.
- Describe lymphoma, its signs and symptoms, and treatment.
- Explain how to promote PRIDE in the person, the family, and yourself.

KEY TERMS

congenital To be born with *(congenitus)*
dysrhythmia An abnormal *(dys)* heart rhythm *(rhythmia)*
high blood pressure See "hypertension"
hypertension The systolic pressure is 140 mm Hg or higher *(hyper)*, or the diastolic pressure is 90 mm Hg or higher; high blood pressure
lymphedema A buildup of lymph in the tissues causing edema (swelling)

pre-hypertension When the systolic pressure is between 120 and 139 mm Hg, or the diastolic pressure is between 80 and 89 mm Hg
sleep apnea Pauses *(a)* in breathing *(pnea)* that occur during sleep

KEY ABBREVIATIONS

CAD	Coronary artery disease	**mm Hg**	Millimeters of mercury
CDC	Centers for Disease Control and Prevention	**O₂**	Oxygen
CO₂	Carbon dioxide	**TB**	Tuberculosis
COPD	Chronic obstructive pulmonary disease	**WBC**	White blood cell
MI	Myocardial infarction		

Cardiovascular and respiratory system disorders are leading causes of death in the United States. Many people have these disorders. Disorders also occur in the lymphatic system. Understanding the disorders in this chapter gives meaning to the care you give.

CARDIOVASCULAR DISORDERS

The circulatory (cardiovascular) system delivers blood to the body's cells. Problems occur in the heart or blood vessels. See Chapter 33 for circulatory ulcers.

See *Body Structure and Function Review: The Circulatory System.*

See *Focus on Children and Older Persons: Cardiovascular Disorders,* p. 698.

BODY STRUCTURE AND FUNCTION REVIEW: THE CIRCULATORY SYSTEM

The circulatory system is made up of the *blood, heart,* and *blood vessels.* The heart pumps blood through the blood vessels.

The Blood
The blood consists of blood cells and *plasma.* Plasma is mostly water. It carries blood cells to other body cells. Plasma also carries substances (food, hormones, and chemicals) that cells need to function.

Red blood cells (RBCs) are called *erythrocytes. Hemoglobin* in the RBCs gives blood its red color. As RBCs circulate through the lungs, hemoglobin picks up oxygen (O_2). Hemoglobin carries O_2 to the cells. When blood is bright red, hemoglobin in the RBCs is filled with O_2. As blood circulates through the body, O_2 is given to the cells. Cells release carbon dioxide (CO_2) (a waste product). It is picked up by the hemoglobin. RBCs filled with CO_2 make the blood look dark red.

Blood also contains *white blood cells (WBCs)* and *platelets (thrombocytes).* WBCs are called *leukocytes.* They protect the body against infection. Platelets are needed for blood clotting.

The Heart
The heart is a muscle. It pumps blood through the blood vessels to the tissues and cells. The heart has four chambers (Fig. 42-1). Upper chambers receive blood and are called *atria.* The *right atrium* receives blood from body tissues. The *left atrium* receives blood from the lungs. Lower chambers are called *ventricles.* Ventricles pump blood. The *right ventricle* pumps blood to the lungs for O_2. The *left ventricle* pumps blood to all parts of the body.

Valves are between the atria and ventricles (see Fig. 42-1). The valves allow blood flow in one direction. They prevent blood from flowing back into the atria from the ventricles. The *tricuspid valve* is between the right atrium and the right ventricle. The *mitral valve (bicuspid valve)* is between the left atrium and left ventricle.

Heart action has two phases:
- *Diastole.* It is the resting phase. Heart chambers fill with blood.
- *Systole.* It is the working phase. The heart contracts. Blood is pumped through the blood vessels when the heart contracts.

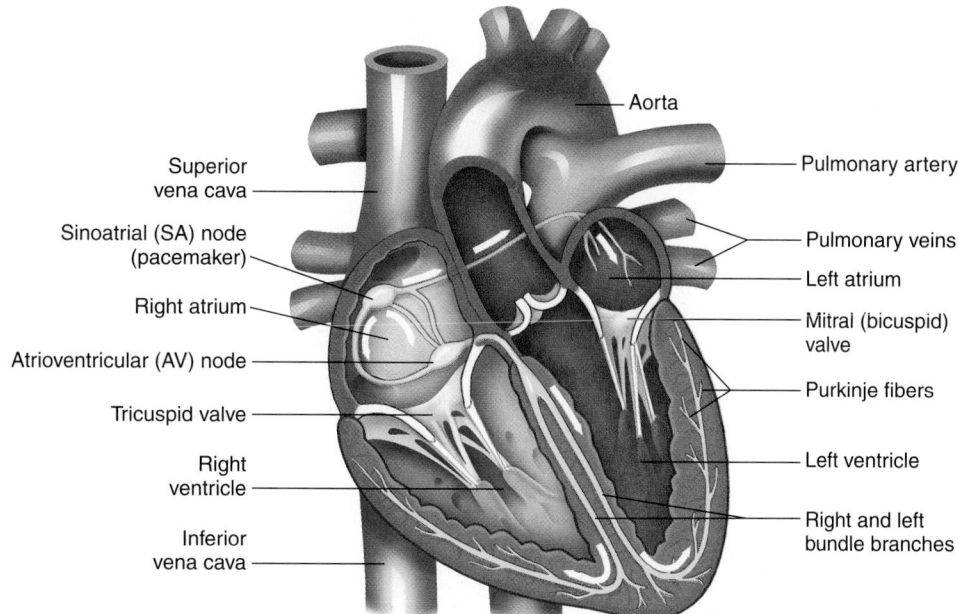

Fig. 42-1 Structures of the heart. Chambers and major vessels that carry blood full of oxygen are shown in red. Chambers and major vessels that carry blood low in oxygen are shown in blue. Valves are white. The heart's electrical system is yellow.

Continued

BODY STRUCTURE AND FUNCTION REVIEW: THE CIRCULATORY SYSTEM—cont'd

The Heart—cont'd

The heart has its own electrical system that stimulates the heart to contract. The electrical signal begins in the sinoatrial (SA) node (see Fig. 42-1). The SA node sets the pace of the heart. It stimulates the heart to beat at 60 to 100 beats per minute. The electrical signal spreads through the heart causing the heart to contract.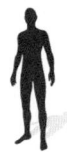

The Blood Vessels

Blood flows to body tissues and cells through the blood vessels. There are three groups of blood vessels: arteries, capillaries, and veins (Fig. 42-2).

Arteries carry blood away from the heart. Arterial blood is rich in O_2. The *aorta* (see Fig. 42-2) is the largest artery. It receives blood directly from the left ventricle. The aorta branches into other arteries that carry blood to all parts of the body. These arteries branch into smaller parts within the tissues. The smallest branch of an artery is an *arteriole*.

Arterioles connect to *capillaries*. Capillaries are very tiny blood vessels. Food, O_2, and other substances pass from capillaries into the cells. The capillaries pick up waste products (including CO_2) from the cells. Veins carry waste products back to the heart.

Veins return blood to the heart. They connect to the capillaries by *venules*. Venules are small veins. Venules branch together to form veins. The many veins also branch together as they near the heart to form two main veins—the *inferior vena cava* and the *superior vena cava* (see Fig. 42-2). Both empty into the right atrium. The inferior vena cava carries blood from the legs and trunk. The superior vena cava carries blood from the head and arms. Venous blood is dark red. It has little O_2 and a lot of CO_2.

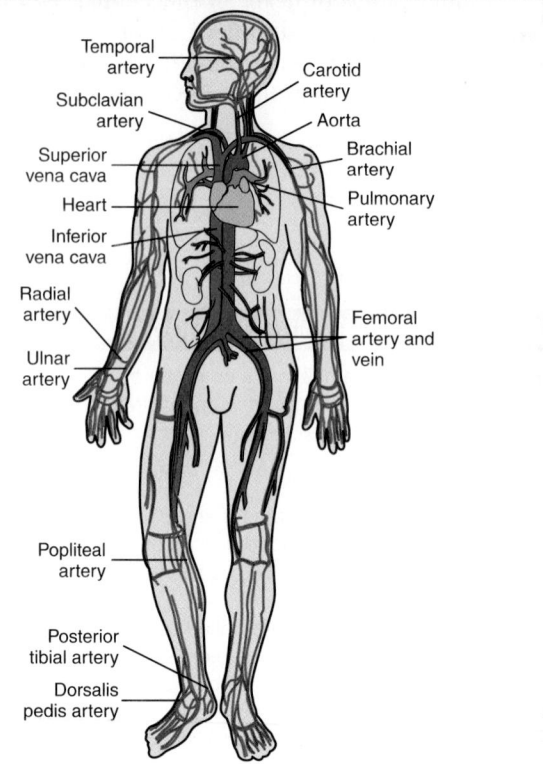

Fig. 42-2 Arterial and venous systems. Arterial system is red. Venous system is blue.

FOCUS ON CHILDREN AND OLDER PERSONS

Cardiovascular Disorders

Children

Some babies are born with congenital heart defects. (*Congenital* comes from the Latin word *congenitus*. *It means to be born with.*) Defects occur during pregnancy as the baby's heart develops. One or more defects can occur in:

* A part of the heart
* The heart valves
* The blood vessels near the heart
  Depending on the defect, blood flow:
* Slows down.
* Goes in the wrong direction.
* Goes to the wrong place.
* Is blocked completely.
  In most cases, the cause is unknown. Risk factors include:
* Heredity. A parent with a congenital heart defect is at risk of having a child with one.
* The mother had a viral infection during pregnancy. German measles (rubella) is a common cause.
* The mother has diabetes.
* The mother took some types of drugs during pregnancy.
* The mother had repeated exposure to some chemicals or x-rays during pregnancy.
* The mother used alcohol or street drugs during pregnancy.

The common signs of congenital heart defects are:

* Heart sounds other than "lub-dub" when you take an apical pulse.
* A bluish tint to the skin, lips, and fingernails.
* Fast breathing or shortness of breath.
* Poor feeding. The infant tires easily while nursing.
* Poor weight gain.
* Tiring easily during exercise or activity. Be alert for this sign in older children.

Some heart defects are found during pregnancy. Others are found when the child is very young. Some defects are not diagnosed until the child is older. Treatment may involve:

* Drugs.
* Correcting the defect by using a catheter. A catheter is inserted into a blood vessel and then into the heart.
* Surgery.
* A heart transplant.

With successful treatment, many children with heart defects grow into healthy adults. Some need life-long treatment.

Factors You *Cannot* Change
- Age—45 years or older for men; 55 years or older for women
- Gender—men are at greater risk than women; risk increases for women after menopause
- Race—African-Americans are at greater risk
- Family history—tends to run in families

Factors You *Can* Change
- Being over-weight
- Stress
- Smoking and tobacco use
- High-salt diet
- Excessive alcohol
- Lack of exercise
- Atherosclerosis
- Blood pressure
- High blood cholesterol
- Diabetes

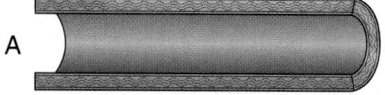

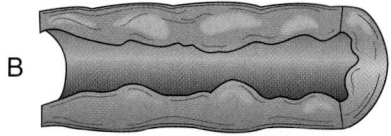

Fig. 42-3 A, Normal artery. **B,** Plaque on the artery wall in atherosclerosis.

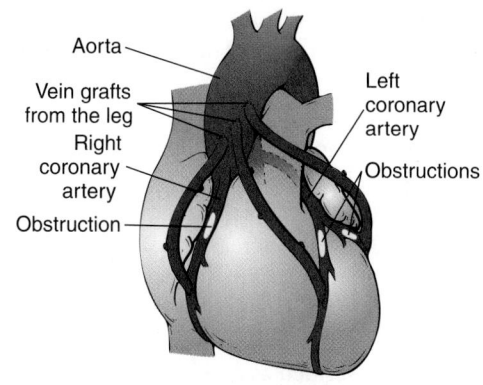

Triple bypass

Fig. 42-4 Coronary artery bypass surgery.

Hypertension

With *hypertension (high blood pressure), the systolic pressure is 140 mm Hg (millimeters of mercury) or higher* (hyper). *Or the diastolic pressure is 90 mm Hg or higher.* The resting blood pressure is too high. Such measurements must occur several times. *Pre-hypertension is when the systolic pressure is between 120 and 139 mm Hg, or the diastolic pressure is between 80 and 89 mm Hg.* Pre-hypertension will likely develop into hypertension in the future. Most people have hypertension some time during their lives. See Box 42-1 for risk factors.

Narrowed blood vessels are a common cause. The heart pumps with more force to move blood through narrowed vessels. Kidney disorders, head injuries, some pregnancy problems, and adrenal gland tumors are causes.

A person can be unaware of hypertension for many years. That is why hypertension is called "the silent killer." Hypertension is found when blood pressure is measured. Signs and symptoms develop over time. Headache, blurred vision, dizziness, and nose bleeds occur. Hypertension can lead to stroke, hardening of the arteries, heart attack, heart failure, kidney failure, and blindness.

Life-style changes can lower blood pressure. A diet low in fat and salt, a healthy weight, and regular exercise are needed. No smoking is allowed. Alcohol and caffeine are limited. Managing stress and sleeping well also lower blood pressure. Certain drugs lower blood pressure.

Coronary Artery Disease

The coronary arteries are in the heart. They supply the heart with blood. In coronary artery disease (CAD), the coronary arteries become hardened and narrow. One or all are affected. The heart muscle gets less blood and oxygen (O_2). CAD also is called *coronary heart disease* and *heart disease.*

The most common cause is *atherosclerosis* (Fig. 42-3). Plaque—made up of cholesterol, fat, and other substances—collects on artery walls. The narrowed arteries block blood flow. Blockage may be total or partial. Blood clots can form along the plaque and block blood flow.

The major complications of CAD are angina, myocardial infarction (heart attack), irregular heartbeats, and sudden death. The more risk factors (see Box 42-1), the greater the chance of CAD and its complications.

CAD can be treated. Treatment goals are to:
- Relieve symptoms (see "Angina," p. 700).
- Slow or stop atherosclerosis.
- Lower the risk of blood clots.
- Widen or bypass clogged arteries.
- Reduce cardiac events (see "Angina" and "Myocardial Infarction," p. 700).

CAD requires life-style changes. The person must quit smoking, exercise, and reduce stress. A healthy diet is needed to lower blood pressure, lower blood cholesterol, and maintain a healthy weight. If over-weight, the person must lose weight.

Some persons need drugs to decrease the heart's work-load and relieve symptoms. Other drugs are given to prevent a heart attack or sudden death. Drugs can delay the need for medical and surgical procedures that open or bypass diseased arteries (Fig. 42-4).

Cardiac Rehabilitation. CAD complications may require cardiac rehabilitation (cardiac rehab). The cardiac rehab team includes doctors (the person's doctor, a heart specialist, a heart surgeon), nurses, exercise specialists, physical and occupational therapists, dietitians, and mental health professionals.

Cardiac rehab has two parts:

* Exercise training. The person learns to exercise safely. Exercises are done to strengthen muscles and improve stamina (staying power, endurance). The exercise plan is based on the person's abilities, needs, and interests.
* Education, counseling, and training. The person learns about:
  * His or her heart condition
  * How to reduce the risk of future problems
  * How to adjust to a new life-style
  * How to deal with fears about the future

Angina

Angina *(pain)* is chest pain from reduced blood flow to part of the heart muscle (myocardium). It occurs when the heart needs more O_2. Normally blood flow to the heart increases when O_2 needs increase. Exertion, a heavy meal, stress, and excitement increase the heart's need for O_2. So does smoking and very hot or cold temperatures. In CAD, narrowed vessels prevent increased blood flow.

Chest pain is described as a tightness, pressure, squeezing, or burning in the chest (Fig. 42-5). Pain can occur in the shoulders, arms, neck, jaw, or back. Pain in the jaw, neck, and down one or both arms is common. The person may be pale, feel faint, and perspire. Dyspnea is common. Nausea, fatigue, and weakness may occur. Some persons complain of "gas" or indigestion. Rest often relieves symptoms in 3 to 15 minutes. Rest reduces the heart's need for O_2. Therefore normal blood flow is achieved. Heart damage is prevented.

Besides rest, a nitroglycerin tablet is taken when angina occurs. It is placed under the tongue. There it dissolves and is rapidly absorbed into the bloodstream. Tablets are kept within the person's reach at all times. The person takes a tablet and then tells the nurse. Some persons have nitroglycerin patches. The nurse applies and removes them.

Things that cause angina are avoided. These include over-exertion, heavy meals and over-eating, and emotional stress. The person stays indoors during cold weather or during hot, humid weather. Cardiac rehabilitation is helpful.

See "Coronary Artery Disease" (p. 699) for the treatment of angina. The goal is to increase blood flow to the heart. Doing so may prevent or lower the risk of heart attack and death. Chest pain lasting longer than a few minutes and not relieved by rest and nitroglycerin may signal heart attack. The person needs emergency care.

Myocardial Infarction

Myocardial refers to the *heart muscle*. *Infarction* means *tissue death*. With myocardial infarction (MI), part of the heart muscle dies. Sudden cardiac death *(sudden cardiac arrest)* can occur (Chapter 51).

MI also is called:

* Heart attack
* Acute myocardial infarction (AMI)
* Acute coronary syndrome (ACS)
* Coronary
* Coronary thrombosis
* Coronary occlusion

In MI, blood flow to the heart muscle is suddenly blocked. A thrombus (blood clot) blocks blood flow in an artery with atherosclerosis. The damaged area may be small or large (Fig. 42-6).

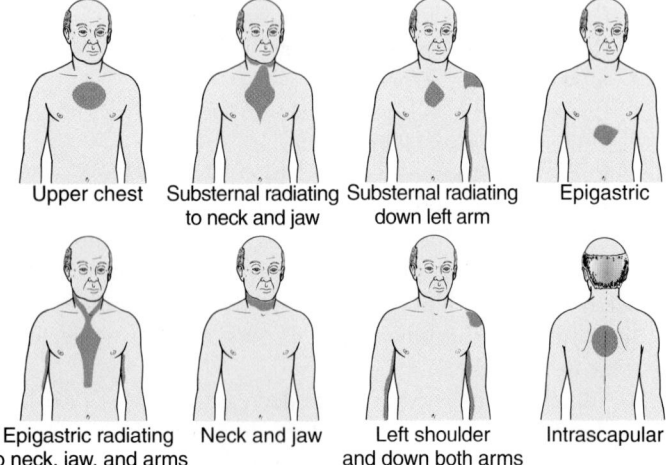

Upper chest   Substernal radiating to neck and jaw   Substernal radiating down left arm   Epigastric

Epigastric radiating to neck, jaw, and arms   Neck and jaw   Left shoulder and down both arms   Intrascapular

Fig. 42-5 *Shaded areas* show where the pain of angina is located.

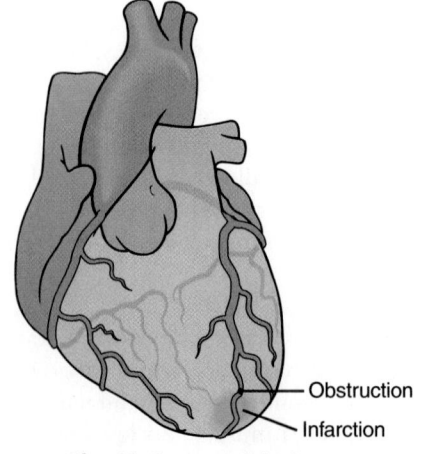

Obstruction

Infarction

Fig. 42-6 Myocardial infarction.

| BOX 42-2 | SIGNS AND SYMPTOMS OF MYOCARDIAL INFARCTION |

- Chest pain
  - Sudden, severe; usually on the left side
  - Described as crushing, stabbing, squeezing, or as someone sitting on the chest
  - More severe and lasts longer than angina
  - Not relieved by rest and nitroglycerin
- Pain or numbness in one or both arms, the back, neck, jaw, or stomach
- Indigestion or "heartburn"

- Dyspnea
- Nausea
- Dizziness
- Perspiration and cold, clammy skin
- Pallor or cyanosis
- Blood pressure: low
- Pulse: weak and irregular
- Fear, apprehension, and a feeling of doom

FOCUS ON LONG-TERM CARE AND HOME CARE
Myocardial Infarction

Home Care
Cardiac rehabilitation continues. The person may go to a gym, health club, or hospital fitness center. Some persons go to indoor malls for walking. Normal activities are increased slowly. The person returns to work with the doctor's approval.

CAD, angina, and previous MI are risk factors. See Box 42-2 for signs and symptoms. MI is an emergency. Efforts are made to:

- Relieve pain.
- Restore blood flow to the heart.
- Stabilize vital signs.
- Give O$_2$.
- Calm the person.
- Prevent death and life-threatening problems.

The person may need medical or surgical procedures to open or bypass the diseased artery. Cardiac rehabilitation is needed. The goals are to:

- Recover and resume normal activities.
- Prevent another MI.
- Prevent complications such as heart failure or sudden cardiac arrest.

See *Focus on Long-Term Care and Home Care: Myocardial Infarction.*

Heart Failure

Heart failure or congestive heart failure (CHF) occurs when the weakened heart cannot pump normally. Blood backs up. Tissue congestion occurs.

When the left side of the heart cannot pump blood normally, blood backs up into the lungs. Respiratory congestion occurs. The person has dyspnea, increased sputum, cough, and gurgling sounds in the lungs. The body does not get enough blood. Signs and symptoms occur from the effects on other organs. Poor blood flow to the brain causes confusion, dizziness, and fainting. The kidneys produce less urine. The skin is pale. Blood pressure falls.

When the right side of the heart cannot pump blood normally, blood backs up into the venous system. Feet and ankles swell. Neck veins bulge. Liver congestion affects liver function. The abdomen is congested with fluid. Less blood is pumped to the lungs. The left side of the heart receives less blood from the lungs. The left side has less blood to pump to the body. As with left-sided heart failure, organs receive less blood. The signs and symptoms of left-sided failure occur.

Pulmonary edema (fluid in the lungs) is a very severe form of heart failure. It is an emergency. The person can die.

A damaged or weak heart usually causes heart failure. CAD, MI, hypertension, diabetes, age, and irregular heart rhythms (p. 702) are common causes. So are damaged heart valves and kidney disease.

Drugs strengthen the heart. They also reduce the amount of fluid in the body. A sodium-controlled diet is ordered. Oxygen is given. Semi-Fowler's position is preferred for breathing. The person must reduce CAD risk factors. If acutely ill, the person needs hospital care.

You assist with these aspects of the person's care:

- Promoting rest and activity as ordered
- Measuring intake and output
- Measuring weight daily
- Assisting with pulse oximetry
- Restricting fluids as ordered
- Promoting a diet that is low in sodium, fat, and cholesterol
- Preventing skin breakdown and pressure ulcers
- Assisting with range-of-motion and other exercises
- Assisting with transfers and ambulation
- Assisting with self-care activities
- Maintaining good alignment
- Applying elastic stockings

Many older persons have heart failure. Skin breakdown is a risk. Tissue swelling, poor circulation, and fragile skin combine to increase the risk of pressure ulcers. Good skin care and regular position changes are needed.

Dysrhythmias

A *dysrhythmia is an abnormal* (dys) *heart rhythm* (rhythmia). The rhythm may be too fast, too slow, or irregular. Dysrhythmias are caused by changes in the heart's electrical system (see Figure 42-1). Changes may result from hypertension, CAD, MI, or heart failure. Weakening and changes in the heart muscle are other causes. So are drug and alcohol abuse, excess caffeine intake, and thyroid problems. Some drugs can cause dysrhythmias.

The person may feel dizzy or light-headed and have fluttering in the chest, chest pain, or dyspnea. The person may faint (Chapter 51). Some dysrhythmias are minor. Others are life-threatening.

Treatment depends on the type of dysrhythmia. Drugs may be given. A procedure may be needed:

- *Defibrillation* (Chapter 51) or *cardioversion*—an electrical shock is given to stop an abnormal rhythm.
- *Ablation*—areas of tissue in the heart sending abnormal electrical signals are destroyed.

Some abnormal rhythms are treated with a *pacemaker* (Fig. 42-7). This device monitors and regulates the heart's rhythm. The device is inserted under the skin near the heart. One or more wires (*leads*) are placed in the heart muscle and connected to the pacemaker. The pacemaker sends signals through the leads to stimulate the heart to beat normally.

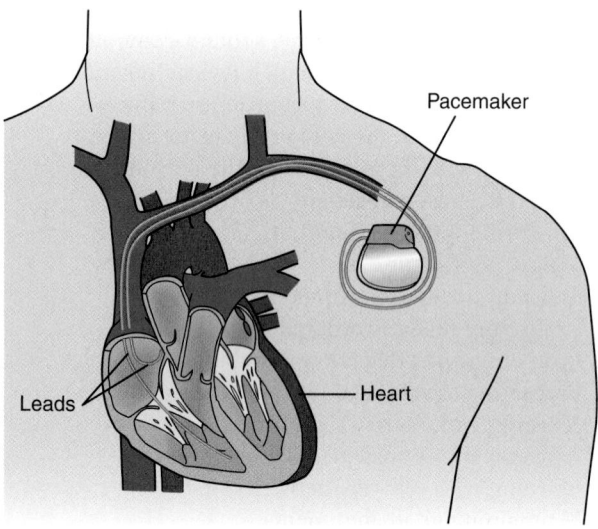

Fig. 42-7 Pacemaker.

For life-threatening dysrhythmias, an *implantable cardioverter defibrillator (ICD)* may be placed. The ICD delivers a shock when the heart is in a life-threatening rhythm. The shock allows the return of a regular heart rhythm. Some devices are both a pacemaker and an ICD.

See *Focus on Long-Term Care and Home Care: Dysrhythmias.*

RESPIRATORY DISORDERS

The respiratory system brings oxygen (O_2) into the lungs and removes carbon dioxide (CO_2) from the body. Respiratory disorders interfere with this function and threaten life.

See *Body Structure and Function Review: The Respiratory System.*

Chronic Obstructive Pulmonary Disease

Chronic obstructive pulmonary disease (COPD) involves two disorders—chronic bronchitis and emphysema. These disorders interfere with O_2 and CO_2 exchange in the lungs. They obstruct airflow. Lung function is gradually lost.

Cigarette smoking is the most important risk factor. Pipe, cigar, and other smoking tobaccos are also risk factors. So is exposure to second-hand smoke. Not smoking is the best way to prevent COPD. COPD has no cure.

COPD affects the airways and alveoli. Less air gets into the lungs; less air leaves the lungs. These changes occur:

- The airways and alveoli (air sacs) become less elastic. They are like old rubber bands.
- The walls between many alveoli are destroyed.
- Airway walls become thick, inflamed, and swollen.
- The airways secrete more mucus than usual. Excess mucus clogs the airways.

BODY STRUCTURE AND FUNCTION REVIEW: THE RESPIRATORY SYSTEM

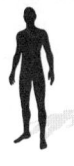

Oxygen is needed to live. Every cell needs oxygen. The respiratory system (Fig. 42-8) brings O_2 into the lungs and removes carbon dioxide. *Respiration* is the process of supplying the cells with O_2 and removing CO_2 from them. Respiration involves breathing in (*inhalation, inspiration*) and breathing out (*exhalation, expiration*).

Air enters the body through the *nose*. Then the air passes into the *pharynx* (throat). It is a tube-shaped passage-way for air and food. Air passes from the pharynx into the *larynx* (voice box). Air passes from the larynx into the *trachea* (windpipe).

The trachea divides at its lower end into the *right bronchus* and the *left bronchus*. Each bronchus enters a *lung*. Upon entering the lungs, the bronchi divide many times into smaller branches (*bronchioles*). Eventually the bronchioles subdivide. They end up in tiny one-celled air sacs called *alveoli*.

O_2 and CO_2 are exchanged between the alveoli and capillaries. Blood in the capillaries picks up O_2 from the alveoli. Then the blood is returned to the left side of the heart and pumped to the rest of the body. Alveoli pick up CO_2 from the capillaries for exhalation.

Each lung is divided into lobes. The right lung has 3 lobes; the left lung has 2. The lungs are separated from the abdominal cavity by a muscle called the *diaphragm*. A bony framework made up of the ribs, sternum, and vertebrae protects the lungs.

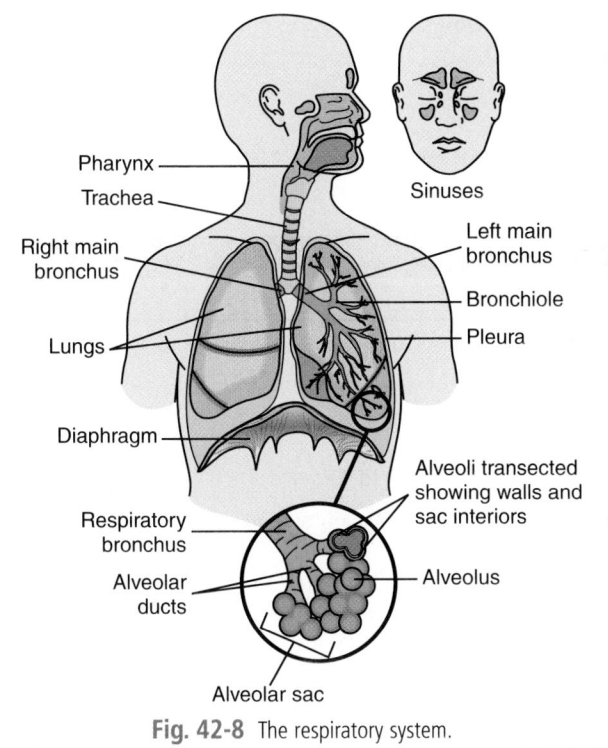

Fig. 42-8 The respiratory system.

Chronic Bronchitis. Chronic bronchitis occurs after repeated episodes of bronchitis. Bronchitis means inflammation (*itis*) of the bronchi (*bronch*). Smoking is the major cause. Infection, air pollution, and industrial dusts are risk factors.

Smoker's cough in the morning is often the first symptom. At first the cough is dry. Over time, the person coughs up mucus. Mucus may contain pus. The cough becomes more frequent. The person has difficulty breathing and tires easily. Mucus and inflamed breathing passages obstruct airflow into the lungs. The body cannot get normal amounts of O_2.

The person must stop smoking. Oxygen therapy and breathing exercises are often ordered. Respiratory tract infections are prevented. If one occurs, the person needs prompt treatment.

Emphysema. In emphysema, the alveoli enlarge. They become less elastic. They do not expand and shrink normally with breathing in and out. As a result, some air is trapped in the alveoli when exhaling. Trapped air is not exhaled. Over time, more alveoli are involved. O_2 and CO_2 exchange cannot occur in affected alveoli. As more air is trapped in the lungs, the person develops a *barrel chest* (Fig. 42-9).

Smoking is the most common cause. Air pollution and industrial dusts are risk factors.

The person has shortness of breath and a cough. At first, shortness of breath occurs with exertion. Over time, it occurs at rest. Sputum may contain pus. Fatigue is common. The person works hard to breathe in and out. And the body does not get enough O_2. Breathing is easier when the person sits upright and slightly forward (Chapter 36).

The person must stop smoking. Respiratory therapy, breathing exercises, oxygen, and drug therapy are ordered.

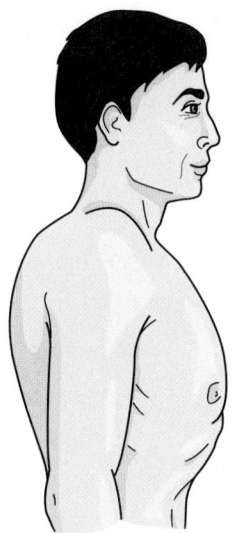

Fig. 42-9 Barrel chest from emphysema.

Asthma

Asthma comes from the Greek word for *panting*. With asthma, the airway becomes inflamed and narrow. Extra mucus is produced. Dyspnea results. Wheezing and coughing are common. So are pain and tightness in the chest. Symptoms are mild to severe.

Asthma usually is triggered by allergies. Other triggers include air pollutants and irritants, smoking and second-hand smoke, respiratory infections, exertion, and cold air.

Sudden attacks (*asthma attacks*) can occur. There is shortness of breath, wheezing, coughing, rapid pulse, sweating, and cyanosis. The person gasps for air and is very frightened. Fear makes the attack worse.

Asthma is treated with drugs. Severe attacks may require emergency care. The person and family learn how to prevent asthma attacks. Repeated attacks can damage the respiratory system.

Sleep Apnea

Apnea is the lack or absence (*a*) of breathing (*pnea*). In *sleep apnea, pauses in breathing occur during sleep.* Pauses last from a few seconds to over a minute and can occur many times during sleep.

The most common cause is blockage of the airway. During sleep, muscles in the throat relax and soft tissues collapse, closing the airway. This is called *obstructive sleep apnea. Central sleep apnea* is less common. This occurs when the brain does not send signals to the muscles to breathe. Some persons have both types.

Signs and symptoms of sleep apnea include:
- Pauses in breathing during sleep
- Loud snoring
- Waking during sleep with a gasp or shortness of breath
- Difficulty staying asleep
- Daytime sleepiness
- Headache in the morning
- Dry mouth or sore throat after sleeping

Life-style changes may help mild sleep apnea. Weight loss, quitting smoking, and avoiding alcohol and sedatives before sleep are examples. For more severe sleep apnea, surgery or the use of a positive airway pressure device may be needed. Two types are common:
- Continuous positive airway pressure (CPAP)—A mask is attached to a pump. Air pressure is forced through the mask. The air keeps the airway open. The same amount of pressure goes through the mask when the person inhales and exhales.
- Bi-level positive airway pressure (BiPAP)—Air pressure is forced through a mask to keep the airway open. The amount of pressure changes when the person inhales and exhales. More pressure is given when breathing in. Less pressure is given when breathing out. The change in pressure is more comfortable for some persons.

Influenza

Influenza (*flu*) is a respiratory infection caused by viruses. Table 42-1 contrasts a *cold* and the *flu*. The flu season is November through March. Older persons are at great risk. Pneumonia is a common complication.

Treatment involves fluids and rest. The doctor orders drugs for symptom relief and to shorten the flu episode. Most people are better in about one week.

Coughing and sneezing spread flu viruses. Follow Standard Precautions. The flu vaccine is the best prevention.

TABLE 42-1	COLD VERSUS THE FLU	
Symptoms	**Cold**	**Flu**
Fever	Rare	Usually high (100°F to 102°F); lasts 3 to 4 days
Headache	Rare	Common
General aches and pains	Slight	Usual; often severe
Fatigue; weakness	Sometimes	Usual; can last 2 to 3 weeks
Extreme exhaustion	Never	Usual; at the beginning of the illness
Stuffy nose	Common	Sometimes
Sneezing	Usual	Sometimes
Sore throat	Common	Sometimes
Chest discomfort; cough	Mild to moderate; hacking cough	Common; can be severe
Complications	Sinus infection; middle ear infection (otitis media); asthma	Bronchitis, pneumonia; can worsen chronic conditions; can be life-threatening

Modified from National Institute of Allergy and Infectious Diseases: *Is it a cold or the flu?* Bethesda, Md, 2008, National Institutes of Health.

Older Persons
Older persons may not have the signs and symptoms listed in Table 42-1. The following may signal flu in older persons:
- Changes in mental status or behavior
- Worsening of other health problems
- A body temperature below the normal range
- Fatigue
- Decreased appetite and fluid intake

BOX 42-3	SIGNS AND SYMPTOMS OF PNEUMONIA

- High fever
- Chills
- Painful cough
- Chest pain on breathing
- Pulse: rapid
- Breathing: rapid, shortness of breath
- Cyanosis
- Sputum: thick and white, green, yellow, or rust-colored
- Nausea and vomiting
- Headache
- Tiredness
- Muscle aches

The Centers for Disease Control and Prevention (CDC) recommends the flu vaccine for persons who:
- Are 6 months to 4 years of age.
- Are 50 years of age and older.
- Have chronic heart, lung, liver, or kidney diseases.
- Have diabetes.
- Have immune system, nervous system, or blood disorders.
- Are pregnant or will be pregnant during the flu season.
- Are 6 months to 18 years of age and receiving long-term aspirin therapy.
- Are nursing center or other long-term care residents.
- Are American Indians or Alaska Natives.
- Are very obese.
- Are in close contact with children under 5 years of age (especially those in contact with children under 6 months).
- Are in close contact with adults 50 years of age and older.
- Are health care workers.
- Have contact with persons at high risk for flu-related complications.
  See *Focus on Children and Older Persons: Influenza.*

Pneumonia

Pneumonia is an inflammation and infection of lung tissue. (*Pneumo* means *lungs.*) Affected tissues fill with fluid. O_2 and CO_2 exchange is affected.

Bacteria, viruses, and other microbes are causes. Microbes reach the lungs by being inhaled, aspirated, or carried in the blood to the lungs from an infection in the body. Children under 2 years of age and adults over 65 years of age are at risk. Smoking, aging, stroke, bedrest, immobility, chronic diseases, and tube feedings increase the risk of pneumonia.

Onset may be sudden. The person is very ill. Signs and symptoms are listed in Box 42-3.

Children
Pneumonia occurs in children of all ages. It is more common in infants and toddlers.

Older Persons
Changes from aging, diseases, and decreased mobility increase the risk of pneumonia in older persons. Decreased mobility after surgery also is a risk factor. Aspiration pneumonia is common in older persons. Dysphagia, decreased cough and gag reflexes, and nervous system disorders are risk factors. So are substances that depress the brain—narcotics, sedatives, alcohol, and drugs for anesthesia. Older adults are at great risk of dying from pneumonia.

Older persons may not have the signs and symptoms listed in Box 42-3. Drugs and other diseases can mask signs and symptoms. Older persons may show signs of confusion, dehydration, and rapid respirations.

Drugs are ordered for infection and pain. Fluid intake is increased because of fever and to thin secretions. Thin secretions are easier to cough up. Intravenous therapy and oxygen may be needed. Semi-Fowler's position eases breathing. Rest is important. Standard Precautions are followed. Isolation precautions are used depending on the cause. Mouth care is important. Frequent linen changes are needed because of fever.

See *Focus on Children and Older Persons: Pneumonia.*

Tuberculosis

Tuberculosis (TB) is a bacterial infection in the lungs. It also can occur in the kidneys, bones, joints, nervous system (including the spine), muscles, and other parts of the body. If TB is not treated, the person can die.

TB is spread by airborne droplets with coughing, sneezing, speaking, singing, or laughing (Chapter 15). Nearby persons can inhale the bacteria. Those who have close, frequent contact with an infected person are at risk. TB is more likely to occur in close, crowded areas. Age, poor nutrition, and HIV (human immunodeficiency virus) infection are other risk factors.

TB can be present in the body but not cause signs and symptoms. An active infection may not occur for many years. Only persons with an active infection can spread the disease to others.

Chest x-rays and TB testing can detect the disease. Signs and symptoms are tiredness, loss of appetite, weight loss, fever, and night sweats. Cough and sputum increase over time. Sputum may contain blood. Chest pain occurs.

Drugs for TB are given. Standard Precautions and isolation precautions are needed (Chapter 15). The person must cover the mouth and nose with tissues when sneezing, coughing, or producing sputum. Tissues are flushed down the toilet, placed in a BIOHAZARD bag, or placed in a paper bag and burned. Hand washing after contact with sputum is essential.

See *Focus on Children and Older Persons: Tuberculosis.*

See *Focus on Long-Term Care and Home Care: Tuberculosis.*

FOCUS ON LONG-TERM CARE AND HOME CARE
Tuberculosis

Long-Term Care

According to the CDC, persons with suspected or confirmed TB should not be treated in long-term care settings. Such settings include skilled nursing facilities and hospices. Persons with suspected or confirmed TB can be treated in long-term care settings if:

- Administrative and environmental controls are in place.
- The agency has a respiratory-protection program.

Cough-inducing procedures are not done unless appropriate infection controls are in place. Or such procedures are done outdoors.

Standard Precautions and Airborne Precautions are followed. See Chapter 15. The person wears a mask during transport to other areas, in waiting areas, and when others are present.

Home Care

The nurse teaches the person with TB and household members about taking drugs, respiratory hygiene and cough etiquette, and the need for proper medical care. The person may have to stay at home until tests are negative for TB or the person is no longer infectious.

Wear a TB respirator to enter the home of a person with suspected or confirmed TB. Also wear a TB respirator to transport the person in a vehicle. The person wears a mask during transport to other areas, in waiting areas, and when others are present.

Cough-inducing procedures are not done unless appropriate infection controls are in place. Or such procedures are done outdoors.

FOCUS ON CHILDREN AND OLDER PERSONS
Tuberculosis

Older Persons

Persons infected long ago can develop active TB when health declines with aging. Other older people with lengthy, extended contact with those infected risk becoming infected. Nursing center residents are examples.

LYMPHATIC DISORDERS

The lymphatic system drains extra fluid from the tissues, helps fight infection, and absorbs and transports fats. Lymphatic disorders affect these functions.

See *Body Structure and Function Review: The Lymphatic System.*

BODY STRUCTURE AND FUNCTION REVIEW: THE LYMPHATIC SYSTEM

The lymphatic (lymph) system transports lymph throughout the body (Fig. 42-10). *Lymph* is a clear, thin, watery fluid. Lymph contains white blood cells (WBCs), proteins, and fats from the intestines.

The lymphatic system:

* Collects extra lymph from the tissues and returns it to the blood. Water, proteins, and other substances normally leak out of the capillaries into surrounding tissues. The lymphatic system drains the extra fluid from the tissues. Otherwise, the tissues swell.
* Defends the body against infection by producing lymphocytes. *Lymphocytes* are a type of WBC that defends the body against microbes that cause infection.
* Absorbs fats from the intestines and transports them to the blood.

Lymph is formed in the tissues. Lymph is transported by *lymphatic vessels.*

Lymph nodes are shaped like beans. They are found in the neck, underarm, groin area, chest, abdomen, and pelvis. Usually, you cannot see or feel lymph nodes. They swell when producing more lymphocytes to fight infection.

Lymph enters lymph nodes through the lymphatic vessels. The lymph nodes filter bacteria, cancer cells, and damaged cells from the lymph. This prevents such substances from entering the blood and circulating throughout the body.

See Figure 42-10 for the location of the *thymus (thymus gland).* Certain lymphocytes—T lymphocytes (T cells)—develop in the thymus. Such lymphocytes are important for immune system function.

The *tonsils* are in the back of the throat. *Adenoids* are behind the nose. These structures trap microbes in the mouth and nose to help prevent infection.

The *spleen* is the largest structure in the lymphatic system. The spleen:

* Filters and removes bacteria and other substances.
* Destroys old RBCs.
* Saves the iron found in hemoglobin when RBCs are destroyed.
* Stores blood. When needed, the blood is returned to the circulatory system.

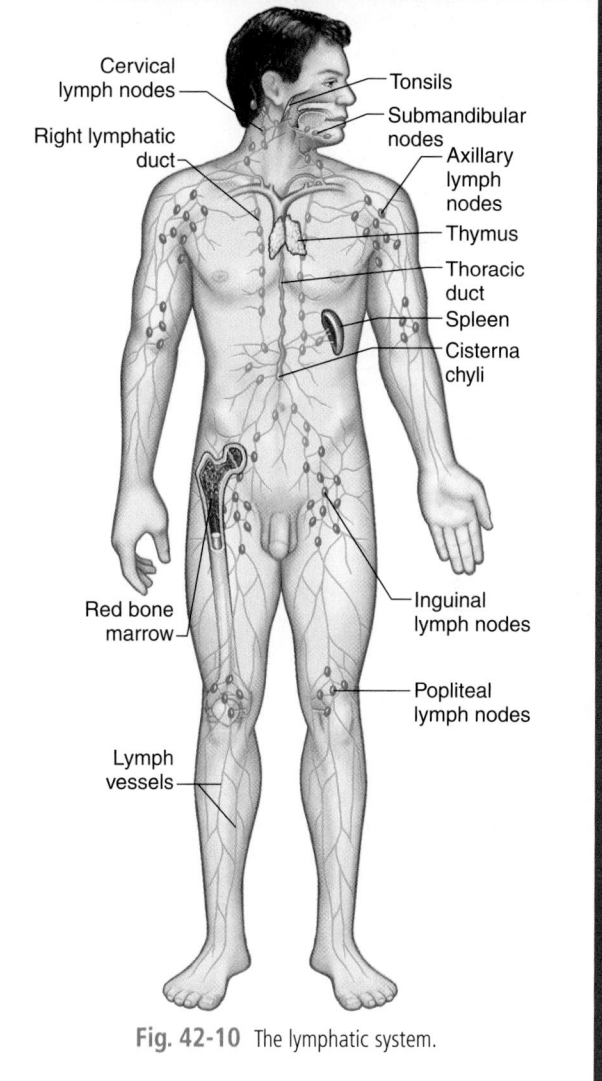

Fig. 42-10 The lymphatic system.

Lymphedema

Lymphedema is a buildup of lymph in the tissues causing edema (swelling). It occurs when there is a blockage or damage to the lymph system. Causes include:

* Cancer
* Infection
* Surgical removal of lymph nodes
* Scar tissue from radiation therapy or surgery
* Absent or abnormal lymph nodes present at birth

Lymphedema usually affects an arm or leg (Fig. 42-11, p. 708). Other body parts can be involved. The person may have a tight or heavy feeling and have trouble moving the body part. Thickening of the skin, pain, itching or burning, and hair loss are also common. Daily activities are often affected.

Damage to the lymph system cannot be reversed. Elastic garments or bandages apply pressure to the area. This helps move fluid and prevents fluid buildup. Treatment also includes exercise, good skin care, and massage therapy. The goals are to control swelling, decrease pain, improve movement and use of the body part, and allow daily activities.

See *Promoting Safety and Comfort: Lymphedema*, p. 708.

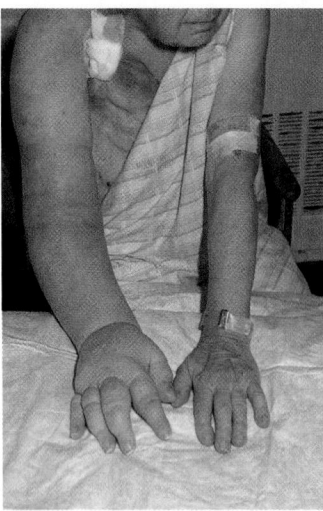

Fig. 42-11 Lymphedema.

Signs and symptoms of lymphoma are also caused by other health problems or infections (Box 42-4). Tests are done for a diagnosis. Treatment may include chemotherapy, radiation, or both (Chapter 40). Psychological, social, and spiritual support are needed.

PROMOTING SAFETY AND COMFORT

Lymphedema

Safety

Actions that block fluid flow or increase fluid buildup can cause lymphedema in persons at risk. Or it can worsen lymphedema. Never apply a blood pressure cuff to an arm with or at risk for lymphedema. For example, lymph nodes are often removed during breast cancer surgery. Do not use the arm on the surgery side to check blood pressure.

If you are unsure which arm to use, ask the nurse. Also, ask the person if he or she has an arm that must not be used.

Comfort

The body part affected by lymphedema can be painful and difficult to move. Handle the person gently. Tell the person before you move the body part. Ask the person to tell you if he or she feels pain. Stop movements that cause pain.

Lymphoma

Lymphoma is cancer involving cells in the immune system (lymphocytes). Lymphocytes are a type of WBC that protects the body from infection. They are found in lymph nodes and other lymph tissues. In lymphoma, these cells do not function normally.

There are two main types of lymphoma—Hodgkin's lymphoma and non-Hodgkin's lymphoma. They differ in the types of cells involved and how they spread and respond to treatment.

Lymphoma begins with an abnormal lymphocyte. The abnormal cell divides and makes more abnormal cells. These cells cannot protect the body. They also live longer than normal. A mass of abnormal cells develops into a tumor (Chapter 40).

FOCUS ON PRIDE

The Person, Family, and Yourself

Personal and Professional Responsibility

Heart disease is a major concern in the United States. You need to know your risk factors and how to reduce your risk. See Box 42-1.

Apply the information in this chapter to your own life. Take pride in making changes to promote a healthy life-style. A healthy life-style benefits you personally and professionally. And you must be healthy and strong to care for others.

Rights and Respect

Persons have the right to make choices for themselves. Some choices are unhealthy. For example, a person with COPD continues to smoke. Or a person with CAD refuses to exercise or make diet changes. The health team teaches the person the risks and encourages healthy changes. The health team cannot force changes. However, they must be sure the person understands the risks.

Some persons believe that unhealthy choices improve their quality of life. They are aware of the risks but choose not to change. Although you may not respect the person's decision, you must respect the person. Treat the person with dignity and respect.

Independence and Social Interaction

Infections like the flu, pneumonia, and TB can spread to others. You must follow Standard Precautions and the Bloodborne Pathogen Standard. Follow isolation precautions as directed. These measures protect you and others from contamination.

The infection and the precautions may cause the person to feel unclean. Family and friends may avoid visiting out of fear of getting the disease. Feelings of loneliness, sadness, and depression can result.

Social and emotional needs are important. As you provide for physical needs, talk with the person. Be polite. Treat the person with kindness and respect. Explain that some precautions are used for all persons. For isolation precautions, explain that they are used for the safety of the person and others. The person should not feel ashamed or dirty. Tell the nurse about any concerns.

Delegation and Teamwork

A person's condition can change very quickly. A person with angina may have an MI. A person with hypertension may have a stroke.

Sudden changes in a person's condition require the nurse's attention. Assist the nurse as directed. You may need to help other patients or residents while the nurse provides care. Always help willingly. The entire nursing team must give that "extra effort" during an emergency.

Ethics and Laws

Performing your job safely and carefully is part of ethical practice. Some agencies use color-coded wristbands to promote safety and prevent harm (Chapter 12). "Limb alert" or "forbidden extremity" wristbands communicate that an arm must not be used for blood pressures, intravenous infusions, or blood draws. These are useful for lymph-edema.

If your agency uses color-coded wristbands, learn the reason for each wristband. Check for wristbands when providing care. Take pride in using such safety measures to prevent harm.

REVIEW QUESTIONS

Circle the BEST answer.

1 A person with a congenital heart defect
   a Needs heart surgery
   b Has damaged heart valves
   c Has blocked coronary arteries
   d Was born with the defect

2 In hypertension, the systolic blood pressure is
   a Over 140 mm Hg   c Over 90 mm Hg
   b Over 120 mm Hg   d Over 80 mm Hg

3 Which is *not* a complication of hypertension?
   a Stroke   c Renal failure
   b Heart attack   d Diabetes

4 Treatment of hypertension may include the following *except*
   a No smoking and regular exercise
   b A high-sodium diet
   c A low-calorie diet if the person is obese
   d Drugs to lower blood pressure

5 A person has angina. Which is *true*?
   a There is heart muscle damage.
   b Pain is described as crushing, stabbing, or squeezing.
   c Pain is relieved with rest and nitroglycerin.
   d Pain is always on the left side of the chest.

6 Cardiac rehabilitation involves
   a Exercise   c Catheter procedures
   b Surgery   d Receiving a vaccine

7 A person is having an MI. Which is *false*?
   a The person is having a heart attack.
   b This is an emergency.
   c The person may have a cardiac arrest.
   d The person does not have enough blood.

8 The pain of MI is usually
   a On the left side of the chest
   b On the right side of the chest
   c In the upper abdomen
   d In the mid-back region

9 A person has heart failure. Which measure should you question?
   a Encourage fluids.
   b Measure intake and output.
   c Measure weight daily.
   d Perform range-of-motion exercises.

10 A person has a dysrhythmia. Tell the nurse at once if
   a You notice a hard, round lump under the skin on the chest
   b The person is dizzy
   c The heart rate is 80
   d The person has a barrel chest

11 The most common cause of COPD is
   a Smoking   c Being over-weight
   b Allergies   d A high sodium diet

12 A person has emphysema. Which is *false*?
   a The person has dyspnea.
   b The person has an infection.
   c Breathing is usually easier sitting upright and slightly forward.
   d Sputum may contain pus.

13 Life-style changes for sleep apnea include the following *except*
   a Weight loss
   b Quitting smoking
   c Avoiding alcohol before sleep
   d Avoiding allergies and irritants

14 The flu virus is spread by
   a Coughing and sneezing
   b The fecal-oral route
   c Blood
   d Needle sharing

15 Pneumonia is
   a An inflammation of the airway
   b Narrowing of the airway
   c Inflammation and infection of lung tissue
   d A bacterial infection in the lungs

16 Which position eases breathing in the person with pneumonia?
   a Supine
   b Prone
   c Semi-Fowler's
   d Trendelenburg's

17 Tuberculosis is spread by
   a Coughing and sneezing
   b Contaminated drinking water
   c Contact with wound drainage
   d The fecal-oral route

18 A person has TB. You had contact with the person's sputum. What should you do?
   a Wash your hands.
   b Put on gloves.
   c Use an alcohol-based hand rub.
   d Tell the nurse.

19 When checking blood pressure
   a Apply the cuff to the arm that is easy to reach
   b Deflate the cuff slowly when using an arm that is swollen
   c Report a blood pressure of 110/70 to the nurse at once
   d Ask if the person has an arm that should not be used for blood pressure

Answers to these questions are on p. 834.

43

Digestive and Endocrine Disorders

OBJECTIVES

- Define the key terms and key abbreviations listed in this chapter.
- Describe gastro-esophageal reflux disease and the care required.
- Describe the care required for vomiting.
- Describe diverticular disease and the care required.

- Describe gallstones and the care required.
- Describe hepatitis and the care required.
- Describe cirrhosis and the care required.
- Describe diabetes and the care required.
- Explain how to promote PRIDE in the person, the family, and yourself.

KEY TERMS

emesis See "vomitus"

heartburn A burning sensation in the chest and sometimes the throat

hyperglycemia High (*hyper*) sugar (*glyc*) in the blood (*emia*)

hypoglycemia Low (*hypo*) sugar (*glyc*) in the blood (*emia*)

jaundice Yellowish color of the skin or whites of the eyes

vomitus Food and fluids expelled from the stomach through the mouth; emesis

KEY ABBREVIATIONS

GERD	Gastro-esophageal reflux disease	**I&O**	Intake and output
HBV	Hepatitis B virus	**IV**	Intravenous

Problems can develop in any part of the digestive system. This includes the liver, gallbladder, and pancreas—the accessory organs of digestion. The pancreas also is part of the endocrine system.

DIGESTIVE DISORDERS

The digestive system breaks down food for the body to absorb. Solid wastes are eliminated. Diarrhea, constipation, flatulence, and fecal incontinence are discussed in Chapter 23. So is ostomy care.

See *Body Structure and Function Review: The Digestive System.*

BODY STRUCTURE AND FUNCTION REVIEW: THE DIGESTIVE SYSTEM

The digestive system *(gastro-intestinal [GI] system)* involves the *alimentary canal (GI tract)* and the accessory organs of digestion (Fig. 43-1). The alimentary canal extends from the mouth to the anus.

Digestion begins in the *mouth (oral cavity)*. Using chewing motions, the *teeth* cut, chop, and grind food into small particles for digestion and swallowing. The *tongue* aids in chewing and swallowing. *Salivary glands* in the mouth secrete *saliva*. Saliva moistens food particles to ease swallowing and begin digestion. During swallowing, the tongue pushes food into the *pharynx* (throat).

Contraction of the pharynx pushes food into the *esophagus*. The esophagus extends from the pharynx to the *stomach*. Involuntary muscle contractions *(peristalsis)* move food down the esophagus through the alimentary canal.

The stomach is a muscular, pouch-like sac. The mucous membrane lining the stomach contains glands that secrete *gastric juices*. Food is mixed and churned with the gastric juices to form a semi-liquid substance called *chyme*. Peristalsis pushes chyme from the stomach into the small intestine.

The first part of the *small intestine* is the duodenum. More digestive juices are added to the chyme. One is called *bile*—a greenish liquid made in the *liver*. Bile is stored in the *gallbladder*. Juices from the *pancreas* and small intestine are added to the chyme. Digestive juices chemically break down food for absorption.

Peristalsis moves the chyme through the two other parts of the small intestine: the *jejunum* and the *ileum*. Most food absorption takes place in the jejunum and the ileum.

Undigested chyme passes from the small intestine into the *large intestine (large bowel* or *colon)*. The colon absorbs most of the water from the chyme. The remaining semi-solid material is called *feces*. Feces contain a small amount of water, solid wastes, and some mucus and germs. These are the waste products of digestion. Feces pass through the colon into the *rectum* by peristalsis. Feces pass out of the body through the *anus*.

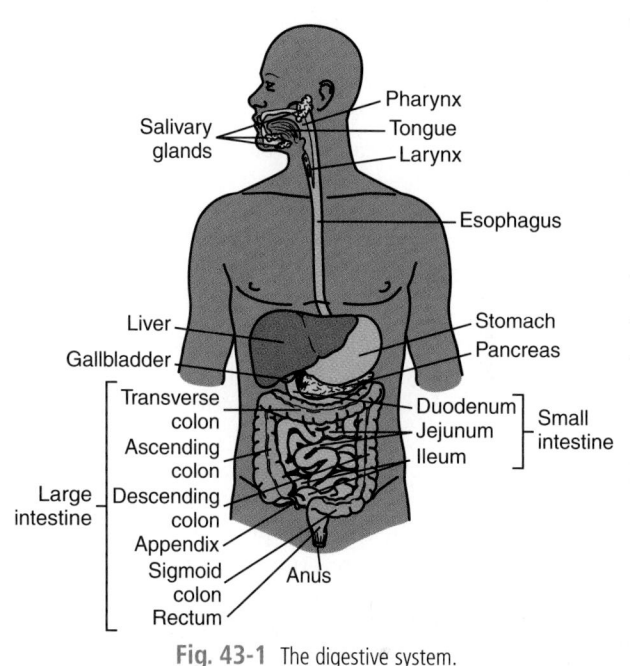

Fig. 43-1 The digestive system.

Gastro-Esophageal Reflux Disease

In gastro-esophageal reflux disease (GERD) stomach contents flow back *(reflux)* from the stomach *(gastro)* into the esophagus *(esophageal)*. Stomach contents contain acid. The acid can irritate and inflame the esophagus lining. This is called *esophagitis*—inflammation *(itis)* of the esophagus.

Heartburn is the most common symptom. *Heartburn is a burning sensation in the chest and sometimes the throat.* The person may have a sour taste in the back of the mouth. If heartburn occurs more than twice a week, the person may have GERD. Besides heartburn, other signs and symptoms include:

* Chest pain, often when lying down
* Hoarseness in the morning
* Dysphagia
* Choking sensation
* Feeling like food is stuck in the throat
* Feeling like the throat is tight
* Dry cough
* Sore throat
* Bad breath

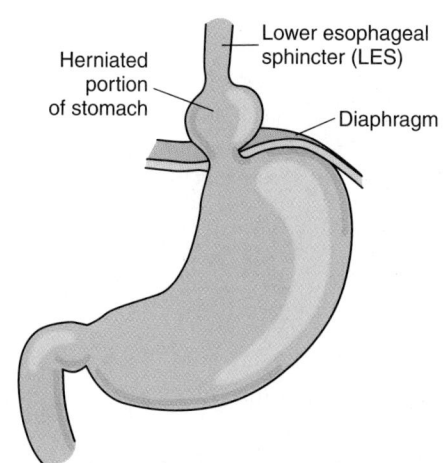

Fig. 43-2 Hiatal hernia.

Risk factors include being over-weight, alcohol use, pregnancy, and smoking. Hiatal hernia is a risk factor. With hiatal hernia, the upper part of the stomach is above the diaphragm (Fig. 43-2). Large meals and lying down after eating can cause gastric reflux. So can citrus fruits, chocolate, caffeine drinks, fried and fatty foods, garlic, onions, spicy foods, and tomato-based foods (pasta sauce, chili, pizza).

The doctor may order drugs to prevent stomach acid production or to promote stomach emptying. Surgery may be needed. Life-style changes include:

- No smoking or drinking alcohol
- Losing weight
- Eating small meals
- Wearing loose belts and loose-fitting clothes
- Not lying down for 3 hours after meals

Vomiting

Vomitus (emesis) is the food and fluids expelled from the stomach through the mouth. Vomiting signals illness or injury. Aspirated vomitus can obstruct the airway. Vomiting large amounts of blood can lead to shock (Chapter 51). These measures are needed:

- Follow Standard Precautions and the Bloodborne Pathogen Standard.
- Turn the person's head well to one side. This prevents aspiration.
- Place a kidney basin under the person's chin.
- Move vomitus away from the person.
- Provide oral hygiene. This helps remove the bitter taste of vomitus.
- Observe vomitus for color, odor, and undigested food. If it looks like coffee grounds, it contains undigested blood. This signals bleeding. Report your observations.
- Measure, report, and record the amount of vomitus.
- Save a specimen for laboratory study.
- Dispose of vomitus after the nurse observes it.
- Eliminate odors.
- Provide for comfort. (See the inside of the front book cover.)

Diverticular Disease

Small pouches can develop in the colon. The pouches bulge outward through weak spots in the colon (Fig. 43-3). Each pouch is called a *diverticulum*. (*Diverticulare* means *to turn inside out.*) *Diverticulosis* is the condition of having these pouches. (*Osis* means *condition of.*) The pouches can become infected or inflamed—*diverticulitis*. (*Itis* means *inflammation.*)

Many people over 60 years of age have diverticulosis. Age, a low-fiber diet, and constipation are risk factors.

When feces enter the pouches, they can become inflamed and infected. The person has abdominal pain and tenderness in the lower left abdomen. Fever, nausea and vomiting, chills, cramping, and constipation are likely. Bloating, rectal bleeding, frequent urination, and pain while voiding can occur.

A ruptured pouch is rare. Feces spill into the abdomen. This causes a severe, life-threatening infection. A pouch also can cause a blockage in the intestine (intestinal obstruction). Feces and gas cannot move past the blocked part.

Diet changes are ordered. Sometimes antibiotics are ordered. Surgery is done for severe disease, obstruction, and ruptured pouches. The diseased part of the bowel is removed. A colostomy may be needed (Chapter 23).

Gallstones

Bile is a liquid made in the liver. It is stored in the gallbladder until needed to digest fat. Gallstones form when the bile hardens into stone-like pieces (Fig. 43-4).

Bile is carried from the liver to the gallbladder through ducts (tubes). The gallbladder contracts and pushes bile through the common bile duct to the small intestine. Gallstones can lodge in any of the ducts (Fig. 43-5). Bile flow is blocked. The gallbladder and ducts become inflamed. Liver and pancreas involvement are possible. Severe infections or damage can cause death.

Gallstones can be as small as a grain of sand or as large as a golf ball. A person may have one large stone. Some people have large and small stones. Persons at risk include those who are:

- Women—especially women who:
  - Are pregnant.
  - Use hormone replacement therapy.
  - Take birth control pills.
- Over age 60
- American Indians
- Mexican Americans
- Over-weight or obese
- Taking cholesterol-lowering drugs
- Diabetics

Signs and symptoms of a "gallbladder attack" or "gallstone attack" occur suddenly (Box 43-1). They often follow a fatty meal. Surgical removal of the gallbladder is common.

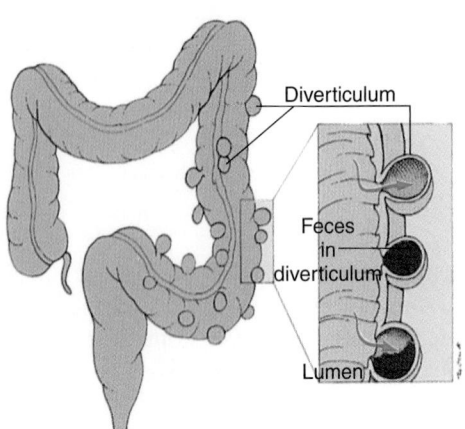

Fig. 43-3 Diverticulosis.

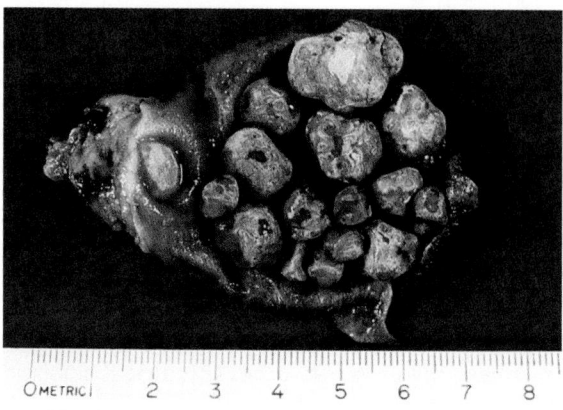

Fig. 43-4 Inflamed gallbladder filled with gallstones.

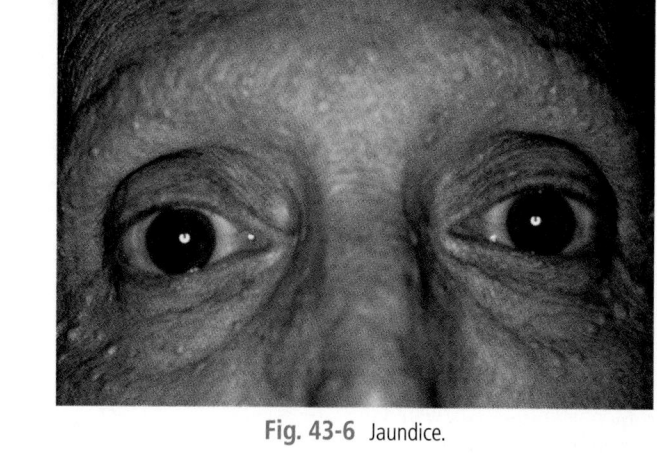

Fig. 43-6 Jaundice.

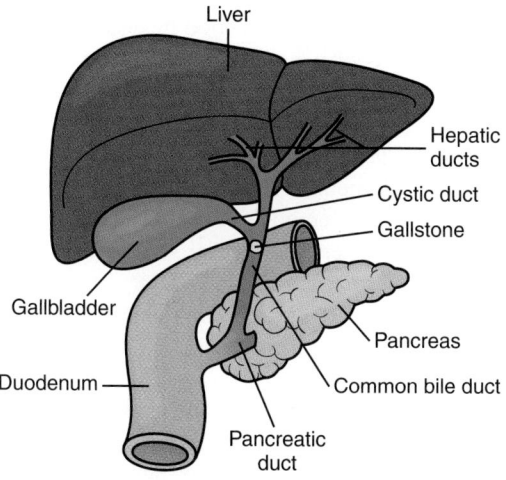

Fig. 43-5 The gallbladder and ducts that carry bile from the liver, gallbladder, and pancreas to the small intestine.

BOX 43-2	SIGNS AND SYMPTOMS OF HEPATITIS

- Jaundice (yellowish color of the skin or whites of the eyes)
- Fatigue, weakness
- Pain and discomfort: abdominal, joint, muscles
- Appetite: loss of
- Nausea and vomiting
- Diarrhea
- Bowel movements: light, clay-colored
- Urine: dark
- Fever and chills
- Headache
- Itching
- Weight loss
- Skin rash

Hepatitis

Hepatitis is an inflammation (*itis*) of the liver (*hepat*). It can be mild or cause death. See Box 43-2 for signs and symptoms. Some people have no symptoms.

Protect yourself and others. Follow Standard Precautions and the Bloodborne Pathogen Standard. Isolation precautions are ordered as necessary (Chapter 15). Assist the person with hygiene and hand washing as needed.

There are five major types of hepatitis. See Box 43-3, p. 714 for persons at risk.

BOX 43-1	SIGNS AND SYMPTOMS OF GALLSTONES

- Steady pain in the upper abdomen
  - Increases rapidly
  - Lasts 30 minutes to several hours
- Pain
  - In the back between the shoulder blades
  - Under the right shoulder
- Prolonged pain—lasting more than 5 hours
- Nausea and vomiting
- Chills
- Fever
- *Jaundice—yellowish color of the skin or whites of the eyes* (Fig. 43-6) (Jaundice comes from the French word *jaune*, meaning *yellow*.)
- Clay-colored stools

Modified from National Digestive Diseases Information Clearinghouse (NDDIC): *Gallstones,* Bethesda, Md, 2007, National Institutes of Health, NIH Publication No. 07-2897.

BOX 43-3   PERSONS AT RISK FOR HEPATITIS

Hepatitis A
- International travelers (especially to developing countries)
- People who live with an infected person
- People who have sex with an infected person
- People living in areas where children are not routinely vaccinated against hepatitis A
- Day-care children and staff (during outbreaks)
- Men who have sex with men
- Users of illegal drugs

Hepatitis B
- People who live with an infected person
- People who have sex with an infected person
- Men who have sex with men
- People who have multiple sex partners
- Injection drug users
- Immigrants from areas with high rates of hepatitis B
- Children of immigrants from areas with high rates of hepatitis B
- Infants born to infected mothers
- Health care workers
- Hemodialysis patients (Chapter 44)
- People who received blood or blood products before 1987
- International travelers

Hepatitis C
- Injection drug users
- People who have sex with an infected person
- People who have multiple sex partners
- Health care workers
- Infants born to infected mothers
- Hemodialysis patients
- People who received blood or blood products before 1992
- People who received blood clotting factors made before 1987

Hepatitis D
- People who have sex with an infected person
- People who received blood or blood products before 1987

Hepatitis E
- International travelers (especially to developing countries)
- People living in areas where hepatitis E outbreaks are common
- People who live with an infected person
- People who have sex with an infected person

Modified from National Digestive Diseases Information Clearinghouse (NDDIC): *Viral hepatitis: A through E and beyond,* Bethesda, Md, 2008, National Institutes of Health, NIH Publication No. 08-4762.

FOCUS ON CHILDREN AND OLDER PERSONS
Hepatitis A

Children

Hepatitis A is more common in pre-school and school-age children. Children in day care are at risk. Poor hygiene after bowel movements leads to contaminated eating and drinking vessels. Also, young children often put their hands in their mouths.

Treatment involves rest, a healthy diet, fluids, and no alcohol. Recovery takes 1 to 2 months.

Persons with fecal incontinence, confusion, and dementia can cause contamination. Carefully look for contaminated items and areas.

Handle bedpans, feces, and rectal thermometers carefully. Good hand washing is needed by everyone, including the person. Assist with hand washing after bowel movements. The hepatitis A vaccine provides protection against the disease.

See *Focus on Children and Older Persons: Hepatitis A.*

Hepatitis B. The hepatitis B virus (HBV) is the cause. It is spread through infected blood or blood products and body fluids (saliva, semen, vaginal secretions) of infected persons. It can be spread by:
- IV (intravenous) drug use and sharing needles and syringes
- Accidental needle-sticks
- Sex without a condom, especially anal sex
- Contaminated tools used for tattoos or body piercings
- Sharing a toothbrush, razor, or nail clippers with an infected person

For the HBV vaccine, see Chapter 15. Drugs are ordered for chronic hepatitis B.

Hepatitis C. This type is spread by blood contaminated with the hepatitis C virus. A person may have no symptoms but can transmit the disease. Serious liver disease and damage may show up years later. Hepatitis C is treated with drugs. The virus can be spread by blood contaminated with the virus through:
- IV drug use and sharing needles and syringes
- Inhaling cocaine through contaminated straws
- Contaminated tools used for tattoos or body piercings
- High-risk sexual activity—sex with an infected person, multiple sex partners
- Sharing a toothbrush, razor, or nail clippers with an infected person

Hepatitis D and Hepatitis E. Hepatitis D occurs only in people infected with hepatitis B. It is spread the same way as HBV.

Hepatitis E is spread through food or water contaminated by feces from an infected person. It is spread by the fecal-oral route. This disease is not common in the United States.

Hepatitis A. This type is spread by food or water contaminated with feces from an infected person. Spread through the fecal-oral route, the hepatitis A virus is ingested when:
- Eating or drinking food or water contaminated with feces
- Eating or drinking from a contaminated vessel

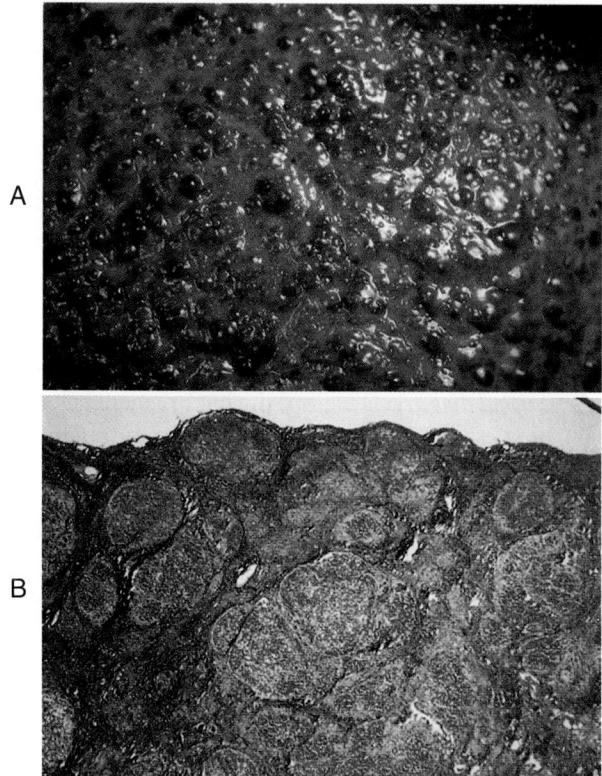

Fig. 43-7 **A** and **B,** Liver damage from alcohol.

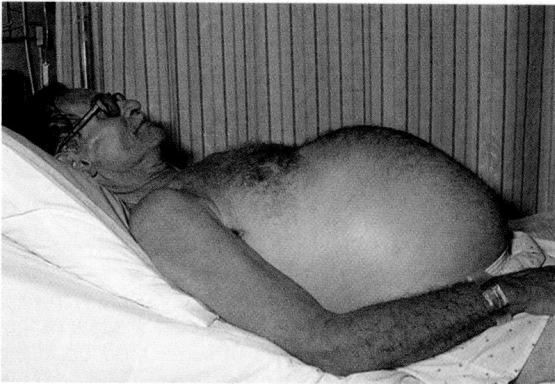

Fig. 43-8 Fluid in the membrane lining the abdominal cavity (ascites).

BOX 43-4	CARE OF THE PERSON WITH CIRRHOSIS

- Use bedrails according to the care plan.
- Keep the signal light within reach.
- Observe vomitus and stools for blood.
- Observe for signs of decreased mental function—confusion, memory loss, behavior changes, and so on.
- Measure vital signs every 2 to 4 hours.
- Measure intake and output (I&O).
- Follow fluid restriction orders.
- Weigh the person daily.
- Provide good skin care.
- Apply lotion to the skin.
- Turn the person at least every 2 hours or as noted on the care plan.
- Provide mouth care every 2 hours.
- Use warm water with baking soda for bathing. This decreases itching.
- Assist with activities of daily living (ADL) as needed.
- Complete a safety check before leaving the room. (See the inside of the front book cover.)

Cirrhosis

Cirrhosis is a liver condition caused by chronic liver damage (Fig. 43-7). (*Cirrho* means *yellow-orange. Osis* means *condition.*) Healthy tissue is replaced by scar tissue. Blood flow through the liver is blocked. Normal liver functions are affected:

- Controlling infection
- Removing bacteria and toxins from the blood
- Processing nutrients, hormones, and drugs
- Making proteins for blood clotting
- Producing bile for fat digestion

Chronic alcohol abuse and chronic hepatitis B and C are common causes. Obesity is becoming a common cause.

Signs and symptoms do not appear early in the disease. These may occur as the disease progresses:

- Weakness and fatigue
- Loss of appetite
- Nausea and vomiting
- Weight loss
- Abdominal pain and bloating when fluid collects in the membrane lining the abdominal cavity (Fig. 43-8)
- Itching
- Spider-like blood vessels on the skin

Cirrhosis has many serious complications. Fluid collects in the legs (edema) and abdomen (ascites). Infection, jaundice, bruising, and bleeding occur. Blood vessels in the esophagus and stomach may enlarge and burst. Gallstones may develop. Toxins build up in the brain causing confusion, personality changes, and memory loss. Diabetes and liver cancer are risks.

Treatment is aimed at preventing scar tissue. Complications are treated. The person needs a healthy diet limited in protein. A low-sodium diet is needed for edema and ascites. Diuretic drugs (water pills) are ordered to remove fluid. Antibiotics are ordered for infection. Drugs and enemas are ordered to remove toxins. The person must avoid alcohol and may need a liver transplant.

The measures listed in Box 43-4 may be part of the person's care plan.

BODY STRUCTURE AND FUNCTION REVIEW: THE ENDOCRINE SYSTEM (PANCREAS)

The endocrine glands (Fig. 43-9) secrete chemical substances called *hormones* into the bloodstream. Hormones regulate the activities of other organs and glands in the body.

The *pancreas* (see Fig. 43-5) secretes *insulin*. Insulin regulates the amount of sugar in the blood available for use by the cells. Insulin is needed for sugar to enter the cells. The cells need glucose for energy. If there is too little insulin, sugar cannot enter the cells. If sugar cannot enter the cells, excess amounts of sugar build up in the blood. This condition is called *diabetes*.

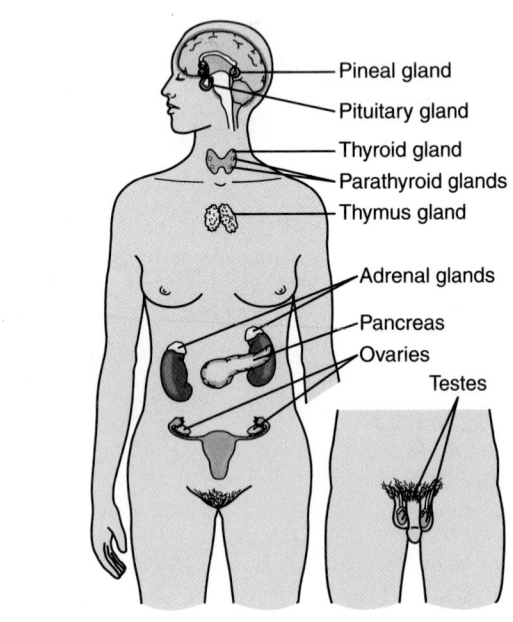

- Pineal gland
- Pituitary gland
- Thyroid gland
- Parathyroid glands
- Thymus gland
- Adrenal glands
- Pancreas
- Ovaries
- Testes

Fig. 43-9 The endocrine system.

ENDOCRINE DISORDERS

The endocrine system is made up of glands. The endocrine glands secrete hormones that affect other organs and glands. Diabetes, the most common endocrine disorder, involves the pancreas.

See *Body Structure and Function Review: The Endocrine System (Pancreas)*.

Diabetes

In diabetes, the body cannot produce or use insulin properly. Without enough insulin, sugar builds up in the blood. Blood glucose (sugar) is high. Cells do not have enough sugar for energy and cannot function.

Types of Diabetes. A family history of the disease is a common risk factor for the three types of diabetes:

- *Type 1 diabetes.* Occurs most often in children. It is more common in whites than in non-whites. The pancreas produces little or no insulin. Onset is rapid.

- *Type 2 diabetes.* This type is more common in older persons. However, it is becoming more common in children, teens, and young adults. Being over-weight, lack of exercise, and hypertension are risk factors. The pancreas secretes insulin. However, the body cannot use it well. Onset is slow. Infections are frequent. Wounds heal slowly. These ethnic groups are at risk:
  - American Indians
  - Blacks
  - African-Americans
  - Hispanics
  - Asians
- *Gestational diabetes.* Develops during pregnancy. (Gestation comes from *gestare*. It means *to bear*.) It usually goes away after the baby is born. However, the mother is at risk for type 2 diabetes later in life.

Signs and Symptoms. Signs and symptoms of diabetes are:

- Being very thirsty
- Urinating often
- Feeling very hungry or tired
- Losing weight without trying
- Having sores that heal slowly
- Having dry, itchy skin
- Tingling or loss of feeling in the feet
- Blurred vision

Complications. Diabetes must be controlled to prevent complications. They include blindness, renal failure, nerve damage, and damage to the gums and teeth. Heart and blood vessel diseases are very serious problems. They can lead to stroke, heart attack, and slow healing. Foot and leg wounds and ulcers are very serious (Chapter 33). Infection and gangrene can occur. Sometimes amputation is necessary.

Treatment. Type 1 diabetes is treated with daily insulin therapy, healthy eating (Chapter 24), and exercise. Type 2 diabetes is treated with healthy eating and exercise. Many persons with type 2 take oral drugs. Some need insulin. Over-weight persons need to lose weight. Types 1 and 2 involve controlling blood pressure, cholesterol, and the risk factors for coronary artery disease.

Good foot care is needed. Corns, blisters, calluses, and other foot problems can lead to an infection and amputation. See Chapters 21 and 33.

The person's blood sugar level can fall too low or go too high. Blood glucose is monitored daily or 3 or 4 times a day for:

- *Hypoglycemia means low* (hypo) *sugar* (glyc) *in the blood* (emia).
- *Hyperglycemia means high* (hyper) *sugar* (glyc) *in the blood* (emia).

See Table 43-1 for the causes, signs, and symptoms of hypoglycemia and hyperglycemia. Both can lead to death if not corrected. You must call for the nurse at once.

See *Focus on Children and Older Persons: Diabetes.*

TABLE 43-1 HYPOGLYCEMIA AND HYPERGLYCEMIA

	Causes	Signs and Symptoms
Hypoglycemia (low blood sugar)	Too much insulin or diabetic drugs Omitting or missing a meal Delayed meal Eating too little food Increased exercise Vomiting Drinking alcohol	Hunger Fatigue; weakness Trembling; shakiness Sweating Headache Dizziness Faintness Pulse: rapid Blood pressure: low Respirations: rapid and shallow Motions: clumsy and jerky Tingling around the mouth Confusion Vision changes Skin: cold and clammy Convulsions Unconsciousness
Hyperglycemia (high blood sugar)	Undiagnosed diabetes Not enough insulin or diabetic drugs Eating too much food Too little exercise Emotional stress Infection or sickness	Weakness Drowsiness Thirst Dry mouth (very) Hunger Urination: frequent Leg cramps Face; flushed Breath odor: sweet Respirations: rapid, deep, and labored Pulse: rapid, weak Blood pressure: low Skin: dry Vision: blurred Headache Nausea and vomiting Convulsions Coma

---

FOCUS ON CHILDREN AND OLDER PERSONS
Diabetes

Children
Your assignment may include preparing meals for a child with diabetes. Follow the child's diet carefully. Also prepare snacks for the child to take to school. The snack is needed in case there is a drop in the child's blood sugar level.

FOCUS ON PRIDE
The Person, Family, and Yourself

Personal and Professional Responsibility
You help the nurse observe patients and residents. You may be the first to notice something wrong. For example, a patient with diabetes is confused, weak, and shaky. You tell the nurse and follow instructions. The person's condition improves.

Your role is important. Take pride in observing the person and reporting concerns.

Rights and Respect
For some health problems, family history is a risk factor. Others result from life-style choices. Poor diet, drug abuse, unsafe sex, and alcohol abuse are examples. So is lack of exercise. Do not judge the person or his or her actions. Always treat the person with dignity and respect.

Independence and Social Interaction
Many digestive and endocrine disorders require life-style changes. Diet changes are common. Adjusting to these changes can be hard. The person and family need support and encouragement.

Delegation and Teamwork
The health team plans care to treat disorders and meet the person's needs. As the person's needs change, the care plan changes. Good communication and teamwork are needed. Assist with the person's care as directed. Follow the person's care plan.

Ethics and Laws
You must protect the person's rights. Privacy, confidentiality, and personal choice are important. So is being free from abuse, mistreatment, and neglect. Provide a safe setting to protect the person from harm and injury.

REVIEW QUESTIONS

Circle the BEST answer.

1 A person has gastro-esophageal reflux disease. Which should you question?
   a Person to wear loose clothing
   b Supine position after meals
   c Person to have small meals
   d No smoking or alcohol

2 A person with gastro-esophageal reflux disease has these food choices. Which is *best* for the person?
   a Baked chicken
   b Pasta with tomato sauce
   c Pizza
   d Salad with orange slices

3 A person is vomiting. Which position is *best*?
   a Supine
   b Prone
   c Semi-Fowler's
   d With the head turned to the side

4 Vomiting is dangerous because of
   a Aspiration
   b Diverticular disease
   c Fluid loss
   d Jaundice

5 Vomitus looks like coffee grounds. This signals
   a Bleeding
   b Gastro-esophageal reflux disease
   c Gallstones
   d A ruptured pouch

6 A person has diverticular disease. You will likely assist with
   a Preventing diarrhea
   b Giving antibiotics
   c Giving enemas
   d Preventing constipation

7 Gallbladder attacks usually occur
   a On awakening
   b During a fast
   c After a fatty meal
   d When the person is lying down

8 Which is *not* a sign of gallstones?
   a Jaundice
   b Pain under the right shoulder
   c Clay-colored stools
   d Hoarseness and choking sensation

9 Hepatitis is an inflammation of the
   a Liver
   b Gallbladder
   c Pancreas
   d Stomach

10 Hepatitis A is spread by
   a Needle sharing
   b IV drug use
   c Contaminated blood
   d The fecal-oral route

11 Hepatitis requires
   a Sterile gloves
   b Double-bagging
   c Standard Precautions
   d Masks, gowns, and goggles

12 Which is a common cause of cirrhosis?
   a Alcohol abuse
   b Diabetes
   c Gallstones
   d GERD

13 A person has cirrhosis. Which should you question?
   a Measure I&O.
   b Weigh the person daily.
   c Use warm water with baking soda for bathing.
   d Encourage fluids.

14 A person has cirrhosis. You should observe stools and vomitus for blood.
   a True
   b False

15 Which is *not* a sign of diabetes?
   a Increased urine production
   b Weight gain
   c Hunger
   d Increased thirst

16 A person with diabetes needs the following *except*
   a Exercise
   b Good foot care
   c A sodium-controlled diet
   d Healthy eating

17 A person with diabetes is vomiting after a meal. The person is at risk for
   a Hypoglycemia
   b Hyperglycemia
   c Jaundice
   d Bleeding

18 A person has diabetes. Blood glucose is monitored daily or
   a 2 or 3 times a day
   b 3 or 4 times a day
   c 4 or 5 times a day
   d 5 or 6 times a day

Answers to these questions are on p. 834.

Urinary and Reproductive Disorders

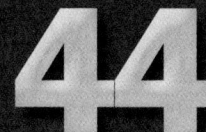

OBJECTIVES

- Define the key terms and key abbreviations listed in this chapter.
- Describe urinary tract infections and the care required.
- Describe prostate enlargement and the care required.
- Describe urinary diversions and the care required.
- Describe renal calculi and the care required.
- Describe acute and chronic kidney failure and the care required.
- Describe sexually transmitted diseases and the care required.
- Explain how to promote PRIDE in the person, the family, and yourself.

KEY TERMS

dialysis The process of removing waste products from the blood

diuresis The process *(esis)* of passing *(di)* urine *(ur)*; large amounts of urine are produced—1000 to 5000 mL (milliliters) a day

dysuria Difficult or painful *(dys)* urination *(uria)*

hematuria Blood *(hemat)* in the urine *(uria)*

oliguria Scant *(olig)* urine *(uria)*

pyuria Pus *(py)* in the urine *(uria)*

urinary diversion A surgically created pathway for urine to leave the body

urostomy A surgically created opening *(stomy)* between a ureter *(uro)* and the abdomen

KEY ABBREVIATIONS

AIDS	Acquired immunodeficiency syndrome	**mL**	Milliliter
BPH	Benign prostatic hyperplasia	**STD**	Sexually transmitted disease
HIV	Human immunodeficiency virus	**UTI**	Urinary tract infection

Urinary and reproductive disorders are common. Understanding the disorders gives meaning to the required care.

URINARY SYSTEM DISORDERS

The kidneys, ureters, bladder, and urethra are the major urinary system structures. Disorders can occur in these structures. Men can develop prostate problems.

See *Body Structure and Function Review: The Urinary System*, p. 720.

BODY STRUCTURE AND FUNCTION REVIEW: THE URINARY SYSTEM

The urinary system (Fig. 44-1):

- Removes waste products from the blood.
- Maintains water balance within the body.
- Maintains electrolyte balance. Electrolytes are substances that dissolve in water—sodium, potassium, and calcium. (See Chapter 9.)
- Maintains acid-base balance. (See Chapter 9.)

The *kidneys* are two bean-shaped organs in the upper abdomen. They lie against the back muscles on each side of the spine.

Each kidney has over a million *nephrons*—the basic working units of the kidney. Each nephron has a cluster of capillaries called a *glomerulus*. Blood passes through the glomerulus and is filtered by the capillaries. Most of the water and other needed substances are re-absorbed by the blood. The rest of the fluid and the waste products form *urine,* which drains into the *renal pelvis* in the kidney.

A *ureter* is attached to the renal pelvis of each kidney. The ureters carry urine from the kidneys to the *bladder*. Urine is stored in the bladder until the need to urinate is felt. Urine passes from the bladder through the *urethra*. The opening at the end of the urethra is the *meatus*. Urine passes from the body through the meatus.

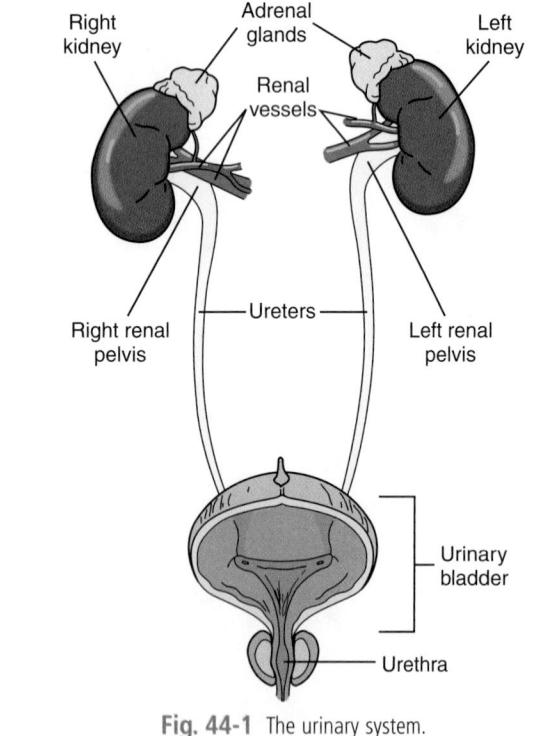

Right kidney
Adrenal glands
Left kidney
Renal vessels
Right renal pelvis
Ureters
Left renal pelvis
Urinary bladder
Urethra

Fig. 44-1 The urinary system.

Urinary Tract Infections

Urinary tract infections (UTIs) are common. Infection in one area can progress through the entire system. Microbes can enter the system through the urethra. Catheterization, urological exams, intercourse, poor perineal hygiene, immobility, and poor fluid intake are common causes. UTI is a common healthcare-associated infection (Chapter 15).

Women are at high risk. Microbes can easily enter the short female urethra. Prostate gland secretions help protect men from UTIs. However, an enlarged prostate increases the risk of UTI.

Older persons are at high risk for UTIs. Incomplete bladder emptying, perineal soiling from fecal incontinence, poor fluid intake, and poor nutrition increase the risk of UTI.

Cystitis. Cystitis is a bladder *(cyst)* infection *(itis)* caused by bacteria. These signs and symptoms are common:

- Urinary frequency
- *Oliguria—scant* (olig) *urine* (uria)
- Urgency
- *Dysuria—difficult or painful* (dys) *urination* (uria)
- Pain or burning on urination
- Foul-smelling urine
- *Hematuria—blood* (hemat) *in the urine* (uria)
- *Pyuria—pus* (py) *in the urine* (uria)
- Fever

Antibiotics are ordered. Fluids are encouraged—usually 2000 mL (milliliters) per day. If untreated, cystitis can lead to pyelonephritis.

Pyelonephritis. Pyelonephritis is inflammation *(itis)* of the kidney *(nephr)* pelvis *(pyelo)*. Infection is the most common cause. Cloudy urine may contain pus, mucus, and blood. Chills, fever, back pain, and nausea and vomiting occur. So do the signs and symptoms of cystitis. Treatment involves antibiotics and fluids.

Prostate Enlargement

The prostate is a gland in men. It lies in front of the rectum and just below the bladder (Fig. 44-2, A). The prostate surrounds the urethra. About the size of a walnut, the prostate grows larger (enlarges) as the man grows older (Fig. 44-2, B). This is called benign prostatic hyperplasia (BPH). *Benign* means *non-malignant. Hyper* means *excessive. Plasia* means *formation or development.* Benign prostatic hypertrophy is another name for enlarged prostate. (*Trophy* means *growth.*)

After age 60, most men have some symptoms of BPH. The enlarged prostate presses against the urethra obstructing urine flow. Bladder function is gradually lost. These problems are common:

- A weak urine stream
- Frequent voidings of small amounts of urine
- Urgency and leaking or dribbling of urine
- Frequent voiding at night
- Urinary retention (The man cannot void. Urine remains in the bladder.)

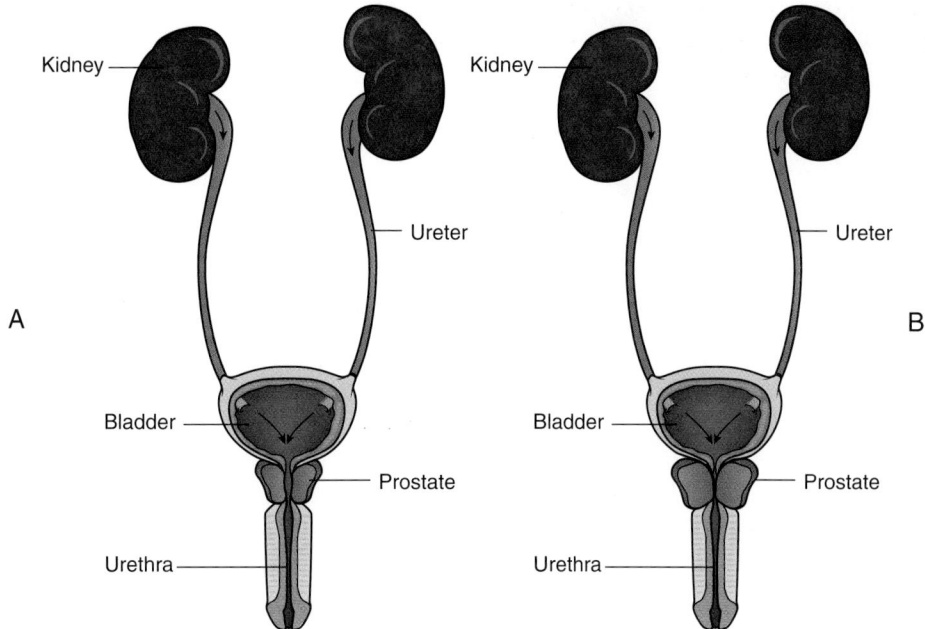

Fig. 44-2 A, Normal prostate size. **B,** Enlarged prostate. The prostate presses against the urethra. Urine flow is obstructed.

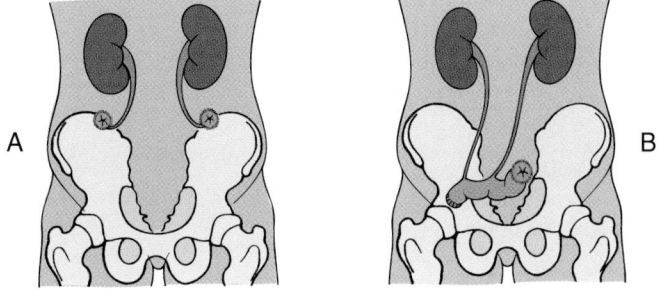

Fig. 44-3 Urostomies. **A,** Both ureters are brought through the skin onto the abdomen. The person has 2 stomas. **B,** The ileal conduit. A small section of the small intestine is removed. One end is sutured closed. The other end is brought through the skin onto the abdomen to form a stoma. The ureters are attached to this part of the small intestine.

Treatment depends on the extent of the problem. For mild BPH, drugs can shrink the prostate or stop its growth. Some microwave and laser treatments destroy excess prostate tissue.

Transurethral resection of the prostate (TURP) is a common surgical procedure. The doctor inserts a lighted scope through the penis. The scope has a wire loop used to cut tissue and seal blood vessels. The removed tissue is flushed out of the bladder. Flushing fluid enters the bladder through a catheter. Urine and the flushing fluid flow out of the bladder through the same catheter. Some bleeding and blood clots are normal. The person's care plan may include:

- No straining or sudden movements
- Drinking at least 8 cups of water daily
- No straining to have a bowel movement
- A balanced diet to prevent constipation
- No heavy lifting

Urinary Diversions

Sometimes the bladder is surgically removed. Cancer and bladder injuries are common reasons. When the bladder is removed, urine must still leave the body. A *urinary diversion is a surgically created pathway for urine to leave the body.*

Often an ostomy is involved. A *urostomy is a surgically created opening* (stomy) *between a ureter* (uro) *and the abdomen* (Fig. 44-3). You may care for persons with long-standing urostomies. The person assists with care as able.

A pouch is applied over the stoma (Fig. 44-4, p. 722). Urine drains from the stoma into the pouch. Pouches are

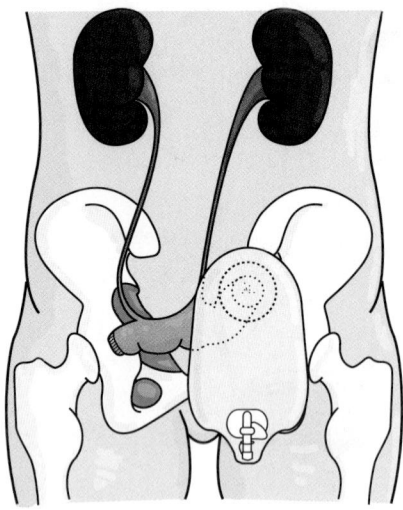

Fig. 44-4 Urostomy pouch.

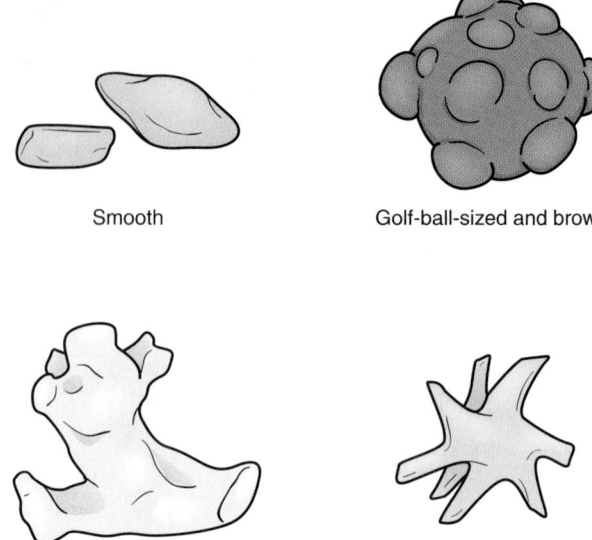

Smooth

Golf-ball-sized and brown

Staghorn

Jagged and yellow

Fig. 44-5 Kidney stones.

PROMOTING SAFETY AND COMFORT
Urinary Diversions

Safety
Microbes can grow in urine. And urine may contain blood. Also, you have contact with mucous membranes. Follow Standard Precautions and the Bloodborne Pathogen Standard.

Comfort
The best time to change a pouch is after sleep and before eating or drinking fluids. Urine flow is less when the person has not had anything to eat or drink for 2 to 3 hours.

The stoma does not have sensation. Touching the stoma does not cause pain or discomfort.

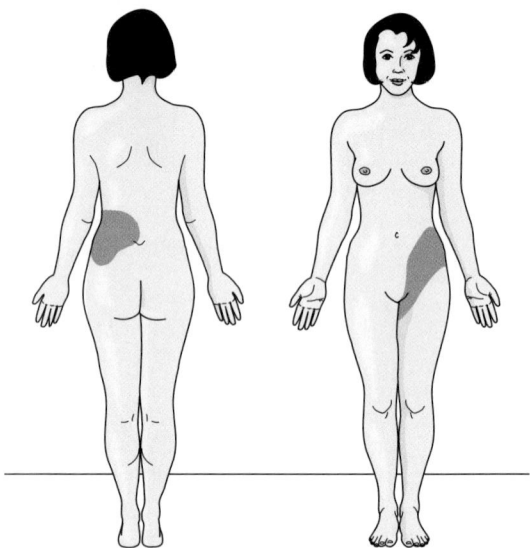

Fig. 44-6 *Shaded areas* show where the pain from kidney stones is located.

changed every 5 to 7 days. A pouch is replaced any time it leaks. Urine on the skin can cause irritation, breakdown, and infection.

Urine drains constantly into the pouch. Empty pouches every 3 to 4 hours. Or empty them when becoming ⅓ (one-third) full. Pouches become heavy as they fill with urine. A heavy pouch can loosen the seal between the pouch and the skin. Urine can leak onto the skin.

Good skin care is needed. You must help prevent skin breakdown. Observe and report skin changes around the stoma. See the "Person With an Ostomy" in Chapter 23.

See *Promoting Safety and Comfort: Urinary Diversions.*

Kidney Stones
Kidney stones (calculi) are most common in white men 40 years of age and older. Bedrest, immobility, and poor fluid intake are risk factors. Stones vary in size from grains of sand to golf-ball-size (Fig. 44-5). Signs and symptoms include:
- Severe, cramping pain in the back and side just below the ribs (Fig. 44-6)
- Pain in the lower abdomen, thigh, and urethra
- Nausea and vomiting
- Fever and chills
- Dysuria—difficult or painful (*dys*) urination (*uria*)
- Urinary urgency
- Burning on urination
- Hematuria—blood (*hemat*) in the urine (*uria*)
- Cloudy urine
- Foul-smelling urine

Drugs are given for pain relief. The person needs to drink 2000 to 3000 mL a day. The fluids help stones pass from the body through the urine. All urine is strained (Chapter 31). Medical or surgical removal of the stone may be necessary. Some diet changes can prevent stones.

Kidney Failure

In kidney failure (renal failure), the kidneys do not function or are severely impaired. Waste products are not removed from the blood. Fluid is retained. Heart failure and hypertension easily result. The person is very ill.

Acute Kidney Failure. Acute kidney failure is sudden. Blood flow to the kidneys is severely decreased. Causes include severe injury or bleeding, heart attack, heart failure, burns, infection, and severe allergic reactions.

At first, *oliguria* (scant amount of urine) occurs. Urine output is less than 400 mL in 24 hours. This phase lasts a few days to 2 weeks. Then *diuresis* occurs—*the process* (esis) *of passing* (di) *urine* (ur). *Large amounts are produced—1000 to 5000 mL a day.* Kidney function improves and returns to normal during the recovery phase. This can take up to 1 year. Some persons develop chronic kidney failure.

Every system is affected when waste products build up in the blood. Death can occur.

Treatment involves drugs, restricted fluids, and diet therapy. The diet is high in carbohydrates and low in protein and potassium. The care plan may include:
- Measuring and recording intake and output.
- Hourly urinary output measurements. Report less than 30 mL per hour at once.
- Restricting fluid intake.
- Measuring weight daily.
- Turning and re-positioning at least every 2 hours.
- Measures to prevent pressure ulcers.
- Frequent oral hygiene.
- Measures to prevent infection.
- Deep-breathing and coughing exercises.
- Measures to meet emotional needs.

Chronic Kidney Failure. The kidneys cannot meet the body's needs. Nephrons are destroyed over many years. Hypertension and diabetes are common causes. Infections, urinary tract obstructions, and tumors are other causes.

Signs and symptoms appear when 75% of kidney function is lost (Box 44-1). Every system is affected as waste products build up in the blood.

Treatment includes fluid restriction, diet therapy, drugs, and dialysis. *Dialysis is the process of removing waste products from the blood.*
- *Hemodialysis* removes waste and fluid by filtering the blood *(hemo)* through an artificial kidney (Fig. 44-7).
- *Peritoneal dialysis* uses the lining of the abdominal cavity *(peritoneal membrane)* to remove waste and fluid from the blood (Fig. 44-8, p. 724).

You will assist in the person's care. See Box 44-2, p. 724.

BOX 44-1	SIGNS AND SYMPTOMS OF CHRONIC KIDNEY FAILURE

- Skin
  - Color: yellow, tan, or dusky
  - Dry, itchy
  - Thin, brittle
- Bruises
- Breath: bad breath *(halitosis)*
- Mouth: inflammation of *(stomatitis)*
- Nausea and vomiting
- Appetite: loss of
- Weight loss
- Diarrhea or constipation
- Urine output: decreased
- Bleeding tendencies
- Infection: susceptible to
- Hypertension
- Heart failure
- Gastric ulcers
- Gastro-intestinal bleeding
- Pulse: irregular
- Breathing: abnormal patterns
- Legs and ankles: swelling
- Legs and feet: burning sensation in
- Muscles: twitching and cramps
- Fatigue
- Sleep disorders
- Headache
- Convulsions
- Confusion
- Coma

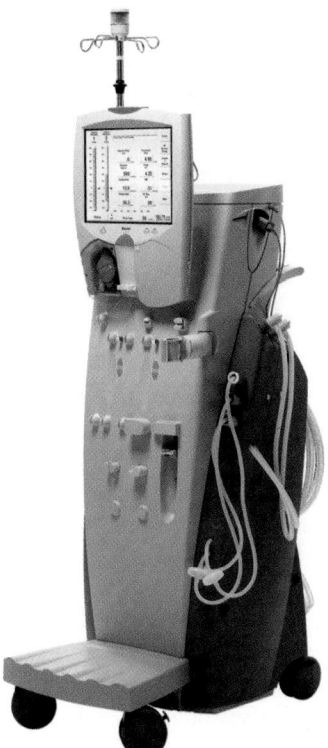

Fig. 44-7 Dialysis machine.

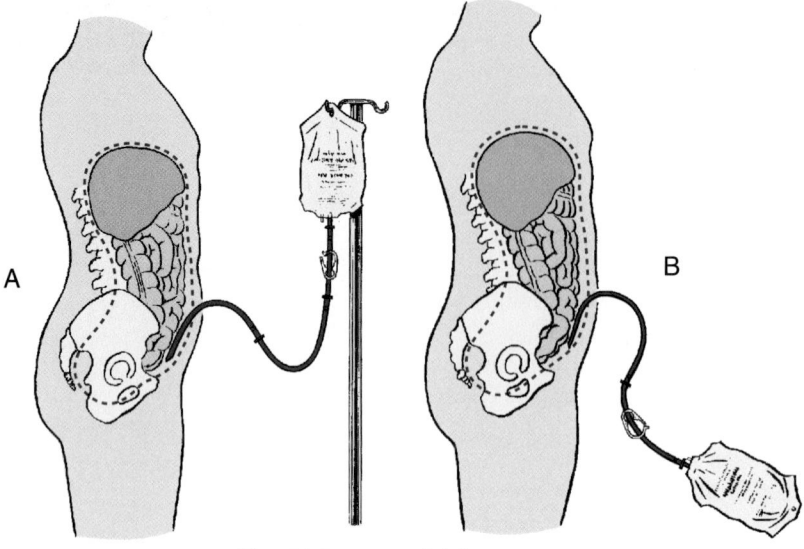

Fig. 44-8 Peritoneal dialysis system.

BOX 44-2	CARE OF THE PERSON IN CHRONIC KIDNEY FAILURE

- A diet low in protein, potassium, and sodium
- Fluid restriction
- Measuring blood pressure in the supine, sitting, and standing positions
- Measuring daily weight
- Measuring and recording intake and output
- Turning and re-positioning
- Measures to prevent pressure ulcers
- Range-of-motion exercises
- Measures to prevent itching (bath oils, lotions, creams)
- Measures to prevent injury and bleeding
- Frequent oral hygiene
- Measures to prevent infection
- Measures to prevent diarrhea or constipation
- Measures to meet emotional needs
- Measures to promote rest

REPRODUCTIVE DISORDERS

Sexual activities involve the structures and functions of the reproductive system. The male reproductive system:

- Produces and transports sperm.
- Deposits sperm in the female reproductive tract.
- Secretes hormones.
  The female reproductive system:
- Produces eggs (ova).
- Secretes hormones.
- Protects and nourishes the fetus during pregnancy.
  Aging affects the reproductive system (Chapters 11 and 48). Many injuries, diseases, and surgeries can affect reproductive structures and functions.

Sexually Transmitted Diseases

A sexually transmitted disease (STD) is spread by oral, vaginal, or anal sex (Table 44-1). Some people do not have signs and symptoms or are not aware of an infection. Others know but do not seek treatment because of embarrassment.

STDs often occur in the genital and rectal areas. They also occur in the ears, mouth, nipples, throat, tongue, eyes, and nose. Condom use helps prevent the spread of STDs, especially the human immunodeficiency virus (HIV) and acquired immunodeficiency syndrome (AIDS). Some STDs are also spread through skin breaks, by contact with infected body fluids (blood, semen, saliva), or by contaminated blood or needles.

Standard Precautions and the Bloodborne Pathogen Standard are followed.

See *Focus on Children and Older Persons: Sexually Transmitted Diseases.*

FOCUS ON CHILDREN AND OLDER PERSONS
Sexually Transmitted Diseases

Older Persons
Many older people are sexually active. They get and can spread STDs in the same ways that younger persons do. However, many do not think they are at risk. Always practice Standard Precautions and the Bloodborne Pathogen Standard. Do not assume that older people are too old to have sex.

TABLE 44-1 SEXUALLY TRANSMITTED DISEASES

Disease	Signs and Symptoms	Treatment
Herpes	Painful, blister-like sores on or near the genitals, mouth, or anus (Fig. 44-9, p. 726) Sores may have a watery discharge Pain, itching, burning, and tingling in the affected area Vaginal discharge Pain during urination or intercourse Fever Swollen glands	No known cure Anti-viral drugs
Genital warts	*Male*—Warts in or on the penis, anus, genitalia, mouth, or throat *Female*—Warts in or on the vagina, cervix, labia, anus, mouth, or throat	Application of an ointment that causes the warts to dry up and fall off Surgical removal may be necessary if the ointment is not effective
HIV/AIDS	See Chapter 40	See Chapter 40
Gonorrhea	Burning and pain on urination Urinary frequency and urgency Genital discharge (vagina, urethra, rectum)	Antibiotic drugs
Chlamydia	May not show symptoms Discharge from the penis or vagina Burning or pain on urination Testicular pain or swelling Vaginal bleeding Rectal inflammation and/or discharge Pain during intercourse Diarrhea Nausea Abdominal pain Fever	Antibiotic drugs
Pubic lice	Intense itching	Over-the-counter or prescription lice treatment Washing or dry-cleaning all exposed clothing, bedding, and towels
Trichomoniasis (occurs in women; men are carriers)	No symptoms in men Frothy, thick, foul-smelling, yellow vaginal discharge Genital itching and irritation Burning and pain on urination Genital swelling	Metronidazole
Syphilis	*Stage 1*—10 to 90 days after exposure • Painless sores (chancres) on the penis, in the vagina, on the genitalia, on the lips or inside of the mouth, or anywhere on the body *Stage 2*—About 3 to 6 weeks after the sores • General fatigue, loss of appetite, nausea, fever, headache, rash, swollen glands, sore throat, bone and joint pain, hair loss, lesions on the lips and genitalia • Symptoms may come and go for many years *Stage 3*—3 to 15 years after infection • Central nervous system damage (including paralysis), heart damage, blindness, liver damage, mental health problems, death	Penicillin and other antibiotic drugs

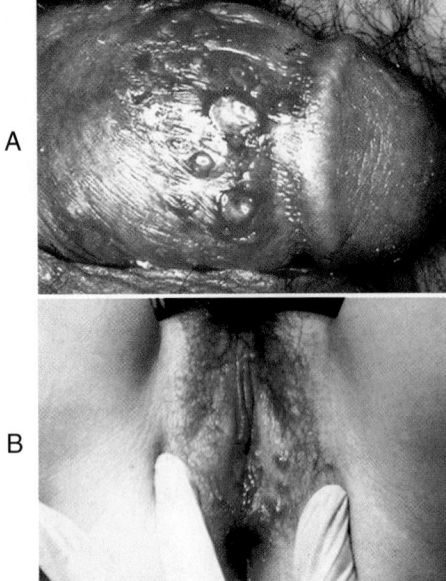

Fig. 44-9 Herpes. **A,** Sores on the penis. **B,** Sores on the female perineum.

FOCUS ON PRIDE

The Person, Family, and Yourself

Personal and Professional Responsibility

UTIs are a common healthcare-associated infection. Females are at high risk. Proper perineal care can prevent UTIs. Always clean females from front to back. Use a clean part of the washcloth for each stroke. Use more than one washcloth if needed.

You are responsible for providing care in a way that protects the person's health and safety. Take pride in performing safe and careful perineal care.

Rights and Respect

An STD can make the person feel embarrassed, ashamed, or guilty. Do not judge the person. Treat the person with dignity and respect.

Independence and Social Interaction

Persons with chronic kidney failure cannot survive without dialysis. Hemodialysis is often done 3 times a week. Each session can take 4 hours or more. Peritoneal dialysis is often done in the home setting. Dialysis is done several times daily, during the night, or both.

Dialysis takes a lot of time. Work, family time, and other activities are limited by the need for dialysis. These social changes affect quality of life. The person and family need support and encouragement.

Delegation and Teamwork

Kidney stone pain is severe. The pain can cause the person to be impatient and rude. Once comfort needs are met, behavior returns to normal. The person is often sorry for the behavior.

Assist in promoting comfort. Be patient, kind, and understanding. Treat the person well, even if he or she does not treat you well. Accept offered apologies. Tell the nurse if you need help dealing with the person's behavior.

Ethics and Laws

Urinary and reproductive disorders are personal. The person does not want information shared with others. Only give information to those directly involved in the person's care. Take pride in protecting the person's right to privacy and confidentiality.

REVIEW QUESTIONS

Circle the BEST answer.

1 A person has cystitis. This is a
   a Kidney infection   c Urinary diversion
   b Kidney stone   d Bladder infection
2 The person with cystitis needs to drink about
   a 500 mL daily   c 1500 mL daily
   b 1000 mL daily   d 2000 mL daily
3 BPH causes urinary problems because
   a The person has a weak urine stream
   b The person voids frequently at night
   c The enlarged prostate presses against the urethra
   d Voidings are in small amounts
4 Mr. Jones had a TURP. Which measure should you question?
   a No sudden movements
   b No heavy lifting
   c No straining to have a bowel movement
   d No oral fluids
5 A person with a urostomy
   a Has a new pathway for urine to exit the body
   b Needs dialysis
   c Had surgery for an enlarged prostate
   d Has pyuria
6 A person has kidney stones. You need to
   a Strain all urine
   b Empty the pouch
   c Collect a urine specimen
   d Change the urinary drainage bag
7 A person has kidney failure. Which is *false*?
   a Waste products are removed from the blood.
   b The body retains fluid.
   c Every body system is affected.
   d Diuresis follows oliguria.
8 For chronic kidney failure, care includes the following *except*
   a A diet low in protein, potassium, and sodium
   b Measuring urine output every hour
   c Measures to prevent pressure ulcers
   d Measuring weight daily
9 These statements are about STDs. Which is *false*?
   a They are usually spread by sexual contact.
   b They affect the genital area and other body parts.
   c Signs and symptoms are obvious.
   d Some result in death.
10 STDs require
   a Masks and protective eyewear
   b Gowns
   c Double-bagging
   d Standard Precautions

Answers to these questions are on p. 834.

Mental Health Problems

OBJECTIVES

- Define the key terms and key abbreviations listed in this chapter.
- Explain the difference between mental health and mental illness.
- List the causes of mental illness.
- Describe four anxiety disorders.
- Explain the defense mechanisms used to relieve anxiety.
- Describe common phobias.

- Explain schizophrenia.
- Describe bipolar disorder and depression.
- Describe personality disorders.
- Describe substance abuse and addiction.
- Describe suicide and the persons at risk.
- Describe the care required by persons with mental health disorders.
- Explain how to promote PRIDE in the person, the family, and yourself.

KEY TERMS

affect Feelings and emotions

anxiety A vague, uneasy feeling in response to stress

compulsion Repeating an act over and over again

conscious Awareness of the environment and experiences; the person knows what is happening and can control thoughts and behavior

defense mechanism An unconscious reaction that blocks unpleasant or threatening feelings

delusion A false belief

delusion of grandeur An exaggerated belief about one's importance, wealth, power, or talents

delusion of persecution A false belief that one is being mistreated, abused, or harassed

emotional illness See "mental disorder"

flashback Reliving a trauma in thoughts during the day and in nightmares during sleep

hallucination Seeing, hearing, smelling, or feeling something that is not real

mental Relating to the mind; something that exists in the mind or is done by the mind

mental disorder A disturbance in the ability to cope with or adjust to stress; behavior and function are impaired; mental illness, emotional illness, psychiatric disorder

mental health The person copes with and adjusts to everyday stresses in ways accepted by society

mental illness See "mental disorder"

obsession A recurrent, unwanted thought, idea, or image

panic An intense and sudden feeling of fear, anxiety, terror, or dread

paranoia A disorder (*para*) of the mind (*noia*); false beliefs (delusions) and suspicion about a person or situation

personality The set of attitudes, values, behaviors, and traits of a person

phobia An intense fear

psychiatric disorder See "mental disorder"

psychosis A state of severe mental impairment

stress The response or change in the body caused by any emotional, physical, social, or economic factor

stressor The event or factor that causes stress

subconscious Memory, past experiences, and thoughts of which the person is not aware; they are easily recalled

suicide To kill oneself

suicide contagion Exposure to suicide or suicidal behaviors within one's family, one's peer group, or media reports of suicide

unconscious Experiences and feelings that cannot be recalled

withdrawal syndrome The person's physical and mental response after stopping or severely reducing the use of a substance that was used regularly

KEY ABBREVIATIONS

BPD	Borderline personality disorder	**OCD**	Obsessive-compulsive disorder
CDC	Centers for Disease Control and Prevention	**PTSD**	Post-traumatic stress disorder
GI	Gastro-intestinal		

The whole person has physical, social, psychological, and spiritual parts. Each part affects the other.

- A physical problem can have social, mental, and spiritual effects.
- A mental health problem can have physical, social, and spiritual effects.
- A social problem can have physical, mental health, and spiritual effects.

BASIC CONCEPTS

Mental relates to the mind. It is something that exists in the mind or is done by the mind. Therefore mental health involves the mind. Mental health and mental disorders involve stress:

- *Stress*—*is the response or change in the body caused by any emotional, physical, social, or economic factor.*
- *Mental health*—*means that the person copes with and adjusts to everyday stresses in ways accepted by society.*
- *Mental disorder*—*is a disturbance in the ability to cope with or adjust to stress. Behavior and function are impaired. Mental illness, emotional illness,* and *psychiatric disorder* are other names.

Causes of mental health disorders include:

- Not being able to cope or adjust to stress
- Chemical imbalances
- Genetics
- Physical, biological, or psychological factors
- Drug or substance abuse
- Social and cultural factors

Personality

Personality is the set of attitudes, values, behaviors, and traits of a person. Personality starts to develop at birth. It is affected by such factors as genes, culture, environment, parenting, and social experiences.

Maslow's theory of basic needs (Chapter 8) affects personality development. Lower-level needs must be met before higher-level needs. Physical needs are met before safety and security, love and belonging, self-esteem, and self-actualization needs. Children who grow up hungry, neglected, cold, or abused will not feel safe and secure. Higher-level needs cannot be met. Unmet needs at any age affect personality development.

Growth and development also affect personality development (Chapter 10). They occur in a sequence, order, and pattern. Certain tasks must be achieved at each stage. Each stage is the basis for the next stage.

Freud's Theory of Personality Development

Freud's theory of personality development involves three levels of awareness:

- *Conscious*—*awareness of the environment and experiences. The person knows what is happening and can control thoughts and behavior.*

- *Subconscious*—*memory, past experiences, and thoughts of which the person is not aware. They are easily recalled.*
- *Unconscious*—*experiences and feelings that cannot be recalled.*

His theory also involves the id, ego, and superego. The *id* is at the unconscious level. Pleasure is the focus. The need for pleasure must be satisfied almost right away. The id deals with hunger, comfort, sex, and warmth. People are not aware that they believe and act in ways to satisfy the id.

The *ego* deals with reality, with what is happening in the person's world. Thoughts, feelings, reasoning, good sense, and problem solving occur in the ego. The ego decides what to do and when.

The *superego* is concerned with right and wrong. Morals and values are in the superego. The superego judges what the ego thinks and does. It is like a parent helping a child look at behaviors.

ANXIETY DISORDERS

Anxiety is a vague, uneasy feeling in response to stress. The person may not know why or the cause. Danger or harm—real or imagined—is sensed. The person acts to relieve the unpleasant feeling. Often anxiety occurs when needs are not met.

Some anxiety is normal. Persons with mental health problems have higher levels of anxiety. Signs and symptoms depend on the degree of anxiety (Box 45-1).

Anxiety level depends on the stressor. A *stressor is the event or factor that causes stress.* It can be physical, emotional, social, or economic. Past experiences and the number of stressors affect how a person reacts. A stressor may cause mild anxiety. Or it can cause higher anxiety at another time.

Coping and defense mechanisms relieve anxiety. Some are healthy. Others are not—eating, drinking, smoking, and fighting are examples. Healthy ways to cope include discussing the problem, exercising, playing music, taking a hot bath, and wanting to be alone.

Defense mechanisms are unconscious reactions that block unpleasant or threatening feelings (Box 45-2). Some use of defense mechanisms is normal. In mental health disorders, they are used poorly.

BOX 45-1	**SIGNS AND SYMPTOMS OF ANXIETY**
• A "lump" in the throat	• Nausea
• "Butterflies" in the stomach	• Diarrhea
• Pulse: rapid	• Urinary frequency and
• Respirations: rapid	urgency
• Blood pressure: increased	• Attention span: poor
• Speech: rapid, voice	• Directions: difficulty
changes	following
• Mouth: dry	• Sleep: difficulty
• Sweating	• Appetite: loss of

BOX 45-2	**DEFENSE MECHANISMS**

Compensation. *Compensate* means to make up for, replace, or substitute. The person makes up for or substitutes a strength for a weakness.

EXAMPLE: Not good in sports, a child develops another talent.

Conversion. *Convert* means to change. An emotion is shown as a physical symptom or changed into a physical symptom.

EXAMPLE: Not wanting to read out loud in school, a child complains of a headache.

Denial. *Deny* means refusing to accept or believe something that is true. The person refuses to face or accept unpleasant or threatening things.

EXAMPLE: After a heart attack, a person continues to smoke.

Displacement. *Displace* means to move or take the place of. An individual moves behaviors or emotions from one person, place, or thing to a safe person, place, or thing.

EXAMPLE: Angry at your boss, you yell at a friend.

Identification. *Identify* means to relate or recognize. A person assumes the ideas, behaviors, and traits of another person.

EXAMPLE: A neighbor is a high school cheerleader. A little girl practices cheerleading in her backyard.

Projection. *Project* means to blame another. An individual blames another person or object for unacceptable behaviors, emotions, ideas, or wishes.

EXAMPLE: Sleeping too long, a worker blames the traffic when late for work.

Rationalization. *Rational* means sensible, reasonable, or logical. An acceptable reason or excuse is given for behaviors or actions. The real reason is not given.

EXAMPLE: Often late for work, an employee does not get a raise. The employee thinks, "My boss doesn't like me."

Reaction formation. A person acts in a way opposite to what he or she truly feels.

EXAMPLE: A worker does not like his boss. He buys the boss a gift.

Regression. *Regress* means to move back or to retreat. The person retreats or moves back to an earlier time or condition.

EXAMPLE: A 3-year-old wants a baby bottle when a new baby comes into the family.

Repression. *Repress* means to hold down or keep back. The person keeps unpleasant or painful thoughts or experiences from the conscious mind. They cannot be recalled or remembered.

EXAMPLE: A child was sexually abused. Now 33 years old, there is no memory of the event.

Panic Disorder

Panic is the highest level of anxiety. *Panic is an intense and sudden feeling of fear, anxiety, terror, or dread.* Onset is sudden with no obvious reason. The person cannot function. Signs and symptoms of anxiety are severe (see Box 45-1). The person may also have:

- Chest pain
- Shortness of breath
- Rapid heart rate ("heart pounding")
- Numbness and tingling in the hands
- Dizziness
- A smothering sensation
- Feeling of impending doom or loss of control

The person may feel that he or she is having a heart attack, losing his or her mind, or on the verge of death. Attacks can occur at any time, even during sleep.

Panic attacks can last for 10 minutes or longer. They can occur often. Panic disorder can last for a few months or for many years.

Many people avoid places where panic attacks occurred. For example, a person had a panic attack in a shopping mall. Malls are avoided.

Phobias

Phobia means an intense fear. The person has an intense fear of an object, situation, or activity that has little or no actual danger. Common phobias are fear of:

- Being in an open, crowded, or public place (agoraphobia—*agora* means *marketplace*)

- Being in pain or seeing others in pain (algophobia—*algo* means *pain*)
- Water (aquaphobia—*aqua* means *water*)
- Being in or being trapped in an enclosed or narrow space (claustrophobia—*claustro* means *closing*)
- The slightest uncleanliness (mysophobia—*myso* means *anything that is disgusting*)
- Night or darkness (nyctophobia—*nycto* means *night* or *darkness*)
- Fire (pyrophobia—*pyro* means *fire*)
- Strangers (xenophobia—*xeno* means *strange*)

The person avoids what is feared. When faced with the fear, the person has high anxiety and cannot function.

Obsessive-Compulsive Disorder

The person with obsessive-compulsive disorder (OCD) has obsessions and compulsions. An *obsession is a recurrent, unwanted thought, idea, or image.* Some people are obsessed with microbes, dirt, violent thoughts, or things forbidden by religion. *Compulsion is repeating an act over and over again* (a ritual). The act may not make sense. Anxiety is great if the act is not done.

Common rituals are hand washing, cleaning, counting things to a certain number, or touching things in a certain order. Such rituals can take over an hour every day. They are very distressing and affect daily life. Some persons with OCD also have depression, eating disorders, substance abuse, and other anxiety disorders.

BOX 45-3	SIGNS AND SYMPTOMS OF POST-TRAUMATIC STRESS DISORDER

- Startles easily
- Emotionally numb—especially to those with whom the person used to be close
- Difficulty trusting or feeling close to people
- Loss of interest in things he or she used to enjoy
- Problems being affectionate
- Feelings of intense guilt
- Irritability
- Avoiding situations that remind the person of the harmful event
- Difficulty around the anniversary of the harmful event
- Gets mad easily

- Outbursts of anger
- Problems sleeping
- Increasingly aggressive and violent
- Physical symptoms:
  - Headache
  - Gastro-intestinal (GI) distress
  - Immune system problems
  - Dizziness
  - Chest pain
  - Discomfort in other body parts

Post-Traumatic Stress Disorder

Post-traumatic stress disorder (PTSD) occurs after a terrifying ordeal. There was physical harm or the threat of physical harm. See Box 45-3 for signs and symptoms. PTSD can develop:
- After being harmed
- After a loved one was harmed
- After seeing a harmful event happen

PTSD can result from many traumatic events. They include:
- War
- A terrorist attack
- Mugging
- Rape
- Torture
- Kidnapping
- Being held captive
- Child abuse
- A crash—vehicle, train, plane
- Bombing
- A natural disaster—flood, tornado, hurricane, earthquake

Flashbacks are common. A *flashback is reliving the trauma in thoughts during the day and in nightmares during sleep.* Flashbacks may involve images, sounds, smells, or feelings. Everyday things can trigger them. A door slamming is an example. During a flashback, the person may believe that the trauma is happening all over again.

Signs and symptoms usually develop about 3 months after the event. Some people recover within 6 months. PTSD lasts longer in other people. The condition may become chronic.

PTSD can develop at any age including childhood. The person may also suffer from depression, substance abuse, and other anxiety disorders.

SCHIZOPHRENIA

Schizophrenia means split *(schizo)* mind *(phrenia).* It is a severe, chronic, disabling brain disorder. It involves:
- *Psychosis—a state of severe mental impairment.* The person does not view the real or unreal correctly.

- *Delusion—a false belief.* For example, the person believes that a radio station is airing the person's thoughts.
- *Hallucination—seeing, hearing, smelling, or feeling something that is not real.* A person may see animals, insects, or people that are not real. "Voices" are a common type of hallucination. "Voices" may comment on behavior, order the person to do things, warn of danger, or talk to other voices.
- *Paranoia—a disorder* (para) *of the mind* (noia). *The person has false beliefs (delusions) and suspicion about a person or situation.* For example, a person believes that others are cheating, harassing, poisoning, spying on, or plotting against him or her.
- *Delusion of grandeur—an exaggerated belief about one's importance, wealth, power, or talents.* For example, a man believes he is Superman. Or a woman believes she is the Queen of England.
- *Delusion of persecution—the false belief that one is being mistreated, abused, or harassed.* For example, a person believes that someone is "out to get" him or her.

The person with schizophrenia has severe mental impairment *(psychosis).* Thinking and behavior are disturbed. The person has false beliefs *(delusions).* He or she also has *hallucinations.* That is, the person sees, hears, smells, or feels things that are not real. The person has problems relating to others. He or she may be *paranoid.* That is, the person is suspicious about a person or situation. The person may have difficulty organizing thoughts. Responses are not appropriate. Communication is disturbed. The person may ramble or repeat what another says. Sometimes speech cannot be understood. He or she may make up words. The person may withdraw. That is, the person lacks interest in others. He or she is not involved with people or society.

Disorders of movement occur. These include:
- Being clumsy and uncoordinated
- Involuntary movements
- Grimacing
- Unusual mannerisms
- Sitting for hours without moving, speaking, or responding

Some persons regress. To *regress* means to retreat or move back to an earlier time or condition. For example, a

BOX 45-4	SIGNS AND SYMPTOMS OF BIPOLAR DISORDER

Mania (Manic Episode)

- Increased energy, activity, and restlessness
- Excessively "high," overly good mood
- Extreme irritability
- Racing thoughts and talking very fast
- Jumping from one idea to another
- Easily distracted; problems concentrating
- Little sleep needed
- Unrealistic beliefs in one's abilities and powers
- Poor judgment
- Spending sprees
- A lasting period of behavior that is different from usual
- Increased sexual drive
- Drug abuse (particularly cocaine, alcohol, and sleeping pills)
- Aggressive behavior
- Denial that anything is wrong

Depression (Depressive Episode)

- Lasting sad, anxious, or empty mood
- Feelings of hopelessness
- Feelings of guilt, worthlessness, or helplessness
- Loss of interest or pleasure in activities once enjoyed
- Loss of interest in sex
- Decreased energy; a feeling of fatigue or being "slowed down"
- Problems concentrating, remembering, or making decisions
- Restlessness or irritability
- Sleeping too much, or unable to sleep
- Change in appetite
- Unintended weight loss or gain
- Chronic pain or other symptoms not caused by physical illness or injury
- Thoughts of death or suicide
- Suicide attempts

5-year-old wets the bed when there is a new baby. This is normal. Healthy adults do not act like infants or children.

In men, the symptoms usually begin in the late teens or early 20s. In women, symptoms usually begin in their 20s and 30s. In rare cases, it can appear in childhood. People with schizophrenia do not tend to be violent. However, if a person with paranoid schizophrenia becomes violent, it is often directed at family members. The violence is usually at home. Some persons with schizophrenia attempt suicide (p. 736).

See *Focus on Communication: Schizophrenia.*

MOOD DISORDERS

Mood or *affect relates to feelings and emotions.* Mood (or affective) disorders involve feelings, emotions, and moods.

Bipolar Disorder

Bipolar means two *(bi)* poles or ends *(polar).* The person with bipolar disorder has severe extremes in mood, energy, and ability to function. There are emotional lows *(depression)* and emotional highs *(mania).* Also called manic-depressive illness, the person may:

- Be more depressed than manic.
- Be more manic than depressed.
- Alternate between depression and mania.

The disorder tends to run in families. It usually develops during the late teens or early adulthood. Life-long management is required.

Signs and symptoms range from mild to severe (Box 45-4). Mood changes are called "episodes." Bipolar disorder can damage relationships and affect school or work performance. Some people are suicidal.

Major Depression

Depression involves the body, mood, and thoughts. Symptoms (see Box 45-4) affect work, study, sleep, eating, and other activities. The person is very sad. Interest in daily activities is lost.

A stressful event such as the death of a partner, parent, or child may cause depression. So can divorce and job loss. Some physical disorders can cause depression. Stroke, heart attack, cancer, and Parkinson's disease are examples. Hormonal factors may cause depression in women—menstrual cycle changes, pregnancy, miscarriage, after childbirth (post-partum depression), and menopause.

Depression in Older Persons. Depression is common in older persons. They have many losses—death of family and friends, loss of health, loss of body functions, loss of independence. Loneliness and side effects from some drugs also are causes. See Box 45-5 (p. 732) for the signs and symptoms of depression in older persons.

Depression in older persons is often overlooked or a wrong diagnosis is made. Often the person is thought to have a cognitive disorder (Chapter 46). Therefore depression is often not treated.

BOX 45-5	SIGNS AND SYMPTOMS OF DEPRESSION IN OLDER PERSONS

- Fatigue and lack of interest
- Inability to experience pleasure
- Feelings of uselessness, hopelessness, and helplessness
- Decreased sexual interest
- Increased dependency
- Anxiety
- Slow or unreliable memory

- Paranoia
- Agitation
- Focus on the past
- Thoughts of death and suicide
- Difficulty completing activities of daily living
- Changes in sleep patterns
- Poor grooming

- Withdrawal from people and interests
- Muscle aches, abdominal pain, and headaches
- Nausea and vomiting
- Dry mouth
- Loss of appetite
- Weight loss

PERSONALITY DISORDERS

Personality disorders involve rigid and maladaptive behaviors. To *adapt* means to *change* or *adjust*. *Mal* means *bad, wrong,* or *ill. Maladaptive* means to *change* or *adjust in the wrong way.* Because of behavior, persons with personality disorders cannot function well in society.

Antisocial Personality Disorder

This is a chronic disorder in which the person's thinking and behaviors show no regard for right and wrong. The person has poor judgment, lacks responsibility, and is hostile. The person is not loyal to any person or group. Morals and ethics are lacking. The rights of others do not matter. The person lies, charms, or cons others for personal gain or pleasure. The person has no guilt and does not learn from experiences or punishment. The person is often in trouble with the police.

Signs and symptoms may include:

- Lying or cheating
- Child abuse or neglect
- Aggressive or violent behaviors
- Poor or abusive relationships
- Blaming others for actions and behaviors
- Problems functioning in work or school

Symptoms tend to peak during the 20s and then decrease. Risk factors include:

- A conduct disorder in childhood
- A family history of antisocial personality disorder
- A family history of mental disorders
- Childhood abuse—verbal, physical, sexual
- Unstable family life during childhood
- Loss of parents during childhood—death, divorce

Borderline Personality Disorder (BPD)

The person has problems with moods, relationships, self-image, behavior, and controlling emotions. Intense bouts of anger, depression, and anxiety may last hours or most of the day. Aggression, self-injury, and drug or alcohol abuse may occur. The person may engage in risky behaviors—unsafe driving, unsafe sex, gambling sprees. The person may greatly admire and love family and friends and then suddenly shift to intense anger and dislike. The person may have thoughts of suicide and other mental health disorders.

BPD is more common in women than in men. Risk factors may include:

- A family history of BPD
- Childhood abuse—sexual, physical
- Childhood neglect or being abandoned
- Changes in the brain
- Brain chemicals that do not function properly

SUBSTANCE ABUSE AND ADDICTION

Substance abuse or addiction occurs when a person overuses or depends on alcohol or drugs. Physical and mental health are affected. So is the welfare of others.

The substances involved affect the nervous system. Some depress the nervous system. Others stimulate it. All affect the mind and thinking.

Alcoholism and Alcohol Abuse

Alcohol slows down brain activity. It affects alertness, judgment, coordination, and reaction time. Over time, heavy drinking damages the brain, central nervous system, liver, kidneys, heart, blood vessels, and stomach. It also can cause forgetfulness and confusion.

Alcoholism (alcohol dependence) includes these symptoms:

- *Craving*—a strong need or urge to drink.
- *Loss of control*—cannot stop drinking once drinking has begun.
- *Physical dependence*—withdrawal symptoms (nausea, sweating, shakiness, anxiety) when drinking is stopped.
- *Tolerance*—greater amounts of alcohol are needed to get "high."

Alcoholism is a chronic disease. It lasts throughout life. Life-style and genetics are risk factors. Some people drink for relief from life stresses—retirement, lowered income, job loss, failing health, loneliness, or the deaths of loved ones. The alcohol craving can be as strong as the need for food or water. An alcoholic continues to drink despite serious family, health, or legal problems.

Alcoholism can be treated but not cured. Counseling and drugs are used to help the person stop drinking. The person must avoid all alcohol to prevent a relapse.

Alcohol abuse is just as harmful as alcoholism. A person who abuses alcohol drinks too much but is not dependent on alcohol.

BOX 45-6	SYMPTOMS OF AN ALCOHOL USE DISORDER

In the past year, the person:
- Drank more or longer than intended.
- Tried more than once to cut down or stop drinking but could not.
- More than once was in situations during or after drinking that increased the chances of getting hurt (driving, swimming, using machines, walking in a dangerous area, unsafe sex).
- Had to drink more to get the desired effect.
- Found that the usual number of drinks had much less effect than before.
- Continued to drink even though he or she felt depressed or anxious or added to another health problem.
- Spent a lot of time drinking, being sick, or getting over the effects of alcohol.
- Continued to drink even though it was causing trouble with family or friends.
- Found that drinking (or being sick from drinking) often interfered with taking care of home or family.
- Gave up or cut back on activities in order to drink.
- More than once got arrested, was held at the police station, or had other legal problems because of drinking.
- Had withdrawal symptoms—trouble sleeping, shakiness, restlessness, nausea, sweating, rapid heart rate, seizure.

Modified from National Institutes of Health: *Rethinking drinking: alcohol and your health,* NIH publication No. 10-3770, revised April 2010.

Problems linked to alcoholism and alcohol abuse include:
- Not being able to meet work, school, or family responsibilities
- Motor vehicle crashes
- Drunk-driving arrests
- Drinking-related medical conditions

Occasional or regular drinking does not mean a drinking problem. Even a few symptoms in Box 45-6 can signal an alcohol use disorder.

See *Focus on Children and Older Persons: Alcoholism and Alcohol Abuse.*

Drug Abuse and Addiction

Drugs interfere with normal brain function. While they create powerful feelings of pleasure, they have long-term effects on the brain. Changes in the brain can turn drug abuse into addiction.

- *Drug abuse*—is the over-use of a drug for non-medical or non-therapy effects.
- *Drug addiction*—is a chronic, relapsing brain disease. The person has an overwhelming desire to take a drug. The person repeatedly takes the drug because of its effect. Usually the effect is altered mental awareness. The person has to have the drug. Often higher doses are needed. The person cannot stop taking the drug without treatment.

FOCUS ON CHILDREN AND OLDER PERSONS
Alcoholism and Alcohol Abuse

Children

According to a 2009 survey, the Centers for Disease Control and Prevention (CDC) reported that:
- 37% of 8th graders had tried alcohol; 15% drank during the past month.
- 72% of 12th graders had tried alcohol; 44% drank during the past month.
- Among high school students during the past 30 days:
  - 42% drank some alcohol.
  - 24% binge drank (5 or more drinks in a row).
  - 10% drove after drinking.
  - 28% rode with a driver who had been drinking.

According to the CDC, underage drinking is more likely to result in:
- School problems—absences, failing grades
- Social problems—fighting, not taking part in youth activities
- Legal problems—driving arrests, hurting someone while drunk
- Physical problems—hang-overs, illness
- Unwanted, unplanned, unprotected sexual activity
- Disrupted normal growth and sexual development
- Physical and sexual assault
- Risk for suicide and homicide
- Alcohol-related car crashes
- Alcohol-related injuries—burns, falls, drowning
- Memory problems
- Drug abuse
- Changes in brain development with life-long effects
- Death from alcohol poisoning

Older Persons

Alcohol effects vary with age. Even small amounts can make older persons feel "high." Older persons are at risk for falls, vehicle crashes, and other injuries from drinking. They have:
- Slower reaction times
- Hearing and vision problems
- A lower tolerance for alcohol

Older people tend to take more drugs than younger persons. Mixing alcohol with some drugs can be harmful, even fatal. Alcohol also makes some health problems worse. High blood pressure is an example.

A diagnosis is based on 3 or more of the following during a 12-month period.
- The drug is often taken in larger amounts. Or it is taken longer than intended.
- The person tries to cut down or stop using the drug.
- Much time is spent using the drug or recovering from its effects. Or a great deal of time is spent trying to obtain the drug. For example, the person visits many doctors to obtain the drug. Or he or she drives long distances to get the drug.
- The person gave up or reduced important social, job, or recreational events because of drug use.
- The person continues to use the drug. The person does so despite knowing that problems are caused by or made worse by using the drug.

- The person has tolerance to the drug:
  - The drug has less and less effect on the person.
  - The person needs more of the drug to get high.
- The person has withdrawal symptoms (*withdraw* means *to stop, remove,* or *take away*):
  - *Withdrawal syndrome is the person's physical and mental response after stopping or severely reducing the use of a substance that was used regularly.* The body responds with anxiety, restlessness, insomnia, irritability, impaired attention, and physical illness.
  - The same (or similar) drug is taken to relieve or avoid withdrawal symptoms.

Drug abuse and addiction affect social and mental function. They are linked to crimes, violence, and car crashes. Physical effects can occur from one use, high doses, or prolonged use—HIV and AIDS (Chapter 40), cardiovascular disease, stroke, sudden death, hepatitis, lung disease, cancer.

Legal and illegal drugs are abused (Table 45-1). Legal drugs are approved for use in the United States. Doctors prescribe them. Illegal drugs are not approved for use. They are obtained through illegal means. Often legal drugs also are obtained through illegal means.

Treatment depends on the drug and the person. A drug treatment program combines various therapies and services to meet the person's needs. The person's age, race, culture, sexual orientation, and gender are considered. So are issues such as pregnancy, parenting, housing, employment, and physical and sexual abuse.

Drug abuse and addiction are chronic problems. Relapses can occur. A short-term, one-time treatment is often not enough. Treatment is a long-term process.

TABLE 45-1 COMMONLY ABUSED DRUGS	
Substance (How Administered)	**Commercial and Street Names**
Cannabinoids	
Effects and potential health problems: euphoria; slowed reaction time; confusion; impaired balance and coordination; frequent respiratory infections; impaired memory and learning; increased heart rate; anxiety; panic attacks; addiction	
hashish *(swallowed; smoked)*	boom, gangster, hash, hash oil, hemp
marijuana *(swallowed; smoked)*	blunt, dope, ganja, grass, herb, joint, Mary Jane, pot, reefer, sinsemilla, skunk, weed, bud, green, trees, smoke
Depressants	
Effects and potential health problems: reduced pain and anxiety; feeling of well-being; lowered inhibitions; slowed pulse and breathing, and lowered blood pressure; poor concentration; fatigue; confusion; impaired coordination, memory, and judgment; addiction; respiratory depression and arrest; death	
barbiturates *(injected; swallowed)*	*Amytal, Nembutal, Seconal, Phenobarbital;* barbs, reds, red birds, phennies, tooies, yellows, yellow jackets
benzodiazepines *(swallowed; injected)* Note: other than flunitrazepam	*Ativan, Halcion, Librium, Valium, Xanax;* candy, downers, sleeping pills, tranks
flunitrazepam *(swallowed; snorted)* Note: drug is associated with sexual assaults; also a "club drug"	*Rohypnol;* forget-me pill, Mexican Valium, R2, Roche, roofies, roofinol, rope, rophies, roach
GHB *(swallowed)* Note: drug is associated with sexual assaults; also a "club drug"	*gamma-hydroxybutyrate;* G, Georgia home boy, grievous bodily harm, liquid ecstasy, soap, scoop, goop, liquid X
Dissociative Anesthetics	
Effects and potential health problems: increased heart rate and blood pressure; impaired motor function; memory loss; feeling of separation from the body and setting; numbness; nausea and vomiting	
ketamine *(injected; snorted; smoked)*	*Ketalar SV;* cat Valium, K, Special K, vitamin K
PCP and analogs *(injected; swallowed; smoked)*	*phencyclidine;* angel dust, boat, hog, love boat, peace pill
Dextromethorphan (DXM) *(swallowed)*	found in some cough and cold medicines; Robotripping, Robo, Triple C
Hallucinogens	
Effects and potential health problems: altered states of perception and feeling; nausea; flashbacks; hallucinations	
LSD *(swallowed; absorbed through mouth tissues);* also see "Dissociative Anesthetics"	*lysergic acid diethylamide;* acid, blotter, cubes, microdot, yellow sunshine, blue heaven
mescaline *(smoked; swallowed);* also see "Dissociative Anesthetics"	buttons, cactus, mesc, peyote
psilocybin *(swallowed)*	magic mushroom, purple passion, shrooms, little smoke

Modified from National Institute on Drug Abuse: *Commonly abused drugs,* Bethesda, Md, National Institutes of Health and National Institute on Drug Abuse: *Prescription drug abuse chart,* Bethesda, Md, National Institutes of Health, updated October 2011.

TABLE 45-1	COMMONLY ABUSED DRUGS—cont'd
Substance (How Administered)	**Commercial and Street Names**

Opioids and Morphine Derivatives

Effects and potential health problems: pain relief; euphoria; drowsiness; nausea; constipation; confusion; sedation; respiratory depression and arrest; tolerance; addiction; unconsciousness; coma; death

codeine *(injected; swallowed)*	*Empirin with Codeine, Fiorinal with Codeine, Robitussin A-C, Tylenol with Codeine;* Captain Cody, schoolboy, doors & fours, loads, pancakes and syrup, Cody
fentanyl *(injected; smoked; snorted)*	*Actiq, Duragesic, Sublimaze;* Apache, China girl, China white, dance fever, friend, goodfella, jackpot, murder 8, TNT, Tango and Cash
heroin *(injected; smoked; snorted)*	*diacetyl-morphine;* brown sugar, dope, H, horse, junk, skag, skunk, smack, white horse, China white, cheese
morphine *(injected; smoked; swallowed)*	*Roxanol, Duramorph;* M, Miss Emma, monkey, white stuff
opium *(swallowed; smoked)*	*laudanum, paregoric;* big O, black stuff, block, gum, hop
oxycodone, meperidine, hydromorphone, hydrocodone, propoxyphene *(swallowed; injected; suppositories; chewed; crushed; snorted)*	*Tylox, OxyContin, Percodan, Percocet;* oxy 80s, oxycotton, oxycet, hillbilly heroin, percs *Demerol, meperidine hydrochloride;* demmies, pain killer *Dilaudid;* juice dillies *Vicodin, Lortab, Lorcet* *Darvon, Darvocet*

Stimulants

Effects and potential health problems: increased pulse, blood pressure, and metabolism; feelings of exhilaration, energy, and increased mental awareness; rapid or irregular heartbeat; reduced appetite; weight loss; heart failure; nervousness; insomnia

amphetamine *(injected; swallowed; smoked; snorted)*	*Biphetamine, Dexedrine;* bennies, black beauties, crosses, hearts, LA turnaround, speed, truck drivers, uppers
cocaine *(injected; smoked; snorted)*	*Cocaine hydrochloride;* blow, bump, C, candy, Charlie, coke, crack, flake, rock, snow, toot
MDMA *(swallowed; snorted; injected)* Note: also a "club drug"	*methylenedioxy-methamphetamine;* Adam, clarity, ecstasy, Eve, lover's speed, peace, uppers
methamphetamine *(injected; swallowed; smoked; snorted)*	*Desoxyn;* chalk, crank, crystal, fire, glass, go fast, ice, meth, speed
methylphenidate *(injected; swallowed; snorted)*	*Ritalin;* JIF, MPH, R-ball, Skippy, the smart drug, vitamin R
nicotine *(smoked; snorted; chewed)*	cigarettes, cigars, bidis, smokeless tobacco (snuff, spit tobacco, chew)

Other Compounds

Anabolic steroids—Effects and potential health problems: hypertension; blood clotting and cholesterol changes; liver cysts; hostility and aggression; acne; premature growth stoppage in adolescents; prostate cancer; reduced sperm production; shrunken testicles; breast enlargement (males); menstrual irregularities; beard and other male characteristics (females)

anabolic steroids *(injected; swallowed; applied to the skin)*	*Anadrol, Oxandrin, Durabolin, Depo-Testosterone, Equipoise;* roids, juice, gym candy, pumpers

Inhalants—Effects and potential health problems: stimulation; loss of inhibition; headache; nausea or vomiting; slurred speech; loss of motor coordination; wheezing; unconsciousness; cramps; muscle weakness; depression; memory impairment; damage to cardiovascular and nervous systems; sudden death

inhalants *(inhaled through the nose or mouth)*	*Solvents (paint thinners, gasoline, glues), gases (butane, propane, aerosol propellants, nitrous oxide), nitrites (isoamyl, isobutyl, cyclohexyl);* laughing gas, poppers, snappers, whippets

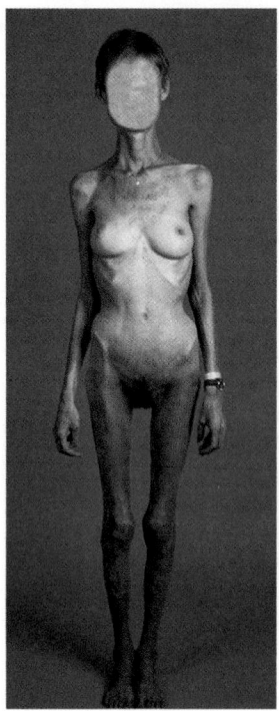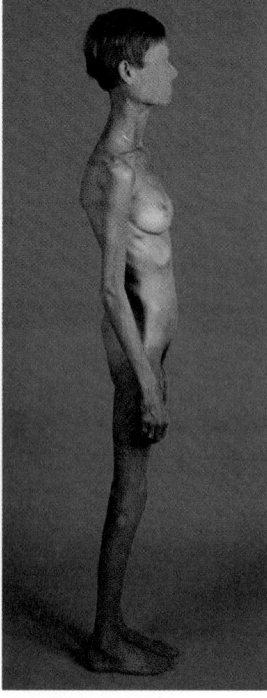

Fig. 45-1 A person with anorexia nervosa.

EATING DISORDERS

An eating disorder involves extremes in eating patterns. Food intake is severely reduced, the person over-eats, or is concerned about body weight and shape. The person has a severe disturbance in eating behavior.

Eating disorders can develop in childhood, the teen years, or young or later adulthood. They are more common in women and girls. Depression, anxiety disorders, and drug abuse may be present.

Anorexia Nervosa

Anorexia means no (*a*) appetite (*orexis*). *Nervosa* relates to *nerves* or *emotions*. Anorexia nervosa occurs when a person has an intense fear of weight gain or obesity.

A fat body image is felt despite being dangerously thin (Fig. 45-1). Poor eating habits include:

- Avoiding food and meals
- Eating a few foods in small amounts
- Weighing and measuring food

Intense exercise and vomiting are common. So is enema and laxative use to rid the body of food. Laxatives are drugs that promote defecation.

Diuretic abuse also may occur. These drugs cause the kidneys to produce large amounts of urine. Extra fluid in the body is lost. Weight loss results.

The person has a poor self-image and may avoid people. Sleep problems and depression may occur. Females may not have monthly menstrual periods. Serious health problems can result. Death is a risk from cardiac arrest or suicide.

Bulimia Nervosa

In bulimia nervosa, binge eating occurs. That is, the person eats large amounts of food. Then the body is purged (rid) of the food to prevent weight gain. Vomiting, laxatives, enemas, diuretics, fasting, and intense exercise are some methods used.

Binge-Eating Disorder

In binge-eating disorder, the person often eats large amounts of food. Eating is out of control. Binge eating is not followed by purging, fasting, or exercise. Often the person is over-weight or obese. Other health problems can occur. They include high blood pressure, heart disease, diabetes, and joint pain.

SUICIDE

Suicide means to kill oneself. According to a 2010 report from the CDC:

- Suicide was the 11th leading cause of death in the United States.
- More than 34,000 people commit suicide each year.
- Firearms are the most common method for men. For women, poison is the most common method.
- Women attempt suicide more often than men.
- More men than women die by suicide.
- American Indians and Alaskan Natives have high rates of suicide.
- Youth, the elderly, and veterans are at risk for suicide.
- The highest rate of suicide was among men aged 75 years and older.
- Suicide was the third leading cause of death among persons aged 15 to 24.

Risk factors for suicide are listed in Box 45-7. *If a person mentions or talks about suicide, take the person seriously. Call for the nurse at once. Do not leave the person alone.*

BOX 45-7 **RISK FACTORS FOR SUICIDE**
• Depression and other mental health disorders • Substance abuse disorder • Prior suicide attempt • Family history of a mental health disorder or substance abuse • Family history of suicide • Family violence (including physical or sexual abuse) • Firearms in the home • Incarceration (prison or jail) • Exposure to the suicidal behavior of others (family, friends, media figures)
Modified from National Institute of Mental Health: *Suicide in the U.S.: statistics and prevention,* National Institutes of Health, NIH publication No. 06-4594, reviewed September 27, 2010.

FOCUS ON COMMUNICATION
Suicide

Persons thinking of suicide may talk about their thoughts. A person may say:
- "I just don't want to live anymore."
- "I wish I was dead."
- "I wish I had never been born."
- "Everyone would be better off without me."

Call for the nurse at once if a person mentions thoughts of suicide.

A person may ask you not to tell anyone about his or her suicidal thoughts. Protecting personal information is important. But the person's safety is the priority. Never promise the person that you will not tell anyone. Report the statements to the nurse at once.

FOCUS ON CHILDREN AND OLDER PERSONS
Suicide

Older Persons

Many older persons suffer from depression (p. 731). Depression often occurs with other serious illnesses. Heart disease, stroke, diabetes, cancer, and Parkinson's disease are examples. The person also may have social and financial problems.

Most older victims did not report depression to their doctors. Or depression was not detected by the doctors.

FOCUS ON LONG-TERM CARE AND HOME CARE
Suicide

Home Care

A firearm in the home is a risk factor for suicide. So are other lethal weapons. If a patient talks about suicide, find out if there are firearms and other weapons in the home. Find out what kind, how many, and where they are located. Report all information to the nurse at once.

If the person is in danger, call 911.

Agencies treating persons with mental health problems must identify persons at risk for suicide. They must:
- Identify specific factors or features that increase or decrease the risk for suicide.
- Meet the person's immediate safety needs.
- Provide the most appropriate setting to treat the person.
- Provide crisis information to the person and family. A crisis "hotline" phone number is an example.

See *Focus on Communication: Suicide.*
See *Focus on Children and Older Persons: Suicide.*
See *Focus on Long-Term Care and Home Care: Suicide.*

Suicide Contagion

Suicide contagion is exposure to suicide or suicidal behaviors within one's family, one's peer group, or media reports of suicide. The exposure has led to more suicides and suicidal behaviors in persons at risk. Adolescents and young adults are at risk for suicide contagion.

Following suicide exposure, those close to the victim should be evaluated by a mental health professional. They include family, friends, peers, and co-workers. Persons at risk for suicide need mental health services.

CARE AND TREATMENT

Treatment of mental health problems involves having the person explore his or her thoughts and feelings. This is done through psychotherapy and behavior, group, occupational, art, and family therapies. Often drugs are ordered.

The care plan reflects the person's needs. The needs of the total person must be met. This includes physical, safety and security, and emotional needs.

Communication is important. Be alert to nonverbal communication. This includes the person's nonverbal communication and your own.

Persons with mental health problems may respond to stress with anxiety, panic, or anger. Some become violent. You must take responsibility for your safety. Your first priority is to protect yourself. Once you are safe, the health team can work together to protect the person and others. To protect yourself:
- Call for help. Do not try to handle the situation on your own.
- Keep a safe distance between you and the person.
- Be aware of your surroundings. Do not let the person between you and the exit.

See *Focus on Communication: Care and Treatment.*

FOCUS ON COMMUNICATION
Care and Treatment

Nonverbal communication involves eye contact, tone of voice, facial expressions, body movements, and posture. Persons with major depression often have little eye contact, poor posture, and speak softly. Some do not speak much at all. Facial expressions may not change. Some persons cry.

Persons with anxiety feel uneasy. They may be restless and unable to sit still. Anxious persons often speak quickly. Eye contact may be prolonged and intense. Others have poor eye contact. The eyes may move quickly from one place to another. Be alert to nonverbal cues. Tell the nurse what you observe.

Your nonverbal communication also is important. When interacting with persons with mental disorders:
- Face the person.
- Maintain eye contact.
- Position yourself near the person but not too close. Do not invade the person's space.
- Crouch, sit, or stand at the person's level if it is safe to do so.
- Show interest and concern through your posture and facial expressions.
- Speak calmly.

FOCUS ON PRIDE

The Person, Family, and Yourself

Personal and Professional Responsibility

People do not choose to have physical or mental health problems. Just as a person does not choose to have diabetes, a person does not choose to have anxiety or depression. How you view the person's illness affects the way you treat the person. Treat the person with kindness, respect, and compassion. Provide quality care. Tell the nurse about any concerns.

Rights and Respect

Persons with mental health disorders may say or do things that seem strange or odd to you. Do not laugh at or insult the person. Do not joke with others about the person. Treat the person with dignity and respect.

Independence and Social Interaction

Social support is important in the treatment of mental illness. Interacting with others offers a healthy way to deal with stress. Family and friends provide a sense of worth and belonging. The care plan includes how they are involved in the person's care.

Providing support for a person with a mental health problem can be demanding. The family needs support. Many communities offer support groups. You can also offer encouragement. Tell the family that you value the support they give.

Delegation and Teamwork

Caring for persons with mental illness requires great teamwork. A person may become hostile or violent. Or the person may threaten or attempt suicide. The team must react quickly to protect the person and others. If someone calls for help, respond at once. Assist as the nurse directs. Take pride in working as a team to ensure safety.

Ethics and Laws

Mental health disorders can affect the person's judgment. Unsafe actions can cause harm. The person must be protected. In the following case, failure to protect the person resulted in patient harm and charges of negligence.

A patient sued a hospital after she set her bed and herself on fire. The patient was in the hospital for alcohol abuse and mental illness. She had a history of mental illness, suicide threats, and alcohol abuse.

While in the hospital:
- *Many packs of cigarettes were taken from her.*
- *Arm, leg, and waist restraints were applied when she became agitated. She was also given a sedative.*
- *After she calmed down, some restraints were removed at her request. They were removed from her right wrist, left ankle, and waist.*
- *She asked to go outside to smoke. A nurse left after asking her to wait a few minutes.*
- *While the nurse was out of the room, the patient set her bed on fire with a cigarette and lighter.*
- *The patient suffered severe burns to her left arm and chest. (The burns required skin grafting. Scars were left at the burn and skin graft sites.)*

The patient's lawsuit claimed negligence because:
- *The nurse left her.*
- *Restraints were removed.*
- *The cigarettes and lighter were not found.*

The jury found in favor of the patient. She was awarded $350,000 for past and future pain, suffering, and disfigurement. (Wilson v Boscobel Area Health Care Center.)

REVIEW QUESTIONS

Circle the BEST answer.

1 Stress is
   a The way a person copes with and adjusts to everyday living
   b A response or change in the body caused by some factor
   c A mental disorder
   d A thought or idea

2 Defense mechanisms are used to
   a Blame others
   b Make excuses for behavior
   c Return to an earlier time
   d Block unpleasant feelings

3 These statements are about defense mechanisms. Which is *false?*
   a Mentally healthy persons use them.
   b They relieve anxiety.
   c They prevent mental disorders.
   d Persons with mental disorders use them.

4 A phobia is
   a The event that causes stress
   b A false belief
   c An intense fear of something
   d Feelings and emotions

5 A person cleans and cleans. This behavior is
   a A delusion
   b A hallucination
   c A compulsion
   d An obsession

6 A person has nightmares about a trauma. The person is having
   a Phobias
   b Panic attacks
   c Flashbacks
   d Anxiety

7 A woman believes she is married to a rock singer. This is called a
   a Fantasy
   b Delusion of grandeur
   c Delusion of persecution
   d Hallucination

8 A man believes that someone is trying to kill him. This is called a
   a Fantasy
   b Delusion of grandeur
   c Delusion of persecution
   d Hallucination

9 These statements are about schizophrenia. Which is *false*?
- a It is a brain disorder.
- b It can be cured with drugs and therapy.
- c Thinking and behavior are disturbed.
- d Suicide is a risk.

10 Bipolar disorder means that the person
- a Is very suspicious
- b Has anxiety
- c Is very unhappy and feels unwanted
- d Has severe mood swings

11 In bipolar disorder, an "emotional high" is called
- a Depression
- b Psychosis
- c An obsession
- d Mania

12 These statements are about antisocial personality disorder. Which is *false*?
- a The person has regard for right and wrong.
- b The person blames others.
- c The person lies or cons others for pleasure.
- d The person is hostile and lacks morals.

13 Substances involved in abuse and addiction affect the
- a Circulatory system
- b Respiratory system
- c Nervous system
- d Immune system

14 These statements are about alcoholism. Which is *false*?
- a The person has a strong craving for alcohol.
- b The disease lasts throughout life.
- c After treatment, the person can have a social drink.
- d The person physically depends on alcohol.

15 These statements are about drug addiction. Which is *false*?
- a It is a chronic brain disease.
- b Higher doses of the drug may be needed.
- c The person has to have the drug.
- d The person can stop taking the drug without treatment.

16 A person has withdrawal syndrome. This means that
- a The person has a physical and mental response when the drug is not taken
- b The person needs higher doses of the drug
- c The effect is reduced with the same amount of drug
- d The person has a relapse after treatment

17 Binge eating followed by purging occurs in
- a Anorexia nervosa
- b Bulimia nervosa
- c Binge-eating disorder
- d The superego

18 For men, the most common method of suicide involves
- a Firearms
- b Suffocation
- c Poisoning
- d Drug overdose

19 Most persons who commit suicide have
- a A mental disorder
- b Schizophrenia
- c A phobia
- d Suicide contagion

20 A person talks about suicide. What should you do?
- a Call for the nurse.
- b Identify factors that increase the risk of suicide.
- c Ask what method the person intends to use.
- d Restrain the person.

21 A person is becoming violent. To protect yourself, you should do the following *except*
- a Call for help
- b Keep a safe distance between you and the person
- c Let the person block the exit
- d Protect yourself

Circle T if the statement is TRUE and F if it is FALSE.

22 T F Personality is how a person copes with stress.
23 T F Some anxiety is normal.
24 T F Anxiety is an intense and sudden feeling of fear or dread.
25 T F Panic is the highest level of anxiety.
26 T F Memories in the subconscious can be recalled.
27 T F Depression is common in older persons.
28 T F Sudden death can occur from one use of a substance.
29 T F The person with binge-eating disorder is at risk for obesity.
30 T F A person is talking about suicide. You can leave the person alone to get the nurse.

Answers to these questions are on p. 834.

46 Confusion and Dementia

OBJECTIVES

- Define the key terms and key abbreviations listed in this chapter.
- Describe confusion and its causes.
- List the measures that help confused persons.
- Explain the differences between delirium, depression, and dementia.
- Describe the signs, symptoms, and behaviors of Alzheimer's disease (AD).

- Explain the care required by persons with AD and other dementias.
- Describe the effects of AD on the family.
- Explain validation therapy.
- Explain how to promote PRIDE in the person, the family, and yourself.

KEY TERMS

cognitive function Involves memory, thinking, reasoning, ability to understand, judgment, and behavior
delirium A state of sudden, severe confusion and rapid changes in brain function
delusion A false belief
dementia The loss of cognitive function that interferes with routine personal, social, and occupational activities
elopement When a person leaves the agency without staff knowledge

hallucination Seeing, hearing, smelling, or feeling something that is not real
paranoia A disorder (*para*) of the mind (*noia*); false beliefs (delusions) and suspicion about a person or situation
pseudodementia False (*pseudo*) dementia
sundowning Signs, symptoms, and behaviors of AD increase during hours of darkness

KEY ABBREVIATIONS

AD	Alzheimer's disease	**NIA**	National Institute on Aging
ADL	Activities of daily living	**OBRA**	Omnibus Budget Reconciliation Act of 1987

Changes in the brain and nervous system occur with aging and certain diseases (Box 46-1). Cognitive function may be affected. (*Cognitive* relates to *knowledge*.) Quality of life is affected. *Cognitive function involves:*

- *Memory*
- *Thinking*
- *Reasoning*
- *Ability to understand*
- *Judgment*
- *Behavior*

CONFUSION

Confusion has many causes. Diseases, infections, hearing and vision loss, and drug side effects are some causes. So is brain injury. With aging, blood supply to the brain is reduced. Personality and mental changes can result. Memory and the ability to make good judgments are lost. A person may not know people, the time, or the place. Over time, some people cannot perform daily activities. Behavior changes are common. The person may be angry, restless, depressed, and irritable.

Acute confusion (delirium—p. 742) occurs suddenly. It is usually temporary. Causes include infection, illness, injury, drugs, and surgery. Treatment is aimed at the cause.

Confusion from physical changes cannot be cured. Some measures help to improve function (Box 46-2). You must meet the person's basic needs.

BOX 46-1 CHANGES IN THE NERVOUS SYSTEM FROM AGING

- Nerve cells are lost.
- Nerve conduction slows.
- Responses and reaction times are slower.
- Reflexes are slower.
- Vision and hearing decrease.
- Taste and smell decrease.
- Touch and sensitivity to pain decrease.
- Blood flow to the brain is reduced.
- Sleep patterns change.
- Memory is shorter.
- Forgetfulness occurs.
- Dizziness can occur.

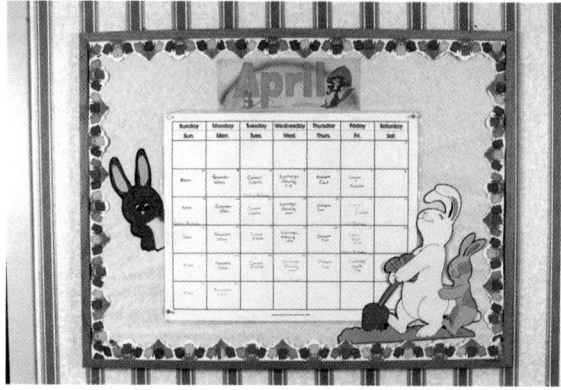

Fig. 46-1 A large calendar can help persons who are confused.

BOX 46-2 CARING FOR PERSONS WITH CONFUSION

- Follow the person's care plan.
- Provide for safety.
- Face the person. Speak clearly.
- Call the person by name every time you have contact with him or her.
- State your name. Show your name tag.
- Give the date and time each morning. Repeat as needed during the day or evening.
- Explain what you are going to do and why.
- Give clear, simple directions and answers to questions.
- Ask clear and simple questions. Give the person time to respond.
- Keep calendars and clocks with large numbers in the person's room and in nursing areas (Fig. 46-1). Remind the person of holidays, birthdays, and other events.
- Have the person wear eyeglasses and hearing aids as needed.
- Use touch to communicate (Chapter 8).
- Place familiar objects and pictures within view.
- Provide newspapers, magazines, TV, and radio. Read to the person if appropriate.
- Discuss current events with the person.
- Maintain the day-night cycle.
  - Open window coverings during the day. Close them at night.
  - Use night-lights at night. Use them in rooms, bathrooms, hallways, and other areas.
  - Have the person wear regular clothes during the day—not sleepwear.
- Provide a calm, relaxed, and peaceful setting. Prevent loud noises, rushing, and congested hallways and dining rooms.
- Follow the person's routine. Meals, bathing, exercise, TV, bedtime, and other activities have a schedule. This promotes a sense of order and what to expect.
- Break tasks into small steps when helping the person.
- Do not re-arrange furniture or the person's belongings.
- Encourage the person to take part in self-care.
- Be consistent.

DEMENTIA

Dementia is the loss of cognitive function that interferes with routine personal, social, and occupational activities. (*De* means *from. Mentia* means *mind.*) The person may have changes in personality, mood, or behavior. Dementia is a group of symptoms that may occur with certain diseases or conditions.

Dementia is not a normal part of aging. Most older people do not have dementia. Early warning signs include:
- Recent memory loss that affects job skills
- Problems with common tasks (for example, dressing, cooking, driving)
- Problems with language; forgetting simple words
- Getting lost in familiar places
- Misplacing things and putting things in odd places (for example, putting a watch in the oven)
- Personality changes
- Poor or decreased judgment (for example, going outdoors in the snow without shoes)
- Loss of interest in life

If brain changes have not occurred, some dementias can be reversed. When the cause is removed, so are the signs and symptoms. Treatable causes include:
- Drugs and alcohol
- Delirium and depression
- Tumors
- Heart, lung, and blood vessel problems
- Head injuries
- Infection
- Vision and hearing problems

Permanent dementias result from changes in the brain. Causes are listed in Box 46-3, p. 742. They have no cure. Function declines over time. Alzheimer's disease is the most common type of permanent dementia.

Pseudodementia means false (pseudo) *dementia.* The person has signs and symptoms of dementia. However, there are no changes in the brain. This can occur with delirium and depression. Both can be mistaken for dementia.

BOX 46-3	CAUSES OF PERMANENT DEMENTIA

- Alcohol-related dementia and Korsakoff's syndrome
- Alzheimer's disease
- AIDS-related dementia
- Brain tumors
- Cerebrovascular disease
- Huntington's disease (a nervous system disease)
- Multi-infarct dementia (MID)—many *(multi)* strokes leave areas of damage *(infarct)*
- Multiple sclerosis
- Parkinson's disease
- Stroke
- Syphilis
- Trauma and head injury

BOX 46-4	SIGNS AND SYMPTOMS OF DELIRIUM

- Alertness: changes in. The person is usually more alert in the morning and less alert at night.
- Sensation: changes in.
- Awareness: changes in.
- Movement: inactive or slow moving.
- Drowsiness.
- Confusion about time or place.
- Memory:
  - Decreased short-term memory and recall. Cannot remember events since the delirium began.
  - Cannot remember past events.
- Thinking and behavior are without purpose.
- Problems concentrating.
- Speech does not make sense.
- Emotional changes:
  - Anger
  - Anxiety
  - Apathy
  - Depression
  - Euphoria
  - Irritability
- Incontinence.
- Restlessness.

Modified from Medline Plus, *Delirium*, Bethesda, Md, August 29, 2011, U.S. National Library of Medicine, National Institutes of Health.

Delirium

Delirium is a state of sudden, severe confusion and rapid changes in brain function. Usually temporary and reversible, it occurs with physical or mental illness. Causes include acute or chronic illness, surgery, drug or alcohol abuse, and infections. Delirium often lasts for about 1 week. However, it may take several weeks for normal mental function to return.

Delirium signals physical illness. It is an emergency. The cause must be found and treated. See Box 46-4 for signs and symptoms.

Depression

Depression is the most common mental health problem in older persons. It is often overlooked. Depression, aging, and some drug side effects have similar signs and symptoms. See Chapter 45 for signs and symptoms of depression in older persons.

Mild Cognitive Impairment

Mild cognitive impairment (MCI) is a type of memory change. The person has problems with memory, language, and other mental functions (attention, judgment, reading, writing). The person or others may notice the problems. However, the problems do not interfere with daily life. The person is at risk for Alzheimer's disease.

ALZHEIMER'S DISEASE

Alzheimer's disease (AD) is a brain disease. Many nerve cells that control intellectual and social function are damaged and die (Fig. 46-2). These functions are affected:

- Memory
- Thinking
- Reasoning
- Judgment
- Language
- Behavior
- Mood
- Personality

The person has problems with work and everyday functions. Problems with family and social relationships occur. There is a slow, steady decline in memory and mental function.

The onset is gradual. Usually symptoms first appear after age 60. The person can live 3 to 4 years or as long as 10 or more years. Nearly half of persons age 85 and older have AD. More women than men have AD. Women live longer than men.

AD is not a normal part of aging. The cause is unknown. A family history of AD increases a person's risk of developing the disease.

Signs of AD

The classic sign of AD is *gradual loss of short-term memory.* At first, the only symptom may be forgetfulness. Box 46-5 lists the warning and other signs of AD. See Box 46-6 for the difference between AD and normal age-related changes.

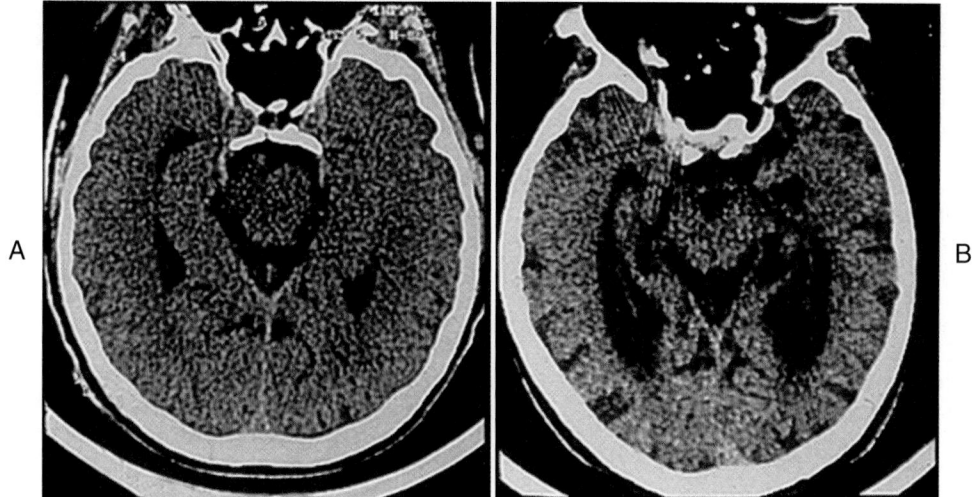

Fig. 46-2 **A,** Normal brain. **B,** Dark patches show damage to brain tissue.

| **BOX 46-5** | **SIGNS OF ALZHEIMER'S DISEASE** |

Warning Signs
- Gradual loss of short-term memory.
- Asking the same question over and over again.
- Repeating the same story—word for word, again and again.
- Forgetting activities that were once done regularly and with ease—cooking, repairs, playing cards, and so on.
- Losing the ability to pay bills or balance a checkbook.
- Getting lost in familiar places.
- Misplacing household items.
- Neglecting to bathe. Or wearing the same clothes over and over again.
- Relying on someone else to make decisions or answer questions that he or she would have handled.

Other Signs
- Forgets recent events, conversations, and appointments.
- Forgets simple directions.
- Forgets names of family members and the names of everyday things (clock, TV, and so on).
- Forgets words, cannot find the right word, loses train of thought.
- Substitutes unusual words and names for what is forgotten.
- Speaks in a native language.
- Curses or swears.

Other Signs—cont'd
- Forgets important dates and events.
- Takes longer to do things.
- Misplaces things. Puts things in odd places.
- Has problems keeping track of bills and writing checks.
- Gives away large amounts of money.
- Does not recognize or understand numbers.
- Has problems following conversations.
- Has problems reading and writing.
- Has problems driving to familiar places.
- Forgets where he or she is.
- Forgets how he or she got to a certain place.
- Does not know how to get back home.
- Wanders from home.
- Cannot tell or understand time or dates.
- Cannot solve everyday problems (iron is left on, stove burners left on, food burning on the stove, and so on).
- Cannot perform everyday tasks (dressing, bathing, brushing teeth, and so on).
- Distrusts others.
- Is stubborn.
- Does not want to do things and withdraws socially.
- Is restless.
- Becomes suspicious and fearful.
- Sleeps more than usual.

Modified from warning signs written by Eric Pfeiffer, MD, founding director of the University of South Florida Suncoast Alzheimer's and Gerontology Center. Reprinted with permission.

| **BOX 46-6** | **ALZHEIMER'S DISEASE AND NORMAL AGE-RELATED CHANGES** |

Signs of AD	Normal Age-Related Changes
• Poor judgment and decision making.	• Makes a bad decision once in a while.
• Cannot manage a budget.	• Misses a monthly payment.
• Loses track of the date or season.	• Forgets which day it is but remembers later.
• Problems having a conversation.	• Sometimes forgets which word to use.
• Misplaces things. Cannot retrace steps to find them.	• Loses things from time to time.

Modified from Alzheimer's Association, *10 signs of Alzheimer's,* updated August 23, 2011.

BOX 46-7   STAGES OF ALZHEIMER'S DISEASE

Mild AD

- Loses spark or zest for life. Does not start anything.
- Loses recent memory. No change in appearance or casual conversation.
- Loses judgment about money.
- Has problems with new learning.
- Has problems making new memories.
- Has trouble finding words. May substitute or make up words. Such words sound like or mean something like the forgotten word.
- May stop talking to avoid mistakes.
- Has a shorter attention span.
- Has less interest in staying with an activity.
- Is easily lost when going to familiar places.
- Resists change or new things.
- Has trouble organizing thoughts and with logical thinking.
- Asks questions over and over again.
- Withdraws from others.
- Loses interest in people and things.
- Is irritable.
- Is less sensitive to the feelings of others.
- Is unusually angry when frustrated or tired.
- Does not make decisions.
- Takes longer to complete routine tasks. Becomes upset if rushed or the unexpected happens.
- Has problems with money. Forgets to pay, pays too much, or forgets how to pay.
- Has problems eating:
  - Forgets to eat or eats constantly.
  - Eats only one kind of food.
- Loses or misplaces things: hides them in odd places; forgets where things go.
- Checks for, searches for, or hoards things of no value.

Moderate AD

- More changes are noticed in:
  - Behavior
  - Concern for appearance
  - Hygiene
  - Sleep
- Has problems recognizing family and friends. For example:
  - Thinks a son is a brother.
  - Thinks a wife is a stranger.

Moderate AD—cont'd

- Creates safety issues from poor judgment:
  - Wandering
  - Poisoning
  - Exploitation
  - Falls
  - Self-neglect
- Has problems recognizing his or her things. May take things that belong to others.
- Repeats stories, words, statements, or motions.
- Is restless in the late afternoon or evening.
- Has problems organizing thoughts.
- Has problems following logical explanations.
- Has problems following written notes or completing tasks.
- Makes up stories to fill in memory gaps.
- Does not respond correctly to a written request.
- Has inappropriate behavior—accuses, threatens, curses, kicks, hits, bites, screams, grabs.
- Becomes sloppy.
- Forgets manners.
- Has hallucinations (p. 746) and delusions (p. 746).
- Naps often.
- Has problems sitting in a chair or on a toilet.
- Needs help with activities of daily living (ADL)—finding the toilet, bathing, drinking, dressing for the weather or an event.
- Has inappropriate sexual behavior:
  - Mistakes another person for his or her spouse or partner.
  - Forgets what is private behavior. May undress or masturbate in public.

Severe AD

- Does not recognize self or family members.
- Speaks in gibberish, is hard to understand, or does not speak.
- Refuses to eat, chokes, or forgets to swallow.
- Cries out repeatedly.
- Cries out when touched or transferred.
- Pats or touches everything.
- Loses bowel and bladder control.
- Loses weight. Skin thins and tears easily.
- Forgets how to walk. Or is too unsteady or weak to stand alone.
- Has seizures.
- Has frequent infections.
- Falls often.
- Groans, screams, or mumbles loudly.
- Sleeps more.
- Needs total assistance with ADL.

Modified from National Institute on Aging: *Understanding stages and symptoms of Alzheimer's disease*, National Institutes of Health, updated February 5, 2009.

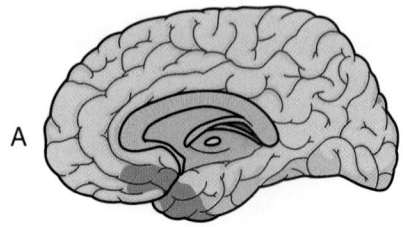
Very Early AD

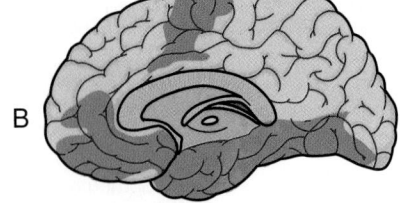
Mild to Moderate AD

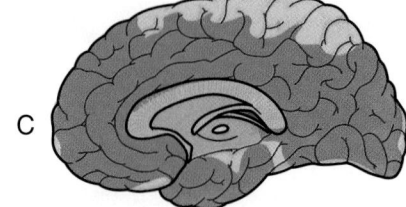
Severe AD

Fig. 46-3   A, Very early AD. **B,** Mild to moderate AD. **C,** Severe AD.

Stages of AD

Signs and symptoms become more severe as the disease progresses. The disease ends in death. AD is often described in terms of 3 stages (Box 46-7; Fig. 46-3). The Alzheimer's Association describes seven stages:

- *Stage 1—No impairment.* The person does not show signs of memory problems.
- *Stage 2—Very mild cognitive decline.* The person thinks that he or she has memory loss or lapses. Familiar words or names are forgotten. The person does not know where to find keys, eyeglasses, or other objects. These problems are not seen by family, friends, or the health team.
- *Stage 3—Mild cognitive decline.* Family, friends, and others notice problems. The person has problems with memory or concentration and with words or names. The person loses or misplaces something valuable. Functioning in social or work settings declines.
- *Stage 4—Moderate cognitive decline (mild or early stage).* Memory of recent or current events declines. There are problems with shopping, paying bills, and managing money. The person may be moody or withdraw in social situations.
- *Stage 5—Moderately severe cognitive decline (moderate or mid-stage).* The person has major memory problems. There may be confusion about the date or day of the week. He or she may need help choosing the correct clothing to wear. The person knows his or her own name, a partner's name, and children's names. Usually help is not needed with eating or elimination.
- *Stage 6—Severe cognitive decline (moderately severe or mid-stage).* Memory problems are worse. Personality and behavior changes develop—delusions, hallucinations, repetitive behavior. The person needs much help with daily activities, including dressing and elimination. Names may be forgotten, but faces may be recognized. Sleep problems, incontinence (urinary and fecal), and wandering are common.
- *Stage 7—Very severe cognitive decline (severe or late stage).* The person cannot respond to his or her setting, speak, or control movement. The person cannot walk without help. Over time, he or she cannot sit up without support or hold the head up. Muscles become rigid. Swallowing is impaired.

Behaviors and Problems

AD changes how a person behaves and acts. These changes are common:

- Getting upset, worried, or angry more easily
- Acting depressed
- Losing interest in things
- Believing other people are hiding things
- Pacing a lot of the time

- Wandering (p. 746)
- Sundowning (p. 746)
- Hallucinations (p. 746)
- Delusions (p. 746)
- Paranoia (p. 747)
- Catastrophic reactions (p. 747)
- Agitation and restlessness (p. 747)
- Aggression and combativeness (p. 747)
- Problems with intimacy and sexuality (p. 748)
- Repetitive behaviors (p. 748)
- Communication problems (p. 748)
- Screaming (p. 749)
- Rummaging and hiding things (p. 749)

Health-related issues can make the problems worse. Examples include illness, infection, drugs, lack of sleep, constipation, hunger, thirst, poor vision or hearing, alcohol, and caffeine. So can problems in the person's setting. According to the National Institute on Aging (NIA), they include:

- A strange setting. The person does not know the setting well.
- Too much noise (TV, radio, people talking at once) can cause confusion and frustration.
- Stepping from one type of flooring to another. With changes in floor color or texture, the person may want to step down.
- Not understanding signs. The person may think that a WET FLOOR sign means to urinate on the floor.
- Mirrors. The person may think that a mirror image is another person in the room.

See *Promoting Safety and Comfort: Behaviors and Problems.*

PROMOTING SAFETY AND COMFORT
Behaviors and Problems

Safety

Some behaviors and problems are not caused by AD. They may be caused by an illness, injury, or drug. If the cause is not treated, it may threaten the person's life. Always report changes in behaviors to the nurse.

Wandering. Persons with AD are not oriented to person, time, and place. They may wander away and not find their way back. Wandering may be by foot, car, bike, or other means. They may be with you one moment and gone the next.

Judgment is poor. They cannot tell what is safe or dangerous. Life-threatening accidents are great risks. They can walk into traffic or into a nearby river, lake, ocean, or forest. If not properly dressed, heat or cold exposure is a risk.

Wandering may have no cause. Or the person may be looking for something or someone—the bathroom, the bedroom, a child, or a partner. Pain, drug side effects, stress, restlessness, and anxiety are possible causes. Sometimes finding the cause prevents wandering.

See *Teamwork and Time Management: Wandering.*

TEAMWORK AND TIME MANAGEMENT
Wandering

Patients and residents may try to wander to another nursing unit or out of the agency. *Leaving the agency without staff knowledge is called elopement.* Serious injury and death have resulted from elopement. State and federal guidelines to prevent elopement are followed.

All staff must be alert to persons who wander. They are allowed to wander in safe areas (Fig. 46-4). However, the person may wander into an unsafe area. Kitchens, shower rooms, and utility rooms are examples.

Tell your team members when you are caring for a person who wanders. You cannot be with the person all the time. The team can assist and monitor the person. Help your team members in the same way. If you see a person wandering into an unsafe area, gently guide the person to a safe place (Fig. 46-5). Report the problem to the nurse.

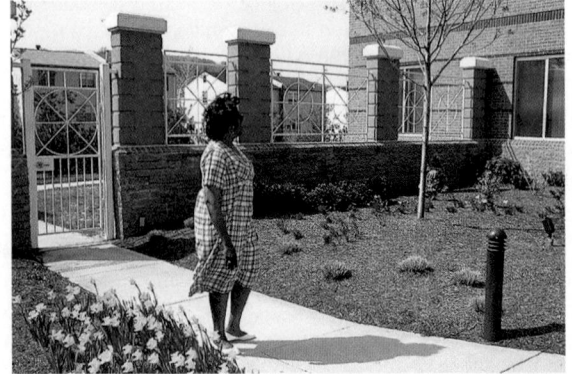

Fig. 46-4 An enclosed garden allows persons with AD to wander in a safe setting.

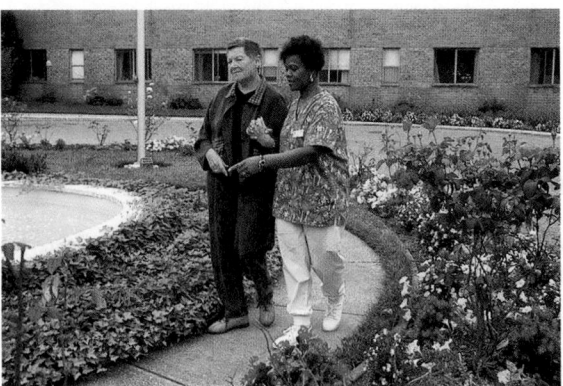

Fig. 46-5 Guide the person who wanders to a safe area.

MedicAlert + Safe Return. *MedicAlert + Safe Return* is a 24-hour emergency service for persons who wander or have a medical emergency. It was formed by the MedicAlert Foundation International and the Alzheimer's Association. The program is nationwide.

The purpose is to identify and safely return persons who wander and become lost. A small fee is charged. A family member completes a form and provides a photo. These are entered into a national database. The person receives an ID (wallet card, bracelet, or necklace).

When reported missing, the person's information is sent to the police. When the person is found, someone calls the toll-free number on the ID. *MedicAlert + Safe Return* then calls the family member or caregiver. The person is returned home safely.

Sundowning. With *sundowning, signs, symptoms, and behaviors of AD increase during hours of darkness.* It occurs in the late afternoon and evening hours. As daylight ends and darkness starts, confusion and restlessness increase. So do anxiety, agitation, and other symptoms. Behavior is worse after the sun goes down. It may continue throughout the night.

Sundowning may relate to being tired or hungry. Poor light and shadows may cause the person to see things that are not there. The person may be afraid of the dark.

Hallucinations and Delusions. A *hallucination is seeing, hearing, smelling, or feeling something that is not real.* Senses are dulled. Affected persons see animals, insects, or people that are not present. Some hear voices. They may feel bugs crawling or feel that they are being touched.

The problem may be caused by poor vision or hearing. The person needs to wear eyeglasses and hearing aids as prescribed.

Delusions are false beliefs. People with AD may think they are some other person. Some believe they are in jail, are being killed, or are being attacked. A person may believe that the caregiver is someone else. Many other false beliefs can occur.

Paranoia. *Paranoia is a disorder* (para) *of the mind* (noia). *The person has false beliefs (delusions) and suspicion about a person or situation.* Paranoia is a type of delusion. The person believes that others are mean, lying, not fair, or "out to get" him or her. The person may be suspicious, fearful, or jealous.

According to the NIA, paranoia may worsen as memory loss gets worse. The NIA uses these examples:

- The person forgets where he or she put something. The person may believe that someone is taking his or her things.
- The person forgets that you are a caregiver. The person may think that you are a stranger and not trust you.
- The person forgets people whom he or she has met. The person may believe that strangers are harmful.
- The person forgets directions that you gave. The person may think that you are trying to trick him or her.

The person may express loss through paranoia. Reasons for the loss do not make sense. Therefore the person blames or accuses others. The NIA offers these helpful measures:

- Do not react if the person blames you for something.
- Do not argue with the person.
- Let the person know that he or she is safe.
- Use touch or gently hug the person. This shows that you care.
- Search for missing things. This helps distract the person. Talk about what you found. For example, you find a photo. Talk about the photo.

See *Promoting Safety and Comfort: Paranoia.*

PROMOTING SAFETY AND COMFORT

Paranoia

Safety

The person's behaviors may not mean paranoia. Fears of harm, strangers, stealing, mistreatment, and so on may be real. Some people take advantage of vulnerable adults (Chapter 4). This includes sexual abuse and financial abuse.

The abuse may be by phone, mail, e-mail, or in person. The abuser may be a friend or family member. The NIA describes financial abuse as including:

- "Scams" such as identity theft, phony prizes, and threats
- Borrowing money and not paying it back
- Giving away or selling the person's property without permission
- Signing or cashing the person's check without permission
- Mis-using bank cards or credit cards
- Forcing the person to sign over property
- Stealing prescription drugs

You must protect the person from harm, abuse, and mistreatment. Report the following at once:

- What the person is saying
- The person seems afraid or worried about money
- Some of the person's items are missing
- The person's behaviors
- Signs and symptoms of problems
- Visitors or family members acting strangely

Catastrophic Reactions. These are extreme responses. The person reacts as if there is a disaster or tragedy. The person may scream, cry, or be agitated or combative. These reactions are common from too many stimuli. Eating, music or TV playing, and being asked questions all at once can overwhelm the person.

Agitation and Restlessness. The person may pace, hit, or yell. Common causes are pain or discomfort, anxiety, lack of sleep, and too many or too few stimuli. Hunger, the need to eliminate, and incontinence also are causes. A calm, quiet setting helps calm the person. So does meeting basic needs.

Caregivers can cause these behaviors. A caregiver may rush the person or be impatient. Or mixed verbal and nonverbal messages are sent. For example, a caregiver talks too fast or too loud. Caregivers always need to look at how their behaviors affect other persons.

The NIA suggests these measures to help with agitation and restlessness:

- Observe for early signs of agitation and restlessness. Try to remove the cause before the behaviors worsen.
- Do not ignore the problem. Try to find the cause.
- Allow personal choice. Let the person decide things to the extent possible.
- Try to distract the person. A snack, safe object, or an activity may help.
- Reassure the person:
  - Speak calmly.
  - Listen to the person's concerns.
  - Try to show that you understand the person's anger or fears.
- Keep personal items within the person's sight. Photos and treasures are examples.
- Reduce noise and clutter.
- Limit the number of people in the room.
- Use gentle touch.
- Provide soothing music.
- Read to the person using a gentle voice.
- Provide quiet times.
- Follow a set routine for ADL.

Aggression and Combativeness. These behaviors include hitting, pinching, grabbing, biting, or swearing. They may result from agitation and restlessness. They frighten others.

Sometimes these behaviors are personality traits. Or pain, fatigue, too much stimulation, caregiver stress, and feeling lost or abandoned are causes. The behaviors can occur during care measures (bathing, dressing) that upset or frighten the person. See Chapter 8 for dealing with the angry person. See Chapter 12 for workplace violence. Also follow the person's care plan. The measures for agitation and restlessness may help.

Intimacy and Sexuality. *Intimacy* is a special bond between people who love and respect each other. It involves the way people talk and act toward each other. *Sexuality* is a type of intimacy. It is the way partners physically express their feelings for each other. AD can affect intimacy and sexuality. The person with AD may:

* Depend on and cling to his or her partner.
* Not remember life with his or her partner.
* Not remember feelings for his or her partner.
* Fall in love with another person.
* Have side effects from drugs that affect sexual interest.
* Have memory loss, brain changes, or depression that affect sexual interest.
* Have abnormal sexual behaviors.

Sexual behaviors are labeled abnormal because of how and when they occur. Persons with AD are not oriented to person, time, and place. Sexual behaviors may involve the wrong person, the wrong place, and the wrong time. Also, persons with AD cannot control behavior.

Healthy persons do not undress or expose themselves in front of others. They do not masturbate or engage in sexual pleasures in public. They know their sexual partners. Persons with AD often mistake someone else for a sexual partner. The person kisses and hugs the other person. Being overly *(hyper)* interested in sex is called *hypersexuality*. The person may try to seduce others. Or the person may masturbate often. These behaviors are symptoms of AD. They may not mean that the person wants to have sex. When a person masturbates in public, lead the person to his or her room. Provide for privacy and safety.

Some behaviors are not sexual. Touching, scratching, and rubbing the genitals can signal infection, pain, or discomfort in the urinary or reproductive systems. Poor hygiene is another cause. So is being wet or soiled from urine or feces. Good hygiene prevents itching. Clean the person quickly and thoroughly after elimination. Do not let the person stay wet or soiled. The nurse assesses the person for urinary or reproductive system problems. The doctor is contacted as necessary.

The nurse encourages the person's partner to show affection. Their normal practices are encouraged. Examples include hand holding, hugging, kissing, touching, and dancing.

Repetitive Behaviors. *Repetitive* means to do over and over again. Persons with AD repeat the same motions over and over again. For example, the person folds the same napkin over and over. Or the person says the same words over and over. Or the same question is asked. Such behaviors do not harm the person. However, they can annoy caregivers and the family.

Harmless acts are allowed. Music, picture books, exercise, and movies are distracting. Taking the person for a walk can help. Such measures help when words or questions are repeated.

Communication Problems. People with AD have trouble remembering things. Communication problems include:

* Struggling to find the right word
* Forgetting what he or she wants to say
* Problems understanding the meaning of words
* Attention problems during conversations
* Losing one's train of thought when talking
* Problems blocking background noises—radio, TV, phones, and so on
* Frustration with problems communicating
* Being sensitive to touch, tone, and voice volume

See *Caring About Culture: Communication Problems.*
See *Focus on Communication: Communication Problems.*

⊛ CARING ABOUT CULTURE
Communication Problems

Some persons with AD learned English as a second language. For example, the first language learned may be Spanish, Italian, French, Russian, Chinese, Japanese, and so on. With AD the person may forget or no longer understand English. He or she may only use and understand the first language learned.

FOCUS ON COMMUNICATION
Communication Problems

Impaired communication is common among persons with AD and other dementias. Communication abilities decline over time. Some persons can have brief conversations. To promote communication, see Box 46-8. Avoid the following:

* *Giving orders.* For example: "Sit down and eat." The statement is bossy. It does not show respect for the person. Instead you can say: "Let me help you sit down."
* *Wanting the truth.* For example, do not say: "Don't you remember?" "What's my name?" "What day is it?" Instead you can say: "Today is Friday."
* *Correcting the person's errors.* For example, do not say: "No, that is your daughter Rose. That's not Mary." Or, "I just told you that it's time to get dressed. You already had breakfast." Instead you can say: "Let me help you get dressed."
* *Pointing out errors.* Instead of saying "You missed a button," say "Let's try it this way."
* *Giving many choices.* For example, "What would you like for dinner?" involves many choices. Instead, limit choices. You can say: "Do you want potatoes or rice?"
* *Asking open-ended questions.* For example, do not say "How did you sleep last night?" Instead, ask "yes" or "no" questions. You can say: "Did you sleep okay last night?"

BOX 46-8	**COMMUNICATION MEASURES FOR PERSONS WITH AD AND OTHER DEMENTIAS**

- Approach the person in a calm, quiet manner.
- Approach the person from the front—not from the side or the back. This avoids startling the person.
- Make eye contact to get the person's attention.
- Have the person's attention before you start speaking.
- Call the person by name.
- Identify other people by name. Avoid pronouns (he, she, them, and so on).
- Follow the rules of communication (Chapters 6 and 8).
- Practice measures to promote communication (Chapter 8).
- Use gestures or cues. Point to objects.
- Speak in a calm, gentle voice.
- Hold the person's hand while you talk.
- Speak slowly. Use simple words and short sentences.
- Ask or say one thing at a time. Present one idea, question, or instruction at a time.
- Do not "baby talk" or use a "baby voice."
- Let the person speak. Do not interrupt or rush the person.

- Give the person time to respond.
- Try other words if the person does not seem to understand.
- Do not criticize, correct, interrupt, argue, or try to reason with the person.
- Give simple, step-by-step instructions.
- Repeat instructions as needed. Give the person time to respond or react.
- Ask simple questions with simple answers. Do not ask complex questions.
- Do not present the person with many questions.
- Provide simple explanations of all procedures and activities.
- Give consistent responses.
- Practice measures to promote hearing (Chapter 39).
- Practice measures to communicate with speech-impaired persons (Chapter 39).
- Practice measures for blind and visually impaired persons (Chapter 39).

Screaming. Persons with AD have communication problems. At first, it is hard to find the right words. As AD progresses, the person speaks in short sentences or in just words. Often speech is not understandable.

The person screams to communicate. This is common in persons who are very confused and have poor communication skills. The person may scream a word or a name. Or the person just makes screaming sounds.

Possible causes include hearing and vision problems, pain or discomfort, fear, and fatigue. Too much or not enough stimulation is another cause. The person may react to a caregiver or family member by screaming. Sometimes these measures are helpful:

- Providing a calm, quiet setting
- Playing soft music
- Having the person wear hearing aids and eyeglasses
- Having a family member or favorite caregiver comfort and calm the person
- Using touch to calm the person

Rummaging and Hiding Things. To *rummage* means to search for things by moving things around, turning things over, or looking through something such as a drawer or closet. The behavior may have no meaning. Or the person may be looking for a certain item but cannot tell you what or why.

The person may hide things, throw things away, or lose something. Some things need to stay with the person. Eyeglasses, hearing aids, and dentures are examples. Always make sure these items are safe. Look for them before discarding linens, returning food trays, or emptying wastebaskets. Money, jewelry, and other important items usually are sent home with the family.

These measures may help with rummaging and hiding behaviors:

- Keep harmful items and products out of the person's sight and reach.
- Remove spoiled items from refrigerators and cabinets. The person may go into a kitchen looking for food and snacks. He or she may not know or be able to taste spoiled food.
- Do not let the person go into the room of another patient or resident.
- Keep wastebaskets covered or out of sight. The person may rummage through a wastebasket or throw things away.
- Check wastebaskets before you empty them. Look for items thrown away or hidden.
- Keep bathroom doors closed and toilet seats down. This helps prevent the person from flushing things down the toilet.
- Allow the person to rummage in a safe place. The agency may have a drawer, closet, bag, box, basket, or chest with safe items.

CARE OF PERSONS WITH AD AND OTHER DEMENTIAS

Usually the person is cared for at home until symptoms are severe. Adult day care may help. Often assisted living or nursing center care is required. Sometimes hospital care is needed for other illnesses. You may care for persons with AD or other dementias in such settings. The person and family need your support and understanding.

People with AD do not choose to be forgetful, incontinent, agitated, or rude. Nor do they choose to have other behaviors, signs, and symptoms of the disease. They cannot control what is happening to them. The disease causes the behaviors. *The disease is responsible, not the person.*

Currently AD has no cure. Symptoms worsen over many years. The rate varies from person to person. Over time, persons with AD depend on others for care. Safety, hygiene, nutrition and fluids, elimination, and activity needs must be met. So must comfort and sleep needs. The person's care plan will include many of the measures listed in Box 46-9.

Comfort and safety are important. Good skin care and alignment prevent skin breakdown and contractures. You must treat these persons with dignity and respect. They have the same rights as persons who are alert and active. Talk to them in a calm voice. Always explain what you are going to do. Massage, soothing touch, music, and aromatherapy are comforting and relaxing. Range-of-motion exercises and touch are also important therapies. The person may need hospice care as death nears (Chapter 52).

The person can have other health problems and injuries. However, the person may not be aware of pain, fever, constipation, incontinence, or other signs and symptoms. Carefully observe the person. Report any change in the person's usual behavior to the nurse.

Infection is a risk. The person cannot fully tend to self-care. Infection can occur from poor hygiene. This includes poor skin care, oral hygiene, and perineal care after bowel and bladder elimination. Inactivity and immobility can cause pneumonia and pressure ulcers.

The person needs to feel useful, worthwhile, and active. This promotes self-esteem. Therapists work with one person, a small group, or a large group. Therapies and activities focus on the person's strengths and past successes. For example:

- A woman used to cook. She helps clean fruit.
- A man was a good dancer. Activities are planned so he can dance.
- A man likes to clean. He helps with dusting.

Supervised activities meet the person's needs and cognitive abilities. The person's interests are considered. Activities are based on what the person enjoys and can do. Some people like crafts, exercise, gardening, and listening and moving to music. Others like sing-alongs, reminiscing, and board games. Some like to string beads, fold towels, or roll dough.

See *Focus on Long-Term Care and Home Care: Care of Persons With AD and Other Dementias*, p. 753.
See *Teamwork and Time Management: Care of Persons With AD and Other Dementias*, p. 753.

Text continued on p. 753

BOX 46-9 CARE OF PERSONS WITH AD AND OTHER DEMENTIAS

Environment
- Follow set routines.
- Avoid changing rooms or roommates.
- Place picture signs by room doors, bathrooms, dining rooms, and other areas (Fig. 46-6, p. 752).
- Keep personal items where the person can see them.
- Stay within the person's sight to the extent possible.
- Place memory aids (large clocks and calendars) where the person can see them.
- Keep noise levels low.
- Play music and show movies from the person's past.
- Select tasks and activities that fit the person's abilities and interests.

Safety
- Reassure the person that you are there to help.
- Remove harmful, sharp, and breakable items from the area. This includes knives, scissors, glass, dishes, razors, and tools.
- Provide plastic eating and drinking utensils. This helps prevent breakage and cuts.
- Place safety plugs in electric outlets. Or cover outlets with safety plates.
- Keep cords and electrical items out of reach.
- Remove electric appliances from the bathroom. Hair dryers, curling irons, make-up mirrors, and electric shavers are examples.
- Store personal care items (shampoo, deodorant, lotion, and so on) in a safe place.
- Keep childproof caps on drug containers and household cleaners.
- Store household cleaners and drugs in locked storage areas.

Safety—cont'd
- Store dangerous equipment and tools in a safe place.
- Remove knobs from stoves or place safety covers on the knobs (Fig. 46-7, p. 752).
- Remove dangerous appliances and power tools from the home.
- Remove firearms from the home.
- Store car keys in a safe place.
- Supervise the person who smokes.
- Store cigarettes, cigars, pipes, matches, and other smoking materials in a safe place.
- Practice safety measures to prevent:
  - Falls (Chapter 13)
  - Fires (Chapter 12)
  - Burns (Chapter 12)
  - Poisoning (Chapter 12)
- Lock all doors to kitchens, utility rooms, and housekeeping closets. Keep them locked.

Wandering
- Follow agency policy for locking doors and windows. Locks are often placed at the top and bottom of doors (Fig. 46-8, p. 752). The person is not likely to look for a lock in such places.
- Keep door alarms and electronic doors turned on. The alarm goes off when the door is opened. Respond to door alarms at once.
- Follow agency policy for fire exits. Everyone must be able to leave the building if there is a fire.
- Make sure the person wears an ID bracelet or *MedicAlert + Safe Return* at all times.

BOX 46-9   CARE OF PERSONS WITH AD AND OTHER DEMENTIAS—cont'd

Wandering—cont'd

- Exercise the person as ordered. Adequate exercise may reduce wandering.
- Involve the person in activities—folding napkins, dusting a table, sorting socks, rolling yarn, sweeping, sanding blocks of wood, or watering plants.
- Do not use restraints. Restraints require a doctor's order. They also tend to increase confusion and disorientation.
- Do not argue with the person who wants to leave. The person does not understand what you are saying.
- Go with the person who insists on going outside. Make sure he or she is properly dressed. Guide the person inside after a few minutes.
- Let the person wander in enclosed areas. The agency may have enclosed areas for walking about. They provide a safe place for the person to wander.

Sundowning

- Complete treatments and activities early in the day.
- Provide a calm, quiet setting late in the day.
- Do not restrain the person.
- Encourage exercise and activity early in the day.
- Meet nutrition needs. Hunger can increase restlessness.
- Promote elimination. The need to eliminate can increase restlessness.
- Do not try to reason with the person. He or she cannot understand what you are saying.
- Do not ask the person to tell you what is bothering him or her. Communication is impaired. The person does not understand what you are asking. He or she cannot think or speak clearly.

Hallucinations and Delusions

- Have the person wear eyeglasses and hearing aids as needed.
- Do not argue with the person. He or she does not understand what you are saying.
- Reassure the person. Tell him or her that you will provide protection from harm.
- Try to comfort the person if he or she is afraid.
- Distract the person with some item or activity. Go to another room. Taking the person for a walk may be helpful.
- Turn off TV or movies when violent and disturbing programs are on. The person may believe that the story is real.
- Use touch to calm and reassure the person (Fig. 46-9, p. 752).
- Eliminate noises that the person could misinterpret. TV, radio, music, furnaces, air conditioners, and other things could affect the person.
- Check lighting. Make sure there are no glares, shadows, or reflections.
- Cover or remove mirrors. The person could misinterpret his or her reflection.
- Make sure the person cannot reach anything that could be used to hurt the self or others.

Sleep

- Develop a regular bedtime. Keep the bedtime at the same time each evening.
- Provide a quiet, peaceful mood in the evening—dim lights, low noise level, and music.

Sleep—cont'd

- Follow bedtime rituals.
- Use night-lights so the person can see. Use them in rooms, hallways, bathrooms, and other areas. They help prevent accidents and disorientation.
- Limit caffeine during the day.
- Discourage naps during the day.
- Follow the person's exercise plan. Play music to the exercise.
- Reduce noises.

Basic Needs

- Follow a daily routine. This helps the person know when certain things will happen.
- Meet food and fluid needs (Chapter 24). Provide finger foods. Cut food and pour liquids as needed.
- Provide good skin care (Chapters 20, 33, and 34). Keep the person's skin free of urine and feces.
- Promote urinary and bowel elimination (Chapters 22 and 23).
- Provide incontinence care as needed (Chapters 22 and 23).
- Promote exercise and activity during the day (Chapter 27). This helps reduce wandering and sundowning behaviors. The person may also sleep better.
- Reduce intake of coffee, tea, and cola drinks. These contain caffeine. Caffeine is a stimulant. It can increase restlessness, confusion, and agitation.
- Provide a quiet, restful setting. Soft music is better than loud TV programs.
- Play music during care activities such as bathing and during meals.
- Promote personal hygiene (Chapter 20). Do not force the person into a shower or tub. People with AD are often afraid of bathing. Try bathing the person when he or she is calm. Use the person's preferred bathing method (tub bath, shower). Provide privacy and keep the person warm. Do not rush the person.
- Provide oral hygiene (Chapter 20).
- Choose clothing that is comfortable and simple to put on. Front opening garments are easy to put on. Pullover tops are harder to put on. And the person may become frightened when his or her head is inside the garment.
- Select clothing that closes with Velcro. Such items are easy to put on and take off. Buttons, zippers, snaps, and other closures can frustrate the person.
- Offer simple clothing choices (Fig. 46-10, p. 752). Let the person choose between 2 shirts or 2 blouses, 2 pants or 2 slacks, and so on.
- Lay clothing out in the order it will be put on. Hand the person one clothing item at a time. Tell or show the person what to do. Do not rush him or her.
- Have equipment ready for any procedure. This reduces the amount of time the person is involved in care measures.
- Observe for signs and symptoms of health problems (Chapter 7).
- Prevent infection (Chapter 15).

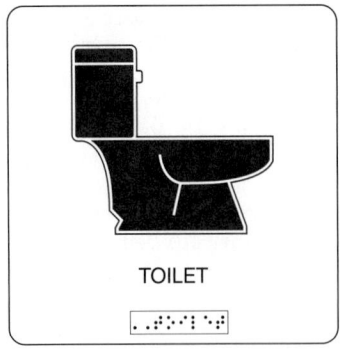

Fig. 46-6 Signs give cues to persons with dementia.

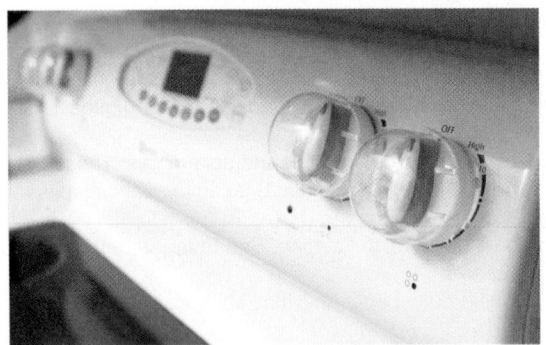

Fig. 46-7 Safety covers are on stove knobs.

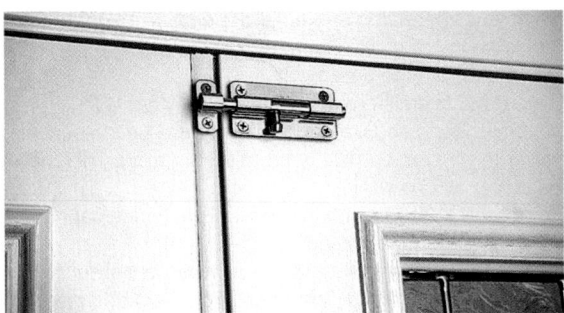

Fig. 46-8 A slide lock is at the top of the door.

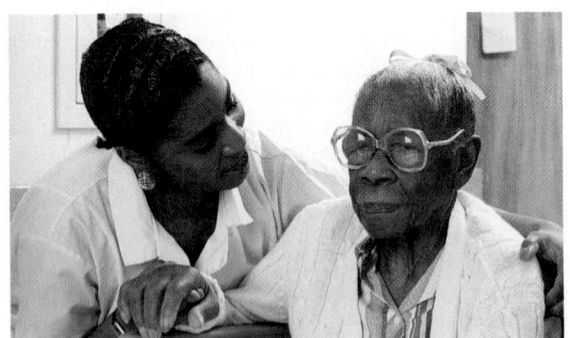

Fig. 46-9 Use touch to calm the person.

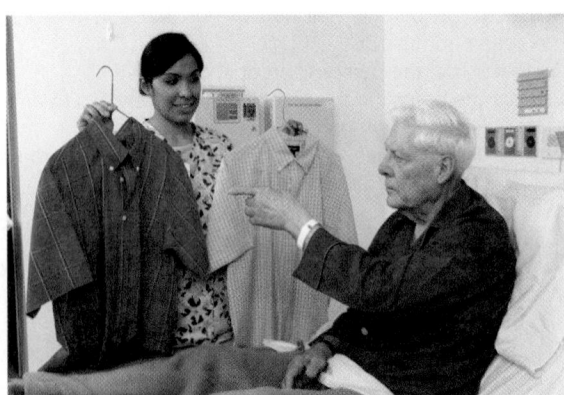

Fig. 46-10 The person with AD is offered simple clothing choices.

Long-Term Care

Many nursing centers have special units for persons with AD and other dementias. Some units are secured. This means that entrances and exits are locked. Persons in these units have a safe setting for moving about. They cannot wander away. Some persons have aggressive behaviors that disrupt or threaten others. They may need a secured unit.

According to the Omnibus Budget Reconciliation Act of 1987 (OBRA), secured units are physical restraints. The center must follow OBRA rules. They must use the least restrictive approach. A dementia diagnosis and a doctor's order are needed to place a person on a secured unit. At least every 90 days, the health team reviews the person's need for a secured unit. The person's rights are always protected.

At some point, the secured unit is no longer needed for safe care. For example, the person's condition progresses to severe AD (see Box 46-7). The person cannot sit or walk. Wandering is not a concern. The person is transferred to another unit.

Licensing and accrediting agencies have standards of care for special care units. Staff must have special training in the care of persons with dementia. The unit must have programs that promote dignity, personal freedom, and safety.

The entire staff must protect the person from harm. Always look for dangers in the person's room and in hallways, lounges, dining areas, and other areas on the nursing unit. Remove the danger if you can, and tell the nurse at once. If you cannot remove the danger, also tell the nurse at once.

The Family

The person may live at home or with a partner, children, or other family members. The family gives care. Or someone stays with the person. Health care is sought when the family cannot deal with the situation or meet the person's needs. Home health care may help for a while. Adult day care is an option. Long-term care is needed when:

- Family members cannot meet the person's needs.
- The person no longer knows the caregiver.
- Family members have health problems.
- Money problems occur.
- The person's behavior presents dangers to self and others.

Diagnostic tests, doctor's visits, drugs, and home care are costly. So is long-term care. The person's medical care can drain family finances.

The family has special needs. Home care and nursing center care are stressful. There are physical, emotional, social, and financial stresses. Adult children are in the *sandwich generation*. They are caught between their own children needing attention and an ill parent needing care. Caring for two families is stressful. Often adult children have jobs too.

Caregivers can suffer from anger, anxiety, guilt, depression, and sleeplessness. Some cannot concentrate or are irritable. Health problems can develop. They need to focus on their own health. They need a healthy diet, exercise, and plenty of rest. Asking family and friends for help is important. However, asking for help is hard for some people. According to the NIA, they may feel that:

- They should do everything themselves.
- It is wrong to leave the person with someone else.
- No one will help if they ask.
- They do not have money to pay someone to help or watch the person for 1 or 2 hours.

Caregivers need much support and encouragement. AD support groups are helpful. They are sponsored by hospitals, nursing centers, and the Alzheimer's Association. The Alzheimer's Association has chapters in cities across the country. Support groups offer encouragement and advice. Members share their feelings, anger, frustration, guilt, and other emotions. They also share coping and caregiving ideas.

The family often feels hopeless. No matter what is done, the person gets worse. Much time, money, energy, and emotion are needed to care for the person. Anger and resentment may result. Guilt feelings are common. The family knows that the person did not choose the disease. They know that the person does not choose to have its signs, symptoms, and behaviors. Sometimes behaviors are embarrassing. The family may be upset and angry that the loved one cannot show love or affection.

The family is an important part of the health team. They help plan care whenever possible. They need to learn how to bathe, feed, dress, and give oral hygiene to the person. They also need to learn how to provide a safe setting. The nurse and support group help the family learn how to give needed care.

Some family members take part in unit activities. For many persons, family members provide comfort. They also need support and understanding from the health team.

The NIA suggests ways that family members can take care of themselves. See Box 46-10, p. 754.

See *Focus on Long-Term Care and Home Care: The Family*, p. 754.

BOX 46-10	FAMILY CAREGIVERS—TAKING CARE OF YOURSELF

- Ask for help when you need it. Asking for something specific may be useful. For example:
  - "Can you make Mom's dinner Sunday night?"
  - "Can you stay with Dad from 2 to 4 Monday afternoon?"
  - "Can Mom stay at your house Saturday afternoon?"
- Join a support group.
- Take breaks every day.
- Spend time with friends.
- Maintain hobbies and interests.
- Eat healthy foods.
- Exercise often.
- See a doctor regularly.
- Keep health, legal, and financial information current.
- Remember that these feelings are normal—being sad, lonely, frustrated, confused, angry. Say the following to yourself:
  - "I'm doing the best I can."
  - "What I'm doing would be hard for anyone."
  - "I'm not perfect, and that's okay."
  - "I can't control some things."
  - "I need to do what works for right now."

- "Even when I do everything that I can, the person with AD will still have problem behaviors. They are caused by the illness, not what I do."
- "I will enjoy the times when we can be together in peace."
- "I will get counseling if caregiving becomes too much for me."
- Meet spiritual needs—attending religious services, believing that larger forces or a higher power is at work.
  - Understand that you may feel powerless and hopeless about what is happening.
  - Understand that you feel a sense of loss and sadness.
  - Understand why you are caring for a person with AD. Was the choice made out of love, loyalty, duty, religious obligation, money concerns, fear, habit, or self-punishment?
  - Let yourself feel "uplifts." Examples include good feelings about the person, support from caring people, time for your own interests.
  - Keep connected to something "higher than yourself." This may be believing in a higher power, religion, or that something good comes from every experience.

Modified from National Institute on Aging: *Caring for a person with Alzheimer's disease: your easy-to-use guide*, NIH Publication No. 09-6173, May 2009.

FOCUS ON LONG-TERM CARE AND HOME CARE

The Family

Home Care

Home care is an option for many families. They may need someone to prepare the person's meals. Help is often needed with bathing and elimination. Someone needs to supervise the person while family members work, do errands, and have time to themselves. The amount and kind of care depend on the person's needs and the family's ability to provide care.

Validation Therapy

Validation therapy may be part of the person's care plan. The therapy is based on these principles:

- All behavior has meaning.
- Development occurs in a sequence, order, and pattern (Chapter 10). Certain tasks must be completed during a stage of development. A stage cannot be skipped. Each stage is the basis of the next stage.
- If a person does not successfully complete a stage of development, unresolved issues and emotions may surface later in life.
- A person may return to the past to resolve such issues and emotions.
- Caregivers need to listen and provide empathy.

- Attempts are not made to correct the person's thoughts or bring the person back to reality. For example:
  - While going from room to room, Mrs. Bell calls for her daughter. In reality, her daughter died 20 years ago. The caregiver does not tell Mrs. Bell that her daughter died. Instead, the caregiver says: "Tell me about your daughter."
  - Mrs. Brown sits all day on a bench by the window. She says that she is at the train station waiting to meet her husband. In reality, her husband was killed during World War II. Buried in England, he never returned home. The caregiver does not remind Mrs. Brown of what happened. Instead, the caregiver encourages Mrs. Brown to talk about her husband.
  - Mr. Garcia was 3 years old when his father died. He holds a ball constantly. He is very upset when anyone tries to remove it from his hand. He calls for his father and repeats "play ball, play ball." The caregiver does not remind Mr. Garcia that he is 80 years old and that his father died many years ago. Instead, the caregiver says: "Tell me about playing ball."

The health team decides if validation therapy might help a person. If so, it will be part of the person's care plan. Proper use of validation therapy requires special training. If the therapy is used in your agency, you will receive the training needed to use it correctly.

FOCUS ON PRIDE

The Person, Family, and Yourself

Personal and Professional Responsibility

Confusion has many causes. The person may have an infection. Or the cause may be hypoglycemia or a drug side effect. You are responsible for reporting changes in the person's condition. If you notice confusion, do not assume the person has AD. Report changes to the nurse at once.

Rights and Respect

The person has the right to privacy and confidentiality. Protect the person from exposure. Only those involved in the person's care are present for care and procedures. The person is allowed to visit in private. Protect confidentiality. Do not share information about the person with others.

The person also has the right to keep and use personal items. Some items provide comfort. A pillow, blanket, afghan, or sweater may have meaning to the person. The person may not know why or even recognize the item. Still, it is important. Keep personal items safe. Protect the person's property from loss or damage.

Independence and Social Interaction

Persons with dementia have problems with ADL. Eating, bathing, dressing, and elimination are examples. Maintaining the person's routines can help the person remain independent as long as possible. For example, Mrs. Lund uses the bathroom, washes hands, brushes teeth, puts on make-up, brushes hair, and dresses in the morning. She is more independent when ADL are done in this order. Changing the order causes confusion. More help is needed.

You may also need to break down tasks into simple steps. Kindly tell the person each step. Repeat directions as needed. Allow extra time for the person to complete a task. Resist the urge to take over. Let the person do as much as is safely possible.

Delegation and Teamwork

Persons with dementia may respond better to certain staff or caregivers. This can vary by day or time of day. Do not be offended if care must be provided by someone else. The team works together to meet the person's needs.

Sometimes the person resists care from all staff and caregivers. Encouraging the person to allow care is often useless. A calm and caring approach is needed. Care may be given at a different time. Force is never used.

Ethics and Laws

Persons with AD often have changes in mood, behavior, and personality. The person may become easily agitated or angry. The person does not have control over words and actions. Some behaviors are hard to deal with. You may become short-tempered. The following case is a real example of a poor response to the person's behavior.

While a licensed nursing assistant (LNA) was feeding a nursing home resident with AD, the resident threw the tray on the floor. The LNA called the resident a degrading name and swore at her.

The Board of Nursing concluded that the LNA abused and improperly cared for the resident. The unprofessional conduct violated the Administrative Rules of the Board of Nursing because of:

- Abusing or neglecting a patient
- Performing unsafe or unacceptable patient care
- Failing to conform to acceptable standards of practice
- Engaging in conduct likely to harm the public

The nursing assistant's license was reprimanded.

(Author note: A reprimand means that the Board considered her conduct to be improper. However, the Board did not limit her right to work as an LNA.)

(State of Vermont Board of Nursing in regard to K. Blaufox, 2000.)

You must control your reactions to stress. Be professional. Tell the nurse if you feel frustrated, angry, or impatient. An assignment change may be needed. Never take out your anger on the person. The person must be protected from physical and verbal abuse and mistreatment.

REVIEW QUESTIONS

Circle the BEST answer.

1 Cognitive function relates to the following *except*
   a Memory loss and personality
   b Thinking and reasoning
   c Ability to understand
   d Judgment and behavior

2 A person is confused after surgery. The confusion is likely to be
   a Permanent
   b Temporary
   c Caused by an infection
   d Caused by a brain injury

3 A person is confused. Which measure should you question?
   a Restrain in bed at night.
   b Give clear, simple directions.
   c Use touch to communicate.
   d Open drapes during the day.

4 A person has delusions. A delusion is
   a A false belief
   b An illness caused by changes in the brain
   c Seeing, hearing, or feeling something that is not real
   d Alzheimer's disease

5 A person has AD. Which is *true*?
   a AD occurs only in older persons.
   b Diet and drugs can cure the disease.
   c AD and delirium are the same.
   d AD ends in death.

Continued

REVIEW QUESTIONS—cont'd

6 The following are common in persons with AD *except*
 a Memory loss, poor judgment, and sleep disturbances
 b Loss of impulse control and the ability to communicate
 c Wandering, delusions, and hallucinations
 d Paralysis, dyspnea, and pain

7 A person leaves the agency without staff knowledge. This is called
 a Elopement
 b Wandering
 c Bad behavior
 d Poor judgment

8 Sundowning means that
 a The person becomes sleepy when the sun sets
 b Behaviors are worse during hours of darkness
 c Behavior improves at night
 d The person goes to bed when the sun sets

9 A person with AD keeps telling you that someone is stealing things. What should you do?
 a Nothing. The person suffers from paranoia.
 b Tell the nurse. Someone could be abusing the person.
 c Replace missing items.
 d Send other items home with the family.

10 A person has AD. To communicate with him or her, you should
 a Give orders
 b Correct the person's mistakes
 c Ask open-ended questions
 d Limit the person's choices

11 A person with AD is screaming. You know that this is
 a An agitated reaction
 b A way to communicate
 c Caused by a delusion
 d A repetitive behavior

12 A person with AD is rummaging in a drawer. Which is *false?*
 a The person may be looking for something.
 b The behavior may have no meaning.
 c The behavior is allowed if items in the drawer are safe.
 d You must distract the person with another activity.

13 Which is the best way to approach a person with AD?
 a From the front
 b From the back
 c From the right side
 d From the left side

14 A person with AD tends to wander. You should do the following *except*
 a Make sure door alarms are turned on
 b Make sure an ID bracelet is worn
 c Assist with exercise as ordered
 d Tell the person where to wander safely

15 Safety is important for the person with AD. Which is *false?*
 a Safety plugs are placed in electrical outlets.
 b Cleaners and drugs are kept locked up.
 c The person can keep smoking materials.
 d Sharp and breakable objects are removed from the person's setting.

16 Which of these can cause delusions in persons with AD?
 a Eyeglasses
 b Hearing aids
 c Mirrors
 d Night-lights

17 You are caring for a person with AD. Which is *false?*
 a You can reason with the person.
 b Touch can calm and reassure the person.
 c A calm, quiet setting is important.
 d Help is needed with ADL.

18 Which helps prevent many of the behaviors and problems of AD?
 a Soothing music
 b Support groups
 c Caffeine
 d Validation therapy

19 AD support groups do the following *except*
 a Provide care
 b Offer encouragement and care ideas
 c Provide support for the family
 d Promote the sharing of feelings and frustrations

Circle T if the statement is TRUE and F if it is FALSE.

20 T F A person with AD is agitated and restless. A caregiver may have caused the behaviors.

21 T F A person with AD may mistake you for a sexual partner. This is called hypersexuality.

22 T F A person with AD keeps moving an empty cup back and forth across the table. The behavior is not harming anyone. The behavior can continue.

23 T F A person with AD hides things. You should check wastebaskets before emptying them.

24 T F The person with AD can control behavior.

25 T F The person with AD can tell you about pain, constipation, and other discomforts.

26 T F The person with AD is at risk for infection from poor hygiene after elimination.

27 T F A set routine is important for the person with AD.

28 T F You can use gestures or point to things to communicate with persons who have AD.

29 T F Restraints help improve the behaviors of AD.

30 T F Family members continue their hobbies and holiday events. They are abusing the person with AD.

Answers to these questions are on p. 835.

Developmental Disabilities

OBJECTIVES

- Define the key terms and key abbreviations listed in this chapter.
- Identify the areas of function limited by a developmental disability.
- Explain how a developmental disability affects the person and family across the life-span.

- Explain when developmental disabilities occur.
- Identify the causes of developmental disabilities.
- Explain how various developmental disabilities affect a person's function.
- Explain how to promote PRIDE in the person, the family, and yourself.

KEY TERMS

birth defect An abnormality present at birth that involves a body structure or function

developmental disability (DD) A disability occurring before 22 years of age

diplegia Similar body parts are affected on both sides of the body

disability Any lost, absent, or impaired physical or mental function

inherited That which is passed down from parents to children

intellectual disability Involves severe limits in intellectual function and adaptive behavior occurring before age 18

spastic Uncontrolled contractions of skeletal muscles

KEY ABBREVIATIONS

ADA	Americans With Disabilities Act of 1990	**FXS**	Fragile X syndrome
CP	Cerebral palsy	**IQ**	Intelligence quotient
DD	Developmental disability	**OBRA**	Omnibus Budget Reconciliation Act of 1987
DS	Down syndrome	**SB**	Spina bifida

Many diseases, illnesses, and injuries cause disabilities in adulthood. A *disability is any lost, absent, or impaired physical or mental function*. A disability occurring before 22 years of age is a *developmental disability (DD)*. DD causes occur before, during, or after birth. Or they are caused by childhood illness and injuries.

A *birth defect is an abnormality present at birth that involves a body structure or function*. It can be inherited (p. 760), occur during pregnancy, or occur during birth. The defect causes disabilities or death. Genetic problems and chromosome problems can cause birth defects. So can problems during pregnancy:

- Rubella (German measles)
- Untreated or uncontrolled diabetes
- Contact with dangerous chemicals
- Using drugs or alcohol
- Smoking

A DD can be a physical or mental impairment or both. It is severe, chronic, and life-long. Function is limited in 3 or more life skills:

* Self-care
* Understanding and expressing language
* Learning
* Mobility
* Self-direction
* Capacity for independent living
* Supporting oneself financially

Developmentally disabled children become adults. They need life-long help, support, and special services for:

* Housing
* Employment
* Education
* Protection of civil and human rights
* Health care

Independence to the extent possible is the goal for these persons. This includes having a job and living in the community. The many resources to assist the person and family include:

* Assistive and self-help devices
* Education and job training
* Personal assistive services
* Home and vehicle changes
* Financial assistance
* Therapies: physical, occupational, speech and language, respiratory, recreation
* Hearing and vision aids

A DD affects the family throughout life. The infant or child becomes a teenager, young adult, middle-age adult, and older adult. Both the child and parents grow older. Often it is hard to care for an older child or adult. It may be hard to handle or move the person. A parent may become ill, injured, or disabled or may die. Still, the disabled person needs care. Older parents may not have the energy or means to care for the aging child.

Changes from aging occur (Chapter 11). Aging may occur earlier when DDs are severe.

Persons with DDs have the same rights as every citizen. They have the right to live, learn, work, and enjoy life. Their rights are also protected by:

* The Americans With Disabilities Act of 1990 (ADA)
* The Developmental Disabilities Assistance and Bill of Rights Act of 2000

Some severely disabled children live in centers for the developmentally disabled. Some adults with DDs need nursing center care. They are further protected by the Omnibus Budget Reconciliation Act of 1987 (OBRA). OBRA requires that centers provide age-appropriate activities. Staff must have special training to meet care needs.

> **FOCUS ON COMMUNICATION**
> **Intellectual Disabilities**
>
> *Mental retardation* was a common term for intellectual disabilities. However, the term is offensive and outdated. *Intellectual disabilities* is the term preferred by the Arc of the United States.
>
> In June 2003, the President's Committee on Mental Retardation was changed to the "President's Committee for People with Intellectual Disabilities." The name was changed to:
> * Update and improve the image of people with intellectual disabilities.
> * Help reduce discrimination against such persons.
> * Reduce confusion between "mental illness" and "mental retardation."
>
> Do not use "mental retardation" and "mentally retarded." Use "intellectual disabilities" or "intellectually disabled."

INTELLECTUAL DISABILITIES

An *intellectual disability involves severe limits in intellectual function and adaptive behavior. It occurs before age 18. Intellectual function* relates to *learning, thinking, reasoning, and solving problems. Adapt* means to *change* or *adjust.* The person has low intellectual function. Adaptive behavior is impaired.

The Arc of the United States is a national organization focused on people with intellectual and related developmental disabilities. The Arc describes an intellectual disability as:

* An IQ score of about 70 or below. (IQ means intelligence quotient.) The person learns at a slower rate than normal. Learning ability is less than normal.
* A significant limit in at least 1 adaptive behavior. Adaptive behaviors are skills needed to function in everyday life—to live, work, and play. They involve communication, reading and writing, and money concepts. Social skills involve interpersonal skills, responsibility, not being tricked by others, following rules, and obeying laws. Practical skills involve personal activities of daily living: eating, dressing, mobility, and elimination. Other personal skills include preparing meals, taking drugs, using the phone, managing money, using transportation, housekeeping, job skills, and maintaining a safe setting.

Brain development is impaired. It can occur before birth, during birth, or before age 18. Causes are listed in Box 47-1. According to the Arc, alcohol is the leading preventable cause of intellectual disabilities.

Intellectual disabilities can be mild to severe. Persons mildly affected are slow to learn in school. As adults, they can function in society with some support. For example, they need help finding a job. Support is not needed every day. Others need much support every day at home and at work. Still others need constant support in all areas.

See *Focus on Communication: Intellectual Disabilities.*

BOX 47-1 CAUSES OF INTELLECTUAL DISABILITIES

Genetic Conditions
- Abnormal genes from parents
- Errors when genes combine
- Gene disorders during pregnancy caused by infections, over-exposure to x-rays, and other factors
- Down syndrome
- Fragile X syndrome (p. 760)

Problems During Pregnancy
- Alcohol use (fetal alcohol syndrome)
- Drug use
- Smoking
- Malnutrition (*mal* means bad)
- Rubella (German measles)
- Diabetes
- Lack of oxygen to the brain
- Syphilis
- Rh blood disease

Problems at Birth
- Prematurity
- Low birth weight
- Head injury
- Lack of oxygen to the brain

Problems After Birth
- Childhood diseases (whooping cough, chicken pox, measles, Hib disease, meningitis, encephalitis)
- Head injuries
- Near drowning
- Lead poisoning
- Poisoning (alcohol, ammonia, bleaches, detergent, household cleaners and polishes, gasoline, kerosene, lighter fluid, drugs, lye, paint thinners and removers, pesticides, turpentine, weed killers, mercury, and so on)
- Shaken baby syndrome
- Malnutrition
- Dehydration
- Reye's syndrome (a disease caused by drugs containing aspirin)
- Poor health care

Modified from *Causes and prevention of intellectual disabilities*, The Arc of the United States, revised March 1, 2011, Silver Spring, Md.

Sexuality

Persons with intellectual and developmental disabilities have physical, emotional, and social needs and desires. Reproductive organs develop. Some have life partners. Others marry and have children. Some persons can control sexual urges. Others cannot. The type and site of sexual responses may be inappropriate. Sometimes persons with intellectual disabilities are sexually abused.

The Arc's beliefs about sexuality include the right to:
- Develop friendships and emotional and sexual relationships. This involves the right to:
  - Love and be loved.
  - End a relationship as he or she chooses.
- Dignity and respect.
- Privacy and confidentiality.
- Freely choose associations.
- Sexual expression.
- Learn about sex, marriage and family, abstinence, safe sex, sexual orientation, sexual abuse, and emotional abuse.
- Be protected from sexual harassment and abuses—physical, sexual, emotional.
- Decide about having and raising children.
- Make birth control decisions.
- Have control over their own bodies.
- Protection from sterilization because of the disability. *Sterilization* means to remove or block sex organs so the person cannot have children.

DOWN SYNDROME

Down syndrome (DS) is named for the doctor who identified the syndrome. DS is a common genetic cause of mild to moderate intellectual disabilities. At fertilization, a male sex cell (sperm) unites with a female sex cell (ovum). Each cell has 23 chromosomes. When they unite, the cell has 46 chromosomes. In DS, an extra 21st chromosome is present. The fertilized cell has 47 chromosomes.

The DS child has certain features caused by the extra chromosome (Fig. 47-1, p. 760):
- Small head
- Eyes that slant upward
- Flat face
- Short, wide neck
- Large tongue
- Wide, flat nose
- Abnormally shaped ears
- Short stature
- Short, wide hands with stubby fingers
- Poor muscle tone

Many children with DS have heart defects and thyroid gland problems. They tend to have hearing and vision problems and to be over-weight. They are at risk for ear and respiratory infections. Leukemia is a risk (Chapter 40). Dementia may appear in adults with DS.

Persons with DS need speech, language, physical, and occupational therapies. Most learn self-care skills. They also need health and sex education. Weight gain and constipation are problems. They need a healthy diet and regular exercise.

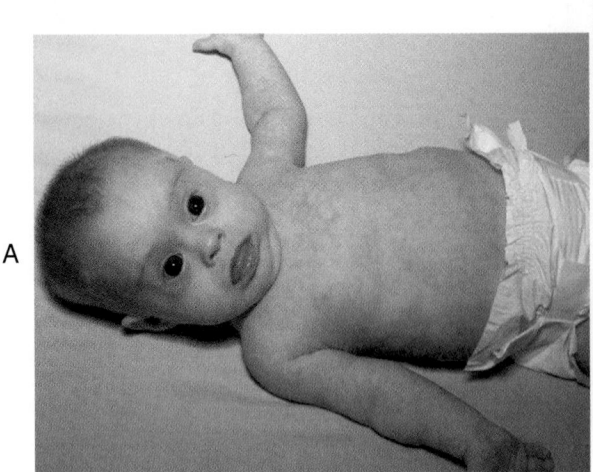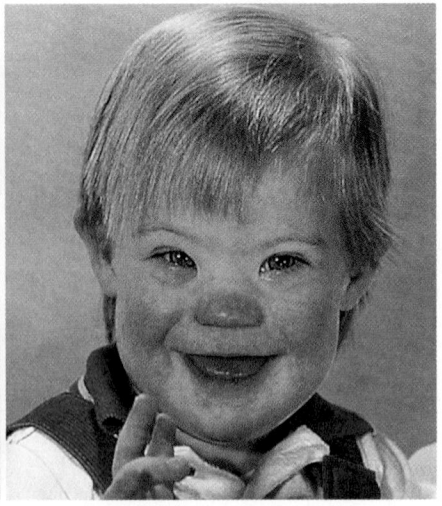

Fig. 47-1 **A,** An infant with Down syndrome. **B,** A child with Down syndrome.

FRAGILE X SYNDROME

Fragile X syndrome (FXS) is inherited. *Inherited means to be passed down from parents to children.* FXS is the most common form of inherited intellectual disabilities. There is a change in the gene that makes a protein needed for brain development. The body makes little or none of the protein.

Girls often have milder symptoms than boys. FXS has no cure. The person needs help to reduce or eliminate these common signs and symptoms:

- *Learning.* Learning disabilities range from mild to severe.
- *Physical.* Teenagers and adults may have long ears, faces, and jaws. Joints may be loose and flexible. This allows extending the elbow, thumb, and knee further than normal.
- *Social and emotional.* Behavior problems are common:
  - Fear and anxiety in new situations
  - Boys: attention problems, aggression
  - Girls: shy around new people
- *Speech and language.* Severe problems are not common in girls. Most boys may have these problems:
  - Speaking clearly
  - Stuttering
  - Leaving out parts of words
  - Understanding "clues" when talking to people (voice tone, body language)
- *Sensory.* Bright lights, loud noises, and how something feels may bother children. Some do like being touched. They may have trouble making eye contact with others.

CEREBRAL PALSY

Cerebral palsy (CP) is a group of disorders involving muscle weakness or poor muscle control *(palsy)*. The defect is in the motor region of the brain *(cerebral)*. Abnormal movements, posture, and coordination result. Problems walking are likely.

The defect is from brain damage before, during, or within a few years after birth. Lack of oxygen to the brain is the usual cause. Or the brain does not develop properly. There is no cure.

Infants at risk include those who:

- Are premature.
- Have low birth weight.
- Do not cry within the first 5 minutes after birth.
- Need mechanical ventilation.
- Have bleeding in the brain.
- Have heart, kidney, or spinal cord defects.
- Have blood problems.
- Have seizures.
- Have fetal alcohol syndrome.

Brain damage in infancy and early childhood also can result in CP. Lack of oxygen to the brain can occur from:

- Poisoning
- Traumatic brain injuries from accidents, falls, or child abuse (including shaken baby syndrome)
- Encephalitis and meningitis
- Rubella (German measles)

Body movements and body parts are affected. These types are the most common:

- *Spastic. Spastic means uncontrolled contractions of skeletal muscles.* Muscles contract or shorten. They are stiff and cannot relax. One or both sides of the body may be involved. Posture, balance, and movement are affected. When arms are affected, there are problems with eating, writing, dressing, and other activities of daily living.
- *Athetoid.* The person cannot control movements. *Athetoid means not fixed.* The person has constant, slow, weaving, or writhing motions. These occur in the trunk, arms, hands, legs, and feet. The tongue, face, and neck muscles may be involved. Drooling and grimacing result.

These terms describe the body parts involved:

- *Hemiplegia.* The arm and leg on one side are paralyzed.
- *Diplegia. Di* means *twice. Diplegia means that similar body parts are affected on both sides of the body.* Both arms or both legs are paralyzed. The legs are commonly involved.
- *Quadriplegia (tetraplegia).* Both arms and both legs are paralyzed. So are the trunk and neck muscles.

The person with CP can have many other impairments. They include:

- Intellectual and learning disabilities
- Hearing, vision, and speech impairments
- Drooling
- Bladder and bowel control problems
- Seizures
- Difficulty swallowing
- Attention deficit hyperactivity disorder (short attention span, poor concentration, increased activity)
- Breathing problems from poor posture
- Pressure ulcers from immobility

Care needs depend on the degree of brain damage. Disabilities range from mild to severe. Some persons are very smart. Others have severe intellectual disabilities. The goal is independence to the extent possible. Physical, occupational, and speech therapies can help. Some persons use braces, walkers, crutches, or wheelchairs. Some need vision and hearing aids. Drugs can control seizures. Surgery and drugs can help some muscle problems.

AUTISM

Autism begins in early childhood. Signs of delayed development are seen at about 18 months of age (Box 47-2). (*Autos* means *self.*) It is a brain disorder with no cure. The child has:

- Problems with social skills
- Verbal and nonverbal communication problems
- Repetitive behaviors and routines and narrow interests (*Repetitive* means *to repeat* or *repeated.*)

Autism is more common in boys than in girls. The cause is unknown. Genetics and environmental factors may be involved.

The disorder ranges from mild to severe. With therapy, the person can learn to change or control behaviors. The therapies include:

- Behavior modification
- Speech and language therapy
- Music therapy
- Auditory therapy
- Sensory therapies
- Physical and occupational therapies
- Drug therapy
- Diet therapy
- Communication therapy
- Recreation therapy

BOX 47-2	**SIGNS OF AUTISM**

Early Signs
- No babbling or pointing by the age of 1
- No single words by 16 months
- No 2-word phrases by age 2
- No response to his or her name
- Loss of language or social skills
- Poor eye contact
- Excessive lining up of toys or objects
- No smiling or social responses

Other Signs
- Shows no interest in other people
- Wants to be alone
- Has trouble understanding the feelings of others
- Has trouble talking about his or her own feelings
- Does not like to be held or cuddled; screams to be put down
- Over-reacts to touch
- Shows little reaction to pain
- Has frequent tantrums for no apparent reason
- Does not notice when others try to talk to him or her
- May not know how to talk, play, or relate to others
- May not talk
- Has slow language development
- Talks later than other children
- Repeats what others say at the moment or later
- Repeats words or phrases
- May not understand gestures (such as waving good-bye)
- Has a voice that sounds flat
- Cannot control voice volume (loudness or softness)
- Does not start or maintain conversations
- Stands too close to people when talking to them
- Stays with one topic of conversation for too long
- Has problems listening to what others say
- May act deaf
- Repeats actions over and over again
- Has routines where things stay the same
- Does not like change
- Repeats body movements (hand flapping, hand twisting, rocking)
- Has strong attachment to one item, idea, activity, or person
- Is very active or very quiet

Social and work skills are needed. Children with autism become adults. Some adults work and live independently. Others need support from family and community services. Some live in group homes or residential facilities.

Other disorders are common with autism. They include FXS and seizures.

SPINA BIFIDA

Spina bifida (SB) is a defect of the spinal column. (*Spina* means *backbone. Bifid* means *split in two parts.*) The defect occurs during the first month of pregnancy. Hydrocephalus often occurs with SB (p. 763).

Spinal column bones *(vertebrae)* protect the spinal cord. In SB, vertebrae do not form properly. This leaves a split in the vertebrae with the spinal cord unprotected. Only a membrane covers the spinal cord, which contains nerves. If the spinal cord is not protected, nerve damage occurs. Affected body parts do not function properly. Paralysis may occur. Bowel and bladder problems are common. Infection is a threat.

SB can occur anywhere in the spine. The lower back is a common site. Types of SB include:

- *Spina bifida occulta. Occult* means *hidden.* Vertebrae are closed. A defect occurs in the vertebrae closure. In other words, the defect is hidden. The spinal cord and nerves are normal. The person has a dimple or tuft of hair on the back (Fig. 47-2). Often there are no symptoms. Foot weakness and bowel and bladder problems can occur.
- *Spina bifida cystica. Cystica* means *pouch* or *sac.* Part of the spinal column is in the pouch or sac. A membrane or a thin layer of skin covers the sac. It looks like a large blister. The pouch is easily injured. Infection is a risk. The two types of spina bifida cystica are (Fig. 47-3):
  - *Meningocele. Meningo* means *membrane. Cele* means *hernia* or *swelling.* Meninges are the connective tissue that cover and protect the brain and spinal cord. Cerebrospinal fluid also protects the brain and spinal cord. The sac contains meninges and cerebrospinal fluid (see Fig 47-3, A and Fig. 47-4). The sac does not contain nerve tissue. The spinal cord and nerves are usually normal. Nerve damage usually does not occur. Surgery corrects the defect.
  - *Myelomeningocele* (or *meningomyelocele*). *Myelo* means *spinal cord.* The pouch contains nerves, spinal cord, meninges, and cerebrospinal fluid (see Fig. 47-3, B). Nerve damage occurs. Loss of function occurs below the level of damage. Leg paralysis and lack of sensation are common. So is the lack of bowel and bladder control. The defect is closed with surgery. Children use braces, crutches, or wheelchairs.

Some children have learning problems. They may have problems with attention, language, reading, and math. They are at high risk for gastro-intestinal disorders and mobility problems. Skin breakdown, depression, and social and sexual issues are other risks.

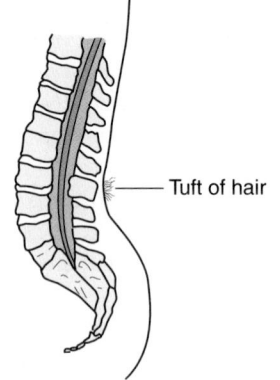

Fig. 47-2 Spina bifida occulta.

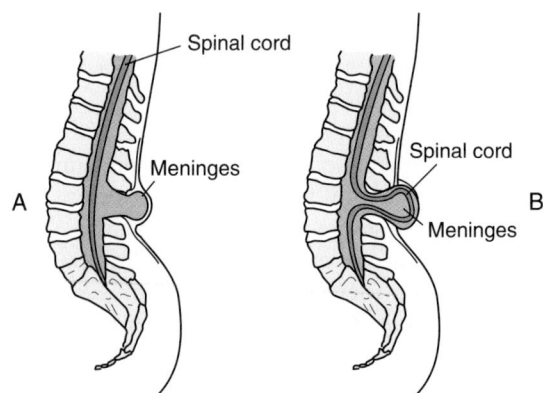

Fig. 47-3 **A,** Meningocele. **B,** Meningomyelocele.

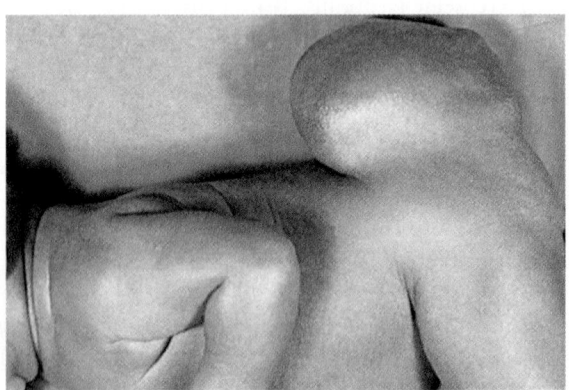

Fig. 47-4 Meningocele.

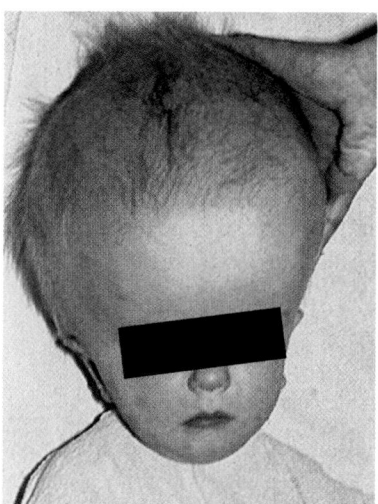

Fig. 47-5 Hydrocephalus.

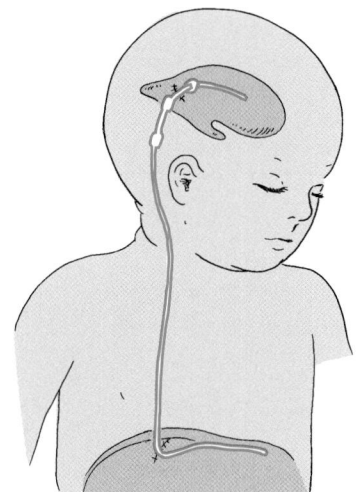

Fig. 47-6 A shunt drains fluid from the brain.

HYDROCEPHALUS

With hydrocephalus, cerebrospinal fluid collects in and around the brain. (*Hydro* means *water*. *Cephalo* means *head*.) The head enlarges (Fig. 47-5). Pressure inside the head increases. Intellectual disabilities and neurological damage occur without treatment. Vision problems, seizures, and learning disabilities can occur.

A shunt is placed in the brain. It allows cerebrospinal fluid to drain from the brain. The shunt is a long flexible tube. It goes from the brain into a body cavity to drain (Fig. 47-6). The shunt must remain open (*patent*). If blocked, the cerebrospinal fluid cannot drain from the brain.

FOCUS ON P R I D E

The Person, Family, and Yourself

Personal and Professional Responsibility

Caring for persons with developmental disabilities is a joy and a challenge. The person may struggle with speech, learning, mobility, or self-care. Care needs can be great. Even with these challenges, the person often has a positive outlook on life and brings joy to others.

Your attitude affects your life and work. A positive attitude brings joy, patience, and kindness. It builds teamwork and work ethics (Chapter 5). And it improves the quality of life of others.

Do not allow challenges to affect your attitude. Instead, let your attitude overcome the challenges. Take pride in your decision to have a positive attitude.

Rights and Respect

Persons with developmental disabilities have the right to enjoy and maintain a good quality of life. Such a life involves friendships, health and safety, and the right to make choices and take risks. Your care affects the person's quality of life. Treat the person with dignity and respect. Allow personal choice. Always provide quality care.

Independence and Social Interaction

The Arc of the United States believes that children with intellectual disabilities should live in a family. They should learn and play with children without disabilities. As adults, they should control their lives as much as possible. They should speak, make choices, and act for themselves. They should live in a home, have friends, do meaningful work, and enjoy adult activities. Independence to the greatest extent possible is the goal.

Delegation and Teamwork

Some persons respond better to care from certain people. For example, Ms. Hawn has cerebral palsy. You are patient and kind, but she refuses to eat. Ms. Hawn's brother comes to visit. He is able to feed Ms. Hawn.

Do not be offended if the person responds better to another person. It does not mean you have done something wrong. And it does not mean the person does not like you. The person may prefer help from a certain person at that time. You may be able to assist the person another day or at another time.

Do not let your pride get in the way of meeting the person's needs. You may need to allow a caregiver, the nurse, or another nursing assistant to assist the person. Learn from the person. Ask for advice. He or she may take a different approach or know the person's preferences. Encourage the caregiver or co-worker. And thank him or her for the help.

Ethics and Laws

Persons with DDs must be protected from abuse, mistreatment, and neglect (Chapters 2 and 4). They may have limited ability to communicate. Or they may fear what will happen if they tell. Changes in mood or behavior, frequent injuries, poor hygiene, weight loss, and anxiety around a caregiver are signs of abuse. See Chapter 4 for others. Tell the nurse right away if you suspect abuse. Take pride in protecting the person's safety and well-being.

REVIEW QUESTIONS

Circle the BEST answer.

1 All developmental disabilities occur
   a At birth
   b From trauma
   c During pregnancy
   d Before 22 years of age
2 These statements are about developmental disabilities. Which is *true*?
   a Self-care, learning, and mobility are always affected.
   b The disability is severe and permanent.
   c Physical and intellectual impairment occur together.
   d The person cannot hold a job.
3 The person with an intellectual disability
   a Has delayed development of sexual organs
   b Does not have the skills to live, work, and play
   c Needs care in a special setting
   d Learns at a slower rate than normal
4 Intellectual disabilities
   a Are always severe
   b Can occur before, during, or after birth
   c Are caused by an extra chromosome
   d Affect the motor region of the brain
5 Down syndrome occurs
   a At fertilization
   b During the first month of pregnancy
   c Any time before, during, or after birth
   d From trauma
6 Down syndrome always involves some degree of
   a Cerebral palsy
   b Autism
   c Impaired mobility
   d Intellectual disability
7 Fragile X syndrome is
   a The result of brain injury
   b Inherited from parents
   c Caused by drug and alcohol use
   d Caused by an infection

8 Cerebral palsy is usually caused by
   a An extra chromosome
   b High fever
   c Lack of oxygen to the brain
   d Infection during pregnancy
9 The spastic type of cerebral palsy involves problems with
   a Learning
   b Drooling
   c Posture, balance, and movement
   d Weaving motions of the trunk, arms, and legs
10 Autism begins
   a At fertilization
   b During pregnancy
   c At birth
   d In early childhood
11 The person with autism has
   a Impaired movement
   b Social and communication problems
   c Diplegia and brain damage
   d Intellectual disabilities
12 Spina bifida involves
   a Nerve damage
   b A defect in the spinal column
   c Seizures
   d Intellectual disabilities
13 Which is common in spina bifida?
   a Short attention span
   b Hearing and vision problems
   c Seizures
   d Bowel and bladder problems
14 Hydrocephalus often occurs with
   a Down syndrome
   b Cerebral palsy
   c Spina bifida
   d Autism
15 Hydrocephalus is treated with
   a Braces and crutches
   b A shunt
   c Drugs
   d Social services

Answers to these questions are on p. 835.

OBJECTIVES

- Define the key terms and key abbreviations listed in this chapter.
- Describe sex, sexuality, and sexual relationships.
- Explain why sexuality is important throughout life.
- Explain how aging, injury, and illness can affect sexuality.
- Explain how the nursing team can promote sexuality.
- Explain why some persons become sexually aggressive.
- Describe how to deal with sexually aggressive persons.
- Explain how to promote PRIDE in the person, the family, and yourself.

KEY TERMS

bisexual A person who is attracted to both sexes

erectile dysfunction (ED) See "impotence"

heterosexual A person who is attracted to members of the other sex

homosexual A person who is attracted to members of the same sex

impotence The inability of the male to have an erection; erectile dysfunction

sex Physical activities involving the reproductive organs; done for pleasure or to have children

sexuality The physical, emotional, social, cultural, and spiritual factors that affect a person's feelings and attitudes about his or her sex

transgender A broad term used to describe people who express their sexuality or gender in other than the expected way; persons who are undergoing hormone therapy or surgery for sexual re-assignment (female to male; male to female)

transsexual A person who believes that he or she is a member of the other sex

transvestite A person who dresses and behaves like the other sex for emotional and sexual relief; cross-dresser

KEY ABBREVIATIONS

ED Erectile dysfunction

OBRA Omnibus Budget Reconciliation Act of 1987

Patients and residents are viewed as whole persons. They have physical and safety needs. They also have love and belonging, self-esteem, and self-actualization needs. Their physical, emotional, social, and spiritual needs are considered.

Sexuality involves the whole person. Illness, injury, and aging can affect sexuality.

See *Body Structure and Function Review: The Reproductive System*, p. 766.

BODY STRUCTURE AND FUNCTION REVIEW: THE REPRODUCTIVE SYSTEM

The Male Reproductive System (Fig. 48-1)

The two *testes (testicles)* are the male sex glands. The testes are suspended between the thighs in a sac called the *scrotum.*

Male sex cells *(sperm)* are produced in the testes. So is *testosterone,* the male hormone. This hormone is needed for reproductive organ function. It also is needed for the development of the male secondary sex characteristics (Chapter 10).

The *prostate gland* lies just below the bladder. The *urethra* runs through the prostate gland. The urethra is contained within the penis.

The *penis* is outside of the body. The penis has *erectile tissue.* When a man is sexually excited, blood fills the erectile tissue. The penis enlarges and becomes hard and erect. The erect penis can enter a female's vagina.

The Female Reproductive System (Figs. 48-2 and 48-3)

The female sex glands are called *ovaries.* An ovary is on each side of the uterus. The ovaries contain *ova* or eggs—the female sex cells. The ovaries secrete the female hormones *estrogen* and *progesterone.* These hormones are needed for reproductive system function. They also are needed for the development of secondary sex characteristics in the female (Chapter 10).

The *uterus* is a hollow, muscular organ. It is behind the bladder and in front of the rectum. Tissue lining the uterus is called the *endometrium.* The uterus serves as a place for the *fetus* (unborn baby) to grow and receive nourishment.

The *cervix* of the uterus projects into a muscular canal called the *vagina.* The vagina opens to the outside of the body. It is just behind the urethra. The vagina receives the penis during intercourse. It also is part of the birth canal. Glands in the vaginal wall keep it moistened with secretions.

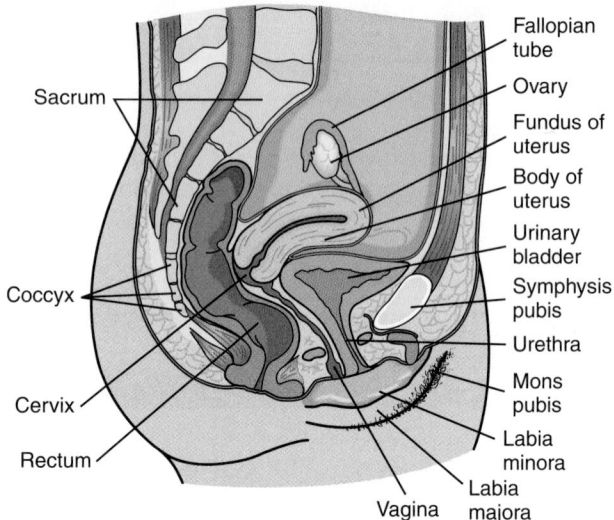

Fig. 48-2 The female reproductive system.

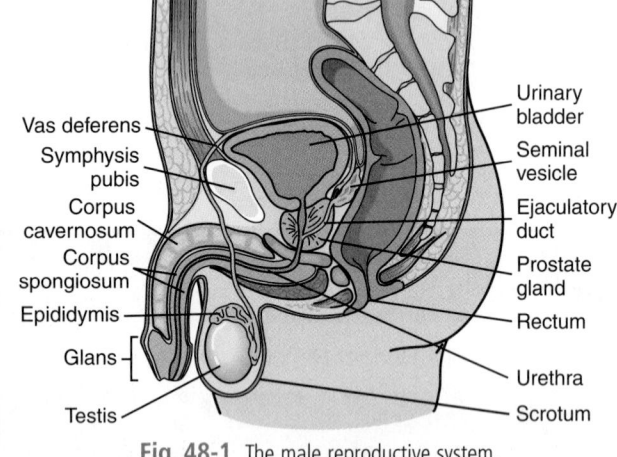

Fig. 48-1 The male reproductive system.

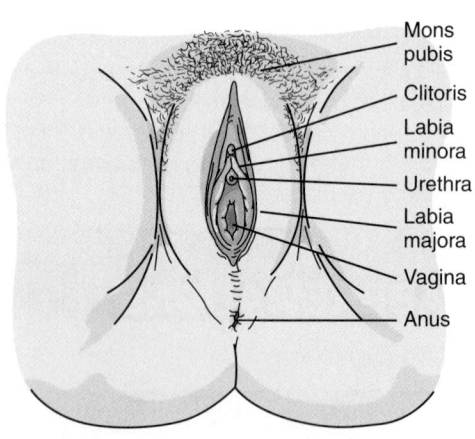

Fig. 48-3 External female genitalia.

SEX AND SEXUALITY

Sex is the physical activities involving the reproductive organs. It is done for pleasure or to have children. Sexuality is the physical, emotional, social, cultural, and spiritual factors that affect a person's feelings and attitudes about his or her sex. Sexuality involves the personality and the body. It affects how a person behaves, thinks, dresses, and responds to others.

Sexuality develops when a baby's sex is known. It is shown in names, colors, and toys. Blue is for boys. Pink is for girls. Dolls are for girls. Trains are for boys. By the age of 2, children know their own sex. Three-year-olds know the sex of other children. They learn male and female roles from adults (Fig. 48-4). Children learn that boys and girls behave in certain ways.

As children grow older, interest increases about the body and how it works. Teens are more aware of sex and the body. Their bodies respond to stimulation. They engage in sexual behaviors. They kiss, embrace, pet, or have intercourse. Pregnancy and sexually transmitted diseases (Chapter 44) are great risks.

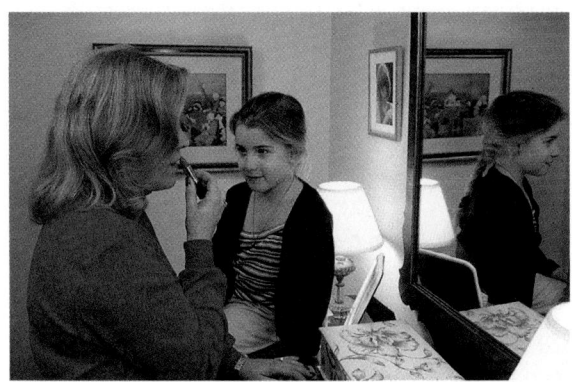

Fig. 48-4 This little girl is learning female roles from her mother.

Sex has more meaning as young adults mature. Attitudes and feelings are important. Partners are selected. They decide about sex before marriage and birth control.

Sexuality is important throughout life. Attitudes and sex needs change with aging. They are affected by life events. These include divorce, death of a partner, injury, illness, and surgery.

SEXUAL RELATIONSHIPS

A *heterosexual is a person who is attracted to members of the other sex.* Men are attracted to women. Women are attracted to men. Sexual behavior is male-female.

A *homosexual is a person who is attracted to members of the same sex.* Men are attracted to men. Women are attracted to women. *Gay* refers to homosexuality. Homosexual men are called *gay men. Lesbian* refers to a female homosexual. Many gay persons openly express their sexual preferences and relationships.

Bisexuals are persons who are attracted to both sexes. Some have same-gender and male-female behaviors. They often marry and have children. They may seek a same-gender relationship or experience outside of marriage.

Transvestites are persons who dress and behave like the other sex for emotional and sexual relief. Commonly called *cross-dressers,* most are men. Often they marry and are heterosexual. They dress as men most of the time. They usually dress as women in private. Some dress completely as women. Others focus on bras and panties. The sex partner may not know about the practice. Some partners take part in cross-dressing activities. Some transvestites have same-gender friends with similar interests.

Transsexuals are persons who believe that they are members of the other sex. A male believes he is a female in a man's body. A female believes she is a male in a woman's body. They often feel "trapped" in the wrong body. Most have always had these feelings. As children they usually behave like the other sex. Some have sex-change operations.

Transgender is a broad term used to describe people who express their sexuality or gender in other than the expected way. The term also describes *persons who are undergoing hormone therapy or surgery for sexual re-assignment (female to male; male to female).*

INJURY, ILLNESS, AND SURGERY

Injury, illness, and surgery can affect sexual function. Sometimes the nervous, circulatory, and reproductive systems are involved. Sexual ability may change. Most chronic illnesses affect sexual function. Heart disease, stroke, diabetes, and chronic obstructive pulmonary disease are examples.

Reproductive system surgeries have physical and mental effects. Removal of the uterus, ovaries, or a breast affects women. Prostate or testes removal affects erections.

Impotence (erectile dysfunction; ED) is the inability of the male to have an erection. The many causes include diabetes, spinal cord injuries, prostate problems, alcoholism, cardiovascular disorders, drug abuse, and psychological factors. Some drugs for high blood pressure cause ED. So do other drugs. Some drugs treat ED.

Emotional changes are common. The person may feel unclean, unwhole, unattractive, or mutilated. The person may feel unfit for closeness and love. Therefore some problems are emotional. Time and understanding are helpful. So is a caring partner. Some persons need counseling.

Changes in sexual function greatly affect the person. Fear, anger, worry, and depression are seen in the person's behavior and comments. The person's feelings are normal and expected. The care plan has measures to help the person deal with his or her feelings.

SEXUALITY AND OLDER PERSONS

Love, affection, and intimacy are needed throughout life (Fig. 48-5, p. 768). Older persons love, fall in love, hold hands, and embrace. Many have intercourse.

Older persons have many losses. Children leave home. Family and friends die. People retire. Health problems occur. Strength decreases. Appearance changes. It helps to feel close to another person.

Reproductive organs change with aging (Chapter 11). Frequency of sex may decrease. Reasons relate to weakness, fatigue, and pain. Reduced mobility, aging, and chronic illness are factors.

Some older people do not have intercourse. This does not mean loss of sexual needs or desires. Often needs are expressed in other ways. They hold hands, touch, caress, and embrace. These bring closeness and intimacy.

Sexual partners are lost through death, divorce, and relationship break-ups. Or a partner needs hospital or nursing center care. These situations occur in adults of all ages.

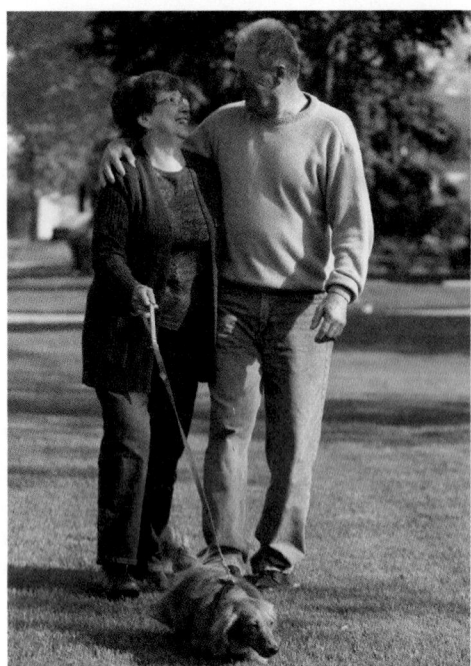

Fig. 48-5 Love and affection are important to persons of all ages.

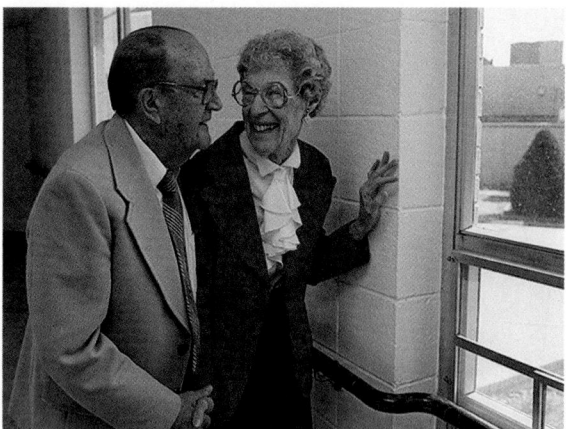

Fig. 48-6 Relationships develop in nursing centers.

MEETING SEXUAL NEEDS

The nursing team promotes the meeting of sexual needs. The measures in Box 48-1 may be part of the person's care plan.

See *Focus on Long-Term Care and Home Care: Meeting Sexual Needs.*

FOCUS ON LONG-TERM CARE AND HOME CARE
Meeting Sexual Needs

Long-Term Care

Married couples in nursing centers can share the same room. This is a requirement of the Omnibus Budget Reconciliation Act of 1987 (OBRA). The couple has lived together a long time. Long-term care is no reason to keep them apart. They can share the same bed if their conditions permit. A double, queen-size, or king-size bed is provided by the couple or the center.

Single persons may develop relationships. They are allowed time together, not kept apart (Fig. 48-6).

BOX 48-1   PROMOTING SEXUALITY

- Let the person practice grooming routines. Assist as needed. For women, this includes applying make-up, nail polish, and cologne. Many women shave their legs and underarms and pluck eyebrows. Men may use after-shave lotion and cologne. Hair care is important to men and women.
- Let the person choose clothing. Hospital gowns can embarrass the person. Street clothes are worn if the person's condition permits.
- Protect the right to privacy. Do not expose the person. Drape and screen the person.
- Accept the person's sexual relationships. The person may not share your sexual attitudes, values, or practices. The person may have a homosexual, premarital, or extramarital relationship. Do not judge or gossip about relationships.
- Allow privacy. If the person has a private room, close the door for privacy. Some agencies have DO NOT DISTURB signs for doors. Let the person and partner know how much time they have alone. For example, remind them about meal times, drugs, and treatments. Tell other staff that the person wants time alone.
- Knock before you enter any room. This simple courtesy shows respect for privacy.
- Consider the person's roommate. Privacy curtains do not block sound. Arrange for privacy when the roommate is out of the room. A roommate may offer to leave for a while. Or the nurse finds a private area.
- Allow privacy for masturbation. It is a normal form of sexual expression. Close the privacy curtain and the door. Knock before you enter any room. This saves you and the person embarrassment. Sometimes confused persons masturbate in public areas. Lead the person to a private area. Or distract him or her with an activity.

THE SEXUALLY AGGRESSIVE PERSON

Some persons want the health team to meet their sexual needs. They flirt or make sexual advances or comments. Some expose themselves, masturbate, or touch the staff. This can anger and embarrass the staff member. These reactions are normal. Often there are reasons for the person's behavior. Understanding this helps you deal with the matter.

Sexually aggressive behaviors have many causes. They include:

- Nervous system disorders
- Confusion, disorientation, and dementia
- Drug side effects
- Fever
- Poor vision

The person may confuse someone with his or her partner. Or the person cannot control behavior. The healthy person controls sexual urges. Changes in the brain and mental function make control difficult. Sexual behavior in these cases is usually innocent.

Sometimes touch is used to gain attention. For example, Mr. Green cannot speak or move his right side. Your buttocks are near him. To get your attention, he touches your buttocks. His behavior is not sexual.

Sometimes masturbation is a sexually aggressive behavior. Some persons touch and fondle the genitals for sexual pleasure. However, urinary or reproductive system disorders can cause genital soreness or itching. So can poor hygiene and being wet or soiled from urine or feces. Touching genitals could signal a health problem.

Touch can have a sexual purpose. For example, a man wants to prove that he is attractive and can perform sexually. You must be professional about the matter.

- Ask the person not to touch you. State the places where you were touched.
- Tell the person that you will not do what he or she wants.
- Tell the person what behaviors make you uncomfortable. Politely ask the person not to act that way.
- Allow privacy if the person is becoming aroused. Provide for safety. Complete a safety check of the room (see the inside of the front book cover). Tell the person when you will return.
- Discuss the matter with the nurse. The nurse can help you understand the behavior.
- Follow the care plan. It has measures to deal with sexually aggressive behaviors. They are based on the cause of the behavior.

See *Focus on Communication: The Sexually Aggressive Person.*

FOCUS ON COMMUNICATION

The Sexually Aggressive Person

Confronting the sexually aggressive person is hard. This is true for young and older staff and for new and experienced staff. Ask yourself these questions:

- Does the person have a health problem that affects impulse control? If yes, the behavior may not have a sexual purpose.
- Is the person's behavior on purpose? Is the intent sexual? If yes, you must confront the behavior. Be direct and matter-of-fact. For example, you can say:
  - "You brushed your hand across my breast (or other body part) two times this morning. Please don't do that again."
  - "No, I cannot kiss you. It would be unprofessional."
  - "You exposed yourself to me again today. Please do not do that again."

The sexually aggressive person needs the nurse's attention. Discuss the matter with the nurse. Report what happened and when. Also report what you said and did. The nurse must deal with the problem. If other staff are reporting such behaviors, the nurse views the problem in a broader way.

Protecting the Person

The person must be protected from unwanted sexual comments and advances. This is sexual abuse (Chapter 4). Tell the nurse right away. No one should be allowed to sexually abuse another person. This includes staff members, patients, residents, family members or other visitors, and volunteers.

SEXUALLY TRANSMITTED DISEASES

Some diseases are spread by sexual contact. They are discussed in Chapter 44.

FOCUS ON PRIDE

The Person, Family, and Yourself

Personal and Professional Responsibility

Touching a person's body without his or her consent is battery (Chapter 4). You must take extra caution when care involves the genitals, buttocks, or breasts. Without consent, you may be accused of sexual abuse.

To obtain consent, explain what you will do at the beginning of procedures and step-by-step. If the person asks you to stop, you must stop. Follow agency policies when caring for persons of the opposite sex. The nurse may need to ask the person's permission or delegate the task to staff of the same gender.

Obtaining consent and explaining procedures are professional responsibilities. The person has control over care, knows what to expect, and is more at ease. The person's rights are protected. And you protect yourself from being accused of battery or sexual abuse.

Continued

Rights and Respect

The person's sexual attitudes, values, or practices may differ from yours. For example, you may not agree with a sexual relationship. Your feelings must not affect the person's care. Do not avoid the person. Do not judge or gossip about the person. Treat the person with dignity and respect.

Independence and Social Interaction

Sexuality includes emotional, social, cultural, spiritual, and physical factors. To promote sexuality:

- Assist the person with hygiene and grooming before visitors arrive.
- Compliment the person on his or her appearance. Comment on a woman's hair, clothing, jewelry, nails, and so on. Compliment men after shaving.
- Talk with the person about his or her family. Years of marriage and number of children are common topics. Respect privacy if the person does not want to talk.
- Use touch to show you care. A touch on the arm, shoulder, or upper back can communicate care without crossing boundaries (Chapter 4).

Delegation and Teamwork

A person may have sexually aggressive behaviors. The team must try to determine the cause. If the cause can be fixed, the behavior may stop. When the cause cannot be fixed, the team follows the care plan to manage the behavior. A professional response is always needed.

Tell the nurse if you notice sexually aggressive behaviors. The problem cannot be ignored. Rely on the nursing team for advice, guidance, and support.

Ethics and Laws

All persons must be protected from sexual abuse. The following is a real case of a nursing assistant who violated the person's right to freedom from abuse and mistreatment.

A certified nursing assistant (CNA) had his certificate revoked by the Arizona State Board of Nursing. The Board found that he violated the state's Nurse Practice Act because of the following actions:

- *He was convicted of "Driving Under the Influence" in April 2002.*
- *In September 2002, he agreed to a $150 penalty on his CNA certificate for several incidents of resident abuse. He also admitted to removing an impaction from a female resident, which he knew was not within the scope of CNA duties.*
- *While employed at a nursing home, the following incidents occurred from November 14 through November 23, 2005:*
  - *A female resident reported that he was "rough with her and 'hurt her groin.'" The resident demanded a transfer to another facility.*
  - *An alert and oriented resident reported that the CNA "'raped' her by placing his hand inside of her private parts." The resident also stated that she "could smell alcohol on his breath."*
  - *His employment was terminated for policy violation and "causing a resident undue stress and fear when he assisted her to expel an impaction."*
- *While employed in a group home, it was reported that he violated agency policy regarding alcohol use. He was employed by the group home during August–December 2005.*

(Arizona State Board of Nursing, May, 18, 2006. NOTE: Names withheld by request of the Arizona State Board of Nursing.)

Sexual abuse is a serious matter. No one is allowed to sexually abuse another person. Report concerns of abuse to the nurse.

REVIEW QUESTIONS

Circle the BEST answer.

1 Sex involves
   a The organs of reproduction
   b Attitudes and feelings
   c Cultural and spiritual factors
   d Masturbation

2 Sexuality is important to
   a Small children
   b Teenagers and young adults
   c Middle-age adults
   d Persons of all ages

3 Impotence is
   a A sexually aggressive behavior
   b A reaction to illness
   c Not being able to achieve an erection
   d No sexual activity

4 Reproductive organs change with aging.
   a True
   b False

5 Mr. and Mrs. Green live in a nursing center. Which will *not* promote their sexuality?
   a Allowing normal grooming routines
   b Having them wear hospital gowns
   c Allowing privacy
   d Accepting their relationship

6 Two residents are holding hands. Nursing staff should keep them apart.
   a True
   b False

7 Mr. and Mrs. Green want some time alone. The nursing team can do the following *except*
   a Close the room door
   b Put a DO NOT DISTURB sign on the door
   c Tell other staff that they want some time alone
   d Close the privacy curtain so no one can hear them

8 Mr. and Mrs. Green should each have a room. This is an OBRA requirement.
   a True
   b False

9 A person is masturbating in the dining room. You should do the following *except*
   a Cover the person
   b Quietly take the person to his or her room
   c Scold the person
   d Tell the nurse

10 A person touches you sexually and asks for a kiss. You should do the following *except*
   a Discuss the matter with the nurse
   b Do what the person asks
   c Explain that the behaviors make you uncomfortable
   d Ask the person not to touch you

Answers to these questions are on p. 835.

Caring for Mothers and Newborns

49

OBJECTIVES

- Define the key terms and key abbreviations listed in this chapter.
- Describe how to meet an infant's safety and security needs.
- Identify the signs and symptoms of illness in infants.
- Explain how to help mothers with breast-feeding.
- Describe three forms of baby formulas.
- Explain how to bottle-feed babies.
- Explain how to burp a baby.

- Describe how to give cord care.
- Describe the purposes of circumcision, needed observations, and the required care.
- Explain how to bathe infants.
- Explain why infants are weighed.
- Describe the care needed by mothers after childbirth.
- Perform the procedures described in this chapter.
- Explain how to promote PRIDE in the person, the family, and yourself.

KEY TERMS

breast-feeding Feeding a baby milk from the mother's breasts; nursing

circumcision The surgical removal of foreskin from the penis

episiotomy Incision *(otomy)* into the perineum

lochia The vaginal discharge that occurs after childbirth

meconium A dark green to black, tarry bowel movement

nursing See "breast-feeding"

postpartum After *(post)* childbirth *(partum)*

umbilical cord The structure that connects the mother and fetus (unborn baby); it carries blood, oxygen, and nutrients from the mother to the fetus

KEY ABBREVIATIONS

C	Centigrade	**F**	Fahrenheit
C-section	Cesarean section	**mm**	Millimeter

Mothers and newborns usually have short hospital stays. Some need home care after discharge. Common reasons for home care include that the mother:
- Has complications before or after childbirth.
- Has health problems.
- Needs help with other young children in the home.
- Had a multiple birth (twins, triplets, and so on).
- Needs help with meals and housekeeping.

Babies depend on others for their basic needs. Babies have physical, safety and security, and love and belonging needs. A review of growth and development will help you care for babies (Chapter 10).

INFANT SAFETY AND SECURITY

Babies cannot protect themselves. They need to feel safe and secure. They feel secure when warm and when wrapped and held snugly. Babies cry to communicate. They cry when wet, hungry, hot or cold, tired, uncomfortable, or in pain. To promote safety and security, respond to their cries—feed them when hungry, change diapers as needed, comfort them, talk to them, and so on. See Chapter 12 for infant safety measures. Also follow the measures in Box 49-1, p. 772.

Nursery equipment must be safe and in good repair. Use the guidelines in Box 49-2, p. 773 to check nursery equipment in an agency or home setting.

BOX 49-1   INFANT SAFETY

General Safety
- Follow the safety measures in Chapters 12 and 19.
- Keep the baby warm. Check windows for drafts. Close windows securely.
- Keep your fingernails short. Do not wear fake nails. Long nails can scratch the baby.
- Do not wear rings or bracelets. Jewelry can scratch the baby.
- Respond to the baby's crying. Babies communicate by crying. Responding to their cries helps them feel safe and secure.
- Keep one hand on the baby at all times when on a changing table or other raised surface.
- Keep pins and small objects out of the baby's reach.
- Do not shake powders directly over the baby. The powder can get into the baby's eyes and lungs. Shake some on your hand away from the baby.
- Use infant seats safely:
  - Restrain the baby in the seat.
  - Do not leave the baby unattended when the seat is on a raised surface.
- Do not tie a pacifier around the baby's neck.

Holding a Baby
- Use both hands to lift a newborn. Use one hand to support the head and upper back. Use your other hand to support the legs. Do not lift a newborn by the arms.
- Hold the baby securely. Use the cradle hold, football hold, or shoulder hold (Fig. 49-1).
- Support the baby's head and neck when lifting or holding the baby. Neck support is necessary for the first 3 months after birth.
- Handle the baby with gentle, smooth movements. Avoid sudden or jerking movements. Do not startle the baby.
- Hold and cuddle infants. It is comforting and helps them learn to feel love and security.

Crib and Furniture Safety
- Tighten all nuts, bolts, and screws on cribs, high chairs, and other infant furniture. Do this often.
- Check mattress hooks to make sure none are bent, broken, or open.
- Make sure the mattress is not covered with plastic.
- Make sure the crib is within hearing distance of the caregivers.
- Place the crib away from heat sources (radiators, registers).
- Place the crib away from other furniture.
- Do not put a pillow, quilts, or soft toys in the crib. They can cause suffocation.
- Do not lay an infant on soft bedding products. This includes fluffy, plush products such as sheepskin, quilts, comforters, pillows, and toys. Soft products can cause suffocation.
- Do not place infants on an adult or child's bed, water bed, bunk bed, or beanbag chair or pillow. Risks include:
  - Death from entrapment. The baby can get trapped between the bed and the wall; between the bed and another object; or between the bed frame, head-board, or foot-board.
  - Death from suffocation in soft bedding. This includes pillows, quilts, and comforters.
  - Death from suffocation after falling onto piles of clothing, plastic bags, pillows, cushions, or other soft materials.
- Do not place the child in a high chair until he or she can sit well with support.

Sleep
- Remove bibs and necklaces before naps and bedtime.
- Lay babies on their backs for sleep. *Do not lay babies on their stomachs for sleep. This can interfere with chest expansion and breathing. The baby can suffocate.* Infants can lie on their sides and stomachs when awake and watched by an adult.
- Make sure there is no soft bedding under the baby.

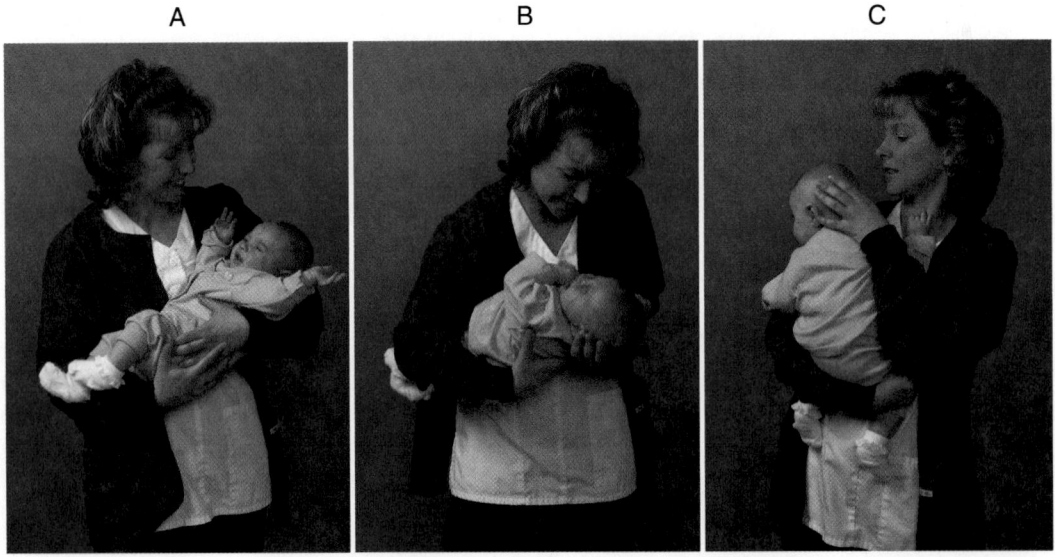

A   B   C

Fig. 49-1 Holding a baby. **A,** The cradle hold. **B,** The football hold. **C,** The shoulder hold.

BOX 49-2 **Safety Guide for Nursery Equipment**

Cribs

- Slats are spaced no more than 2⅜ inches (60 mm [millimeters]) apart.
- No slats are missing, loose, or cracked.
- The mattress fits snugly—less than a 2-finger width between the edge of the mattress and crib side.
- The mattress support is securely attached to the head and footboards.
- Corner posts are no higher than 1/16 inch (1.5 mm). This prevents entanglement of clothing or other objects worn by the child.
- There are no cutouts in the headboard and footboard. Cutouts allow head entrapment.
- All screws, bolts, and other hardware are present and tight.
- The crib meets federal safety standards for strength, durability, and testing.
- See Chapters 12 and 19.

Crib Toys

- Strings or cords do not dangle into the crib.
- A crib gym or mobile has a label warning to remove the device from the crib when one of the following occurs:
  - The child can push on the hands and knees.
  - The child reaches 5 months of age.
- Toy parts are too large to be a choking hazard.

Gates and Enclosures

- Gate openings are too small to entrap a child's head or neck.
- The gate has a pressure bar or other fastener that will resist forces exerted by a child.

High Chairs

- The high chair has a "crotch" strap that must be used when restraining a child in a high chair.
- The high chair has restraining straps that are independent of the tray.
- The tray locks securely.
- Buckles on straps are easy to fasten and unfasten.
- The high chair has a wide, stable base.
- Caps or plugs on tubing are firmly attached and cannot be pulled off and choke a child.
- A folding high chair has an effective locking device. The locking device keeps the chair from collapsing.

Playpens

- Playpens or travel cribs have top rails that automatically lock when lifted into the normal use position.
- The playpen does not have a rotating hinge in the center of the top rails.
- A drop-side mesh playpen or mesh crib has a label about never leaving a side in the down position.
- Playpen mesh has small weave (less than ¼ inch openings).
- The mesh has no tears, holes, or loose threads.
- The mesh is securely attached to the top rail and floor-plate.
- A wooden playpen has slats spaced no more than 2⅜ inches (60 mm) apart.

Rattles, Squeeze Toys, and Teethers

- Rattles, squeeze toys, and teethers have handles too large to lodge in the baby's throat.
- Squeeze toys do not contain a squeaker that could detach and choke a baby.
- Rattles do not have ball-shaped ends.

Toy Chests

- The toy chest has no latch to entrap the child within the chest.
- The toy chest has a spring-loaded lid support that will not require frequent adjustment. It supports the lid in any position to prevent lid slam.
- The chest has ventilation holes or spaces. The ventilation holes are in case the child gets caught inside.

Walkers

- The walker has safety features to help prevent a fall down stairs.

Back Carriers

- Leg openings are small enough to prevent the child from slipping out but large enough to prevent chafing.
- The folding mechanism has frame joints.
- There is a padded covering over the metal frame near the baby's face.

Bassinets and Cradles

- The item has a sturdy bottom and a wide base for stability.
- The item has smooth surfaces—no protruding staples or other hardware that could injure the baby.
- Legs have strong, effective locks to prevent folding while in use.
- The mattress is firm and fits snugly.
- Wood or metal cradles have slats spaced no more than 2⅜ inches (60 mm) apart.

Carrier Seats

- The item has a wide, sturdy base for stability.
- The item has non-skid feet to prevent slipping.
- Supporting devices lock securely.
- The seat has a crotch and waist strap.
- The buckle or strap is easy to use.

Changing Tables

- The table has safety straps to prevent falls.
- The table has drawers or shelves that are easy to reach without leaving the baby unattended.

Hook-on Chairs

- The chair has a restraining strap.
- The chair has a clamp that locks onto the table for added security.
- Caps or plugs on tubing are firmly attached and cannot be pulled off and choke a child.
- The hook-on chair has a warning never to place the chair where the child can push off with the feet.

Pacifiers

- The item has no ribbons, strings, cords, or yarn attached.
- The shield is large and firm enough so it cannot fit into the child's mouth.
- The guard or shield has ventilation holes to allow the baby to breathe if the shield does get into the mouth.
- The pacifier nipple has no holes or tears that might cause it to break off in the baby's mouth.

Modified from U.S. Consumer Product Safety Commission: *The safe nursery,* CPSC 202, Washington, DC.

Continued

BOX 49-2	Safety Guide for Nursery Equipment—cont'd

Strollers and Carriages
- There is a wide base to prevent tipping.
- The seat belt and crotch strap securely attach to the frame.
- The seat belt buckle is easy to use.
- Brakes securely lock the wheels.

- The shopping basket is low on the back. It is located directly over or in front of the rear wheels.
- When used in the carriage position, the leg openings can be closed.

BOX 49-3	SIGNS AND SYMPTOMS OF ILLNESS IN BABIES

- The baby has jaundice—a yellowish color to the skin and whites of the eyes.
- The baby looks sick.
- The baby has redness or drainage around the cord stump (p. 782) or circumcision (p. 783).
- The baby has a fever (Chapter 26).
- The baby is limp and slow to respond.
- The baby is hard to wake up.
- The baby is less active than usual.
- The baby cries all the time or does not stop crying.
- The baby is flushed, pale, or perspiring.
- The baby has noisy, rapid, difficult, or slow respirations.

- The baby is coughing or sneezing.
- The baby has reddened or irritated eyes.
- The baby turns his or her head to one side or puts a hand to one ear (signs of an earache).
- The baby screams for a long time.
- The baby is feeding poorly or has skipped feedings.
- The baby has vomited most of the feeding or vomits between feedings.
- The baby has watery stools or hard, formed stools.
- Stools are light-colored, green, or foul-smelling.
- The baby has fewer wet diapers.
- The baby has a rash.

Signs and Symptoms of Illness

Babies can become ill quickly. Signs and symptoms may be sudden. You must be very alert. Report any of the signs and symptoms in Box 49-3 to the nurse at once. Be alert to any change in the baby's behavior—sleep pattern, cry, appetite, or activity.

Tell the nurse when a sign or symptom began. You may need to measure the child's temperature, pulse, and respirations (Chapter 26). The nurse tells you what temperature site to use—tympanic, rectal, temporal artery, or axillary. Apical pulses are taken on infants and young children.

HELPING MOTHERS BREAST-FEED

Breast-feeding (nursing) is feeding a baby milk from the mother's breasts.
- The baby can feed at the mother's breast.
- The mother can pump milk from her breasts. The baby is fed breast milk from a bottle.

Babies usually breast-feed every 2 to 3 hours during the first month (8 to 12 times a day). They are fed on demand. That is, they are fed when hungry, not on a schedule.

Breast milk is digested faster than formula. Therefore breast-feeding is needed more often.

Babies nurse for a short time the first few days (5 to 10 minutes at each breast). Eventually nursing time takes 10 to 20 minutes at each breast. The rate varies for each baby. The following signal the end of the feeding:
- The baby's sucking slows.
- The baby pulls off the breast.
- The baby is no longer interested in feeding.

Nurses help new mothers learn to breast-feed. They also teach breast care. Mothers and babies learn how to nurse in a very short time. Tell the nurse if the mother or baby is having problems breast-feeding.

Mothers may need help getting ready to breast-feed. They may need help with hand washing and positioning. Assist as needed. Make sure the signal light is within reach before you leave the room. Also provide for privacy. Follow the care plan and the measures in Box 49-4 to help with breast-feeding.

See *Focus on Long-Term Care and Home Care: Helping Mothers Breast-Feed*, p. 776.

BOX 49-4 HELPING WITH BREAST-FEEDING

- Practice hand hygiene and Standard Precautions. Remember, HIV can be transmitted through breast milk (Chapter 40).
- Place milk, juice, or water near the mother. Most mothers become thirsty while breast-feeding.
- Help the mother wash her hands. She needs clean hands before handling her breasts.
- Help the mother to a comfortable position. The cradle position, side-lying position, and football hold are the basic positions for breast-feeding (Fig. 49-2).
- Change the baby's diaper if necessary. Bring the baby to the mother.
- Make sure the mother holds the baby close to her breast.
- Have the mother use her nipple to stroke the baby's cheek or lower lip. This stimulates the *rooting reflex*. The baby turns his or her head toward the breast and starts to suck.
- Make sure the baby's nose is not blocked by the mother's breast. One nostril must be clear for breathing. If the nose seems blocked, have mother do one of the following:
  - Re-position the baby. She can raise the baby's hips. Or she can move the baby's head back slightly.
  - Use her thumb to keep breast tissue away from the baby's nose (Fig. 49-3, p. 776).
- Give her a baby blanket to cover the baby and her breast. This promotes privacy.
- Encourage nursing from both breasts at each feeding. If the last feeding ended at the right breast, the next feeding is started at the right breast. The mother can use a ribbon or diaper pin on her bra strap to remind her which breast to start with.
- Remind her how to remove the baby from the breast. To break the suction between the baby and the breast, she can insert a finger into a corner of the baby's mouth (Fig. 49-4, p. 776).
- Help the mother burp the baby (p. 779). The baby is burped after nursing at one breast. Then the baby is burped after nursing at the other breast.
- Remind the mother to air-dry her nipples after a feeding.
- Change the baby's diaper after the feeding.
- Lay the baby in the crib if he or she has fallen asleep. *Lay the baby on his or her back. Do not lay the baby on the stomach.*
- Help the mother prevent dry and cracked nipples. Follow the nurse's directions and the care plan.
  - Milk is left on the nipple after a feeding. The milk is allowed to air-dry.
  - The mother applies prescribed cream after each feeding if the nipples are cracked. Remind her to wash her breasts with water before a feeding to remove the cream.
  - Soap is not used to clean the breasts and nipples.
  - Breasts and nipples are washed and allowed to air dry.
- Help the mother straighten clothing after the feeding if necessary.
- Remind the mother to wash her breasts with a clean washcloth and warm water. Soap is not used. It can cause the nipples to dry and crack. Nipples are air-dried after washing to prevent cracking and soreness.
- Encourage the mother to wear a nursing bra day and night. The bra supports the breasts and promotes comfort.
- Encourage the mother to place nursing pads in the bra. The pads absorb leaking milk.

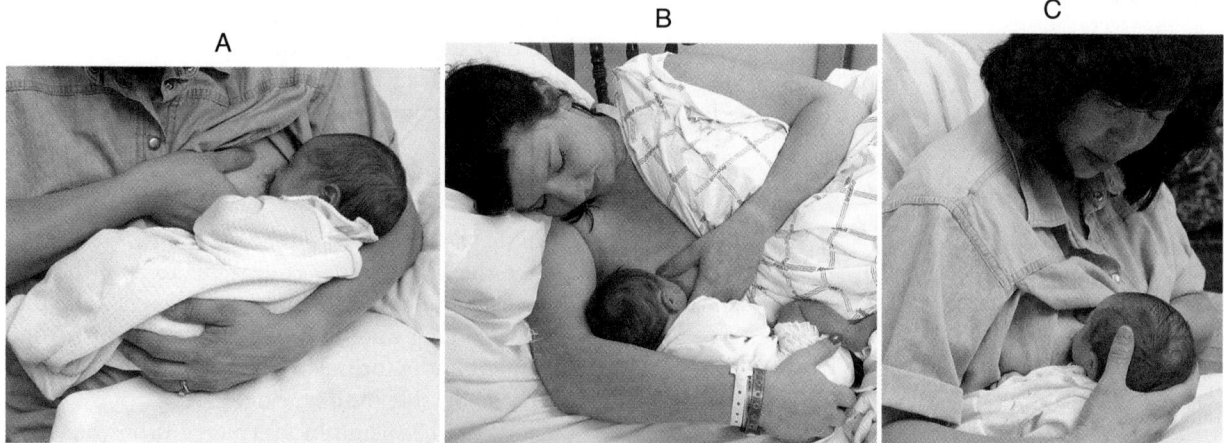

Fig. 49-2 Basic breast-feeding positions. **A,** Cradle position. **B,** Side-lying position. **C,** Football hold.

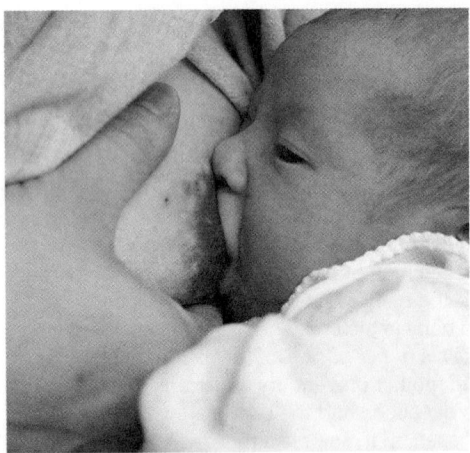

Fig. 49-3 The mother supports her breast with one hand. The thumb is on top of the breast to keep breast tissue away from the baby's nose.

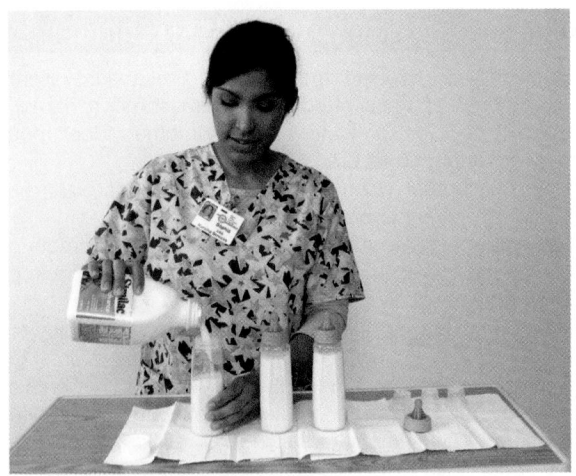

Fig. 49-5 Ready-to-feed formula is poured from the can into the bottle.

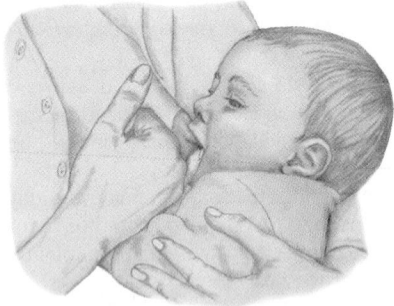

Fig. 49-4 The mother inserts a finger into the corner of the baby's mouth to remove the baby from the breast.

BOTTLE-FEEDING BABIES

Formula is given to babies who are not breast-fed. The doctor prescribes the formula. It provides the nutrients the infant needs.

Formula comes in 3 forms.

- *Ready-to-feed.* It is ready to use. It is poured from the can into the baby bottle (Fig. 49-5). The can may have more than 1 feeding. Refrigerate the can after opening it. Use the contents within 24 hours.
- *Powdered.* Container directions tell how much powder and water to use.
- *Liquid concentrate.* Container directions tell you how much liquid and water to use.

Bottles are prepared one at a time or in batches for the whole day. To prepare a bottle:

- Boil water as directed by the nurse.
- Follow the container directions carefully. Measure exact amounts.
- Pour the correct amount of water and formula into the bottle.
- Gently shake or swirl the bottle to mix.
- Place the bottle under cold water to cool the formula. Or place the bottle in cold or ice water. Keep the level of the cooling water below the bottle's lid to avoid contaminating the formula.
- Dry the outside of the bottle.
- Check the temperature by placing drops on the inside of your wrist. The formula should feel warm, not hot.
- Cap extra bottles (Fig. 49-6). Store them in the refrigerator. Use stored bottles within 24 hours.

FOCUS ON LONG-TERM CARE AND HOME CARE

Helping Mothers Breast-Feed

Home Care

When the mother is nursing, stay within hearing distance in case she needs help.

The nursing mother needs good nutrition. When planning meals or grocery shopping, remember that:

- Calorie intake may increase. The nurse tells you what the mother's calorie intake needs to be.
- She should have 3 servings a day from the milk, yogurt, and cheese group. She can drink whole, 2%, or skim milk. The nurse tells you if more servings are needed.
- She needs foods high in calcium.
- She can eat the foods she likes. The baby may become fussy or gassy or have cramping or diarrhea after she eats a certain food. She should avoid that food for a while. Onions, garlic, spices, cabbage, brussel sprouts, asparagus, and beans are examples.
- Chocolate, cola beverages, coffee, and tea contain caffeine. They are used in moderation. Caffeine can cause the baby to be fussy or gassy. The baby may become agitated or have sleep problems.
- She should not drink alcohol.

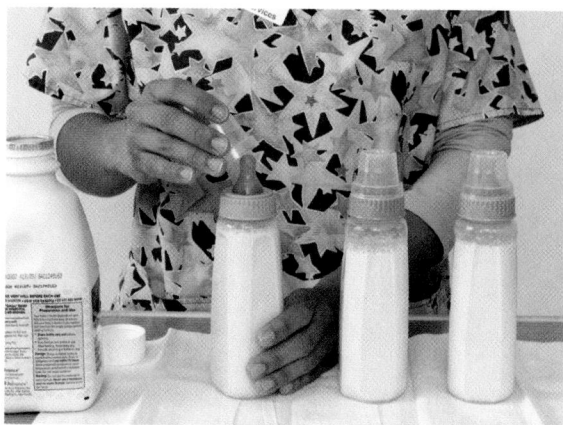

Fig. 49-6 Bottles are capped for storage in the refrigerator.

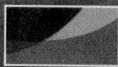 **Cleaning Baby Bottles**

Protect the baby from infection. Baby bottles, caps, nipples, and other items must be as clean as possible. Disposable equipment is used in hospitals. Re-usable equipment is common in homes. It is carefully washed in hot, soapy water or in a dishwasher. Complete rinsing is needed to remove all soap. Some bottles have plastic liners that are discarded after one use.

See *Focus on Long-Term Care and Home Care: Cleaning Baby Bottles.*
See *Promoting Safety and Comfort: Cleaning Baby Bottles.*

CLEANING BABY BOTTLES

PRE-PROCEDURE

1 See *Promoting Safety and Comfort: Cleaning Baby Bottles.*
2 Practice hand hygiene.
3 Collect the following:
- Bottles, nipples, and caps
- Funnel
- Can opener
- Bottle brush
- Dishwashing soap
- Other items used to prepare formula
- Towel

PROCEDURE

4 Wash the bottles, nipples, caps, funnel, and can opener in hot, soapy water. Wash other items used to prepare formula.
5 Clean inside baby bottles with the bottle brush (Fig. 49-7, p. 778).
6 Squeeze hot, soapy water through the nipples (Fig. 49-8, p. 778). This removes formula.
7 Rinse all items thoroughly in hot water. Squeeze hot water through the nipples to remove soap.
8 Lay a clean towel on the counter.
9 Stand bottles upside down to drain. Place nipples, caps, and other items on the towel. Let the items dry.

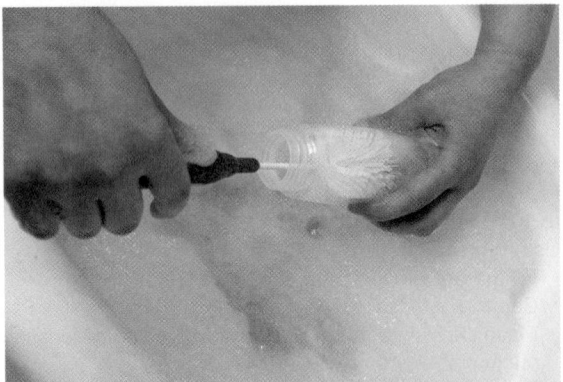

Fig. 49-7 A bottle brush is used to clean inside a baby bottle.

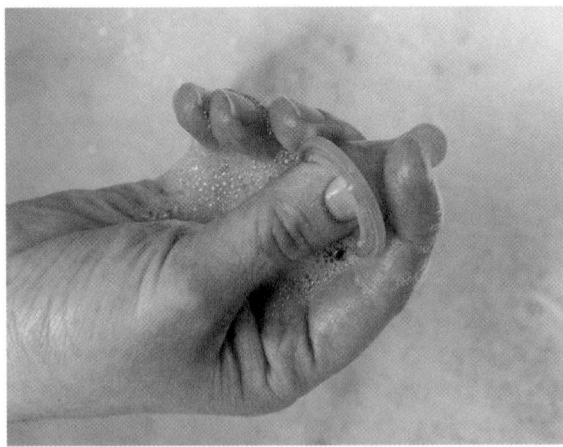

Fig. 49-8 Water is squeezed through the nipple during washing and rinsing.

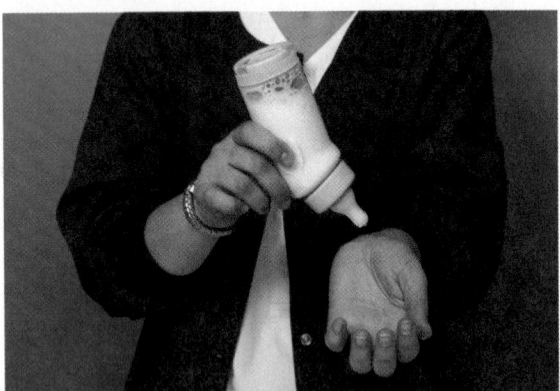

Fig. 49-9 Formula should feel warm on the inside of your wrist.

| BOX 49-5 | BOTTLE-FEEDING BABIES |

- Warm a refrigerated bottle. The formula should feel warm to the inside of your wrist.
- Assume a comfortable position for the feeding.
- Hold the baby close to you. Relax and snuggle the baby.
- Stroke the baby's cheek or lip with the nipple. The baby's head will turn to the nipple.
- Tilt the bottle so that the neck of the bottle and the nipple are always full (Fig. 49-10). Otherwise some air is in the neck or nipple. The baby sucks air into the stomach. The air causes cramping and discomfort.
- Do not prop the bottle and lay the baby down for the feeding (Fig. 49-11).
- Burp the newborn after every ½ to 1 ounce of formula. Older babies are burped less often—after every 2 to 3 ounces. Also burp the baby at the end of the feeding.
- Do not leave the baby alone with a bottle.
- Do not force the baby to finish the bottle.
- Discard remaining formula. Do not save or reheat it for another feeding.
- Wash the bottle, cap, and nipple after the feeding (see procedure: *Cleaning Baby Bottles*, p. 777).

Feeding the Baby

Bottle-fed babies usually want to be fed every 2 to 4 hours. They are fed on demand. The amount of formula taken increases as they grow older. The nurse or the mother tells you how much formula a baby needs at each feeding. Babies usually take as much formula as they need. The baby stops sucking and turns away from the bottle when satisfied.

Most babies do not like cold formula out of the refrigerator. Warm a bottle before the feeding. Do one of the following:

- Warm it in a pan of water on the stove. Use low heat. Turn the bottle often.
- Hold the bottle under warm running tap water or in a container of warm water. Turn the bottle to warm the formula evenly.

The formula should feel warm. To test the temperature, sprinkle a few drops on the inside of your wrist (Fig. 49-9). Allow the formula to cool if it is hot. The guidelines in Box 49-5 will help you bottle-feed babies.

Solid foods are given at 4 to 6 months. Usually baby rice cereal is the first solid food given. The cereal is mixed with breast milk or formula to a thin consistency. Other solid foods are added as the baby grows. The nurse tells you what foods the baby can have.

See *Promoting Safety and Comfort: Feeding the Baby*.

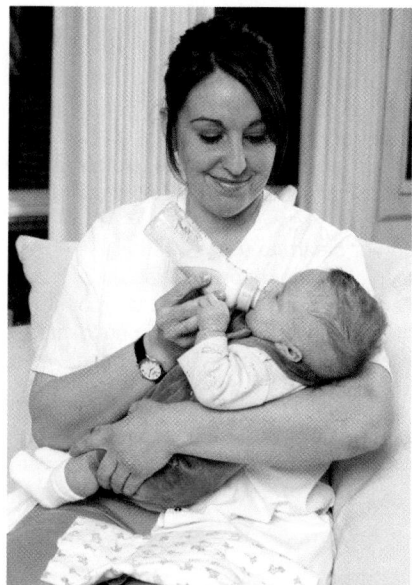

Fig. 49-10 The bottle is tilted so that formula fills the bottle neck and nipple.

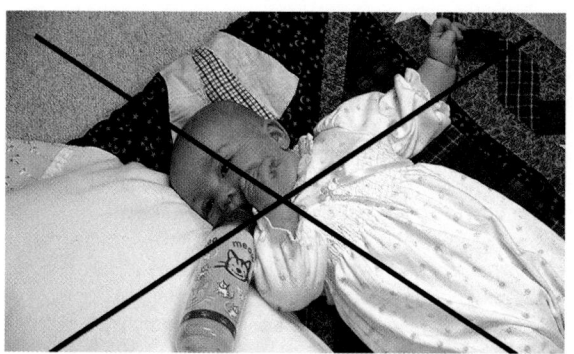

Fig. 49-11 Do NOT prop the bottle to feed the baby.

BURPING THE BABY

Babies take in air during feedings. Air in the stomach and intestines causes cramping and discomfort. This can lead to vomiting. Burping helps to get rid of the air. Most babies burp mid-way and after a feeding.

Burping a baby also is called *bubbling*. You pat or rub the baby's back with circular motions. Do this for 2 or 3 minutes. Figure 49-12 shows how to position the baby for burping.

- *Over the shoulder.* First place a clean diaper or towel over your shoulder. This protects your clothing if the baby "spits up." Then hold the infant over your shoulder.
- *On your lap.* Support the baby in a sitting position on your lap. Hold the towel or diaper in front of the baby. *Remember to support the infant's head and neck for the first 3 months after birth.*
- *On the baby's stomach.* First place a clean diaper or towel on your lap where the baby's head will be. Position the baby on your lap with his or her stomach down.

A   B   C

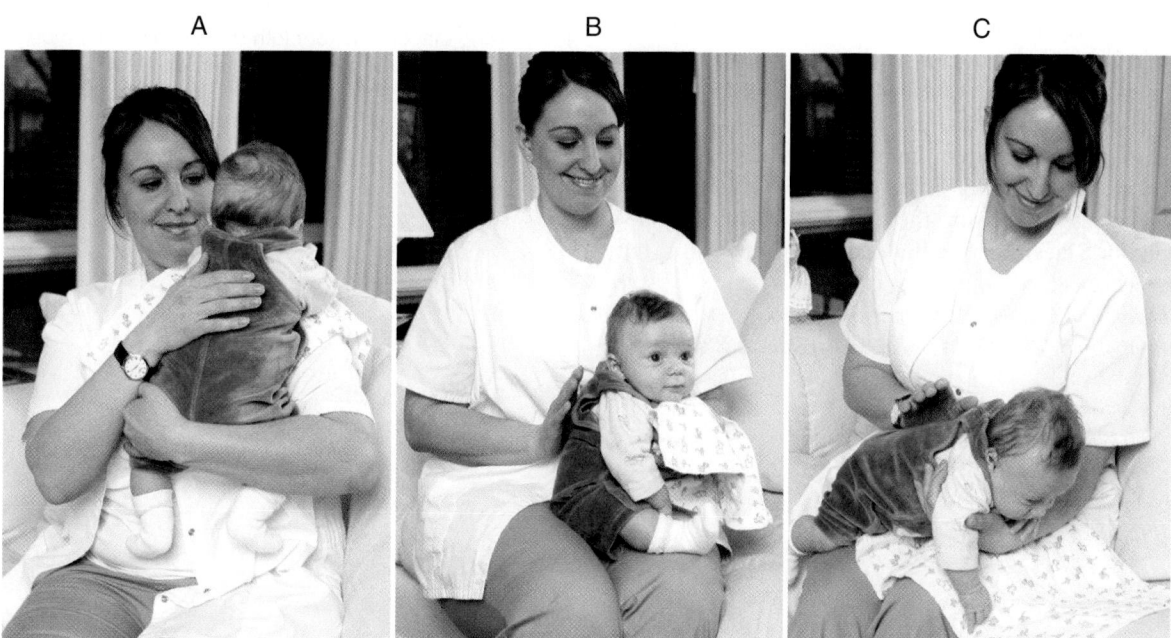

Fig. 49-12 Burping a baby. **A,** The baby is held over the shoulder. **B,** The baby is supported in the sitting position. **C,** The baby is laid on the stomach.

DIAPERING

In the first 1 or 2 days after birth, newborns have meconium stools. *Meconium is a dark green to black, tarry bowel movement.* By day 3 or 4, stools are greenish brown to yellowish brown in color and less sticky. By day 4 or 5:

- Breast-fed babies—have yellow and seedy-looking stools. They are soft or runny. Breast-fed babies usually have a bowel movement with every feeding.
- Bottle-fed babies—have yellow to brown stools. Bottle-fed babies have fewer stools than breast-fed babies, and their stools are firmer. They may have 1 or 2 stools a day.

Over time, an elimination pattern develops. Some babies have 1, 2, or 3 stools a day. Stools are usually soft and unformed. Hard, formed stools signal constipation. Watery stools mean diarrhea. Diarrhea is very serious in infants. Their fluid balance is upset quickly (Chapter 24). Tell the nurse at once if you suspect constipation or diarrhea.

Babies wet at least 6 to 8 times a day. Diapers are changed when wet or when stools are present.

Cloth diapers are re-used. With Velcro fasteners, no diaper pins are needed. The danger of sticking the baby or yourself with a diaper pin is avoided. To care for cloth diapers:

- Rinse a soiled cloth diaper in the toilet.
- Store soiled diapers in a diaper pail.
- Wash them daily or every 2 days.
- Do not wash them with other laundry items.
- Wash them in hot water. Use a baby laundry detergent.
- Put them through the wash cycle a second time without detergent. This helps remove all soap.
- Hang them outside to dry if possible. This gives them a fresh, clean smell. Otherwise, dry them in the dryer.

Disposable diapers are secured with Velcro or tape strips. Fold soiled diapers so the soiled area is on the inside. Then discard the diaper in the trash container. Do not flush it down the toilet. Using disposable diapers costs more than using cloth ones.

Changing diapers often helps prevent diaper rash. Moisture, stools, and urine irritate the baby's skin. When changing diapers, make sure the baby is clean and dry before applying a clean diaper. If a diaper rash develops, tell the nurse at once.

See *Delegation Guidelines: Diapering a Baby.*
See *Promoting Safety and Comfort: Diapering a Baby.*

DELEGATION GUIDELINES
Diapering a Baby

Before changing a baby's diaper, you need this information from the nurse and the care plan:

- The size and type of diaper to use (cloth or disposable)
- If you need to give cord care (p. 782) or circumcision care (p. 783)
- What lotion or cream to use
- What observations to report and record:
  - Color, amount, consistency, and odor of stools
  - Condition of the baby's skin and genital area
  - Redness or irritation of the skin or genital area
  - Blood or discharge on the diaper
- When to report observations
- What concerns to report at once

PROMOTING SAFETY AND COMFORT
Diapering a Baby

Safety

Disposable diapers present safety hazards to babies. Babies can choke on tab papers that cover tape strips. Keep tab papers away from the baby. Discard them as soon as possible.

Older babies can tear and pull disposable diapers apart. They can choke or suffocate on the plastic if they put the plastic in their noses or mouths. Observe babies closely. Change any torn or damaged diaper at once.

You must keep the baby safe during diapering. The baby may squirm, wiggle, or kick and cry. To prevent falls:

- Gather all needed supplies before you begin.
- Place the baby on a firm surface. If the baby is on a table, make sure it is sturdy.
- Always keep one hand on a baby who is on a table or other raised surface.
- Never look away from the baby.

If using diaper pins for cloth diapers, the pins must point away from the abdomen. If a pin opens toward the abdomen, it can pierce the skin and damage organs.

DIAPERING A BABY

PRE-PROCEDURE

1. Follow *Delegation Guidelines: Diapering a Baby*. See *Promoting Safety and Comfort: Diapering a Baby*.
2. Practice hand hygiene.
3. Collect the following:
   - Gloves
   - Clean diaper
   - Waterproof changing pad
   - Washcloth
   - Disposable wipes or cotton balls
   - Basin of warm water
   - Baby soap
   - Baby lotion or cream

PROCEDURE

4. Put on the gloves.
5. Place the changing pad under the baby.
6. Unfasten the dirty diaper. Place diaper pins out of the baby's reach.
7. Wipe the genital area with the front of the diaper (Fig. 49-13). Wipe from the front to the back.
8. Fold the diaper so urine and feces are inside. Set the diaper aside.
9. Clean the genital area from front to back. Use a wet washcloth, disposable wipes, or cotton balls. Wash with mild soap and water for a large amount of feces or if the baby has a rash. Rinse thoroughly and pat the area dry.
10. Clean the circumcision (p. 783). Give cord care (p. 782).
11. Apply cream or lotion to the genital area and buttocks. Do not use too much. Caking can occur.
12. Raise the baby's legs. Slide a clean diaper under the buttocks.

13. Fold a cloth diaper as follows:
    a. For a boy: the extra thickness is in the front (Fig. 49-14, A, p. 782).
    b. For a girl: the extra thickness is at the back (Fig. 49-14, B, p. 782).
    c. Bring the diaper between the baby's legs.
14. Make sure the diaper is snug around the hips and abdomen.
    a. It is loose near the penis if the circumcision has not healed.
    b. It is below the umbilicus if the cord stump has not healed.
15. Secure the diaper in place. Use the tape strips or Velcro on disposable diapers (Fig. 49-15, A, p. 782). Make sure the tabs stick in place. Use baby pins or Velcro for cloth diapers. Pins point away from the abdomen (Fig. 49-15, B, p. 782).
16. Apply a diaper cover or plastic pants if cloth diapers are worn.
17. Put the baby in the crib, infant seat, or other safe location.

POST-PROCEDURE

18. Rinse feces from the cloth diaper in the toilet.
19. Store used cloth diapers in a covered pail. Put a disposable diaper and paper tabs in the trash.
20. Remove and discard the gloves. Practice hand hygiene.
21. Put on clean gloves.
22. Clean, rinse, dry, and return other items to their proper location.
23. Remove and discard the gloves. Practice hand hygiene.
24. Report and record your observations.

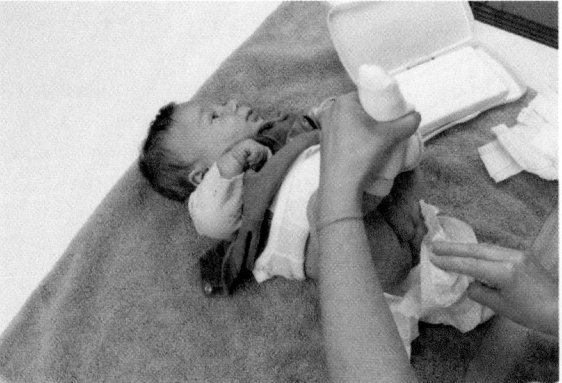 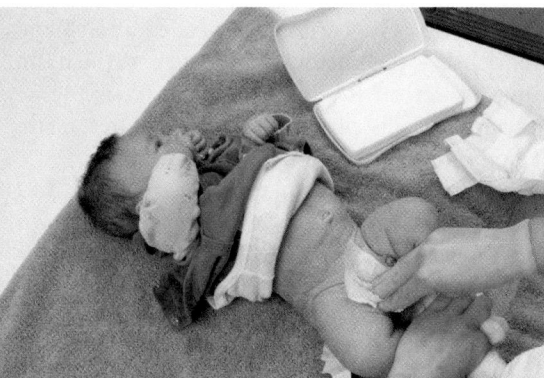

Fig. 49-13 The front of the diaper is used to clean the genital area from front to back.

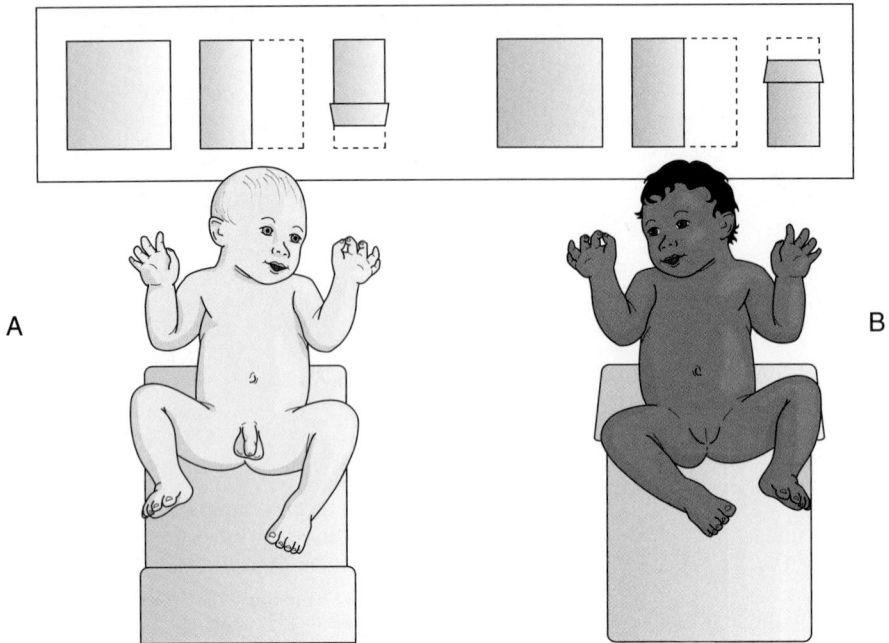

Fig. 49-14 A, A cloth diaper is folded in front for boys. **B,** The diaper has a fold in the back for girls.

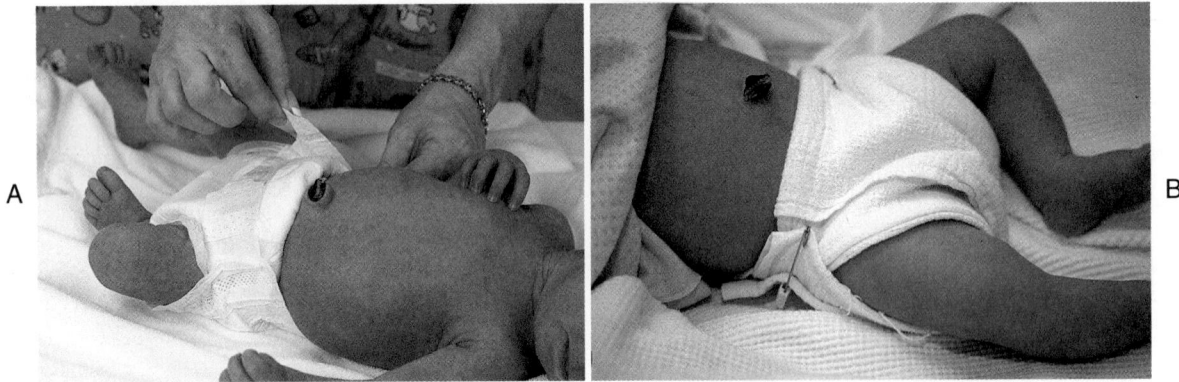

Fig. 49-15 Securing a diaper. **A,** A disposable diaper is secured in place with tape strips. **B,** Diaper pins secure a cloth diaper. Pins point away from the abdomen. NOTE: The diapers in A and B are below the cord.

CARE OF THE UMBILICAL CORD

The *umbilical cord connects the mother and the fetus (unborn baby). It carries blood, oxygen, and nutrients from the mother to the fetus* (Fig. 49-16). The cord is not needed after birth. Shortly after delivery, the doctor clamps and cuts the cord. A cord stump is left on the baby (see Fig. 49-15). The stump dries up and falls off within 2 weeks after birth. Slight bleeding can occur when the cord comes off.

The cord provides a place for microbes to grow. You need to keep it clean and dry. Cord care is done at each diaper change. Cord care is continued for 1 or 2 days after the cord comes off. It involves the following:

- Keep the stump clean and dry. Do not get the stump wet.

- Keep the diaper below the cord as in Figure 49-15. This prevents the diaper from irritating the stump. It also keeps the cord from becoming wet from urine.
- Give sponge baths until the cord falls off. Then the baby can have a tub bath.
- Do not pull the cord off—even if looks ready to fall off.
- Report the following to the nurse:
  - Swelling, redness, odor, or drainage from the stump
  - Bleeding from the cord or navel area
  - Fever

See *Promoting Safety and Comfort: Care of the Umbilical Cord.*

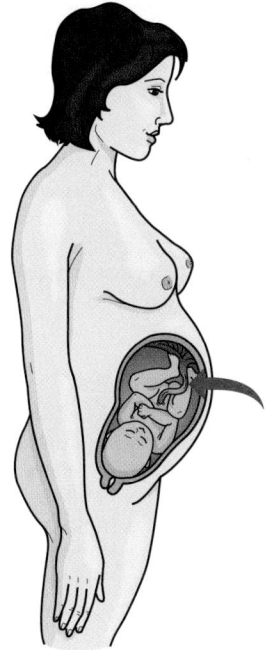

Fig. 49-16 The umbilical cord connects the mother and fetus.

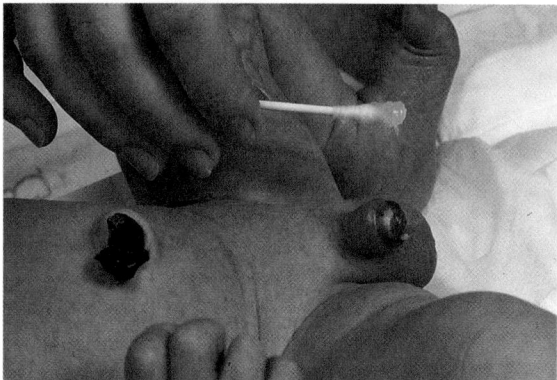

Fig. 49-17 Petrolatum jelly is applied to the circumcised penis.

CARE OF THE CIRCUMCISION

Boys are born with foreskin on the penis. *The surgical removal of foreskin from the penis is called a circumcision* (Chapter 20). The procedure allows good hygiene. It is thought to:

* Prevent urinary tract infections in infants.
* Lower the risk of cancer of the penis.
* Decrease the risk of sexually transmitted diseases.

The procedure is usually done before the baby leaves the hospital. Circumcision is a religious ceremony in the Jewish faith.

The tip of the penis will look red, swollen, and sore. However, the entire penis should not be swollen. And the circumcision should not interfere with voiding. Carefully observe for signs of bleeding and infection. There should be no odor, drainage, or fever. A slight yellowish discharge or crust at the tip of the penis is normal. It does not signal infection. Report any concerns to the nurse at once. The area should heal in 7 to 10 days.

Circumcision care involves the following:
* Clean the penis at each diaper change. This is very important after a bowel movement.
* Use mild soap and water, plain water, or commercial wipes as the nurse directs.
* Apply a petrolatum gauze dressing or petrolatum jelly to the penis as the nurse directs. This protects the penis from urine and feces. It also prevents the penis from sticking to the diaper. Use a cotton swab to apply the petrolatum jelly (Fig. 49-17).
* Apply the diaper loosely. This prevents the diaper from irritating the penis.

BATHING AN INFANT

A bath is important for hygiene. Though babies do not get very dirty, they need good skin care. Baths comfort and relax babies. They also provide a wonderful time to hold, touch, and talk to babies. Stimulation is important for development. Being touched and held helps babies learn safety, security, and love and belonging.

Planning for the bath is important. You cannot leave the baby alone if you forget something. Gather needed equipment, supplies, and the baby's clothes before you start the bath. Everything you need must be within your reach.

There are two bath procedures for babies. Sponge baths are given until the cord stump falls off and the umbilicus and circumcision heal. *The cord must not get wet.* The tub bath is given after the cord site and circumcision heal (Fig. 49-18, p. 784).

See *Focus on Long-Term Care and Home Care: Bathing an Infant*, p. 784.
See *Delegation Guidelines: Bathing an Infant*, p. 784.
See *Promoting Safety and Comfort: Bathing an Infant*, p. 784.

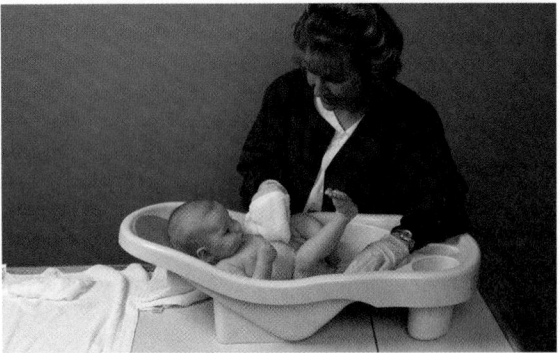

Fig. 49-18 The baby is given a tub bath in a baby bath tub.

FOCUS ON LONG-TERM CARE AND HOME CARE
Bathing an Infant

Home Care
Bath time is part of the baby's routine. Some mothers bathe their babies in the morning. Others do so in the evening. Evening baths have important advantages.
- The bath is comforting and relaxing. This helps some babies sleep longer at night.
- Working fathers are usually home in the evening. The evening bath lets them be involved.

Sometimes fathers bathe babies so mothers can rest or tend to other children. Follow the family's routine when working in the home.

DELEGATION GUIDELINES
Bathing an Infant

Before bathing an infant, you need this information from the nurse and the care plan:
- How often to bathe the baby. Babies do not need baths every day.
- What type of bath to give—sponge bath or tub bath.
- What water temperature to use—usually 100°F to 105°F (Fahrenheit) (37.7°C to 40.5°C [centigrade]).
- When to bathe the infant.
- If you should use baby soap or plain water. Usually soap is not used unless the baby is dirty or smells.
- If you should apply lotion after the bath.
- What observations to report and record:
  - Bruising
  - Rashes
  - Skin irritation
  - Redness
  - Swelling
  - Open skin areas
  - See "Care of the Umbilical Cord," p. 782
  - See "Care of the Circumcision," p. 783
- When to report observations.
- What concerns to report at once.

PROMOTING SAFETY AND COMFORT
Bathing an Infant

Safety
To protect an infant during a bath, follow these safety measures.
- Turn up the thermostat and close windows and doors about 20 minutes before the bath. Room temperature should be 75°F to 80°F for the bath. The room may be too warm for you. Remove a sweater or lab coat or roll up your sleeves before starting the bath.
- Measure bath water temperature with a bath thermometer. The nurse tells you what temperature to use (usually 100°F to 105°F [37.7°C to 40.5°C]). Or test water temperature with the inside of your wrist (Fig. 49-19). The water should feel warm and comfortable to your wrist. Babies have delicate skin and are easily burned.
- Never leave the baby alone on a table or in the bath tub.
- Always keep one hand on the baby if you must look away for a moment.
- Hold the baby securely during the bath. Babies are slippery when they are wet. A wet, squirming baby is hard to hold.

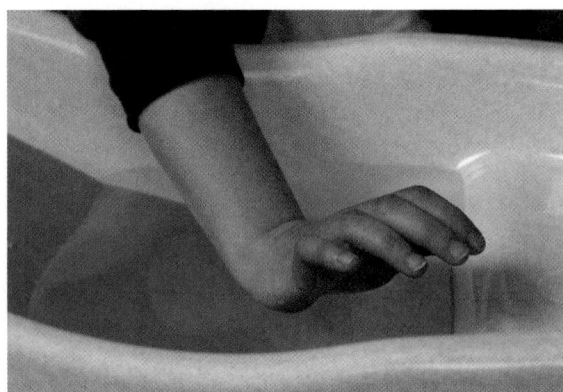

Fig. 49-19 The inside of the wrist is used to test bath water temperature.

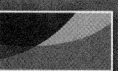 **GIVING A BABY A SPONGE BATH**

QUALITY OF LIFE

Remember to:
- Knock before entering the baby's room.
- Address the baby and parents by name.
- Introduce yourself by name and title.
- Explain the procedure to the parents before beginning and during the procedure.
- Protect the baby's rights during the procedure.
- Handle the baby gently during the procedure.

PRE-PROCEDURE

1 Follow *Delegation Guidelines: Bathing an Infant*. See *Promoting Safety and Comfort: Bathing an Infant*.
2 Practice hand hygiene.
3 Place the following items in your work area:
   - Bath basin
   - Bath thermometer
   - Bath towel
   - Two hand towels
   - Receiving blanket
   - Washcloth
   - Clean diaper
   - Clean clothing for the baby
   - Cotton balls
   - Baby soap (if needed)
   - Baby shampoo
   - Baby lotion
   - Gloves

PROCEDURE

4 Fill the bath basin with warm water. Water temperature should be 100°F to 105°F (37.7°C to 40.5°C). Measure water temperature with the bath thermometer or use the inside of your wrist. The water should feel warm and comfortable.
5 Provide for privacy.
6 Identify the baby following agency policy.
7 Put on gloves.
8 Undress the baby. Leave the diaper on.
9 Wash the baby's eye lids (Fig. 49-20, p. 786):
   a Dip a cotton ball into the water.
   b Squeeze out excess water.
   c Wash one eye lid from the inner part to the outer part.
   d Repeat this step for the other eye with a new cotton ball.
10 Moisten the washcloth and make a mitt (Chapter 20). Clean the outside of the ear and then behind the ear. Repeat this step for the other ear. Be gentle.
11 Rinse and squeeze out the washcloth. Make a mitt with the washcloth.
12 Wash the baby's face (Fig. 49-21, p. 786). Clean inside the nostrils with the washcloth. *Do not use cotton swabs to clean inside the nose.* Pat the face dry.
13 Pick up the baby. Hold the baby over the bath basin using the football hold. Support the baby's head and neck with your wrist and hand.

14 Wash the baby's head (Fig. 49-22, p. 786):
   a Squeeze a small amount of water from the washcloth onto the baby's head. Or bring water to the baby's head using a cupped hand.
   b Apply a small amount of baby shampoo to the head.
   c Wash the head with circular motions.
   d Rinse the head by squeezing water from a washcloth over the baby's head. Or bring water to the baby's head using a cupped hand. Rinse thoroughly. Do not get soap in the baby's eyes.
   e Use a small hand towel to dry the head.
15 Lay the baby on the table.
16 Remove the diaper.
17 Wash the front of the body. Also wash the arms, hands, fingers, legs, feet, and toes. Use a washcloth. Or wash the baby with your hands. Do not get the cord wet. Rinse thoroughly. Pat dry. Be sure to wash and dry all creases and folds.
18 Turn the baby to the prone position. Wash the back and buttocks. Use a washcloth or your hands. Rinse thoroughly. Pat dry.
19 Give cord care. Clean the circumcision.
20 Apply baby lotion as directed by the nurse.
21 Remove and discard the gloves. Practice hand hygiene.
22 Put a clean diaper and clean clothes on the baby.
23 Wrap the baby in the receiving blanket. Put the baby in the crib or other safe area.

POST-PROCEDURE

24 Practice hand hygiene. Put on gloves.
25 Clean, rinse, dry, and return equipment and supplies to the proper place. Do this step when the baby is settled.
26 Remove and discard the gloves. Practice hand hygiene.
27 Complete a safety check of the room. (See the inside of the front book cover.)
28 Report and record your observations.

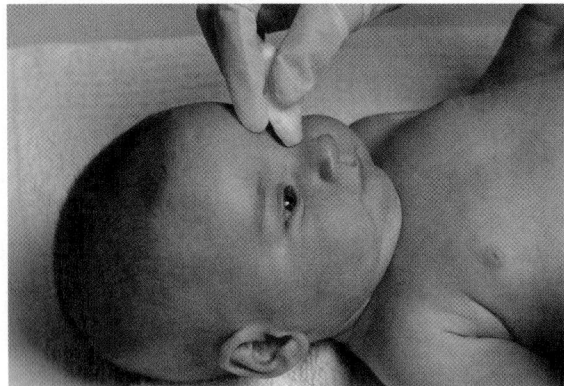

Fig. 49-20 Wash the baby's eyes with cotton balls. The eye lids are cleaned from the inner to the outer part.

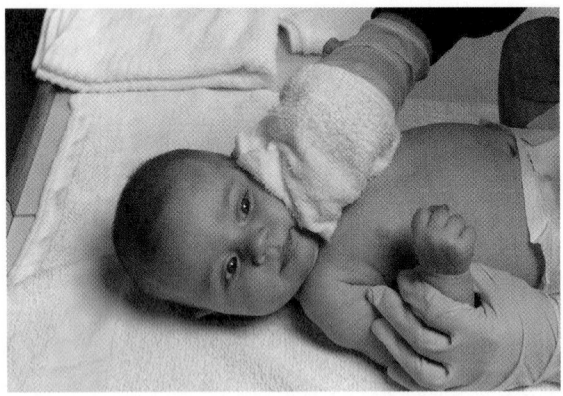

Fig. 49-21 The baby's face is washed with a mitted washcloth.

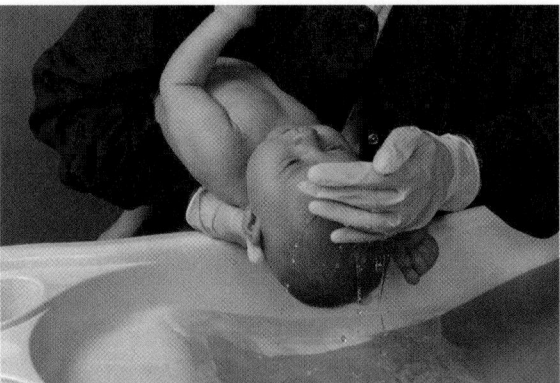

Fig. 49-22 The baby's head is washed over the bath basin.

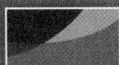

GIVING A BABY A TUB BATH

QUALITY OF LIFE

Remember to:
- Knock before entering the baby's room.
- Address the baby and parents by name.
- Introduce yourself by name and title.

- Explain the procedure to the parents before beginning and during the procedure.
- Protect the baby's rights during the procedure.
- Handle the baby gently during the procedure.

PROCEDURE

1 Follow steps 1 through 16 in procedure: *Giving a Baby a Sponge Bath* (p. 785).
2 Hold the baby as in Figure 49-23:
  a Place one hand under the baby's shoulders. Your thumb should be over the baby's shoulder. Your fingers should be under the arm.
  b Support the buttocks with your other hand. Slide your hand under the thighs. Hold the far thigh with your other hand.
3 Lower the baby into the water feet first.
4 Wash the front of the baby's body. Also wash the arms, hands, fingers, legs, feet, and toes. Wash all folds and creases.

5 Wash the genital area. Rinse thoroughly.
6 Reverse your hold. Use your other hand to hold the baby.
7 Wash the baby's back and buttocks. Rinse thoroughly.
8 Reverse your hold again. Hold the baby with your other hand.
9 Lift the baby out of the water and onto a towel.
10 Wrap the baby in the towel. Also cover the baby's head.
11 Pat the baby dry. Dry all folds and creases.
12 Follow steps 20 through 28 in procedure: *Giving a Baby a Sponge Bath* (p. 785).

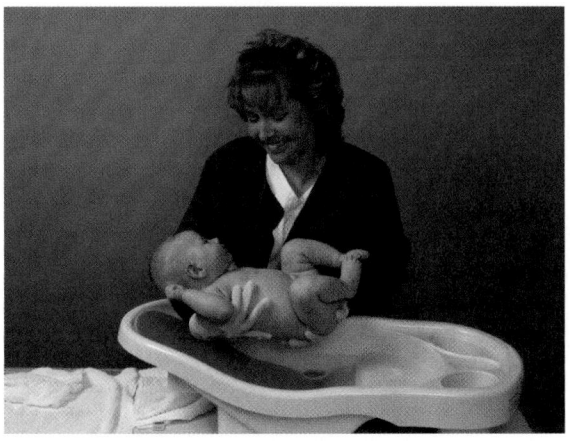

Fig. 49-23 The baby is held for the tub bath.

NAIL CARE

The baby's fingernails and toenails are kept short. Otherwise, the baby can scratch himself or herself and others. Nails are best cut when the baby is sleeping. The baby is quiet and will not squirm or fuss. Use infant nail clippers and a soft emery board.

- Hold the finger or toe with one hand.
- Press the skin under the nail. This moves the skin out of the way to avoid pinching or cutting the skin.
- Trim the nails with an infant nail clipper:
  - Fingernails: clip following the natural shape of the nail.
  - Toenails: clip straight across as for an adult (Chapter 21).
- Smooth rough or sharp edges with a soft emery board.

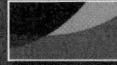 WEIGHING INFANTS

The infant's birth weight is the baseline for measuring growth. The nurse uses weight measurements in the assessment step of the nursing process. They also are used to measure the amount of breast milk taken during breast-feeding. The baby is weighed before and after breast-feeding. The difference in the weights is the amount of milk taken in during breast-feeding. It tells the nurse if the baby is getting enough milk.

See *Delegation Guidelines: Weighing Infants.*
See *Promoting Safety and Comfort: Weighing Infants.*

DELEGATION GUIDELINES
Weighing Infants

Before weighing an infant, you need this information from the nurse and the care plan:
- When to weigh the baby.
- If the baby is breast-fed or bottle-fed. Breast-fed babies wear the same diaper for "before" and "after" feeding weight measurements. The clothes and blanket are removed.
- When to report the weight measurement.
- What concerns to report at once.

PROMOTING SAFETY AND COMFORT
Weighing Infants

You must meet the baby's safety needs. Protect the baby from chills. Keep the room warm and free of drafts. Also protect the baby from falling. Always keep a hand over the baby when taking the weight measurement. Remember to keep one hand on the baby if you need to look away.

WEIGHING AN INFANT

QUALITY OF LIFE

Remember to:
- Knock before entering the baby's room.
- Address the baby and parents by name.
- Introduce yourself by name and title.

- Explain the procedure to the parents before beginning and during the procedure.
- Protect the baby's rights during the procedure.
- Handle the baby gently during the procedure.

PRE-PROCEDURE

1 Follow *Delegation Guidelines: Weighing Infants.* See *Promoting Safety and Comfort: Weighing Infants.*
2 Practice hand hygiene.

3 Collect the following:
- Baby scale (Fig. 49-24, p. 788)
- Paper for the scale
- Items for diaper changing (see procedure: *Diapering a Baby,* p. 781)
- Gloves

Continued

WEIGHING AN INFANT—cont'd

PROCEDURE

4 Identify the baby following agency policy.
5 Place the paper on the scale. Adjust the scale to zero (0).
6 Put on the gloves.
7 Undress the baby and remove the diaper. Clean the genital area.
8 Remove and discard the gloves and practice hand hygiene. Put on clean gloves.
9 Lay the baby on the scale. Keep one hand over the baby to prevent falling.

10 Read the digital display or move the weights until the scale is balanced.
11 Note the measurement.
12 Take the baby off of the scale.
13 Diaper and dress the baby. Lay the baby in the crib.
14 Discard the paper and soiled diaper.
15 Disinfect the scale following agency policy.
16 Remove and discard the gloves. Practice hand hygiene.

POST-PROCEDURE

17 Return the scale to its proper place.
18 Practice hand hygiene.

19 Report and record your observations.

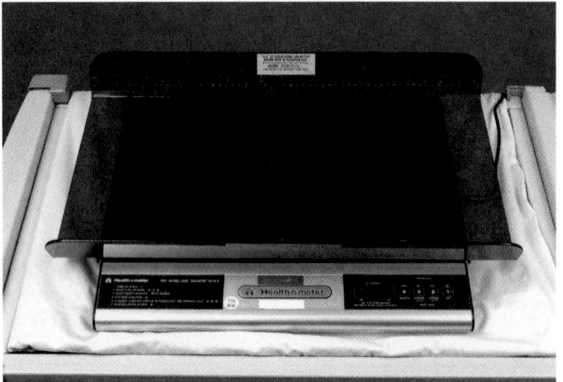

Fig. 49-24 Digital infant scale.

CARE OF THE MOTHER

Postpartum means *after* (post) *childbirth* (partum). The postpartum period starts with birth of the baby. It ends 6 weeks later. The mother's body returns to its normal state during this time. The mother adjusts physically and emotionally to childbirth.

The uterus returns almost to its pre-pregnant size. This is called *involution of the uterus.* If the mother does not breast-feed, she can expect a menstrual period within 3 to 8 weeks. Breast-feeding is not an effective method of birth control. Without birth control measures, the mother can get pregnant again.

After childbirth, a vaginal discharge called lochia *occurs.* (Lochia comes from the Greek word *lochos.* It means *childbirth.*) Lochia consists of blood and other matter left in the uterus from childbirth. The lochia changes color and decreases in amount during the postpartum period.

- *Lochia rubra*—is dark or bright red *(rubra)* discharge. Mainly blood, it is seen during the first 3 to 4 days.
- *Lochia serosa*—is pinkish-brown *(serosa)* drainage. It lasts until about 10 days after birth.
- *Lochia alba*—is whitish *(alba)* drainage. It continues for 2 to 6 weeks after birth.

Lochia increases with breast-feeding and activity. When she stands after lying or sitting, the mother may feel a gush of lochia. She wears a sanitary napkin to absorb the lochia. Normally lochia smells like menstrual flow. Foul-smelling lochia signals infection.

Good perineal care is important. Sanitary pads are changed often. When wiping after elimination, the mother wipes from front to back. Sanitary napkins are applied and removed from front to back. Good hand washing is essential after perineal care, changing sanitary napkins, and elimination. Standard Precautions and the Bloodborne Pathogen Standard are followed.

Some mothers have episiotomies. An *episiotomy is an incision* (otomy) *into the perineum.* (*Episeion* means *pubic region.*) The doctor performs this procedure during childbirth. It increases the size of the vaginal opening for the baby. The incision is sutured after delivery. The doctor may order sitz baths for comfort and hygiene (Chapter 35). Like other incisions, complications can develop. These include infection and wound separation *(dehiscence).* Tell the nurse at once if the mother complains of pain, discomfort, or a discharge.

Some mothers deliver by *cesarean section (C-section)*. The doctor makes an incision into the abdominal wall. The baby is delivered through the incision. This is done when:

- The baby must be delivered to save the baby's or mother's life.
- The baby is too large to pass through the birth canal.
- The mother has a vaginal infection that could be transmitted to the baby.
- A normal vaginal delivery will be difficult for the baby or mother.

The C-section incision needs to heal. See Chapter 33 for wound healing and wound care.

The mother has emotional reactions after childbirth. Hormone changes, life-style changes, and lack of sleep can cause mood swings. So can frequent visits and telephone calls from family and friends. Some interfere or offer advice and opinions about parenting. The mother can help herself by resting when the baby sleeps. She needs time for herself and her partner. She may feel better after a shower, washing and styling her hair, and getting dressed. These can be done while the baby sleeps.

Complications can occur during pregnancy, labor, and delivery. They also can occur in the postpartum period. Report any sign or symptom listed in Box 49-6 to the nurse at once.

BOX 49-6	**SIGNS AND SYMPTOMS OF POSTPARTUM COMPLICATIONS**

- Temperature of 100.4°F or greater
- Pain: abdominal or perineal
- Discharge:
  - Foul smelling from the vagina
  - From an episiotomy
  - From a C-section incision
- Bleeding from an episiotomy or C-section incision
- Redness, swelling: episiotomy or C-section incision
- Saturating a sanitary napkin within 1 hour of application
- Lochia:
  - Red lochia after lochia has changed color to pinkish-brown or white
  - Lochia with large clots
- Urination: burning
- Leg pain, tenderness, or swelling
- Sadness or feelings of depression
- Breast pain, tenderness, or swelling

FOCUS ON **PRIDE**

The Person, Family, and Yourself

Personal and Professional Responsibility

Newborns do not spend every moment in the mother's room. A newborn may go to the nursery while the mother rests. Or a test or procedure is needed. A circumcision is an example.

Identification of the newborn is important. You must return the baby to the correct parent. You must not rely on the parent to identify the baby. Safe identification of the baby is a professional responsibility. Follow agency policy for identifying the mother and newborn.

Rights and Respect

A parent's preferences for newborn care may differ from yours. For example, a mother wants to bottle-feed. You believe babies should be breast-fed. You do not need to agree with the person. However, your opinion must not affect the care you give. Respect the person's preferences.

Independence and Social Interaction

Parents must learn to care for their newborn. The nurse teaches parents about newborn care. They watch the nurse. Then they try it on their own. Parents gain confidence by performing care independently.

Parents who rely on the staff may not know how to provide care once at home. Avoid doing everything for the parents. Tell the nurse if the parents rely on the staff too much.

Delegation and Teamwork

Many agencies use alarm systems to protect the security of newborns. The newborn wears an electronic security bracelet. An alarm activates when the baby is carried toward an exit. Alarms and exits are checked at once. All staff members respond. If a baby is missing, security sends out a message to the entire agency. Procedures are followed to find the baby. The entire agency works as a team to protect the newborn.

Ethics and Laws

Having a baby is usually a happy time. However, this is not always the case. The health team must monitor closely for signs of mistreatment. A parent may not be interested in the baby. Or the parent may be unwilling to learn to care for the baby. The baby must be protected from abuse and neglect. Tell the nurse about any concerns at once.

REVIEW QUESTIONS

Circle the BEST answer.

1 A baby's head and neck are supported for the first
   a 7 to 10 days
   b Month
   c 3 months
   d 6 months

2 When holding a newborn, do the following *except*
   a Hold the infant securely
   b Cuddle the infant
   c Use two hands
   d Lift the infant by the arms

3 You observe the following. Which is normal?
   a The baby looks flushed and is perspiring.
   b The baby has watery stools.
   c The baby's eyes are red and irritated.
   d The baby spits up a small amount when burped.

4 A baby is breast-fed. The mother should do the following *except*
   a Wash her hands
   b Hold the baby close to her breast
   c Stimulate the rooting reflex
   d Clean her breasts with soap and water

5 A breast-fed baby is burped
   a Every 5 minutes
   b After nursing from each breast
   c After 1 ounce of breast milk
   d After half the formula is taken

6 You are shopping for baby formula. Which should you buy?
   a The one that is on sale
   b The ready-to-feed type
   c The one ordered by the doctor
   d The powdered form

7 When warming a baby bottle,
   a Warm the bottle in the microwave
   b Leave the formula out to warm at room temperature
   c Check that the formula is warm on the inside of your wrist
   d Boil the formula in a pan for 5 minutes

8 When bottle-feeding a baby,
   a Tilt the bottle so the formula fills the neck of the bottle and the nipple
   b Save remaining formula for the next feeding
   c Burp the baby every 5 minutes
   d Leave the baby alone with the bottle

9 A newborn's cord has not yet healed. The diaper should be
   a Loose over the cord
   b Snug over the cord
   c Below the cord
   d Disposable

10 A circumcision is cleaned
   a Once a day
   b When the baby has a bowel movement
   c Three times a day
   d At every diaper change

11 Bath water for a newborn should be
   a 85°F to 90°F
   b 90°F to 95°F
   c 95°F to 100°F
   d 100°F to 105°F

12 Which should you use to wash a baby's nose?
   a A mitted washcloth
   b Alcohol wipes
   c A cotton swab
   d Cotton balls

13 A mother has a red vaginal discharge the first few days after childbirth. This
   a Is a menstrual period
   b Signals a postpartum complication
   c Is lochia rubra
   d Is from her episiotomy

14 A cesarean delivery involves
   a A vaginal incision
   b A perineal incision
   c An abdominal incision
   d A normal delivery through the birth canal

Circle T if the statement is TRUE and F if it is FALSE.

15 T F   A baby's crib should be within hearing distance of caregivers.

16 T F   A baby needs a pillow for sleep.

17 T F   A baby is placed on his or her back for sleep.

18 T F   A yellowish crust at the tip of a circumcised penis is a sign of infection.

19 T F   A baby's diapers are changed whenever they are wet.

20 T F   A baby's cord and circumcision have not healed. The baby should have a sponge bath.

21 T F   Cotton swabs are used to clean a baby's ears.

22 T F   A breast-fed baby needs a "before" and "after" feeding weight. The baby is weighed with the diaper on.

Answers to these questions are on p. 835.

Assisted Living 50

OBJECTIVES

- Define the key terms and key abbreviations listed in this chapter.
- Identify the purpose of assisted living.
- Identify the person's rights.
- Identify the types of assisted living residences and the living areas offered.
- Describe the physical and environmental requirements for assisted living.
- Describe the requirements for assisted living staff.
- Describe the requirements for persons who want to live in an assisted living residence.
- Explain the purpose of a service plan.
- Explain how to assist with housekeeping and laundry.
- Identify food safety measures.
- Explain how to assist with drugs.
- Identify the reasons for transferring, discharging, or evicting a person.
- Explain how to promote PRIDE in the person, the family, and yourself.

KEY TERMS

assisted living A housing option for older persons who need help with activities of daily living yet wish to remain independent as long as possible

medication reminder Reminding the person to take drugs, observing them being taken as prescribed, and charting that they were taken

service plan A written plan listing the services needed, how much help is needed, and who provides the services

KEY ABBREVIATIONS

AD Alzheimer's disease
ADL Activities of daily living

ALR Assisted living residence

Many older people cannot or do not want to live alone. Some need help with self-care. Some have physical or cognitive problems and disabilities. Still others need help taking drugs. Yet they do not need constant care.

Assisted living is a housing option for older persons who need help with activities of daily living (ADL) yet wish to remain independent as long as possible. It offers quality of life with independence, companionship, and social involvement. Little or no medical care is provided. A home-like setting is provided. Assisted living residences (ALRs) usually offer:

- 3 meals a day
- Help with ADL—bathing, dressing, grooming, toileting, eating, walking

- Housekeeping and maintenance
- Linen and personal laundry
- A 24-hour communication system for an emergency or to call for help
- 24-hour security
- 24-hour supervision
- Transportation
- Social, educational, recreational, and spiritual services
- Help with shopping, banking, and money management
- Some health services
- Exercise and wellness programs
- Medication (drug) management or help taking drugs
- Supervision for persons with Alzheimer's disease (AD), dementia, and other disabilities

Living areas vary. A small apartment has a bedroom, bathroom, living area, kitchen, and laundry area (Figs. 50-1 and 50-2). Some people just want a bedroom and bathroom. Box 50-1 lists the requirements and features of assisted living units. Box 50-2 lists environment requirements.

ALRs also are called *assisted living facilities (ALFs)*. Some are part of retirement communities. State laws and licensing requirements for ALRs vary. Residents' rights are part of such laws.

See *Promoting Safety and Comfort: Assisted Living*.

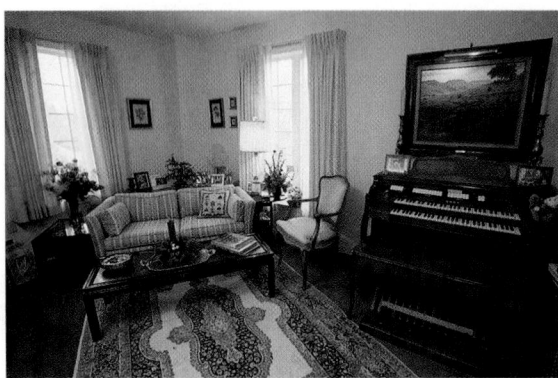

Fig. 50-1 A living area in an assisted living apartment.

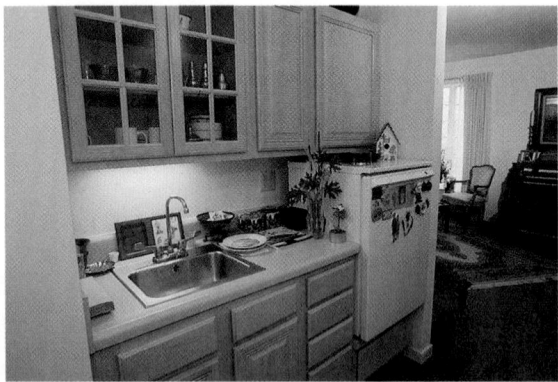

Fig. 50-2 A kitchen in an assisted living apartment.

PROMOTING SAFETY AND COMFORT
Assisted Living

Safety
Residents have the same diseases and illnesses as persons at home, in hospitals, and in nursing centers. Infections are risks. This includes sexually transmitted and other communicable diseases. Follow Standard Precautions and the Bloodborne Pathogen Standard when contact with blood, body fluids, secretions, excretions, or potentially contaminated items and surfaces is likely.

BOX 50-1	REQUIREMENTS AND FEATURES OF ASSISTED LIVING UNITS

- A door that locks; the person keeps a key
- A telephone jack
- A 24-hour emergency communication system in the person's room
- A window or door that provides natural light
- Wheelchair access
- Lighted common areas
- A window or door that allows safe exit in an emergency
- A mailbox for each person
- A bathroom that provides privacy:
  - A sink in the bathroom or in the next room
  - A bathtub or shower that has a shower curtain and non-slip surfaces
  - Ventilation or a window that opens
  - Grab bars for the toilet and bathtub or shower
  - Other assistive devices needed for safety and identified in the service plan (p. 794)
- Smoke detectors and a fire sprinkler system
- A bed (frame and mattress) that is clean and in good repair
- General and task lighting
- An easy chair
- A table and chair for meals
- Adjustable window covers that provide privacy
- A dresser or storage space for clothing and personal items
- Appliances for food—sink, stove, refrigerator with freezer, and storage for food and cooking items

---

BOX 50-2	ENVIRONMENT REQUIREMENTS

- The ALR is clean, safe, orderly, odor-free, and in good repair.
- The ALR is free of insects and rodents.
- Garbage is stored in covered containers lined with plastic bags. Bags are removed at least once a week.
- Hot water temperatures are no higher than 120°F (Fahrenheit).
- The hot and cold water supply meets hygiene needs.
- Bathrooms have toilet paper, soap, and cloth towels, paper towels, or a dryer.
- Clean linens are handled, transported, and stored to prevent contamination.
- Soiled linen and clothing are stored in closed containers away from food, kitchen, and dining areas.
- Oxygen containers are stored according to the manufacturer's instructions.
- Cleaning solutions, insecticides, and other hazardous substances are stored in their original containers. They are in locked cabinets in rooms separate from food, dining areas, and drugs.
- Pets or animals are controlled to protect residents and maintain sanitation.
- Employees have access to a first aid kit.

PURPOSE

People are living longer, and there are more older people than before. Life partners are lost through death or divorce. Some remarry; others do not. Some persons have never married. Today's older persons had some birth control options. Many had small families. And the United States is a mobile society. Children grow up and move away from their families. For these reasons, many older persons live alone. Often there is no family nearby to help them.

ALR RESIDENTS

ALR residents usually need some help with one or more ADL:

- Personal care—bathing, dressing, grooming, elimination
- Meals—cooking, eating
- Taking drugs
- Housekeeping
- Personal safety
- Transportation

ALR residents do not need 24-hour nursing care. They are not bedridden. Some have chronic illnesses or are cognitively impaired. However, they do not have complex medical problems.

Mobility is often a requirement. The person walks or uses a wheelchair or motor scooter. The person must be able to leave the building in an emergency. Stable health is another requirement. Only limited health care or treatment is needed.

RESIDENT RIGHTS

ALR residents have rights and liberties as United States citizens. They also gain special rights under state laws and rules (Box 50-3). If unable to exercise his or her rights, family members, legal representatives, or ombudsmen act on the person's behalf.

BOX 50-3 | ASSISTED LIVING RESIDENTS' RIGHTS

Quality of Life

Residents have the right to:

- Receive a list of current resident rights. Language barriers or disabilities will not interfere.
- Current phone numbers of state and local agencies protecting the rights of older persons.
- Be treated with dignity and respect.
- Make choices about how to live one's everyday life.
- Make choices about how to receive care.
- Receive needed care and services for the highest level of physical, mental, and social well-being.
- Take part in deciding services.

Self-Determination

Residents have the right to:

- A setting that promotes dignity, individuality, independence, self-determination, privacy, and choice.
- Free choice to select a primary care provider, pharmacy, or other services and assume related costs.
- Submit grievances to employees and outside agencies.
- Take part in developing a written service plan.
- Receive a copy of service plans.
- Receive services specified in the service plan.
- Review and revise the service plan at any time.
- Refuse services, unless:
  - They are court-ordered.
  - Refusing endangers the health, safety, or welfare of others.
- Free choice to select activities, schedules, and daily routines.
- Have the same civil and human rights as other persons.
- Terminate living at an ALR without notice if a government agency proves:
  - Neglect
  - Exploitation
  - Conditions that are an immediate threat to life, health, or safety

Self-Determination—cont'd

- Terminate living at an ALR after 14 days written notice if the ALR failed to comply with the service plan or residency agreement.
- Receive written notice from the ALR when it terminates the person's residency. The notice shall include:
  - The effective date
  - The right to submit a grievance
  - The grievance procedure
  - The ALR's refund policy

Transfer and Discharge

Residents have the right to:

- Ask to locate or refuse to re-locate within the ALR.
- Know the reasons why the ALR may terminate residency.
  - Without notice:
    - If behavior is an immediate threat to the health and safety of others
    - For urgent medical or health needs requiring transfer to another health care agency
    - If care and service needs exceed the level of care provided by the ALR
  - Within 14 days of written notice for:
    - Failure to pay fees or charges
    - Not following the residency agreement or ALR requirements

Personal and Privacy Rights

Residents have the right to:

- Take part in or refuse to take part in activities.
- Perform or refuse to perform work for the ALR.
- Privacy in correspondence, communication, visits, and financial and personal matters.

Modified from Assisted Living Residents' Rights, Arizona Administrative Code R9-Chapter 10-Article 7.

Continued

BOX 50-3	ASSISTED LIVING RESIDENTS' RIGHTS—cont'd

Personal and Privacy Rights—cont'd
- Privacy in hygiene and health-related services.
- Receive visitors.
- Make private phone calls.
- Maintain and use personal items, unless the health, safety, or welfare of others is affected.
- Have financial and other records kept in confidence.
- Be treated with consideration and respect.
- Have access to common areas in the ALR.

Rights Against Restraints and Abuse
Residents have the right to:
- Be free from physical, mental, and sexual abuse and sexual assault.
- Be free from involuntary seclusion.
- Not be deprived of the care and services needed for physical or mental health.

Rights Against Restraints and Abuse—cont'd
- Not have one's resources used for another's profit or advantage.
- Be free from the use of physical restraints used for discipline or staff convenience.
- Be free from chemical restraints used to control behavior.
- Be free from discrimination in regard to race, color, national origin, sex, sexual orientation, and religion.

Right to Information
Residents have the right to:
- Review the ALR's most recent state survey.
- Review a copy of the state's code for ALRs.
- Receive written notice of fee or charge changes at least 30 days before the change. (Does not apply to service plan changes.)
- Review records during business hours or other set time.

STAFF REQUIREMENTS

Staff requirements vary among states. Some require a nursing assistant training and competency evaluation program for staff. Others require training in these areas:
- The needs and goals of ALR residents
- Promoting dignity, independence, and resident rights
- Using service plans
- Ethics, privacy, and confidentiality of records and information
- Hygiene and infection control
- Nutrition and menu planning
- Food preparation, service, and storage
- Housekeeping and sanitation
- Preventing and reporting abuse and neglect
- Incident reports
- Fire, emergency, and disaster plans
- Assisting with drugs
- Early signs of illness and the need for health care
- Safety measures
- Communication skills
- Special needs of persons with AD and other dementias
- Cardiopulmonary resuscitation and first aid (Chapter 51)

Criminal background and fingerprint checks are common requirements. The ALR cannot employ a person with a criminal record.

SERVICE PLAN

A *service plan is a written plan listing:*
- *The services needed*
- *How much help is needed*
- *Who provides the services*

The plan relates to ADL, activities and social services, dietary needs, taking drugs, and special needs. Health services are included.

For example, a person needs help getting dressed. The service plan states that you will assist the person. The service plan also states that a nurse will replace the person's catheter. The person needs physical therapy after a hip fracture. The service plan states a physical therapist will visit. And the person needs help taking drugs. A family member will assist the person.

The plan is reviewed when the person's condition, wants, or service needs change. Services are added or reduced as the person's needs change.

Meals

Three meals a day and snacks are provided. The time between the evening meal and breakfast is usually no more than 14 hours. It can be longer if there is a nutritious evening snack. Special dietary needs are met. Menus are posted for residents to see.

Residents eat in the dining room with others. Or they eat in their rooms. Assistive devices are provided. So is help with eating, opening cartons, buttering bread, cutting meat, and so on (Chapter 24).

Housekeeping

Housekeeping measures help prevent infection. And they keep living units neat and clean.

- Dust furniture at least weekly.
- Vacuum floors at least weekly and as needed.
- Wipe up spills right away.
- Use a dust mop or broom to sweep. Use a dustpan to collect dust and crumbs.
- Sweep daily or more often as needed.
- Make sure toilets are flushed after each use.
- Rinse the sink after washing, shaving, or oral hygiene.
- Clean the tub or shower after each use.
- Remove and dispose of hair from the sink, tub, or shower.
- Hang towels to dry. Or place them in a hamper.
- Clean bathroom surfaces every day. Use a disinfectant or water and detergent to clean all surfaces:
  - The toilet bowl, seat, and outside areas of the toilet
  - The floor
  - The sides, walls, and curtain or door of the tub or shower
  - Towel racks and toilet tissue, toothbrush, and soap holders
  - The sink and mirror
  - Window sills
- Mop or vacuum the bathroom floor every day.
- Empty bathroom wastebaskets every day.
- Put out clean towels and washcloths every day.
- Wash bath mats, the wastebasket, and laundry hamper every week.
- Replace toilet and facial tissue as needed.
- Open bathroom windows for a short time. Also use air fresheners.

Food Safety

Certain measures are needed to handle, prepare, and store food. They protect against infection. See Chapter 24. Also practice these measures:

- Follow the safe handling instructions on food labels (Fig. 50-3).
- Place left-over food in small containers. Cover containers with lids, foil, or plastic wrap. Date and refrigerate containers as soon as possible.
- Use left-over food within 2 or 3 days.
- Use liquid detergent and hot water to wash eating and cooking items. Wash glasses and cups first. Follow with silverware, plates, bowls, and then pots and pans. Rinse well with hot water.
- Place washed items in a drainer to dry. Air-drying is more aseptic than towel drying.

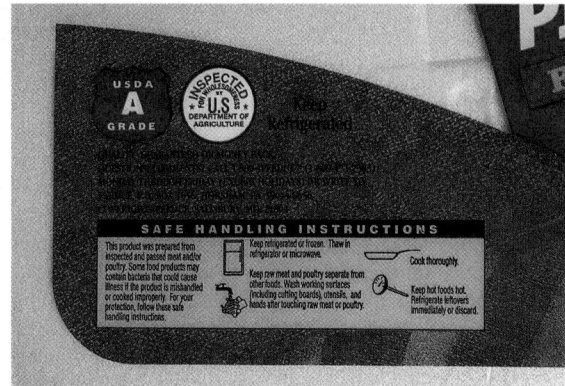

Fig. 50-3 Safe handling instructions for meat and poultry. They are required by the U.S. Department of Agriculture.

- Rinse dishes before loading them into a dishwasher. Use dishwasher soap.
- Do not wash pots and pans and cast iron, wood, and some plastic items in a dishwasher.
- Clean appliances, counters, tables, and other surfaces after each meal. Use hot, soapy water and paper towels or clean cloths.
- Remove grease spills and splashes. Use a liquid surface cleaner.
- Clean sinks with a sink cleaner.
- Dispose of garbage, left-overs, and other soiled supplies after each meal. Use a garbage disposal for food and liquid garbage but not bones.
- Recycle paper, boxes, cans, and plastic containers according to the ALR policy.
- Empty garbage at least once a day.

Laundry

Clean linens are provided. Residents can use a washer, dryer, iron, and ironing board. When assisting with laundry:

- Wear gloves to handle soiled laundry (see *Promoting Safety and Comfort: Assisted Living*, p. 792).
- Separate white, colored, and dark items. Separate sturdy and delicate fabrics.
- Empty pockets.
- Fasten buttons, zippers, snaps, hooks, and other closures.
- Wash heavily soiled items separately.
- Follow detergent directions.
- Follow care label directions and the person's preferences for the correct:
  - Wash cycle and water temperature
  - Drying temperature and cycle
- Fold, hang, or iron clothes as the person prefers. See *Teamwork and Time Management: Laundry*, p. 796.

Residents may share washers and dryers. If assisting with laundry, remove clothes from washers and dryers promptly. Others may want to use them. You may find someone's laundry left in a washer or dryer. First, try to find the person who left the laundry. Politely tell the person that the machine is done and that you have laundry to do. Offer to remove laundry if the other person is busy. If you cannot find that person, do the following:

- If left in a washer—place the wet laundry on a clean surface, not in the dryer. Some items may need to dry flat or hang to dry. Some fabrics may need certain dryer settings. Or the resident may have drying preferences.
- If left in a dryer—fold and place the laundry on a clean surface.

While laundry is in the washer or dryer, tend to other tasks. Assist with ADL, do housekeeping tasks, prepare meals, and so on.

Nursing Services

Some ALRs provide limited nursing services. The nurse assesses each person and monitors health. The nurse supervises tasks delegated to you. If a person cannot manage his or her own drugs, the nurse gives them.

Medication Assistance

Drugs must be taken as prescribed. The six rights of drug administration are:

- The right drug
- The right dose (amount)
- The right route (by mouth, injection, applied to the skin, inhalation, vaginally, or rectally)
- The right time
- The right person
- The right documentation

How you assist with drugs depends on your state's laws, ALR policy, and your training and education. *Remember, you do not give drugs (Chapter 3). Also remember that the person has the right to refuse to take prescribed drugs.* Your role may involve:

- Reminding the person it is time to take a drug
- Reading the drug label to the person
- Opening containers for persons who cannot do so
- Checking the dosage against the drug label
- Providing water, juice, milk, crackers, applesauce, or other food and fluids as needed
- Making sure the person takes the right drug, the right amount, at the right time, and in the right way
- Charting that the person took or refused to take the drug (right documentation)
- Storing drugs

Residents manage and take their own drugs if able. This is called *self-directed medication management.* The person knows drugs by name, color, or shape. The person knows what drugs to take, the correct doses, and when and how to take them. The person is able to question changes in the usual drug routine. For example, the person comments that a pill is not broken in half. Or the person says that a pill looks different. Report comments or questions to the nurse.

Pill organizers (Fig. 50-4) have sections for days and times. They are for a week or month. The person, a family member or legal representative, or a nurse prepares the pill organizer. The person then takes the drugs on the right day and at the right time.

You may need to remind some people. A *medication reminder means reminding the person to take drugs, observing them being taken as prescribed, and charting that they were taken.*

See *Focus on Communication: Medication Assistance.*

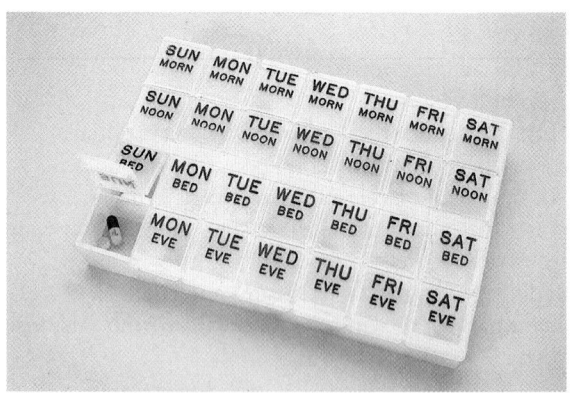

Fig. 50-4 Pill organizer.

To remind a person to take his or her drugs, you can say:

- "Ms. Parks, it's time for your 8 o'clock pills."
- "Mr. Ladd, you need to take your pills in about 10 minutes."
- "Mrs. Young, are you ready to take your medicine?"
  To read a drug label to a person, read the following:
- The name of the person on the drug label
- The name of the drug
- How to take the drug (by mouth, with food, with a full glass of water, apply to the skin, rectally, and so on)
- The dosage
- When to take the drug (before meals, with meals, after meals, and so on)
- How often to take the drug
- Warnings and other information on the drug label

Medication Record. A medication record is kept. The record includes:

* The person's name
* Drug name, dose, directions, and route of administration
* Date and time to take the drug
* Date and time help was given
* Signature or initials of the person assisting

Drug Errors. Report any drug error to the nurse. Also complete an incident report. An error means one or more of the following:

* Taking another person's drugs
* Taking the wrong drug
* Taking the wrong dose
* Taking an extra dose
* Missing or skipping a dose
* Taking a drug at the wrong time
* Taking a drug by the wrong route
* Not taking a drug when ordered
* Not recording that a drug was taken

Storing Drugs. Drugs are kept in a secure place. This prevents others from taking them. If the ALR stores the drugs, they are kept in a locked place.

Some persons store their own drugs. This is on the service plan. If sharing a room, each person's ability to safely have drugs is assessed. Drugs are kept in a locked container if safety is a factor.

Drugs must have the original pharmacy label. They are stored as directed on the label. For example, some drugs are refrigerated. Others are kept away from light. The label also has an expiration date. The ALR has procedures for disposing of expired or discontinued drugs.

Activities and Recreation

Residents are urged to take part in activity and recreational programs. Social, physical, and community activities promote well-being and independence. An activities director plans, organizes, and conducts the ALR's activity program. These activities are on a calendar. The calendar also tells about community events and activities.

Special Services and Safety Needs

Sometimes emergencies occur. Some people need help getting out of bed or transferring to a wheelchair. Then they can leave the building with little or no help.

Other people cannot walk or use a wheelchair. They need attendants 24 hours a day. The ALR and the person agree on how and who will meet the person's needs.

TRANSFER, DISCHARGE, AND EVICTION

Residents can be transferred, discharged, or evicted. State laws require that the ALR tell the person about the action. Reasons for such action are:

* The ALR can no longer meet the person's needs. The person is a threat to the health and safety of self or others. Or the ALR cannot provide needed care.
* The person fails to pay for services as agreed upon.
* The person fails to comply with ALR policies or rules.
* The person wants to transfer.
* The ALR closes.

FOCUS ON PRIDE

The Person, Family, and Yourself

Personal and Professional Responsibility

Moving into assisted living can bring mixed emotions. The person may be happy and excited. Fear, anxiety, and uncertainty are also common. The move may bring peace of mind for the family. The person is in a clean, safe setting. Needs are met. Healthy meals are provided. And the person has supervision.

Help the resident and family adapt to the change. Greet them kindly. Be professional and caring. Your interactions should assure the resident and family that you will provide safe, dignified care.

Rights and Respect

ALR residents have rights. Federal and state laws protect the person's rights. The person has the right to quality of life, self-determination, privacy, protection against restraint and abuse, and access to information. The person also has rights regarding transfer and discharge from the ALR. See Box 50-3. Take pride in protecting the person's rights.

Independence and Social Interaction

People choose assisted living for many reasons. Most need some help. But they want to live independently with dignity and respect. Many like the social interaction with other residents. The ALR's activities and services offer other benefits.

To promote independence, assist as needed while allowing as much privacy and personal choice as possible. Follow the resident's service plan.

Delegation and Teamwork

Residents are allowed to bring personal belongings into their rooms. This helps the room feel home-like. The family will need help moving the person's belongings. More help means less work for all involved. Good teamwork is needed when new residents arrive. The person and family should see that the staff is helpful and works together to meet the person's needs.

Continued

FOCUS ON PRIDE—cont'd

Ethics and Laws

Some ALR residents need assistance with drugs. How you assist with drugs depends on your state's laws, ALR policy, and your training. Nursing assistants do not give drugs. In some states, nursing assistants with advanced training can give drugs.

There are legal limits to your role. If you act beyond those limits, you could be practicing nursing without a license. You can lose your job and your ability to work as a nursing assistant. Follow the limits for your state and agency.

REVIEW QUESTIONS

Circle the BEST answer.

1 ALRs provide the following *except*
   a Nursing care
   b Housing
   c Help with ADL
   d Support services

2 These statements are about ALRs. Which is *false?*
   a Each person has a private apartment.
   b Some residents have Alzheimer's disease.
   c 24-hour security is provided.
   d Three meals a day are provided.

3 Which statement is *false?*
   a Residents can refuse care.
   b Residents must organize their own activities.
   c Residents are able to lock their doors.
   d An emergency communication system is provided.

4 Which violates an ALR resident's rights?
   a Covering the person during personal care
   b Giving the person unopened mail
   c Keeping information confidential
   d Choosing activities for the person

5 A person wants to attend a concert. Which is *true?*
   a The ALR must approve the concert.
   b The person must return by 10 PM.
   c An attendant must go with the person.
   d The ALR must respect the person's choice.

6 Assisted living staff must
   a Complete a nursing assistant training and competency evaluation program
   b Meet state requirements
   c Assist with drugs
   d Provide transportation

7 ALRs often require the following *except*
   a That persons be mobile
   b That persons have stable health
   c That persons require only limited care
   d That persons speak English

8 A service plan
   a Describes nursing care needs
   b Describes needed services and who provides them
   c Lists the drugs the person needs to take
   d Lists service fees and charges

9 ALR residents are encouraged to eat
   a In their rooms
   b In the dining room
   c At home
   d At community events

10 You assist with housekeeping. Which is *false?*
   a Dusting and vacuuming are done at least weekly.
   b Spills are wiped up right away.
   c Bathroom surfaces are cleaned daily.
   d Spills and splashes are wiped up after meals.

11 You assist with food. Which is *false?*
   a Safe handling instructions are followed.
   b Left-over food is used in 3 to 5 days.
   c Garbage is emptied at least once a day.
   d Pots and pans are washed by hand.

12 You assist with laundry. Which is *true?*
   a Care label directions are followed.
   b Clothes are washed in hot water.
   c Clothes are ironed.
   d All white fabrics are washed together.

13 Usually ALR staff are allowed to
   a Give drugs
   b Give medication reminders
   c Refill drugs
   d Prepare pill organizers

14 Drugs are kept
   a In the person's closet
   b In the person's drawer
   c In a locked place
   d By the family

15 The ALR cannot provide a person with all needed services. Which is *true?*
   a The ALR must hire more staff.
   b The family must provide the needed care.
   c The ALR can ask the person to transfer.
   d The person's service plan needs to change.

Answers to these questions are on p. 835.

Basic Emergency Care

51

OBJECTIVES

- Define the key terms and key abbreviations listed in this chapter.
- Describe the rules of emergency care.
- Identify the signs of sudden cardiac arrest and the emergency care required.
- Describe the signs, symptoms, and emergency care for hemorrhage.
- Identify the common causes and emergency care for fainting.
- Identify the signs, symptoms, and emergency care for shock.

- Describe the signs, symptoms, and emergency care for stroke.
- Explain the causes and types of seizures and how to care for a person during a seizure.
- Identify the causes, types, and emergency care for burns.
- Perform the procedures described in this chapter.
- Explain how to promote PRIDE in the person, the family, and yourself.

KEY TERMS

anaphylaxis A life-threatening sensitivity to an antigen

cardiac arrest See "sudden cardiac arrest"

convulsion See "seizure"

fainting The sudden loss of consciousness from an inadequate blood supply to the brain

first aid Emergency care given to an ill or injured person before medical help arrives

hemorrhage The excessive loss of blood in a short time

respiratory arrest Breathing stops but heart action continues for several minutes

seizure Violent and sudden contractions or tremors of muscle groups; convulsion

shock Results when tissues and organs do not get enough blood

sudden cardiac arrest (SCA) The heart stops suddenly and without warning; cardiac arrest

KEY ABBREVIATIONS

AED	Automated external defibrillator		**RRT**	Rapid Response Team
AHA	American Heart Association		**SCA**	Sudden cardiac arrest
BLS	Basic Life Support		**VF**	Ventricular fibrillation
CPR	Cardiopulmonary resuscitation		**V-fib**	Ventricular fibrillation
EMS	Emergency Medical Services			

Emergencies can occur anywhere. Sometimes you can save a life if you know what to do. You are encouraged to take a first aid course and a Basic Life Support (BLS) course. These courses prepare you to give emergency care.

The BLS procedures in this chapter are given as basic information. They do not replace certification training. You need a BLS course for health care providers.

EMERGENCY CARE

First aid is the emergency care given to an ill or injured person before medical help arrives. The goals of first aid are to:
- Prevent death.
- Prevent injuries from becoming worse.

In an emergency, the Emergency Medical Services (EMS) system is activated. Emergency personnel (paramedics, emergency medical technicians) rush to the scene. They treat, stabilize, and transport persons with life-threatening problems. Their ambulances have emergency drugs, equipment, and supplies. They have guidelines for care and communicate with doctors in hospital emergency departments. The doctors can tell them what to do. To activate the EMS system, do one of the following:
- Dial 911.
- Call the local fire or police department.
- Call the phone operator.

Each emergency is different. The rules in Box 51-1 apply to any emergency. Hospitals and other agencies have procedures for emergencies. Rapid Response Teams (RRTs) are called to the bedside when a person shows warning signs of a life-threatening condition. An RRT may include a doctor, an RN, and a respiratory therapist. The RRT's goal is to prevent death.

See *Focus on Communication: Emergency Care.*
See *Focus on Long-Term Care and Home Care: Emergency Care.*
See *Promoting Safety and Comfort: Emergency Care.*

FOCUS ON COMMUNICATION
Emergency Care

Some illnesses and injuries are life-threatening. To find out what happened and the person's condition, you can say:
- "Are you okay?"
- "Tell me what's wrong."
- "Where does it hurt?"
- "If you can, please point to where it hurts."
- "Can you move your arms and legs?"

BOX 51-1   RULES OF EMERGENCY CARE

- Know your limits. Do not do more than you are able. Do not perform an unfamiliar procedure. Do what you can under the circumstances.
- Stay calm. This helps the person feel more secure.
- Know where to find emergency supplies.
- Follow Standard Precautions and the Bloodborne Pathogen Standard to the extent possible.
- Check for life-threatening problems. Check for breathing, a pulse, and bleeding.
- Keep the person lying down or as you found him or her. Moving the person could make an injury worse.
- Move the person only if the setting is unsafe. Examples include:
  - A burning building or car
  - A building that might collapse
  - Stormy conditions with lightning
  - In water
  - Near electrical wires
- Wait for help to arrive if the scene is not safe enough for you to approach.
- Perform necessary emergency measures.

- Call for help. Or have someone activate the EMS system. *Do not hang up until the operator has hung up.* Give the operator the following information:
  - Your location: street address and city, cross streets or roads, and landmarks
  - Phone number you are calling from
  - What seems to have happened (for example: heart attack, crash, fire)—police, fire equipment, and ambulances may be needed
  - How many people need help
  - Conditions of victims, obvious injuries, and life-threatening situations
  - What aid is being given
- Do not remove clothes unless you have to. If you must remove clothing, tear or cut garments along the seams.
- Keep the person warm. Cover the person with a blanket, coats, or sweaters.
- Reassure the person. Explain what is happening and that help was called.
- Do not give the person food or fluids.
- Keep onlookers away. They invade privacy and tend to stare, give advice, and comment about the person's condition. The person may think the situation is worse than it really is.

BASIC LIFE SUPPORT FOR ADULTS

When the heart and breathing stop, the person is clinically dead. Blood is not circulated through the body. Heart, brain, and other organ damage occurs within minutes. The American Heart Association's (AHA) BLS procedures support circulation and breathing.

Chain of Survival for Adults

The AHA's BLS courses teach the adult *Chain of Survival.* These actions are taken for heart attack (Chapter 42), sudden cardiac arrest, respiratory arrest, stroke (Chapter 41 and p. 817), and choking (p. 816). They also apply to other life-threatening problems. They are done as soon as possible. Any delay reduces the person's chance of surviving.

Chain of Survival actions for the adult are:

- Recognizing cardiac arrest and activating the EMS system at once.
- Early cardiopulmonary resuscitation (CPR).
- Early defibrillation. See p. 806.
- Early advanced care. This is given by EMS staff, doctors, and nurses. They give drugs and perform life-saving measures.
- Organized post–cardiac arrest care. This is care given to improve survival following cardiac arrest.

See *Focus on Communication: Chain of Survival for Adults.*

Sudden Cardiac Arrest

Sudden cardiac arrest (SCA) or cardiac arrest is when the heart stops suddenly and without warning. Within moments, breathing stops as well. Permanent brain and other organ damage occurs unless circulation and breathing are restored. There are 3 major signs of SCA:

- No response.
- No breathing or no normal breathing. The person may have *agonal gasps* or *agonal respirations* early during SCA. (*Agonal* comes from the Greek word that means *to struggle.* Agonal is used in relation to death and dying.) Agonal gasps do not bring enough oxygen into the lungs. Gasps are not normal breathing.
- No pulse.

The person's skin is cool, pale, and gray. The person is not coughing or moving.

SCA is a sudden, unexpected, and dramatic event. It can occur anywhere and at any time—while driving, shoveling snow, playing golf or tennis, watching TV, eating, or sleeping. Common causes include heart disease, drowning, electric shock, severe injury, choking (Chapter 12), and drug over-dose. These causes lead to an abnormal heart rhythm called ventricular fibrillation (p. 806). The heart cannot pump blood. A normal rhythm must be restored. Otherwise the person will die.

Respiratory Arrest

Respiratory arrest is when breathing stops but heart action continues for several minutes. If breathing is not restored, cardiac arrest occurs. Causes of respiratory arrest include:

- Drowning
- Stroke
- Choking
- Drug over-dose
- Electric shock (including lightning strikes)
- Smoke inhalation
- Suffocation
- Heart attack
- Coma
- Other injuries

Rescue Breathing. Rescue breaths are given when there is a pulse but no breathing or only gasping. To give rescue breaths:

- Open the airway (p. 804).
- Give 1 breath every 5 to 6 seconds for adults.
- Give 1 breath every 3 to 5 seconds for infants and children.
- Give each breath over 1 second. The chest should rise when breaths are given.
- Check the pulse every 2 minutes. If there is no pulse, begin CPR. If the pulse is lower than 60 in an infant or child, begin CPR (p. 810).

Cardiopulmonary Resuscitation for Adults

When the heart and breathing stop, blood and oxygen are not supplied to the body. Brain and other organ damage occurs within minutes.

CPR must be started at once when a person has SCA. CPR supports circulation and breathing. It provides blood and oxygen to the heart, brain, and other organs until advanced emergency care is given. CPR involves:

- Chest compressions
- Airway
- Breathing
- Defibrillation

CPR procedures require speed, skill, and efficiency. Chest compressions and airway and breathing procedures are done until a defibrillator arrives. The defibrillator is used as soon as possible.

See *Promoting Safety and Comfort: Cardiopulmonary Resuscitation for Adults.*

Chest Compressions. The heart, brain, and other organs must receive blood. Otherwise, permanent damage results. In cardiac arrest, the heart has stopped beating. Blood must be pumped through the body in some other way. Chest compressions force blood through the circulatory system.

Before starting chest compressions, check for a pulse. Use the carotid artery on the side near you. To find the carotid pulse, place 2 or 3 fingertips on the trachea (windpipe). Then slide your fingertips down off the trachea to the groove of the neck (Fig. 51-1). Check for a pulse for at least 5 seconds but no more than 10 seconds. While checking for a pulse, look for signs of circulation. See if the person has started breathing or is coughing or moving.

The heart lies between the sternum (breastbone) and the spinal column. When pressure is applied to the sternum, the sternum is depressed. This compresses the heart between the sternum and spinal column (Fig. 51-2). For effective chest compressions, the person must be supine on a hard, flat surface—floor or back-board. You are positioned at the person's side.

Hand position is important for effective chest compressions (Fig. 51-3). You use the heels of your hands—one on top of the other—for chest compressions. For proper placement:

- Expose the person's chest. Remove clothing or move it out of the way. You need to be able to see the person's bare skin for proper hand position.
- Place the heel of one hand (usually your dominant hand) in the center of the bare chest. The heel of this hand is placed on the sternum between the nipples.
- Place the heel of your other hand on top of the heel of the first hand.

PROMOTING SAFETY AND COMFORT
Cardiopulmonary Resuscitation for Adults

Safety
The discussion and procedures that follow assume that the person does not have injuries from trauma (Chapter 33). If injuries are present, special measures are needed to position the person and open the airway. Such measures are learned during a BLS certification course.

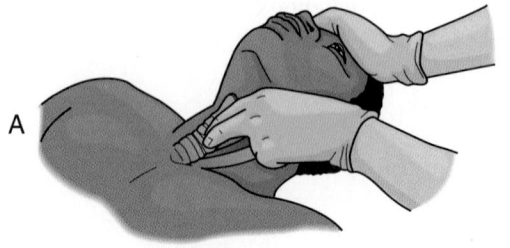
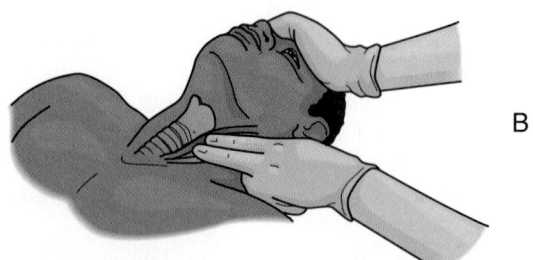

Fig. 51-1 Locating the carotid pulse. **A,** Two fingers are placed on the trachea. **B,** The fingertips are moved down into the groove of the neck to the carotid artery.

To give chest compressions, your arms are straight. Your shoulders are directly over your hands. And your fingers are interlocked (Fig. 51-4). Exert firm downward pressure to depress the adult sternum at least 2 inches. Then release pressure without removing your hands from the chest. Releasing pressure allows the chest to recoil—to return to its normal position. Recoil lets the heart fill with blood.

The AHA recommends that you:

- Give compressions at a rate of at least 100 per minute.
- Push hard, and push fast.
- Push deeply into the chest.
- Interrupt chest compressions only when necessary. Interruptions should be less than 10 seconds. When there are no chest compressions, blood does not flow to the heart, brain, and other organs.

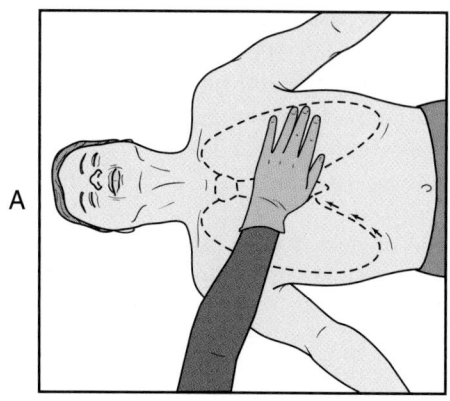

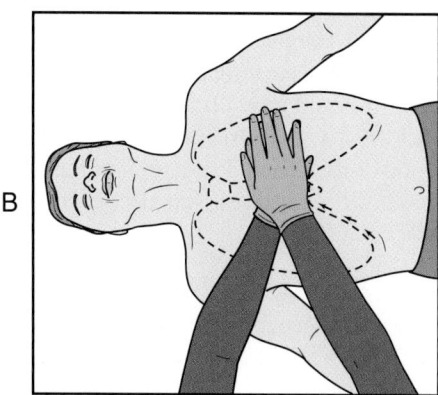

Fig. 51-3 Proper hand position for CPR. **A,** The heel of the dominant hand is placed in the center of the chest between the nipples. **B,** The heel of the non-dominant hand is placed on top of the dominant hand.

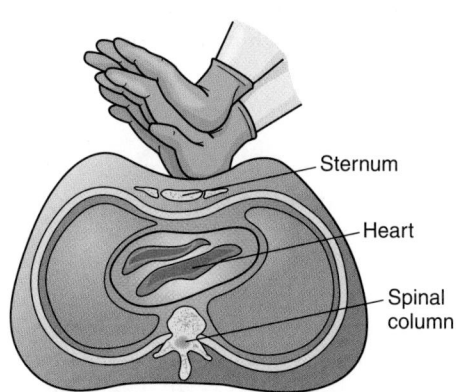

Fig. 51-2 The heart lies between the sternum and the spinal column. The heart is compressed when pressure is applied to the sternum.

Sternum

Heart

Spinal column

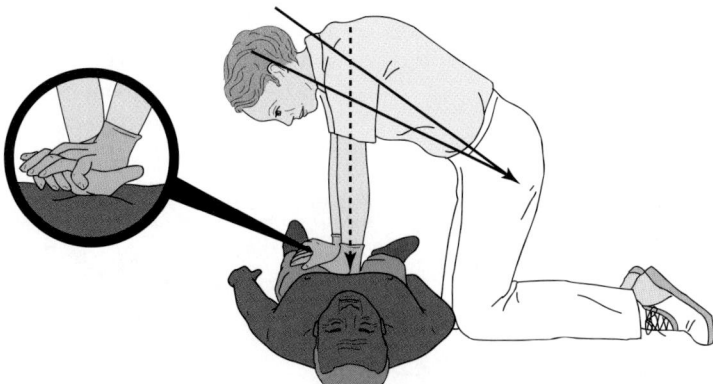

Fig. 51-4 Giving chest compressions. The arms are straight. The shoulders are over the hands. The fingers are interlocked.

Airway. The respiratory passages (airway) must be open to restore breathing. The airway is often obstructed (blocked) during SCA. The person's tongue falls toward the back of the throat and blocks the airway. The head tilt–chin lift method opens the airway (Fig. 51-5):

- Place the palm of one hand on the forehead.
- Tilt the head back by pushing down on the forehead with your palm.
- Place the fingers of your other hand under the lower jaw. Use your index and middle fingers. Do not use your thumb.
- Lift the jaw. This brings the chin forward.
- Do not close the person's mouth. The mouth should be slightly open unless you need to do mouth-to-nose breathing.

Breathing. Air is not inhaled when breathing stops. The person must get oxygen. If not, permanent heart, brain, and other organ damage occurs. The person is given *breaths*. That is, a rescuer inflates the person's lungs.

Each breath should take 1 second. *You should see the chest rise with each breath.* Two breaths are given after every 30 chest compressions. When 2 rescuers perform CPR on an infant or child, 2 breaths are given after every 15 compressions (p. 810).

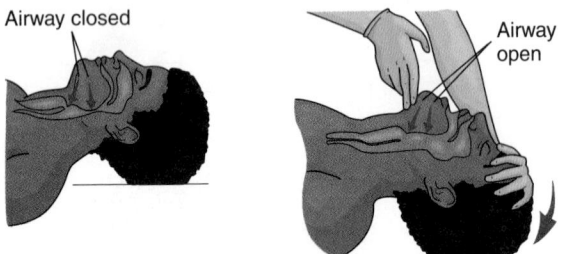

Fig. 51-5 The head tilt–chin lift method opens the airway. One hand is on the person's forehead. Pressure is applied to tilt the head back. The chin is lifted with the fingers of the other hand.

Mouth-to-mouth breathing. Mouth-to-mouth breathing (Fig. 51-6) is one way to give breaths. You place your mouth over the person's mouth. Contact with the person's blood, body fluids, secretions, or excretions is likely. To give mouth-to-mouth breathing:

- Keep the airway open with the head tilt–chin lift method.
- Pinch the person's nostrils shut. Use your thumb and index finger. Use the hand on the forehead. Shutting the nostrils prevents air from escaping through the nose.
- Take a breath. A regular breath is needed, not a deep breath.
- Place your mouth tightly over the person's mouth. Seal the person's mouth with your lips.
- Blow air into the person's mouth. You should see the chest rise as the lungs fill with air. You should also hear air escape when the person exhales.
- Repeat the head tilt–chin lift method if the person's chest did not rise.
- Remove your mouth from the person's mouth. Then take in a quick breath.
- Give another breath. You should see the chest rise.

Barrier device breathing. A barrier device is used for giving breaths whenever possible. The device prevents contact with the person's mouth and blood, body fluids, secretions, or excretions. A face shield may be used (Fig. 51-7). A face shield is replaced with a face mask as soon as possible (Fig. 51-8, A). The mask is placed over the person's mouth and nose (Fig. 51-8, B). When using a barrier device, seal the device against the person's face. The seal must be tight. Then open the airway with the head tilt–chin lift method.

A bag valve mask (Fig. 51-9) is another device used to give rescue breaths. The device consists of a hand-held bag attached to a mask. The mask is held securely to the person's face. And the bag is squeezed to give breaths. The bag can be connected to an oxygen source.

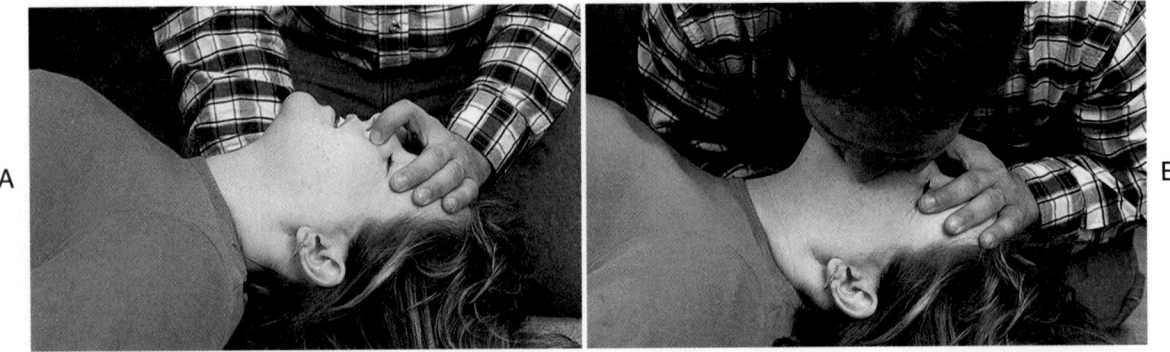

Fig. 51-6 Mouth-to-mouth breathing. **A,** The person's airway is opened. The nostrils are pinched shut. **B,** The person's mouth is sealed by the rescuer's mouth.

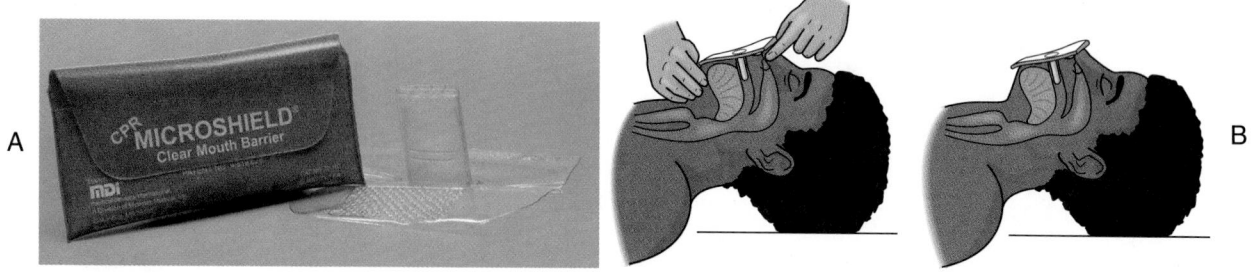

Fig. 51-7 A, Face shield. **B,** The face shield is in place.

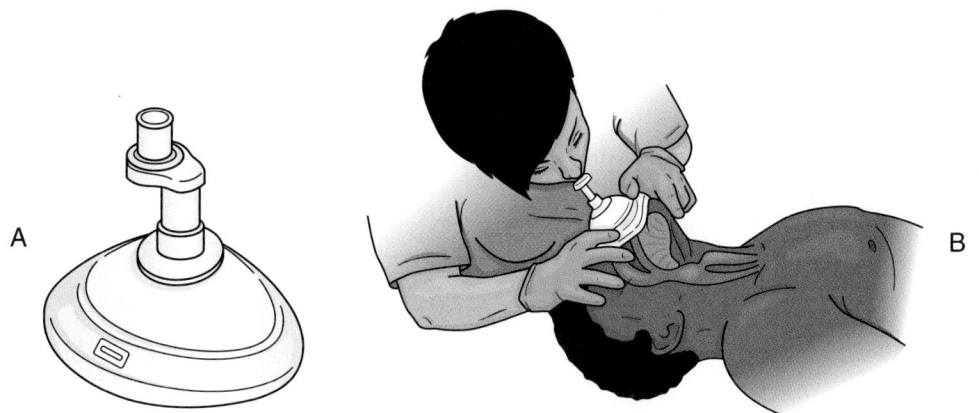

Fig. 51-8 A, Mask for giving breaths. **B,** The mask is in place.

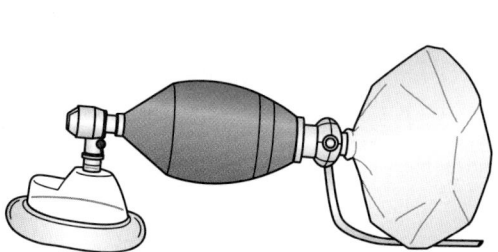

Fig. 51-9 A bag valve mask.

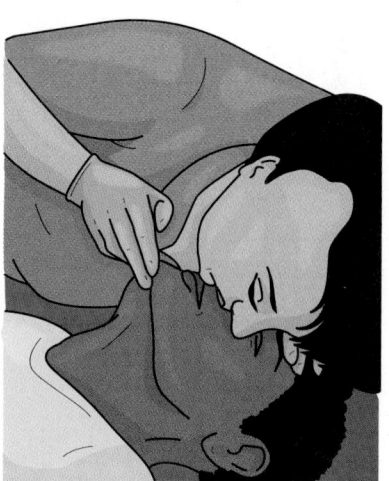

Fig. 51-10 Mouth-to-nose breathing.

Mouth-to-nose breathing. Mouth-to-nose breathing is used when:

- You cannot breathe through the person's mouth.
- You cannot open the mouth.
- Your mouth is too small to make a tight seal for mouth-to-mouth breathing.
- The mouth or jaw is severely injured.
- The person is bleeding from the mouth.

The mouth is closed for mouth-to-nose breathing. The head tilt–chin lift method opens the airway. Pressure is placed on the chin to close the mouth. To give a breath, place your mouth over the person's nose and blow air into the nose (Fig. 51-10). After giving a breath, remove your mouth from the person's nose.

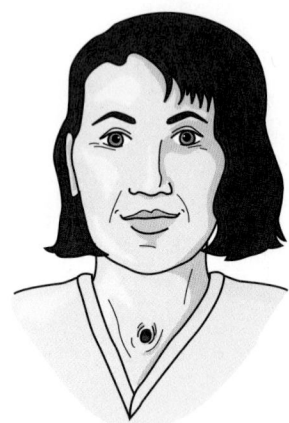

Fig. 51-11 A stoma in the neck. The person breathes in and out of the stoma.

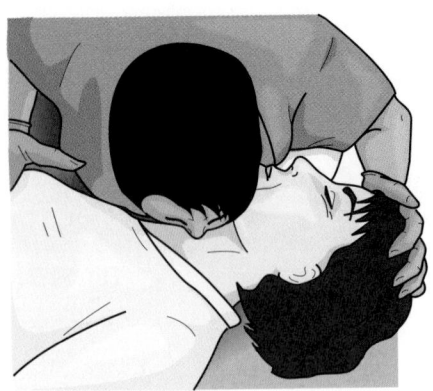

Fig. 51-12 Mouth-to-stoma breathing.

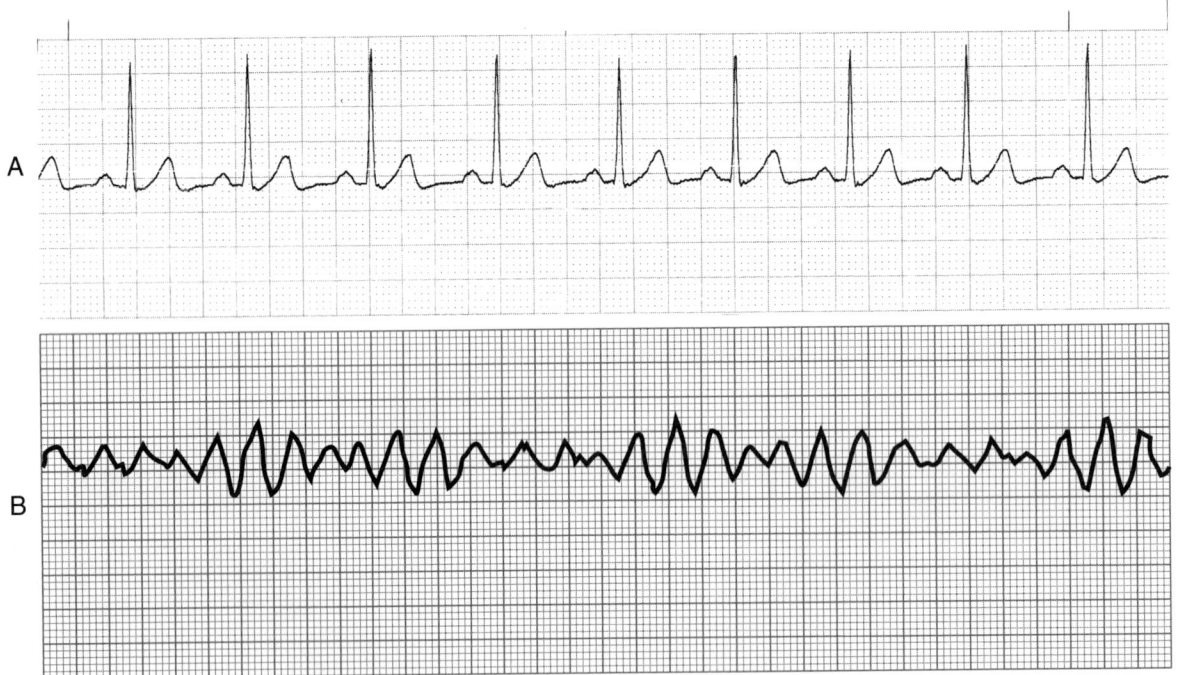

Fig. 51-13 **A,** Normal rhythm. **B,** Ventricular fibrillation.

Mouth-to-stoma breathing. Some people breathe through *stomas* (openings) in their necks (Fig. 51-11). To give mouth-to-stoma breathing:

- Keep the person's mouth closed.
- Do not tilt the person's head back.
- Seal your mouth around the stoma.
- Blow air into the stoma (Fig. 51-12).

If the person's chest does not rise, you may need to pinch the nostrils shut.

Before giving mouth-to-mouth or mouth-to-nose breathing, always check to see if the person has a stoma. Other rescue breathing methods are not effective if the person has a stoma.

Defibrillation. Ventricular fibrillation (VF, V-fib) is an abnormal heart rhythm (Fig. 51-13). It causes sudden cardiac arrest. Rather than beating in a regular rhythm, the heart shakes and quivers like a bowl of Jell-O. The heart does not pump blood. The heart, brain, and other organs do not receive blood and oxygen.

A *defibrillator* is used to deliver a shock to the heart. The shock stops the VF (V-fib). This allows the return of a regular heart rhythm. Defibrillation as soon as possible after the onset of VF (V-fib) increases the person's chance of survival.

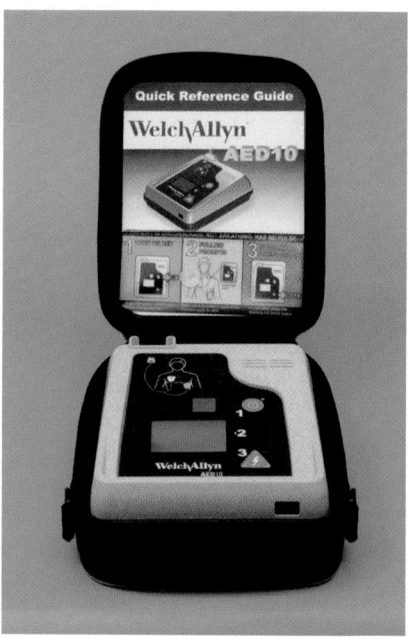

Fig. 51-14 An automated external defibrillator (AED).

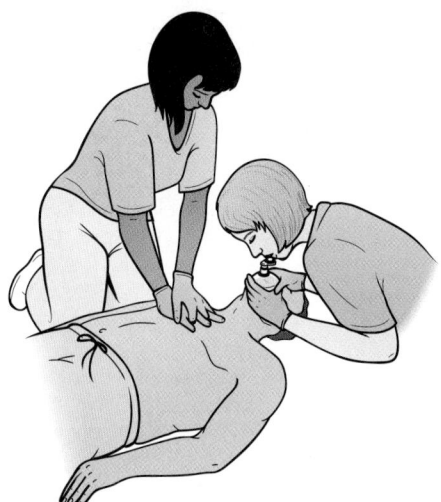

Fig. 51-15 Two people perform CPR.

For adults, the AHA recommends that rescuers:
* Attach and use the automated external defibrillator (AED) as soon as it is available.
* Minimize interruptions in chest compressions before and after a shock is delivered.
* Give one shock. Then resume CPR at once. Begin with compressions. Do 5 cycles of 30 compressions and 2 breaths.
* Check for a heart rhythm.

AEDs are found in hospitals, nursing centers, dental offices, and other health care agencies (Fig. 51-14). They are on airplanes and in airports, health clubs, malls, and many other public places. Many people have them in their homes.

You will learn more about using an AED in the AHA's *BLS for Healthcare Providers* course.

See *Focus on Children and Older Persons: Defibrillation.*

Performing Adult CPR. CPR is done only for cardiac arrest. You must determine if cardiac arrest or fainting (p. 817) has occurred. *CPR is done if the person does not respond, is not breathing (or has no normal breathing), and has no pulse.*

CPR is done alone or with another person. When done alone, chest compressions and rescue breathing are done by 1 rescuer. With 2 rescuers, 1 person gives chest compressions and the other does rescue breathing (Fig. 51-15). Rescuers switch tasks about every 2 minutes to avoid fatigue and inadequate compressions. The second rescuer uses the AED if one is available.

See *Focus on Communication: Performing Adult CPR.*
See *Promoting Safety and Comfort: Performing Adult CPR.*

FOCUS ON COMMUNICATION
Performing Adult CPR

Good communication is needed when 2 rescuers perform CPR. The rescuer giving compressions must count out loud so the other rescuer is ready to give breaths. Clear communication prevents delays and minimizes interruptions in chest compressions.

FOCUS ON CHILDREN AND OLDER PERSONS
Defibrillation

Children

Some AEDs are designed for adults and children. A key or switch is used to change the dosage. Or child pads are used. Always follow the manufacturer's instructions.

The shock dosage for children 8 years and older is the same as the adult dosage. Lower shock dosages are used for children younger than 8 years. For infants, a manual defibrillator is best. Trained staff and EMS personnel use the defibrillator. If one is not available, an AED with child dosages may be used. If neither is available, adult dosages may be used. If adult pads are used, the pads must not touch or overlap.

PROMOTING SAFETY AND COMFORT
Performing Adult CPR

Safety

Never practice CPR on another person. Serious damage can be done. Mannequins are used to learn and practice CPR.

Make sure you have a safe setting for CPR. Move the person only if the setting is unsafe (see Box 51-1). Do not approach the person if the scene is unsafe for you.

The person must be on a hard, flat surface for CPR. If the person is in bed, place a board under the person. Or move the person to the floor.

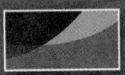

ADULT CPR—ONE RESCUER

PROCEDURE

1 Make sure the scene is safe.
2 Take 5 to 10 seconds to check for a response and breathing:
   a Check if the person is responding. Tap or gently shake the person. Call the person by name, if known. Shout, "Are you okay?"
   b Check for no breathing or no normal breathing (gasping).
3 Call for help. Activate the EMS system or the agency's RRT if the person is not responding and not breathing or not breathing normally (gasping).
4 Get or ask someone to bring an AED if available.
5 Position the person supine on a hard, flat surface. Logroll the person so there is no twisting of the spine. Place the arms alongside the body.
6 Check for a carotid pulse. This should take 5 to 10 seconds. Start chest compressions if you do not feel a pulse.
7 Expose the person's chest.

8 Give chest compressions at a rate of at least 100 per minute. Push hard and fast. Establish a regular rhythm. Count out loud. Press down at least 2 inches. Allow the chest to recoil between compressions. Give 30 chest compressions.
9 Open the airway. Use the head tilt–chin lift method.
10 Give 2 breaths. Each breath should take only 1 second. Each breath must make the chest rise. (If the first breath does not make the chest rise, try opening the airway again. Use the head tilt–chin lift method.)
11 Continue the cycle of 30 chest compressions followed by 2 breaths. Limit interruptions in compressions to less than 10 seconds. Continue CPR cycles until the AED arrives. See procedure: *Adult CPR With AED—Two Rescuers*. Or continue until help arrives or the person begins to move. If movement occurs, place the person in the recovery position.

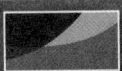

ADULT CPR WITH AED—TWO RESCUERS

PROCEDURE

1 Make sure the scene is safe.
2 *Rescuer 1*—Take 5 to 10 seconds to check for a response and breathing:
   a Check if the person is responding. Tap or gently shake the person. Call the person by name, if known. Shout, "Are you okay?"
   b Check for no breathing or no normal breathing (gasping).
3 *Rescuer 2:*
   a Activate the EMS system or the agency's RRT if the person is not responding and not breathing or not breathing normally (gasping).
   b Get a defibrillator (AED) if one is available.
4 *Rescuer 1:*
   a Position the person supine on a hard, flat surface. Logroll the person so there is no twisting of the spine. Place the arms alongside the body.
   b Check for a carotid pulse. This should take 5 to 10 seconds. Start chest compressions if you do not feel a pulse.
   c Expose the person's chest.
   d Give chest compressions at a rate of at least 100 per minute. Push hard and fast. Establish a regular rhythm. Count out loud. Press down at least 2 inches. Allow the chest to recoil between compressions. Give 30 chest compressions.
   e Open the airway. Use the head tilt–chin lift method.
   f Give 2 breaths. Each breath should take only 1 second. Each breath must make the chest rise. (If the first breath does not make the chest rise, try opening the airway again. Use the head tilt–chin lift method.)
   g Continue the cycle of 30 chest compressions followed by 2 breaths. Limit interruptions in compressions to less than 10 seconds.

5 *Rescuer 2:*
   a Open the case with the AED.
   b Turn on the AED (Fig. 51-16, A).
   c Apply adult electrode pads to the person's chest (Fig. 51-16, B). Follow the instructions and diagram provided with the AED. Attach the connecting cables to the AED (Fig. 51-16, C).
   d Attach the connecting cables to the AED (Fig. 51-16, C).
   e Clear away from the person. Make sure no one is touching the person (Fig. 51-16, D).
   f Let the AED check the person's heart rhythm.
   g Make sure everyone is clear of the person if the AED advises a "shock" (see Fig. 51-16, D). Loudly instruct others not to touch the person. Say: "I am clear, you are clear, everyone is clear!" Look to make sure no one is touching the person.
   h Press the "SHOCK" button if the AED advises a "shock" (Fig. 51-16, E).
6 *Rescuers 1 and 2:*
   a Perform 2-person CPR:
      (1) Begin with compressions. One rescuer gives chest compressions at a rate of at least 100 per minute. Push hard and fast. Establish a regular rhythm. Count out loud. Allow the chest to recoil between compressions. Give 30 chest compressions. Pause to allow the other rescuer to give 2 breaths.
      (2) The other rescuer gives 2 breaths after every 30 chest compressions.
7 Repeat step 5, e, f, g, and h after 2 minutes of CPR (5 cycles of 30 compressions and 2 breaths). Change positions and continue CPR beginning with compressions.
8 Continue until help takes over or the person begins to move. If movement occurs, place the person in the recovery position.

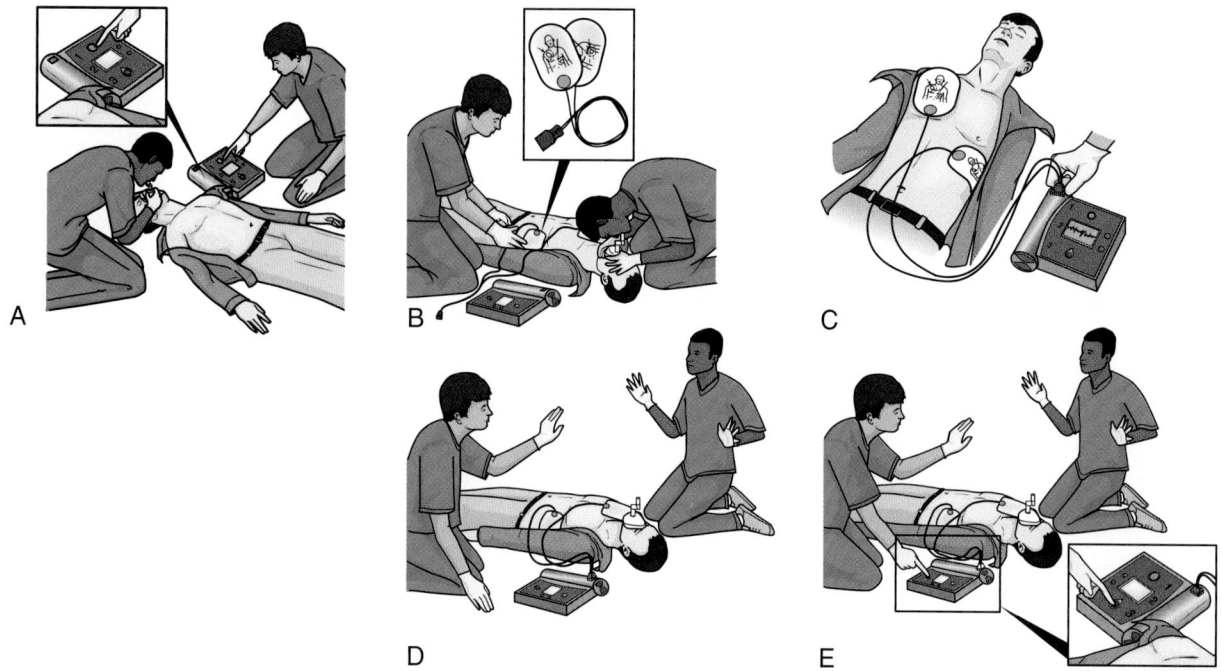

Fig. 51-16 A, The rescuer turns on the AED. **B,** Electrode pads are placed on the person's chest. **C,** The cables are connected to the AED. **D,** The rescuer "clears" the person. The rescuer makes sure no one is touching the person. **E,** The "SHOCK" button is pressed to deliver a shock.

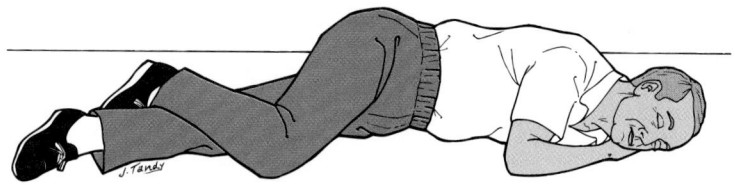

Fig. 51-17 Recovery position.

Hands-Only CPR. When an adult has sudden cardiac arrest, the person's survival depends on others nearby. Outside of the health care setting, persons trained in BLS are often not available. Bystanders may worry that they will not do CPR correctly or that they may injure the person.

The AHA developed "Hands-Only CPR" to improve the response of bystanders who witness an adult collapse suddenly in the out-of-hospital setting. In "Hands-Only CPR," CPR is simplified to 2 steps:

1 Call 911.

2 Push hard and fast in the center of the chest.

"Hands-Only CPR" is used to educate persons not trained in BLS. As a health care provider, use the CPR method presented in this chapter and in a BLS course.

Recovery Position

The recovery position is used when the person is breathing and has a pulse but is not responding (Fig. 51-17). The position helps keep the airway open and prevents aspiration.

Logroll the person into the recovery position. Keep the head, neck, and spine straight. A hand supports the head. *Do not use this position if the person might have neck injuries or other trauma.*

BASIC LIFE SUPPORT FOR CHILDREN AND INFANTS

The AHA defines a child and an infant as follows:

* *Child*—from 1 year of age to puberty. Puberty is marked by secondary sex characteristics in males and females (Chapter 10).
* *Infant*—from birth (outside of the delivery room) until 1 year (12 months) of age.

Chain of Survival for Children and Infants

Sudden infant death syndrome (SIDS) is the sudden, unexplained death of an infant younger than 1 year old. It is the leading cause of death in children between 1 month and 1 year of age. Most SIDS deaths occur in babies between 2 months and 4 months of age. It usually occurs during sleep.

Cardiac arrest caused by heart disease is rare in children. More common causes involve respiratory diseases or injuries that lead to respiratory arrest or circulatory failure. Motor vehicle crashes, drowning, burns, smoke inhalation, and guns are major death-producing injuries.

The AHA's pediatric *Chain of Survival* involves these steps:

* Preventing cardiac arrest
* Early and effective CPR
* Rapid activation of the EMS system or the agency's RRT
* Early and effective advanced life support
* Organized post–cardiac arrest care

CPR for Children and Infants

The AHA's CPR guidelines for children and infants differ from adult guidelines (Box 51-2). The procedures also differ. Remember to use barrier devices for breathing whenever possible.

Text continued on p. 814

BOX 51-2	CPR RULES FOR CHILDREN AND INFANTS

Children

* If you are alone:
  * Perform 5 cycles of CPR. Then activate the EMS system or the agency's RRT if the arrest was not witnessed.
  * Activate the EMS system or the agency's RRT first if the arrest was sudden and witnessed. Then begin CPR.
* Count the pulse for at least 5 seconds but no more than 10 seconds. For the heart rate per minute:
  * 5 seconds: multiply the number by 12
  * 10 seconds: multiply the number by 6
* Start CPR if the child's heart rate is less than 60 beats per minute with signs of poor circulation. For example, the child's skin color is poor.
* Use the same hand position for chest compressions as for adults (p. 802).
* Use 2 hands for chest compressions. Use 1 hand if the child is very small (Fig. 51-18).
* Give chest compressions with enough pressure to press down at least ⅓ the depth of the chest (about 2 inches).
* Release pressure and allow the chest to recoil after each compression.
* Give compressions at the rate of at least 100 per minute. Push hard and fast.
* Change chest compressions and breathing when 2 rescuers are present:
  * 1 rescuer—30 compressions followed by 2 breaths
  * 2 rescuers—15 compressions followed by 2 breaths
* Give only enough air to make the child's chest rise. If the child is very small, use less air than for larger children and adults.
* Give 2 breaths that make the child's chest rise. If a breath does not make the chest rise:
  * Try again to open the airway.
  * Give a breath. The breath should make the chest rise.
* Use an AED as soon as possible. Use child pads and a child system for children younger than 8 years if possible.

Infants

* If you are alone:
  * Perform 5 cycles of CPR. Then activate the EMS system or the agency's RRT and get the AED if the arrest was not witnessed.
  * Activate the EMS system or the agency's RRT first if the arrest was sudden and witnessed. Then begin CPR.
* Use the brachial artery to check for a pulse (Fig. 51-19):
  * Place the index and middle fingers on the inside of the infant's upper arm. Finger placement is between the elbow and shoulder.
  * Press gently for 5 to 10 seconds.
* Count the pulse for at least 5 seconds but no more than 10 seconds. For the heart rate per minute:
  * 5 seconds: multiply the number by 12
  * 10 seconds: multiply the number by 6
* Start CPR if the infant's heart rate is less than 60 beats per minute with signs of poor circulation. For example, the infant's skin color is poor.
* Locate hand position for chest compressions (Fig. 51-20, p. 812):
  * Draw an imaginary line between the nipples. Find the sternum (breastbone).
  * Place 2 fingers on the sternum just below the imaginary line.
* Give chest compressions as follows:
  * Press on the lower half of the sternum. Do not press on the bottom of the sternum.
  * Use enough pressure to press down at least ⅓ the depth of the chest (about 1½ inches).

Adapted from *BLS for Healthcare Providers*, copyright 2011, American Heart Association.

BOX 51-2 CPR RULES FOR CHILDREN AND INFANTS—cont'd

Infants—cont'd

- Use the 2 thumb-encircling hands method for chest compressions when there are 2 rescuers (Fig. 51-21, p. 812):
  - Draw an imaginary line between the nipples. Find the sternum (breastbone).
  - Place both thumbs just below the imaginary line. The thumbs are side by side in the center of the chest. (Thumbs may overlap. The infant may be small. Or you may have large hands.)
  - Encircle the infant's chest with your hands.
  - Support the infant's back with your fingers. Use both hands.
  - Press down on the sternum with your thumbs. Squeeze the chest with your fingers. Press down at least ⅓ the depth of the chest (about 1½ inches).
- Release pressure and allow the chest to recoil after each compression.
- Give compressions at a rate of at least 100 per minute:
  - 1 rescuer—30 compressions followed by 2 breaths
  - 2 rescuers—15 compressions followed by 2 breaths
- Use the head tilt–chin lift method to open the airway. Often the tongue obstructs the airway when it falls into the throat (Fig. 51-22, p. 812).
  - Place one hand on the infant's forehead.
  - Use your palm to push the head back.
  - Place the fingers of your other hand under the bony part of the lower jaw. This is near the chin. Do not press in deep.
  - Use your fingers (not your thumb) to lift the jaw to bring the chin forward. The head should be in a neutral ("sniffing") position.
  - Do not close the infant's mouth completely.

Infants—cont'd

- Use the mouth-to-mouth-and-nose method to give breaths (Fig. 51-23, p. 813). This is the preferred method. Use the mouth-to-mouth method if you cannot cover the infant's nose and mouth with your mouth. To give mouth-to-mouth-and-nose breaths:
  - Keep the airway open with the head tilt–chin lift method.
  - Cover the infant's nose and mouth with your mouth. Make sure you have a tight seal.
  - Blow air into the infant's nose and mouth.
- Give 2 breaths that make the infant's chest rise. If a breath does not make the chest rise:
  - Try again to open the airway.
  - Give a breath. The breath should make the chest rise.
- Use an AED as soon as possible. Use child pads and a child system if possible.

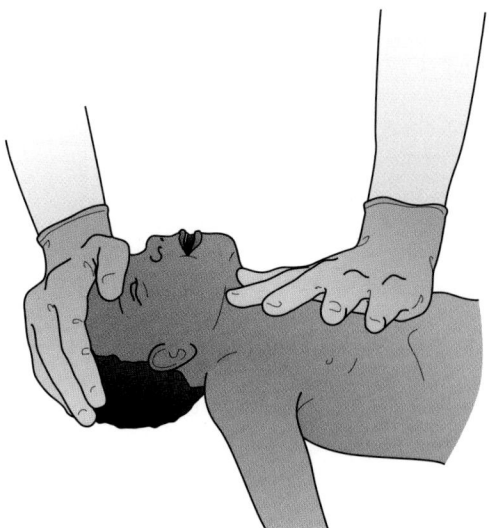

Fig. 51-18 The heel of one hand can be used for CPR if the child is very small. The fingers are off the chest.

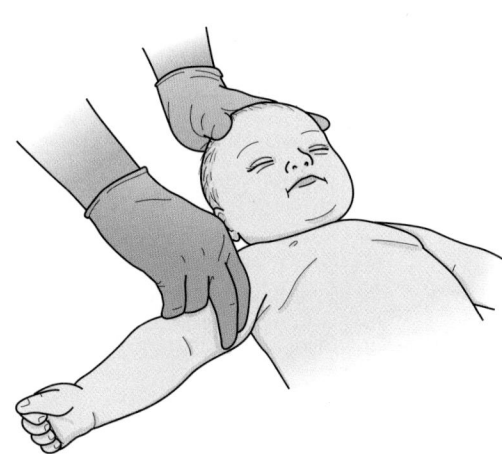

Fig. 51-19 Locating the infant's brachial pulse.

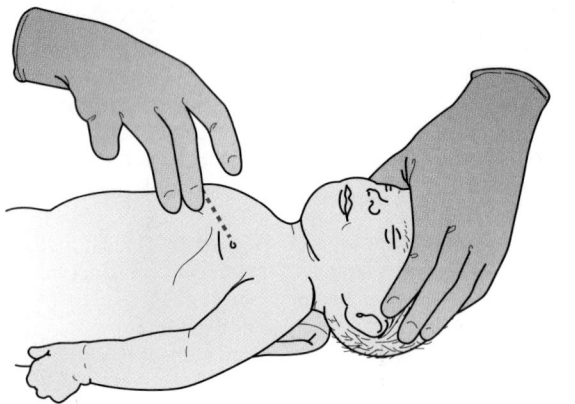

Fig. 51-20 Locating hand position for infant chest compressions. Draw an imaginary line between the nipples. Find the sternum (breastbone). Place 2 fingers on the sternum just below the imaginary line.

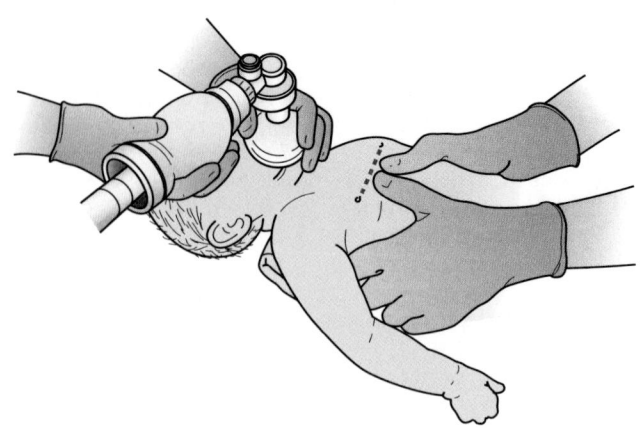

Fig. 51-21 The 2 thumb-encircling hands method for chest compressions.

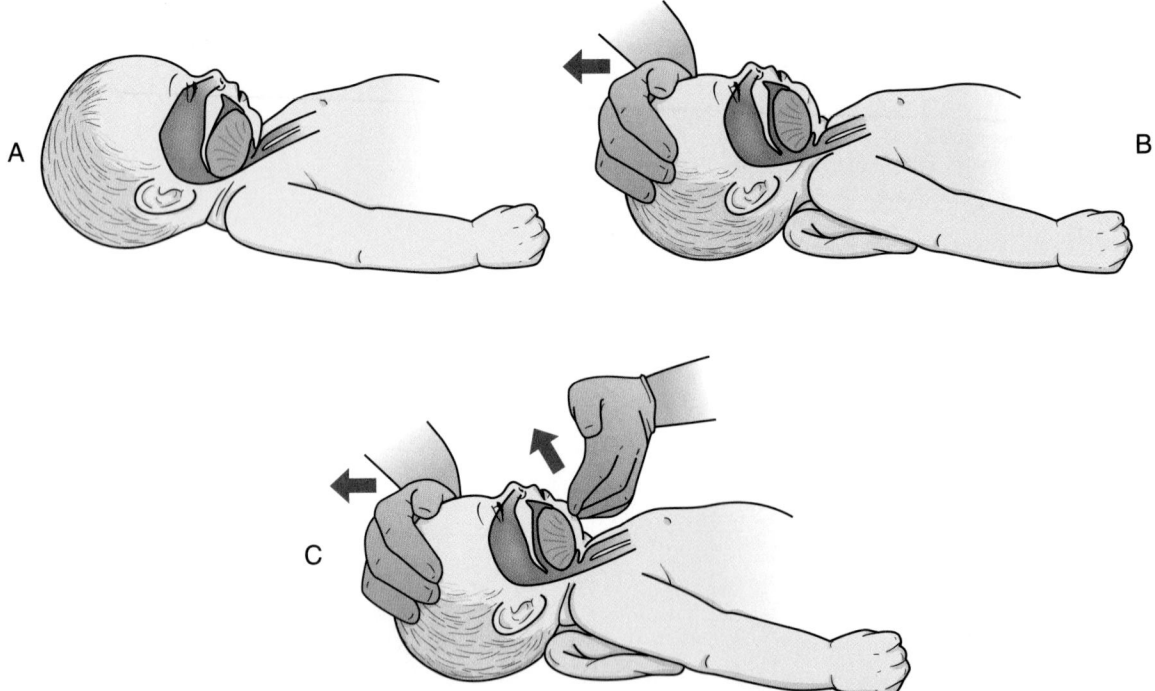

Fig. 51-22 The head tilt–chin lift method for infants. **A,** The tongue is at the back of the throat, obstructing the airway. **B,** One hand is on the infant's forehead. The palm is used to push the head back. **C,** The fingers of the other hand are under the bony part of the lower jaw. This is near the chin. The fingers are used to lift the jaw to bring the chin forward. The head is in a neutral ("sniffing") position.

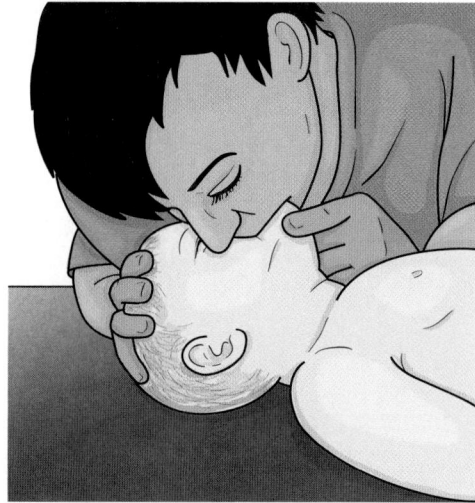

Fig. 51-23 Mouth-to-mouth-and-nose breathing. The infant's nose and mouth are covered to give breaths.

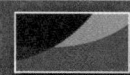 **CHILD CPR—ONE RESCUER**

PROCEDURE

1 Make sure the scene is safe.
2 Take 5 to 10 seconds to check for a response and breathing:
   a Check if the child is responding. Tap or gently shake the child. Call the child by name, if known. Shout, "Are you okay?"
   b Check for no breathing or no normal breathing (gasping).
3 Call for help if the child is not responding and not breathing or not breathing normally (gasping). If someone responds, ask the person to do the following. You do the following before beginning CPR if the arrest was sudden and witnessed:
   a Activate the EMS system or the agency's RRT.
   b Get an AED.
4 Position the child supine on a hard, flat surface. Logroll the child so there is no twisting of the spine. Place the arms alongside the body.
5 Check for a carotid pulse. This should take 5 to 10 seconds. Start CPR if you do not feel a pulse or if the pulse is less than 60 with signs of poor circulation.
6 Expose the child's chest.
7 Give chest compressions at a rate of at least 100 per minute. Push hard and fast. Establish a regular rhythm. Count out loud. Press down at least ⅓ the depth of the chest (about 2 inches). Allow the chest to recoil between compressions. Give 30 chest compressions.

8 Open the airway. Use the head tilt–chin lift method.
9 Give 2 breaths. Each breath should take only 1 second. Each breath must make the chest rise. If the first breath does not make the chest rise:
   a Open the airway again. Use the head tilt–chin lift method.
   b Give another breath.
10 Continue the cycle of 30 chest compressions followed by 2 breaths. Limit interruptions in compressions to less than 10 seconds.
11 Do the following after 5 cycles (2 minutes) of CPR if not already done:
   a Activate the EMS system or the agency's RRT.
   b Get a defibrillator (AED).
   c Use the AED.
12 See step 5 in the procedure: *Child CPR With AED—Two Rescuers,* p. 814.
   a Give 1 shock if advised. Then start CPR beginning with compressions.
   b If the rhythm is not shockable, start CPR beginning with compressions.
13 Check the rhythm after 5 cycles of CPR.
14 Continue CPR and use of the AED until help arrives or the child starts to move.

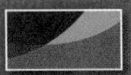 **Child CPR—Two Rescuers.** When two rescuers give child CPR, 15 compressions are given followed by 2 breaths. Use the following procedure if an AED is available.

Infant CPR. The guidelines and procedures for infant CPR differ from adult and child CPR. See Box 51-2.

CHILD CPR WITH AED—TWO RESCUERS

PROCEDURE

1 Make sure the scene is safe.
2 *Rescuer 1*—Take 5 to 10 seconds to check for a response and breathing:
  a Check if the child is responding. Tap or shake the child. Call the child by name if known. Shout, "Are you okay?"
  b Check for no breathing or no normal breathing (gasping).
3 *Rescuer 2:*
  a Activate the EMS system or the agency's RRT if the child is not responding and not breathing or not breathing normally (gasping).
  b Get a defibrillator (AED) if one is available.
4 *Rescuer 1:* Position the child supine on a hard, flat surface. Logroll the child so there is no twisting of the spine. Place the arms alongside the body. Begin 1-rescuer CPR until the second rescuer returns. (See procedure: *Child CPR—One Rescuer*, steps 5–10, p. 813.)
5 *Rescuer 2:*
  a Open the case with the AED.
  b Turn on the AED.
  c Apply child electrode pads if available. Or use the key or switch to change to the child setting. If neither is available, use the adult pads and settings. The pads must not touch or overlap. Follow the instructions and diagram provided with the AED.

  d Attach the connecting cables to the AED.
  e Clear away from the child. Make sure no one is touching the child.
  f Let the AED check the child's heart rhythm.
  g Make sure everyone is clear of the child if the AED advises a "shock." Loudly instruct others not to touch the child. Say: "I am clear, you are clear, everyone is clear!" Look to make sure no one is touching the child.
  h Press the "SHOCK" button if the AED advises a "shock."
6 *Rescuers 1 and 2:*
  a Perform 2-rescuer CPR:
    (1) Begin with compressions. One rescuer gives chest compressions at a rate of at least 100 per minute. Push hard and fast. Establish a regular rhythm. Count out loud. Allow the chest to recoil between compressions. Give 15 chest compressions. Pause to allow the other rescuer to give 2 breaths.
    (2) The other rescuer gives 2 breaths after every 15 chest compressions.
7 Repeat step 5, e, f, g, and h after 2 minutes of CPR (10 cycles of 15 compressions and 2 breaths). Change positions and continue CPR beginning with compressions.
8 Continue CPR and use of the AED until help arrives or the child starts to move.

INFANT CPR—ONE RESCUER

PROCEDURE

1 Make sure the scene is safe.
2 Take 5 to 10 seconds to check for a response and breathing:
  a Check if the infant is responding. Tap the infant's foot. Shout, "Are you okay?" (NOTE: Infants cannot answer you. However, shouting should startle the responsive infant.)
  b Check for no breathing or no normal breathing (gasping).
3 Call for help if the infant is not responding and not breathing or not breathing normally (gasping). If someone responds, ask the person to do the following. You do the following before beginning CPR if the arrest was sudden and witnessed:
  a Activate the EMS system or the agency's RRT.
  b Get a defibrillator (AED) if one is available.

4 Position the infant supine on a hard, flat surface.
5 Check for a brachial pulse. See Box 51-2 and Figure 51-19. This should take 5 to 10 seconds. Start CPR if you do not feel a pulse or if the pulse is less than 60 with signs of poor circulation.
6 Expose the infant's chest.
7 Place 2 fingers on the sternum just below the nipple line. See Box 51-2 and Figure 51-20. Give chest compressions at a rate of at least 100 per minute. Push hard and fast. Establish a regular rhythm. Count out loud. Press down at least $\frac{1}{3}$ the depth of the chest (about $1\frac{1}{2}$ inches). Allow the chest to recoil between compressions. Give 30 chest compressions.

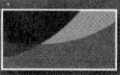 **INFANT CPR—ONE RESCUER—cont'd**

PROCEDURE—cont'd

8 Open the airway. Use the head tilt–chin lift method. The head should be in a neutral ("sniffing") position. See Box 51-2 and Figure 51-22.

9 Give 2 breaths. Each breath should take only 1 second. Each breath must make the chest rise. If the first breath does not make the chest rise:
   a Open the airway again. Use the head tilt–chin lift method.
   b Give another breath.

10 Continue the cycle of 30 chest compressions followed by 2 breaths. Limit interruptions in compressions to less than 10 seconds.

11 Do the following after 5 cycles (2 minutes) of CPR if not already done:
   a Activate the EMS system or the agency's RRT.
   b Get a defibrillator (AED).
   c Use the AED.

12 See step 5 in the procedure: *Infant CPR With AED—Two Rescuers.*
   a Give 1 shock if advised. Then start CPR beginning with compressions.
   b If the rhythm is not shockable, start CPR beginning with compressions.

13 Check the rhythm after 5 cycles of CPR.

14 Continue CPR and use of the AED until help arrives or the infant starts to move.

 **INFANT CPR WITH AED—TWO RESCUERS**

PROCEDURE

1 Make sure the scene is safe.

2 *Rescuer 1*—Take 5 to 10 seconds to check for a response and breathing:
   a Check if the infant is responding. Tap the infant's foot. Shout, "Are you okay?" (NOTE: Infants cannot answer you. However, shouting should startle the responsive infant.)
   b Check for no breathing or no normal breathing (gasping).

3 *Rescuer 2:*
   a Activate the EMS system or the agency's RRT if the infant is not responding and not breathing or not breathing normally (gasping).
   b Get a defibrillator (AED) if one is available.

4 *Rescuer 1:* Position the infant supine on a hard, flat surface. Begin 1-rescuer CPR until the second rescuer returns. (See procedure: *Infant CPR—One Rescuer*, steps 5–10.)

5 *Rescuer 2:*
   a Open the case with the AED.
   b Turn on the AED.
   c Apply child electrode pads if available. Or use the key or switch to change to the child setting. If neither is available, use the adult pads and settings. The pads must not touch or overlap. Follow the instructions and diagram provided with the AED.
   d Attach the connecting cables to the AED.

   e Clear away from the infant. Make sure no one is touching the infant.
   f Let the AED check the infant's heart rhythm.
   g Make sure everyone is clear of the infant if the AED advises a "shock." Loudly instruct others not to touch the infant. Say: "I am clear, you are clear, everyone is clear!" Look to make sure no one is touching the infant.
   h Press the "SHOCK" button if the AED advises a "shock."

6 *Rescuers 1 and 2:*
   a Perform 2-rescuer CPR:
      (1) Begin with compressions. One rescuer uses the 2 thumb-encircling hands method to give compressions at a rate of at least 100 per minute. See Box 51-2 and Figure 51-21. Push hard and fast. Establish a regular rhythm. Count out loud. Allow the chest to recoil between compressions. Give 15 chest compressions. Pause to allow the other rescuer to give 2 breaths.
      (2) The other rescuer gives 2 breaths after every 15 chest compressions.

7 Repeat step 5, e, f, g, and h after 2 minutes of CPR (10 cycles of 15 compressions and 2 breaths). Change positions and continue CPR beginning with compressions.

8 Continue CPR and use of the AED until help arrives or the infant starts to move.

CHOKING

Foreign bodies can obstruct the airway. This is called *choking* or *foreign-body airway obstruction (FBAO)*. Air cannot pass through the airways into the lungs. The body does not get enough oxygen. It can lead to cardiac arrest.

Airway obstruction can be mild or severe. With severe airway obstruction, air does not move in and out of the lungs. If the obstruction is not removed, the person will die. Abdominal thrusts are used to relieve severe airway obstruction. See Chapter 12 for emergency care of the choking person.

HEMORRHAGE

Life and body functions require an adequate blood supply. If a blood vessel is cut or torn, bleeding occurs. The larger the blood vessel, the greater the bleeding and blood loss. *Hemorrhage is the excessive loss of blood in a short time.* If bleeding is not stopped, the person will die.

Hemorrhage is internal or external. You cannot see internal hemorrhage. The bleeding is inside body tissues and body cavities. Pain, shock, vomiting blood, coughing up blood, and loss of consciousness signal internal hemorrhage. There is little you can do for internal bleeding.

- Follow the rules in Box 51-1. This includes activating the EMS system.
- Keep the person warm, flat, and quiet until help arrives.
- Do not give fluids.

If not hidden by clothing, external bleeding is usually seen. Bleeding from an artery occurs in spurts. There is a steady flow of blood from a vein. To control external bleeding:

- Follow the rules in Box 51-1. This includes activating the EMS system.
- Do not remove any objects that have pierced or stabbed the person.
- Elevate the affected part—hand, arm, foot, or leg.
- Place a sterile dressing directly over the wound. Or use any clean material (handkerchief, towel, cloth, or sanitary napkin).
- Apply pressure with your hand directly over the bleeding site (Fig. 51-24). Do not release pressure until the bleeding stops.
- If direct pressure does not control bleeding, apply pressure over the artery above the bleeding site (Fig. 51-25). For example, if bleeding is from the lower arm, apply pressure over the brachial artery.
- Bind the wound when bleeding stops. Tape or tie the dressing in place. You can tie the dressing with such things as clothing, a scarf, a necktie, or a belt.

See *Promoting Safety and Comfort: Hemorrhage.*

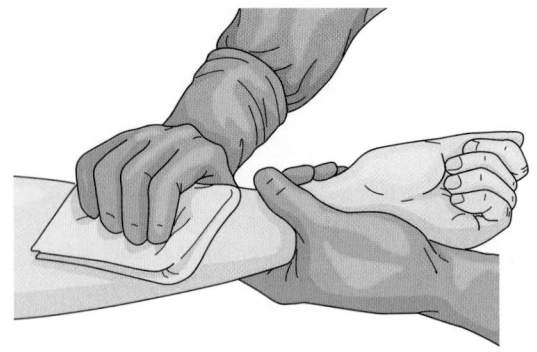

Fig. 51-24 Direct pressure is applied to the wound to stop bleeding.

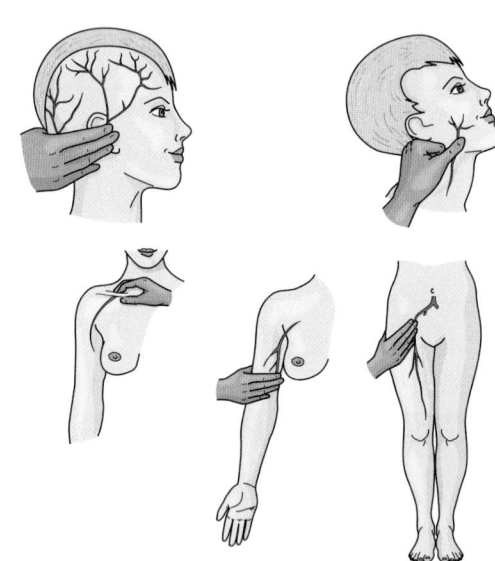

Fig. 51-25 Pressure points to control bleeding.

PROMOTING SAFETY AND COMFORT
Hemorrhage

Safety
Contact with blood is likely with hemorrhage. Follow Standard Precautions and the Bloodborne Pathogen Standard to the extent possible. Wear gloves if possible. Practice hand hygiene as soon as you can.

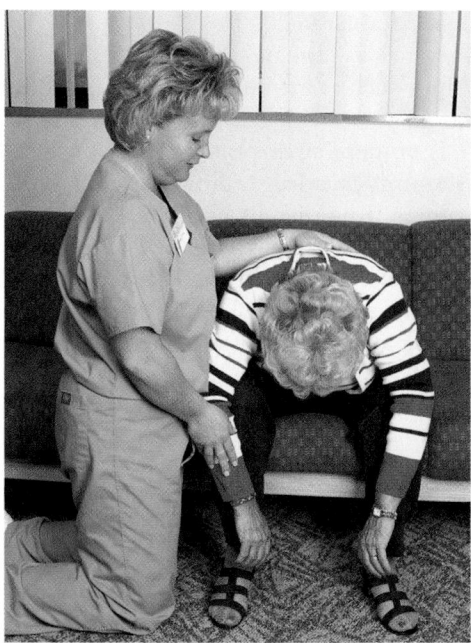

Fig. 51-26 The person bends forward and lowers her head between her knees to prevent fainting.

FAINTING

Fainting is the sudden loss of consciousness from an inadequate blood supply to the brain. Hunger, fatigue, fear, and pain are common causes. Some people faint at the sight of blood or injury. Standing in one position for a long time and being in a warm, crowded room are other causes. Dizziness, perspiration (sweating), and blackness before the eyes are warning signals. The person looks pale. The pulse is weak. Respirations are shallow if consciousness is lost. Emergency care includes the following:

* Have the person sit or lie down before fainting occurs.
* If sitting, the person bends forward and places the head between the knees (Fig. 51-26).
* If the person is lying down, raise the legs.
* Loosen tight clothing (belts, ties, scarves, collars, and so on).
* Keep the person lying down if fainting has occurred. Raise the legs.
* Do not let the person get up until symptoms have subsided for about 5 minutes.
* Help the person to a sitting position after recovery from fainting. Observe for fainting.

SHOCK

Shock results when organs and tissues do not get enough blood. Blood loss, heart attack (myocardial infarction), burns, and severe infection are causes. Signs and symptoms include:

* Low or falling blood pressure
* Rapid and weak pulse
* Rapid respirations
* Cold, moist, and pale skin
* Thirst
* Restlessness
* Confusion and loss of consciousness as shock worsens

Shock is possible in any person who is acutely ill or severely injured. Follow the rules in Box 51-1. Keep the person lying down, maintain an open airway, and control bleeding. Begin CPR if cardiac arrest occurs.

Anaphylactic Shock

Some people are allergic or sensitive to foods, insects, chemicals, and drugs. For example, many people are allergic to the drug *penicillin*. An *antigen* is a substance that the body reacts to. The body releases chemicals to fight or attack the antigen. The person may react with an area of redness, swelling, or itching. Or the reaction can involve the entire body.

Anaphylaxis is a life-threatening sensitivity to an antigen. (*Ana* means *without. Phylaxis* means *protection.*) The reaction can occur within seconds. Signs and symptoms include:

* Sweating
* Shortness of breath
* Low blood pressure
* Irregular pulse
* Respiratory congestion
* Swelling of the larynx (laryngeal edema)
* Hoarseness
* Dyspnea

Anaphylactic shock is an emergency. The EMS system must be activated. The person needs special drugs to reverse the allergic reaction. Keep the person lying down and the airway open. Start CPR if cardiac arrest occurs.

STROKE

Stroke (cerebrovascular accident) occurs when the brain is suddenly deprived of its blood supply (Chapter 41). Usually only part of the brain is affected. A stroke may be caused by a thrombus, an embolus, or hemorrhage if a blood vessel in the brain ruptures.

Signs of stroke vary (Chapter 41). They depend on the size and location of brain injury. Loss of consciousness or semi-consciousness, rapid pulse, labored respirations, high blood pressure, facial drooping, and hemiplegia (paralysis on one side of the body) are signs of a stroke. The person may have sudden confusion, numbness on one side of the body or in a body part, slurred speech, and aphasia (the inability to have normal speech). Loss of vision in one or both eyes, sudden and severe headache, unsteadiness, and falling also are signs. Seizures may occur.

Emergency care includes the following:
- Follow the rules in Box 51-1. This includes activating the EMS system.
- Find out when the symptoms began. Tell the EMS staff the time.
- Position the person in the recovery position (see Fig. 51-17).
- Raise the head without flexing the neck.
- Loosen tight clothing (belts, ties, scarves, collars, and so on).
- Keep the person quiet and warm.
- Reassure the person.
- Provide CPR if necessary.
- Provide emergency care for seizures if necessary.

SEIZURES

Seizures (convulsions) are violent and sudden contractions or tremors of muscle groups. Movements are uncontrolled. The person may lose consciousness. Seizures are caused by an abnormality in the brain. Causes include head injury during birth or from trauma, high fever, brain tumors, poisoning, and nervous system disorders or infections. Lack of blood flow to the brain, seizure disorders, and epilepsy are other causes.

Epilepsy

Epilepsy is a brain disorder in which clusters of nerve cells sometimes signal abnormally. There are brief changes in the brain's electrical function. The person can have strange sensations, emotions, and behavior. Sometimes there are seizures, muscle spasms, and loss of consciousness.

A single seizure does not mean epilepsy. In epilepsy, seizures recur. The person has a permanent brain injury or defect.

Children and young adults are commonly affected. However, epilepsy can develop at any time in a person's life. It can occur with any problem affecting the brain. Such causes include:
- Brain injury before, during, or after birth (Chapter 47)
- Problems with brain development before birth
- The mother having an injury or infection during pregnancy
- Head injury (accidents, gunshot wounds, sports injuries, falls, blows to the head)
- Poor nutrition
- Brain tumor

- Childhood fevers
- Poison—such as lead and alcohol
- Infection—such as meningitis and encephalitis
- Stroke

There is no cure at this time. Doctors order drugs to prevent seizures. The drugs control seizures in many people. For others, drug therapy does not work.

When controlled, epilepsy usually does not affect learning and activities of daily living. Activity and job limits occur in severe cases. For example, a person has seizures at any time. The person may not be allowed to drive. This may limit job choices. Also, the person is at risk for accidents and injuries. Safety measures are needed. They are needed for the home, workplace, transportation, and recreation.

Types of Seizures

The major types of seizures are:
- *Partial seizure.* Only one part of the brain is involved. A body part may jerk. Or the person has a hearing or vision problem or stomach discomfort. The person does not lose consciousness.
- *Generalized tonic-clonic seizure (grand mal seizure).* This type has two phases. In the *tonic phase*, the person loses consciousness. If standing or sitting, the person falls to the floor. The body is rigid because all muscles contract at once. The *clonic phase* follows. Muscle groups contract and relax. This causes jerking and twitching movements. Urinary and fecal incontinence may occur. A deep sleep is common after the seizure. Confusion and headache may occur on awakening.
- *Generalized absence (petit mal) seizure.* This type usually lasts a few seconds. There is loss of consciousness, twitching of the eyelids, and staring. No first aid is necessary. However, you should guide the person away from dangers—stairs, streets, a hot stove, fireplaces, and so on.

Emergency Care for Seizures

You cannot stop a seizure. However, you can protect the person from injury:
- Follow the rules in Box 51-1. This includes activating the EMS system.
- Do not leave the person alone.
- Lower the person to the floor. This protects the person from falling.
- Note the time the seizure started.
- Place something soft under the person's head (Fig. 51-27). It prevents the person's head from striking the floor. You can use a pillow, a cushion, or a folded blanket, towel, or jacket. Or cradle the person's head in your lap.

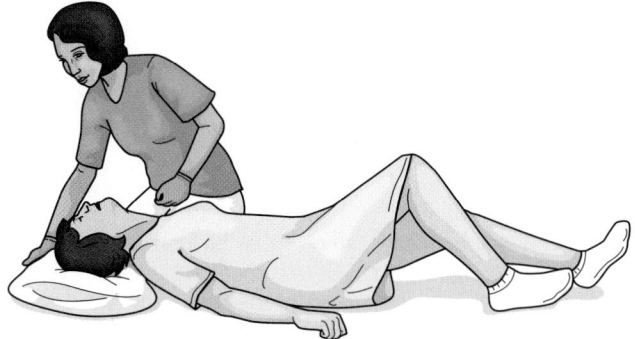

Fig. 51-27 A pillow protects the person's head during a seizure.

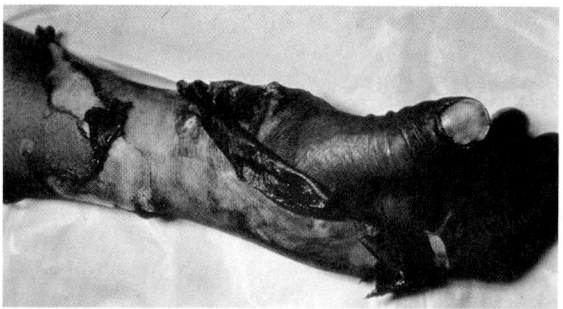

Fig. 51-28 Full thickness burn.

- Loosen tight jewelry and clothing around the person's neck. Ties, scarves, collars, and necklaces are examples.
- Turn the person onto his or her side. Make sure the head is turned to the side.
- Do not put any object or your fingers between the person's teeth. The person can bite down on your fingers during the seizure.
- Do not try to stop the seizure or control the person's movements.
- Move furniture, equipment, and sharp objects away from the person. He or she may strike these objects during the seizure.
- Note the time when the seizure ends.
- Make sure the mouth is clear of food, fluids, and saliva after the seizure.
- Provide BLS if the person is not breathing after the seizure.

BURNS

Burns can severely disable a person (Fig. 51-28). They can also cause death. Most burns occur in the home. Infants, children, and older persons are at risk. Common causes of burns and fires are:

- Scalds from hot liquids
- Playing with matches and lighters
- Electrical injuries (Fig. 51-29)
- Cooking accidents (barbecues, microwave ovens, stoves, ovens)
- Falling asleep while smoking
- Fireplaces
- Space heaters
- No smoke detectors or non-functioning smoke detectors
- Sunburn
- Chemicals

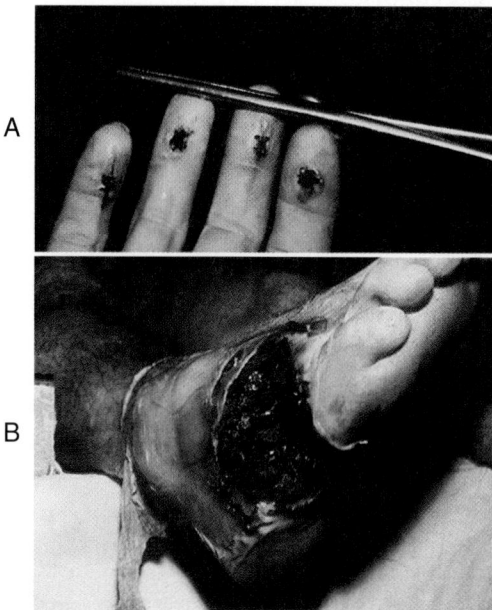

Fig. 51-29 An electrical burn. **A,** The electrical current enters through the hand. **B,** The electrical current exits through the foot.

The skin has two layers: the epidermis and dermis. Burns are described as:

- *Superficial (first degree) burns*—involve the epidermis only. They are painful, but the burn is not severe.
- *Partial thickness (second degree) burns*—involve the epidermis and part of the dermis. They are very painful. Nerve endings are exposed.
- *Full thickness (third degree) burns*—involve the entire epidermis and dermis. Fat, muscle, and bone may be injured or destroyed. These burns are not painful. Nerve endings are destroyed.

Some burns are minor; others are severe. Severity depends on burn size and depth, the body part involved, and the person's age. Burns to the face, eyes, ears, hands, and feet are more serious than burns to an arm or leg. Infants, young children, and older persons are at high risk for death.

Emergency care for severe burns includes the following:
- Follow the rules in Box 51-1. This includes activating the EMS system.
- Do not touch the person if he or she is in contact with an electrical source. Have the power source turned off, or remove the electrical source. Use an object that does not conduct electricity (rope or wood) to remove the electrical source.
- Remove the person from the fire or burn source.
- Stop the burning process. Put out flames with water or roll the person in a blanket. Or smother flames with a coat, sheet, or towel.
- Do not remove burned clothing.
- Remove hot clothing that is not sticking to the skin. If you cannot remove hot clothing, cool the clothing with water.
- Remove jewelry and any tight clothing that is not sticking to the skin.
- Provide rescue breathing and CPR as needed.
- Cover burns with sterile, cool, moist coverings. Or use towels, sheets, or any other clean cloth. Keep the covering wet.
- Do not put oil, butter, salve, or ointments on the burns.
- Cover the person with a blanket or coat to prevent heat loss.

FOCUS ON PRIDE

The Person, Family, and Yourself

Personal and Professional Responsibility

Having an understanding of emergency care is a professional responsibility. This knowledge allows you to safely assist in an emergency situation. This chapter includes basic information on emergency care. BLS courses for health care providers offer further training. The courses allow you to practice emergency procedures. CPR and the use of an AED are examples.

Most agencies require nursing assistants to be certified in BLS. Certification courses often involve a written and skills test. During the skills test, you demonstrate your ability to provide BLS. Take the course seriously. And take pride in receiving this training. What you learn can save a life.

Rights and Respect

During emergencies, protect the right to privacy. Do not expose the person unnecessarily. You may be in a place where you cannot close doors or window coverings. The person may be in a lounge, dining area, or public place. Do what you can to provide privacy. As always, treat the person with dignity and respect.

Independence and Social Interaction

Promoting quality of life and independence in an emergency is important. Choices may be few. However, they are given when possible. Hospital care may be required. The person has the right to choose a hospital.

Sometimes the person may want to refuse care. The EMS staff has guidelines to follow for persons refusing care. For example, the person must be competent and able to legally make his or her own medical decisions. The person must also be informed of the risks, benefits, and alternatives to the care recommended.

Delegation and Teamwork

Onlookers can threaten privacy and confidentiality. During an emergency, your main concern is the person's illness or injuries. You cannot give care and manage onlookers at the same time. Ask a team member to deal with onlookers. If someone else is giving care, keep onlookers away from the person. Take pride in working as a team to protect the person's privacy in an emergency situation.

Ethics and Laws

People are curious. They want to know what happened, the extent of injuries or illness, and if the person will be okay. Do not discuss the situation. Do not offer ideas of what is wrong with the person. Information about the person's care, treatment, and condition is confidential. Keep the person's information private. It is the right thing to do.

REVIEW QUESTIONS

Circle the BEST answer.

1 The goals of first aid are to
  a Call for help and keep the person warm
  b Prevent death and prevent injuries from becoming worse
  c Stay calm and give emergency care
  d Calm the person and keep bystanders away
2 When giving first aid, you should
  a Know your own limits
  b Move the person
  c Give the person fluids
  d Keep the person cool
3 Sudden cardiac arrest is
  a The same as stroke
  b The sudden stopping of heart action
  c The sudden loss of consciousness
  d When organs and tissues do not get enough blood
4 The signs of sudden cardiac arrest are
  a No response, no normal breathing, and no pulse
  b Restlessness, rapid breathing, and a weak pulse
  c Confusion, hemiplegia, and slurred speech
  d Dizziness, pale skin, and rapid breathing
5 Rescue breathing for an adult involves
  a Giving each breath over 2 seconds
  b Watching the abdomen rise with each breath
  c Giving a breath every 3 to 5 seconds
  d Giving a breath every 5 to 6 seconds

6 In adult CPR, the chest is compressed
   a 1½ inches with the index and middle fingers
   b 2 inches with the heel of one hand
   c At least 2 inches with two hands
   d At least 1 inch with two hands
7 When checking for breathing,
   a Use the head tilt–chin lift method to open the airway
   b Look for no breathing or gasping
   c Look, listen, and feel for air moving in and out of the lungs
   d Take 10 to 15 seconds to listen for breathing
8 Which pulse is used during adult CPR?
   a The apical pulse
   b The brachial pulse
   c The carotid pulse
   d The femoral pulse
9 Which compression rate is used for adult, child, and infant CPR?
   a At least 150 compressions per minute
   b At least 100 compressions per minute
   c At least 30 compressions per minute
   d At least 15 compressions per minute
10 When doing adult CPR,
   a Give 2 breaths after every 15 compressions
   b Give 2 breaths after every 30 compressions
   c Give 1 breath after every 5 compressions
   d Give 2 breaths when you are tired from giving compressions
11 Two rescuers are giving child CPR. Rescue breaths are given
   a After every compression
   b After every 5 compressions
   c After every 15 compressions
   d After every 30 compressions
12 Arterial bleeding
   a Cannot be seen
   b Oozes from the wound
   c Is dark red
   d Occurs in spurts
13 A person is hemorrhaging from the left forearm. Your first action is to
   a Lower the arm
   b Apply pressure to the brachial artery
   c Apply direct pressure to the wound
   d Tape a dressing in place

14 A person is about to faint. What should you do?
   a Take the person outside for fresh air.
   b Have the person sit or lie down.
   c Have the person stand very still.
   d Raise the head if the person is lying down.
15 Which is *not* a sign of shock?
   a High blood pressure
   b Rapid pulse
   c Rapid respirations
   d Cold, moist, and pale skin
16 A person in shock needs
   a Rescue breathing
   b To be kept lying down
   c Clothes removed
   d The recovery position
17 A person is having a stroke. Emergency care involves the following *except*
   a Asking when the person's symptoms began
   b Giving the person sips of water
   c Activating the EMS system
   d Keeping the person quiet and warm
18 These statements relate to tonic-clonic seizures. Which is *false*?
   a There is contraction of all muscles at once.
   b Incontinence may occur.
   c The seizure lasts 5 seconds.
   d There is loss of consciousness.
19 A person was burned. There are no complaints of pain. You know that
   a The burn is minor
   b The burn is partial thickness
   c The burn is full thickness
   d Nerve endings are exposed
20 Burns are covered with
   a A clean, moist cloth or dressing
   b Butter, oil, or salve
   c Water
   d Nothing

Answers to these questions are on p. 835.

52 End-of-Life Care

OBJECTIVES

- Define the key terms and key abbreviations listed in this chapter.
- Describe terminal illness.
- Describe the factors that affect attitudes about death.
- Describe how different age-groups view death.
- Describe the five stages of dying.
- Explain how to meet the needs of the dying person and family.
- Describe palliative care and hospice care.
- Explain the purpose of the Patient Self-Determination Act.
- Explain what is meant by a "Do Not Resuscitate" order.
- Identify the signs of approaching death and the signs of death.
- Explain how to assist with post-mortem care.
- Perform the procedure described in this chapter.
- Explain how to promote PRIDE in the person, the family, and yourself.

KEY TERMS

advance directive A document stating a person's wishes about health care when that person cannot make his or her own decisions

autopsy The examination of the body after death

end-of-life care The support and care given during the time surrounding death

palliative care Care that involves relieving or reducing the intensity of uncomfortable symptoms without producing a cure

post-mortem care Care of the body after (*post*) death (*mortem*)

reincarnation The belief that the spirit or soul is reborn in another human body or in another form of life

rigor mortis The stiffness or rigidity (*rigor*) of skeletal muscles that occurs after death (*mortis*)

terminal illness An illness or injury from which the person will not likely recover

KEY ABBREVIATIONS

DNR	Do Not Resuscitate
ID	Identification

OBRA	Omnibus Budget Reconciliation Act of 1987

End-of-life care *describes the support and care given during the time surrounding death.* Sometimes death is sudden. Often it is expected. Some people gradually fail. End-of-life care may involve days, weeks, or months.

According to the National Institute on Aging, most people die in hospitals or nursing centers. Hospice care is becoming a common option. Therefore the health team sees death often. Many team members are not sure of their feelings about death. Dying persons and the subject of death cause discomfort. Death and dying mean helplessness and failure to cure. They also remind us that our loved ones and we will die.

Your feelings about death affect the care you give. You will help meet the dying person's physical, psychological, social, and spiritual needs. Therefore you must understand the dying process. Then you can approach the dying person with caring, kindness, and respect.

See *Teamwork and Time Management: End-of-Life Care.*

TERMINAL ILLNESS

Many illnesses and diseases have no cure. The body cannot function after some injuries. Recovery is not expected. The disease or injury ends in death. *An illness or injury from which the person will not likely recover is a terminal illness.*

Doctors cannot predict the time of death. A person may have days, months, weeks, or years to live. People expected to live for a short time have lived for years. Others have died sooner than expected.

Modern medicine has found cures or has prolonged life in many cases. Research will bring new cures. However, hope and the will to live strongly influence living and dying. Many people have died for no apparent reason when they have lost hope or the will to live.

Types of Care

Persons with terminal illnesses can choose palliative care or hospice care. The person may opt for palliative care and then change to hospice care.

- *Palliative care. Palliate* means to *soothe* or *relieve. Palliative care involves relieving or reducing the intensity of uncomfortable symptoms without producing a cure.* The focus is on relief of symptoms. The illness also is treated. The intent is to improve the person's quality of life and provide family support. This care is for anyone with a long-term illness that will cause death. Settings include hospitals, nursing centers, and the person's home.
- *Hospice care.* The focus is on the physical, emotional, social, and spiritual needs of dying persons and their families (Chapter 1). Often the person has less than 6 months to live. Hospice care is not concerned with cure or life-saving measures. Pain relief and comfort are stressed. The goal is to improve quality of life. Hospitals, nursing centers, and home care agencies offer hospice care. Or a hospice may be a separate agency. Follow-up care and support groups for survivors are hospice services. Hospice also provides support for the health team to help deal with a person's death.

ATTITUDES ABOUT DEATH

Experiences, culture, religion, and age influence attitudes about death. Many people fear death. Others do not believe they will die. Some look forward to and accept death. Attitudes about death often change as a person grows older and with changing circumstances.

Dying people often need hospital, nursing center, hospice, or home care. The family is often involved in the person's care. They usually gather at the bedside to comfort the person and each other. When death occurs, the funeral director is called. The body is taken to the funeral home to prepare it for funeral practices.

Many adults and children have had no contact with a dying person. Nor have they been present at the time of death. Some have not attended a visitation (wake) or funeral. They have not seen the process of dying and death. Therefore it is frightening, morbid, and a mystery.

Culture and Spiritual Needs

Practices and attitudes about death differ among cultures. See *Caring About Culture: Death Rites*, p. 824. In some cultures, dying people are cared for at home by the family. Some families prepare the body for burial.

Spiritual needs relate to the human spirit and to religion and religious beliefs. They do not involve material or physical things. Rather they involve finding meaning in one's life. Some people need to resolve issues with family and friends. Many people strengthen their religious beliefs when dying. Religion provides comfort for the dying person and the family.

Attitudes about death are closely related to religion. Some believe that life after death is free of suffering and hardship. They also believe in reunion with loved ones. Many believe sins and misdeeds are punished in the afterlife. Others do not believe in the afterlife. To them, death is the end of life.

There also are religious beliefs about the body's form after death. Some believe the body keeps its physical form. Others believe that only the spirit or soul is present in the afterlife. *Reincarnation is the belief that the spirit or soul is reborn in another human body or in another form of life.*

Many religions practice rites and rituals during the dying process and at the time of death. Prayers, blessings, scripture readings, and religious music are common and sources of comfort. So are visits from a minister, priest, rabbi, or other cleric.

See *Focus on Communication: Culture and Spiritual Needs,* p. 824.

CARING ABOUT CULTURE
Death Rites

In *Vietnam*, dying persons are helped to recall past good deeds and to achieve a fitting mental state. Death at home is preferred. In some areas, a coin or jewels (a wealthy family) and rice (a poor family) are put in the dead person's mouth. This is from the belief that they will help the soul go through encounters with gods and devils and the soul will be born rich in the next life.

The *Chinese* have an aversion to death and anything concerning death. Autopsy and disposal of the body are not prescribed by religion. Donating body parts is encouraged. The eldest son makes all arrangements. The body is buried in a coffin. After 7 years, the body is exhumed and cremated. The urn, containing the ashes, is buried in the family tomb. White, yellow, or black clothing is worn for mourning.

In *India,* Hindu persons are often accepting of God's will. The person's desire to be clear-headed as death nears must be assessed in planning treatment. A time and place for prayer are essential for the family and the person. Prayer helps them deal with anxiety and conflict. The Hindu priest reads from Holy Sanskrit books. Some priests tie strings (meaning a blessing) around the neck or wrist. After death, the son pours water into the mouth of the deceased. Blood transfusions, organ transplants, and autopsies are allowed. Cremation is preferred.

From D'Avanzo CE: *Pocket guide to cultural health assessment,* ed 4, St Louis, 2008, Mosby.

FOCUS ON COMMUNICATION
Culture and Spiritual Needs

You may have different cultural or religious practices and beliefs about death. You must not judge the person by your standards. Do not make negative comments or insult the person's beliefs. Respect the person as a whole. This includes his or her beliefs and customs.

Age

Adults fear pain and suffering, dying alone, and the invasion of privacy. They also fear loneliness and separation from loved ones. They worry about the care and support of those left behind. Adults often resent death because it affects plans, hopes, dreams, and ambitions.

See *Focus on Children and Older Persons: Age.*

FOCUS ON CHILDREN AND OLDER PERSONS
Age

Children

Infants and toddlers do not understand the nature or meaning of death. They know or sense that something is different. They sense a caregiver's absence or a different caregiver. They also sense changes in when and how their needs are met. They may feel a sense of loss.

Between 2 and 6 years old, children think death is temporary. It can be reversed. The dead person continues to live and function in some ways and can come back to life. These ideas come from fairy tales, cartoons, movies, video games, and TV. For example, a cartoon character is injured and dies. Later the character comes back to life, whole and intact. Children this age often blame themselves when someone or something dies. To them, death is punishment for being bad. They know when family members or pets die. They notice dead birds or bugs. Answers to questions about death often cause fear and confusion. Children who are told "He is sleeping" may be afraid to go to sleep.

Between 6 and 11 years, children learn that death is final. They do not think that they will die. Death happens to others, especially adults. It can be avoided. Children relate death to punishment and body mutilation. It also involves witches, ghosts, goblins, and monsters.

By age 11, death is more fully understood. Death is still viewed as something that happens to other people. One's own death is an event in the distant future. Without correct information, they may have some wrong ideas. However, understanding increases as they grow older and have more experiences with death.

Older Persons

Older persons usually have fewer fears than younger adults. They know death will occur. They have had more experiences with dying and death. Many have lost family and friends. Some welcome death as freedom from pain, suffering, and disability. Death also means reunion with those who have died. Like younger adults, many fear dying alone.

THE STAGES OF DYING

Dr. Elisabeth Kübler-Ross described five stages of dying. They also are known as the "stages of grief." *Grief* is the person's response to loss.

- *Stage 1: Denial.* The person refuses to believe that he or she is dying. "No, not me" is a common response. The person believes a mistake was made. Information about the illness or injury is not heard. The person cannot deal with any problem or decision about the matter. This stage can last for a few hours, days, or much longer. Some people are still in denial when they die.

- *Stage 2: Anger.* The person thinks: "Why me?" There is anger and rage. Dying persons envy and resent those with life and health. Family, friends, and the health team are often targets of anger. The person blames others and finds fault with those who are loved and needed the most. It is hard to deal with the person during this stage. Anger is normal and healthy. Do not take the person's anger personally. Control any urge to attack back or avoid the person.
- *Stage 3: Bargaining.* Anger has passed. The person now says: "Yes, me, but. . . ." Often the person bargains with God or a higher power for more time. Promises are made in exchange for more time. The person may want to see a child marry, see a grandchild, have one more Christmas, or live for some other event. Usually more promises are made as the person makes "just one more" request. You may not see this stage. Bargaining is usually private and spiritual.
- *Stage 4: Depression.* The person thinks "Yes, me" and is very sad. The person mourns things that were lost and the future loss of life. The person may cry or say little. Sometimes the person talks about people and things that will be left behind.
- *Stage 5: Acceptance.* The person is calm and at peace. The person has said what needs to be said. Unfinished business is completed. The person accepts death. This stage may last for many months or years. Reaching the acceptance stage does not mean death is near.

Dying persons do not always pass through all five stages. A person may never get beyond a certain stage. Some move back and forth between stages. For example, Mr. Jones reached acceptance but moves back to bargaining. Then he moves forward to acceptance. Some people stay in one stage.

COMFORT NEEDS

Comfort is a basic part of end-of-life care. It involves physical, mental and emotional, and spiritual needs. For spiritual needs, see "Culture and Spiritual Needs" on p. 823. Comfort goals are to:

- Prevent or relieve suffering to the extent possible.
- Respect and follow end-of-life wishes.

Dying persons may want family and friends present. They may want to talk about their fears, worries, and anxieties. Some want to be alone. Often they need to talk during the night. Things are quiet, distractions are few, and there is more time to think. You need to listen and use touch.

- *Listening.* The person needs to talk and share worries and concerns. Let the person express feelings and emotions in his or her own way. Do not worry about saying the wrong thing or finding comforting words. You do not need to say anything. Being there for the person is what counts.
- *Touch.* Touch shows care and concern when words cannot. Sometimes the person does not want to talk but needs you nearby. Do not feel that you need to talk. Silence, along with touch, is a powerful and meaningful way to communicate.

Some people may want to see a spiritual leader. Or they want to take part in religious practices. Provide privacy during prayer and spiritual moments. Be courteous to the spiritual leader. The person has the right to have religious objects nearby—medals, pictures, statues, writings, and so on. Handle these valuables with care and respect.

See *Focus on Communication: Comfort Needs.*
See *Focus on Children and Older Persons: Comfort Needs.*

FOCUS ON COMMUNICATION
Comfort Needs

You may not know what to say to the dying person. That is hard for many experienced health team members. Unless you have been near death yourself, do not say: "I understand what you are going through." The statement is a communication barrier. Instead you can say:

- "Would you like to talk? I have time to listen."
- "You seem sad. How can I help?"
- "Is it okay if I quietly sit with you for a while?"

FOCUS ON CHILDREN AND OLDER PERSONS
Comfort Needs

Older Persons

Persons with Alzheimer's disease (AD) become more and more disabled. Those with advanced AD cannot share their concerns, discomforts, or problems. And it is hard to provide emotional and spiritual comfort.

Focusing on the person's senses—hearing, touch, sight—can promote comfort. Comforting touch or massage can be soothing. So can soft music or sounds from nature—birds chirping, gentle breezes, ocean waves, and so on.

Physical Needs

Dying may take a few minutes, hours, days, or weeks. Body processes slow. The person is weak. Changes occur in levels of consciousness. To the extent possible, independence is allowed. As the person weakens, basic needs are met. The person may depend on others for basic needs and activities of daily living. Every effort is made to promote physical and psychological comfort. The person is allowed to die in peace and with dignity.

Pain. Some dying persons do not have pain. Others may have severe pain. Always report signs and symptoms of pain at once (Chapter 28). Pain management is important. The nurse can give pain-relief drugs. Preventing and controlling pain is easier than relieving pain.

Skin care, personal and oral hygiene, back massages, and good alignment promote comfort. So do frequent position changes and supportive devices. Turn the person slowly and gently. Follow the care plan to prevent and control pain.

Breathing Problems. Shortness of breath and difficulty breathing (dyspnea) are common end-of-life problems. Semi-Fowler's position and oxygen (Chapter 36) are helpful. An open window for fresh air may help some people. For others, a fan circulating air is helpful.

Noisy breathing—called the *death rattle*—is common as death nears. This is due to mucus collecting in the airway. These may help:

- The side-lying position
- Suctioning by the nurse
- Drugs to reduce the amount of mucus

Vision, Hearing, and Speech. Vision blurs and gradually fails. The person turns toward light. A darkened room may frighten the person. The eyes may be half-open. Secretions may collect in the eye corners.

Because of failing vision, explain who you are and what you are doing to the person or in the room. The room should be well lit. However, avoid bright lights and glares.

Good eye care is needed (Chapter 20). If the eyes stay open, a nurse may apply a protective ointment. Then the eyes are covered with moist pads to prevent injury.

Hearing is one of the last functions lost. Many people hear until the moment of death. Even unconscious persons may hear. Always assume that the person can hear. Speak in a normal voice. Provide reassurance and explanations about care. Offer words of comfort. Avoid topics that could upset the person. Do not talk about the person.

Speech becomes harder. It may be hard to understand the person. Sometimes the person cannot speak. Anticipate the person's needs. Do not ask questions needing long answers. Ask "yes" or "no" questions. These should be few in number. Despite speech problems, you must talk to the person.

Mouth, Nose, and Skin. Oral hygiene promotes comfort. Give routine mouth care if the person can eat and drink. Give frequent oral hygiene as death nears and when taking oral fluids is difficult. Oral hygiene is needed if mucus collects in the mouth and the person cannot swallow. A lip balm may help dry lips.

Crusting and irritation of the nostrils can occur. Nasal secretions, an oxygen cannula, and a naso-gastric tube are common causes. Carefully clean the nose. Apply lubricant as directed by the nurse and the care plan.

Circulation fails and body temperature rises as death nears. The skin is cool, pale, and mottled (blotchy). Perspiration increases. Skin care, bathing, and preventing pressure ulcers are necessary. Linens and gowns are changed as needed. Although the skin feels cool, only light bed coverings are needed. Blankets may make the person feel warm and cause restlessness. However, observe for signs of cold. Shivering, hunching the shoulders, and pulling covers up may signal that the person is cold. Prevent drafts and provide more blankets.

Nutrition. Nausea, vomiting, and loss of appetite are common at the end of life. The doctor can order drugs for nausea and vomiting.

Some persons are too tired or too weak to eat. You may need to feed them. Favorite foods may help loss of appetite. So may small, frequent meals.

As death nears, loss of appetite is common. The person may choose not to eat or drink. Do not force the person to eat or drink. Doing so may add to discomfort. Report refusal to eat or drink to the nurse.

Elimination. Urinary and fecal incontinence may occur. Use incontinence products or bed protectors as directed. Give perineal care as needed. Constipation and urinary retention are common. Enemas and catheters may be needed. Follow the care plan for catheter care.

The Person's Room. Provide a comfortable and pleasant room. It should be well lit and well ventilated. Remove unnecessary equipment. Some equipment is upsetting to look at (suction machines, drainage containers). If possible, keep these items out of the person's sight.

Mementos, pictures, cards, flowers, and religious items provide comfort. Arrange them within the person's view. The person and family arrange the room as they wish. This helps meet love, belonging, and esteem needs. The room should reflect the person's choices.

Mental and Emotional Needs

Mental and emotional needs are very personal. Some persons are anxious or depressed. Others have specific fears and concerns. Examples include:

- Severe pain
- When and how death will occur
- What will happen to loved ones
- Dying alone

The doctor may order drugs for anxiety or depression. Simple measures may soothe the person—touch, holding a hand, back massage, soft lighting, music at a low volume.

THE FAMILY

This is a hard time for the family. You may find it hard to find comforting words. To show you care, be available, courteous, and considerate. Use touch to show your concern.

Family members usually can stay as long as they wish. Sometimes they keep a *vigil*. That is, someone is with the person at all times including at night. They watch over or pray for the person. Help make them as comfortable as possible.

Respect the right to privacy. The person and family need time together. However, do not neglect care because the family is present. Most agencies let family members help give care. Or you can suggest that they take a break for a beverage or meal.

The family may be very tired, sad, and tearful. Watching a loved one die is very painful. So is dealing with the eventual loss of that person. The family goes through stages like the dying person. They need support, understanding, courtesy, and respect. A spiritual leader may provide comfort. Communicate this request to the nurse at once.

LEGAL ISSUES

Much attention is given to the right to die. Many people do not want machines or other measures keeping them alive. Consent is needed for any treatment. When able, the person makes care decisions. Some people make end-of-life wishes known.

The Patient Self-Determination Act

The Patient Self-Determination Act and the Omnibus Budget Reconciliation Act of 1987 (OBRA) give persons the right to accept or refuse treatment. They also give the right to make advance directives. An *advance directive is a document stating a person's wishes about health care when that person cannot make his or her own decisions.* It lets others know the type of care he or she wants if seriously ill or dying. Advance directives usually forbid certain care if there is no hope of recovery. Living wills and durable power of attorney for health care are common advance directives.

These laws protect quality of care. Quality of care cannot be less because of the person's advance directives.

Agencies must inform all persons of the right to advance directives on admission. This information is in writing. The medical record documents whether or not the person has made them.

Living Wills. A living will is about measures that support or maintain life when death is likely. Tube feedings, ventilators, and resuscitation are examples. A living will may instruct doctors:

- Not to start measures that prolong dying
- To remove measures that prolong dying

Durable Power of Attorney for Health Care. This advance directive gives the power to make health care decisions to another person. That person is often called a *health care proxy.* Usually this is a family member, friend, or lawyer. When a person cannot make health care decisions, the health care proxy can do so. This advance directive does not cover property or financial matters.

"Do Not Resuscitate" Orders

When death is sudden and unexpected, efforts are made to save the person's life. See Chapter 51.

For terminally ill persons, doctors often write "Do Not Resuscitate" (DNR) or "No Code" orders. The person will not be resuscitated. The person is allowed to die with peace and dignity. The orders are written after consulting with the person and family. The family and doctor make the decision if the person is not mentally able to do so. Some advance directives address resuscitation.

You may not agree with care and resuscitation decisions. However, you must follow the person's or family's wishes and the doctor's orders. These may be against your personal, religious, and cultural values. If so, discuss the matter with the nurse. You may need an assignment change.

SIGNS OF DEATH

In the weeks before death, the following may occur:

- Restlessness and agitation
- Shortness of breath; pauses in breathing
- Depression
- Anxiety
- Drowsiness
- Confusion
- Constipation or incontinence
- Nausea and loss of appetite
- Healing problems
- Swelling in the hands, feet, or other body areas

As death nears, these signs may occur fast or slowly:

- Movement, muscle tone, and sensation are lost. This usually starts in the feet and legs. When mouth muscles relax, the jaw drops. The mouth may stay open. The facial expression is often peaceful.
- Peristalsis and other gastro-intestinal functions slow down. Abdominal distention, fecal incontinence, nausea, and vomiting are common.
- Body temperature rises. The person feels cool or cold, looks pale, and perspires heavily.
- Circulation fails. The pulse is fast or slow, weak, and irregular. Blood pressure starts to fall.
- The respiratory system fails. Slow or rapid and shallow respirations are observed. Mucus collects in the airway. Breathing sounds are noisy and gurgling—commonly called the *death rattle.*
- Pain decreases as the person loses consciousness. However, some people are conscious until the moment of death.

The signs of death include no pulse, no respirations, and no blood pressure. The pupils are fixed and dilated. A doctor determines that death has occurred. He or she pronounces the person dead. The cause, time, and place are noted for the death certificate.

CARE OF THE BODY AFTER DEATH

Care of the body after (post) *death* (mortem) *is called post-mortem care.* You may be asked to assist the nurse. Post-mortem care begins when the doctor pronounces the person dead.

Post-mortem care is done to maintain a good appearance of the body. Discoloration and skin damage are prevented. Valuables and personal items are gathered for the family. The right to privacy and the right to be treated with dignity and respect apply after death.

Within 2 to 4 hours after death, rigor mortis develops. *Rigor mortis is the stiffness or rigidity* (rigor) *of skeletal muscles that occurs after death* (mortis). The body is positioned in normal alignment before rigor mortis sets in. The family may want to see the body. The body should appear in a comfortable and natural position.

In some agencies, the body is prepared for viewing only by the family. The funeral director completes post-mortem care.

Sometimes an autopsy is done. An *autopsy is the examination of the body after death.* (*Autos* means *self. Opsis* means *view.*) It is done to determine the cause of death. The coroner or medical examiner can order an autopsy. Or the family can request one. Follow agency procedures for an autopsy. Post-mortem care is not done. Doing so could remove or destroy evidence.

Post-mortem care involves moving the body. For example, soiled areas are bathed and the body is placed in good alignment. Moving the body can cause remaining air in the lungs, stomach, and intestines to be expelled. When air is expelled, sounds are produced. Do not let these sounds alarm or frighten you. They are normal and expected.

See *Delegation Guidelines: Care of the Body After Death.*

See *Promoting Safety and Comfort: Care of the Body After Death.*

DELEGATION GUIDELINES

Care of the Body After Death

To assist with post-mortem care, you need this information from the nurse:

- If dentures are inserted or placed in a denture cup
- If tubes and dressings are removed or left in place
- If rings are removed or left in place
- If the family wants to view the body
- Special agency policies and procedures

PROMOTING SAFETY AND COMFORT

Care of the Body After Death

Safety

Standard Precautions and the Bloodborne Pathogen Standard are followed. You may have contact with blood, body fluids, secretions, or excretions.

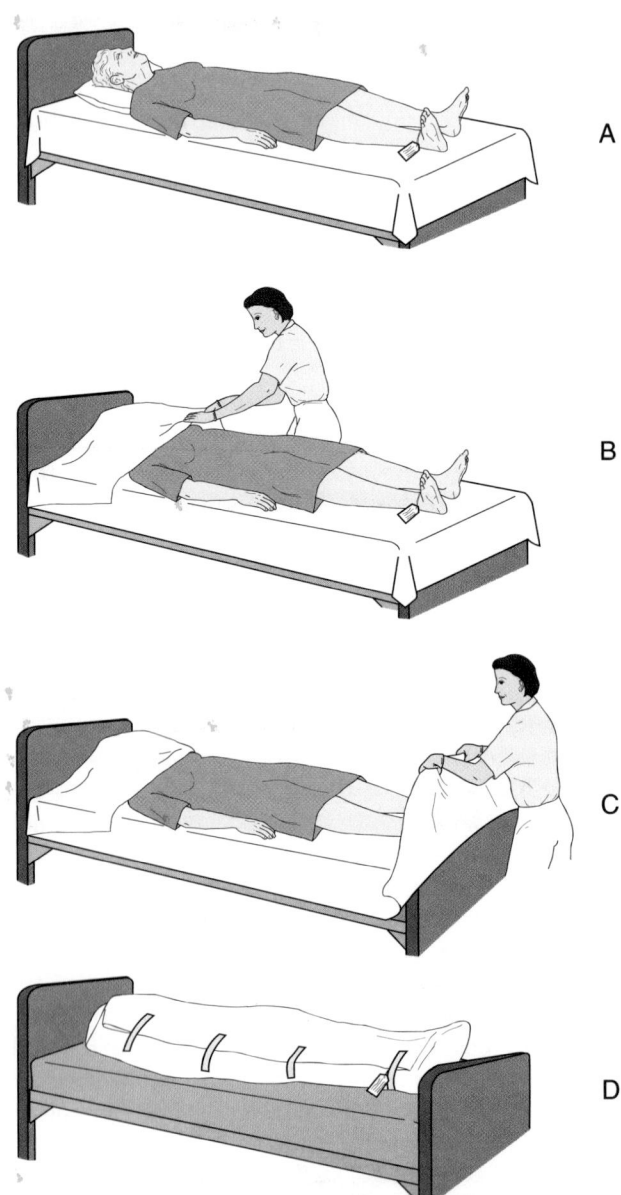

Fig. 52-1 Applying a shroud. **A,** Position the shroud under the body. **B,** Bring the top of the shroud down over the head. **C,** Fold the bottom up over the feet. **D,** Fold the sides over the body. Tape or pin the sides together. Attach the ID tag.

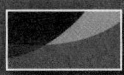 **ASSISTING WITH POST-MORTEM CARE**

PRE-PROCEDURE

1 Follow *Delegation Guidelines: Care of the Body After Death.* See *Promoting Safety and Comfort: Care of the Body After Death.*
2 Practice hand hygiene.
3 Collect the following:
   • Post-mortem kit (shroud or body bag, gown, ID [identification] tags, gauze squares, safety pins)
   • Bed protectors
   • Wash basin
   • Bath towel and washcloths
   • Denture cup
   • Tape
   • Dressings
   • Gloves
   • Cotton balls
   • Valuables envelope
4 Provide for privacy.
5 Raise the bed for body mechanics.
6 Make sure the bed is flat.

PROCEDURE

7 Put on the gloves.
8 Position the body supine. Arms and legs are straight. A pillow is under the head and shoulders. Or raise the head of the bed 15 to 20 degrees if this is agency policy.
9 Close the eyes. Gently pull the eyelids over the eyes. Apply moist cotton balls gently over the eyelids if the eyes will not stay closed.
10 Insert dentures if it is agency policy to do so. If not, put them in a labeled denture cup.
11 Close the mouth. If necessary, place a rolled towel under the chin to keep the mouth closed.
12 Follow agency policy for jewelry. Remove all jewelry, except for wedding rings if this is agency policy. List the jewelry that you removed. Place the jewelry and the list in a valuables envelope.
13 Place a cotton ball over the rings. Tape them in place.
14 Remove drainage containers.
15 Remove tubes and catheters. Use the gauze squares as needed.
16 Bathe soiled areas with plain water. Dry thoroughly.
17 Place a bed protector under the buttocks.
18 Remove soiled dressings. Replace them with clean ones.
19 Put a clean gown on the body. Position the body as in step 8.
20 Brush and comb the hair if necessary.
21 Cover the body to the shoulders with a sheet if the family will view the body.
22 Gather the person's belongings. Put them in a bag labeled with the person's name. Make sure you include eyeglasses, hearing aids, and other valuables.
23 Remove supplies, equipment, and linens. Straighten the room. Provide soft lighting.
24 Remove and discard the gloves. Practice hand hygiene.
25 Let the family view the body. Provide for privacy. Return to the room after they leave.
26 Practice hand hygiene. Put on gloves.
27 Fill out the ID tags. Tie one to the ankle or to the right big toe.
28 Place the body in the body bag or cover it with a sheet. Or apply the shroud (Fig. 52-1).
   a Position the shroud under the body.
   b Bring the top down over the head.
   c Fold the bottom up over the feet.
   d Fold the sides over the body.
   e Pin or tape the shroud in place.
29 Attach the second ID tag to the shroud, sheet, or body bag.
30 Leave the denture cup with the body.
31 Pull the privacy curtain around the bed. Or close the door.

POST-PROCEDURE

32 Remove and discard the gloves. Practice hand hygiene.
33 Strip the unit after the body has been removed. Wear gloves for this step.
34 Remove and discard the gloves. Practice hand hygiene.
35 Report the following:
   • The time the body was taken by the funeral director
   • What was done with jewelry, other valuables, and personal items
   • What was done with dentures

FOCUS ON PRIDE

The Person, Family, and Yourself

Personal and Professional Responsibility

You may assist with the dying person's care. To give quality care:

- Promote comfort. Report the person's complaints or signs of pain to the nurse at once. Follow the comfort measures in the care plan.
- Protect the person's privacy.
- Provide support to the person and family. Be kind. Show compassion and respect.
- Offer the family time alone with the person.
- Take pride in supporting the person and family during a difficult time.

Rights and Respect

A person has the right to die in peace and with dignity. Box 52-1 contains the dying person's bill of rights. Respect the person's last rights.

Independence and Social Interaction

The person is encouraged to take part in his or her care to the extent possible. Some days the person can do more than on other days. Follow the nurse's directions and the care plan. Do not force the person to do more than he or she can physically or mentally do.

Delegation and Teamwork

Over time, the health team often bonds with the person. This is common in hospice and long-term care. The person's death is difficult for the staff. Sadness and grief may occur.

Tell the nurse if you have trouble coping with a person's death. Support others who need help. A kind word, a hug, or taking time to listen show concern. Take pride in being a part of a caring and supportive team.

Ethics and Laws

The dying person has rights under OBRA:

- *The right to privacy before and after death.* The person has the right not to have his or her body seen by others. Proper draping and screening are important.
- *The right to visit others in private.* If the person is too weak to leave the room, the roommate may have to do so. The nurse and social worker develop a plan that satisfies everyone. Moving the dying person to a private room provides privacy. The family can also stay as long as they like.
- *The right to confidentiality before and after death.* The final moments and cause of death are kept confidential. So are statements, conversations, and family reactions.
- *The right to be free from abuse, mistreatment, and neglect.* The person has the right to receive kind and respectful care before and after death. Report signs of abuse, mistreatment, or neglect to the nurse at once.
- *Freedom from restraint.* Restraints are used only if ordered by the doctor. Dying persons are often too weak to be dangerous to themselves or others.
- *The right to have personal possessions.* The person may want photos and religious items nearby. Protect the person's property from loss or damage before and after death. They may be family treasures or mementos.
- *The right to a safe and home-like setting.* Dying persons depend on others for safety. Everyone must keep the setting safe and home-like. The center is the person's home. Try to keep equipment and supplies out of view. The room also should be free from unpleasant odors and noises. Do your best to keep the room neat and clean.
- *The right to personal choice.* The person has the right to be involved in treatment and care. The dying person may refuse treatment. Advance directives are common. The health team must respect choices to refuse treatment or not prolong life.

BOX 52-1	A DYING PATIENT'S BILL OF LAST RIGHTS

- *The Right to BE IN CONTROL.* Grant me the right to make as many decisions as possible regarding my care. Please do not take choices from me. Let me make my own decisions.
- *The Right to HAVE A SENSE OF PURPOSE.* I have lost my job. I can no longer fulfill my role in my family. Please help me find some sense of purpose in my last days.
- *The Right to REMINISCE.* There has been pleasure in my life, moments of pride, moments of love. Please give some time to recollect those moments. And please listen to my recollections.
- *The Right to TOUCH AND BE TOUCHED.* Sometimes I need distance. Yet sometimes I have a strong need to be close. When I want to reach out, please come to me and hold me as I hold you.
- *The Right to LAUGH.* People often—far too often—come to me wearing masks of seriousness. Although I am dying, I still need to laugh. Please laugh with me and help others to laugh as well.
- *The Right to BE ANGRY AND SAD.* It is difficult to leave behind all my attachments and all that I love. Please allow me the opportunity to be angry and sad.
- *The Right to HAVE A RESPECTED SPIRITUALITY.* Whether I am questioning or affirming, doubting or praising, I sometimes need your ear, a non-judging ear. Please let my spirit travel its own journey, without judging its direction.
- *The Right to HEAR THE TRUTH.* If you withhold the truth from me, you will treat me as if I am no longer living. I am still living, and I need to know the truth about my life. Please help me find that truth.
- *The Right to BE IN DENIAL.* If I hear the truth and choose not to accept it, that is my right.

Honor these Rights. One day you too will want the same Rights.

Modified from *The Hospice RN: Patient's bill of rights: a dying patient's bill of last rights.*

REVIEW QUESTIONS

Circle the BEST answer.

1 Which is *true*?
   a Death from terminal illness is sudden.
   b Doctors know when death will occur.
   c An illness is terminal when recovery is not likely.
   d All severe injuries end in death.

2 These statements relate to attitudes about death. Which is *false*?
   a Dying people are often cared for in health care agencies.
   b Religion influences attitudes about death.
   c Infants and toddlers understand death.
   d Young children often blame themselves when someone dies.

3 Reincarnation is the belief that
   a There is no afterlife
   b The spirit or soul is reborn into another human body or another form of life
   c The body keeps its physical form in the afterlife
   d Only the spirit or soul is present in the afterlife

4 A 5-year-old views death as
   a Temporary
   b Final
   c Adults do
   d Going to sleep

5 Adults and older persons usually fear
   a Dying alone
   b Reincarnation
   c The five stages of dying
   d Advance directives

6 Persons in the stage of denial
   a Are angry
   b Are calm and at peace
   c Are sad and quiet
   d Refuse to believe they are dying

7 A person tries to gain more time during the stage of
   a Anger
   b Bargaining
   c Depression
   d Acceptance

8 When caring for the dying person, you should
   a Use touch and listen
   b Do most of the talking
   c Keep the room darkened
   d Speak in a loud voice

9 As death nears, the last sense lost is
   a Sight
   b Taste
   c Smell
   d Hearing

10 The dying person's care includes the following *except*
   a Eye care
   b Mouth care
   c Active range-of-motion exercises
   d Position changes

11 The dying person is positioned in
   a The supine position
   b The Fowler's position
   c Good body alignment
   d The dorsal recumbent position

12 A "DNR" order means that
   a CPR will not be done
   b The person has a living will
   c Life-prolonging measures will be carried out
   d The person is kept alive as long as possible

13 Which are *not* signs of approaching death?
   a Increased body temperature and rapid pulse
   b Loss of movement and muscle tone
   c Increased pain and blood pressure
   d Slow or rapid and shallow respirations

14 The signs of death are
   a Convulsions and incontinence
   b No pulse, respirations, or blood pressure
   c Loss of consciousness and convulsions
   d The eyes stay open, no muscle movements, and the body is rigid

15 Post-mortem care is done
   a After rigor mortis sets in
   b After the doctor pronounces the person dead
   c When the funeral director arrives for the body
   d After the family has viewed the body

Answers to these questions are on p. 835.

REVIEW QUESTION ANSWERS

CHAPTER 1
1 d
2 b
3 a
4 b
5 b
6 a
7 a
8 a
9 b
10 a
11 a
12 a
13 c
14 d

CHAPTER 2
1 a
2 d
3 b
4 b
5 c
6 d
7 b
8 a
9 a
10 a
11 b
12 a
13 d
14 d
15 b
16 a
17 b
18 d
19 F
20 T
21 T
22 F
23 F
24 T
25 F
26 T
27 F
28 F

CHAPTER 3
1 b
2 c
3 c
4 d
5 c
6 b
7 c
8 c

9 c
10 b
11 a
12 a
13 b
14 c
15 b

CHAPTER 4
1 b
2 c
3 d
4 a
5 b
6 c
7 d
8 a
9 d
10 c
11 b
12 a
13 d
14 b
15 d
16 a
17 a
18 a
19 b
20 a
21 c
22 b
23 c
24 c

CHAPTER 5
1 T
2 T
3 F
4 T
5 T
6 T
7 F
8 F
9 T
10 F
11 c
12 c
13 a
14 d
15 b
16 d
17 c
18 b
19 c
20 d

21 c
22 b
23 a
24 a
25 b
26 d
27 d
28 c
29 a
30 a
31 d
32 d

CHAPTER 6
1 F
2 F
3 T
4 F
5 F
6 F
7 a
8 c
9 d
10 a
11 c
12 c
13 d
14 d
15 b
16 b
17 d
18 a
19 d
20 b

CHAPTER 7
1 a
2 d
3 b
4 c
5 d
6 b
7 a
8 c
9 c
10 b
11 c
12 d

CHAPTER 8
1 c
2 d
3 b
4 a
5 d

6 a
7 a
8 c
9 b
10 d
11 c
12 a
13 c
14 a
15 d
16 a
17 d
18 c
19 d
20 b
21 b
22 c

CHAPTER 9
1 a
2 b
3 d
4 c
5 c
6 a
7 b
8 c
9 d
10 d
11 b
12 a
13 b
14 b
15 b
16 c
17 d
18 a
19 d
20 a
21 b

CHAPTER 10
1 b
2 c
3 b
4 a
5 b
6 c
7 b
8 a
9 c
10 c
11 c
12 c
13 a

14 b
15 c
16 a
17 d
18 c

CHAPTER 11
1 c
2 c
3 a
4 d
5 c
6 b
7 c
8 a
9 b
10 a
11 b
12 d
13 c
14 d
15 c
16 a
17 d
18 b
19 a
20 b
21 d
22 c
23 c
24 a

CHAPTER 12
1 a
2 d
3 c
4 a
5 a
6 c
7 a
8 d
9 b
10 c
11 d
12 a
13 a
14 c
15 c
16 d
17 b
18 a
19 b
20 b
21 c
22 b

23 d
24 b
25 b
26 a
27 b
28 c
29 c
30 c
31 b
32 d

CHAPTER 13
1 a
2 d
3 c
4 a
5 a
6 c
7 d
8 c
9 a
10 b
11 a
12 c
13 c
14 a

CHAPTER 14
1 F
2 T
3 T
4 F
5 F
6 T
7 T
8 T
9 F
10 F
11 T
12 F
13 F
14 T
15 F
16 a
17 c
18 b
19 c
20 a
21 d
22 c
23 c
24 d

CHAPTER 15
1 F
2 T
3 T
4 F
5 F
6 F
7 F
8 T
9 T
10 F
11 F
12 b
13 d
14 d
15 b
16 a
17 b
18 a
19 d
20 c
21 a
22 d
23 c
24 a
25 d
26 b
27 d
28 c
29 b
30 a

CHAPTER 16
1 d
2 b
3 a
4 a
5 a
6 c
7 c
8 b
9 a
10 b
11 c
12 a

CHAPTER 17
1 b
2 a
3 a
4 b
5 a
6 b
7 a
8 a
9 a
10 a
11 b
12 a
13 d
14 b
15 c
16 c

CHAPTER 18
1 c
2 d
3 a
4 b
5 d
6 a
7 b
8 d
9 c
10 b
11 c
12 c
13 T
14 T
15 F
16 T
17 T
18 T
19 T
20 T
21 F
22 F

CHAPTER 19
1 F
2 F
3 F
4 F
5 T
6 F
7 T
8 T
9 F
10 T
11 d
12 b
13 a
14 b
15 a
16 d
17 c

CHAPTER 20
1 T
2 T
3 F
4 T
5 F
6 F
7 F
8 T
9 F
10 T
11 F
12 F
13 F
14 F
15 F
16 T
17 T
18 T
19 d
20 d
21 d
22 b
23 b
24 b
25 c
26 c
27 b
28 d
29 b
30 c

CHAPTER 21
1 d
2 b
3 c
4 a
5 d
6 d
7 b
8 d
9 b
10 F
11 T
12 T
13 F
14 F

CHAPTER 22
1 b
2 d
3 a
4 b
5 a
6 b
7 d
8 c
9 a
10 a
11 a
12 a
13 b
14 a
15 d
16 d
17 a

CHAPTER 23
1 a
2 b
3 d
4 a
5 c
6 c
7 b
8 a
9 a
10 c
11 d
12 d

CHAPTER 24
1 b
2 a
3 a
4 d
5 d
6 c
7 a
8 c
9 a
10 c
11 d
12 a
13 c
14 c
15 c
16 b
17 b
18 c
19 d
20 b
21 c
22 d
23 T
24 F
25 F
26 T
27 F
28 F
29 F
30 F
31 T
32 T

CHAPTER 25
1 c
2 a
3 a
4 b
5 d
6 a
7 a
8 a
9 a
10 c
11 a
12 b
13 a
14 d
15 b
16 b
17 b
18 a

CHAPTER 26
1 c
2 b
3 a
4 c
5 b
6 a
7 a
8 b
9 b
10 c
11 b
12 d
13 a
14 b
15 b

CHAPTER 27
1 b
2 b
3 c
4 b
5 c
6 b
7 c
8 a
9 c
10 a
11 c
12 b
13 F
14 F
15 T
16 T

CHAPTER 28
1 a
2 c
3 d
4 c
5 a
6 b
7 c
8 d
9 b
10 c
11 d
12 a
13 b
14 T
15 F
16 T

CHAPTER 29
1 F
2 T
3 F
4 T
5 T
6 F
7 F
8 F
9 T
10 F
11 F
12 T
13 T
14 T
15 F
16 T
17 T
18 T

CHAPTER 30
1 b
2 d
3 c
4 b
5 c

CHAPTER 31
1 d
2 b
3 a
4 c
5 b
6 a
7 d
8 a
9 b
10 c
11 a
12 a

CHAPTER 32
1 c
2 b
3 b
4 a
5 a
6 c
7 c
8 a
9 b
10 c
11 d
12 a
13 b
14 a
15 d
16 a
17 F
18 T
19 F
20 F
21 F
22 T
23 T
24 F
25 T
26 T

CHAPTER 33
1 a
2 c
3 a
4 c
5 a
6 d
7 b
8 d
9 c
10 b
11 d

12 c
13 b
14 d
15 a
16 c

CHAPTER 34
1 b
2 a
3 a
4 a
5 d
6 c
7 b
8 b
9 d
10 a
11 b
12 a
13 d
14 c
15 d
16 d
17 b
18 F
19 T
20 T
21 T
22 T
23 T
24 F
25 T
26 F
27 T
28 F
29 F
30 T

CHAPTER 35
1 d
2 b
3 b
4 b
5 c
6 b
7 d
8 a
9 d
10 c
11 a
12 b

CHAPTER 36
1 a
2 c
3 c
4 b
5 b
6 d
7 c
8 d
9 a
10 a
11 a
12 b
13 a
14 c
15 d
16 b
17 b
18 c

CHAPTER 37
1 a
2 d
3 d
4 b
5 b
6 a
7 d
8 c
9 d
10 b
11 c
12 d

CHAPTER 38
1 c
2 b
3 a
4 d
5 c
6 c
7 T
8 T
9 T
10 F
11 T
12 T
13 F
14 T
15 T
16 T

CHAPTER 39
1 b
2 b
3 a
4 c
5 b
6 b
7 a
8 c
9 c
10 a
11 c
12 b
13 a
14 b
15 a
16 b
17 c
18 a
19 b
20 a
21 d
22 c

CHAPTER 40
1 b
2 a
3 a
4 a
5 a
6 a
7 a
8 d
9 d
10 b
11 T
12 T
13 T
14 T
15 T
16 F
17 T
18 T

CHAPTER 41
1 a
2 b
3 d
4 b
5 c
6 b
7 a
8 b
9 d

10 a
11 b
12 a
13 c
14 a
15 c
16 a
17 a
18 a
19 d
20 c
21 a
22 a

CHAPTER 42
1 d
2 a
3 d
4 b
5 c
6 a
7 d
8 a
9 a
10 b
11 a
12 b
13 d
14 a
15 c
16 c
17 a
18 a
19 d

CHAPTER 43
1 b
2 a
3 d
4 a
5 a
6 d
7 c
8 d
9 a
10 d
11 c
12 a
13 d
14 a
15 b
16 c
17 a
18 b

CHAPTER 44
1 d
2 d
3 c
4 d
5 a
6 a
7 a
8 b
9 c
10 d

CHAPTER 45
1 b
2 d
3 c
4 c
5 c
6 c
7 b
8 c
9 b
10 d
11 d
12 a
13 c
14 c
15 d
16 a
17 b
18 a
19 a
20 a
21 c
22 F
23 T
24 F
25 T
26 T
27 T
28 T
29 T
30 F

CHAPTER 46
1 a
2 b
3 a
4 a
5 d
6 d
7 a
8 b
9 b
10 d
11 b
12 d
13 a
14 d
15 c
16 c
17 a
18 a
19 a
20 T
21 F
22 T
23 T
24 F
25 F
26 T
27 T
28 T
29 F
30 F

CHAPTER 47
1 d
2 b
3 d
4 b
5 a
6 d
7 b
8 c
9 c
10 d
11 b
12 b
13 d
14 c
15 b

CHAPTER 48
1 a
2 d
3 c
4 a
5 b
6 b
7 d
8 b
9 c
10 b

CHAPTER 49
1 c
2 d
3 d
4 d
5 b
6 c
7 c
8 a
9 c
10 d

11 d
12 a
13 c
14 c
15 T
16 F
17 T
18 F
19 T
20 T
21 F
22 T

CHAPTER 50
1 a
2 a
3 b
4 d
5 d
6 b
7 d
8 b
9 b

10 d
11 b
12 a
13 b
14 c
15 c

CHAPTER 51
1 b
2 a
3 b
4 a
5 d
6 c
7 b
8 c
9 b
10 b
11 c
12 d
13 c
14 b
15 a

16 b
17 b
18 c
19 c
20 a

CHAPTER 52
1 c
2 c
3 b
4 a
5 a
6 d
7 b
8 a
9 d
10 c
11 c
12 a
13 c
14 b
15 b

NATIONAL NURSE AIDE ASSESSMENT PROGRAM (NNAAP®) WRITTEN EXAMINATION CONTENT OUTLINE

The NNAAP® Written Examination is comprised of seventy (70) multiple choice questions. Ten (10) of these questions are pre-test (non-scored) questions on which statistical information will be collected.

I. Physical Care Skills
A. Activities of Daily Living   **14% of exam**
1. Hygiene
2. Dressing and Grooming
3. Nutrition and Hydration
4. Elimination
5. Rest/Sleep/Comfort

B. Basic Nursing Skills   **39% of exam**
1. Infection Control
2. Safety/Emergency
3. Therapeutic/Technical Procedures
4. Data Collection and Reporting

C. Restorative Skills   **7% of exam**
1. Prevention
2. Self Care/Independence

II. Psychosocial Care Skills
A. Emotional and Mental Health Needs   **11% of exam**
B. Spiritual and Cultural Needs   **2% of exam**

III. Role of the Nurse Aide
A. Communication   **8% of exam**
B. Client Rights   **7% of exam**
C. Legal and Ethical Behavior   **3% of exam**
D. Member of the Health Care Team   **9% of exam**

NATIONAL NURSE AIDE ASSESSMENT PROGRAM (NNAAP®) SKILLS EVALUATION

List of Skills
1. Hand Hygiene (Hand Washing)
2. Applies one knee-high elastic stocking
3. Assists to ambulate using transfer belt
4. Assists with use of bedpan
5. Cleans upper or lower denture
6. Counts and records radial pulse
7. Counts and records respirations
8. Donning and removing PPE (gown and gloves)
9. Dresses client with affected (weak) right arm
10. Feeds client who cannot feed self
11. Gives modified bed bath (face and one arm, hand and underarm)
12. Measures and records blood pressure
13. Measures and records urinary output
14. Measures and records weight of ambulatory client
15. Performs modified passive range of motion (PROM) for one knee and one ankle
16. Performs modified passive range of motion (PROM) for one shoulder
17. Positions on side
18. Provides catheter care for female
19. Provides foot care on one foot
20. Provides mouth care
21. Provides perineal care (peri-care) for female
22. Transfers from bed to wheelchair using transfer belt

MINIMUM DATA SET: SELECTED PAGES

Sample Page from Functional Status Form

Resident _____ Identifier _____ Date _____

Section G	Functional Status

G0110. Activities of Daily Living (ADL) Assistance
Refer to the ADL flow chart in the RAI manual to facilitate accurate coding

Instructions for Rule of 3
- When an activity occurs three times at any one given level, code that level.
- When an activity occurs three times at multiple levels, code the most dependent, exceptions are total dependence (4), activity must require full assist every time, and activity did not occur (8), activity must not have occurred at all. Example, three times extensive assistance (3) and three times limited assistance (2), code extensive assistance (3).
- When an activity occurs at various levels, but not three times at any given level, apply the following:
  - When there is a combination of full staff performance, and extensive assistance, code extensive assistance.
  - When there is a combination of full staff performance, weight bearing assistance and/or non-weight bearing assistance code limited assistance (2).

If none of the above are met, code supervision.

1. ADL Self-Performance
Code for **resident's performance** over all shifts - not including setup. If the ADL activity occurred 3 or more times at various levels of assistance, code the most dependent - except for total dependence, which requires full staff performance every time

Coding:

Activity Occurred 3 or More Times
0. **Independent** - no help or staff oversight at any time
1. **Supervision** - oversight, encouragement or cueing
2. **Limited assistance** - resident highly involved in activity; staff provide guided maneuvering of limbs or other non-weight-bearing assistance
3. **Extensive assistance** - resident involved in activity, staff provide weight-bearing support
4. **Total dependence** - full staff performance every time during entire 7-day period

Activity Occurred 2 or Fewer Times
7. **Activity occurred only once or twice** - activity did occur but only once or twice
8. **Activity did not occur** - activity (or any part of the ADL) was not performed by resident or staff at all over the entire 7-day period

2. ADL Support Provided
Code for **most support provided** over all shifts; code regardless of resident's self-performance classification

Coding:
0. **No** setup or physical help from staff
1. **Setup** help only
2. **One** person physical assist
3. **Two+** persons physical assist
8. ADL activity itself **did not occur** during entire period

	1. Self-Performance	2. Support
	↓ Enter Codes in Boxes ↓	
A. Bed mobility - how resident moves to and from lying position, turns side to side, and positions body while in bed or alternate sleep furniture	☐	☐
B. Transfer - how resident moves between surfaces including to or from: bed, chair, wheelchair, standing position (**excludes** to/from bath/toilet)	☐	☐
C. Walk in room - how resident walks between locations in his/her room	☐	☐
D. Walk in corridor - how resident walks in corridor on unit	☐	☐
E. Locomotion on unit - how resident moves between locations in his/her room and adjacent corridor on same floor. If in wheelchair, self-sufficiency once in chair	☐	☐
F. Locomotion off unit - how resident moves to and returns from off-unit locations (e.g., areas set aside for dining, activities or treatments). **If facility has only one floor**, how resident moves to and from distant areas on the floor. If in wheelchair, self-sufficiency once in chair	☐	☐
G. Dressing - how resident puts on, fastens and takes off all items of clothing, including donning/removing a prosthesis or TED hose. Dressing includes putting on and changing pajamas and housedresses	☐	☐
H. Eating - how resident eats and drinks, regardless of skill. Do not include eating/drinking during medication pass. Includes intake of nourishment by other means (e.g., tube feeding, total parenteral nutrition, IV fluids administered for nutrition or hydration)	☐	☐
I. Toilet use - how resident uses the toilet room, commode, bedpan, or urinal; transfers on/off toilet; cleanses self after elimination; changes pad; manages ostomy or catheter; and adjusts clothes. Do not include emptying of bedpan, urinal, bedside commode, catheter bag or ostomy bag	☐	☐
J. Personal hygiene - how resident maintains personal hygiene, including combing hair, brushing teeth, shaving, applying makeup, washing/drying face and hands (**excludes** baths and showers)	☐	☐

Sample Page from Care Assessment (CAA) Summary

Resident _____   Identifier _____   Date _____

Section V	**Care Area Assessment (CAA) Summary**

V0200. CAAs and Care Planning

1. Check column A if Care Area is triggered.
2. For each triggered Care Area, indicate whether a new care plan, care plan revision, or continuation of current care plan is necessary to address the problem(s) identified in your assessment of the care area. The Addressed in Care Plan column must be completed within 7 days of completing the RAI (MDS and CAA(s)). Check column B if the triggered care area is addressed in the care plan.
3. Indicate in the Location and Date of CAA Information column where information related to the CAA can be found. CAA documentation should include information on the complicating factors, risks, and any referrals for this resident for this care area.

A. CAA Results

Care Area	A. Care Area Triggered	B. Addressed in Care Plan	Location and Date of CAA Information
	↓ Check all that apply ↓		
01. Delirium	☐	☐	
02. Cognitive Loss/Dementia	☐	☐	
03. Visual Function	☐	☐	
04. Communication	☐	☐	
05. ADL Functional/Rehabilitation Potential	☐	☐	
06. Urinary Incontinence and Indwelling Catheter	☐	☐	
07. Psychosocial Well-Being	☐	☐	
08. Mood State	☐	☐	
09. Behavioral Symptoms	☐	☐	
10. Activities	☐	☐	
11. Falls	☐	☐	
12. Nutritional Status	☐	☐	
13. Feeding Tube	☐	☐	
14. Dehydration/Fluid Maintenance	☐	☐	
15. Dental Care	☐	☐	
16. Pressure Ulcer	☐	☐	
17. Psychotropic Drug Use	☐	☐	
18. Physical Restraints	☐	☐	
19. Pain	☐	☐	
20. Return to Community Referral	☐	☐	

B. Signature of RN Coordinator for CAA Process and Date Signed

1. Signature   2. Date ☐☐ - ☐☐ - ☐☐☐☐
                                                       Month   Day   Year

C. Signature of Person Completing Care Plan and Date Signed

1. Signature   2. Date ☐☐ - ☐☐ - ☐☐☐☐
                                                       Month   Day   Year

KEY RECOMMENDATIONS FROM DIETARY GUIDELINES 2010

Balancing Calories to Manage Weight

- Prevent and/or reduce overweight and obesity through improved eating and physical activity behaviors.
- Control total calorie intake to manage body weight. For people who are overweight or obese, this will mean consuming fewer calories from foods and beverages.
- Increase physical activity and reduce time spent in sedentary behaviors.
- Maintain appropriate calorie balance during each stage of life—childhood, adolescence, adulthood, pregnancy and breastfeeding, and older age.

Food and Food Components to Reduce

- Reduce daily sodium intake to less than 2300 milligrams (mg) and further reduce intake to 1500 mg among persons who are 51 and older and those of any age who are African-American or have hypertension, diabetes, or chronic kidney disease. The 1500 mg recommendation applies to about half of the U.S. population, including children and the majority of adults.
- Consume less than 10% of calories from saturated fatty acids by replacing them with monounsaturated and polyunsaturated fatty acids.
- Consume less than 300 mg per day of dietary cholesterol.
- Keep *trans* fatty acid consumption as low as possible by limiting foods that contain synthetic sources of *trans* fats, such as partially hydrogenated oils, and by limiting other solid fats.
- Reduce the intake of calories from solid fats and added sugars.
- Limit the consumption of foods that contain refined grains, especially refined grain foods that contain solid fats, added sugars, and sodium.
- If alcohol is consumed, it should be consumed in moderation—up to one drink per day for women and two drinks per day for men—and only by adults of legal drinking age.*

Food and Nutrients to Increase

Individuals should meet the following recommendations as part of a healthy eating pattern while staying within their calorie needs.

- Increase vegetable and fruit intake.
- Eat a variety of vegetables, especially dark-green, red, and orange vegetables and beans and peas.
- Consume at least half of all grains as whole grains. Increase whole-grain intake by replacing refined grains with whole grains.
- Increase intake of fat-free or low-fat milk and milk products, such as milk, yogurt, cheese, or fortified soy beverages.*
- Choose a variety of protein foods, which include seafood, lean meat, poultry, eggs, beans, peas, soy products, and unsalted nuts and seeds.
- Increase the amount and variety of seafood consumed by choosing seafood in place of some meat and poultry.
- Replace protein foods that are higher in solid fats with choices that are lower in solid fats and calories and/or are sources of oils.
- Use oils to replace solid fats where possible.
- Choose foods that provide more potassium, dietary fiber, calcium, and vitamin D, which are nutrients of concern in American diets. These foods include vegetables, fruits, whole grains, and milk and milk products.

Recommendations for Specific Population Groups

Women capable of becoming pregnant*

- Choose foods that supply heme iron, which is more readily absorbed by the body, additional iron sources, and enhancers of iron absorption such as vitamin C-rich foods.
- Consume 400 micrograms (mcg) per day of synthetic folic acid (from fortified foods and/or supplements) in addition to food forms of folate from a varied diet.*

Women who are pregnant or breastfeeding*

- Consume 8 to 12 ounces of seafood per week from a variety of seafood types.
- Due to their high methyl mercury content, limit white (albacore) tuna to 6 ounces per week and do not eat the following four types of fish: tilefish, shark, swordfish, and king mackerel.
- If pregnant, take an iron supplement, as recommended by an obstetrician or other health care provider.

Individuals ages 50 years and older

- Consume foods fortified with vitamin B_{12}, such as fortified cereals, or dietary supplements.

Building healthy eating patterns

- Select an eating pattern that meets nutrient needs over time at an appropriate calorie level.
- Account for all foods and beverages consumed and assess how they fit within a total healthy eating pattern.
- Follow food safety recommendations when preparing and eating foods to reduce the risk of foodborne illnesses.

*For complete information go to http://www.cnpp.usda.gov/publications/dietaryguidelines/2010/policydoc/execsumm.pdf.

ILLUSTRATION CREDITS

Chapter 1 1-2: Courtesy Anne Arundel Health System, Inc, Annapolis, Md.

Chapter 3 3-2: Provided by MCN Healthcare, Denver, Colo. www.MCNHealthcare.com. All rights reserved.

Chapter 4 4-1: Modified from the National Council of State Boards of Nursing, Inc.: *Professional boundaries: a nurse's guide to the importance of appropriate professional boundaries*, Chicago, 1996, Author.

Chapter 5 5-3: Courtesy ADP Screening and Selections Services, Ft. Collins, Colo.

Chapter 6 6-2: Courtesy OSF St. Joseph Medical Center, Bloomington, Ill. **6-5:** Courtesy Briggs Corporation, Des Moines, Iowa. **6-11:** Courtesy Abraham Lincoln Memorial Hospital, Lincoln, Ill.

Chapter 8 8-2: From Maslow AH, Frager RD, Fadiman J: *Motivation and personality*, ed 3. Reprinted by permission of Pearson Education, Inc., Upper Saddle River, NJ.

Chapter 9 9-9: Redrawn from Thibodeau GA, Patton KT: *The human body in health and disease*, ed. 5, St. Louis, 2010, Mosby. **9-18:** From Thibodeau GA, Patton KT: *The human body in health and disease*, ed. 5, St. Louis, 2010, Mosby. **9-28:** From Thibodeau GA, Patton KT: *Structure and Function of the Body*, ed 11, St. Louis, 2000, Mosby.

Chapter 10 10-1: Thibodeau GA, Patton KT: *The human body in health and disease*, ed. 5, St. Louis, 2010, Mosby. **10-2:** Courtesy Marjori M Pyle for LifeCircle, Costa Mesa, Calif. **10-3, 10-6:** Courtesy Paul Vincent Kuntz, Texas Children's Hospital, as found in Hockenberry MJ, Wilson D: *Wong's nursing care of infants and children*, ed 9, St. Louis, 2011, Mosby. **10-4:** From Seidel HM and others: *Mosby's guide to physical examination*, ed 3, St. Louis, 1995, Mosby. **10-10:** From James SR, Ashwill JW, Droske SC: *Nursing care of children: principles and practices*, ed 3, Philadelphis, 2007, Saunders.

Chapter 12 12-12: Courtesy Children's Hospital, Pittsburgh Poison Center, Pittsburgh, Pa.

Chapter 13 13-2, 13-3, 13-10, 13-11: Images provided courtesy Posey Company, Arcadia, Calif.

Chapter 14 14-1, 14-2, 14-4, 14-7, 14-8, 14-9, 14-11, 14-12, 14-13, 14-14, 14-15, 14-18, 14-21: Images provided courtesy Posey Company, Arcadia, Calif. **14-16:** Modified from Briggs Corp., Des Moines, Iowa.

Chapter 15 15-1: Redrawn from Potter PA, Perry AG: *Fundamentals of nursing: concepts, process, and practice*, ed 7, St. Louis, 2009, Mosby. **15-14:** Siegel JD, Rhinehart E, Jackson M, Chiarello L, and the Healthcare Infection Control Practices Advisory Committee, 2007 *Guideline for Isolation Precautions: Preventing Transmission of Infectious Agents in Healthcare Settings* http://www.cdc.gov/ncidod/dhqp/pdf/isolation2007.pdf.

Chapter 16 16-13, 16-14: Images provided courtesy Posey Company, Arcadia, Calif.

Chapter 17 17-1, 17-2: Courtesy ARJO, Inc., Roselle, Ill. (800)323-1245. **17-25:** Courtesy MedCare Products, Burnsville, Minn.

Chapter 18 18-11, 18-12: Redrawn from Food and drug Administration: *Guidance for industry and FDA staff: hospital bed system dimensional and assessment guidance to reduce entrapment*, 2006. **18-13, 18-15:** © Hill-Rom Services, Inc. Reprinted with permission. All rights reserved. **18-16:** Courtesy Oriental Furniture, Cambridge Mass.

Chapter 20 20-3: Courtesy ElderStore, Alpharetta, Ga. **20-4:** From Eisen D, Lynch DP: The Mouth: Diagnosis and Treatment. St. Louis, 1998, Mosby. **20-23, 20-27:** Courtesy ARJO, Inc., Roselle, Ill. (800)323-1245.

Chapter 21 21-1: From North Coast Medical Inc., Morgan Hill, Calif. **21-3:** Redrawn from MedlinePlus: Head lice. Bethesda, Md., National Institutes of Health. **21-4:** From Marks JG, Miller JJ: *Lookingbill & Marks' principles of dermatology*, ed 4, St. Louis, 2006, Saunders. **21-5:** From Adkinson NF: *Middleton's allergy: principles and practice*, ed 7, St. Louis, 2008, Mosby.

Chapter 22 22-5: Courtesy AliMed, Inc., Dedham, Mass. **22-10C:** Courtesy Medical Depot, Inc., Port Washington, NY. **22-11B:** Courtesy Hartmann USA Inc, Rock Hill, S.C. **22-11C:** Courtesy Hartmann Inc., Heidenheim, Germany. **22-11D:** Courtesy Principle Business Enterprises, Dunbridge, Oh. **22-22:** From Potter PA, Perry AG: *Fundamentals of nursing*, ed 7, St. Louis, 2009, Mosby.

Chapter 23 23-4: Modified from deWit SC: *Fundamental concepts and skills for nursing*, ed 3, Philadelphia, 2009, Saunders.

Chapter 24 24-2: From U.S. Food and Drug Administration, 2011. **24-3:** Courtesy U.S. Department of Agriculture, Center for Nutrition and Policy Promotion, April 2005, CNPP-15. **24-4:** Courtesy ElderStore, Alpharetta, Ga. **24-5:** Modified from OSF St. Joseph Medical Center, Bloomington, Ill. **24-12:** Redrawn from U.S. Department of Health and Human Services and U.S. Department of Agriculture: Dietary Guidelines for Americans 2010.

Chapter 25 25-7, 25-11: From Potter PA, Perry AG, Stockert PA, Hall A: *Basic nursing*, ed 7, St. Louis, 2011, Mosby. **25-9:** Modified from *Mosby's dictionary of medicine, nursing, and health professions*, ed 8, St. Louis, 2009, Mosby. **25-13:** From James SR, Ashwill JW: *Nursing care of children: principles and practice*, ed 3, St. Louis, 2007, Saunders. **25-15:** Courtesy Baxter Healthcare Corporation, Round Lake, Illinois. **25-17, 25-18:** From Elkin MK, Perry AG, Potter PA: *Nursing interventions & clinical skills*, ed 4, St. Louis, 2007, Mosby. **25-19:** Courtesy I.V. House, St. Louis, Mo.

Chapter 26 26-21: From Jarvis C: *Physical examination and health assessment*, ed 4, Philadelphia, 2004, Saunders. **26-23D:** Courtesy Briggs Medical Service Company, Des Moines, Iowa.

Chapter 27 27-7, 27-8: Images provided courtesy Posey Company, Arcadia, Calif.

Chapter 28 28-3: From deWit SC: *Fundamental concepts and skills for nursing*, ed 3, St. Louis, 2009, Saunders. **28-4:** From Hockenberry MJ and others: *Wong's nursing care of infants and children*, ed 8, St. Louis, 2007, Mosby.

Chapter 29 29-2: Courtesy Briggs Corp., Des Moines, Iowa. **29-4D:** Courtesy Arjo, Morton Grove, Ill.

Chapter 31 31-1: Courtesy Welcon, Inc., Fort Worth, Tex. **31-3:** From Hockenberry MJ, Wilson D: *Wong's nursing care of infants and children*, ed 9, St. Louis, 2011, Mosby. **31-9:** From Potter PA, Perry AG: *Fundamentals of nursing*, ed 7, 2009, Mosby. **31-11:** From Bonewit-West, K: *Clinical procedures for medical assistants*, ed 7, St. Louis, 2008, Saunders. **31-12:** From Bonewit-West, K: *Clinical procedures for medical assistants*, ed 5, Philadelphia, 2000, Saunders. **31-13:** From James SR, Ashwill JW, Droske SC: *Nursing care of children: principles and practice*, ed 3, Philadelphia, 2007, Saunders.

Chapter 32 **32-6:** Courtesy Illinois Valley Community Hospital, Peru, Ill. **32-11:** From deWit SC: Fundamental concepts and skills for nursing, Philadelphia, 2001, Saunders.

Chapter 33 **33-1:** From Kumar V, Abbas AK, Fausto N: *Robbins and Cotran pathologic basis of disease,* ed 7, Philadelphia, 2005 Saunders. **33-2:** From Habif TP: *Clinical dermatology: a color guide to diagnosis and therapy,* ed 4, St. Louis, 2004, Mosby. **33-3:** From Finkbeiner W, Ursell P, Davis R: *Autopsy pathology: a manual and atlas,* London, 2004, Churchill Livingstone. **33-4:** From Elkin MK, Perry AG, Potter PA: *Nursing intervention and clinical skills,* ed 4, St. Louis, 2007, Mosby. **33-5:** From Roberts JR, Hedges JR: *Clinical procedures in emergency medicine,* ed 5, St. Louis, 2009, Saunders. **33-6, 33-7:** Penetrating wound. From McCance KL, Huether SE: *Pathophysiology: the biologic basis for disease in adults and children,* ed 6, St. Louis, 2010, Mosby. **33-8:** Used with permission from Rosemary Kohr, RN, PhD, ACNP (cert), www.lhsc.on.ca/wound, Rosemary.Kohr@lhsc.on.ca. **33-10:** From Belch J and others: *Color atlas of peripheral vascular diseases,* ed 2, London, 1996, Wolfe Medical Publishers. **33-11:** From Black JM, Hawks JH: *Medical-surgical nursing: clinical management for positive outcomes,* ed 7, St. Louis, 2005, WB Saunders. **33-12:** Redrawn from *Prevent diabetes problems: keep your feet and skin healthy,* National Diabetes Information Clearinghouse [NDIC]: NIH Publication No. 08-4282, May 2008, Bethesda Md. **33-13:** Modified from Ignatavicius DD, Workman ML: *Medical-surgical nursing: critical thinking for collaborative care,* ed 5, St. Louis, 2006, Saunders. **33-14:** Courtesy KCI Licensing, Inc., San Antonio, Tex. **33-15:** From Ignatavicius DD, Workman ML: *Medical-surgical nursing: critical thinking for collaborative care,* ed 5, St. Louis, 2006, Saunders. **33-16, 33-17, 33-18, 33-19, 33-20, 33-24:** From Potter PA, Perry AG, Stockert PA, Hall A: *Basic nursing,* ed 7, St. Louis, 2011, Mosby. **33-21:** From deWit SC: *Fundamental concepts and skills for nursing,* ed 3, St. Louis, 2000, Saunders.

Chapter 34 **34-2:** From Proceedings from the November National V.A.C.®, *Ostomy wound management,* Feb 2005, Vol. 51, [2A,[Supp]: 7S, HMP Communications. **34-3:** Redrawn from *Understanding your body: what are pressure ulcers?* U.S. Department of Health & Human Services, Agency for Healthcare Research and Quality, September 2009. **34-4A (parts 1 & 2), 34-4B–F (part 1):** From National Pressure Ulcer Advisory Panel, 2011. **34-4B–E (part 2):** Courtesy Laurel Wiersema-Bryant, RN, MSN, Clinical Nurse Specialist, Barnes-Jewish Hospital, St. Louis, Mo. **34-4F (part 2):** From Bryant RA, Nix DP: *Acute & chronic wounds: current management concepts,* ed 3, St. Louis, 2007, Mosby. **34-7, 34-8, 34-9, 34-10:** Images provided courtesy Posey Company, Arcadia, Calif. **34-13:** Braden, B. and Bergstrom, N. © 1988. All rights reserved. Reprinted with permission.

Chapter 36 **36-2:** Modified from Talbot L, Meyers-Marquardt M: *Pocket guide to critical care assessment,* ed 3, St. Louis, 1997, Mosby. **36-3:** Modified from Monahan FD, Neighbors M: *Foundations for clinical practice,* ed 2, Philadelphia, 1998, Saunders. **36-17:** Image used by permission from Nellcor Puritan Bennet LLC, Boulder, Colo; part of Covidien. **36-24:** From Hockenberry MJ, Wilson D: *Wong's nursing care of infants and children,* ed 9, St. Louis, 2011, Mosby.

Chapter 37 **37-6:** Modified from Hockenberry MJ, Wilson D: *Wong's nursing care of infants and children,* ed 9, St. Louis, 2011, Mosby. **37-8:** Courtesy VIASYS Respiratory Care, Yorba Linda, Calif. **37-9, 37-10:** Modified from Elkin MK, Perry

AG, Potter PA: *Nursing interventions and clinical skills,* ed 4, St. Louis, 2007, Mosby. **37-11:** From Lewis SM and others: *Medical-surgical nursing: assessment and management of clinical problems,* ed 6, St. Louis, 2004, Mosby.

Chapter 38 **38-2A, C, D:** Courtesy of Parsons ADL, Inc., Tottenham, Ontario. **38-2B:** Courtesy OXO International, Inc., New York, NY.

Chapter 39 **39-2:** Courtesy National Association of the Deaf, Silver Spring, Md. **39-4:** Courtesy Siemens Hearing Instruments, Inc. Piscataway NJ. **39-7:** From Swartz NH: Textbook of physical diagnosis, ed 5, Philadelphia, 2006, Saunders. **39-8:** From National Eye Institute: *Cataract: what you should know,* National Institutes of Health, Bethesda, Md. **39-9:** From National Eye Institute: *Age-related macular degeneration: what you should know,* National Institutes of Health, Bethesda, Md. **39-10:** From National Eye Institute: *Diabetic retinopathy: what you should know,* National Institutes of Health, Bethesda, Md. **39-13:** From Lewis SM, Heitkemper MM, Dirksen SR: *Medical-surgical nursing: assessment and management of clinical problems,* ed 5, St. Louis, 2000, Mosby.

Chapter 40 **40-2, 40-3:** From Belcher AE: *Cancer nursing,* St. Louis, 1992, Mosby. **40-4:** From Belchetz PE, Hammond P: *Diabetes and endocrinology,* London, 2003, Mosby. **40-5:** Redrawn from National Institute of Arthritis and Musculoskeletal and Skin Diseases: *Do I have lupus?* Bethesda, Md, National Institutes of Health. **40-7:** Courtesy of the Department of Dermatology, School of Medicine, University of Utah.

Chapter 41 **41-3:** Modified from Thibodeau GA, Patton KT: *The human body in health & disease,* ed 5, St. Louis, 2010, Mosby. **41-4, 41-11:** From Thibodeau GA, Patton KT: *The human body in health & disease,* ed 5, St. Louis, 2010, Mosby. **41-7, 41-8:** From Swartz MH: *Textbook of physical diagnosis,* ed 5, Philadelphia, 2006, Saunders. **41-9:** Courtesy Zimmer, Inc., a Bristol-Meyers Squibb Company, Warsaw, Ind. **41-10:** Modified from Monahan FD and others: *Phipps' medical-surgical nursing: health and illness perspectives,* ed 8, St. Louis, 2007, Mosby. **41-12:** Modified from Beare PG, Meyers JL: *Adult health nursing,* ed 3, St. Louis, 1998, Mosby. **41-13:** From Lewis SM, Heitkemper MM, Dirksen SR: *Medical-surgical nursing: assessment and management of clinical problems,* ed 7, St. Louis, 2007, Mosby. **41-15:** Modified from Harkness GA, Dincher JR: *Medical-surgical nursing: total patient care,* ed 10, St. Louis, 1999, Mosby. **41-17, 41-19, 41-21, 41-24:** From Monahan FD and others: *Phipps' medical-surgical nursing: health and illness perspectives,* ed 8, St. Louis, 2007, Mosby. **41-18:** From Christensen BL, Kockrow EO: *Adult health nursing,* ed 6, St. Louis, 2011, Mosby. **41-20:** Modified from Christensen BL, Kockrow EO: *Adult health nursing,* ed 6, St. Louis, 2011, Mosby. **41-22:** Courtesy Cameron Bangs, MD. From Auerbach PS: *Wilderness medicine, management of wilderness and environmental emergencies,* ed 3, St. Louis, 1995, Mosby. **41-23:** Courtesy Otto Bock Health Care, Minneapolis, Minn.

Chapter 42 **42-1, 42-10:** From Thibodeau GA, Patton KT: *The human body in health & disease,* ed 5, St. Louis, 2010, Mosby. **42-4:** Modified from Thibodeau GA, Patton KT: *The human body in health & disease,* ed 3, St. Louis, 2002, Mosby. **42-5:** From Lewis SM, Heitkemper MM, Dirksen SR: *Medical-surgical nursing: assessment and management of clinical problems,* ed 7, St. Louis, 2007, Mosby. **42-6:** Modified from Lewis SM, Heitkemper MM, Dirksen SR: *Medical-surgical nursing: assessment and management of clinical problems,* ed 7, St. Louis, 2007,

Mosby. **42-11:** From Swartz MH: *Textbook of physical diagnosis,* ed 5, Philadelphia, 2006, Saunders.

Chapter 43 43-2: From Monahan FD and others: *Phipps' medical-surgical nursing: health and illness perspectives,* ed 8, St. Louis, 2007, Mosby. **43-3:** From Christensen BL, Kockrow EO: *Adult health nursing,* ed 6, St. Louis, 2011, Mosby. **43-4:** From Thompson JM, Wilson SF: *Health assessments for nursing practice,* St. Louis, 1996, Mosby. **43-5:** Modified from National Digestive Diseases Information Clearinghouse (NDDIC): Gallstones, National Institutes of Health, NIH Publication No. 07-2897, Bethesda Md, July 2007. **43-6:** From Lebwohl MG (ed): *Atlas of the skin and systemic diseases,* ed 1, New York, 1995, Churchill Livingstone. **43-7A:** From Thibodeau GA and Patton KT: *The human body in health & disease,* ed 5, St. Louis, 2010, Mosby. **43-7B:** From Kumar V and others: *Robbins basic pathology,* ed 8, Philadelphia, 2007, Saunders. **43-8** From Swartz MH: *Textbook of physical diagnosis,* ed 5, Philadelphia, 2006, Saunders.

Chapter 44 44-2B: From National Kidney and Urologic Diseases Information Clearinghouse, *Prostate enlargement: benign prostatic hyperplasia,* National Institues of Health, NIH Publication No. 07-3012, Bethesda, Md, June 2006, National Institutes of Health. **44-3:** From Beare PA, Myers JL: *Principles and practices of adult health nursing,* ed 3, St. Louis, 1998, Mosby. **44-7:** Courtesy Baxter Heatlhcare Corp., Deerfield, Ill. **44-8:** From Tucker S et al: Patient care standards: collaborative practice planning guides, ed 6, St. Louis, 1996, Mosby. **44-9:** Courtesy United States Public Health Service, Washington, DC.

Chapter 45 45-1: Courtesy George D. Comerci, MD, Tuscon, Arizona. In Jarvis C: *Physical examination and health assessment,* ed 4, Philadelphia, 2004, Saunders.

Chapter 46 46-2A, B: From Thibodeau GA and Patton KT: *The human body in health & disease,* ed 5, St. Louis, 2010, Mosby. **46-3:** From Alzheimer's Disease Education & Referral (ADEAR) Center, *Alzheimer's disease fact sheet,* National Institutes of Health, NIH publication No. 08-6423, updated February 19, 2010.

Chapter 47 47-1A, 47-6: From Hockenberry MJ, Wilson D: *Wong's nursing care of infants and children,* ed 9, St. Louis, 2011, Mosby. **47-1B:** From Thibodeau GA, Patton KT: *The human body in health & disease,* ed 5, St. Louis, 2010, Mosby. **47-4:** From Zitelli BJ, Davis HW: *Atlas of pediatric physical diagnosis,* St. Louis, 1987, Gower Medical Publishing. **47-5:** From Hart CA, Broadhead RL, *Color atlas of pediatric infectious diseases,* London, 1992, Mosby-Wolfe.

Chapter 49 49-2, 49-3: From James SR & Ashwill JW: *Nursing care of children: principles and practice,* ed 3, St. Louis, 2007, WB Saunders. **49-4:** From James SR, Ashwill JW, Droske SC: *Nursing care of children: principles and practice,* ed 2, Philadelphia, 2002, WB Saunders.

Chapter 51 51-28: From Ignatavicius DD, Workman ML: *Medical-surgical nursing: critical thinking for collaborative care,* ed 6, St. Louis, 2010, Saunders. **51-29:** From Sanders M: *Mosby's paramedic textbook,* ed 3, St. Louis, 2007, Mosby.

abbreviation A shortened form of a word or phrase

abduction Moving a body part away from the mid-line of the body

abrasion A partial-thickness wound caused by the scraping away or rubbing of the skin

abuse The willful infliction of injury, unreasonable confinement, intimidation, or punishment that results in physical harm, pain, or mental anguish; depriving the person (or the person's caregiver) of the goods or services needed to attain or maintain well-being

accountable Being responsible for one's actions and the actions of others who performed the delegated tasks; answering questions about and explaining one's actions and the actions of others

acetone See "ketone"

activities of daily living (ADL) The activities usually done during a normal day in a person's life

acute illness A sudden illness from which a person is expected to recover

acute pain Pain that is felt suddenly from injury, disease, trauma, or surgery

adduction Moving a body part toward the mid-line of the body

admission Official entry of a person into a health care setting

adolescence The time between puberty and adulthood; a time of rapid growth and physical, sexual, emotional and social changes

advance directive A document stating a person's wishes about health care when that person cannot make his or her own decisions

affect Feelings and emotions

allergy A sensitivity to a substance that causes the body to react with signs and symptoms

alopecia Hair loss

ambulation The act of walking

AM care See "early morning care"

amputation The removal of all or part of an extremity

anaphylaxis A life-threatening sensitivity to an antigen

anesthesia The loss of feeling or sensation produced by a drug

anorexia The loss of appetite

anterior At or toward the front of the body or body part; ventral

antibiotic A drug that kills certain microbes that cause infections

anticoagulant A drug that prevents or slows down (*anti*) blood clotting (*coagulate*)

anxiety A vague, uneasy feeling in response to stress

aphasia The total or partial loss (*a*) of the ability to use or understand language (*phasia*); a language disorder resulting from damage to parts of the brain responsible for language

apical-radial pulse Taking the apical and radial pulses at the same time

apnea The lack or absence (*a*) of breathing (*pnea*)

arterial ulcer An open wound on the lower legs or feet caused by poor arterial blood flow

artery A blood vessel that carries blood away from the heart

arthritis Joint (*arthr*) inflammation (*itis*)

arthroplasty The surgical replacement (*plasty*) of a joint (*arthro*)

asepsis Being free of disease-producing microbes

aspiration Breathing fluid, food, vomitus, or an object into the lungs

assault Intentionally attempting or threatening to touch a person's body without the person's consent

assessment Collecting information about the person; a step in the nursing process

assisted living A housing option for older persons who need help with activities of daily living yet wish to remain independent as long as possible

assisted living residence (ALR) Provides housing, personal care, support services, health care, and social activities in a home-like setting to persons needing help with daily activities

atelectasis The collapse of a portion of the lung

atrophy Shrink; the decrease in size or the wasting away of tissue

autopsy The examination of the body after death

avoidable pressure ulcer A pressure ulcer that develops from the improper use of the nursing process

bariatrics The field of medicine focused on the treatment and control of obesity

base of support The area on which an object rests

battery Touching a person's body without his or her consent

bedfast Confined to bed

bed rail A device that serves as a guard or barrier along the side of the bed; side rail

benign tumor A tumor that does not spread to other body parts; it can grow to a large size

biohazardous waste Items contaminated with blood, body fluids, secretions, or excretions; *bio* means *life*, and *hazardous* means *dangerous* or *harmful*

Biot's respirations Rapid and deep respirations followed by 10 to 30 seconds of apnea

birth defect An abnormality present at birth that involves a body structure or function

bisexual A person who is attracted to both sexes

blindness The absence of sight

blood pressure (BP) The amount of force exerted against the walls of an artery by the blood

body alignment The way the head, trunk, arms, and legs are aligned with one another; posture

body language Messages sent through facial expressions, gestures, posture, hand and body movements, gait, eye contact, and appearance

body mechanics Using the body in an efficient and careful way

body temperature The amount of heat in the body that is a balance between the amount of heat produced and the amount lost by the body

bony prominence An area where the bone sticks out or projects from the flat surface of the body

boundary crossing A brief act or behavior outside of the helpful zone

boundary sign An act, behavior, or thought that warns of a boundary crossing or violation

boundary violation An act or behavior that meets your needs, not the person's

bradycardia A slow *(brady)* heart rate *(cardia)*; less than 60 beats per minute

bradypnea Slow *(brady)* breathing *(pnea)*; respirations are fewer than 12 per minute

braille A touch reading and writing system that uses raised dots for each letter of the alphabet; the first 10 letters also represent the numbers 0 through 9

breast-feeding Feeding a baby milk from the mother's breasts; nursing

Broca's aphasia See "expressive aphasia"

calorie The fuel or energy value of food

cancer See "malignant tumor"

capillary A tiny blood vessel; food, oxygen, and other substances pass from the capillaries into the cells

cardiac arrest See "sudden cardiac arrest"

carrier A human or animal that is a reservoir for microbes but does not develop the infection

case management A nursing care pattern; a case manager (an RN) coordinates a person's care from admission through discharge and into the home or long-term care setting

catheter A tube used to drain or inject fluid through a body opening

catheterization The process of inserting a catheter

cell The basic unit of body structure

cerumen Earwax

chairfast Confined to a chair

chart See "medical record"

chemical restraint Any drug that is used for discipline or convenience and not required to treat medical symptoms

Cheyne-Stokes respirations Respirations gradually increase in rate and depth and then become shallow and slow; breathing may stop *(apnea)* for 10 to 20 seconds

cholesterol A soft, waxy substance found in the bloodstream and all body cells

chronic illness An ongoing illness, slow or gradual in onset; it has no known cure; it can be controlled and complications prevented with proper treatment

chronic pain Pain that continues for a long time (months or years) or occurs off and on; persistent pain

chronic wound A wound that does not heal easily

circadian rhythm Daily rhythm based on a 24-hour cycle; the day-night cycle or body rhythm

circulatory ulcer An open sore on the lower legs or feet caused by decreased blood flow through the arteries or veins; vascular ulcer

circumcision The surgical removal of foreskin from the penis

civil law Laws concerned with relationships between people

clean-contaminated wound Occurs from the surgical entry of the reproductive, urinary, respiratory, or gastrointestinal system

clean technique See "medical asepsis"

clean wound A wound that is not infected

clinical record See "medical record"

closed fracture The bone is broken but the skin is intact; simple fracture

closed wound Tissues are injured but the skin is not broken

cognitive function Involves memory, thinking, reasoning, ability to understand, judgment, and behavior

colonized The presence of bacteria on the wound surface or in wound tissue; the person does not have signs and symptoms of an infection

colostomy A surgically created opening *(stomy)* between the colon *(colo)* and abdominal wall

coma A state of being unaware of one's setting and being unable to react or respond to people, places, or things

comatose Being unable to respond to stimuli

comfort A state of well-being; the person has no physical or emotional pain and is calm and at peace

communicable disease A disease caused by pathogens that spread easily; a contagious disease

communication The exchange of information—a message sent is received and correctly interpreted by the intended person

compound fracture See "open fracture"

compress A soft pad applied over a body area

compulsion Repeating an act over and over again

confidentiality Trusting others with personal and private information

conflict A clash between opposing interests or ideas

congenital To be born with *(congenitus)*

conscious Awareness of the environment and experiences; the person knows what is happening and can control thoughts and behavior

constipation The passage of a hard, dry stool

constrict To narrow

contagious disease See "communicable disease"

contaminated wound A wound with a high risk of infection

contamination The process of becoming unclean

contracture The lack of joint mobility caused by abnormal shortening of a muscle

contusion A closed wound caused by a blow to the body; a bruise

convulsion See "seizure"

cotton drawsheet A drawsheet made of cotton; it helps keep the mattress and bottom linens clean

courtesy A polite, considerate, or helpful comment or act

crime An act that violates a criminal law

criminal law Laws concerned with offenses against the public and society in general

culture The characteristics of a group of people—language, values, beliefs, habits, likes, dislikes, customs—passed from one generation to the next

cyanosis Bluish color; bluish color to the skin, lips, mucous membranes, and nail beds

Daily Value (DV) How a serving fits into the daily diet; expressed in a percent (%) based on a daily diet of 2000 calories

dandruff Excessive amounts of dry, white flakes from the scalp

deafness Hearing loss in which it is impossible for the person to understand speech through hearing alone

deconditioning The loss of muscle strength from inactivity

defamation Injuring a person's name and reputation by making false statements to a third person

defecation The process of excreting feces from the rectum through the anus; a bowel movement

defense mechanism An unconscious reaction that blocks unpleasant or threatening feelings

dehiscence The separation of wound layers

dehydration The excessive loss of water from tissues; a decrease in the amount of water in body tissues

delegate To authorize another person to perform a nursing task in a certain situation

delirium A state of sudden, severe confusion and rapid changes in brain function

delusion A false belief

delusion of grandeur An exaggerated belief about one's importance, wealth, power, or talents

delusion of persecution A false belief that one is being mistreated, abused, or harassed

dementia The loss of cognitive and social function caused by changes in the brain; the loss of cognitive function that interferes with routine personal, social, and occupational activities

denture An artificial tooth or a set of artificial teeth

development Changes in mental, emotional, and social function

developmental disability (DD) A disability occurring before 22 years of age

developmental task A skill that must be completed during a stage of development

diabetic foot ulcer An open wound on the foot caused by complications from diabetes

dialysis The process of removing waste products from the blood

diaphoresis Profuse (excessive) sweating

diarrhea The frequent passage of liquid stools

diastole The period of heart muscle relaxation; the heart is at rest

diastolic pressure The pressure in the arteries when the heart is at rest

digestion The process that breaks down food physically and chemically so that it can be absorbed for use by the cells

dilate To expand or open wider

diplegia Similar body parts are affected on both sides of the body

dirty wound See "infected wound"

disability Any lost, absent, or impaired physical or mental function

disaster A sudden catastrophic event in which people are injured and killed and property is destroyed

discharge Official departure of a person from a health care setting

discomfort See "pain"

disinfection The process of destroying pathogens

distal The part farthest from the center or from the point of attachment

distraction To change the person's center of attention

diuresis The process (*esis*) of passing (*di*) urine (*ur*); large amounts of urine are produced—1000 to 5000 mL (milliliters) a day

dorsal See "posterior"

dorsal recumbent position The back-lying or supine position; the supine position with the legs together; horizontal recumbent position

dorsiflexion Bending the toes and foot up at the ankle

drawsheet A small sheet placed over the middle of the bottom sheet

dysphagia Difficulty (*dys*) swallowing (*phagia*)

dyspnea Difficult, labored, or painful (*dys*) breathing (*pnea*)

dysrhythmia An abnormal (*dys*) heart rhythm (*rhythmia*)

dysuria Painful or difficult (*dys*) urination (*uria*)

early morning care Routine care given before breakfast; AM care

edema The swelling of body tissues with water; swelling caused by fluid collecting in tissues

ejaculation The release of semen

elder abuse Any knowing, intentional, or negligent act by a caregiver or any other person to an older adult; the act causes harm or serious risk of harm

elective surgery Surgery done by choice to improve the person's life or well-being

electrical shock When electrical current passes through the body

elopement When a person leaves the agency without staff knowledge

embolus A blood clot that travels through the vascular system until it lodges in a blood vessel

emergency surgery Surgery done at once to save life or function

emesis See "vomitus"

emotional illness See "mental disorder"

enabler A device that limits freedom of movement but is used to promote independence, comfort, or safety

end-of-life care The support and care given during the time surrounding death

end-of-shift report A report that the nurse gives at the end of the shift to the on-coming shift

enema The introduction of fluid into the rectum and lower colon

enteral nutrition Giving nutrients into the gastro-intestinal (GI) tract (*enteral*) through a feeding tube

enuresis Urinary incontinence in bed at night

epidermal stripping Removing the epidermis (outer skin layer) as tape is removed from the skin

episiotomy Incision (*otomy*) into the perineum

erectile dysfunction (ED) See "impotence"

ergonomics The science of designing a job to fit the worker

eschar Thick, leathery dead tissue that may be loose or adhered to the skin; it is often black or brown

esteem The worth, value, or opinion one has of a person

ethics Knowledge of what is right conduct and wrong conduct

evaluation To measure if goals in the planning step were met; a step in the nursing process

evening care Care given in the evening at bedtime; PM care

evisceration The separation of the wound along with the protrusion of abdominal organs

excoriation Loss of the epidermis (top skin layer) caused by scratching or when skin rubs against skin, clothing, or other material

expressive aphasia Difficulty expressing or sending out thoughts; motor aphasia, Broca's aphasia

expressive-receptive aphasia Difficulty expressing or sending out thoughts and difficulty understanding language; global aphasia, mixed aphasia

extension Straightening a body part

external rotation Turning the joint outward

fainting The sudden loss of consciousness from an inadequate blood supply to the brain

false imprisonment Unlawful restraint or restriction of a person's freedom of movement

fecal impaction The prolonged retention and buildup of feces in the rectum

fecal incontinence The inability to control the passage of feces and gas through the anus

feces The semi-solid mass of waste products in the colon that is expelled through the anus

fever Elevated body temperature

first aid Emergency care given to an ill or injured person before medical help arrives

flashback Reliving a trauma in thoughts during the day and in nightmares during sleep

flatulence The excessive formation of gas or air in the stomach and intestines

flatus Gas or air passed through the anus

flexion Bending a body part

flow rate The number of drops per minute (*gtt/min*) or milliliters per hour (*mL/hr*)

Foley catheter See "indwelling catheter"

footdrop The foot falls down at the ankle; permanent plantar flexion

Fowler's position A semi-sitting position; the head of the bed is raised between 45 and 60 degrees

fracture A broken bone

fraud Saying or doing something to trick, fool, or deceive a person

freedom of movement Any change in place or position of the body or any part of the body that the person is able to control

friction The rubbing of one surface against another

full-thickness wound The dermis, epidermis, and subcutaneous tissue are penetrated; muscle and bone may be involved

full visual privacy Having the means to be completely free from public view while in bed

functional incontinence The person has bladder control but cannot use the toilet in time

functional nursing A nursing care pattern focusing on tasks and jobs; each nursing team member has certain tasks and jobs to do

gait belt See "transfer belt"

gangrene A condition in which there is death of tissue

gastrostomy tube A feeding tube inserted through a surgically created opening (*stomy*) in the stomach (*gastro*); stomach tube

gavage The process of giving a tube feeding

general anesthesia The loss of consciousness and all feeling or sensation

genupectoral position See "knee-chest position"

geriatrics The branch of medicine concerned with the problems and diseases of old age and older persons; the care of aging people

gerontology The study of the aging process

global aphasia See "expressive-receptive aphasia"

glucosuria Sugar (*glucos*) in the urine (*uria*); glycosuria

glycosuria Sugar (*glycos*) in the urine (*uria*); glucosuria

goal That which is desired for or by a person as a result of nursing care

gossip To spread rumors or talk about the private matters of others

graduate A measuring container for fluid

ground That which carries leaking electricity to the earth and away from an electrical item

growth The physical changes that are measured and that occur in a steady, orderly manner

guided imagery Creating and focusing on an image

hallucination Seeing, hearing, smelling, or feeling something that is not real

harassment To trouble, torment, offend, or worry a person by one's behavior or comments

hazard Any thing in the person's setting that may cause injury or illness

hazardous substance Any chemical in the workplace that can cause harm

healthcare-associated infection (HAI) An infection that develops in a person cared for in any setting where health care is given; the infection is related to receiving health care

health team The many health care workers whose skills and knowledge focus on the person's total care; interdisciplinary health care team

hearing loss Not being able to hear the normal range of sounds associated with normal hearing

heartburn A burning sensation in the chest and sometimes the throat

hematoma A swelling (oma) that contains blood (hemat)

hematuria Blood (hemat) in the urine (uria)

hemiplegia Paralysis (plegia) on one side (hemi) of the body

hemoglobin The substance in red blood cells that carries oxygen and gives blood its red color

hemoptysis Bloody (hemo) sputum (ptysis means to spit)

hemorrhage The excessive loss of blood in a short time

hemothorax Blood (hemo) in the pleural space (thorax)

heterosexual A person who is attracted to members of the other sex

high blood pressure See "hypertension"

high-Fowler's position A semi-sitting position, the head of the bed is raised 60 to 90 degrees

hirsutism Excessive body hair

holism A concept that considers the whole person; the whole person has physical, social, psychological, and spiritual parts that are woven together and cannot be separated

homosexual A person who is attracted to members of the same sex

horizontal recumbent position See "dorsal recumbent position"

hormone A chemical substance secreted by the endocrine glands into the bloodstream

hospice A health care agency or program for persons who are dying

hyperextension Excessive straightening of a body part

hyperglycemia High (hyper) sugar (glyc) in the blood (emia)

hypertension When the systolic pressure is 140 mm Hg or higher (hyper), or the diastolic pressure is 90 mm Hg or higher; high blood pressure

hyperthermia A body temperature (thermia) that is much higher (hyper) than the person's normal range

hyperventilation Breathing (ventilation) is rapid (hyper) and deeper than normal

hypoglycemia Low (hypo) sugar (glyc) in the blood (emia)

hypotension When the systolic pressure is below (hypo) 90 mm Hg, or the diastolic pressure is below 60 mm Hg

hypothermia A very low (hypo) body temperature (thermia)

hypoventilation Breathing (ventilation) is slow (hypo), shallow, and sometimes irregular

hypoxemia A reduced amount (hypo) of oxygen (ox) in the blood (emia)

hypoxia Cells do not have enough (hypo) oxygen (oxia)

ileostomy A surgically created opening (stomy) between the ileum (small intestine [ileo]) and the abdominal wall

immunity Protection against a disease or condition; the person will not get or be affected by the disease

implementation To perform or carry out nursing measures in the care plan; a step in the nursing process

impotence The inability of the male to have an erection; erectile dysfunction

incident Any event that has harmed or could harm a patient, resident, visitor, or staff member

incision A cut produced surgically by a sharp instrument; it creates an opening into an organ or body space

indwelling catheter A catheter left in the bladder so urine drains constantly into a drainage bag; retention or Foley catheter

infancy The first year of life

infected wound A wound containing large amounts of microbes that shows signs of infection; a dirty wound

infection A disease state resulting from the invasion and growth of microbes in the body

infection control Practices and procedures that prevent the spread of infection

inherited That which is passed down from parents to children

insomnia A chronic condition in which the person cannot sleep or stay asleep all night

intake The amount of fluid taken in

intellectual disability Involves severe limits in intellectual function and adaptive behavior occurring before age 18

intentional wound A wound created for therapy

internal rotation Turning the joint inward

intravenous (IV) therapy Giving fluids through a needle or catheter inserted into a vein; IV and IV infusion

intubation Inserting an artificial airway

invasion of privacy Violating a person's right not to have his or her name, photo, or private affairs exposed or made public without giving consent

involuntary seclusion Separating a person from others against his or her will, keeping the person to a certain area, or keeping the person away from his or her room without consent

jaundice Yellowish color of the skin or whites of the eyes

jejunostomy tube A feeding tube inserted into a surgically created opening *(stomy)* in the *jejunum* of the small intestine

job description A document that describes what the agency expects you to do

Kardex A type of card file that summarizes information found in the medical record—drugs, treatments, diagnoses, routine care measures, equipment, and special needs

ketone A substance that appears in urine from the rapid breakdown of fat for energy; acetone, ketone body

ketone body See "ketone"

knee-chest position The person kneels and rests the body on the knees and chest; the head is turned to one side, the arms are above the head or flexed at the elbows, the back is straight, and the body is flexed about 90 degrees at the hips; genupectoral position

Kussmaul respirations Very deep and rapid respirations

laceration An open wound with torn tissues and jagged edges

laryngeal mirror An instrument used to examine the mouth, teeth, and throat

lateral Away from the mid-line; at the side of the body or body part

lateral position The person lies on one side or the other; side-lying position

law A rule of conduct made by a government body

libel Making false statements in print, writing, or through pictures or drawings

lice See "pediculosis"

licensed practical nurse (LPN) A nurse who has completed a 1-year nursing program and has passed a licensing test; called *licensed vocational nurse (LVN)* in some states

licensed vocational nurse (LVN) See "licensed practical nurse (LPN)"

lithotomy position The woman lies on her back with her hips at the edge of the exam table, her knees are flexed, her hips are externally rotated, and her feet are in stirrups

local anesthesia The loss of feeling or sensation in a small area

lochia The vaginal discharge that occurs after childbirth

logrolling Turning the person as a unit, in alignment, with one motion

low vision Eyesight that cannot be corrected with eyeglasses, contact lenses, drugs, or surgery

lymphedema A buildup of lymph in the tissues causing edema (swelling)

malignant tumor A tumor that invades and destroys nearby tissues and can spread to other body parts; cancer

malpractice Negligence by a professional person

mechanical ventilation Using a machine to move air into and out of the lungs

meconium A dark green to black, tarry bowel movement

medial At or near the middle or mid-line of the body or body part

medical asepsis Practices used to remove or destroy pathogens and to prevent their spread from one person or place to another person or place; clean technique

medical diagnosis The identification of a disease or condition by a doctor

medical record A written or electronic account of a person's condition and response to treatment and care; chart or clinical record

medical symptom An indication or characteristic of a physical or psychological condition

medication reminder Reminding the person to take drugs, observing them being taken as prescribed, and charting that they were taken

melena A black, tarry stool

menarche The first menstruation and the start of menstrual cycles

menopause The time when menstruation stops and menstrual cycles end

menstruation The process in which the lining of the uterus (endometrium) breaks up and is discharged from the body through the vagina

mental Relating to the mind; something that exists in the mind or is done by the mind

mental disorder A disturbance in the ability to cope with or adjust to stress; behavior and function are impaired; mental illness, emotional illness, psychiatric disorder

mental health The person copes with and adjusts to everyday stresses in ways accepted by society

mental illness See "mental disorder"

mentor See "preceptor"

metabolism The burning of food for heat and energy by the cells

metastasis The spread of cancer to other body parts

microbe See "microorganism"

microorganism A small *(micro)* living thing *(organism)* seen only with a microscope; a microbe

micturition See "urination"

mite A very small spider-like organism

mixed aphasia See "expressive-receptive aphasia"

mixed incontinence The combination of stress incontinence and urge incontinence

morbid obesity The person weighs 100 pounds or more over his or her normal weight

morning care Care given after breakfast; hygiene measures are more thorough at this time

motor aphasia See "expressive aphasia"

nasal speculum An instrument used to examine the inside of the nose

naso-enteral tube A feeding tube inserted through the nose (*naso*) into the small bowel (*enteral*)

naso-gastric (NG) tube A feeding tube inserted through the nose (*naso*) into the stomach (*gastro*)

need Something necessary or desired for maintaining life and mental well-being

neglect Failure to provide the person with the goods or services needed to avoid physical harm, mental anguish, or mental illness

negligence An unintentional wrong in which a person did not act in a reasonable and careful manner and a person or the person's property was harmed

nocturia Frequent urination (*uria*) at night (*noct*)

non-pathogen A microbe that does not usually cause an infection

nonverbal communication Communication that does not use words

normal flora Microbes that live and grow in a certain area

NREM sleep The phase of sleep when there is *no rapid eye movement*; non-REM sleep

nursing See "breast-feeding"

nursing assistant A person who has passed a nursing assistant training and competency evaluation program; performs delegated nursing tasks under the supervision of a licensed nurse

nursing care plan A written guide about the person's nursing care; care plan

nursing diagnosis Describes a health problem that can be treated by nursing measures; a step in the nursing process

nursing intervention An action or measure taken by the nursing team to help the person reach a goal

nursing process The method nurses use to plan and deliver nursing care; its five steps are assessment, nursing diagnosis, planning, implementation, and evaluation

nursing task Nursing care or a nursing function, procedure, activity, or work that can be delegated to nursing assistants when it does not require an RN's professional knowledge or judgment

nursing team Those who provide nursing care—RNs, LPNs/LVNs, and nursing assistants

nutrient A substance that is ingested, digested, absorbed, and used by the body

nutrition The processes involved in the ingestion, digestion, absorption, and use of foods and fluids by the body

obesity Having an excess amount of total body fat; a person is said to be obese when his or her weight is 20% or more above what is considered normal for that person's height and age

objective data Information that is seen, heard, felt, or smelled by an observer; signs

observation Using the senses of sight, hearing, touch, and smell to collect information

obsession A recurrent, unwanted thought, idea, or image

obstetrics The branch of medicine concerned with the care of women during pregnancy, labor, and childbirth and for 6 to 8 weeks after birth

oliguria Scant amount (*olig*) of urine (*uria*); less than 500 mL in 24 hours

ombudsman Someone who supports or promotes the needs and interests of another person

open fracture The broken bone has come through the skin; compound fracture

open wound The skin or mucous membrane is broken

ophthalmoscope A lighted instrument used to examine the internal eye structures

optimal level of function A person's highest potential for mental and physical performance

oral hygiene Mouth care

organ Groups of tissues with the same function

orthopnea Breathing (*pnea*) deeply and comfortably only when sitting (*ortho*)

orthopneic position Sitting up (*ortho*) and leaning over a table to breathe (*pneic*)

orthostatic hypotension Abnormally low (*hypo*) blood pressure when the person suddenly stands up (*ortho* and *static*); postural hypotension

ostomy A surgically created opening for the elimination of body wastes; see "colostomy" and "ileostomy"

otoscope A lighted instrument used to examine the external ear and the eardrum (tympanic membrane)

output The amount of fluid lost

overflow incontinence Small amounts of urine leak from a full bladder

oxygen concentration The amount (percent) of hemoglobin containing oxygen

pack Wrapping a body part with a wet or dry application

pain To ache, hurt, or be sore; discomfort

palliative care Care that involves relieving or reducing the intensity of uncomfortable symptoms without producing a cure

panic An intense and sudden feeling of fear, anxiety, terror, or dread

paralysis Loss of muscle function, sensation, or both

paranoia A disorder (*para*) of the mind (*noia*); false beliefs (delusions) and suspicion about a person or situation

paraphrasing Restating the person's message in your own words

paraplegia Paralysis in the legs and lower trunk (*para* means *beyond*; *plegia* means *paralysis*)

parenteral nutrition Giving nutrients through a catheter inserted into a vein; *para* means *beyond*; *enteral* relates to the *bowel*

partial-thickness wound The dermis and epidermis of the skin are broken

patent Open and unblocked

pathogen A microbe that is harmful and can cause an infection

patient-focused care A nursing care pattern; services are moved from departments to the bedside

pediatrics The branch of medicine concerned with the growth, development, and care of children; they range in age from newborns to teenagers

pediculosis Infestation with wingless insects; lice

pediculosis capitis Infestation of the scalp (*capitis*) with lice; head lice

pediculosis corporis Infestation of the body (*corporis*) with lice

pediculosis pubis Infestation of the pubic (*pubis*) hair with lice

peer A person of the same age-group and background

penetrating wound An open wound that breaks the skin and enters a body area, organ, or cavity

percussion hammer An instrument used to tap body parts to test reflexes; reflex hammer

percutaneous endoscopic gastrostomy (PEG) tube A feeding tube inserted into the stomach (*gastro*) through a small incision (*stomy*) made through (*per*) the skin (*cutaneous*); a lighted instrument (*scope*) is used to see inside a body cavity or organ (*endo*)

pericare See "perineal care"

perineal care Cleaning the genital and anal areas; pericare

peristalsis Involuntary muscle contractions in the digestive system that move food down the esophagus through the alimentary canal; the alternating contraction and relaxation of intestinal muscles

persistent pain See "chronic pain"

personality The set of attitudes, values, behaviors, and traits of a person

phantom pain Pain felt in a body part that is no longer there

phlebitis Inflammation (*itis*) of a vein (*phleb*)

phobia An intense fear

physical restraint Any manual method or physical or mechanical device, material, or equipment attached to or near the person's body that he or she cannot remove easily and that restricts freedom of movement or normal access to one's body

planning Setting priorities and goals; a step in the nursing process

plantar flexion The foot (*plantar*) is bent (*flexion*); bending the foot down at the ankle

plaque A thin film that sticks to the teeth; it contains saliva, microbes, and other substances

pleural effusion The escape and collection of fluid (*effusion*) in the pleural space

PM care See "evening care"

pneumothorax Air (*pneumo*) in the pleural space (*thorax*)

poison Any substance harmful to the body when ingested, inhaled, injected, or absorbed through the skin

pollutant A harmful chemical or substance in the air or water

polyuria Abnormally large amounts (*poly*) of urine (*uria*)

posterior At or toward the back of the body or body part

post-mortem care Care of the body after (*post*) death (*mortem*)

post-operative After surgery

postpartum After (*post*) childbirth (*partum*)

postural hypotension See "orthostatic hypotension"

posture See "body alignment"

preceptor A staff member who guides another staff member; mentor

prefix A word element placed before a root; it changes the meaning of the word

pre-hypertension When the systolic pressure is between 120 and 139 mm Hg, or the diastolic pressure is between 80 and 89 mm Hg

pre-operative Before surgery

pressure ulcer A localized injury to the skin and/or underlying tissue usually over a bony prominence resulting from pressure or pressure in combination with shear and/or friction; any lesion caused by unrelieved pressure that results in damage to underlying tissues

primary caregiver The person mainly responsible for providing or assisting with the child's basic needs

primary nursing A nursing care pattern; an RN is responsible for the person's total care

priority The most important thing at the time

professional boundary That which separates helpful behaviors from behaviors that are not helpful

professionalism Following laws, being ethical, having good work ethics, and having the skills to do your work

professional sexual misconduct An act, behavior, or comment that is sexual in nature

progress note Describes the care given and the person's response and progress

pronation Turning the joint downward

prone position Lying on the abdomen with the head turned to one side

prosthesis An artificial replacement for a missing body part

protected health information Identifying information and information about the person's health care that is maintained or sent in any form (paper, electronic, oral)

proximal The part nearest to the center or to the point of origin

pseudodementia False (*pseudo*) dementia

psychiatric disorder See "mental disorder"

psychiatry The branch of medicine concerned with mental health problems

psychosis A state of severe mental impairment

puberty The period when reproductive organs begin to function and secondary sex characteristics appear

pulse The beat of the heart felt at an artery as a wave of blood passes through the artery

pulse deficit The difference between the apical and radial pulse rates

pulse rate The number of heartbeats or pulses felt in 1 minute

puncture wound An open wound made by a sharp object

purulent drainage Thick green, yellow, or brown drainage

pyuria Pus *(py)* in the urine *(uria)*

quadriplegia Paralysis in the arms, legs, and trunk *(quad* means *four; plegia* means *paralysis);* tetraplegia

radiating pain Pain felt at the site of tissue damage and in nearby areas

range of motion (ROM) The movement of a joint to the extent possible without causing pain

receptive aphasia Difficulty understanding language; Wernicke's aphasia

recording The written account of care and observations; charting

reflex An involuntary movement

reflex incontinence Urine is lost at predictable intervals when the bladder is full

regional anesthesia The loss of feeling or sensation in a large area of the body

registered nurse (RN) A nurse who has completed a 2-, 3-, or 4-year nursing program and has passed a licensing test

regurgitation The backward flow of stomach contents into the mouth

rehabilitation The process of restoring the person to his or her highest possible level of physical, psychological, social, and economic function

reincarnation The belief that the spirit or soul is reborn in another human body or in another form of life

relaxation To be free from mental and physical stress

religion Spiritual beliefs, needs, and practices

remove easily The manual method, device, material, or equipment used to restrain the person that can be removed intentionally by the person in the same manner it was applied by the staff

REM sleep The phase of sleep when there is *rapid eye movement*

reporting The oral account of care and observations

representative Any person who has the legal right to act on the resident's behalf when he or she cannot do so for himself or herself

reservoir The environment in which a microbe lives and grows; host

respiration The process of supplying the cells with oxygen and removing carbon dioxide from them; breathing air into *(inhalation)* and out of *(exhalation)* the lungs

respiratory arrest When breathing stops; breathing stops but heart action continues for several minutes

respiratory depression Slow, weak respirations at a rate of fewer than 12 per minute

responsibility The duty or obligation to perform some act or function

rest To be calm, at ease, and relaxed with no anxiety or stress

restorative aide A nursing assistant with special training in restorative nursing and rehabilitation skills

restorative nursing care Care that helps persons regain health, strength, and independence

retention catheter See "indwelling catheter"

reverse Trendelenburg's position The head of the bed is raised and the foot of the bed is lowered

rigor mortis The stiffness or rigidity *(rigor)* of skeletal muscles that occurs after death *(mortis)*

root A word element containing the basic meaning of the word

rotation Turning the joint

sanguineous drainage Bloody *(sanguis)* drainage

sedation A state of quiet, calmness, or sleep produced by a drug

seizure Violent and sudden contractions or tremors of muscle groups; convulsion

self-actualization Experiencing one's potential

self-esteem Thinking well of oneself and seeing oneself as useful and having value

self-neglect A person's behaviors and way of living that threaten his or her health, safety, and well-being

semi-Fowler's position The head of the bed is raised 30 degrees; or the head of the bed is raised 30 degrees and the knee portion is raised 15 degrees

semi-prone side position See "Sims' position"

serosanguineous drainage Thin, watery drainage *(sero)* that is blood-tinged *(sanguineous)*

serous drainage Clear, watery fluid *(serum)*

service plan A written plan listing the services needed, how much help is needed, and who provides the services

sex Physical activities involving the reproductive organs; done for pleasure or to have children

sexuality The physical, emotional, social, cultural, and spiritual factors that affect a person's feelings and attitudes about his or her sex

sexual orientation Sexual arousal or romantic attraction to persons of the other gender (heterosexual), the same gender (homosexual), or both genders (bisexual)

shear When layers of the skin rub against each other; when the skin remains in place and underlying tissues move and stretch and tear underlying capillaries and blood vessels causing tissue damage

shearing When skin sticks to a surface while muscles slide in the direction the body is moving

shock Results when tissues and organs do not get enough blood

side-lying position See "lateral position"

signs See "objective data"

simple fracture See "closed fracture"

Sims' position A left side-lying position in which the upper leg (right leg) is sharply flexed so it is not on the lower leg (left leg) and the lower arm (left arm) is behind the person; semi-prone side position

skin tear A break or rip in the outer layers of the skin; the epidermis (top skin layer) separates from the underlying tissues

slander Making false statements orally

sleep A state of unconsciousness, reduced voluntary muscle activity, and lowered metabolism

sleep apnea Pauses (a) in breathing (pnea) that occur during sleep

slough Dead tissue that is shed from the skin; it is usually light colored, soft, and moist; may be stringy at times

spastic Uncontrolled contractions of skeletal muscles

sphygmomanometer A cuff and measuring device used to measure blood pressure

spore A bacterium protected by a hard shell

sputum Mucus from the respiratory system that is expectorated (expelled) through the mouth

standard of care The skills, care, and judgments required by a health team member under similar conditions

stasis ulcer See "venous ulcer"

sterile The absence of all microbes

sterile field A work area free of all pathogens and non-pathogens (including spores)

sterile technique See "surgical asepsis"

sterilization The process of destroying all microbes

stethoscope An instrument used to listen to sounds produced by the heart, lungs, and other body organs

stoma A surgically created opening seen through the abdominal wall; see "colostomy" and "ileostomy"

stomatitis Inflammation (itis) of the mouth (stomat)

stool Excreted feces

straight catheter A catheter that drains the bladder and then is removed

stress The response or change in the body caused by any emotional, physical, social, or economic factor

stress incontinence When urine leaks during exercise and certain movements that cause pressure on the bladder

stressor The event or factor that causes stress

subconscious Memory, past experiences, and thoughts of which the person is not aware; they are easily recalled

subjective data Things a person tells you about that you cannot observe through your senses; symptoms

suction The process of withdrawing or sucking up fluid (secretions)

sudden cardiac arrest (SCA) The heart stops suddenly and without warning; cardiac arrest

suffix A word element placed after a root; it changes the meaning of the word

suffocation When breathing stops from the lack of oxygen

suicide To kill oneself

suicide contagion Exposure to suicide or suicidal behaviors within one's family, one's peer group, or media reports of suicide

sundowning Signs, symptoms, and behaviors of Alzheimer's disease increase during hours of darkness

supination Turning the joint upward

supine position The back-lying or dorsal recumbent position

suppository A cone-shaped, solid drug that is inserted into a body opening; it melts at body temperature

surgical asepsis The practices that keep items free of all microbes; sterile technique

symptoms See "subjective data"

syncope A brief loss of consciousness; fainting

system Organs that work together to perform special functions

systole The period of heart muscle contraction; the heart is pumping blood

systolic pressure The pressure in the arteries when the heart contracts

tachycardia A rapid (tachy) heart rate (cardia); more than 100 beats per minute

tachypnea Rapid (tachy) breathing (pnea); respirations are more than 20 per minute

tartar Hardened plaque

team nursing A nursing care pattern; a team of nursing staff is led by an RN who decides the amount and kind of care each person needs

teamwork Staff members work together as a group; each person does his or her part to provide safe and effective care

terminal illness An illness or injury from which the person will not likely recover

tetraplegia See "quadriplegia" (tetra means four; plegia means paralysis)

thermometer A device used to measure (meter) temperature (thermo)

thrombus A blood clot

tinnitus A ringing, roaring, hissing, or buzzing sound in the ears or head

tissue A group of cells with similar functions

tort A wrong committed against a person or the person's property

tracheostomy A surgically created opening (stomy) into the trachea (tracheo)

transfer Moving the person from one place to another; moving the person to another health care setting; moving the person to a new room

transfer belt A device used to support a person who is unsteady or disabled; gait belt

transgender A broad term used to describe people who express their sexuality or gender in other than the expected way; persons who are undergoing hormone therapy or surgery for sexual re-assignment (female to male; male to female)

transient incontinence Temporary or occasional incontinence that is reversed when the cause is treated

transsexual A person who believes that he or she is a member of the other sex

transvestite A person who dresses and behaves like the other sex for emotional and sexual relief; cross-dresser

trauma An accident or violent act that injures the skin, mucous membranes, bones, and organs

treatment The care provided to maintain or restore health, improve function, or relieve symptoms

Trendelenburg's position The head of the bed is lowered and the foot of the bed is raised

tumor A new growth of abnormal cells; tumors are benign or malignant

tuning fork An instrument vibrated to test hearing

ulcer A shallow or deep crater-like sore of the skin or a mucous membrane

umbilical cord The structure that connects the mother and fetus (unborn baby); it carries blood, oxygen, and nutrients from the mother to the fetus

unavoidable pressure ulcer A pressure ulcer that occurs despite efforts to prevent one through proper use of the nursing process

unconscious Experiences and feelings that cannot be recalled

unintentional wound A wound resulting from trauma

urge incontinence The loss of urine in response to a sudden, urgent need to void; the person cannot get to a toilet in time

urgent surgery Surgery needed for the person's health; it is done soon to prevent further damage or disease

urinary diversion A surgically created pathway for urine to leave the body

urinary frequency Voiding at frequent intervals

urinary incontinence The involuntary loss or leakage of urine

urinary retention The inability to void

urinary urgency The need to void at once

urination The process of emptying urine from the bladder; micturition or voiding

urostomy A surgically created opening (*stomy*) between a ureter (*uro*) and the abdomen

vaccination Giving a vaccine to produce immunity against an infectious disease

vaccine A preparation containing dead or weakened microbes

vaginal speculum An instrument used to open the vagina to examine it and the cervix

vascular ulcer See "circulatory ulcer"

vector A carrier (animal, insect) that transmits disease

vehicle Any substance that transmits microbes

vein A blood vessel that returns blood to the heart

venous ulcer An open sore on the lower legs or feet caused by poor venous blood flow; stasis ulcer

ventral See "anterior"

verbal communication Communication that uses written or spoken words

vertigo Dizziness

vital signs Temperature, pulse, respirations, and blood pressure; and pain in some agencies

voiding See "urination"

vomitus Food and fluids expelled from the stomach through the mouth; emesis

vulnerable adult A person 18 years old or older who has a disability or condition that makes him or her at risk to be wounded, attacked, or damaged

waterproof drawsheet A drawsheet made of plastic, rubber, or absorbent material used to protect the mattress and bottom linens from dampness and soiling

Wernicke's aphasia See "receptive aphasia"

will A legal document of how a person wants property distributed after death

withdrawal syndrome The person's physical and mental response after stopping or severely reducing the use of a substance that was used regularly

word element A part of a word

work ethics Behavior in the workplace

workplace violence Violent acts (including assault and threat of assault) directed toward persons at work or while on duty

wound A break in the skin or mucous membrane

AD	Alzheimer's disease		F	Fahrenheit
ADA	Americans With Disabilities Act of 1990		FBAO	Foreign-body airway obstruction
ADL	Activities of daily living		FDA	Food and Drug Administration
AE	Anti-embolism, anti-embolic		FXS	Fragile X syndrome
AED	Automated external defibrillator			
AHA	American Heart Association; American Hospital Association		GERD	Gastro-esophageal reflux disease
			GI	Gastro-intestinal
AIDS	Acquired immunodeficiency syndrome		gtt	Drops
AIIR	Airborne infection isolation room		gtt/min	Drops per minute
ALR	Assisted living residence			
ALS	Amyotrophic lateral sclerosis		HAI	Healthcare-associated infection
AMD	Age-related macular degeneration		HBV	Hepatitis B virus
ASL	American Sign Language		Hg	Mercury
			HIPAA	Health Insurance Portability and Accountability Act of 1996
BLS	Basic Life Support			
BM	Bowel movement		HIV	Human immunodeficiency virus
BP	Blood pressure		HMO	Health maintenance organization
BPD	Borderline personality disorder			
BPH	Benign prostatic hyperplasia		I&O	Intake and output
			ID	Identification
C	Centigrade		IDCP	Interdisciplinary care planning
CAA	Care Area Assessment		IQ	Intelligence quotient
CAD	Coronary artery disease		IV	Intravenous
CBC	Complete blood count			
CCRC	Continuing care retirement community		JRA	Juvenile rheumatoid arthritis
CDC	Centers for Disease Control and Prevention		lb	Pound
cm	Centimeter		L/min	Liters per minute
CMS	Centers for Medicare & Medicaid Services		LNA	Licensed nursing assistant
			LPN	Licensed practical nurse
CNA	Certified nursing assistant; certified nurse aide		LVN	Licensed vocational nurse
CNS	Central nervous system		MDRO	Multidrug-resistant organism
CO	Carbon monoxide		MDS	Minimum Data Set
CO_2	Carbon dioxide		mg	Milligram
COPD	Chronic obstructive pulmonary disease		MI	Myocardial infarction
CP	Cerebral palsy		mL	Milliliter
CPR	Cardiopulmonary resuscitation		mL/hr	Milliliters per hour
C-section	Cesarean section		mm	Millimeter
CVA	Cerebrovascular accident		mm Hg	Millimeters of mercury
			MRSA	Methicillin-resistant *Staphylococcus aureus*
DD	Developmental disability		MS	Multiple sclerosis
DNR	Do Not Resuscitate		MSD	Musculo-skeletal disorder
DON	Director of nursing		MSDS	Material safety data sheet
DS	Down syndrome			
DUS	Doppler ultrasound stethoscope		NANDA-I	North American Nursing Diagnosis Association International
DV	Daily Value		NATCEP	Nursing assistant training and competency evaluation program
ECG	Electrocardiogram		NCSBN	National Council of State Boards of Nursing
ED	Erectile dysfunction			
EKG	Electrocardiogram		NG	Naso-gastric
EMS	Emergency Medical Services		NIA	National Institute on Aging
EPA	Environmental Protection Agency		NPO	*Non per os;* nothing by mouth
EPHI; ePHI	Electronic protected health information		NREM	No rapid eye movement
ET	Endotrachial			

O_2	Oxygen
OASIS	Outcome and Assessment Information Set
OBRA	Omnibus Budget Reconciliation Act of 1987
OCD	Obsessive-compulsive disorder
OPIM	Other potentially infectious materials
OR	Operating room
OSHA	Occupational Safety and Health Administration
oz	Ounce
PACU	Post anesthesia care unit
PASS	*Pull* the safety pin, *aim* low, *squeeze* the lever, *sweep* back and forth
PEG	Percutaneous endoscopic gastrostomy
PHI	Protected health information
PPE	Personal protective equipment
PPO	Preferred provider organization
PT	Physical therapist
PTSD	Post-traumatic stress disorder
PVS	Persistent vegetative state
RA	Rheumatoid arthritis
RACE	Rescue, alarm, confine, extinguish
RBC	Red blood cell
REM	Rapid eye movement
RN	Registered nurse
RNA	Registered nurse aide
ROM	Range of motion
RRT	Rapid Response Team
RT	Respiratory therapist
SARS	Severe acute respiratory syndrome
SB	Spina bifida
SCA	Sudden cardiac arrest
SCD	Sequential compression device
SNF	Skilled nursing facility
SpO_2	Saturation of peripheral oxygen; oxygen concentration
SSE	Soapsuds enema
STD	Sexually transmitted disease
STNA	State tested nurse aide
TB	Tuberculosis
TBI	Traumatic brain injury
TED	Thrombo-embolic disease
TIA	Transient ischemic attack
TJC	The Joint Commission
TPN	Total parenteral nutrition
USDA	United States Department of Agriculture
UTI	Urinary tract infection
VF	Ventricular fibrillation
V-fib	Ventricular fibrillation
VRE	Vancomycin-resistant *Enterococci*
WBC	White blood cell

Page numbers followed by *b*, *t*, and *f* indicate boxes, tables, and figures, respectively.